Health Information Management Technology

An Applied Approach

Fourth Edition

Nanette B. Sayles, EdD, RHIA,
CHPS, CCS, CPHIMS, FAHIMA
Editor

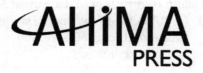

ISBN: 978-1-58426-352-4
AHIMA Product No.: AB103112

18 17 16 15 14   2 3 4 5

Jessica Block, MA, Assistant Editor
June E. Bronnert, RHIA, CCS, CCS-P
Jill S. Clark, MBA, RHIA
Kathryn A. DeVault, RHIA, CCS
Angela K. Dinh, MHA, RHIA, CHPS
Melanie A. Endicott, MBA, RHIA, CCS, CCS-P
Katie Greenock, MS, Production Development Editor
Karen M. Kostick, RHIT, CCS, CCS-P
Jason O. Malley, Vice President, Business and Innovation
Diana M. Warner, MS, RHIA, CHPS
Lou Ann Wiedemann, MS, RHIA
Pamela Woolf, Director of Publications

American Health Information Management Association
233 North Michigan Avenue, 21st Floor
Chicago, Illinois 60601-5809
ahima.org

Contents

Part 1 Healthcare Data Management

Part 2 Health Statistics, Biomedical Research, and Quality Management

Detailed Table of Contents

Part 1 Healthcare Data Management

Part 2   Health Statistics, Biomedical Research, and Quality Management

Part 3   Health Services Organization and Delivery

Part 4   Information Technology and Systems

Part 5   Organizational Resources

Chapter 18   Principles of Organization and Work Planning 1073

Appendices, Glossary, and Index

Nanette B. Sayles, EdD, RHIA, CCS, CHP, CPHIMS, FAHIMA, an associate professor in the Health Information Management Program at East Central College in Union, Missouri, has a BS in medical record administration, an MS in health information management, a master's in public administration, and a doctorate of education in adult education. Dr. Sayles has more than 10 years of experience as a health information management practitioner with experience in hospitals, a consulting firm, and a computer vendor. She was the 2005 American Health Information Management Association Triumph Educator award winner. She has held numerous volunteer roles for the American Health Information Management Association (AHIMA), the Georgia Health Information Management Association (GHIMA), the Alabama Association of Health Information Management (AAHIM), Middle Georgia Health Information Management Association (MGHIMA), and Birmingham Regional Health Information Management Association (BRHIMA). These positions include: AHIMA Educational Strategies Committee, AHIMA co-chair RHIA Workgroup, GHIMA director, and president of MGHIMA. Dr. Sayles has published two books: *Professional Review Guide for the CHP, CHS, and CHPS Examinations* and *Case Studies for Health Information Management*. She is an editor for two chapters in the *PRG Professional Review Guide* for the RHIA and RHIT Examinations.

Margret K. Amatayakul, MBA, RHIA, CHPS, CPHIT, CPEHR, FHIMSS, is president of Margret\A Consulting, LLC, in Schaumburg, Illinois, a consulting firm specializing in computer-based patient records and associated HIM standards and regulations, such as HIPAA. She has more than 30 years of experience in national and international HIM. A leading authority on electronic health record (EHR) strategies for healthcare organizations, she has extensive experience in EHR selection and project management, and she formed and served as executive director of the Computer-based Patient Record Institute (CPRI). Other positions held include associate executive director of AHIMA, associate professor at the University of Illinois, and director of medical record services at the Illinois Eye and Ear Infirmary. She is a much sought-after speaker, has published extensively, and has earned several professional service awards. Amatayakul also serves as an adjunct faculty member of the College of St. Scholastica and the University of Illinois at Chicago.

Sheila Carlon, PhD, RHIA, FAHIMA, CHPS, has served as the director of the Division of Health Services Administration at Regis University in Denver for twelve years. Prior to that she was the HIM program director at Dakota State University in Madison, South Dakota. Her industry experience includes consulting with Deloitte & Touche, HIM management at Stanford Hospital and Dominican Hospital in California, practice management in California and additional HIM experience in various hospitals in Colorado. She has a PhD in organization development from the Fielding Graduate Institute, an MS in health services from San Jose State University, and bachelor's degrees in health care management and broadcast journalism and communications. She has served as chair of Education Strategy Committee for AHIMA, is on the CAHIIM Panel of Reviewers, and is a reviewer for *Perspectives in HIM,* and received the Educator's Award in 2006. She is a frequent speaker on health information management and technology at the local, national, and international levels and is involved in international implementation of HIT in several countries.

Bonnie S. Cassidy, MPA, RHIA, FAHIMA, FHIMSS, was the 2011 President of AHIMA, serving as the Chairman of the AHIMA Board of Directors, and continues to serve on the Board as the 2012 Past President Director. Bonnie previously served on the AHIMA Board as a Director from 2006 to 2008. Bonnie is the Vice President of HIM Innovation for QuadraMed and previously served as the Vice President of HIM Product Management for QuadraMed. Bonnie is an AHIMA Academy ICD-10-CM/PCS Certificate Holder and Ambassador.

Prior to joining QuadraMed, Bonnie served as an executive with the Certification Commission for Healthcare Information Technology (CCHIT). Bonnie is an experienced healthcare consultant and advisor, having worked for the national management consulting firms of Price Waterhouse and Ernst & Young, and she was an HIM administrator at two major teaching hospitals, including the Cleveland Clinic Foundation.

Bonnie was the president of the Ohio Health Information Management Association (OHIMA) and was honored to receive the OHIMA Distinguished Member Award. Ms. Cassidy is the recipient of three AHIMA awards: Legacy Award, Volunteer Excellence Award, and Professional Achievement Award.

Lisa A. Cerrato, MS, RHIA, is the program coordinator of the health information management technology department at Columbus State Community College (CSCC), in Columbus, Ohio. She received a BS in health information management administration from The Ohio State University. Upon graduation, Lisa became the director of the medical records department at Meridia Huron Hospital, part of the Cleveland Clinic Health System in Cleveland. She then earned an MS in allied health education. Lisa is now a full-time faculty member at CSCC. She led the development of CSCC's online courses and certificate programs in medical coding and medical transcription.

Chris Elliott, MS, RHIA, holds a master's degree in information systems and has pursued significant graduate study in medical informatics at the University of Utah. He recently retired as director of health information services and privacy officer designee at San Francisco General Hospital Medical Center after 40 years of public service in hospitals and health profession education settings.

Kathy Giannangelo, MA, RHIA, CCS, CPHIMS, is a medical informaticist with Language and Computing, Inc. In this position, she supports the ontology, modeling, sales, and product development activities related to the creation and implementation of natural language-processing applications where clinical terminology and classification systems are utilized. Kathy has a comprehensive background in the field of clinical terminologies and classification, with more than 30 years of experience in the health information management (HIM) field. Prior to joining L&C, she was director of practice leadership with AHIMA in Chicago. Kathy has served as senior nosologist for a health information services company and worked in various HIM roles, including vice president of product development, education specialist, director of medical records, quality assurance coordinator, and manager of a Centers for Disease Control and Prevention research team. Kathy has developed classification, grouping, and reimbursement systems products for healthcare providers; conducted seminars; and provided consulting assessments throughout the United States as well as in Canada, Australia, the United Kingdom, Ireland, and Bulgaria. In addition, she has authored numerous articles and created online continuing education courses on clinical terminologies. As adjunct faculty at the College of St. Scholastica, she teaches the graduate-level course, Clinical Vocabularies and Classification Systems. In addition, she is actively involved as a volunteer in the HIM profession at the international, national, state, and local levels. Kathy holds a master's degree in HIM from the College of St. Scholastica.

Laurinda B. Harman, PhD, RHIA, FAHIMA, Associate Professor Emeritus, Department of Health Information Management in the College of Health Professions and Social Work at Temple University in Philadelphia, has been an HIM professional and educator for over 40 years. She has directed HIM baccalaureate programs at Temple University, George Washington University in Washington, DC, and The Ohio State University in Columbus. Dr. Harman was a faculty member in the health information technology program at Northern Virginia Community College and served as director of education and human resource development for the Department of Health Care Sciences at George Washington University. She edited *Ethical Challenges in the Management of Health Information* in 2001, the 2nd edition was published in 2006 and the 3rd edition is in progress. She contributed chapters to *Health Informatics Research: Practices and Innovative Approaches*; *Health Information Management: Concepts, Principles, and Practice;* and *Health Information Technology: An Applied Approach* for the American Health Information Management Association. Dr. Harman is on the editorial board of *Perspectives in Health Information Management*, has contributed articles to the *Journal of American Health Information Management Association* and has delivered presentations at international, national, state and local association meetings on topics related to HIM and ethics. She received a BS in biology with a concentration in medical record administration from Daemen College in Buffalo, New York, an MS in education at Virginia Polytechnic and State University in Blacksburg, Virginia, and a PhD in human and organizational systems at Fielding Graduate University in Santa Barbara, California. Dr. Harman received the AHIMA 2001 Triumph Legacy Award for *Ethical Challenges in the Management of Health Information*, the 2011 Triumph Legacy Educator Award, and the 2011 Dorland Peoples Ethicist Award for her textbook and its contribution to helping healthcare professionals deal with ever-increasing ethical health information issues.

Anita C. Hazelwood, MLS, RHIA, FAHIMA, is a professor in the Health Information Management Department at the University of Louisiana at Lafayette and has been a credentialed registered health information administrator (RHIA) for more than 30 years. Anita has actively consulted in hospitals, nursing homes, physician's offices, clinics, facilities for the mentally retarded, and in other educational institutions. She has conducted numerous ICD-9-CM and CPT coding workshops throughout Louisiana for hospitals and physicians' offices and has written numerous articles and coauthored chapters in several HIM textbooks. Anita has coauthored two books titled *ICD-9-CM Coding and Reimbursement for Physicians' Services* and *ICD-10-CM Preview* for which she won AHIMA's Legacy Award in 2003. Anita has been a member of AHIMA for 32 years and has served on various committees and boards. Anita is a member of the Louisiana Health Information Management Association (LHIMA) and was selected as its 1997 Distinguished Member. She has served throughout the years as president, president-elect, treasurer, strategy manager, and board member and has directed numerous committees and projects.

Cheryl V. Homan, MBA, RHIA, is administrative director of information systems and biomedical engineering for the Lima Memorial Health System, located in Lima, Ohio. She also serves as adjunct faculty for the Health Management Program at The Ohio State University at Lima. She received her MBA from Ashland University in Ashland, Ohio, and her BS in allied health professions from The Ohio State University. She has been an HIM professional for more than 30 years, served on AHIMA's Board of Directors from 1997 to 1999, and is a former president of the Ohio Health Information Management Association.

Loretta A. Horton, MEd, RHIA, FAHIMA, received a medical record technician certificate from Research Hospital and Medical Center and a bachelor's degree in psychology from Rockhurst College, both in Kansas City, Missouri; a post-baccalaureate certificate in health information administration from Stephens College in Columbia, Missouri; and a master's in education with an emphasis in curriculum and instruction from Wichita State University in Wichita, Kansas. She also has completed graduate work in sociology at the University of Nebraska in Omaha. Currently, Loretta is cochair of the Allied Health Department and coordinator of the Health Information Technology Program at Hutchinson Community College in Hutchinson, Kansas. Previously, she worked in a variety of health information settings, including acute care and mental health, and she has consulted with long-term care, mental retardation, home health, hospice, and prison systems. She is an AHIMA fellow.

Donald W. Kellogg, PhD, RHIA, CPEHR, is an assistant professor at University of Saint Mary in Leavenworth, Kansas, and is the coordinator of the bachelor of health science program as well as a faculty member in the health information technology program. He earned a bachelor's degree in health information management at the University of Kansas Medical Center and his doctorate at the University of Kansas in higher education administration. Kellogg has served the Kansas Health Information Management Association (KHIMA) as a director for three years, a delegate to the AHIMA House of Delegates for four years, and as President-Elect/President/Past-President as well as chairing multiple committees. He is a recipient of KHIMA's Volunteer, Champion, and Achievement Awards. He was Kansas's first liaison to the AHIMA Foundation and Community Education Coordinator (CEC), a state association leadership position on personal health record public outreach and education efforts. Kellogg has also served on AHIMA's Educational Strategies Committee (ESC), for which he was chair in 2008; the "Increasing the RHIA-Credentialed Workforce" task force; and is currently a commissioner with the Commission on Accreditation for Health Informatics and Information Management Education (CAHIIM).

Bonnie J. Petterson, PhD, RHIA, recently formed HIM Educational Consulting after retirement as director of HIM programs at Phoenix College, part of the Maricopa Community Colleges in Phoenix, Arizona. She has been a full-time HIM educator for over 25 years, serving first at the health information administration level and then working with health information technology and certificate students. In addition, she has held full-time positions as a health information manager in an acute care hospital, a home health care agency, and in a psychiatric care setting and consulted in ambulatory care, home health care, and long-term care. Petterson is coauthor of a textbook titled *Using the Electronic Health Record in the Healthcare Provider Practice* from Cengage Learning. She is a past Chair of AHIMA's Commission on Certification for Informatics and Information Management (CCHIIM), its Research Committee and the AOE Program Committee, and has served on the Education Strategy Committee as well as several AHIMA task forces. She has volunteered for a variety of roles in state health information associations, including election as an AHIMA delegate from both Wisconsin and Arizona. Petterson was the recipient of the mentor and the lifetime achievement awards from the state of Arizona. She holds a PhD in educational leadership and policy studies from Arizona State University and an MS in educational psychology and a BS in health information administration from the University of Wisconsin-Milwaukee.

Laurie A. Rinehart-Thompson, JD, RHIA, CHP, is an associate professor of clinical allied medicine in the Health Information Management and Systems program at The Ohio State University in Columbus. She earned her BS in medical record administration and her law degree from The Ohio State University. In addition to education, her professional experiences include behavioral health, home health, and acute care. She has served as an expert witness in civil litigation testifying as to the privacy and confidentiality of health information. She has served and continues to serve on AHIMA committees and is on the Board of Directors of the Ohio Health Information Management Association. A frequent speaker on the HIPAA privacy rule, she is a contributing author of *Ethical Challenges in the Management of Health Information* (AHIMA and Jones and Bartlett 2006) and *Documentation in Medical Practices* (AHIMA 2011). She is a coeditor of *Fundamentals of Law for Health Informatics and Information Management* (AHIMA 2009).

Jane Roberts, MS, RHIA, is an associate professor in health information management technology at Columbus State Community College, in Columbus, Ohio. She received a BS degree from The Ohio State University in 1988 and an MS degree in 2004. Her prior work experience includes director of medical records in acute care facilities, supervisor of medical records in a long-term care facility, and office manager in a physician office setting.

Karen S. Scott, MEd, RHIA, CCS-P, CPC, has more than 20 years' experience in the healthcare field. Karen is the sole proprietor of Karen Scott Seminars and Consulting. She has been an educator for many years, including teaching in the health information management programs at the University of Tennessee Health Science Center and Arkansas Tech University. She has worked as an HIM director in an acute care hospital setting, training director for a national transcription company, and reimbursement specialist for a regional physicians' group. She holds a BS degree in health information management and a master's degree of education in instructional technology from Arkansas Tech University in Russellville. She is past president of both the Tennessee and Arkansas Health Information Management Associations and is past chair of the AHIMA Council on Certification. Karen has won several awards, including the Tennessee Innovator Award. In 2005, THIMA recognized Karen for her achievements with its Distinguished Member Award. Karen teaches seminars on coding, reimbursement, medical terminology, and management throughout the country for physician and hospital audiences. She has published numerous articles on various healthcare topics including chapters in HIM and coding textbooks. The 3rd edition of her textbook, *Coding and Reimbursement for Hospital Inpatient Services,* was published in 2010.

Marcia Y. Sharp, EdD, MBA, RHIA, is an assistant professor in the Department of Health Informatics and Information Management at the University of Tennessee Health Sciences Center. She has had an outstanding career in health information management and in human resource management. She is an active member of the Memphis Health Information Management Association, serving as former treasurer, and the Tennessee Health Information Management Association, serving as TN delegate to the AHIMA House of Delegates, and former member of the TN Nominating Committee. She is currently a member of the editorial review panel for *Perspectives in Health Information Management* (PHIM). She has contributed chapters to several AHIMA publications, *Health Information Management Technology: An Applied Approach,* and *Fundamentals of Law for Health Informatics and Information Management.*

Martin Smith, Med, RHIT, CCA has served as a professor in the HIM programs at Hodges University in Naples, Florida, the Allen school in Brooklyn, New York, and St. Petersburg College in St. Petersburg, Florida, for more than nine years. He has managed several HIM programs in addition to serving as faculty. Prior to this he was a police constable in London, working for New Scotland Yard, and a combat medic in the US Army. He received his undergraduate degrees from St. Petersburg College and American Intercontinental University (AIU) before earning a master's degree in education with a concentration in instructional technology from AIU. He completed the healthcare informatics graduate certificate program at the College of St. Scholastica in Duluth, Minnesota, and is currently completing his master's degree in health information management at the same school. He has authored several articles on healthcare topics and in 2011 completed his service as the cochair of the Florida Health Information Management Association (FHIMA) legislative committee after being voted to the board of directors in 2009. He has attended several Hill Day events in Tallahassee, Florida, and is a vocal advocate of the HIM profession. He has served at the local level on FHIMA's bridging the gap and find, inspire, recruit, educate (FIRE) mentoring committees and regularly visits local middle and high schools to talk about the profession. He is currently teaching and mentoring the next generation of HIM professionals at Hodges University.

Carol A. Venable, MPH, RHIA, FAHIMA, is a professor and department head of HIM at the University of Louisiana at Lafayette and has been an HIM professional for nearly 30 years. She is actively involved with AHIMA's Assembly on Education (AOE), Panel of Accreditation Surveyors, and several other committees, as well as the Louisiana Health Information Management Association, where she has held many leadership positions and was selected as Distinguished Member in 1991. In addition, she is a member of the Society for Clinical Coding (SCC). Previously, she was director of medical records at Lafayette General Medical Center, has consulted in a variety of healthcare facilities and educational institutions, and conducts coding workshops for hospitals and physician offices. Venable has written, coauthored, and edited numerous publications, including AHIMA's *ICD-9-CM Diagnostic Coding and Reimbursement for Physician Services* and *ICD-10-CM Preview*, for which she was awarded AHIMA's Legacy Award in 2003. She frequently serves as a reviewer for publishers of HIM-related textbooks, certification exams, and electronic materials.

Health information management (HIM) professionals are an integral part of the healthcare team. They serve the healthcare industry and the public by using best practices in managing healthcare information to support quality healthcare delivery. Whether stored on paper or in electronic file form, reliable health information is critical to high-quality healthcare. Enhancing individual patient care through timely and relevant information is one of the primary goals for the HIM profession.

The American Health Information Management Association (AHIMA) represents more than 64,000 HIM professionals who work throughout the healthcare industry. AHIMA has a long history of commitment to HIM education. Among other contributions, AHIMA has developed and maintained a rigorous accreditation process for academic programs, continuously developed up-to-date curriculum models, supported faculty development, and continued to research and study the needs and future directions of HIM education.

This text, specifically developed for associate degree programs in health information technology (HIT), is an outgrowth of AHIMA's ongoing effort to provide rich resources for the education and training of new HIM professionals. In addition, it offers a ready resource for current practitioners. Its subject matter is based on AHIMA's HIM Associate Degree Program Entry-Level Competencies and Knowledge Clusters and AHIMA's RHIT certification examination content domains. Following the prescribed curricular content found in the HIM Associate Degree Entry-Level Competencies, the text covers information and topics considered essential for every entry-level HIT practitioner. Although the text is directed primarily at students enrolled in two-year HIT programs, students in other HIM disciplines and allied health programs also will find its content highly useful.

The fundamental organization of the text is built on the curricular content of the HIM Associate Degree Entry-Level Competencies and Knowledge Clusters. Each of the content areas is represented in the book except those relating to the biomedical sciences and to technical aspects of classification systems such as ICD. To provide maximum flexibility for instructional delivery, the content of each chapter is designed to stand on its own, providing maximum coverage of specific domains and competencies. Because of the interdependency of content areas that support knowledge and skills for performing many of the competencies, this approach has necessitated duplication of some material throughout the text. In these cases, the predominant content is covered in depth and is supplemented by a high-level overview of other supporting knowledge. Where appropriate, students are referred to other chapters for additional information or detail to round out necessary knowledge.

The organizing framework for content of the text is arranged in order by the five domains contained in the HIM Associate Degree Entry-Level Competencies and the RHIT certification examination. This organization does not presuppose a pedagogical progression of presenting basic foundations and then progressing to advanced concepts.

Therefore, given its student population, mission and goals, and other variables, each academic program must assess the appropriate sequence of presentation of the chapters within its curriculum. Additional information and models of chapter sequencing can be found in the instructor's manual.

The book's underlying structure is to translate basic theory into practice. A review of the cognitive and competency levels of the Entry Level Competencies reveals that HIT programs are applied in nature. Outcome expectations are that students understand theory at a basic level with a major emphasis on skill building to perform day-to-day operational tasks in health information management.

Therefore, the features used throughout the book focus on translating basic theory into practice. To accomplish this, each chapter contains the following sections:

- **Theory into Practice:** Located at the beginning of each chapter, this section presents a case study that serves as an organizing framework for the theory presented in the chapter. This instructional design strategy "sets the stage" and "gains the learner's attention," two of the first and most basic steps in instructional design.

- **Check Your Understanding:** These sections are content review exercises. These exercises are positioned throughout each chapter so that students can reinforce their understanding of the concepts they have just read before going on to the following concepts. Multiple-choice, matching, and true-and-false formats are used.

- **Real-World Case:** Located near the end of each chapter, this section presents an actual situation faced by healthcare enterprises as reported in current literature and periodicals. The case supports the preceding instruction and moves toward selective perception.

Features in the accompanying workbook include:

- **Real-World Case Discussion Questions:** The questions in this section are designed to initiate discussion of and elaboration on the concepts presented in the Real-World Case.

- **Application Exercises:** The purpose of these exercises is to give students the opportunity to put theory into practice. Because skill building is an important part of the expected outcomes for HIT students, these exercises will bring the real world into their sphere.

- **Review Quizzes:** The review quizzes are in multiple-choice format and test chapter content knowledge.

The text is divided into five parts that correspond with the domains from the AHIMA Associate Degree Competencies and the RHIT certification examination content outline. Where appropriate, chapter content is expanded in the fourth edition to prepare students for transitional and changing roles in an electronic health information environment. All chapters in the fourth edition have been updated to reflect current trends, practices, standards, and legal issues.

Part 1, Healthcare Data Management, concentrates on the roles of the health information manager; the content, function, structure, and uses of health information; and how health information is managed. Chapter 1 introduces the concept of health information management. The discussion focuses on the history of the HIM profession and the evolution of the roles and functions of HIM professionals over the years. Particular emphasis is placed on HIM future roles and their relationship to the movement toward an electronic health record (EHR). Chapter 2, Purpose and Function of the Health Record, and chapter 3, Content and Structure of the Health Record, discuss the general components of the content, use, and structure of healthcare data. Content of the health record and documentation requirements are covered. The formats of paper and electronic record systems are investigated in chapter 3. Chapter 4, Healthcare Data Sets and Standards, builds on the basic knowledge presented in the previous chapters and discusses prominent healthcare data sets and their purposes and uses. Chapter 5, Clinical Vocabularies and Classification Systems, provides an introduction to clinical vocabularies and classification systems. Its purpose is to introduce the characteristics of prominent systems and help students understand how they are used throughout the healthcare system. Chapter 6, Reimbursement Methodologies, is an introduction to the uses of coded data and healthcare payment systems. It is meant to help students understand the process of reimbursement, billing procedures, use of chargemasters, and auditing. Part 1 concludes with chapter 7, Health Information Functions, which explains the typical functions associated with managing paper-based, hybrid, and EHR systems.

Part 2, Health Statistics, Biomedical Research, and Quality Management, introduces the timely topics of healthcare service evaluation. Consisting of three chapters, part 2 looks at the effective use, collection, arrangement, presentation, and verification of healthcare data. Chapter 8, Secondary Data Sources, reviews various types of secondary data sources, such as registries and indexes, that are used in healthcare service evaluation. Chapter 9, Healthcare Statistics, presents fundamental concepts of descriptive, vital, and facility statistics. It also discusses external and internal uses of statistics and patient data for research and the protection of patients and patient data in research. Chapter 10, Clinical Quality Performance Improvement and Management, addresses quality of patient care and the tools used. It also covers risk management, utilization management, and performance principles.

Part 3, Health Services Organization and Delivery, looks at the environment in which HIT professionals work, essentially, the US healthcare delivery system. It further demonstrates the complexity of the current delivery mechanisms, systems, and regulations involving healthcare. Chapter 11 introduces the history, organization, financing, and delivery of health services in the United States. Chapter 12 discusses the ethical issues associated with health information management and presents the concepts of stewardship and the HIM professional's core ethical obligations. Chapter 13 covers concepts basic to the US legal system as they relate to the work of the HIT professional, with a focus on updated federal privacy and confidentiality rules and regulations applied to health information.

Part 4, Information Technology and Systems, introduces information technology (IT) concepts and provides a broad view of how IT supports the functions of healthcare delivery. Chapter 14 provides a comprehensive discussion of information system concepts, components, and resources. The chapter helps students to conceptualize the various components necessary for development of a total health information system. Chapter 15 builds on the previous chapter and provides an overview of the application of technology to healthcare information systems and the EHR and ancillary feeder systems. Chapter 16 covers the EHR, health information exchange, and meaningful use. Chapter 17 provides a thorough discussion of information security program development and implementation and contains a review of recent updates in federal requirements for the protection of healthcare information.

Finally, **Part 5, Organizational Resources,** consists of two chapters, chapter 18, which introduces concepts and principles of organization and supervision, and chapter 19, on the future direction of the health information management profession.

A complete glossary of HIM terms is provided at the end of the book. **Boldface** type is used in the text chapters to indicate the first substantial reference to each glossary term.

Appendices and a detailed content index complete the book.

AHIMA provides supplemental materials for educators who use this book in their classes. Instructor materials for this book include lesson plans, lesson slides, an RHIT competency map, and other useful resources. Please visit http://www.ahima.org/publications/educators.aspx for further instruction. If you have any questions regarding the instructor materials, please contact AHIMA Customer Relations at (800) 335-5535 or submit a customer support request at https://secure.ahima.org/contact/contact.aspx.

Acknowledgments

Many individuals contributed to the development of the fourth edition of this landmark textbook. First, the editor and AHIMA publications staff extend their sincere thanks to all the chapter authors for sharing their expertise with new entrants into the HIM profession. Developing the rich content of this text along with searching for the best examples and resources was a time-consuming process for these very busy professionals.

Second, no text is ever complete without the diligent work of the content reviewers. Their careful review and insightful suggestions ensure the essential quality of any effort of this kind. We also would like to thank the following reviewers who lent a critical eye to this endeavor:

- Janie Batres, RHIT, CCS
- June E. Bronnert, RHIA, CCS, CCS-P
- Jill S. Clark, MBA, RHIA
- Kathryn A. DeVault, RHIA, CCS
- Angela K. Dinh, MHA, RHIA, CHPS
- Julie A. Dooling, RHIT
- Melanie A. Endicott, MBA, RHIA, CCS, CCS-P
- Karen M. Kostick, RHIT, CCS, CCS-P
- Theresa A. Rihanek, RHIA, CCS
- Diana M. Warner, MS, RHIA, CHPS
- Lou Ann Wiedemann, MS, RHIA

We would also like to acknowledge students from the College of DuPage, under the supervision of Cheryl P. Jackson, RHIA, CCS, who reviewed the Check Your Understanding (CYU) exercises in each of the 4th edition chapters. Their help is greatly appreciated.

- Katherine Anderson
- Nancy Bauer
- Maryana Bodnar
- Patricia Cady
- Elizabeth Campbell
- Elaine Caravello

- Nartanong Harte
- Diana Henselman
- Tracey Johnson
- Carol Klein
- Carol Kritselis
- Monika Krol
- Amber Mack
- Monika Mihali
- Vaishali Patel
- Luisa Perez
- Peterine Svoboda
- Tiffany Vogel
- John Wallace
- Krista Walters
- Emily Wernsman
- William Wojtyla

Additionally, the editor would like to acknowledge authors who contributed chapters to each edition of this book. Their work served as the basis for several chapters that were revised by new authors:

- Sandra Bailey, RHIA
- Cathleen A. Barnes, RHIA, CCS
- Mary Jo Bowie, MS, RHIA
- Elizabeth D. Bowman, MPA, RHIA
- Bonnie S. Cassidy, MPA, RHIA, FAHIMA, FHIMSS
- Michelle L. Dougherty, RHIA, CHP
- Sandra R. Fuller, MA, RHIA
- Michelle A. Green, MPS, RHIA, CMA, CHP
- Terrill Herzig, MSHI
- Beth M. Hjort, RHIA
- Joan Hicks, MSHI, RHIA
- Merida Johns, PhD, RHIA

- Kathleen M. LaTour, MA, RHIA, FAHIMA
- Joan Ludwig, RHIA
- Carol E. Osborn, PhD, RHIA
- Harry B. Rhodes, MBA, RHIA
- Karen A. Wager, DBA, RHIA
- Frances Wickham Lee, DBA, RHIA
- Susan B. Willner, RHIA
- Andrea Weatherby White, PhD, RHIA

To Tomorrow's Health Information Management Professionals

As healthcare evolves in response to healthcare reform, technology, and new models of patient care, the role of the health information (HI) professional must evolve. Health information management (HIM) is the profession that collects, maintains, and processes patient information for the healthcare providers, payers, and the government. With widespread adoption of electronic health records and other technology-based information sources and the use of the electronically available data for healthcare management, the role of the AHIMA professional will continue to evolve. It is estimated that the demand for HIM professionals will far exceed the supply of trained workers. An analysis by Hersch and Wright estimates that approximately 40,000 more healthcare IT staff and professionals are needed for broad adoption of healthcare IT than currently exist. The HIM and HIT workforce is expected to grow more than 27 percent through 2020.

We must become savvy in our use of technology and data analytic tools to better serve patients, inform policy leaders, and move the HIM profession into the 21st century. To meet the needs of various healthcare organizations in their use of emerging technologies, we need to be proactive in better understanding our new roles. As new health information professionals, you must be able to define your future in the HIM marketplace.

This textbook is intended to help guide you in your career as an HIM professional. Current work on the HIM core model suggests that your role in tomorrow's healthcare organizations will expand into areas of data management, data integrity, fraud and abuse, revenue cycle, and managing across the healthcare organization.

Health Information Management Technology: An Applied Approach, Fourth Edition brings together an impressive array of HIM professionals that will provide direction as to how the future of HIM will look. Topical areas covered in the book cover the HIM field of the future and will provide you with an understanding of the knowledge and skill necessary to succeed. It is essential that you as a student understand the content and purpose of the health record and how it is used for purposes of data integrity, reimbursement, research, the foundation for standards, quality improvement, privacy and security, and in the delivery of safe healthcare to the patient.

This textbook will help to serve as your guide to help you better understand both the complexities of healthcare and your role in not only meeting those demands but in shaping your future.

You are the future.

William J Rudman, PHD, RHIA
Executive Director AHIMA Foundation and
Vice President of Education Visioning

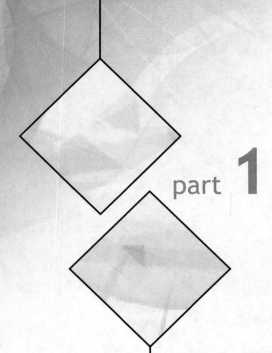

part **1**

Healthcare Data Management

chapter 1

Introduction to the HIM Profession

Nanette B. Sayles, EdD, RHIA, CCS, CHPS, CPHIMS, FAHIMA

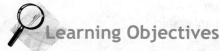

Learning Objectives

- Summarize the development of the health information management profession from its beginnings to the present
- Discuss how professional practice must evolve to accommodate changes in the healthcare environment
- Identify the responsibilities of health information management professionals
- Describe the purpose and structure of the American Health Information Management Association
- Explain the certification processes of the American Health Information Management Association
- Discuss the accreditation process of the Commission on Accreditation for Health Informatics and Information Management Education (CAHIIM)
- Identify the appropriate professional organizations for the various specializations of health information management

Key Terms

Accreditation

Active membership

American Academy of Professional Coders

American Association of Medical Record Librarians (AAMRL)

American College of Surgeons (ACS)

American Health Information Management Association (AHIMA)

American Medical Record Association (AMRA)

American Recovery and Reinvestment Act of 2009

Association for Healthcare Documentation Integrity (AHDI)

Association of Record Librarians of North America (ARLNA)

Certification

Certified Documentation Improvement Practitioner (CDIP)

Code of Ethics

Commission on Accreditation for Health Informatics and Information Management Education (CAHIIM)

Commission on Certification for Health Informatics and Information Management (CCHIIM)

Communities of Practice (CoP)

Community College Consortia to Educate Health Information Technology Professionals

Component state associations (CSAs)

Credentialing

Curriculum

Fellowship Program

Health information management (HIM)

Hospital Standardization Program

House of Delegates

National Cancer Registrars Association (NCRA)

Registered Health Information Administrator (RHIA)

Registered Health Information Technician (RHIT)

Registration

Student membership

Introduction

Health information management (HIM) has been recognized as an allied health profession since 1928. The **Association of Record Librarians of North America** (ARLNA) was formed only 10 years after the beginning of the hospital standardization movement. The association's original objective was to elevate the standards of clinical recordkeeping in hospitals, dispensaries, and other healthcare facilities.

The first annual meeting of the professional organization was held in Chicago in 1929. Since then, the organization and the professionals affiliated with it have been advocates for the effective management of clinical records.

The name of the organization has changed several times throughout the years to reflect the changing healthcare environment. Today, the association is known as the **American Health Information Management Association** (AHIMA). Still, the association's underlying purpose remains the same: to ensure the quality, confidentiality, and availability of health information across diverse organizations, settings, and disciplines.

This chapter provides an introduction to the history of the HIM profession. The chapter offers insights into the current and future roles and functions of health information managers. The mission of the original organization is no less important today than it was in 1928. In fact, the role of HIM professionals is even more important and complex in today's information- and technology-driven healthcare environment.

Those entering the HIM profession benefit from the commitment and hard work of previous visionaries in the field, who understood what it takes to develop and maintain a profession. Thus, to carry on with this legacy, today's HIM professionals must be equally committed to the original goal of "elevating standards for clinical records" as well as fulfilling the obligations of healthcare professionals.

Theory into Practice

This is the era of e-HIM. The HIM director at Community Hospital, a multifacility healthcare organization, is responsible for ensuring the quality and availability of health information to facilitate real-time healthcare delivery and critical health-related decision making for multiple purposes across the organization. The organization's information systems are completely electronic, and HIM is a virtual department. The director still oversees traditional HIM functions that existed in a paper-based medical record environment such as record processing, analysis and completion, release of information, medical transcription, and forms management. While the purpose of the functions has remained the same in the electronic environment, the way in which they are carried out has dramatically changed. This means that the HIM director has increased knowledge and skills in the capture, use, and management of information. Among these are skills in terminology mapping, data modeling, data governance, data flow design and improvement, data mining, and workflow coordination and management.

In the virtual HIM department, maintaining a large staff of file clerks is no longer necessary because information is generated at the point of care and stored electronically. Release of information processes have been transformed and electronic authentication has shortened record completion turnaround time.

Many functions are performed by personnel associated not only with HIM but also with other departments. For example, the HIM director at Community Hospital supervises several data steward positions that are physically located in departments such as clinical laboratory, radiology, admitting, billing, and dietary management. Furthermore, the virtual HIM department consists of employees who are located remotely away from the organization. Among these are medical transcriptionists and clinical coders.

A major part of the HIM director's work involves monitoring and reconciling interfaces, running electronic data integrity audits, attending design sessions for new EHR applications, and resolving health information exchange, privacy, and security issues. Among the automated systems that the HIM director and her staff works with are: the master patient index (MPI), the healthcare information system (HIS), the clinical information system (CIS), the electronic health record system (EHR), the electronic document management system (EDMS), the HIM department information system (HIMIS), the revenue cycle management system (RCM), the voice/text/speech (VTS) system, and the registry information system (RIS).

In the world of e-HIM, automation now influences every aspect of traditional HIM functions (table 1.1).

Table 1.1. HIM functions automated by line-of-business information systems

Function	Automated by Line-of-Business Information Systems								
Master patient index management	MPI								
Medical record processing (e.g., chart assembly)		HIS	CIS	EHR	EDMS				
Medical record analysis and completion		HIS		EHR	EDMS	HIMIS			
Medical record coding and abstracting	MPI					HIMIS	RCM		
Medical record report dictation and transcription								VTS	
Release of information		HIS		EHR	EDMS	HIMIS			
Medical record file services		HIS		EHR	and/or EDMS				
Medical record data collection and analysis		HIS	CIS	and/or EHR		HIMIS			
Department organization and management		HIS		EHR	EDMS	HIMIS			
Registry management						and/or HIMIS			RIS
Forms management (format and content)		HIS		EHR	and/or EDMS				
Information confidentiality and security	MPI	HIS	CIS	EHR	EDMS	HIMIS			

Adapted from Servais 2009, 38–42.

Early History of Health Information Management

Today's HIM professionals are the benefactors of the wisdom, insight, and fortitude of pioneers whose untiring commitment is reflected in today's dynamic profession. The history of the HIM profession is witness to how a small group of dedicated individuals can come together and make a difference for decades to come.

The early history of the health information profession was summarized by Edna K. Huffman in an article appearing in the March 1941 issue of the *Bulletin of the American Association of Medical Record Librarians* (Huffman 1941). Three distinct steps influenced development of the profession. These included the hospital standardization movement, the organization of records librarians, and the approval of formal educational processes, and a curriculum for medical record librarians.

Hospital Standardization

Before 1918, the creation and management of hospital medical records were the sole responsibility of the attending physician. Physicians in the early 20th century, like many physicians today, often disliked doing paperwork. Unless the physician was interested in medical research, the medical records in the early 20th century were "practically worthless and consisted principally of nurse's notes" (Huffman 1941, 101).

Medical records of that time did not contain graphical records or laboratory reports. Because there was no general management of medical record processes, the incomplete records were often filed as received on discharge of the patient. Hospitals made no effort to ensure that the deficient portions were completed. Furthermore, no standardized vocabulary was used to document why the patient was admitted to the hospital or what the final diagnosis upon discharge was.

In 1918, the hospital standardization movement was inaugurated by the **American College of Surgeons** (ACS). The purpose of the **Hospital Standardization Program** was to raise the standards of surgery by establishing minimum quality standards for hospitals. The ACS realized that one of the most important items in the care of any patient was a complete and accurate report of the care and treatment provided during hospitalization. Specifically, the standard required the following:

> Accurate and complete medical records [must] be written for all patients and filed in an accessible manner in the hospital, a complete medical record being one which includes identification data; complaint; personal and family history; history of the present illness; physical examination; special examinations such as consultations, clinical laboratory, x-ray and other examinations; provisional or working diagnosis; medical or surgical treatment; gross or microscopical pathological findings; progress notes; final diagnosis; condition on discharge; follow-up; and, in case of death, autopsy findings (Huffman 1941, 101).

It was not long before hospitals realized that to comply with the hospital standards, new medical record processes had to be implemented. In addition, new staff had to be hired to ensure that the new processes were appropriately carried out. Furthermore, hospitals recognized that medical records must be maintained and filed in an orderly manner and that cross-indexes of disease, operations, and physicians must be compiled. Thus, the job position of medical record clerk was established.

Organization of the Association of Record Librarians

A nucleus of 35 members of the Club of Record Clerks met at the Hospital Standardization Conference in Boston in 1928. Near the close of the meeting, the Association of Record Librarians of North America (ARLNA) was formed. During its first year, the association had a charter membership of 58 individuals. Members were admitted from 25 of the 48 states, the District of Columbia, and Canada (Huffman 1985). The ARLNA was the predecessor of the American Health Information Management Association (AHIMA).

Approval of Formal Education and Certification Programs

Early HIM professionals understood that for an occupation to be recognized as a profession there must be preliminary training. They also understood that such training needed to be distinguished from mere skill. That is, it needed to be intellectual in character, involving knowledge and, to some extent, learning. Therefore, work began on the formulation of a prescribed course of study as early as 1929. In 1932, the association adopted a formal **curriculum.**

The first schools for medical record librarians were surveyed and approved by the ARLNA in 1934. By 1941, 10 schools had been approved to provide training for medical record librarians. This formal **accreditation** process of academic programs was the precursor to the current accreditation program, **Commission on Accreditation for Health Informatics and Information Management Education** (CAHIIM).

The Board of Registration was instituted in 1933. The founders of the profession recognized that the existence of unqualified workers in the field lowered the standards of their profession. Therefore, they organized a **certification** board so that there would be a baseline by which to measure qualified medical record librarians. The Board of Registration established criteria for eligibility for **registration.** The board also developed and administered the qualifying examination. Today, the role of the Board of Registration is played by AHIMA's **Commission on Certification for Health Informatics and Information Management** (CCHIIM).

Development of the HIM profession coincided with the professionalization of other healthcare disciplines such nursing, x-ray technology, and laboratory technology. All these disciplines established registration and/or training programs around the same time.

The professional membership of the association of HIM professionals grew steadily over the subsequent decades. Although the names of the association and the credentials have changed several times during the past decades, the fundamental elements of the profession—formal training requirements and certification by examination—have remained the same.

Evolution of Practice

The various names given to the medical record association and its associated credentials reveal a lot about the evolution of the profession and its practice. In 1928, the organization's name was the Association of Record Librarians of North America (ARLNA). In 1944, Canadian members formed their own organization, and the name of the organization was changed to the **American Association of Medical Record Librarians** (AAMRL). In 1970, the organization changed its name again to eliminate the term *librarian.* The organization's name became the **American Medical Record Association** (AMRA). The organization underwent another name change in 1991 to become the American Health Information Management Association (AHIMA).

The organization's title changes in 1970 and 1991 reflected the changing nature of the roles and functions of the association's professional membership. In 1970, the term *administrator* mirrored the work performed by members more accurately than the term *librarian.* Similarly, in 1991, association leaders believed that the management of information, rather than the management of records, would be the primary function of the profession in the future.

The names of the credentials conferred by the organization changed as the association's name changed. In 1999, the AHIMA House of Delegates approved a credential name change. Registered record administrator (RRA) became **registered health information administrator** (RHIA), and accredited record technician (ART) became **registered health information technician** (RHIT).

What does the changing of the organization and credential names say about the profession? Probably one of the most significant things that it indicates is a major shift in what professionals do and how they fit within their environment. The combined forces of new information technologies and the demands for increased, better, and more timely information require the profession to change radically.

Traditional Practice

The original practice of health information management was based on the Hospital Standardization Program, initiated in 1918. The program emphasized the need to ensure that complete and accurate medical records were compiled and maintained for every patient. Accurate records were needed to support the care and treatment provided to the patient as well as to conduct various types of clinical research. This emphasis remained fundamental to the profession through 1990. For example, a review of the professional practice standards published by AMRA in 1984 and updated in 1990 shows a model of practice that was highly quantitative and department based (Johns 1991, 57).

Further evaluation of the 1990 professional practice standards discloses that the tasks of medical record practitioners at that time involved planning, developing, and implementing systems designed to control, monitor, and track the quantity of record content and the flow, storage, and retrieval of medical records. In other words, activities primarily centered on the medical record or reports within the record as a physical unit rather than on the data elements that make up the information within the medical record.

At that time, very few standards "addressed issues relating to determination of the completion, significance, organization, timeliness, or accuracy of information contained in the medical record or its usefulness to decision support" (Johns 1991, 57). Figure 1.1 illustrates how traditional practice focused on the management of medical records as objects.

Figure 1.1.   Traditional model of practice

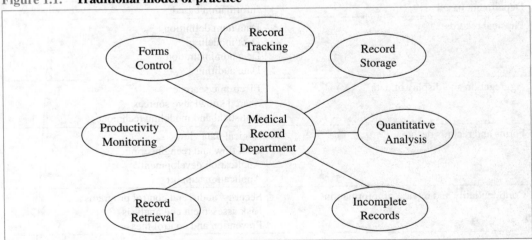

Source: Johns 1991, p. 55.

Information-oriented Management Practice

The traditional model of practice shown in figure 1.1 would not be appropriate for today's information-intensive and automated healthcare environment. The traditional model of practice is department focused. Tasks are devoted primarily to processing and tracking records rather than processing and tracking information.

Studies have consistently shown that 25 to 40 percent of a hospital's operating costs are devoted to information handling. Obviously, information management has become a top priority for healthcare institutions (Blum 1986; Protti 1984). In today's information age, information crosses departmental boundaries and is broadly disseminated throughout the organization and beyond. In fact, information grows out of data manipulation from a variety of shared data sources. An information-oriented management model includes tasks associated with a broad range of information services. Therefore, the tasks performed as a health information manager—in contrast to tasks performed as a medical record manager—are information based, "emphasizing data manipulation and information management tasks and focusing on the provision of an extensive range of information services" (Johns 1991, 59).

Visioning the Future of HIM

What are the information services and functions that are being performed by health information managers? For many years AHIMA has been planning for and envisioning the future of the HIM profession. In 1996, AHIMA embarked on an initiative called Vision 2006 that identified many new roles that information managers would likely assume in the upcoming information-focused decades. Moreover, it demonstrated the difference between traditional practice and information-oriented practice. Table 1.2 shows the differences

Table 1.2.   Comparison of traditional HIM and Vision 2006 roles

Traditional HIM	Vision 2006
Department based	Information based
Physical records	Data item definition Data modeling Data administration Data auditing
Aggregation and display of data	Electronic searches Shared knowledge sources Statistical and modeling techniques
Forms and records design	Logical data views Data flow and reengineering Application development Application support
Confidentiality and release of information	Security, audit, and control programs Risk assessment and analysis Prevention and control measures

between tasks in traditional and information-focused practice (as envisioned through AHIMA's Vision 2006 initiative).

As table 1.2 shows, the traditional model of practice is department based and the health information manager's activities were usually performed in the medical record department. In the new model, tasks are information based and many of the health information manager's activities are performed outside the HIM department as the Theory into Practice example at the beginning of this chapter describes. Indeed, many health information managers today work entirely in other areas of the facility and in other settings. They work in a variety of functional areas, such as quality improvement, decision support, information systems, utilization management, data privacy, data security, and so on. Instead of working primarily in hospitals, many work in ambulatory care facilities, information systems vendors, consulting companies, and other nontraditional settings. In fact, as shown by table 1.3, 52 percent of HIM professionals work in acute care facilities (HIcareers).

A second important difference is that the traditional model of practice is based on creating, tracking, and storing physical records. In today's information-intense environment, the physical (paper-based) health record is being replaced by the electronic health record. The information in EHRs is created, compiled, and stored in many different areas within the enterprise and is brought together electronically only when needed. The tasks performed by a health information manager focus on such activities as maintaining data dictionaries, developing data models, performing data administration tasks, and ensuring data quality through a variety of auditing tasks.

Another difference between the two models of practice centers on tasks associated with data analysis and interpretation. In the traditional model of practice, the tasks involve the aggregation and display of data. However, today's information world is much more complicated than it was two or three decades ago and contains more enabling technologies to search and analyze data. Thus, the health information manager who works in decision support or quality improvement today uses sophisticated computer-based tools to analyze data from a variety of data sources.

Table 1.3.   HIM profession's job settings

Acute care hospital	52%
Integrated healthcare delivery system	9%
Other provider setting	9%
Clinic/provider setting	8%
Nonprovider setting	6%
Educational institution	4%
Consulting	3%
Behavorial/mental health	3%
Long-term care or nursing facility	3%
Home health or hospice	2%

Source: http://HIcareers.com.

With more emphasis being placed on the development of an electronic record, health information managers find that the tasks they perform are less concerned with paper forms design and focus instead on developing good user interfaces for electronic medical records.

Finally, health information practitioners have always been concerned with the privacy and confidentiality of data. The tasks in the traditional model of practice were confined principally to issues involving release of information. However, in today's more technologically sophisticated world, these tasks are shifting to include enterprise-wide responsibilities for computer data security and privacy programs as well as functions in health information exchange organizations.

AHIMA's e-HIM Task Force in 2003 confirmed the information-handling focus of HIM practice where the state of health information is described as electronic, patient-centered, comprehensive, longitudinal, accessible, and credible (AHIMA 2003).

From Traditional Roles to New Opportunities

In the Vision 2006 initiative, AHIMA identified several new roles as opportunities for health information managers in 2006 and beyond. These new roles are based on the information model of practice and include the following (AHIMA 1999, 5–6):

- The health information manager for integrated systems is responsible for the organization-wide direction of health information functions.

- The clinical data specialist is responsible for data management functions, including clinical coding, outcomes management, and maintenance of specialty registries and research databases.

- The patient information coordinator assists consumers in managing their personal health information, including personal health histories and release of information.

- The data quality manager is responsible for data management functions that involve formalized continuous quality improvement activities for data integrity throughout the organization, such as data dictionary and policy development and data quality monitoring and audits.

- The information security manager is responsible for managing the security of electronically maintained information, including the promotion of security requirements, policies, privilege systems and performance auditing.

- The data resource administrator manages the data resources of the organization, such as data repositories and data warehouses.

- The research and decision support specialist provides senior managers with information for decision making and strategy development.

Figure 1.2 illustrates the interrelationships among these roles with the patient as the center and primary focus of all information management tasks. As predicted, HIM professionals are working in all of these types of roles and in a variety of organizations and the

Figure 1.2. **Vision 2006 roles**

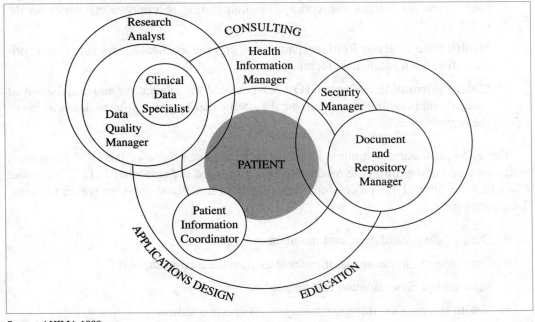

Source: AHIMA 1999.

profession has truly evolved to e-HIM. More recently the following new and revised jobs are among those that demonstrate the trends changing HIM and the opportunities that lie ahead (Dimick 2008):

- **Terminology modeler:** Creates digital links among various terminologies and classification systems

- **Personal health record (PHR) liaison or consultant:** Assists individuals in compilation of their personal health records

- **Physician group consultant:** Aids in EHR system implementation, auditing documentation practices, or assisting with revenue cycle management

- **Privacy officer:** Creates the rules for exchange of health information and ensures that the health information remains confidential

- **Health record reviewer:** Responsible for monitoring quality of health information and reconciling information within health record banks and monitoring records for quality

- **HIM director:** Works with the design, development, and implementation of the EHR monitoring and reconciling interfaces, running electronic data integrity audits, and supervising a staff of individuals in a "virtual" HIM department

- **Enterprise content and information manager:** Manages an organization's nonclinical paper and electronic documents including developing systems to index and track the location of content and information within the enterprise

- **Revenue cycle manager:** Oversees all of the processes that make up the revenue cycle from documentation, coding, through billing to improve efficiency in the cycle
- **Health data analyst:** Retrieves, analyzes, and reports health data using appropriate software and statistical techniques
- **Chief information officer (CIO):** Responsible for evaluation and acquisition of clinical and nonclinical technological systems that best meet the business needs of the organization

The HIM profession continues to evolve with the latest view of the HIM profession being described in the draft core model that was published in September 2011. This model shows that the future HIM professional has five main functional areas on which to focus. These areas are:

- Data capture, validation, and maintenance
- Data/information analysis, transformation, and decision support
- Information dissemination and liaison
- Health information resource management and innovation
- Information governance and stewardship (AHIMA 2011)

The model is shown in figure 1.3.

Figure 1.3.   The HIM Professional Core Model

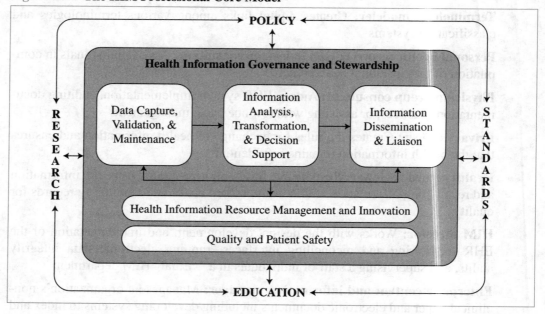

The roles of HIM professionals will continue to evolve to meet the needs of the health-care delivery system. The future of the HIM profession is positive due to the growth in opportunities. However, for individual members of the profession to be successful, each must engage in a program of lifelong learning. This means that change is an everyday occurrence. Health information professionals must commit themselves to continually upgrade their skills so that they can successfully address a constantly changing and challenging environment.

Check Your Understanding 1.1

1. HIM has been recognized as an allied health profession since:

    A. 1910
    B. 1918
    C. 1928
    D. 2006

2. The hospital standardization movement was inaugurated by the:

    A. American Health Information Management Association
    B. American College of Surgeons
    C. Record Librarians of North America
    D. American College of Physicians

3. Critique this statement. The HIM professional's role in privacy and security has not changed.

    A. This is a true statement as the HIM professional's role in privacy and security is still limited to release of information.
    B. This is a false statement as the HIM professional's role has diminished.
    C. This is a false statement as the HIM professional role is more enterprise focused.
    D. This is a true statement as the HIM professional's role in privacy and security is still limited to the paper record.

4. The traditional model of HIM practice was:

    A. Department based
    B. Information based
    C. Electronically based
    D. Analytically based

5. The new model of HIM practice is:

    A. Information focused
    B. Record focused
    C. Department focused
    D. Traditionally focused

6. What evolving role oversees the revenue cycle from documentation through billing?

   A. HIM director
   B. Health record reviewer
   C. Health data analyst
   D. Revenue cycle manager

7. The organization that accredits HIM education programs is:

   A. Joint Commission
   B. CAHIIM
   C. AHIMA
   D. CCHIIM

8. What evolving role assesses quality in health record banking?

   A. Physician group consultant
   B. Health record reviewer
   C. Health data analyst
   D. Terminology manager

Today's Professional Organization

The health information management profession began with establishment of the ARLNA in 1928. As previously described, the organization's name has changed several times. The last name change occurred in 1991, when the professional organization assumed the name of AHIMA. The most recent name change reflects the requirements of the information age and, subsequently, the needs of the healthcare delivery system and the new roles of health information managers.

Mission

Before studying AHIMA's structure, it is important to understand why the organization exists and what contributions it makes to both its members and the healthcare system in general. The mission of an organization explains what the organization is and what it does. In other words, it describes the organization's distinctive purpose. Figure 1.4 shows AHIMA's current mission, values, and vision statements.

AHIMA is a membership organization. The majority of its members are credentialed HIM professionals who work throughout the healthcare industry. These professionals serve the healthcare industry and the public by managing, analyzing, and utilizing information vital for patient care and making it accessible to healthcare providers when and where it is needed.

The primary focus of the organization is to foster the professional development of its members through education, certification, and lifelong learning. By doing this, AHIMA promotes the development of high-quality information that benefits the public, the healthcare

Figure 1.4.   **AHIMA mission, values, and vision**

The Mission of the American Health Information Management Association

To be the professional community that improves healthcare by advancing best practices and standards for health information management and the trusted source for education, research, and professional credentialing.

AHIMA Values:

- The public's right to accurate and confidential personal health information
- Innovation and leadership in advancing health information management practices and standards worldwide
- Adherence to the AHIMA Code of Ethics
- Advocacy and interdisciplinary collaboration with other professional organizations

Vision

Quality healthcare through quality information

---

consumer, healthcare providers, and other users of clinical data. The organization has certification programs that set high standards to ensure the qualifications of the individuals who practice as health information managers and technicians. In addition, it supports numerous continuing education (CE) programs to help its credentialed members and others maintain their knowledge base and skills.

To accomplish its mission, AHIMA expects that all its members will follow a code of professional ethics. (A complete discussion of ethical principles and the AHIMA Code of Ethics is provided in chapter 12.) As the **Code of Ethics** stipulates, all members of AHIMA are expected to act in an ethical manner and comply with all laws, regulations, and standards governing the practice of health information management. As professionals, members are expected to continually update their knowledge base and skills through CE and lifelong learning. HITs and managers are expected to promote high standards of HIM practice, education, and research. Additionally, they are expected to promote and protect the confidentiality and security of health records and health information.

Membership

Today, AHIMA has more than 63,000 members. To accommodate the diversity in membership, the organization has two membership categories.

Active membership is open to all individuals interested in the AHIMA purpose and willing to abide by the Code of Ethics. Active members in good standing are entitled to all membership privileges including the right to vote and to serve in the House of Delegates. Active membership provides HIM professionals the opportunity to participate in the organization and to offer input to the current and future practices of the profession.

Student membership includes any student who does not have an AHIMA credential, has not previously been an active member of AHIMA, and who is formally enrolled in an AHIMA-approved coding program or in a CAHIIM-accredited health information management program. The student membership category gives entry-level professionals an opportunity to participate on a national level in promoting sound HIM practices. Student members can serve on committees and subcommittees in designated student positions with voice, but no vote.

Structure and Operation

Every organization needs a management structure to operate effectively and efficiently. AHIMA is made up of two components: a volunteer component and a staff component. The volunteer structure establishes the organization's mission and goals, develops policy, and provides oversight for the organization's operations. Figure 1.5 shows the AHIMA volunteer structure. The staff component of the organization carries out the operational tasks necessary to support the organization's mission and goals. The staff works within the policies established by the volunteer component.

Association Leadership

As a nonprofit membership association, AHIMA depends on the participation and direction of volunteer leaders from the HIM community. AHIMA's members elect the delegates who serve in the governing bodies of the organization.

AHIMA's Board of Directors leads the volunteer structure. It has responsibility for managing the property, affairs, and operations of AHIMA. This body is charged with tremendous responsibility. Its members include the president, the president-elect, the past president, nine elected directors, and the chief executive officer of the organization. Except for the chief executive officer, who is selected by the Board, all members of the Board are elected by the membership and serve three-year terms of office. Members of the Board must be active members of the association.

In addition to the Board of Directors, two other groups are elected directly by the overall membership. These include the Commission on Certification for Health Informatics and Information Management (CCHIIM) and the Commission on Accreditation for Health Informatics and Information Management Education (CAHIIM). The CCHIIM is responsible for overseeing AHIMA's certification process and for setting policies and procedures. Similarly, CAHIIM is responsible for overseeing accreditation of college programs in health information technology and health information administration and graduate programs in health informatics.

Communities of Practice

The **Communities of Practice** (CoP) make up a virtual network of AHIMA members who communicate via a web-based program managed by AHIMA. The CoP is open only to AHIMA members and provides the following benefits:

- Provides opportunities for members to contact other members for quick problem-solving, support, advice, and career-building tips and opportunities. It also makes it possible to share best practices.

Figure 1.5.   AHIMA volunteer organizational structure

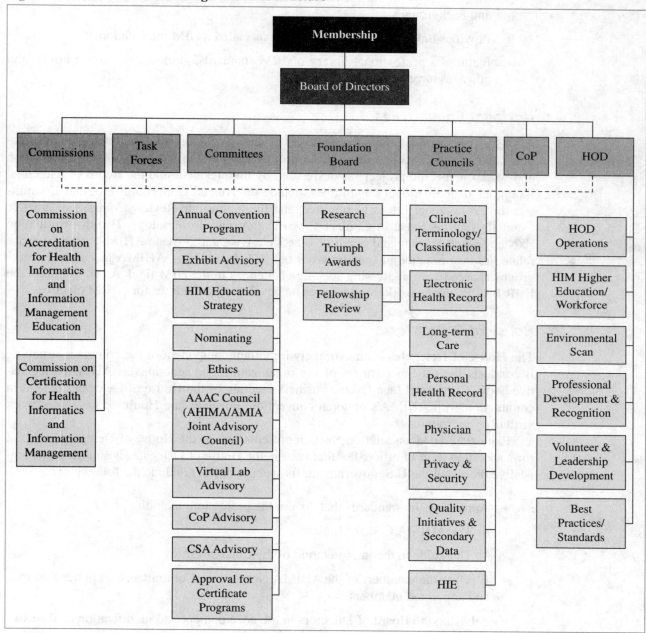

- Makes it possible for members to search for other members with similar interests and backgrounds.

- Provides links to other sites that have specialized HIM information.

- Includes a professional library of HIM standards, guidelines, practice briefs, and other resources.

National Committees

AHIMA's president appoints the members of the association's national committees, practice councils, and workgroups. These groups support the mission of the organization and work on specific projects as designated by the president and the Board of Directors. Examples of the national committees include the Annual Convention Program Committee, the Professional Ethics Committee, and the Fellowship Review Committee. Practice Councils such as those in Clinical Classification and Terminology, Health Information Exchange, and Privacy and Security Practice advise and provide AHIMA with expertise related to best practice in specific areas of HIM. In addition, AHIMA has several workgroups charged with addressing specific challenges in the HIM field. As an example, the EHR Best Practices workgroup focuses on developing guidelines for e-HIM practice.

House of Delegates

The **House of Delegates** is an extremely important component of the volunteer structure. It conducts the official business of the organization and functions as AHIMA's legislative body. The annual face-to-face business meeting of the House of Delegates is held in conjunction with AHIMA's national convention, however, the House of Delegates work virtually year round.

Each state HIM association elects representatives to the House of Delegates to serve for a specified term of office. For that reason, the House of Delegates is similar to the legislative branch of the U.S. government. Its specific powers include the following:

- Approving the standards that govern the profession, including:

  — The AHIMA Code of Ethics

  — The guide to the interpretation of the Code of Ethics

- Electing the members of the AHIMA Nominating Committee, except the chairman and appointed members

- Advising the Board of Directors in the development and modification of the association's plans

- Levying special assessments

- Approving amendments to AHIMA's bylaws

- Approving the standing rules of the House of Delegates

- Approving resolutions

Each Component State Association (CSA) assigns a member to each of the House of Delegates six House Teams. The House Teams are where the business before the House is discussed and problems are resolved. The six House Teams are:

- **Best Practices/Standards**: advances the health industry by collaborating and vetting the development of HIM practice guidance, professional guidelines, and research initiatives

- **Environmental Scan**: conducts environmental scanning with CSAs and delegates to discover trends and long-term change in forces shaping the future

- **HIM Higher Education and Workforce**: supports and promotes the robust academic network of programs and faculty that produce and place graduates prepared for future roles

- **House Operations**: provides the general oversight for the operations of the House of Delegates and ensures the effectiveness of each House Team

- **Professional Development and Recognition**: identifies the learning needs of health information and information management professionals and suggests resources to increase competence and promote their value

- **Volunteer and Leadership Development**: increase the number of qualified volunteers involved in leadership activities in collaboration with AHIMA's Nominating Committee and CSAs (AHIMA nd)

State and Local Associations

In addition to its national volunteer organization, AHIMA supports a system of component organizations in every state, plus Washington, DC, and Puerto Rico. **Component state associations** (CSAs) provide their members with local access to professional education, networking, and representation. CSAs also serve as an important forum for communicating information relevant to national issues and keeping members informed of regional affairs that affect health information management.

Many states also have local or regional organizations. For newly credentialed professionals, the state and local organizations are ideal avenues for becoming involved with volunteer work within the professional organization. Most HIM professionals who serve in the House of Delegates or serve on AHIMA's Board of Directors got their start in volunteer services with local, regional, and state associations.

Staff Structure

AHIMA's headquarters are located in Chicago. The staff required to run the day-to-day operations of the organization is organized into a number of divisions. The executive director is the individual responsible for overseeing day-to-day operations. A team of executives, managers, and staff support the chief executive officer. Examples of the staff departments include, among others, member services, education, professional practice services, publications, marketing, and policy and government relations.

Accreditation of Educational Programs

AHIMA has a long tradition of commitment to HIM education. As discussed previously, the first prescribed curriculum for the training of medical record professionals was proposed in 1929. The first educational programs were accredited in 1934. Since that time, the association has developed and maintained a rigorous accreditation process for academic programs, continuously developed up-to-date curriculum models, and supported educational programs in a variety of ways.

In 2004, the AHIMA House of Delegates voted to establish an independent accreditation commission (CAHIIM) with sole and independent authority in all matters pertaining to accreditation of educational programs in health informatics and information management. CAHIIM is the accrediting agency for degree-granting programs in health informatics and information management. CAHIIM serves the public interest by establishing quality standards for the educational preparation of future HIM professionals. When a program is accredited by CAHIIM, it means that it has voluntarily undergone a rigorous review process and has been determined to meet or exceed the standards established by the CAHIIM. CAHIIM accreditation is a way to recognize and publicize best practices for HIM education programs.

CAHIIM reviews formal applications from college programs that apply for Candidacy status. After a successful review of the application documentation, a program may be deemed a Candidate for Accreditation for up to two years. Students enrolled in programs that are placed in Candidacy status are eligible to join AHIMA as student members. Within an agreed upon time frame, the college program prepares a self-assessment document and a campus site visit occurs. A report of the site visit is reviewed by the CAHIIM Board of Commissioners and a final determination is made as to the ability of the college program to meet the accreditation standards for curriculum, facility, resources, and other requirements. The accreditation of educational programs is important because only those individuals who graduate from an approved program may sit for the national **credentialing** examinations for registered health information technician (RHIT) or registered health information administrator (RHIA).

Certification and Registration Program

The founding members of the organization recognized early on the necessity of setting standards for medical record practitioners. In 1933, the association organized a certifying board known as the Board of Registration. This board was developed "so that there might be a yard-stick by which qualified medical record librarians could be determined" (Huffman 1941, 101). To become a registered record librarian (RRL) in 1940, a candidate needed to:

- Be at least 21 years of age
- Be a graduate of a school for record librarians approved by AAMRL
- Be currently employed in medical records work
- Pass a qualifying credentialing examination

As the field of health information management became more complex, the association recognized the need to expand its credentialing program. In 2008, the Commission on Certification for Health Informatics and Information Management (CCHIIM) was established. CCHIIM is dedicated to assuring the competency of professionals practicing HIM. CCHIIM serves the public by establishing, implementing, and enforcing standards and procedures for certification and recertification of HIM professionals. CCHIIM provides strategic oversight of all AHIMA certification programs. This standing commission of AHIMA is empowered with the sole and independent authority in all matters pertaining to both the initial certification and ongoing recertification (certification maintenance) of HIM professionals.

Today, the AHIMA certification program encompasses several different types of credentials, including:

- Health Information Technician (RHIT)
- Registered Health Information Administrator (RHIA)
- Certified Coding Associate (CCA)
- Certified Coding Specialist (CCS)
- Certified Coding Specialist—Physician based (CCS-P)
- Certified in Healthcare Privacy and Security (CHPS)
- Certified Health Data Analyst (CHDA)
- Clinical Documentation Improvement Practitioner (CDIP)

Each of these credentials has specific eligibility requirements and a certification examination. To achieve certification from AHIMA, individuals must meet the eligibility requirements for certification and successfully complete the certification examination.

Because the HIM profession is constantly changing, certified individuals must demonstrate that they are continuing to maintain their knowledge and skill base. Therefore, to maintain their certification, individuals who hold any of AHIMA's credentials must complete a designated set of CE credits. Activities that qualify for CE credits include such things as attending workshops and seminars, taking college courses, participating in independent study activities, and engaging in self-assessment activities. AHIMA's website provides information on the most recent requirements for maintenance of certification.

Fellowship Program

The AHIMA **Fellowship Program** is a program of earned recognition for AHIMA members who have made significant and sustained contributions to the HIM profession through meritorious service, excellence in professional practice, education, and advancement of the profession through innovation and knowledge sharing. Individuals who earn fellowship use the designation Fellow of the American Health Information Management Association (FAHIMA).

Fellowship is open to any individual who is an active or senior member of AHIMA and who meets the eligibility requirements. Fellows must have a minimum of 10 years full-time professional experience in HIM or a related field; a minimum of 10 years continuous AHIMA membership at the time of application (excluding years as a student member); and hold a minimum of a master's degree and provide evidence of sustained and substantial professional achievement that shows professional growth and use of innovative and creative solutions. Once conferred, the fellowship is a lifetime recognition, subject to continuing AHIMA membership and compliance with the AHIMA Code of Ethics.

The AHIMA Foundation

The AHIMA Foundation actively promotes education and research in the HIM field. Founded in 1962, the AHIMA Foundation is a separately incorporated philanthropic and charitable arm of AHIMA.

The HIM profession is based on the belief that high-quality healthcare requires high-quality information. Historically the Foundation has provided the knowledge, research, and education infrastructure for this industry. Its role is to envision the future direction and needs of the field and to respond with strategies, information, planning, and programs that will keep the HIM profession on the cutting edge.

Some of the initiatives that have been spearheaded by the Foundation include the Leadership Recognition Program, the benchmarking and best practices research initiative, the legal and regulatory clearinghouse and curriculum, and various faculty support initiatives. In addition, the foundation administers a number of programs, including the scholarship and research programs. The AHIMA Foundation strives to be the premiere resource for HIM professionals and the leader in advancing the field for the betterment of the HIM profession and healthcare consumers.

Health Information Management Specialty Professional Organizations

HIM professionals frequently specialize in an area of the HIM profession. Examples of these specialties include coding, tumor registry, medical transcription, and information systems. A number of specialty organizations support these areas.

Healthcare Information and Management Systems Society

HIMSS is a not-for-profit organization whose goal is "to lead healthcare transformation through the effective use of health information technology" (HIMSS nd). HIMSS sponsors the Certified Professional in Healthcare Information and Management Systems (CPHIMS) certification for healthcare information and management systems professionals. The exam covers topics such as healthcare, technology, system analysis, system design, privacy and security, and administration (HIMSS nd).

Association for Healthcare Documentation Integrity

The **Association for Healthcare Documentation Integrity** (AHDI) is a professional organization dedicated to the capture of health data and documentation. It was formerly known as the American Academy of Medical Transcription but changed its name to fit their broadened scope. AHDI sponsors the Certified Medical Transcription and Registered Medical Transcriptionist certifications. The RMT exam content includes topics such as transcription standards and styles, clinical medicine, and health information technology. The CMT exam covers clinical medicine and health information technology (AHDI nd).

American Academy of Professional Coders

The **American Academy of Professional Coders** (AAPC) educates and certifies medical coders. They sponsor certifications in coding, medical compliance and medical auditing. The certifications include: Certified Professional Coder (CPC), Certified Professional Coder—Hospital Outpatient (CPC-H), Certified Professional Coder—Payer (CPC-P), Certified Interventional Radiology Cardiovascular Coder (CIRCC), Certified Professional Medical Auditor (CPMA), Certified Professional Compliance Officer (CPCO) as well as many specialty coding certifications (AAPC nd).

National Cancer Registrars Association

The **National Cancer Registrars Association** (NCRA) represents cancer registrar professionals. Their mission is to "serve as the premier education, credentialing and advocacy resource for cancer data professionals" (NCRA nd). The NCRA sponsors the Certified Tumor Registrar (CTR) certification. This exam includes information on registry organization and operations, abstracting, coding, follow-up, data analysis, and interpretation as well as coding and staging.

American Recovery and Reinvestment Act of 2009— Community College Consortia to Educate Health Information Technology Professionals

The advent of the electronic health record has increased the need for HIM professionals. Because of the shortage of HIM professionals, there is a need to supplement the workforce. One of the ways that this has been done is through the **American Recovery and Reinvestment Act of 2009** (ARRA). This federal law funded several grants including the **Community College Consortia to Educate Health Information Technology Professionals** (Consortia) program. This Community College Consortia Program divided the country into five regional groups. Eighty-two colleges received funding through the Office of the National Coordinator for Health IT to create nondegree academic programs, which can be completed by information technology or healthcare professionals in six months or less. The grant required the colleges to implement programs to train people in six roles that are needed for the implementation of the electronic health record. These roles are:

- Practice workflow and information management redesign specialists
- Clinician/practitioner consultants
- Implementation support specialists
- Implementation managers
- Technical/software support
- Trainers (Office of the National Coordinator for Health Information Technology nd)

Another component of the ARRA grants is a competency exam for each of these roles. These HIT Pro Exams are available to graduates of the Consortia programs as well as to other professionals with health information technology skills (HITP nd).

Check Your Understanding 1.2

1. The primary focus of AHIMA is to:
   A. Ensure that health records are complete
   B. Implement an electronic record in hospitals
   C. Foster professional development of its members
   D. Set and implement standards

2. The Consortia's educational program is designed to be completed in what amount of time?

   A. 1 year
   B. 6 months
   C. 3 months
   D. 9 months

3. Which of the following functions as the legislative body of AHIMA?

   A. Board of Directors
   B. House of Delegates
   C. CCHIIM
   D. CAHIIM

4. Which of the following promotes education and research?

   A. CCHIIM
   B. CAHIIM
   C. AHIMA
   D. AHIMA Foundation

5. The virtual network used by AHIMA members is:

   A. Certification
   B. Fellowship
   C. House of Delegates
   D. Communities of Practice

Real-World Case

The following case is adapted from an article by Diana Warner that appeared in the *Journal of AHIMA*, September 2011.

With the advent of the EHR, staffing patterns are changing. More and more HIM staff members are working from home which improves job satisfaction. Many of these employees will no longer perform many of the traditional HIM roles. With these changes, many functions no longer requrie 24/7/365 coverage. At Vanderbilt University Medical Center, the HIM staff need utilize a different skill set than ever before. They must be able to correct errors in the EHR, solve problems, understand health record content, and be able to analyze data. Other skills include data mapping, strong interpersonal skills and advanced understanding of the EHR.

Summary

The health information management profession has a rich history. It continues to prosper today as it takes advantage of new opportunities and accommodates the changes ushered in by the information age. At the beginning of the organization's inception in 1928, founding members realized the need to direct the field of medical records toward professional standing. This required the development of a formal organization devoted to establishing standards and best practices for the discipline, including the creation of a prescribed training curriculum and the launch of a formal certification program. Amazingly, all this was accomplished in only six short years from the formation of the organization in 1928, to the establishment of a credentialing program in 1933, to the first accreditation of academic programs in 1934.

The professional association, beginning first as the Association of Record Librarians of North America and continuing today as the American Health Information Management Association, has demonstrated remarkable resilience in an ever-changing healthcare delivery system. Thanks to the foresight and insight of health information professionals through the decades, the organizational structure of the association has adapted to the membership's changing needs:

- Credentialing programs have been expanded to represent the diversity of work tasks in the discipline.

- Accreditation standards for academic programs have continued to become more rigorous through monitoring program outcomes, which is important because of the growing need for better-trained and qualified graduates.

- Advocacy for confidentiality and patients' rights continues to be a fundamental objective as AHIMA's expertise and input are sought in the development of federal policy.

- The role and definition of professional practice have been studied and changed to meet new demands.

The new generation of HIM professionals has inherited a powerful legacy from HIM pioneers. The growth and viability of the profession in years to come will depend on the dedication of current professionals to actively participate in the professional organization at the local, state, and national levels and to commit to continually updating their knowledge base and skills through lifelong learning.

References

AHIMA. (nd). http://www.ahima.org

AHIMA. 1999. *Evolving HIM Roles: Seven Roles for the Future.* Chicago: AHIMA.

AHIMA. 2003. *A Vision of the e-Him Future: A Report from the AHIMA e-Him Task Force.* Chicago: AHIMA.

AHIMA. 2011. A new view of HIM: Introducing the Core Model Review Draft. Chicago. http://library.ahima.org/xpedio/groups/public/documents/ahima/bok1_049283.pdf#xml=http://library.ahima.org/xpedio/idcplg?IdcService=GET_XML_HIGHLIGHT_INFO&QueryText=xPublishSite+%3csubstring%3e+%60BoK%60+%3cAND%3e+%28xCategory+%3csubstring%3e+%60HIM+Career%60%29&SortField=xPubDate&SortOrder=Desc&dDocName=bok1_049283&HighlightType=PdfHighlight

American Academy of Professional Coders (nd). http://www.aapc.com/

Association for Healthcare Documentation Integrity (nd). http://www.ahdionline.org/

Blum, B.I. 1986. *Clinical Information Systems.* New York: Springer-Verlag.

Dimick, C. 2008. HIM jobs of tomorrow: Eleven new and revised jobs illustrate the trends changing HIM and the opportunities that lie ahead. *Journal of AHIMA* 79(10):26–34.

Health Information Careers (nd). http://www.hicareers.com/Toolbox/salarystudy.aspx

Health Information Technology Professional (nd). http://HITproexams.org

Healthcare Information Management Systems Society. (nd). http://www.himss.org/ASP/aboutHimssHome.asp

Huffman, E.K. 1941. Requirements and advantages of registration for medical record librarians. *Bulletin of the American Association of Medical Record Librarians.*

Huffman, E.K. 1985. *Medical Record Management,* 8th ed. Berwyn, IL: Physicians' Record Company.

Johns, M.L. 1991. Information management: A shifting paradigm for medical record professionals? *Journal of the American Medical Record Association* 62(8).

National Cancer Registrars Association (nd). http://www.ncra-usa.org/

Office of the National Coordinator for Health Information Technology (nd). http://healthit.hhs.gov/portal/server.pt?open=512&objID=1804&mode=2

Protti, D.J. 1984. Knowledge and skills expected of health information scientists: A sample survey of prospective employers. *Methods of Information in Medicine* 23:204–208.

Servais, C. 2009. Virtual HIM: Considering the transition to remote departments. *Journal of AHIMA* 80(3):38–42.

Warner, D. 2011. The EHR's impact on staffing models. *Journal of AHIMA* 82(9):44–45.

Additional Resources

AHIMA. 2004. *Data for Decisions: The HIM Workforce and Workplace.* Chicago: AHIMA.

American Medical Record Association. 1984. *Professional Practice Standards.* Chicago: AMRA.

American Medical Record Association. 1990. *Professional Practice Standards.* Chicago: AMRA.

chapter 2

Purpose and Function of the Health Record

Cheryl V. Homan, MBA, RHIA

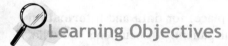

Learning Objectives

- Define the term *health record*
- Understand the purposes of the health record
- Identify the different users of the health record and its importance to each user
- Explain the functions of the health record
- Apply quality characteristics to the collection and maintenance of health data and databases
- Clarify the differences in paper-based, hybrid, and electronic methods in fulfilling the functions of the health record
- Discuss the attributes of security, access, flexibility, connectivity, and efficiency in fulfilling the functions of the health record
- Identify the roles and responsibilities of health information management professionals in the development and maintenance of health record systems

Key Terms

Accreditation organization
Aggregate data
Allied health professional
Centers for Medicare and Medicaid
    Services (CMS)

Coding specialist
Confidentiality
Data
Data accessibility
Data accuracy

Data comprehensiveness
Data consistency
Data currency
Data definition
Data granularity
Data precision
Data quality management
Data relevancy
Data timeliness
Diagnostic codes
Electronic health record (EHR)
Health record
Hybrid health record
Information

Integrated health record format
Interoperability
Personal health record (PHR)
Privacy
Problem-oriented health record format
Procedural codes
Quality improvement organization (QIO)
Reimbursement
Security
Source-oriented health record format
Third-party payers
Transcriptionist
Utilization management organization

Introduction

The **health record** is the principal repository (storage place) for **data** and **information** about the healthcare services provided to an individual patient. It documents the who, what, when, where, why, and how of patient care. The health record also records the health status of the patient.

Healthcare providers have created and maintained records of the medical care provided to individual patients for centuries. However, modern documentation standards for the health record did not begin to appear until the early 20th century.

Today, almost every person in the United States has at least one health record maintained by the healthcare system with his or her identification on it. Moreover, every time a person consults a new healthcare provider, another health record is created. Thus, it is very likely that any given patient may have multiple health records.

The health record is known by different names in different healthcare settings. The records of acute care patients who receive services as hospital inpatients are often called *patient records.* Physicians and physicians' office personnel typically use the term *medical record.* The records of patients in long-term care facilities are often called *resident records.* Facilities that provide ambulatory behavioral health services sometimes refer to *client records.* Paper-based health records are also sometimes called *charts,* especially in hospital settings. No matter what term is used, however, the primary function of the health record is to document and support patient care services.

Although sometimes used interchangeably, the terms *data* and *information* do not mean the same thing. *Data* represent the basic facts about people, processes, measurements, conditions, and so on. They can be collected in the form of dates, numerical measurements and statistics, textual descriptions, checklists, images, and symbols. After data have been collected and analyzed, they are converted into a form that can be used for a specific purpose. This useful form is called *information.* In other words, data represent facts and information represents meaning.

Today, the management of health record systems and services is the primary responsibility of health information management (HIM) professionals. As discussed in chapter 1, the HIM profession has evolved as healthcare delivery has changed since individual patient records were first created almost a hundred years ago. The ongoing development and implementation of electronic healthcare applications and standards continues to bring change to the profession.

The traditional practice of health record management was based on the collection of data on paper forms stored in paper file folders. Today, paper-based documentation systems are being replaced with electronic systems. Thus, many HIM professionals are challenged with managing hybrid record environments that are partially electronic and partially paper based. Future professional practice will be based on the electronic collection, storage, and analysis of healthcare information created and maintained in interactive **electronic health record** (EHR) systems.

In recent years, the term **personal health record** (PHR) has been used to describe a health record initiated and maintained by an individual. The PHR is owned by the individual and is comprised of data and information from healthcare providers and the individual. PHRs may be paper-based or electronic. Paper-based PHRs are the files containing information from doctors, insurance companies, pharmacies, hospitals, and other healthcare entities that patients keep around their homes. The ideal PHR is electronic, contains the complete health history of an individual, and is accessible online to anyone that has been given access by the individual (AHIMA 2010c). The electronic PHR may be personal-computer-based or web-based. Personal-computer-based PHRs are created by patients on their personal computers by typing or scanning their personal health information into generic software or into a specific PHR application. The personal-computer-based PHR generally lacks the ability to exchange information electronically with healthcare providers as it resides on the patient's PC. On the other hand, the web-based PHR allows patients to maintain their personal health information in private online accounts that provide around-the-clock access from any Internet-connected device. Today, many healthcare providers and third-party payers offer web-based PHRs (sometimes called patient portals) to encourage patients to be active participants in their medical care.

It is important to note that the PHR and EHR are not the same thing. EHRs are electronic systems designed for use by healthcare providers and support the legal mandate providers have to document care. Currently, there is no legal mandate for an individual to maintain a PHR. However, the patient-centric healthcare delivery model revolves around the PHR. PHR best practices recommend that PHR information be integrated into the EHR (AHIMA 2009).

Theory into Practice

Until recently, most healthcare providers documented their services directly in the paper-based records of their patients. That is, they handwrote or dictated their clinical notes and orders and filled out paper data-collection forms. Dictated reports were typewritten by

transcriptionists and then checked by clinicians for accuracy. All these paper-based materials were then filed in paper folders or clipped together in paper charts.

Today, information technology is revolutionizing the way healthcare data and information are created, collected, and stored. Speech recognition and natural language processing are changing the role of the transcriptionist from one of typist to one of medical editor. Virtually every healthcare organization uses computer technology to collect, store, or retrieve all or portions of a patient's healthcare data. For example, the results of laboratory tests have been routinely reported via computer printouts for some time. In most environments, healthcare providers access these results via computer workstations and other electronic output devices such as personal digital assistants, smartphones, and even iPads,

Movement to implement EHRs is part of the national agenda in the United States. Eventually, every healthcare organization and provider will adopt a paperless health record system. In 2001, the National Committee on Vital and Health Statistics (NCVHS) issued a report and recommendations detailing how to build a national health information infrastructure (NCVHS 2001). Based on these recommendations and in an effort to reduce healthcare costs, improve care, and avoid medical errors, then President George W. Bush outlined a plan to achieve EHRs for most Americans by 2014. The Office of the National Coordinator for Health Information Technology (ONC), a sub-Cabinet-level post at the Department of Health and Human Services (HHS), was formed and charged with coordinating this national effort. During the Bush Administration, the ONC focused on development of the Nationwide Health Information Network (NHIN) along with promotion and development of fundamental infrastructure standards, protocols, and profiles to enable EHR interoperability (NCVHS 2008).

In 2009, President Barack Obama signed into law the American Recovery and Reinvestment Act (ARRA), an economic stimulus package that provides reimbursement incentives to providers and hospitals that are "meaningful users" of certified EHR technology. These reimbursement incentives have accelerated EHR adoption in the United States. At the end of 2011, HHS reported that the adoption of EHR technology by providers in the United States doubled from 17 to 34 percent between 2008 and 2011 (HHS 2011). This focus on "meaningful use" of the technology promises better healthcare for all Americans as EHRs can improve access to care, help coordinate treatment, measure outcomes, and reduce costs.

In making EHRs a reality, healthcare organizations and providers experience significant challenges. Replacing the paper record requires a thorough understanding of current organizational processes. Problems with the current paper-based system need to be outlined and fixed with implementation of the EHR. To ensure quality of electronic patient data, standardized documentation procedures related to definition, content, and structure need to be developed as part of the implementation process. Quality checkpoints should be established throughout the data capture process to enable effective and efficient electronic exchange of data between providers. Overall, the success of an EHR is dependent on its ability to provide accurate patient data in a timely manner.

Purposes of the Health Record

Health records are used for a number of purposes related to patient care. The primary purposes of the health record are associated directly with the provision of patient care services as well as the documentation of the patient's health status. The secondary purposes of the health record are related to the environment in which healthcare services are provided. The secondary purposes are not related directly to specific patient care encounters (Dick et al. 1997, 77–79).

Primary Purposes

According to the Institute of Medicine (Dick et al. 1997, 77–78), the primary purposes of the health record can be classified into the following categories:

- *Patient care delivery:* The health record documents the services provided by clinical professionals and **allied health professionals** working in a variety of settings. Health record documentation helps physicians, nurses, and other clinical care professionals make informed decisions about diagnoses and treatments. The health record is also a tool for communication among the individual patient's different caregivers. Effective communication ensures the continuity of patient services. Moreover, the detailed information stored in health records allows healthcare providers to assess and manage risk. Finally, the health record represents legal evidence of the services received by the individual patient and represents the business record of the organization.

- *Patient care management:* Patient care management refers to all the activities related to managing the healthcare services provided to patients. The health record assists providers in analyzing various illnesses, formulating practice guidelines, and evaluating the quality of care.

- *Patient care support processes:* Patient care support encompasses the activities related to the handling of the healthcare organization's resources, the analysis of trends, and the communication of information among different clinical departments.

- *Financial and other administrative processes:* Because the health record documents the patient's course of illness and treatment, the information in it determines the payment the provider will receive in every type of reimbursement system. Health record data elements are trended to assist in managing and reporting costs.

- *Patient self-management:* Individuals have become more actively involved in managing their own health and healthcare and are therefore becoming a primary user of the health record (IOM 2003, 5).

Figure 2.1 lists examples of the primary uses of the health record.

Figure 2.1.   Primary purposes of the health record

Patient Care Delivery (Patient)
- To document services received
- To constitute proof of identity
- To self-manage care
- To verify billing

Patient Care Delivery (Provider)
- To foster continuity of care (that is, to serve as a communication tool)
- To describe diseases and causes (that is, to support diagnostic work)
- To support decision making about diagnosis and treatment of patients
- To assess and manage risk for individual patients
- To facilitate care in accordance with clinical practice guidelines
- To document patient risk factors
- To assess and document patient expectations and patient satisfaction
- To generate care plans
- To determine preventive advice or health maintenance information
- To provide reminders to clinicians
- To support nursing care
- To document services provided

Patient Care Management
- To document case mix in institutions and practices
- To analyze severity of illness

- To formulate practice guidelines
- To manage risk
- To characterize the use of services
- To provide the basis for utilization review
- To perform quality assurance

Patient Care Support
- To allocate resources
- To analyze trends and develop forecasts
- To assess workload
- To communicate information among departments

Financial and Other Administrative Processes
- To document services for payments
- To bill for services
- To submit insurance claims
- To adjudicate insurance claims
- To determine disabilities (for example, workmen's compensation)
- To manage costs
- To report costs
- To perform actuarial analysis

Source: Adapted from Dick et al. 1997, 78, and IOM 2003, 5. Reprinted with permission from *The Computer-Based Patient Record: An Essential Technology for Health Care*, Revised Edition, 1997, by the National Academy of Sciences. Courtesy of the National Academies Press, Washington, D.C.

Secondary Purposes

The secondary purposes of the health record are not associated with specific encounters between patient and healthcare professional. Rather, they are related to the environment in which patient care is provided. According to the Institute of Medicine (IOM), education, research, regulation, and policy making are all considered secondary purposes of the health record (Dick et al. 1997, 76–77). Figure 2.2 lists some examples of the secondary purposes of the health record. In 2003, public health and homeland security were added to the list of secondary purposes (IOM 2003, 5).

Figure 2.2. Secondary purposes of the health record

Education

- To document the experience of healthcare professionals
- To prepare conferences and presentations
- To teach healthcare students

Regulation

- To serve as evidence in litigation
- To foster postmarketing surveillance
- To assess compliance with standards of care
- To accredit professionals and hospitals
- To compare healthcare organizations

Research

- To develop new products
- To conduct clinical research
- To assess technology

- To study patient outcomes
- To study effectiveness and cost-effectiveness of patient care
- To identify populations at risk
- To develop registries and databases
- To assess the cost-effectiveness of record systems

Public Health and Homeland Security

- To monitor public health
- To monitor bioterrorism activity

Policy Making and Support

- To allocate resources
- To conduct strategic planning

Industry

- To conduct research and development
- To plan marketing strategy

Source: Adapted from Dick et al. 1997, 79, and IOM 2003, 5. Reprinted with permission from *The Computer-Based Patient Record: An Essential Technology for Health Care*, Revised Edition, 1997, by the National Academy of Sciences. Courtesy of the National Academies Press, Washington, D.C.

Check Your Understanding 2.1

1. We had 324 Medicare patients last month. This statement represents which of the following:

   A. Information
   B. Data
   C. Content of the PHR
   D. Patient-specific information

2. I am a patient. My medical history including information from myself and my physicians is stored on the Internet. This is an example of which of the following:

   A. Health record
   B. EHR
   C. PHR
   D. Data

3. Which of the following is an example of a primary purpose of the medical record?

   A. Education
   B. Policy making
   C. Research
   D. Patient care management

4. Examples of patient care delivery usage of the medical record include which of the following uses?

   A. Developing of practice guidelines
   B. Communication between caregivers
   C. Reimbursement for patient care
   D. Getting patients involved in their own care

5. Critique this statement: The PHR and EHR are synonyms.

   A. This is a true statement; both are controlled by the patient.
   B. This is a false statement as the PHR is controlled by the care providers and the EHR is controlled by the patient.
   C. This is a false statement as the PHR is controlled by the patient and the EHR is controlled by the care providers.
   D. This is a true statement; both are controlled by the healthcare provider.

Instructions: Indicate whether the following statements are true or false (T or F).

6. ____ The health record is the principal repository for data and information about the healthcare services provided to individual patients.

7. ____ The lab test "hemoglobin: 14.6 gm/110 ml" is considered information.

8. ____ The primary purposes of the health record are associated directly with the provision of patient care services, as well as the documentation of the patient's health status.

9. ____ Submitting health record documentation to a third-party payer for the purpose of substantiating a patient bill is considered a secondary purpose of the health record.

10. ____ Use of the health record to study the effectiveness of a given drug is considered a primary use of the health record.

Users of the Health Record

The primary users of health records are patient care providers. However, many other individuals and organizations also use the information in health records. Managed care organizations, integrated healthcare delivery systems, regulatory and **accreditation organizations,** licensing bodies, educational organizations, **third-party payers,** and research facilities all use information that was originally collected to document patient care.

The IOM broadly defines the users of health records as "those individuals who enter, verify, correct, analyze, or obtain information from the record, either directly or indirectly through an intermediary" (Dick et al. 1997, 75). All the users of health records influence clinical care in some way, but they use the information from health records for various reasons and in different ways. Some users (for example, nurses, physicians, and **coding specialists**) refer to the health records of specific patients as a part of their daily work. Many other users, however, never have direct access to the records of individual patients. Instead, they use clinical and demographic information collected from the records. Figures 2.3 and 2.4 list examples of the individual and institutional users of health records (Dick et al. 1997, 76–77).

Individual Users

As already noted, many individuals depend on the information in health records to perform their jobs. Some of these individual users are identified in the following paragraphs.

Patient Care Providers

The individuals who provide direct patient care services include physicians, nurses, nurse practitioners, allied health professionals, and other clinical personnel. Allied health professionals include physician assistants, physical therapists, respiratory therapists, occupational therapists, radiology technicians, and medical laboratory technicians. Other medical

Figure 2.3. Representative individual users of health records

Patient Care Delivery (Providers)	**Patient Care Management and Support**
• Chaplains	• Administrators
• Dental hygienists	• Financial managers and accountants
• Dentists	• Quality managers
• Dietitians	• Records professionals
• Laboratory technologists	• Risk managers
• Nurses	• Unit clerks
• Occupational therapists	• Utilization review managers
• Optometrists	**Patient Care Reimbursement**
• Pharmacists	• Benefit managers
• Physical therapists	• Insurers (federal, state, and private)
• Physician assistants	**Other**
• Physicians	• Accreditors
• Podiatrists	• Government policy makers and legislators
• Psychologists	• Lawyers
• Radiology technologists	• Healthcare researchers and clinical investigators
• Respiratory therapists	• Health sciences journalists and editors
• Social workers	
Patient Care Delivery (Consumers)	
• Patients	
• Families	

Source: Adapted from Dick et al. 1997, 76. Reprinted with permission from *The Computer-Based Patient Record: An Essential Technology for Health Care*, Revised Edition, 1997, by the National Academy of Sciences. Courtesy of the National Academies Press, Washington, D.C.

Figure 2.4. Representative institutional users of health records

Healthcare Delivery (Inpatient and Outpatient)
- Alliances, associations, networks, and systems of providers
- Ambulatory surgery centers
- Donor banks (blood, tissue, organs)
- Health maintenance organizations
- Home care agencies
- Hospices
- Hospitals (general and specialty)
- Nursing homes
- Preferred provider organizations
- Physician offices (large and small group practices, individual practitioners)
- Psychiatric facilities
- Public health departments
- Substance abuse programs

Management and Review of Care
- Medicare peer review organizations
- Quality management companies
- Risk management companies
- Utilization review and utilization management companies

Reimbursement of Care
- Business healthcare coalitions
- Employers
- Insurers (federal, state, and private)

Research
- Disease registries
- Healthcare technology developers and manufacturers (equipment and device firms, pharmaceutical firms, and computer hardware and software vendors for patient record systems)
- Health data organizations
- Research centers

Education
- Allied health professional schools and programs
- Schools of medicine
- Schools of nursing
- Schools of public health

Accreditation
- Accreditation organizations
- Institutional licensure agencies
- Professional licensure agencies

Policy Making
- Federal government agencies
- Local government agencies
- State government agencies

Source: Adapted from Dick et al. 1997, 77. Reprinted with permission from *The Computer-Based Patient Record: An Essential Technology for Health Care*, Revised Edition, 1997, by the National Academy of Sciences. Courtesy of the National Academies Press, Washington, D.C.

professionals also provide clinical services. These individuals include pharmacists, social workers, dietitians, psychologists, podiatrists, and chiropractors.

Direct patient care providers document their services directly in their patients' health records. Other service providers (for example, medical laboratory technicians, radiology technicians, and EKG technicians) do not directly document within the health record, but provide reports that become part of individual health records.

Healthcare providers offer services to a number of patients during any given period of time. For providers, the health record serves as a device for communicating vital information among departments and across disciplines and settings.

Patient Care Managers and Support Staff

Patient care managers and support staff oversee the services provided to patients within their organizations. The health record provides the data they need to evaluate the performance of individual patient care providers and to determine the effectiveness of the services provided. The patient care manager refers to the documentation in the health record when questions arise about a specific patient's course of treatment or about the services the patient received.

Patient care managers also are responsible for the overall evaluation of services rendered for their particular area of responsibility. To identify patterns and trends, they take details from individual health records and then put all the information together in one place. On the basis of these combined **aggregate data,** the managers recommend changes to patient care processes, equipment, and services. Aggregate data is "extracted from individual health records and combined to form de-identified information about groups of patients that can be compared and analyzed" (AHIMA 2012, 12). The goal of the changes is to improve the future outcomes of patient care.

Coding and Billing Staff

Healthcare **reimbursement** is based on the documentation contained in the health record. By referring to the records of individual patients, coding specialists identify the patients' diagnoses as well as the therapeutic procedures they underwent and the services they received. Using this information, coding specialists assign appropriate **diagnostic** and **procedural codes.** The coded information is then used to generate a patient bill and/or a claim for reimbursement to a third-party payer, such as a commercial health insurance company or government-sponsored health program such as Medicare.

Some third-party payers require billers to submit copies of portions of the health record along with the claims. The health record documentation substantiates the need for services and the fact that such services were provided. Please see chapter 6 for more information on coding and reimbursement.

Patients

Today, patients are taking an active interest in their own health and in the preventive and therapeutic healthcare they receive. Federal legislation—the Health Insurance Portability and Accountability Act (HIPAA) of 1996—includes health record security and privacy provisions. HIPAA grants most patients the right to access their health records. In addition, they have the right to request an amendment to the information in their records and to add missing information. Patients can also review their records for documentation of services provided to verify and substantiate billed charges. Many patients obtain copies of their health records to incorporate into their PHR.

Other Individual Users

Many other individuals may use the health record as a source of information provided they can demonstrate appropriate authorization granting access.

Employers

Employers use information based on the health records of their employees to determine the extent and effects of occupational hazards. They also use health record information to manage healthcare, worker's compensation, and disability insurance benefits for their employees. Moreover, individual employees' disability claims must be supported by the information in their health records.

Lawyers

The health record is considered legal documentation of the healthcare services provided to patients. Attorneys for healthcare organizations use it as a tool to protect the legal interests of the facility and its patient care providers. The legal representatives of physicians and their malpractice insurance carriers also depend on the documentation in the health record. Attorneys for patients who bring civil suits use health records to support claims for compensation of medical malpractice, accident settlements, and more. Attorneys also use information from the health record to determine the mental competency of individuals.

Law Enforcement Officials

Law enforcement officials, such as police officers, agents of the Federal Bureau of Investigation (FBI), sheriffs, and marshals, also may use the health record in limited situations. For example, health records are used in the investigation of gunshot injuries, child abuse and neglect, domestic violence, and other crimes. Law enforcement officials also use information contained in health records to identify and locate suspects, fugitives, material witnesses, and missing persons.

Congress passed two bills following the September 11, 2001 attacks, the USA Patriot Act (2001) and The Homeland Security Act (2002) which granted law enforcement additional rights to private information. In an effort to deter and punish terrorist attacks in the United States, the USA Patriot Act reduced law enforcement restrictions to search telephone records, e-mail communication, and health records. The Homeland Security Act established the US Department of Homeland Security and expanded and centralized the data gathering permitted by the USA Patriot Act. These acts permit law enforcement agencies access to any and all information deemed necessary to protect the nation, including health records, provided that appropriate identification of the law enforcement or governmental official is obtained and verified (AHIMA 2010a).

Healthcare Researchers and Clinical Investigators

Clinical research is the process by which the effectiveness of treatment methods is evaluated and improved methods for future care are developed. Researchers review health records for the particular population being studied and extract data. The data help them to evaluate and make decisions about disease processes and treatments. Healthcare researchers and clinical investigators also use aggregate health record data.

Health Science Publishers and Journalists

Healthcare consumers continue to seek more and more information about developments in clinical research, alternative medicine, preventive medicine, and public health. The Internet offers extensive healthcare information to Americans. Radio, television, and print journalists also look for legitimate sources of information on healthcare topics. Publishers and journalists use patient care information aggregated by researchers and investigators to generate these consumer reports.

Government Policy Makers

Local, state, and federal government policy makers are responsible for evaluating the overall health and well-being of the populations they serve. Government agencies establish the requirements for reporting cases of certain communicable diseases. They also require the reporting of information relevant to health-related social issues such as gunshot wounds, teenage pregnancies, and drug abuse. The health record is the source for the information needed to meet such reporting requirements. Policy makers develop aggregate information, which serves as the basis for investigations of the health patterns and trends in a given population. Using this information, policy makers can develop and fund community programs.

Institutional Users

A number of organizations depend on access to healthcare-related information. The health record is the most reliable source of such information.

Healthcare Delivery Organizations

Healthcare delivery organizations include physicians' practices, ambulatory clinics, blood and tissue donor banks, home care agencies, hospices, acute care hospitals, rehabilitation hospitals, psychiatric hospitals, long-term care facilities, and public health departments and clinics. Such organizations use data from health records in providing services, evaluating and monitoring the use of resources, seeking reimbursement for the services provided, and planning and marketing services.

Third-Party Payers

Third-party payers are organizations responsible for the reimbursement of healthcare services covered by some kind of insurance program. Third-party payers include commercial health insurance companies, managed care organizations, self-insured employers, and the fiscal (or financial) intermediaries representing Medicare and Medicaid. Third-party payers review individual health records to determine whether the documentation supports the provider's claim for reimbursement. Claims that are not supported by adequate health record documentation are often denied. Many third-party payers enter into contractual arrangements with medical review organizations to perform the actual review of health records.

Medical Review Organizations

Quality improvement organizations (QIOs) and **utilization management organizations** evaluate the adequacy and appropriateness of the care provided by healthcare organizations. These medical review organizations work under contract with the federal government and examine individual health records for specific episodes of care to determine whether services were medically necessary. Depending on the organization, this process may take place on a concurrent basis while the patient is still under treatment or on a retrospective basis after the patient has received services. The results of the medical reviews are usually linked directly to the level of reimbursement paid to the provider.

Research Organizations

Organizations performing healthcare-related research study the current healthcare environment to prove or disprove hypotheses related to disease processes and treatments. Research organizations include disease registries, research centers, and health data companies. In some instances, the law may require healthcare providers to provide aggregate data from health records on specific disease processes. In other instances, participation is voluntary. Healthcare providers committed to health education and research work closely with research organizations to develop and test experimental patient care protocols and to provide the relevant data from the health record.

Educational Organizations

Healthcare professionals undergo rigorous professional education based on classroom and hands-on training. Medical schools, dental schools, nursing schools, and allied health training programs frequently use health records as sources of case study information.

Accreditation Organizations

The mission of healthcare accreditation organizations is to improve the quality of services offered in healthcare facilities. Participation in accreditation programs is voluntary. Accreditation organizations, to name a few, include:

- The Joint Commission
- Healthcare Facilities Accreditation Program
- Commission on Accreditation of Rehabilitation Facilities

- American College of Surgeons
- National Committee on Quality Assurance
- Accreditation Association for Ambulatory Health Care

Every participating healthcare organization is subject to a periodic accreditation survey. Surveyors visit each facility and compare its programs, policies, and procedures to a pre-published set of performance standards. A key component of every accreditation survey is a review of the facility's health records. Surveyors review the documentation of patient care services to determine whether the standards for care are being met. They then use the results of the review to make the overall accreditation decision. The surveys usually involve the direct review of a sample of health records from recent and current patients along with a review of aggregate statistics related to expected patient outcomes. Additional information on accreditation can be found in chapter 3.

Government Licensing Agencies

The goal of local, state, and federal licensing agencies is to make sure that the healthcare facilities in their areas provide effective and appropriate care to healthcare consumers. Licensing agencies include state licensing bureaus and federal and state departments responsible for certifying facilities that receive funding from the federal, state, and local governments. As part of the licensing process, health records are reviewed to determine whether the facility is complying with the licensing regulations in that geographic area.

Policy-making Bodies

The **Centers for Medicare and Medicaid Services** (CMS) is a division of the US Department of Health and Human Services. (Until 2001, it was known as the Health Care Financing Administration, or HCFA.) CMS is responsible for administering the federal Medicare program and the federal portion of the Medicaid program.

Data taken from health records and supplied by healthcare organizations as part of the Medicare billing and reimbursement process are kept in a national database. The database is used to make decisions related to healthcare reimbursement mechanisms, the effectiveness of healthcare services, and the general health of the Medicare population. Although the content and sources of data differ, similar information databases are maintained at the state level.

In addition to the information kept in federal and state databases, policy-making bodies rely on the support of various health-related organizations that have been created to support high standards of healthcare in the United States. Although their overall mission varies, organizations such as the American Medical Association, the American Psychiatric Association, the American Hospital Association, the American Health Information Management Association, the American College of Surgeons, and the American College of Physicians all develop healthcare standards. They also make recommendations to the federal and state governments on healthcare policy issues.

Check Your Understanding 2.2

1. Which of the following users of the health record is an example of an institutional user?

   A. Third-party payer
   B. Patient
   C. Physician
   D. Employer

2. Which of the following users would utilize aggregate data?

   A. Patient care providers
   B. Coding and billing staff
   C. Law enforcement officers
   D. Patient care managers and support staff

3. I work for an organization that utilizes health record data to prove or disprove hypotheses related to disease. I must work for what type of organization?

   A. Healthcare delivery
   B. Medical review
   C. Research
   D. Education

4. Critique the following statement: A user of health records includes only care providers who document in the health record or refer to it for patient care.

   A. This is a true statement as defined by the IOM.
   B. This is a false statement as the information is used for other purposes such as analysis.
   C. This is a true statement as defined by AHIMA.
   D. This is a false statement as the information contained in the health record is also used for patients to document in their own health record.

5. I work for CMS; how would I use the health record?

   A. Make decisions on healthcare reimbursement
   B. Medical research
   C. Issuing hospital and medical staff licenses
   D. Accrediting healthcare organizations

Instructions: Indicate whether the following statements are true or false (T or F).

6. _____ A physical therapist documenting in the health record is an institutional health record user.

7. _____ An auditor who is employed by Medicare is reviewing a health record for a mortality study. This auditor is an individual health record user.

8. ____ CMS uses data to accredit hospitals.

9. ____ A researcher uses data to determine the recommended treatment.

10. ____ Patients do not have the right to add missing information to the health record.

Functions of the Health Record

The primary function of the health record is to store patient care documentation. A number of systems, policies, and processes make it possible to collect patient care documentation efficiently and to store it in easily accessible and secure formats of high quality.

Besides storage of patient care documentation, the health record has other equally important functions. These include helping physicians, nurses, and other caregivers make diagnoses and choose treatment options. Paper-based health record formats limit these types of clinical decision-making functions due to lack of linkages to evidence-based research and treatment protocols. With the implementation of EHR systems, the use of the health record as an interactive tool for clinical problem solving and decision making is increasing.

Storage of Patient Care Documentation

As noted earlier, the main function of the health record is to store patient care data and information. According to the IOM (Dick et al. 1997, 81–93), the attributes associated with the storage function are quality, accessibility, security, flexibility, connectivity, and efficiency.

Quality

Clinicians, patients, administrators, researchers, and many other individuals and organizations rely on the quality of the information in the health record. In large part, the quality of such information depends on the design of the organization's systems and processes for collecting the original information.

Health record information is collected in different ways and from numerous sources. Patients and their families provide information to healthcare providers. Healthcare providers retrieve information from the documentation of previous patient encounters. Physicians and other providers make direct observations about the patient, assess clinical problems, provide diagnostic and therapeutic services, and evaluate the results of therapy. The data generated by electronic diagnostic and monitoring equipment such as laboratory results and tracings from heart monitors are also included in the health record. All this information is recorded on paper forms or in electronic formats to become part of the health record.

To accomplish the primary and secondary purposes of the health record, the data in it must be of the highest quality. Incomplete or missing data (for example, unrecorded lab results) could compromise patient care in that a patient could be treated for a condition that he or she does not have. Likewise, a patient may end up not being treated for a condition he or she has. Poor quality data could also contribute to incorrect assumptions made by policy makers. For example, policymakers might provide funding for a preventative heathcare initiative that didn't apply to that locale because their decision was based on data that were incorrect. Further, incomplete or missing data could result in inaccurate research findings, thus subjecting patients to inappropriate and/or ineffective treatment protocols. The need for high-quality data has been magnified with the implementation of EHRs. A single electronic error has the potential of being passed on to the entire population of health record users and can threaten patient safety as well as create inaccuracies in the myriad number of databases used to support healthcare. In November 2011, the Institute of Medicine (IOM) released recommendations from the Committee on Patient Safety and Health Information Technology. The Committee's findings related to EHRs were inconclusive. Some findings suggested EHRs have improved patient safety while others found no effect (IOM 2011, 2). Future monitoring and assessment needs to be conducted to ensure EHRs are improving the patient care experience and not creating additional hazards in the already complex care delivery system. Needless to say, the old adage, "garbage in equals garbage out" applies here. One of the HIM professional's most important roles is to ensure that the health record contains the highest-quality data possible.

In 1998, the American Health Information Management Association (AHIMA) developed a **data quality management** model (figure 2.5), which is based on four domains (Cassidy et al. 1998):

- *Data applications:* The purposes for which data are collected

- *Data collection:* The processes by which data are collected

- *Data warehousing:* The processes and systems by which data are archived (saved for future use)

- *Data analysis:* The processes by which data are translated into information that can be used for designated application

The data quality management model applies the following quality characteristics to the four quality management domains:

- Accuracy

- Accessibility

- Comprehensiveness

- Consistency

- Currency

- Definition

Figure 2.5. Data quality management model

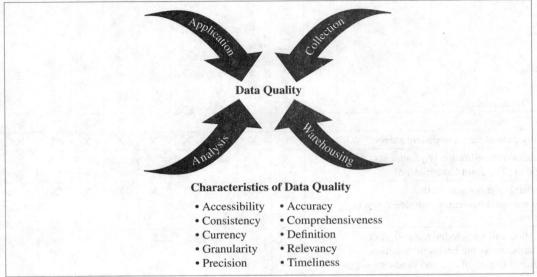

Source: Cassidy et al. 1998.

- Granularity

- Precision

- Relevancy

- Timeliness

Figure 2.6 demonstrates how each of the data quality characteristics are incorporated with health information management responsibilities.

Data accuracy means that data are correct. The data should represent what was intended or defined by the original source of the data. For example, the patient's emergency contact information recorded in a paper record or a database should be the same as what the patient said it was. Results of laboratory testing for a particular patient should reflect the results generated by the laboratory equipment. Data related to the medication provided to a particular patient should reflect the actual date, time, and medication administered. The accuracy of the data placed in the health record depends on a number of factors, including:

- The patient's physical health and emotional state at the time the data were collected

- The provider's interviewing skills

- The provider's recording skills

- The availability of the patient's clinical history

- The dependability of the automated equipment

- The reliability of the electronic communications media

Figure 2.6. HIM principles related to data quality attributes

	Data Quality Attributes / Principles	Accuracy	Accessibility	Comprehensiveness	Currency	Consistency	Definition	Granularity	Precision	Relevancy	Timeliness
		1	2	3	4	5	6	7	8	9	10
A	Support quality patient care and patient safety	X	X	X	X	X	X	X	X	X	X
B	Support regulatory/accreditation requirements (HIPAA, CFR 21, The Joint Commission)		X		X						X
C	Advocate leadership endorsement that standardization of data content is a strategic aim of the organization			X		X	X	X	X	X	
D	Provide education and knowledge transfer of data content standards across the health information exchange member organizations and vendors					X	X				
E	Support cooperative initiatives related to data standardization efforts, such as selection criteria for purchasing (or designing) new applications						X				
F	Lead health information exchange in data dictionary development and data mapping						X				
G	Provide leadership for development of data content standards					X	X	X	X	X	
H	Provide leadership in ongoing management of the data dictionary						X	X	X	X	
I	Coordinate data integration between and among systems		X		X	X					X
J	Work with vendors toward standards compliance	X	X	X	X	X	X	X	X	X	X
K	Liaison with clinical staff to facilitate adoption of data content standards			X			X				
L	Provide support for interoperability efforts among participants in health information exchange			X		X		X	X	X	
M	Bridge clinical and technological knowledge domains	X	X	X	X	X	X	X	X	X	X
N	Be the domain expert for health information standards						X	X	X	X	
O	Ensure security of data		X		X						X
P	Ensure privacy of data		X	X	X						X
Q	Provide quality data to support confidence in clinical decision making	X	X		X			X	X	X	X

Source: AHIMA e-HIM Workgroup on Health Information Management in Health Information Exchange 2007.

Data accessibility means that the data are easily obtainable. Any organization that maintains health records for individual patients must have systems in place that identify each patient and support efficient access to information on each patient. Authorized users of the health record must be able to access information easily when and where they need it. For example, an emergency room physician should be able to review the documented past medical history of a patient prior to or while examining the patient. A radiologist should be able to access the radiology images and reports remotely to provide immediate diagnosis and/or consultation with care providers. A family practice provider should be able to quickly access health records for an individual patient no matter where the various records are located (that is, the hospital, the emergency room, home health agency, specialty clinic, and so forth). Every health record system should allow record access 24 hours a day regardless of the format in which the record is stored.

The following factors affect the accessibility of health record data and information:

- Whether previous health records are available when and where they are needed
- Whether dictation equipment is accessible and working properly
- Whether transcription of dictation is accurate, timely, and readily available to healthcare providers
- Whether computer data-entry devices are working properly and are readily available to healthcare providers
- Whether the computer network and servers are accessible and working properly

In paper-based health record systems, access control is relatively straightforward. The records are stored in locked storage areas that are accessible only to authorized HIM staff. When needed for patient care purposes, the health record is retrieved from the file and forwarded to the appropriate service area. The record is then logged out according to a prescribed procedure. In this way, the HIM staff knows where to find the record in the event it is needed by another department or provider.

EHR systems have the same access control requirements that paper-based systems do. However, the mechanisms for controlling access to confidential information are different. Access control mechanisms are built in to EHRs. Technology-based access control mechanisms include the use of passwords, access cards or tokens, biometric devices, workstation restrictions, and role-based restrictions. (See chapter 17 for additional information on access control.)

Data comprehensiveness means that all the required data elements are included in the health record. In essence, comprehensiveness means that the record is complete. In both paper-based and electronic systems, having a complete health record is critical to the organization's ability to provide excellent patient care and to meet all regulatory, legal, and reimbursement requirements. In general, the health record must include the following data elements:

- Patient identification
- Consents for treatment

- Advance directives
- Problem list
- Diagnoses
- Clinical history
- Diagnostic test results
- Treatments and outcomes
- Conclusions and follow-up requirements

Data consistency means that the data are reliable. Reliable data do not change no matter how many times or in how many ways they are stored, processed, or displayed. Data values are consistent when the value of any given data element is the same across applications and systems. Related data items also should be reliable. For example, the clinical history for a male patient would not likely include a hysterectomy as a past surgical procedure.

Legitimate documentation inconsistencies do occur in health records. Any given health record may contain numerous references to the patient's diagnosis in terms of:

- The admitting diagnosis
- The diagnostic impression upon physical examination
- The postoperative diagnosis
- The pathology diagnosis
- The discharge diagnosis

Any inconsistencies among the various types of diagnoses would be legitimate. The different diagnoses incorporate the results of tests and findings not available at the time the previous documentation took place.

In other instances, however, data inconsistencies in the health record are not acceptable. For example, a nursing assessment might indicate that the patient is deaf when there is no documentation by the physician that the patient's hearing is compromised. Another unacceptable inconsistency occurs when different healthcare providers use different terminology. For example, different providers might use the words *cyst, lesion,* and *abscess* interchangeably in documenting a skin condition for the same patient. Such inconsistencies create difficulties for other caregivers and can be very confusing to external users of the health record.

Data currency means that healthcare data should be up-to-date.

Data timeliness refers to data being recorded at or near the time of the event or observation. Because care and treatment rely on accurate and current data, an essential characteristic of data quality is the timeliness of the documentation or data entry. For example, the dictation or recording of findings by the clinician during the performance of a physical exam will provide the most reliable information about the patient.

Data definition means that the data and information documented in the health record are defined. Users of the data must understand what the data mean and represent. Every data element should have a clear definition and a range of acceptable values. For example, the data element of race in healthcare is used to describe variations in the human population. The range of acceptable values for race may include white, black, Asian, Hispanic, and other. The data element of provider specialty may be used to describe the branch of medical science in which a provider is licensed to practice. The range of acceptable values might include family practice, emergency medicine, surgery, internal medicine, cardiology, urology, obstetrics, gynecology, radiology, pathology, or other.

Data granularity requires that the attributes and values of data be defined at the correct level of detail for the intended use of the data. For example, numerical values for laboratory results should be recorded to the appropriate decimal place as required for the meaningful interpretation of test results—or in the collection of demographic data, data elements should be defined appropriately to determine the differences in outcomes of care among various populations.

Data precision is the term used to describe expected data values. As part of data definition, the acceptable values or value ranges for each data element must be defined. For example, a precise data definition related to gender would include three values: male, female, and unknown. Or year of birth should be recorded with a 4-digit numeric value such as 1965 rather than the shortcut 65.

Precise data definition yields accurate data collection. In paper-based health records, much of the documentation and data are collected in narrative format and it is difficult to apply the concept of data precision to narrative text. However, electronic health records provide an opportunity to improve data precision.

Data relevancy means that the data in the health record are useful. The reason for collecting the data element must be clear to ensure the relevancy of the data collected. In paper-based health records, the volume of narrative detail provided often limits the usefulness of the data and information. For example, nursing documentation can be lengthy and physicians and other caregivers may not have sufficient time to review it. However, key data elements must be collected to assist in quantifying quality of care provided and care outcomes. For example, one of the 2011 Joint Commission National Hospital Inpatient Quality Measures for the management of acute myocardial infarction looks for evidence that aspirin was prescribed at discharge. Electronic and paper health records must provide this information in an easily interpretable format. Today, initiatives to improve patient safety and quality of care have spawned the development of hundreds of measurement criteria for which data must be captured in the health record during the care delivery process.

Data Quality Improvement

Traditional approaches to data quality improvement in the paper-based health record involve retrospective audits and corrective actions. Given that the EHR is shared with multiple constituencies on a real-time basis, EHR quality is dependent upon accurate data collection at the time of observation or rendering of treatment. Standardized documentation procedures are required to improve and ensure the quality of data within EHRs. To assist HIM professionals in quality improvement of EHR data, AHIMA's e-HIM work group developed a model to assist in improving data quality at the time the data is being created and recorded. The model is based on the 10 data quality characteristics just reviewed and requires that data quality checkpoints be established. These checkpoints are the critical points in the EHR documentation process where safeguards need to be built within the system to check for data quality (AHIMA e-HIM Workgroup 2007). Designing the registration data entry screen to require that the patient's date of birth be captured in MM/DD/YYYY format and that the registrar cannot complete the registration unless a valid date in this format is entered is an example of a quality safeguard built within the EHR. Figure 2.7 provides an example of how the model is applied to a patient encounter.

Security

Healthcare organizations and the clinical professionals who provide patient care services depend on the accuracy and accessibility of the information collected and stored in the health record. In addition, healthcare administrators, third-party payers, government agencies, accreditation organizations, and medical researchers all must have access to detailed healthcare information in order to fulfill their functions. However, these legitimate needs for access to information must be balanced against the public's expectation that healthcare providers will respect and protect the **privacy** of their patients.

Privacy, **confidentiality,** and **security** are related, but distinct, concepts. In the context of healthcare, *privacy* can be defined as the right of individuals to control access to their personal health information. *Confidentiality* refers to the expectation that the personal information shared by an individual with a healthcare provider during the course of care will be used only for its intended purpose. *Security* is the protection of the privacy of individuals and the confidentiality of health records. In other words, security allows only authorized users to access health records. In the broader sense, security also includes the protection of healthcare information from damage, loss, and unauthorized alteration. Additional information on privacy is found in chapter 13 and security in chapter 17.

Flexibility

For the health record to fulfill its intended purposes, health record data should be flexible enough to meet the needs of all the record's different users. In paper-based health record systems, this characteristic cannot be fully realized. Standardized forms are designed to make data readily available and meaningful to those caring for the patient. However, these forms may not support the needs of everyone who uses the health record. For example, individual physicians may wish to view laboratory results in ways that a single standard display does not permit such as trending with a line graph, bar graph, or pie chart.

When designed appropriately, EHR systems are extremely flexible in the way they display and present information. Authorized caregivers and other legitimate health record users display the information they need in the formats they prefer. For example, caregivers may wish to see views of the data by source, encounter, problem, date, or any number of

Figure 2.7. **EHR Documentation Improvement Model applied to a patient encounter**

Data Characteristics	Registration[1]	Assessment[2]	Treatment[3]	Follow-up[4]	Information Management[5]	Information Exchange (external)[6]
	Data Quality Checkpoint: Identification (ID) Validation (identity proofing)	Data Quality Checkpoint: History and physical (H&P)	Data Quality Checkpoint: Medication reconciliation	Data Quality Checkpoint: Discharge/Transfer/Referral (DTR) record with patient instructions	Data Quality Checkpoint: Audit log of unauthorized access to the patient record	Data Quality Checkpoint: Information from external sources
Accuracy—Ensures data have the correct value, are valid, and attached to the correct patient record.	Photo ID or two other forms of identification used.	Authentication by author licensed by the state. Patient demographics—five core data elements (i.e., name [first, middle initial, last], date of birth, gender, Social Security number, medical record number) checked against that of the record.	List is current and the source of information is noted.	Policies exist defining the components of the DTR record (e.g., correct patient ID, location for follow-up/ongoing care, patient instructions for self-care, diet, activity, and current medication regimen and allergies).	Periodic system security audits conducted to prevent unauthorized alteration or loss of data.	Incoming records matched against requests for information and validated.
Accessibility—Data items should be easily obtainable and legal to access with strong protections and controls built into the process.	Record of ID validation for each patient encounter exists (i.e., mandatory flag indicating the ID was validated and checked against the master person index).	Available to the right person, in the right place, at right time, for the right purpose as allowed by state and federal law.	Clinical history that pulls the data from previous encounters is available for verification and usage in patient care (e.g., check and verify patient meds with prior record).	Information is made available to patient and patient-authorized organization/ individual responsible for ongoing care at conclusion of visit/ stay.	End user authentication achieved by system signature, date/time stamp.	Data available in PDF format only and linked to appropriate patient record by note in system.

(continued on next page)

Figure 2.7.   **EHR Documentation Improvement Model applied to a patient encounter** (*continued*)

Data Characteristics	Registration[1]	Assessment[2]	Treatment[3]	Follow-up[4]	Information Management[5]	Information Exchange (external)[6]
Comprehensiveness— All required data items are included. Ensure that the entire scope of the data is collected and document intentional limitations.	Source and date of ID validation noted. Flags addressed. Multiple discriminations that would further ID the patient such as mother's maiden name included.	Includes all components required by regulatory/accrediting agencies, medical staff rules, and bylaws.	Data needed for treatment as defined by regulatory/accrediting agencies, medical staff rules, and bylaws is available at the point of service (e.g., for each medication the name, dosage, route, timing, duration are documented).	Record includes all components required by regulatory agencies/accrediting bodies, medical staff rules, and bylaws. Verification of patient understanding of instructions is documented by licensed author.	Includes user's login ID and date and time of access and the content accessed.	Policies note external data cannot be certified as comprehensive.
Consistency— The value of the data should be reliable and the same across applications.	Standards exist for ID search criteria (e.g., full name search, partial name search).	Required content is the same and available across the encounter and between applications (e.g., the allergy stated in the H&P should be the same throughout the patient stay).	Data values are coordinated across the continuum of care (e.g., the translation of a patient's medication list to a required formulary is verified each time a translation occurs).	Process exists ensuring DTR data is consistent with data in other parts of the medical record.	A plan and schedule exists for audits and follow-up.	Policies address the use of external data because it may not meet internal definitions.
Currency—The data should be up-to-date.	Policies exist ensuring the latest ID data is entered and validated.	Information is updated in real-time or within a certain time frame (i.e., information is synchronized every 30 minutes). When autopopulation of data occurs, author validates and updates as necessary and a notation is captured by the system of this occurrence.	Medications taken by the patient are verified against the previous record and updated as necessary.	Policies exist to ensure the most current data are entered and verified for each component.	Verify data classes are clearly and appropriately defined and consistent with current business needs and requirements (e.g., public, sensitive, private, confidential).	Policies note data from external source will not be current. Relying on dates within documentation is suspect in electronic form.

Figure 2.7.   EHR Documentation Improvement Model applied to a patient encounter (*continued*)

Data Characteristics	Registration[1]	Assessment[2]	Treatment[3]	Follow-up[4]	Information Management[5]	Information Exchange (external)[6]
Definition— Clear definitions should be provided so that current and future data users will know what the data mean. Each data element should have clear meaning and acceptable values.	A policy and procedure for updating, communicating, disseminating, and implementing the data dictionary exists (e.g., standards exist to ensure the same patient name and ID flows across all modules of the system including use of hyphens, apostrophes, etc.).	Guidelines defining H&P content (e.g., those by an accrediting agency) are available to authors and noted in the application user guide.	Standardized formulary exists.	Standardized data definitions for each required component of DTR are clearly defined.	A storage security assessment and audit procedure integrated with other security practices once the major elements of storage security have been defined appropriately for your organizations.	Policies note any agreements with other providers as to definitions of the data.
Granularity— The attributes and values of data should be defined at the correct level of detail.	A policy and procedure for updating, communicating, disseminating, and implementing the data dictionary exists (e.g., truncation does not occur and values are clearly understood).	Components of the H&P as defined by the chosen standard (e.g., CMS E&M guidelines) are documented.	Attributes for each medication (e.g., dosage, form, route, etc.) are defined.	Content of the DTR is defined so all required information for each component is captured (e.g., for medications: brand/generic name, dosage, route, frequency; for activities allowed description of examples).	A storage security assessment and audit procedure integrated with other security practices once the major elements of storage security have been defined appropriately for your organizations.	Policies note beyond what would be expected from the current standards there is no assurance of the values assigned to data (e.g., laboratory values from another source may not be expressed in the same manner as receiving facility).

(continued on next page)

Figure 2.7.   **EHR Documentation Improvement Model applied to a patient encounter** (*continued*)

Data Characteristics	Registration[1]	Assessment[2]	Treatment[3]	Follow-up[4]	Information Management[5]	Information Exchange (external)[6]
Precision—Data values should be just large enough to support the application or process.	Standard policies exist ensuring the same set of rules apply to the ID data values for capture, storage, display, and reporting.	Data obtained by the provider support the degree of patient complexity.	Checks are done to ensure what is ordered is what is given to the patient.	Policies exist to allow prepopulated fields (e.g., discharge medication list, instructions) as well as free text to facilitate data capture (e.g., name/location of organization to provide ongoing care).	Changes are identified and potential security impact assessed.	As directed by HIPAA, the sending organization sends only the minimum necessary information upon request.
Relevancy—The data are meaningful to the performance of the process or application for which they are collected.	Standard policies exist requiring the capture of all demographic data that reflects the information needed for ID validation. Standard algorithm for pulling up the patient.	Data obtained by the provider support the plan of care (e.g., significant positive/negative findings).	Express relationships to established standards, meet the patient/client needs, achieve the organization's goals and produce benefits.	Policies exist requiring the DTR to contain data relevant and necessary for coordination of ongoing care of the patient.	Compliance with specified controls and procedures verified.	Policies note beyond what would be expected from the current standards there is no assurance of the receipt of meaningful data.
Timeliness—Timeliness is determined by how the data are being used and their context.	Real-time updates of ID are performed.	Documented at the time of encounter by the authorized provider and available for patient care.	Patient's medications are noted for patient care.	Record is documented at the conclusion of the patient encounter and made available to the patient and patient-authorized organization/individual responsible for ongoing care.	Conduct audits on a regularly scheduled routine and as needed.	Policies note data from external source will never be timely in the sense of context because the receiver would not be defining the context.

Source: AHIMA e-HIM Workgroup on Assessing and Improving Healthcare Data Quality in the EHR 2007.

other variables. Further, the user may need data in detail or in summary form. Some users may only need to know the presence or absence of certain data, not necessarily the nature of the data. In these instances, the EHR has the potential to accommodate these needs and enhance the confidentiality of patient-identifiable health information.

Connectivity

Connectivity refers to the capacity of health record systems to provide electronic communication linkages and allow the exchange of health record data among information systems. Communications technology can be used within individual organizations to connect the various information systems that contain electronic components of the health record. For example, in organizations with disparate information systems, connectivity would allow the user access to lab tests, radiology reports, and EKGs in one location rather than acessing three different systems. Health record information that is not stored in an electronic format, however, must be transferred from place to place within the organization in a paper-based format.

In recent years, the concept of connectivity has evolved into what is known as system **interoperability** today. Interoperability standards that permit the electronic exchange of patient information within a region and within the nation are being developed. Health information exchanges are currently being created at the regional and state levels. Implementation of EHR systems will not be complete until patient information can be exchanged electronically among all healthcare providers throughout the United States.

Efficiency

Efficiency is another component of health record storage that is improved in electronic systems. As noted earlier, providing access to paper-based health records is an inefficient process, especially when information must be transferred between providers and facilities. Even internal transfers of health records can be troublesome because paper records may be needed in more than one place at a time. Moreover, paper records can be easily misplaced by users or misfiled by staff rendering them unavailable when needed.

Another factor related to efficiency is the structure of the data. Today, much of the information entered into an electronic system for storage has been scanned in from paper forms. Thus, the information available is in an image format rather than discrete data elements and cannot be used to make meaningful comparisons. For example, transcribed reports and data obtained from electronic document management systems provide electronically stored images. Such information cannot be analyzed efficiently. In fully functional EHR systems, structured data capture processes use controlled vocabularies and code sets which allow the data to be turned into information that can be used for patient care and the other purposes described earlier. Data collected in standard forms and housed within a database management system can be analyzed efficiently and compared using computer software database analysis and reporting applications designed for the database management system in use (i.e. Oracle, SQL Server, Sybase, etc.).

Guidance in Clinical Problem Solving

Physicians, nurses, and other caregivers use the information in individual health records as the basis for making diagnoses and choosing treatment options. A properly formatted health record can guide clinicians through the process of solving clinical problems. *Health record format* refers to the organization of electronic information or paper forms within the individual health record.

Paper Records

Three types of formats are commonly used in paper-based record systems: source-oriented, problem-oriented, and integrated. The **source-oriented health record format** organizes the information according to the patient care department that provided the care. For example, all lab tests are filed together, progress notes are filed together and so forth. This format is mostly used by acute care hospitals that are still using a paper record. The **problem-oriented health record format** is a documentation approach in which the physician defines each clinical problem individually and all documentation related to that clinical problem is stored together. Information about the problems is organized into four components: the database, the problem list, initial plans, and progress notes. The **integrated health record format** organizes all the paper forms in strict chronological order and mixes the forms created by different departments. Chapter 3 discusses health record formats in more detail.

Over the years, there has been debate about which record format is most useful for clinical problem solving. In 1991, the IOM's Committee on Improving the Patient Record studied various formats. The committee could not agree on which format would be the most useful in improving patient care. It felt that a mere translation of current record formats from paper media to electronic media would not result in meaningful improvements.

Hybrid Records

As healthcare organizations make the transition from paper-based records to electronic records, most HIM professionals are faced with working in a **hybrid health record** environment. It is rare for an organization to be able to be paper-based one day and totally electronic the next. In most healthcare organizations, providers, clinicians, and HIM professionals must find ways to work with and manage health records maintained in both paper-based and electronic formats while the electronic record of the future is being developed and implemented. Hybrid record environments are especially challenging when it comes to locating all components of a health record for a particular individual. Parts of the record will be found in traditional paper file storage while other portions of the record that are electronic need to be viewed and/or printed from one or more computer systems. Due to the disparate record creation and completion processes that are characteristic of hybrid records, organizations have found that the same information can be produced from several systems in a variety of formats, thus creating a need for organizations to identify the location for the source of truth for each piece of required documentation. Hybrid record environments are also very costly to manage as duplicate processes must be maintained (i.e., processes for handling the paper record as well as processes for handling the portion of the record that is electronic).

In November 2010, AHIMA issued a practice brief to assist HIM managers with the transition from paper records to hybrid records, and from hybrid records to electronic records. All HIM processes must be examined and revised to accommodate the hybrid record. High priority activities for the hybrid record environment include the definition of the legal record; archive, purge, retention, and destruction guidelines; forms management; access management; confidentiality; security; print control; spoliation mitigation; disclosure; e-discovery; and documentation inventories (AHIMA 2010b).

Electronic Records

A study (Dick et al. 1997) of paper-based record systems noted that such systems rely on clinician behaviors and record forms produced substantial waste, imprecision, and complexity. The study concluded that the movement toward EHR systems gives healthcare organizations and providers the opportunity to study and improve clinical approaches. Improvements in clinical care then will be reflected in the health record format (Dick et al. 1997). EHR systems are introducing new formats and functionality. Results management, order entry, and order management were added to the EHR functional model by the IOM in 2003 (IOM 2003, 7–8).

Results Management. Having timely access to all types of results, including laboratory results, radiology results, and other test results, over a period of time helps providers make informed choices for diagnoses and treatment and increases quality of care. With EHRs, both current and previous electronic results can be displayed automatically for care providers to improve effectiveness and efficiency of treatment while reducing the cost of care by eliminating duplicate testing. Formats for trending and comparing results over time are not available in paper-based systems.

Order-Entry/Order Management. Computerized provider order-entry (CPOE) systems have been developed to improve quality of care. Whereas paper-based health records capture handwritten orders, CPOE provides physicians and other providers the ability to place orders via the computer from any number of locations and adds decision support capability to enhance patient safety. Early adopters of this technology have been able to eliminate lost orders, eliminate issues with illegible handwriting, eliminate duplicate orders, reduce medication errors, and reduce the time to fill orders (IOM 2003, 8). CPOE provides another health record functionality that is unique to the EHR.

Clinical Decision Support. Effective and efficient patient care requires a great deal of complex information. To be an effective tool in clinical decision support, the health record needs to be more than a simple repository of patient care data (Dick et al. 1997). Fully functional EHR systems provide a number of decision-making tools that are not currently available in paper-based health record systems.

Clinical decision support tools review structured electronic data and alert practitioners to out-of-range laboratory values or dangerous trends before problems become evident.

The tools can recall relevant diagnostic criteria and treatment options on the basis of the data in the record. This supports the physician as he or she considers various diagnostic and treatment alternatives. Because the human memory is imperfect, such tools provide a consistent, supplementary knowledge base grounded in the latest clinical research.

In addition, electronic clinical decision support tools give clinicians instant access to pharmaceutical formularies, referral databases, and reference literature. This type of ready access provides clinicians with updates to information that they may use infrequently. Further, these applications help healthcare professionals learn about new developments because the bibliographic information in the decision support databases is always up-to-date.

Standard commercial software packages also can be included in health information systems so that descriptive, graphical, and statistical analyses of clinical data can be carried out. Such analyses may be limited to a specific case or performed on aggregate data to identify trends in a larger patient population. This functionality is not readily accomplished in paper-based record systems without a significant investment in staff time.

As the EHR continues to evolve and the delivery of healthcare changes, new formats and functionalities will be developed. Some will be more effective than others in encouraging the use of efficient, scientific problem-solving methods in the clinical process.

Check Your Understanding 2.3

1. A physician just received notification from an EHR system that a patient's lab test had a dangerously high value. This is an example of what kind of clinical tool?

    A. Clinical decision support
    B. Electronic records
    C. Results management
    D. Order-entry/order management

2. I just told my physician something embarrassing about myself. I told him because I expect him to use the information for my care only. This concept is called:

    A. Data relevancy
    B. Security
    C. Privacy
    D. Confidentiality

3. Someone suggested that we collect a patient's eye color. This was not implemented. What quality characteristic would be the justification for not collecting this information?

    A. Accuracy
    B. Consistency
    C. Granularity
    D. Relevancy

4. It was suggested that we enter the patient's age manually in all of our information systems rather than having it entered once in one system and interfaced to the other systems. What quality characteristic would be the justification for not doing this manual entry into each information system,

   A. Accuracy
   B. Consistency
   C. Granularity
   D. Relevancy

5. According to the AHIMA data quality model, what is the term that is used to describe how data is translated into information?

   A. Data applications
   B. Data collection
   C. Data warehousing
   D. Data analysis

Instructions: Match the following terms with the correct definitions.

6. _____ Data granularity

7. _____ Security

8. _____ Privacy

9. _____ Data comprehensiveness

10. _____ Data relevancy

a. A characteristic of data whose values are defined at the appropriate level of detail

b. A program designed to protect patient privacy and to prevent unauthorized access, alteration, or destruction of health records

c. A characteristic of data where the data are useful

d. An individual's right to control access to his or her personal information

e. A characteristic of data that includes every required data element

Real-World Case #1

The following case study is adapted from a journal article by Chris Dimick published in June 2008 in the *Journal of AHIMA*.

The innovation of the EHR has made it easier to reuse previously documented patient information. Previous information can be easily recalled and pasted into current documentation with a single click. While these shortcuts make documentation easier and faster for busy clinicians, such cut-and-paste practices can have serious repercussions for patient care and reimbursement, as illustrated in the scenario below.

As the patient's health worsened, a hospital stay of days turned to weeks. But through the various tests and physician visits, the progress notes generated in the hospital's electronic record system looked similar. Past notes were being electronically copied and pasted into current records. Old services rendered were being documented over and over again, with additions to reflect any new services. This pulling forward of information from past visits, was meant to save time on the busy hospital floor. It resulted in misrepresentation of the patient's stay and a fraudulent submission for reimbursement (Dimick 2008a, 40).

Real-World Case #2

The following case study is adapted from a journal article by Chris Dimick published in the November–December 2008 *Journal of AHIMA*.

HIM professionals face a number of challenges when working in a hybrid health record environment. One of the most significant obstacles relates to the difficulty in quickly locating all documents that belong in an individual's health record. In the paper-based world, health record documents for an individual patient are stored together in a paper file. In a hybrid situation, some documents are in a paper file while others are found in various electronic systems. HIM professionals must find ways to manage the where-abouts of the hybrid record.

OU Medical Center in Oklahoma City has created databases and spreadsheets to list the location of different pieces of the health record. The medical center also attaches a sheet called "hybrid record" to every paper record that lists all of the pieces of the record that are located in an electronic system. The grid also notes the date that certain documents were no longer printed and started to be stored in electronic form. This assists HIM staff in their process to compile the complete record when requested (Dimick 2008b).

Summary

The health record is the principal repository of data and information about the healthcare services provided to patients. A number of individuals and institutions use it as a source of information, but the primary users are the clinical professionals who provide direct patient care. Secondary users include healthcare managers and administrators, government agencies and policy makers, third-party payers, researchers, educators, and accreditation organizations.

The primary function of the health record is the storage of patient care information. The most important attributes of record storage include accessibility, quality, security, flexibility, connectivity, and efficiency. The importance of quality data within EHRs cannot be underestimated. Poor documentation, inaccurate data, and insufficient communication can result in errors and adverse events. The full implementation of interactive electronic health record systems adds more functionality to the health record than provided by traditional paper-based records. In addition to storing health information, EHRs provide knowledge resources to help clinicians solve diagnostic problems, support clinical decision making and administrative processes, and provide support for electronic reporting for population health management.

The concepts of privacy, confidentiality, and security are central to health information management. They are also on the forefront of the current healthcare industry landscape. Patients have the right to expect that healthcare providers will respect their privacy and guard their healthcare information against unauthorized access. Confidentiality forms the basis of meaningful patient–provider relationships. Without the protection of confidentiality, patients would be reluctant to be honest and open about issues related to their health. Security ensures that the information stored in a health record is protected from unauthorized alteration, damage, and loss.

References

AHIMA. 2009. Current state of PHRs. *Journal of AHIMA* 80(6):59–60.

AHIMA. 2010a. "Homeland Security Act, Patriot Act, Freedom of Information Act, and HIM." (Updated November 2010).

AHIMA. 2010b. "Managing the Transition from Paper to EHRs." (Updated November 2010).

AHIMA. 2010c. "Role of the Personal Health Record in the EHR (Updated)." Updated November 2010.

AHIMA. 2012. *Pocket Glossary of Health Information Management and Technology.* Chicago: AHIMA.

AHIMA e-HIM Workgroup on Assessing and Improving Healthcare Data Quality in the EHR. 2007. FORE Library HIM Body of Knowledge. http://library.ahima.org/xpedio/groups/public/documents/ahima/bok1_034032.hcsp?dDocName=bok1_034032

AHIMA e-HIM Workgroup on Health Information Management in Health Information Exchange. 2007. Practice brief: HIM Principles in Health Information Exchange. *Journal of AHIMA* 78(8):69–74.

Cassidy, B., et al. 1998. Practice brief: Data quality management model. *Journal of AHIMA* 69(6).

Dick, R.S., E.B. Steen, and D.E. Detmer, eds. 1997. *The Computer-Based Patient Record: An Essential Technology for Health Care,* rev. ed. Washington, DC: National Academies Press.

Dimick, C. 2008a. Documentation bad habits: Shortcuts in electronic records pose risk. *Journal of AHIMA* 79(6):40–43.

Dimick, C. 2008b. Record limbo: Hybrid systems add burden and risk to data reporting. *Journal of AHIMA* 79(11):28–32.

Institute of Medicine. 2003. *Key capabilities of an electronic health record system: Letter report.* http://www.nap.edu/catalog.php?record_id=10781

Institute of Medicine. 2011. *Health IT and Patient Safety: Building Safer Systems for Better Care.* http://www.iom.edu/Reports/2011/Health-IT-and-Patient-Safety-Building-Safer-Systems-for-Better-Care.aspx

National Committee on Vital and Health Statistics. 2001. *A strategy for building the health information infrastructure.* Washington, DC: US Department of Health and Human Services.

National Committee on Vital and Health Statistics/Subcommittee on Quality. 2008. *23 building blocks for quality: The view from 2008.* Washington, DC: US Department of Health and Human Services. http://www.ncvhs.hhs.gov/080717rpt.pdf

US Department of Health & Human Services HHS.gov. 2011. *We Can't Wait: Obama Administration takes new steps to encourage doctors and hospitals to use health Information technology to lower costs, improve quality, create jobs.* http://www.hhs.gov/news/press/2011pres/11/20111130a.html

Additional Resources

AHIMA. 2011. "Security Audits of Electronic Health Information (Updated)." *Journal of AHIMA* 82(3):46–50.

Amatayakul, M.K. 2009. *Electronic Health Records: A Practical Guide for Professionals and Organizations,* 4th ed. Chicago: AHIMA Press.

Cofer, J., ed. 1994. *Health Information Management,* 10th ed. Berwyn, IL: Physicians' Record Company.

Fernandez, L., et al. 1997. Practice brief: Master patient (person) index (MPI)—recommended core data elements. *Journal of AHIMA* 68(7).

Joint Commission National Hospital Inpatient Quality Measures. 2012. http://www.jointcommission.org/specifications_manual_for_national_hospital_inpatient_quality_measures/

Odom-Wesley, B., and D. Brown. 2009. Edited by C.L. Meyers. *Documentation for Medical Records.* Chicago: AHIMA Press.

Welch, J. 2000. Practice brief: Authentication of health record entries. *Journal of AHIMA* 71(3).

chapter 3

Content and Structure of the Health Record

Bonnie J. Petterson, PhD, RHIA

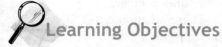

Learning Objectives

- Identify the content of health records in various healthcare settings

- Describe the purpose, use, and documentation requirements for customary reports, observations, orders, notes, authorizations, and consents included in a health record

- Explain documentation best practices as applied to the content of health records in paper-based, hybrid, and electronic environments

- Summarize the documentation requirements of accreditation organizations and state and federal government agencies

- Describe the clinical documentation improvement process

- Describe the different formats used for health records in healthcare organizations and the strengths and weaknesses of each

- Discuss the core capabilities of an electronic health record

- Identify the advantages of electronic health records over paper-based and hybrid records

- Explain the purpose and elements of a personal health record

Key Terms

Accreditation

Accreditation Association for Ambulatory Health Care (AAAHC)

Accreditation Commission for Health Care (ACHC)

Advance directive

American Association for Accreditation
of Ambulatory Surgery Facilities
(AAAASF)
American Correctional Association
American Osteopathic Association (AOA)
Anesthesia report
Authorization to disclose information
Autopsy report
Care area assessments (CAAs)
Care plan
Centers for Medicare and Medicaid
Services (CMS)
Certification
Commission for the Accreditation of Birth
Centers
Commission on Accreditation of
Rehabilitation Facilities (CARF)
Community Health Accreditation Program
Computer-based patient record (CPR)
Conditions for Coverage
Conditions of Participation
Consent to treatment
Consultation report
Deemed status
Discharge summary
DNV (Det Norske Veritas)
Electronic health record (EHR)
Electronic medical record (EMR)
Expressed consent
Hybrid record
Implied consent
Integrated health record
Joint Commission

Licensure
Medical history
Medical staff privileges
Medicare Conditions of Participation or
Conditions for Coverage
Minimum Data Set (MDS) for Long-Term
Care
National Commission on Correctional
Health Care
National Committee for Quality Assurance
(NCQA)
Operative report
Outcomes and Assessment Information
Set (OASIS)
Palliative care
Pathology report
Patient assessment instrument (PAI)
Patient history questionnaire
Patient Self-Determination Act (PSDA)
Patient's bill of rights
Personal health record (PHR)
Physical examination report
Physician's orders
Problem list
Problem-oriented health record
Progress notes
Recovery room report
Resident assessment instrument (RAI)
Source-oriented health record
Subjective, objective, assessment, plan
(SOAP)
Transfer record

Introduction

Chapter 2 introduced both primary and secondary purposes of a health record. One primary purpose is the documentation of patient care. A record represents the main communication mechanism used by healthcare providers in the delivery of patient treatment. Without it, providers would be unable to deliver safe and effective care. The record is the legal document that provides evidence of the interventions of healthcare professionals. This chapter will focus on the primary uses of a healthcare record. Meeting regulatory requirements, a secondary purpose, will be shown to have significant impact as well. Content of a record must meet the needs of all of its potential users, however, so all purposes of a health record become factors either in healthcare record content or documentation practices at one time or another.

For more than a century health records were created and maintained in paper-based formats. In recent years, however, many healthcare providers have implemented electronic records. As the demand for health information increases and incentives encourage healthcare facilities to adopt advanced information technology, electronic records are replacing most paper-based systems. A number of different terms have been used to describe electronic records. Today, **electronic health record** (EHR) is the term used most widely by the federal government and other entities. It refers to a health record available electronically, allowing communication across providers and permitting real-time decision making. It also allows for efficient reporting mechanisms. Other terms that reflect the evolution of the concept include **electronic medical record** (EMR) and **computer-based patient record** (CPR). When a facility is transitioning from paper to electronic systems and uses components of both, the record is referred to as a **hybrid record.** Chapter 16 discusses the EHR in more detail and chapter 7 provides an overview of best practices for managing hybrid and electronic health records.

This chapter describes the basic content of acute care health records and then provides specialized information requirements of other healthcare settings. It also introduces the documentation methods required by government and accreditation organizations. Finally, the chapter discusses the formats of paper-based, hybrid, and electronic health records, compares their strengths and weaknesses, and introduces the clinical documentation improvement process.

Theory into Practice

Major shifts in the way physicians, organizations, hospitals, and other health settings manage health records are appearing throughout the United States. The following real-life case is an example of the steps an organization takes in the transition from paper-based health record formats to computer-based systems.

Mayo Clinic Hospital, a 244-bed acute care hospital located in Phoenix, Arizona, has nearly 350 physicians from more than 65 medical and surgical specialties on its medical staff.

The Phoenix hospital opened in the fall of 1998 with a hybrid health record, and has transitioned over the past decade to using more electronic entry and less hardcopy records. Much of the care record is entered and accessed via vendor-purchased, site-edited software. The conditions of admission, consents and authorizations, physician progress notes, and patient discharge instructions and referrals are paper documents. All dictated physician reports (history and physicals, operative reports, consultations, and discharge summaries) are immediately viewable in the electronic record after transcription, and available for electronic signature in the provider's in-box. All other documentation, including that done by nursing, therapists, and other health professionals, and diagnostic or therapeutic testing, including imaging, are recorded and reported electronically.

Discharge record analysis (reviewing the record upon patient discharge for missing elements) is done by health information personnel using a computer. The system filters documents so that only those needing review are accessed. Electronic signatures are used and physicians can enter the system from any workstation. E-mail notices to physicians on record deficiencies are generated automatically upon completion of analysis. Although the parts of the record generated on paper are stored for a very short period of time after scanning, all release of information and other processes, including coding, use the computer-based record.

About 14 miles away, Mayo Clinic's outpatient clinic practice uses the same electronic record. Computers are located in each examination room and in stations outside the rooms. Information such as current medications, immunizations, and allergies can be entered directly. Progress notes from all patient visits at the clinic and from the two primary care practice sites located elsewhere in the metropolitan area are dictated immediately after each visit. Similar to hospital-dictated reports, they are transcribed and made immediately available as part of the electronic record. Paper documents in the outpatient setting include consents, insurance cards, outside information, and miscellaneous specialty-specific documentation. All paper documents are picked up hourly by health information personnel, scanned and indexed into the imaging system, and reviewed for quality and accuracy. The scanned material is available in the electronic record within two hours of the pickup time.

Kathie Falk, manager of Health Information Management Services at Mayo Clinic in Arizona, notes that the Mayo facilities in Rochester, Minnesota, Jacksonville, Florida, and the Mayo Clinic Health Systems (MCHS) currently have site-specific electronic records. Information is shared; for example, Arizona and Florida and the MCHS share the same EMR and database, and all sites use the same registration and radiology system. Improving interoperability across the enterprise is a Mayo Clinic priority.

Documentation Standards

First and foremost, the health record is a tool for documenting patient care. The information in the health record is provided directly by the healthcare professionals who participate in the patient's care to record what has been or is to be accomplished and to share information with other care providers.

The health record generally contains two types of data: clinical and administrative. *Clinical data* document the patient's medical condition, diagnosis, and procedures performed as well as the healthcare treatment provided. *Administrative data* include demographic and financial information as well as various consents and authorizations related to the provision of care and the handling of confidential patient information.

Types of Standards

The content of the health record varies, depending on the healthcare setting and the provider's medical specialty. Record content is determined primarily by practice needs and pertinent standards. Standards are statements of expected behavior or reference points against which structures, processes, or outcomes can be measured. Standards for documentation can be found in the following four main sources:

- *Facility-specific standards:* Standards might be found in facility policies and procedures and, when a facility has an organized medical staff, in the medical staff bylaws, rules, and regulations. Facility-specific guidelines govern the practice of physicians and others within a specific organization.

- *Licensure requirements:* Before they can provide services, most healthcare organizations must be licensed by government entities such as the state or county in which they are located and must maintain a license as long as care is provided.

- *Certification standards:* Government reimbursement program standards are applied to facilities that choose to participate in federal programs such as Medicare and Medicaid. These standards are titled **Conditions of Participation** or **Conditions for Coverage.** Facilities are said to be certified if the standards are met.

- *Accreditation standards:* Accreditation is the end result of an intensive external review process that indicates a facility has voluntarily met the standards of the independent accrediting organization.

The standards of these groups not only address content but often also outline time limits for completion of particular portions of the health record. Healthcare data sets also help determine elements of record content. For example, the Uniform Ambulatory Care Data Set outlines what data should be documented in facilities where ambulatory care is delivered. Data sets are discussed in chapter 4.

Significant overlap exists among the documentation requirements of accrediting bodies and federal and state regulations and laws. Although overlap may exist, differences among the standards must be recognized. When determining its policies, the organization must evaluate all relevant standards. Generally, following the strictest directives that apply ensures adequate compliance. In all cases, the ultimate goal is quality of care for patients in every healthcare environment.

Standards Organizations

As noted above, there are four main sources for documentation guidelines. Facility-specific standards vary widely and are beyond the scope of this text. A description of alternatives available in the remaining categories follows.

State Regulating Agencies

Individual states pass legislation and mandate regulations that affect how healthcare organizations within them operate and care for patients. The nature of these regulations varies from state to state.

Compliance with state licensing laws is required in order for healthcare organizations to begin or remain in operation within their states. To continue licensure, organizations must demonstrate their knowledge of, and compliance with, documentation regulations.

Medicare and Medicaid Programs

Administered by the federal government **Centers for Medicare and Medicaid Services (CMS)**, the **Medicare Conditions of Participation or Conditions for Coverage** apply to a variety of healthcare organizations that participate in the Medicare program. In other words, participating organizations receive federal funds from the Medicare program for services provided to patients and thus must follow the Medicare Conditions of Participation. The regulations vary according to setting and address documentation conditions that must be met to continue participation. Standards currently exist for hospitals, including rural hospitals and hospitals with swing beds, long-term care facilities, home health agencies, hospices, some rehabilitation facilities, qualified health centers, some outpatient or independent therapy services, and some behavioral health providers including those focused on substance abuse. Additionally, services provided by Suppliers of End Stage Renal Disease (ESRD), rural health clinics, transplant centers, portable x-ray suppliers, and ambulatory surgery centers are covered by standards.

Medicare recognizes some accreditation organizations as having standards that sufficiently cover the related Conditions of Participation. After reviewing the standards of accrediting groups that seek this recognition, Medicare may identify them as a Medicare recognized Accreditation Organization (AO) and award them **deemed status.** As long as a healthcare setting maintains active accreditation by an accreditation program with deemed status, separate Medicare surveys are not required. In 2011, there were seven organizations holding deemed status for each of several specified types of settings: the Joint Commission, Det Norske Veritas Healthcare, American Osteopathic Association's Healthcare Facilities Accreditation Program, American Association for Accreditation of Ambulatory Surgical Facilities, Accreditation Association for Ambulatory Health Care, Community Health Accreditation Program, and the Accreditation Commission for Health Care, Inc. The deemed programs of each organization are identified in their descriptions below. For all other facilities and programs, surveys are performed. This task is often contracted to state government health reviewers who may combine Medicare surveys with state standards compliance surveys.

Medicaid programs are funded jointly by federal and state governments but are administered by individual states. Thus, some Medicaid guidelines may vary from state to state. Similar to Medicare participation, however, facilities are required to meet federal Conditions of Participation or Conditions for Coverage to receive these funds.

Accreditation Organizations

Many healthcare organizations seek public recognition through accreditation by recognized accrediting bodies. This status signifies that the facility has met patient care and other standards for providing high-quality care. In some cases, it also allows facilities to participate in programs that affect their financial status, such as Medicare and Medicaid, Medical Resident Programs, and other training programs. Organizations seeking accreditation must meet specific documentation standards. Periodic surveys and detailed record review by the accrediting body evaluate how well the organization is complying with documentation standards. Standards are reviewed by the sponsoring body on a regular basis, usually every one to three years, with updates made as needed.

Healthcare organizations voluntarily seek accreditation from a variety of private, not-for-profit accreditation organizations. Different types of organizations are accredited by different accreditation organizations.

The Joint Commission

A number of healthcare settings are eligible for the **Joint Commission's** accreditation programs, including hospitals (acute, critical access, children's, psychiatric, and rehabilitation), ambulatory care organizations, behavioral health organizations, home care including hospice providers, long-term care facilities, clinical laboratories, and office-based surgery practices. Additional specialty certifications are available to accredited organizations for some disease-specific or advanced disease programs, advanced critical palliative care, and the healthcare staffing function. As an additional benefit for its accredited organizations, the Joint Commission has earned CMS deemed status for its hospital, critical access hospital, psychiatric hospital, ambulatory surgery center, home health agency, and hospice accreditation programs.

Beginning with its acute hospital standards in 2004, the Joint Commission initiated a process that moved from survey monitors every three years to a philosophy of continuous improvement and continuous standard compliance. In support of this philosophy, unannounced on-site surveys were implemented in 2006 along with a priority focus process that assists surveyors in conducting reviews on issues that are important for safety and quality of care. Annual submission of a Periodic Performance Review helps facilities evaluate compliance internally and requires development of a Plan of Action when a deficiency is found. The Joint Commission implements most changes in standards or the accreditation process with its hospital accreditation program, but eventually adopts the new methods in most of its accreditation programs.

The Joint Commission recognizes the appropriateness of applying documentation standards consistently across the healthcare continuum and has identified a number of common standards that apply to all healthcare settings. Frequently, these core expectations are supplemented by additional standards that represent the specific requirements of different settings and services. For example, a teaching hospital that hosts medical education programs for residents would be evaluated on its compliance with standards for supervision of residents, in addition to common standards and standards specific to acute care settings.

Most standards that apply to health records are found in Information Management chapters. However, to ensure compliance with all health information-related standards, review of all sections and monitoring of all pertinent standards that are found is important.

This concept applies to standards of other accreditation organizations as well. The Joint Commission also has addressed errors in interpretation of abbreviations commonly used in health records by publishing a prohibited abbreviation list. The abbreviations noted on the list should not be found in the patient health records of their accredited health providers.

American Osteopathic Association

American Osteopathic Association (AOA) first initiated its hospital accreditation program to ensure the quality of residency programs for doctors of osteopathy. Today, its Healthcare Facilities Accreditation Program (HFAP) accredits a number of additional healthcare organizations and facilities, including acute, specialty, and critical access hospitals; clinical laboratories; and ambulatory care/ambulatory and office-based surgery, behavioral and mental health, and primary stroke centers. Documentation standards are both broad (as they pertain to common documentation requirements) and specific (as they address specialty services). The HFAP also holds Medicare deemed status for its hospital, critical access hospital, and ambulatory surgery center programs.

Accreditation Association for Ambulatory Health Care

Accreditation Association for Ambulatory Health Care (AAAHC) has established ambulatory care core standards for all organizations and adjunct standards that only pertain to specific types of services. Health record documentation standards are core standards. When a patient has multiple visits or care is complex, standards require summaries for enhancing continuity of care including summaries of past surgeries, diagnoses, and problems. A wide variety of ambulatory care facilities including dental group and surgical practices, managed care organizations, and ambulatory surgical centers qualify for specific AAAHC accreditation programs. The latter two programs hold CMS deemed status.

Commission on Accreditation of Rehabilitation Facilities

Commission on Accreditation of Rehabilitation Facilities (CARF) accredits rehabilitation programs and services in medical rehabilitation, a variety of rehabilitation focused care programs for the aging, behavioral health, children and youth services, employment and community services, opioid treatment, vision rehabilitation, durable medical equipment, and business/service management networks. Health record documentation is used to evaluate procedural issues surrounding special circumstances in the treatment and handling of patients and clients.

National Committee for Quality Assurance

National Committee for Quality Assurance (NCQA) began accrediting managed care organizations in 1991. The NCQA standards focus on patient safety, confidentiality, consumer protection, access to services, service quality, and continuous improvement efforts. Proof of compliance for the organizations is dependent on documentation of patient services provided and their outcomes. More recently, NCQA expanded its programs to include other types of health plans and specialty certifications for non-comprehensive programs such as ones focusing on multicultural healthcare or disease management.

Other Accreditation Groups

A number of other organizations accredit specific types of healthcare facilities. **The Commission for the Accreditation of Birth Centers** and the **American Association for Accreditation of Ambulatory Surgery Facilities** focus on specific ambulatory or managed healthcare settings. The latter holds CMS deemed status for ambulatory surgery centers and outpatient rehabilitation therapy services. **The Accreditation Commission for Health Care** and the **Community Health Accreditation Program** accredit home health and hospice organizations. CMS deemed status has been awarded to both accrediting bodies for their home health and hospice programs. Correctional institutions can choose to have health services reviewed by the **National Commission on Correctional Health Care** and the **American Correctional Association**. Standards that affect health record content can be found in the guidelines for all accreditation programs.

Beginning in 2008, the **DNV (Det Norske Veritas)**, an international accrediting organization, began a hospital accreditation program in the United States. The DNV standards program, referred to as the National Integrated Accreditation for Healthcare Organizations (NIAHO), incorporates international quality management standards (ISO 9001) and the Medicare hospital Conditions of Participation. Although still in its infancy in the United States, its CMS hospital and critical access hospital deemed status and quality focus have been positively received.

Although this is not a comprehensive listing, figure 3.1 provides the accrediting agencies for the practice settings discussed in this chapter and includes each organization's website.

Standards of each of the organizations mentioned above have an important impact on health record content. In addition, the evolution of the practice of healthcare and each health care profession's specific body of knowledge helps determine other elements. New technology, procedures, and advancing knowledge of disease processes also must be reflected in documentation that may vary by type of healthcare provided. Thus, a description of the content of health records in each major type of care setting follows.

Figure 3.1.   Organization contacts

- Accreditation Association for Ambulatory Health Care (AAAHC) http://www.aaahc.org/
- American Association for Accreditation of Ambulatory Surgery Facilities (AAAASF) http://aaaasf.org/
- Accreditation Commission for Health Care (ACHC) http://www.achc.org/
- American Correctional Association (ACA) http://www.aca.org/
- American Osteopathic Association (AOA) http://www.osteopathic.org/
- Centers for Medicare and Medicaid Services (CMS) http://www.cms.hhs.gov/CFCsAndCoPs/
- Commission for the Accreditation of Birth Centers (CABC) http://www.birthcenteraccreditation.org
- Commission on Accreditation of Rehabilitation Facilities (CARF) http://www.carf.org/
- Community Health Accreditation Program (CHAP) http://www.chapinc.org/
- DNV (Det Norske Veritas) http://www.dnv.com/industry/healthcare/hospital_accreditation/
- National Commission on Correctional Health Care (NCCHC) http://www.ncchc.org/
- National Committee for Quality Assurance (NCQA) http://www.ncqa.org/
- The Joint Commission http://www.jointcommission.org/

Check Your Understanding 3.1

1. Which two major types of data are contained in the health record?

   A. Nursing and physician
   B. Administrative and clinical
   C. Demographic and financial
   D. Surgical and medical

2. Which of the following terms refers to state or county regulations that healthcare facilities must meet to be permitted to provide care?

   A. Accreditation
   B. Bylaws
   C. Certification
   D. Licensure

3. Which of the following is an accrediting organization?

   A. State regulating agencies
   B. American Health Information Management Association
   C. Det Norske Veritas Healthcare
   D. Centers for Medicare and Medicaid Services

4. An accrediting organization is awarded deemed status by Medicare for one of its programs. This means that facilities receiving accreditation under its guidelines do not need to:

   A. Meet licensure standards
   B. Undergo Medicare certification surveys
   C. Undergo accreditation surveys
   D. Meet Medicare certification standards

5. Which group focuses on accreditation of managed care?

   A. Accreditation Association for Ambulatory Healthcare
   B. National Committee for Quality Assurance
   C. Commission on Accreditation of Rehabilitation Facilities
   D. The Joint Commission

6. Which group focuses on accreditation of rehabilitation programs and services?

   A. CARF
   B. AOA
   C. AAAHC
   D. HFAP

7. Which of these accreditation organizations provides standards for the widest variety of healthcare facilities?

   A. American Correctional Association
   B. The Joint Commission
   C. Accreditation Commission for Health Care
   D. American Osteopathic Association

Acute Care Health Record Documentation

Programs addressing uniformity in the content of records and quality of documentation began almost a century ago with the general hospital setting. In addition, acute care hospitals provide the most intensive, critical care services. Acute hospital records provide the foundation for content and practices for other healthcare settings. Thus the discussion of record documentation practices will begin with acute care health records.

Basic Acute Care Content

The basic components of health records maintained by acute care hospitals described in this section will be found in a record whether it is paper-based, hybrid, or electronic. (See table 3.1 for a summary of the basic components of an acute care health record.) However, the actual location of data elements, whether found on a paper form or across computer screens, will vary. A number of groups provide standards for acute care hospital documentation from all four major sources previously described. Federal government Conditions of Participation for Hospitals and for critical access hospitals (facilities in rural settings meeting special criteria) both include record content requirements. Accreditation standards from the Joint Commission, the Healthcare Facilities Accreditation Program of the

Table 3.1. **Basic components of the acute care health record**

Component	Function
Registration record	Documents demographic information about the patient
Medical history	Documents the patient's current and past health status
Physical examination	Contains the provider's findings based on an examination of the patient
Clinical observations	Provide a chronological summary of the patient's illness and treatment as documented by physicians, nurses, and allied health professionals
Physician's orders	Document the physician's instructions to other parties involved in providing the patient's care, including orders for medications and diagnostic and therapeutic procedures
Reports of diagnostic and therapeutic procedures	Describe the procedures performed and give the names of clinicians and other providers; include the findings of x-rays, mammograms, ultrasounds, scans, laboratory tests, and other diagnostic procedures
Consultation reports	Document opinions about a patient's condition furnished by providers other than the attending physician
Discharge summary	Concisely summarizes the patient's stay in a hospital
Patient instructions	Document the instructions for follow-up care that the provider gives to the patient or the patient's caregiver
Consents, authorizations, and acknowledgments	Document the patient's agreement to undergo treatment or services, permission to release confidential information, or recognition that information has been received

American Osteopathic Association (AOA), or the DNV's (Det Norske Veritas) NIAHO standards provide hospitals with options for voluntary external review.

Clinical Data

The patient's attending or primary physician usually gives the hospital some preliminary information about the patient before he or she is admitted to the hospital. (Admission is the process of formal registration for hospital services.) Such information includes an admitting or working diagnosis, also called a provisional diagnosis. The admitting diagnosis identifies the condition or illness, as understood at the time of admission, for which the patient needs medical care. This information is recorded on an admission or registration record, also referred to as a face sheet in paper-based systems. The admission record also includes demographic and financial data about the patient. (See the administrative data section later in this chapter.)

The following types of clinical data are documented in the health record during the patient's hospital stay:

- Patient's medical history and pertinent family history
- Report of the patient's initial physical examination
- Attending physician's diagnostic and therapeutic orders
- Clinical observations of the providers who care for the patient
- Reports and results of every diagnostic and therapeutic procedure performed
- Reports of consulting physicians
- Patient's discharge summary
- Final instructions to the patient upon discharge

Medical History

A complete **medical history** documents the patient's current complaints and symptoms and lists his or her past medical, personal, and family history. In acute care, the medical history is usually the responsibility of the attending physician. Medical histories obtained by specialists such as gynecologists and cardiologists concentrate on the organ systems involved in the patient's current illness. Table 3.2 shows the information that is usually included in a medical history.

Physical Examination Report

The **physical examination report** represents the attending physician's assessment of the patient's current health status after evaluating the patient's physical condition. This report should document information on all the patient's major organ systems. Table 3.3 lists the components that are usually included in this report.

Table 3.2. **Information usually included in a complete medical history**

Components of the History	Complaints and Symptoms
Chief complaint	Nature and duration of the symptoms that caused the patient to seek medical attention as stated in his or her own words
Present illness	Detailed chronological description of the development of the patient's illness, from the appearance of the first symptom to the present situation
Past medical history	Summary of childhood and adult illnesses and conditions, such as infectious diseases, pregnancies, allergies and drug sensitivities, accidents, operations, hospitalizations, and current medications
Social and personal history	Marital status; dietary, sleep, and exercise patterns; use of coffee, tobacco, alcohol, and other drugs; occupation; home environment; daily routine; and so on
Family medical history	Diseases among relatives in which heredity or contact might play a role, such as allergies, cancer, and infectious, psychiatric, metabolic, endocrine, cardiovascular, and renal diseases; health status or cause of and age at death for immediate relatives
Review of systems	Systemic inventory designed to uncover current or past subjective symptoms that includes the following types of data: • *General:* Usual weight, recent weight changes, fever, weakness, fatigue • *Skin:* Rashes, eruptions, dryness, cyanosis, jaundice; changes in skin, hair, or nails • *Head:* Headache (duration, severity, character, location) • *Eyes:* Glasses or contact lenses, last eye examination, glaucoma, cataracts, eyestrain, pain, diplopia, redness, lacrimation, inflammation, blurring • *Ears:* Hearing, discharge, tinnitus, dizziness, pain • *Nose:* Head colds, epistaxis, discharges, obstruction, postnasal drip, sinus pain • *Mouth and throat:* Condition of teeth and gums, last dental examination, soreness, redness, hoarseness, difficulty in swallowing • *Respiratory system:* Chest pain, wheezing, cough, dyspnea, sputum (color and quantity), hemoptysis, asthma, bronchitis, emphysema, pneumonia, tuberculosis, pleurisy, last chest x-ray • *Neurological system:* Fainting, blackouts, seizures, paralysis, tingling, tremors, memory loss • *Musculoskeletal system:* Joint pain or stiffness, arthritis, gout, backache, muscle pain, cramps, swelling, redness, limitation in motor activity • *Cardiovascular system:* Chest pain, rheumatic fever, tachycardia, palpitation, high blood pressure, edema, vertigo, faintness, varicose veins, thrombophlebitis • *Gastrointestinal system:* Appetite, thirst, nausea, vomiting, hematemesis, rectal bleeding, change in bowel habits, diarrhea, constipation, indigestion, food intolerance, flatus, hemorrhoids, jaundice • *Urinary system:* Frequent or painful urination, nocturia, pyuria, hematuria, incontinence, urinary infections • *Genitoreproductive system:* Male—venereal disease, sores, discharge from penis, hernias, testicular pain, or masses; female—age at menarche, frequency and duration of menstruation, dysmenorrhea, menorrhagia, symptoms of menopause, contraception, pregnancies, deliveries, abortions, last Pap smear • *Endocrine system:* Thyroid disease; heat or cold intolerance; excessive sweating, thirst, hunger, or urination • *Hematologic system:* Anemia, easy bruising or bleeding, past transfusions • *Psychiatric disorders:* Insomnia, headache, nightmares, personality disorders, anxiety disorders, mood disorders

Table 3.3.   Information usually documented in the report of a physical examination

Report Components	Content
General condition	Apparent state of health, signs of distress, posture, weight, height, skin color, dress and personal hygiene, facial expression, manner, mood, state of awareness, speech
Vital signs	Pulse, respiration, blood pressure, temperature
Skin	Color, vascularity, lesions, edema, moisture, temperature, texture, thickness, mobility and turgor, nails
Head	Hair, scalp, skull, face
Eyes	Visual acuity and fields; position and alignment of the eyes, eyebrows, eyelids; lacrimal apparatus; conjunctivae; sclerae; corneas; irises; size, shape, equality, reaction to light, and accommodation of pupils; extraocular movements; ophthalmoscopic exam
Ears	Auricles, canals, tympanic membranes, hearing, discharge
Nose and sinuses	Airways, mucosa, septum, sinus tenderness, discharge, bleeding, smell
Mouth	Breath, lips, teeth, gums, tongue, salivary ducts
Throat	Tonsils, pharynx, palate, uvula, postnasal drip
Neck	Stiffness, thyroid, trachea, vessels, lymph nodes, salivary glands
Thorax, anterior and posterior	Shape, symmetry, respiration
Breasts	Masses, tenderness, discharge from nipples
Lungs	Fremitus, breath sounds, adventitious sounds, friction, spoken voice, whispered voice
Heart	Location and quality of apical impulse, trill, pulsation, rhythm, sounds, murmurs, friction rub, jugular venous pressure and pulse, carotid artery pulse
Abdomen	Contour, peristalsis, scars, rigidity, tenderness, spasm, masses, fluid, hernia, bowel sounds and bruits, palpable organs
Male genitourinary organs	Scars, lesions, discharge, penis, scrotum, epididymis, varicocele, hydrocele
Female reproductive organs	External genitalia, Skene's glands and Bartholin's glands, vagina, cervix, uterus, adnexa
Rectum	Fissure, fistula, hemorrhoids, sphincter tone, masses, prostate, seminal vesicles, feces
Musculoskeletal system	Spine and extremities, deformities, swelling, redness, tenderness, range of motion
Lymphatics	Palpable cervical, axillary, inguinal nodes; location; size; consistency; mobility and tenderness
Blood vessels	Pulses, color, temperature, vessel walls, veins
Neurological system	Cranial nerves, coordination, reflexes, biceps, triceps, patellar, Achilles, abdominal, cremasteric, Babinski, Romberg, gait, sensory, vibratory
Diagnosis(es)	

Diagnostic and Therapeutic Orders

Physician's orders are the instructions the physician gives to the other healthcare professionals who actually perform diagnostic tests and treatments, administer medications, and provide specific services to a particular patient. Admission and discharge orders should be found for every patient unless the patient leaves the facility against medical advice (AMA), but other orders will vary from patient to patient. All orders must be legible and include the date and the physician's signature. In electronic systems, signatures are attached via an authentication process. See figure 3.2 for an example of a physician's order in an electronic format.

Standing orders are orders the medical staff or an individual physician have established as routine care for a specific diagnosis or procedure. Standing orders are commonly used in hospitals, ambulatory surgery facilities, and long-term care facilities (figure 3.3). Usually, standing orders are preprinted on a single sheet of paper or available via a standard computer screen. Like other physician's orders, they must be signed/verified and dated.

Physicians may communicate orders verbally or via the telephone when the hospital's medical staff rules allow. State law and medical staff rules specify which practitioners, for example only registered nurses, are allowed to accept and execute verbal and telephone orders. How the orders are to be signed as well as the time period allowed for authentication also may be specified. In this age of electronic communications, it is notable that the Joint Commission currently specifically prohibits orders sent via text message.

Figure 3.2.   Example of a physician's order in electronic format

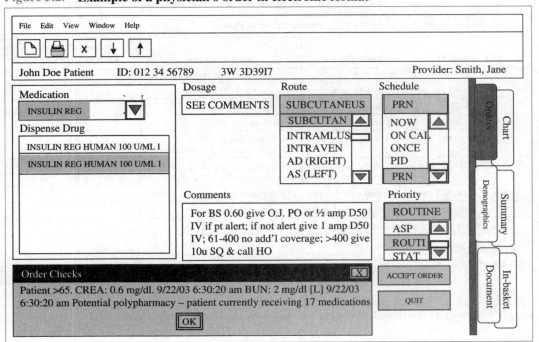

Figure 3.3.   **Example of a physician's standing order in paper format**

Midwest Medical Center

**HEPARIN ORDER: REGULAR UNFRACTIONATED
HEPARIN FOR ADULTS**

PATIENT LABEL

Diagnosis: _____

Allergies: _____

Total Body Weight: _____lb = _____kg

Warning: Due to an increased risk of serious bleeding, patients should not receive both regular heparin and low-molecular-weight heparin.

Patients should also be evaluated for continuance of other medications such as aspirin, clopidogrel, and NSAID therapy.

---

1. Check baseline PTT, PT/INR, heme panel

---

2. Check the appropriate bolus regimen according to diagnosis/disease
   a. ☐ No initial bolus
   b. ☐ Acute coronary syndrome—heparin bolus 75 units/kg = _____ units IV
      (round to the nearest 1000 units—maximum bolus = 10,000 units)
   c. ☐ In combination with thrombolytic therapy for acute MI (TNKase, Retavase, TPA)
      ☐ 5000 units bolus if 65 kg or greater
      ☐ 4000 units bolus if less than 65 kg
   d. ☐ Treatment of DVT/PE—heparin bolus 80 units/kg = _____ units IV
      (round to the nearest 1000 units—maximum bolus = 10,000 units)

---

3. Following bolus, begin IV heparin infusion (check the appropriate regimen):
   • Premixed IV bag contains heparin 25,000 units in 250 ml of D5W (100 units/ml)
   • Maximum initial infusion rate not to exceed 2000 units/h
   ☐ All cardiology regimens: 16 units/kg/h = _____ ml/h
   ☐ Treatment of DVT or PE: 18 units/kg/h = _____ ml/h

---

4. Check PTT 6 hours after initiation of heparin infusion

---

5. Adjust heparin based on guidelines below
   (document all changes on MAR and physician's orders sheet):

PTT (seconds)	Bolus Dose	Rate Changes	Repeat PTT after Each Dosage Change
PTT <35	Bolus 4000 units	Increase rate 200 units/h	6 h
PTT 35–45	Bolus 3000 units	Increase rate 200 units/h	6 h
PTT 46–70	No bolus	No rate change	Next a.m.
PTT 71–90	No bolus	Decrease rate 100 units/h	6 h
PTT 91–100	No bolus	Hold infusion 1 h, then decrease rate by 200 units/h	6 h
PTT >100	No bolus	Hold infusion 1 h, then decrease rate by 300 units/h	6 h

---

6. Check PTT and heme panel every morning (while patient is on heparin protocol).

---

7. Check stools daily for occult blood and notify physician if positive.

---

8. Notify physician for bleeding, hematoma, or heart rate above 120 bpm.

Physician Signature: _____ Date/Time: _____

RN Signature: _____ Date/Time: _____

HEPARIN ORDER
000013 (11/2002)

Clinical Observations

In acute care hospitals, the documentation of clinical observations is usually provided in **progress notes.** The purpose of documenting the clinical observations of physicians, nurses, and other caregivers is to create a chronological report of the patient's condition and response to treatment during his or her hospital stay. Progress notes serve to justify further acute care treatment in the facility. In addition, they document the appropriateness and coordination of the services provided. The patient's condition determines the frequency of the notes.

Physician Notes

The rules and regulations of the hospital's medical staff specify which healthcare providers are allowed to enter progress notes in the health record. Typically, the patient's attending physician, consulting physicians who have **medical staff privileges,** house medical staff, nurses, nutritionists, social workers, and clinical therapists are authorized to enter progress notes. Depending on the record format used by the hospital, each discipline may maintain a separate section of the health record or the observations of all the providers may be combined in the same chronological or integrated health record. (Source-oriented and integrated health records are discussed later in this chapter.) Guidelines for the frequency of notations may also be found in the Medical Staff Rules and Regulations.

Special types of notes are frequently found in a record. For example, prior to the administration of anything other than local anesthesia, the anesthesiologist visits the patient and documents important factors about the patient's condition that may have an impact on the anesthesia chosen or its administration. Allergies and drug reactions would be noted. A post-anesthesia note also should be found describing the patient's recovery from the anesthetic. Similarly, the surgeon responsible for a major procedure must document both pre- and post-surgical patient evaluations.

Despite the best efforts of hospital caregivers and physicians, some patients die while they are hospitalized. In such cases, the attending physician should add a summary statement to the patient's health record to document the circumstances surrounding the patient's death. The statement can take the form of a final progress note or a separate report. The statement should indicate the reason for the patient's admission, his or her diagnosis and course in the hospital, and a description of the events that led to his or her death.

Nursing and Allied Health Notes and Assessments

Just as physician documentation begins with the history and physical examination, nurses and allied health professionals (for example, occupational, physical, respiratory, and speech therapists; dieticians; and social workers) may begin their care with assessments focused on understanding the patient's condition from the perspective of their specialized body of knowledge. Figure 3.4 provides an example of an admission nursing assessment. Often a **care plan** may then follow the assessment. A care plan is a summary of the patient's problems from the nurse or other professional's perspective with a detailed plan for interventions. In addition, nurses are responsible for specific patient admission and discharge notes and for documenting the patient's condition at regular intervals throughout the patient's stay. If a patient should die while hospitalized, nursing notes regarding the circumstances leading to and of death are important.

Figure 3.4.   Example of initial nursing assessment in paper format

Midwest Medical Center

INITIAL NURSING ASSESSMENT

PATIENT LABEL

Baseline Information

Date:	Time:	Age:	Arrived: AMB WC Stretcher EMS Carried Other:	Primary MD:

Initial/Chief Complaint/History of Present Illness:

T: PO R TM	P:	R:	BP: R L	⊕ O₂ Sats %	Sex: M F	Height:	Weight: Actual: Stated:

⊕ Tetanus/Immunizations:		Pneumococcal Vaccine	☐ No ☐ Yes Most Recent Date:

⊕ Pregnant ☐ No ☐ Yes	LNMP:	Influenza Vaccine ☐ No ☐ Yes Most Recent Date:

Allergies:	☐ None	☐ Medications	☐ Latex	☐ Food	☐ Anesthesia	☐ Other

List Names and Reactions:

TB Assessment (Initiate airborne isolation if 4 or more criteria are checked yes)

Persistent Cough > 2 weeks	☐ No ☐ Yes	Abnormal Chest X-Ray	☐ No ☐ Yes	Respiratory Isolation
Fever > 100.4 (night sweats)	☐ No ☐ Yes	Physician Order for AFB (smear/culture)	☐ No ☐ Yes	Ordered ☐ No ☐ Yes
Unexplained Weight Loss	☐ No ☐ Yes	Recent Exposure to Person with Suspected TB or +PPD	☐ No ☐ Yes	

RN/LPN Signature: _____

☐ See Home Medication Orders	Medication/Over the Counter/Herbal History			☐ Investigation Drugs/Devices		
Medication	Dose	Freq	Last Dose	Medication	Dose	Freq	Last Dose

Hospitalizations/Surgeries:

Medical History

Neurological	☐ No	☐ Yes		Sensory Impairment	☐ No	☐ Yes	
Cardiovascular	☐ No	☐ Yes		Endocrine	☐ No	☐ Yes	
Hypertension	☐ No	☐ Yes		Blood Disorder	☐ No	☐ Yes	
Respiratory	☐ No	☐ Yes		Cancer	☐ No	☐ Yes	
Gastrointestinal	☐ No	☐ Yes		Psychological	☐ No	☐ Yes	
Renal/Urological	☐ No	☐ Yes		Tobacco Use	☐ No	☐ Yes	
Gynecological	☐ No	☐ Yes		Alcohol/Drug Use	☐ No	☐ Yes	
Musculoskeletal	☐ No	☐ Yes		Infectious Disease	☐ No	☐ Yes	
Integumentary	☐ No	☐ Yes		Cough/Cold Past 2 Weeks	☐ No	☐ Yes	
EENT	☐ No	☐ Yes		Anesthesia	☐ No	☐ Yes	

Source of Information	☐ Patient	☐ Family	☐ Unable to Obtain	☐ Other	☐ Medications Sent Home with Patient: _____

Arrival Date:	Arrival Time:	T: PO R TM	P:	R:	BP: R L	O₂ Sats %: (If applicable)

RN Initial: _____   RN Signature: _____   Date: _____   Time: _____   Unit: _____

RN Initial: _____   RN Signature: _____   Date: _____   Time: _____   Unit: _____

INITIAL NURSING ASSESSMENT
000039 (10/2002)

Figure 3.5. **Electronic plotted vital signs**

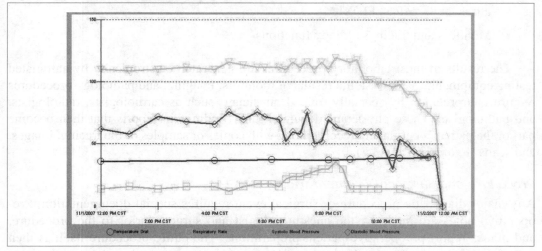

Nursing professionals also maintain chronological records of the patient's vital signs (blood pressure, heart rate, respiration rate, and temperature) and documentation of medications ordered and administered. Other chronological monitors such as measures of a patient's fluid input and output may be ordered and recorded depending on the patient's diagnosis. Sometimes these records are referred to as flow records because they show trends over time, or the data may be represented in graphic form for ease of communication. (See figure 3.5 for an example of monitors in electronic format.) Special interventions such as the use of restraints also require documentation. For example, restraint information must include the type of restraint used, time frame used, and regular vital signs monitors and descriptions of the patient's physical condition while restrained.

After an initial assessment, documentation by other allied health professionals varies by specialty. Each facility will define appropriate content and frequency of recording using specific regulations and standards in addition to the profession's practice guidelines. For example, respiratory therapy treatments may be documented via samples of graphic monitors with interpretations and social work interventions may appear as dictated reports.

Reports of Diagnostic and Therapeutic Procedures

The results of all diagnostic and therapeutic procedures become part of the patient's health record.

Diagnostic Reports

Diagnostic procedures include the following:

- Laboratory tests performed on blood, urine, and other samples from the patient
- Pathological examinations of tissue samples and tissues or organs removed during surgical procedures

- Imaging procedures of the patient's body and specific organs (radiology, scans, ultrasounds, MRIs, PETs)

- Monitors and tracings of body functions

The results of most laboratory procedures are generated electronically by automated testing equipment. In contrast, the results of monitors, imaging, and pathology procedures require interpretation by specially trained physicians such as cardiologists, radiologists, and pathologists. These physicians document their findings in reports that then become part of the patient's permanent record, along with copies or samples of the tracing, images, and scans (figures 3.6 and 3.7).

Procedure and Surgical Documentation

Any major diagnostic procedure or surgical event requires special documentation. Preoperative notes are made by the anesthesiologist and surgeon prior to the procedure, and nurses report preoperative patient preparations. The entire procedure itself is then recorded, along with an anesthesia record, an operative report, and a post-anesthesia or recovery room report. When tissue is removed for evaluation, a pathology report also must be present.

Patient Consent Documentation

The patient must consent to a procedure after an explanation and an opportunity to ask questions. This is called an informed consent. Often special documents or screens are designed to provide evidence of consent, including the appropriate signature. The need to obtain the patient's consent before medical and surgical procedures is based on the legal concept of battery. Battery is the unlawful touching of a person without his or her implied or expressed consent.

Figure 3.6. Electronic lab report

Navigator	Lab View	8/6/200 6 5:28	8/5/200 6 1:36	8/5/200 6 1:35	8/5/200 6 12:35	8/5/200 6 5:30	8/4/200 6 6:00	8/1/200 6 2:00	7/31/20 06 5:35	7/31/20 06 3:35
☑ CBC	☐ FiO2		100	100	100		100			
☑ Routine Coag	**Routine Chem**									
☑ Blood Gases	☐ Sodium Level	136				134				141
☑ Routine Chem	☐ Potassium Level	3.3				3.6				4.0
☑ Lipids	☐ Chloride					96				109
	☐ CO2					25				27
	☐ BUN	37				35				20
	☐ Creatinine	1.1				1.4				0.9
	☐ Glucose Level					291				119
	☐ Calcium Level	8.5				8.8				
	☐ Phos	2.4				3.7			3.1	
	☐ Albumin Level					3.1			3.6	
	☐ Alk Phos					42			42	
	☐ AST					12			17	
	☐ Bili Total					1.5			1.5	
	☐ Total Protein					7.1			7.8	
	Lipids									
	☐ Chol					133			217	

Figure 3.7. **Example of an electrocardiography report in paper format**

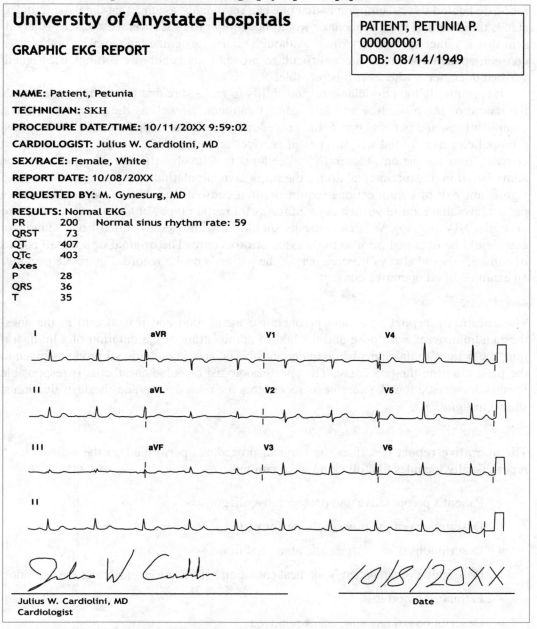

University of Anystate Hospitals

GRAPHIC EKG REPORT

PATIENT, PETUNIA P.
000000001
DOB: 08/14/1949

NAME: Patient, Petunia

TECHNICIAN: SKH

PROCEDURE DATE/TIME: 10/11/20XX 9:59:02

CARDIOLOGIST: Julius W. Cardiolini, MD

SEX/RACE: Female, White

REPORT DATE: 10/08/20XX

REQUESTED BY: M. Gynesurg, MD

RESULTS: Normal EKG

PR	200	Normal sinus rhythm rate: 59
QRST	73	
QT	407	
QTc	403	
Axes		
P	28	
QRS	36	
T	35	

Julius W. Cardiolini, MD
Cardiologist

10/8/20XX
Date

Implied consent is assumed when a patient voluntarily submits to treatment. The rationale behind this assumption is that one can reasonably assume that the patient understands the nature of the treatment or would not submit to it. **Expressed consent** is a consent that is either spoken or written. Although courts recognize both spoken and written consent, spoken consent is more difficult to prove. Thus healthcare settings use signed/verified documents whenever it is possible.

It is primarily the physician's responsibility to make sure that the patient understands the nature of the procedure and alternative treatments as well as the procedure's risks, complications, and benefits before the procedure is performed. Medical staff rules or hospital policies usually list which types of services and procedures always require written consent from the patient. Generally, procedures that involve the use of anesthetics, the administration of experimental drugs, the surgical manipulation of organs and tissues, and significant risk of complications require written consent. In addition, some states have passed laws that require written consent forms for certain types of testing procedures (for example, HIV testing). Written consents should be witnessed by at least one individual and should be obtained prior to the service or procedure. The original or scanned copies of consents should always become part of the patient's health record. Figure 3.8 provides an example of an operative consent.

Anesthesia Report

The **anesthesia report** notes any preoperative medication and response to it, the anesthesia administered with dose and method of administration, the duration of administration, the patient's vital signs while under anesthesia, and any additional products given to the patient during the procedure. The anesthesiologist or nurse anesthetist is responsible for this documentation. An anesthesia record that includes the pre-anesthesia evaluation is shown in figure 3.9.

Procedure and Operative Reports

The **operative report** describes the surgical procedures performed on the patient. Each report usually includes the following information:

- Patient's preoperative and postoperative diagnosis
- Descriptions of the procedures performed
- Descriptions of all normal and abnormal findings
- Description of the patient's medical condition before, during, and after the operation
- Estimated blood loss
- Descriptions of any specimens removed
- Descriptions of any unique or unusual events during the course of the surgery
- Names of the surgeons and their assistants
- Date and duration of the surgery

Figure 3.8.   Example of informed consent for operation with blood products

University of Anystate Hospitals

┌─────────────────────────┐
│   │
│   PATIENT LABEL   │
│   │
└─────────────────────────┘

**INFORMED CONSENT FOR OPERATION/
PROCEDURE/ANESTHESIA INCLUDING
BLOOD AND BLOOD PRODUCTS**

1. I give permission to Dr.(s) _____ to perform

   the following procedure(s): _____

   _____

   _____ on _____ (patient's name).

2. I understand that during the procedure(s), new findings or conditions may appear and require an additional procedure(s) for proper care.

3. My physician has explained the following items:
   * the nature of my condition
   * the nature and purpose of the procedure(s) that I am now authorizing
   * the possible complications and side effects that may result, problems that may be experienced during recuperation, and the likelihood of success
   * the benefits to be reasonably expected from the procedure(s)
   * the likely result of no treatment
   * the available alternatives, including the risks and benefits
   * the other possible risks that accompany any surgical and diagnostic procedure (in addition to those already discussed). I acknowledge that neither my physician nor anyone else involved in my care has made any guarantees or assurances to me as to the result of the procedure(s) that I am now authorizing.

4. I know that other clinical staff may help my physician during the procedure(s).

5. I understand that the procedure(s) may require that I undergo some form of anesthesia, which may have its own risks.

6. Any tissue or specimens taken from my body as a result of the procedure(s) may be examined and disposed of, retained, preserved, or used for medical, scientific, or teaching purposes by the hospital.

7. I understand that my procedure(s) may be photographed or videotaped and that observers may be present in the room for the purpose of advancing medical care and education.

8. I understand that during or after the procedure(s) my physician may find it necessary to give me a transfusion of blood or blood products. My physician has explained the alternatives to, and possible risks of, transfusion.

9. I understand what my physician has explained to me and have had all my questions fully answered.

10. Additional comments: _____

    _____

After talking with my physician and reading this form, I give my consent to the procedure(s) described above.

Signature of Patient or
Legal Representative: _____ Date: _____ Time: _____

If Legal Representative, Relationship to Patient: _____

Witness: _____

Verbal or Telephone Consent

Name of Legal Representative: _____ Date: _____ Time: _____

Relationship to Patient: _____

Witness: _____ Witness: _____

I have explained the risks, benefits, potential complications, and alternatives of the treatment to the patient and have answered all questions to the patient's satisfaction, and he/she has granted consent to proceed.

Physician Signature: _____ Date: _____ Time: _____

INFORMED CONSENT FOR OPERATION
000015 (11/2002)

Figure 3.9.   Example of a pre-anesthesia and anesthesia record in paper format

University of Anystate Hospitals

ANESTHESIA RECORD
PAGE 1 OF 2

PATIENT LABEL

Date: _____   Time: _____
Age: ____ Sex: ____ Height: _____ Weight: _____ BP: ____ P: ____ R: ____ T: _____
Lab: _____   Status: _____
Allergies: _____   Last Intake: _____
Premedication: _____

☐ **Patient reassessed immediately prior to induction. Condition satisfactory for planned anesthesia.**

Vital Signs

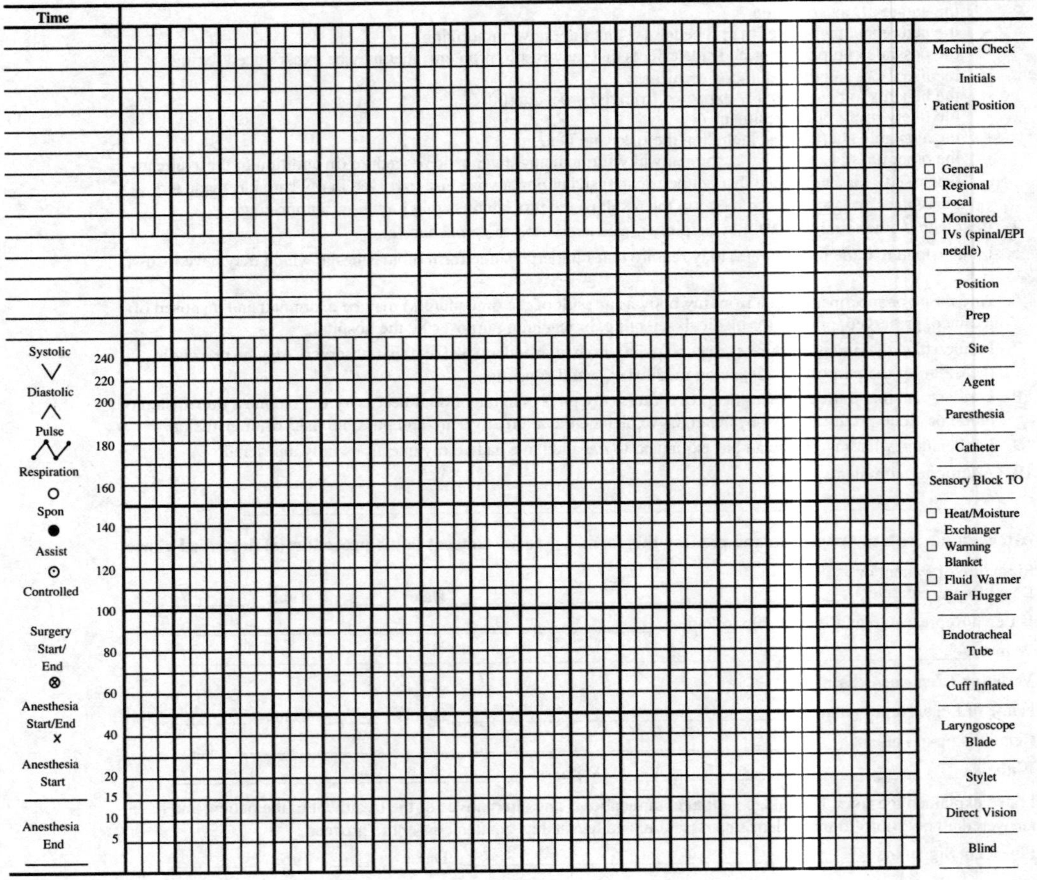

Time		Machine Check

Initials

Patient Position

☐ General
☐ Regional
☐ Local
☐ Monitored
☐ IVs (spinal/EPI needle)

Position

Prep

Site

Agent

Paresthesia

Catheter

Sensory Block TO

☐ Heat/Moisture Exchanger
☐ Warming Blanket
☐ Fluid Warmer
☐ Bair Hugger

Endotracheal Tube

Cuff Inflated

Laryngoscope Blade

Stylet

Direct Vision

Blind

Systolic
∨
Diastolic
∧
Pulse
∿
Respiration
○
Spon
●
Assist
⊙
Controlled

Surgery Start/End
⊗
Anesthesia Start/End
×
Anesthesia Start
___
Anesthesia End

240
220
200
180
160
140
120
100
80
60
40
20
15
10
5

Figure 3.9. **Example of a pre-anesthesia and anesthesia record in paper format** *(continued)*

University of Anystate Hospitals

ANESTHESIA RECORD
PAGE 2 OF 2

PATIENT LABEL

Monitors
☐ NIBP ☐ R ☐ L
☐ APB ☐ R ☐ L
☐ T (site): _____
☐ Pulse oximeter (site): _____
☐ ECG (lead): _____
☐ Airway gas monitor
☐ FiO₂ analyzer
☐ Pulmonary artery
☐ CVP
☐ EEG
☐ Stethoscope (site): _____
☐ SSEP
☐ Peripheral nerve stimulator
☐ Capnography

Remarks

Fluid		Fluid		Fluid		Fluid		Fluid		Fluid	
Start	Finish	Start	Finish	Start	Finish	Start	Finish	Start	Finish	Start	Finish

Operation

Surgeon   Anesthesiologist   Date

Recovery Room   Time: _____
BP
P   T   °F   Endotracheal
                                   In ☐   Out ☐
Condition   SpO₂   %

Preanesthesia Evaluation

Review of Clinical Data

☐ Yes ☐ No Patient Medical History Reviewed
☐ Yes ☐ No Current Medications Reviewed
☐ Yes ☐ No Allergies Reviewed
☐ Yes ☐ No ☐ N/A Lab Results Reviewed
☐ Yes ☐ No ☐ N/A CXR Results Reviewed
☐ Yes ☐ No ☐ N/A EKG Results Reviewed

Anesthesia History

☐ Yes ☐ No Past Hx of Anesthesia Complications
☐ Yes ☐ No Family Hx of Anesthesia Complications
☐ Yes ☐ No History of Malignant Hyperthermia

Pertinent Physical Exam

	Normal	Abnormal	Comments
EENT			
Respiratory			
Cardiac			
Mental Status			

ASA Classification

1   2   3   4   5   E

Airway Evaluation

Dentures: ☐ None ☐ Upper ☐ Lower
Capped Teeth: ☐ None ☐ Yes
Condition of Teeth: ☐ Good ☐ Fair ☐ Poor
Estimated Intubation Difficulty:
☐ Normal ☐ Moderately Difficult ☐ Difficult

Anesthesia Plan

☐ General   ☐ Rapid Sequence Intubation
☐ Spinal   ☐ MAC
☐ Epidural   ☐ Epidural for POPM
☐ Regional Block

☐ Alternatives, risks of anesthesia, and potential complications were discussed. Patient and/or guardian state understanding and acceptance of anesthesia plan.

Comments:

_____   _____
Anesthesiologist   Date

ANESTHESIA RECORD
000017 (11/2002)

Figure 3.10. **Electronic operative report**

SURGEON: CHANDLER BLOCK, DO

PRE-OPERATIVE DIAGNOSIS:
Painful Swallowing

POST-OPERATIVE DIAGNOSIS:
Significant Barrett's esophagus, acute GE junction inflammation secondary to reflux. Moderate gastritis.

OPERATION: Gastroscopy, biopsy, and Clo test.

According to his wife, this male is being seen at the request of Dr. Swenson, after developing painful swallowing. The patient and his wife were told the reasons for the procedure and the possible esophageal dilation including other risks.

PROCEDURE: Following local anesthesia with Cetacaine, 25 mg of Demerol and 1 mg of Versed IV, the GIF-100 was with some difficulty passed into the esophagus where starting at about 28 cm to the GE junction, scattered area of what looked like typical Barrett's esophagus. It was a little more prominent distally at the GE junction where there was no stricturing process. The scope was easily passed into the small hiatus hernia into the stomach where the gastric mucosa and the body and the antrum were significantly inflamed and, therefore, Clo test was taken of pyloric ring and duodenum which was negative. The scope was then withdrawn back up into the esophagus where random biopsy from the inflamed area was taken.

IMPRESSION: I wonder if the patient has had a greater degree of reflux during hospitalization when he has had more bed rest.

PLAN: Anti-reflux program, Prevacid.

Figure 3.10 shows an operative report in electronic format. The operative report should be written or dictated by the surgeon immediately after surgery and become part of the health record as soon as possible. When there is a delay in dictation or transcription, a progress note describing the surgery should be entered into the patient's record. Reports of other procedures or treatments may or may not be associated with surgery. For example, administration of blood transfusions may occur prior to, during, or after surgery, but chemotherapy documentation is usually separate from that of other procedures.

Recovery Room Report

Immediately after the procedure, the patient is usually evaluated for a period of time in a special unit called a recovery room. Monitoring is important to make sure the patient sufficiently recovers from the anesthesia and is stable enough to be moved to another location. The **recovery room report** includes the post-anesthesia note (if not found elsewhere), nurses' notes regarding the patient's condition and surgical site, vital signs, and intravenous fluids, and other medical monitoring.

Pathology Report

A **pathology report** is dictated by a pathologist after examination of tissue received for evaluation. This report usually includes descriptions of the tissue from a gross or macroscopic (with the eye) level and representative cells at the microscopic level along with interpretive findings. Sometimes an initial tissue evaluation occurs while the surgery is in progress to give the surgeon information important to the remainder of the operation. A full written report would follow (figure 3.11).

Figure 3.11.   **Electronic surgical pathology report**

SURGICAL PATHOLOGY REPORT

SPECIMEN STATED TO BE:
Distal esophageal bx's

CLINICAL DIAGNOSIS:
Dysphagia

MACROSCOPIC:
The specimen consists of tan soft tissue fragments aggregating 0.3 cm - all embedded.

MICROSCOPIC:
Sections show benign ulcerated/inflammatory squamous mucosa, nonspecific features.

DIAGNOSIS:
Benign ulcerated/inflammatory squamous mucosa.

Consultation Reports

The **consultation report** documents the clinical opinion of a physician other than the primary or attending physician. The consultation is usually requested by the primary or attending physician, but occasionally may be the request of the patient or the patient's family. The report is based on the consulting physician's examination of the patient and a review of his or her health record.

Some organizations allow consultation requests by telephone and provide the consultant with selected information from the patient's record. The consultant then dictates his or her findings and returns them to the requesting physician.

Discharge Summary

The **discharge summary** is a concise account of the patient's illness, course of treatment, response to treatment, and condition at the time of patient discharge (official release) from the hospital. The summary also includes instructions for follow-up care to be given to the patient or his or her caregiver at the time of discharge. Because it provides an overview of the entire medical encounter, it is used for a variety of purposes:

- Ensures the continuity of future care by providing information to the patient's attending physician, referring physician, and any consulting physicians

- Provides information to support the activities of the medical staff review committee

- Provides concise information that can be used to answer information requests from authorized individuals or entities

The discharge summary is the responsibility of, and must be signed by, the attending physician. A paper-based record summary is found in figure 3.12. If the patient's stay is

Figure 3.12.   Example of a discharge summary in paper format

Midwest Medical Center

DISCHARGE SUMMARY

SAYLORMEN, POPEYE T.
333333333
DOB: 02/09/1961

PHYSICIAN/SURGEON: Philip P. Heartstopper, MD

DATE OF DISCHARGE: 05/18/20XX

PRINCIPAL OPERATION AND PROCEDURE: OPCAB × 3, left internal mammary artery of the LAD, saphenous vein graft to D-1, and saphenous vein graft to OM-1

HISTORY OF PRESENT ILLNESS: Mr. Saylormen was seen at the request of Dr. Doctor regarding surgical treatment of ischemic heart disease. He is a 42-year-old male with a family history of coronary artery disease. He smokes a pipe and had a previous myocardial infarction approximately three years ago. His current status is postangioplasty. While working on a construction project, he developed anginal-type symptoms and was seen in the emergency room and then admitted to the hospital for further evaluation.

ADMITTING DIAGNOSIS: Coronary artery disease

HOSPITAL COURSE: The patient underwent cardiac catheterization and was found to have significant three-vessel coronary artery disease. It was felt that he would benefit from undergoing an OPCAB procedure. On 05/14/XX, the patient underwent OPCAB × 3 as described above. The patient tolerated the procedure well and returned to the Cardiothoracic Intensive Care Unit hemodynamically stable. On postoperative day one, he was weaned from mechanical ventilation, extubated, and transferred to the Cardiothoracic Step-Down Unit, where he continued on a progressive course of recovery. On postoperative day four, he was up and about in his room and the halls without difficulty. Upon discharge, he was tolerating his diet well. His lungs were clear. His abdomen was soft, and his incisions were unremarkable. His vital signs were stable. He was in normal sinus rhythm. His heart rate was in the 70s and 80s. Blood pressure had been running consistently in the low 110s/60s. He was afebrile. Oxygen saturations on room air were reported at 97%.

LABORATORY DATA AT DISCHARGE: BUN 14, Creatinine 0.9, H&H 8.8 and 25.4

MEDICATIONS AT DISCHARGE: Lisinopril 5 mg q.d.; Lipitor 80 mg q.d.; metoprolol 50 mg q.d.; aspirin 81 mg q.d.; Darvocet-N 100—one to two tablets every 4–6 hours as needed for pain; iron sulfate 325 mg q.d. × 30 days; and Colace 100 mg b.i.d. × 30 days

DIET: He may follow a regular diet.

FINAL DIAGNOSIS: Coronary artery disease

DISPOSITION: No lifting greater than 10 pounds. No driving for 4–6 weeks. He may shower but he should not take a tub bath. Follow up with Dr. Doctor in 1–2 weeks.

Philip P. Heartstopper, MD   5/18/20XX
_____   _____
Philip P. Heartstopper, MD   Date

d: 05/18/20XX
t: 05/19/20XX
PPH, MD/mb

not complicated and lasts less than 48 hours or involves an uncomplicated delivery or normal newborn, a discharge note in place of a full summary is often acceptable.

Patient Instructions and Transfer Records

It is vital that the patient be given clear, concise instructions upon discharge so that the recovery progress begun in the hospital continues. Ideally, patient instructions are communicated both verbally and in writing. The healthcare professional who delivers the instructions to the patient or caregiver should sign the record to indicate that he or she has issued them. In addition, the person receiving the instructions should sign to verify that he or she has received and understands them. A copy of the instructions becomes part of the health record (figure 3.13).

When someone other than the patient assumes responsibility for the patient's aftercare, the record should indicate that the instructions were given to the responsible party. Documentation of patient education may be accomplished by using formats that prompt the person providing instruction to cover important information.

When a patient is being transferred from the acute setting to another healthcare organization, a **transfer record** may be initiated. This record is also called a referral form. A brief review of the patient's acute stay along with current status, discharge and transfer orders, and any additional instructions will be noted. Social service and nursing personnel often complete portions of the transfer record.

Autopsy Reports

An **autopsy report** is a description of the examination of a patient's body after he or she has died. Also called necropsies, autopsies are usually conducted when there is some question about the cause of death or when information is needed for educational or legal purposes. The purpose of the autopsy is to determine or confirm the cause of death or to provide more information about the course of the patient's disease.

The autopsy report is completed by a pathologist and becomes part of the patient's permanent health record. Because reports from tissue examination or laboratory testing can take extended time such as weeks or even months, a preliminary report including preliminary diagnoses is often documented until findings are received and the final report is completed. The authorization for the autopsy, signed by the patient's next of kin or by law enforcement authorities, must be obtained prior to the autopsy and also should become part of the record.

Obstetrics and Newborn Documentation

Each individual that is admitted to a healthcare setting must have a health record. A record on a newborn is generated upon live birth. The mother's hospital obstetric record

Figure 3.13.   Example of patient instructions provided at discharge

University of Anystate Hospitals

PATIENT/FAMILY INSTRUCTIONS
PAGE 1 OF 2

PATIENT LABEL

This is a guide for your care. Call your doctor for any problems or changes that concern you.

Diet

Diet: _____   If on a special diet and have questions, call dietitian.

Managing Your Meds Discussed
(Place a checkmark if medication handouts given)   ↓

Medications (list all medications)

Name/Dose	How to Take	

Activities/Special Care

Activities (Check as indicated)
- ☐ Crutches/walker
- ☐ Walk with assistance
- ☐ Gradually resume normal activity
- ☐ Bedrest
- ☐ Other _____

Dressing and Wound Care
(Report increased pain, redness, swelling, drainage, or fever)
- ☐ Doctor to change dressing
- ☐ Keep dressing dry
- ☐ If no dressing, keep incision clean and dry
- ☐ Clean wound and change dressing

Additional Instructions (PEARLS)

Follow-Up (appointments/ equipment/referrals)

Agency	Phone	Arrangements (Instructions provided by agency)

Dr. _____   Date/Time _____   ☐ Call for an appointment
Dr. _____   Date/Time _____   ☐ Call for an appointment
Dr. _____   Date/Time _____   ☐ Call for an appointment

I understand the above instructions and have the ability to carry these out after discharge. I am aware of the importance of medical follow-up with my doctor.

Patient/Patient Rep. Signature: _____   Date: _____

RN Signature: _____   Date: _____

Figure 3.13. Example of patient instructions provided at discharge *(continued)*

University of Anystate Hospitals

PATIENT/FAMILY INSTRUCTIONS
PAGE 2 OF 2

PATIENT LABEL

Discharge Date: _____ Time: _____ Mode: _____

Discharged With:

☐ Family member   ☐ Friend   ☐ By self   ☐ Other: _____

Escorted by: ☐ Hospital Attendant   ☐ Ambulance Attendant

RN Discharge Assessment

Continuing Care Assessment		
Care Plan	☐ All goals resolved on IPOC/clinical path/plan of care. Exceptions documented.	
Discharge with:	☐ Self/family care	• Patient and/or family verbalized an understanding of instructions. Person(s) to assist if needed: _____
Discharge with:	☐ Support services	• Patient will receive follow-up with a referral agency or extended care facility. See front of form.
Discharge to:	☐ Home ☐ Home with home health ☐ Extended care facility ☐ Other: _____	

☐ Patient Expired   Date: _____   Time: _____   Valuables Given to: ☐ Family   ☐ Funeral home   ☐ Security
☐ Patient Left without Permission   Date: _____   Time: _____

RN Signature: _____ Date: _____

PATIENT INSTRUCTIONS
5435680 (03/2002)

is separate from the infant's record and actually begins in her practitioner's office. In the case of a baby born deceased, however, all information about the baby and the mother is maintained in the mother's health record. (See also information pertaining to obstetric/gynecologic care later in this chapter.)

Obstetric delivery records include a prenatal care summary provided by the practitioner's office, an admission evaluation by the attending physician to update the summary, and a record of labor, including information on contractions, fetal heart tones, an examination of the birth canal, medications given, and vital signs. The delivery record includes type of delivery; medications administered, including anesthesia; description of the birth process, and any blood loss; evaluation of the placenta and cord; and information about any other delivery interventions. Data about the baby also will be recorded in the mother's record, including sex, weight, length, Apgar scores, any abnormal findings, and any treatments given. Postpartum care records begin after the birth and contain progress notes by physicians and nurses and other care providers in addition to the results of any diagnostic tests, treatments, and medications received by the mother.

The newborn record begins with the birth history, which may be the same as or similar to the mother's labor and delivery data noted above. Newborn identification generally includes bands worn by both the mother and baby, which are regularly checked for matching information, and the infant's footprints. A thorough newborn physical examination is completed shortly after the baby's birth with periodic updates throughout hospitalization. Head and chest measurements are part of an evaluation of all body systems. Nursing documentation includes information on the baby's feeding and elimination status, weight, vital signs, appearance, response to environment, sleeping patterns, and condition of the cord stump. Any special tests, treatments, and medications will also be noted. More extensive documentation will be found if a baby is born prematurely or requires intensive care services. Figure 3.14 provides an example of a prenatal summary.

Administrative Data

As noted earlier in this section, an acute care health record contains the patient's demographic and financial information as well as information about care provided. Commonly, the administrative information is collected by hospital admitting personnel who personally ask the patient or the patient's representative for the information needed to complete the admissions documentation. For elective admissions (ones that can be planned in advance) some information may be gathered in advance via a secure facility website or a telephone interview.

Today, most hospitals record admissions information electronically. For hospitals that maintain a paper-based health record system, a printout of the admissions information is placed in the health record. In both paper-based and electronic health record systems, the admissions information becomes a permanent part of the patient's record. The admissions information may be referred to as a face sheet, a registration form, or a registration record.

Figure 3.14.   Maternal/prenatal care summary in paper format

Anytown Community Hospital

MATERNAL/PRENATAL CARE SUMMARY

PATIENT LABEL

Mother's Name: _____

Mother's Age: _____ Gravida: _____ Term: ____

Premature: _____ Abnormal: ____ Living: ____

Expected Delivery Date: _____

Prenatal Labs: _____

Maternal/Prenatal/Family History: _____

_____

_____

Social Problems: _____

_____

Type of Delivery: □ Vaginal

                     □ C-Section

Type of Anesthesia: _____

Tubal Ligation: □ Yes   □ No

Apgars: 1 min __ 5 min __ 10 min __

Complications of Labor and Delivery: _____

_____

_____

Transfer From: _____

Date: _____

Delivery Weight: _____

Last Weight: _____

Service Notified: _____

Date and Time: _____

Person Notified: _____

Examined: _____

Void: □

Stool: □

Circumcision: □ Yes □ No

Done: _____

Date: _____

Metabolic Screen: □ Yes □ No

Done: _____

Date: _____

Hearing Screen: □ Yes □ No

Done: _____

Date: _____

Pass/Refer: _____

Follow-up Appointment

Made: _____

Vitals: _____

Glucoses: _____

Breast: _____

Formula: _____

IVF _____ @ _____

UAC _____ @ _____

UVC _____ @ _____

Mother's Blood Type and RH: ____

Cord Blood: _____

COOMBS: _____

Cord Bili: _____

Baby Safe Signed: □

Gift Bags Given: □

Hepatitis B Vaccine:

□ Yes   □ No

Orders: _____

_____

_____

_____

_____

Medications: _____

_____

Messages: _____

_____

Obstetrician	Delivery Date	Delivery Time	Baby's Gender
Mother's Room Number		Pediatrician	

Demographic and Financial Information

Demographics is the study of the statistical characteristics of human populations. In the context of healthcare, demographic information includes the following elements:

- Patient's full name
- Patient's facility identification or account number
- Patient's address
- Patient's telephone number
- Patient's date and place of birth
- Patient's gender
- Patient's race or ethnic origin
- Patient's marital status
- Name and address of patient's next of kin
- Date and time of admission
- Hospital's name, address, and telephone number

The financial information maintained in the acute care health record is limited to any third party payment information collected from the patient at the time of admission. This information includes the name of the expected payer, the name of the policyholder (or insured), the gender of the policyholder, the patient's relationship to the policyholder, the employer of the policyholder, individual and group insurance policy numbers, and possibly the patient's Social Security number (figure 3.15).

Other Administrative Information

Some healthcare facilities place property lists and birth and death certificates in health records. When a patient brings personal property and valuables to the healthcare facility, the facility may document them in the health record. Items such as eyeglasses, hearing aids, prostheses, and other special medical equipment should be documented. When items are kept in a secure location by the facility, that fact should be documented on the property/ valuables list.

State governments use birth and death certificates to collect vital information and health statistics. The content requirements vary somewhat according to state law. In some states, the certificates are prepared by hospital personnel. Copies of the certificates are often included in patients' health records.

Figure 3.15. **Electronic admissions records**

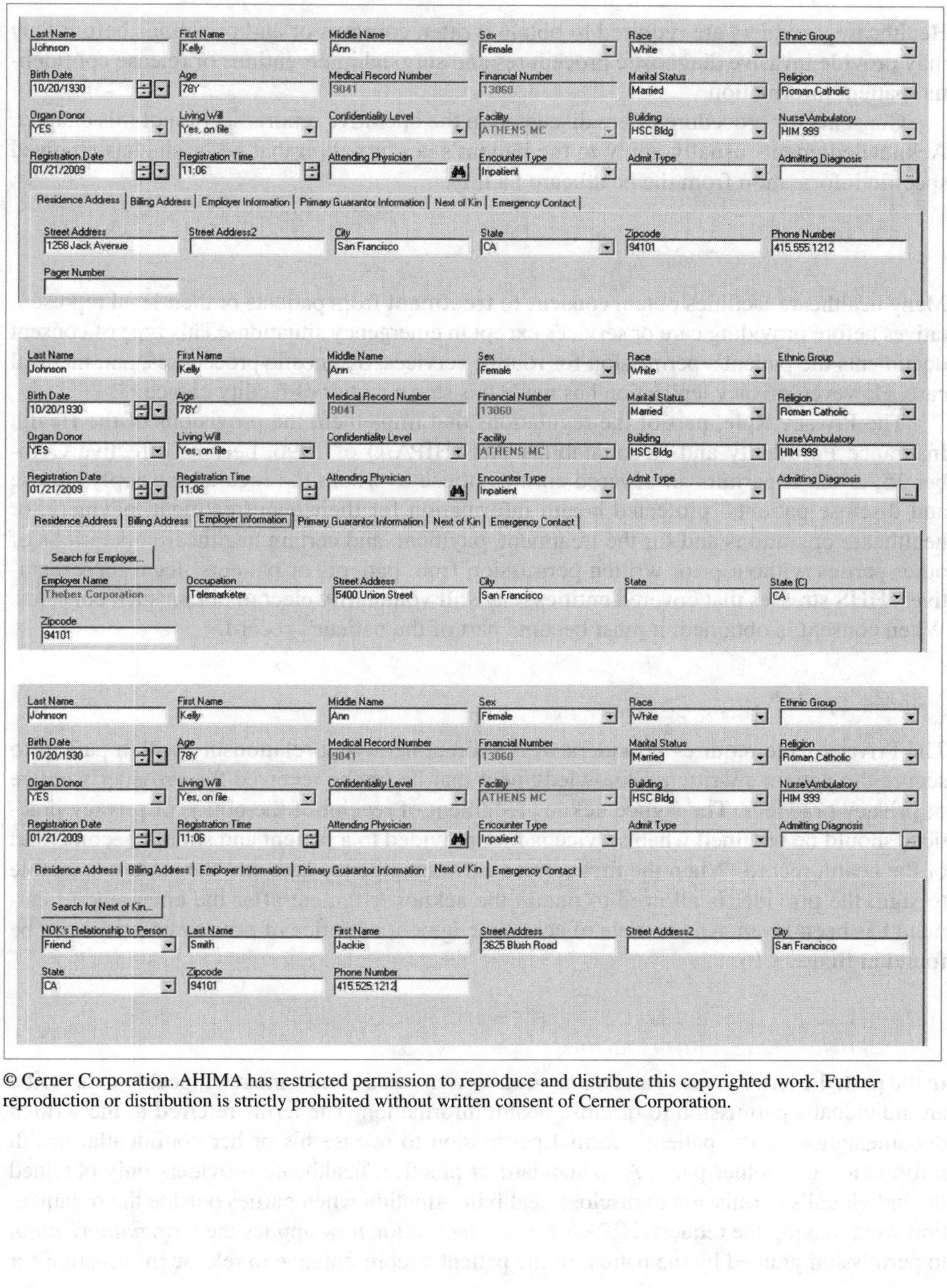

Consents, Authorizations, and Acknowledgments

Healthcare providers are required to obtain written consents or authorizations before they may provide invasive diagnostic procedures and surgical interventions or release confidential patient information.

Consents for procedures were discussed in the operative reports section of this chapter. Acknowledgments usually apply to the patient's confirmation that he or she has received specific information from the healthcare facility.

Consent to Treatment

Many healthcare facilities obtain **consent to treatment** from patients or their legal representatives before providing care or services except in emergency situations. This type of consent documents the patient's permission for routine services, diagnostic procedures, and medical care. However, privacy legislation has made this step a matter of facility choice.

The Privacy Rule, part of the regulations that implement the provisions of the Health Insurance Portability and Accountability Act (HIPAA) of 1996, became effective October 15, 2002. It permits all covered entities (those to whom the regulations apply) to use and disclose patients' protected health information for their own treatment, payment, or healthcare operations and for the treatment, payment, and certain healthcare operations of other parties without prior written permission from patients or patients' legal representatives. HHS stresses that covered entities may still voluntarily elect to obtain such consents. When consent is obtained, it must become part of the patient's record.

Notice of Privacy Practices

The Privacy Rule requires providers with a direct treatment relationship with a patient to secure the patient's written acknowledgment that he or she received the provider's notice of privacy practices. The signed acknowledgment of receipt of the notice of privacy practices should be obtained when service is first provided to a patient and should become part of the health record. When the first service is for emergency care and the patient is unable to sign, the provider is allowed to obtain the acknowledgment after the emergency treatment has been given. An example of acknowledgment of notice of privacy practices can be found in figure 3.16.

Authorizations Related to the Release and Disclosure of Confidential Health Information

In the past, the terms *consent* and *authorization* were used almost interchangeably to describe an individual's permission to disclose health information. The terms referred to the written documentation of the patient's formal permission to release his or her confidential health information to another party. As a standard of practice, healthcare providers only obtained the individual's permission to disclose health information when parties outside the organization were making the request. HIPAA privacy legislation now applies the term *authorization* to permission granted by the patient or the patient's representative to release information for

Figure 3.16. **Notice of privacy practices acknowledgment**

Anytown Community Hospital

**ACKNOWLEDGMENT OF NOTICE
OF PRIVACY PRACTICES**

PATIENT LABEL

I understand that as part of my healthcare, this organization originates and maintains health records describing my health history, symptoms, examination and test results, diagnoses, treatment, and any plans for future care or treatment. I understand that this information serves as:

- A basis for planning my care and treatment
- A means of communication among the many health professionals who contribute to my care
- A source of information for applying my diagnosis and surgical information to my bill
- A means by which a third-party payer can verify that services billed were actually provided
- And a tool for routine healthcare operations such as assessing quality and reviewing the competence of healthcare professionals

I understand and have been provided with a *Notice of Information Practices* that provides a more complete description of information uses and disclosures. I understand that I have the right to review the notice prior to signing this consent. I understand that the organization reserves the right to change their notice and practices and prior to implementation will mail a copy of any revised notice to the address I've provided. I understand that I have the right to object to the use of my health information for directory purposes. I understand that I have the right to request restrictions as to how my health information may be used or disclosed to carry out treatment, payment, or healthcare operations and that the organization is not required to agree to the restrictions requested. I understand that I may revoke this consent in writing, except to the extent that the organization has already taken action in reliance thereon.

☐ I request the following restrictions to the use or disclosure of my health information:

_____

_____

_____

Signature of Patient or Legal Representative	Date

Witness	Date

_____
Notice Effective Date or Version

☐ Accepted   ☐ Denied

Signature	Title	Date

ACKNOWLEDGMENT OF PRIVACY NOTICE
100093 (1/2002)

reasons other than treatment, payment, or healthcare operations. The term *consent* is used when the permission is for treatment, payment, or healthcare operations.

An **authorization to disclose information** allows the healthcare facility to verbally disclose or send health information to other organizations. The patient or his or her legal representative signs the authorization. This authorization is retained to document why health information was disclosed.

Advance Directives

An **advance directive** is a written document that provides directions about a patient's desires in relation to care decisions for use by healthcare workers if the patient is incapacitated or not capable of communicating. One type of advance directive, a durable power of attorney for healthcare, names the patient's choice of legal representative for healthcare purposes. The person designated by the patient is then empowered to make healthcare decisions on behalf of the patient in the event that the patient is no longer capable of expressing his or her preferences. A second type of advance directive, a living will, describes what types of care the patient does and/or does not desire if he/she is not capable of communicating the information or of making decisions. Physician orders for "do not resuscitate" (DNR) and "do not attempt intubation" (DNI) should be consistent with the patient's advance directives.

The federal **Patient Self-Determination Act** (PSDA) went into effect in 1991. The PSDA requires healthcare facilities to provide written information on the patient's right to execute advance directives and to accept or refuse medical treatment. Healthcare organizations that accept Medicare or Medicaid patients are required to follow these provisions of the PSDA:

- Develop policies that meet the requirements of state law regarding the patient's right to accept or refuse medical treatment and to develop advance directives.

- Upon admission, provide written information to the patient that describes the treatment decisions that patients may make and the hospital's related policies.

- Document the fact that the patient has an advance directive in his or her health record. However, organizations are not required to make a copy of the directive a permanent part of the patient's health record.

Acknowledgments of Patient's Rights

Acknowledgment forms are used to document the fact that information about the patient's rights while under care was provided to the patient. Referred to as the **patient's bill of rights,** Medicare Conditions of Participation or Conditions for Coverage require hospitals to provide patients this information. The information must include the right to:

- Know who is providing treatment
- Confidentiality
- Receive information about treatment

- Refuse treatment
- Participate in care planning
- Be safe from abusive treatment

There are two common ways to document the receipt of rights information in the health record. First, the patient or his or her legal representative can sign a document to indicate that the patient received the bill of rights. Second, the facility can have the patient sign and date the actual bill of rights and place it in the health record.

Check Your Understanding 3.2

1. Which of the following would not be found in a medical history?

   A. Chief complaint
   B. Vital signs
   C. Present illness
   D. Review of systems

2. An attending physician requests the advice of a second physician who then reviews the health record and examines the patient. The second physician records impressions in what type of report?

   A. Consultation
   B. Progress note
   C. Operative report
   D. Discharge summary

3. Which specialized type of progress note provides healthcare professionals impressions of patient problems with detailed treatment action steps?

   A. Flow record
   B. Vital signs record
   C. Care plan
   D. Surgical note

4. Written or spoken permission to proceed with care is classified as:

   A. Expressed consent
   B. Acknowledgment
   C. Advance directive
   D. Implied consent

5. Which of the following reports provides information on tissue removed during a procedure?

   A. Operative report
   B. Laboratory report
   C. Pathology report
   D. Anesthesia report

6. Sleeping patterns, head and chest measurements, feeding and elimination status, weight, and Apgar scores are recorded in which of the following records?

   A. Obstetric
   B. Newborn
   C. Surgical
   D. Emergency

7. Which of the following is not considered patient demographic information?

   A. Patient's date of birth
   B. Name of next of kin
   C. Type of admission
   D. Admitting diagnosis

8. Which of the following administrative documents provides information on the patient's desires for healthcare for use if he/she is incapacitated?

   A. Advance directive
   B. Patient's bill of rights
   C. Notice of privacy practices
   D. Authorization for release of information

Specialized Health Record Documentation

There are differences as well as similarities among the health records maintained by various healthcare settings. The type of care provided is one factor. For example, the records of residents in long-term care facilities often contain immunization records and must contain documentation of communication of patient's rights. Acute care records, in contrast, do not usually contain immunization records but do contain acknowledgment of receipt of a bill of rights.

The content also depends on external factors such as which accreditation or regulatory standards apply. For example, the Joint Commission issues specific health information standards for acute care hospitals. However, the standards of the Commission on Accreditation of Rehabilitation Facilities (CARF) are more frequently used by rehabilitation hospitals.

The type and complexity of medical services the patient requires also impacts record content. For example, the content of the record for an obstetrics patient would be different from the content of the record for a neurosurgical patient. Content also depends in part on the duration of medical services. For example, the content of a long-term rehabilitation record would be different from the content of an emergency services record. Traits of individual patients such as age or functional status are additional factors.

Emergency Care Documentation

The delivery of emergency care services occurs primarily in hospital-based emergency departments and in some freestanding urgent care centers. Emergency care documentation is limited to information about the patient's presenting problem and the diagnostic and therapeutic services provided during the episode of care. The services provided in emergency situations concentrate on diagnosing the medical problem and stabilizing the patient. Although minor injuries and illnesses may require no further medical treatment, emergency patients often must be referred to ambulatory care providers for follow-up care. Seriously ill or injured patients are admitted to a hospital for ongoing acute care treatment.

The following information should be entered into the patient's health record for each emergency care visit:

- Patient identification (or the reason it could not be obtained)
- Time and means of the patient's arrival at the facility
- Pertinent history of the illness or injury and physical findings, including the patient's vital signs
- Emergency care given to the patient prior to and after arrival
- Presenting condition and initial assessment
- Diagnostic and therapeutic orders
- Clinical observations, including the results of treatment
- Reports and results of procedures and tests
- Diagnostic impression
- Medications administered
- Conclusion at the termination of evaluation/treatment, including final disposition, the patient's condition on discharge or transfer, and any instructions given to the patient, the patient's representative, or another healthcare facility for follow-up care
- Documentation of cases when the patient left the facility against medical advice

Ambulatory Care Documentation

Ambulatory care includes care provided in physicians' offices, group practices, and clinics, as well as hospital outpatient, neighborhood health, public health, industrial health, and urgent care settings. Documentation required by those providing care through managed care organizations or under managed care contracts such as through health maintenance organizations (HMOs), preferred provider organizations (PPOs), or independent physician associations (IPAs) is also included in this discussion.

Basic Ambulatory Documentation

Many of the data found in ambulatory care setting records are similar to those found in acute care hospitals. The registration record used in a physician's office, for example, includes the same demographic and financial information as a hospital admissions record. However, for special ambulatory patients, such as those referred as outpatients to a hospital for special diagnostic testing that is only available there, or those visiting a public health setting for immunizations, records may have much more limited content. In general, documentation in ambulatory care patient records typically includes the following materials:

- Registration forms including patient identification data
- Problem lists
- Medication lists
- Patient history questionnaires
- History and physicals
- Progress notes
- Results of consultations
- Diagnostic test results
- Miscellaneous flow sheets (for example, pediatric growth charts and immunization records and specialty-specific flow sheets)
- Copies of records of previous hospitalizations or treatment by other healthcare practitioners
- Correspondence
- Consents to disclose information
- Advance directives

Ambulatory care records, however, do include several elements unique to the ambulatory setting. For example, ambulatory records usually contain a **problem list** whose function is to facilitate ongoing patient care management. The problem list describes any significant current and past illnesses and conditions as well as the procedures the patient has undergone. Sometimes problems are separated into acute (short-term, such as otitis media) and chronic (such as diabetes mellitus) categories. The problem list also may include information on the patient's previous surgeries, allergies, and drug sensitivities. Some physician practices place information on the patient's current prescription medications on the problem list. Others maintain a separate medication list. (See figure 3.17 for an example of a problem list.) Some ambulatory practices also use a structured format to collect past medical history information from the patient. This is called a **patient history questionnaire.**

Most ambulatory care settings can earn accreditation from the Accreditation Association for Ambulatory Health Care (AAAHC), the Joint Commission, or the AOA. All have health information documentation standards. Accreditation by the National Committee for Quality Assurance (NCQA) focuses on managed care organizations. Most physician practices do not participate in voluntary accreditation programs, but some clinics, outpatient settings, and managed care organizations choose to do so.

Figure 3.17. **Example of a problem list in paper format**

PROBLEM LIST				
Identification Number				
Medical Record Number				
Last Name		First Name		Middle Initial
Date of Birth				
PROBLEM NUMBER	DATE ENTERED	LIST SIGNIFICANT ACUTE AND CHRONIC CONDITIONS INCLUDING SURGICAL PROCEDURES	PROBLEM RESOLVED	DATE RESOLVED
1				
2				
3				
4				
5				
6				
7				
8				
9				
10				
11				
12				
13				
14				
15				
16				
17				
18				
19				
20				

Obstetric/Gynecologic Care Documentation

Some ambulatory care records have unique requirements because of the specialized services provided. Specifically, the following kinds of information should be maintained for both obstetric and gynecologic patients in addition to other ambulatory care documents:

- Medical history to include history of abuse or neglect and sexual practices
- Periodic laboratory testing, including Pap tests and mammography, cholesterol levels, and fecal blood tests
- Additional laboratory testing needed for high-risk groups such as tuberculosis skin testing and testing for sexually transmitted diseases

As an additional resource, a physician specialty group, the American College of Obstetricians and Gynecologists (ACOG) provides guidelines to members for perinatal and women's healthcare that have implications for record content. Another group whose voluntary accreditation process includes perinatal documentation standards is the Commission for the Accreditation of Birth Centers.

Pediatric Care Documentation

The records of infants, children, and adolescents also require special content. These ambulatory care records should include the following special documentation:

- Birth history
- Nutritional history
- Personal, social, and family history
- Growth and development record
- Immunizations

In addition, the records should include documentation of well-child visits as well as visits for medical concerns, including any medications prescribed.

Ambulatory Surgical Care Documentation

The operating room (OR) records maintained by freestanding ambulatory surgery centers are very similar to those maintained by hospital-based surgery departments. Specifically, Medicare regulations require that ambulatory surgery records include the following information:

- Registration forms including patient identification data
- Documentation of the patient's informed consent to surgical treatment
- Significant medical history and physical examination

- Preoperative studies (studies performed before surgery)
- Operative report
- Pathology report for tissue removed
- Allergies and abnormal drug reactions
- Record of anesthesia administration
- Recovery room record
- Discharge diagnosis

Many ambulatory surgery centers also telephone patients at home after their surgery as a routine follow-up procedure. The patient's record should include records of any follow-up calls. In addition to the Joint Commission, the AOA, and the AAAHC, the American Association for Accreditation of Ambulatory Surgery Facilities (AAAASF) has standards that apply to this type of setting. Conditions of Coverage for ambulatory surgical centers govern those that seek Medicare reimbursement.

Long-term Care Documentation

Long-term care is provided in a variety of facilities, including the following:

- Skilled nursing facilities (SNFs) or units, subacute care facilities
- Nursing facilities (NFs) (nursing homes, long-term care facilities)
- Assisted-living facilities

The regulations that govern long-term care facilities vary among these settings. Most SNFs and NFs are governed by both federal and state regulations, including the Medicare Conditions of Participation. Assisted-living facilities are usually governed only by state regulations. Most long-term care providers do not participate in voluntary accreditation programs, although the Joint Commission does have long-term care facility standards.

Because the stay for a patient or resident in long-term settings can be lengthy, health records are based on ongoing assessments and reassessments of the patient's (or resident's) needs. An interdisciplinary team develops a plan of care for each patient upon admission to the facility, and the plan is updated regularly over the patient's stay. The team includes the patient's physician and representatives from nursing services, nutritional services, social services, and other specialty areas (such as physical therapy), as appropriate.

In SNFs, the care plan is based on a format required by federal regulations. The care plan format is called the **resident assessment instrument** (RAI). The RAI is based on the **Minimum Data Set (MDS) for Long-Term Care.** The overall RAI framework includes the MDS, triggers, utilization guidelines, and **care area assessments** (CAAs). The patient is assessed and reassessed at defined intervals as well as whenever there is a significant change in his or her condition.

The RAI is a critical component of the health record. In addition to development of the care plan, Medicare uses the form to determine reimbursement. Many states also use it to determine Medicaid payments, and accreditation surveyors use information from it during the survey process. (Chapters 4 and 6 also discuss the MDS, RAIs, and CAAs in detail.)

The RAI is submitted electronically to each state health department and then on to the Centers for Medicare and Medicaid Services (CMS). At CMS, demographic and quality indicator information is compiled and provided as feedback to each facility.

The physician's role in a long-term care facility is not as visible as it is in other care settings. The physician develops a plan of treatment, which includes the medications and treatments to be provided to the resident. He or she then visits the resident in the facility on a 30- or 60-day schedule unless the resident's condition requires more frequent visits. At each visit, the physician reviews the plan of care and physician's orders and makes changes as necessary. Between visits, the physician is contacted when nursing personnel identify changes in the resident's condition.

The following list identifies the most common components of long-term care records:

- Registration forms including resident identification data
- Personal property list, including furniture and electronics
- History and physical and hospital records
- Advance directives, bill of rights, and other legal records
- Clinical assessments
- RAI/MDS and care plan
- Physician's orders
- Physician's progress notes/consultations
- Nursing notes
- Rehabilitation therapy notes (physical therapy, occupational therapy, and speech therapy)
- Social services, nutritional services, and activities documentation
- Medication and records of monitors, including administration of restraints
- Laboratory, radiology, and special reports
- Discharge or transfer documentation

If paper-based records are found in a long-term setting, a process called record thinning may occur at intervals during the patient's stay. Records of patients whose stay extends to months or years become cumbersome to handle. Selected material may be removed and filed elsewhere according to facility guidelines. Any material removed must remain accessible when needed for patient care and service evaluation.

Home Healthcare Documentation

Home health agencies provide medical and nonmedical services in the patient's home or place of residence. Growth in the aged population, the desire of Americans to live at home as long as possible, and cost savings over residential settings such as long-term care facilities have resulted in an increase in this type of care.

Federal regulations govern the home care agencies that accept Medicare enrollees. States also have licensure regulations for home care agencies. Organizations such as the Joint Commission, the Community Health Accreditation Program, and the Accreditation Commission for Health Care (ACHC) also provide accreditation services for some home health agencies.

For Medicare certified agencies, the home health certification/plan of care is a central component of documentation. This document is a plan of treatment established by a physician. It details the patient's diagnoses, impairments, goals, rehabilitation potential, and the type and frequency of services to be provided. The physician reviews and renews the home health certification/plan of care at least once during a 60-day episode. Between renewals, certification is updated via the physician's telephone orders. There are no requirements for physician visits in home care; patients are responsible for seeing their physicians as necessary.

Medicare-certified home healthcare also uses a standardized patient assessment instrument called the **Outcomes and Assessment Information Set** (OASIS). OASIS items are a component of the comprehensive assessment that is the foundation for the plan of care and, for Medicare, reimbursement of services. OASIS is completed at the start or resumption of care, with each 60-day episode, with a significant change in condition, and upon patient transfer or discharge. The most recent version, referred to as OASIS-C, is submitted electronically to the state health department and then to CMS. (Chapters 4 and 6 discuss OASIS in additional detail.)

Unique to home care is a service agreement that details the type and frequency of services, the charges for the services, and the parties responsible for payment. Home health aides may assist the patient with activities of daily living such as bathing and housekeeping, which allows the patient to remain at home. Documentation of this type of intervention is also necessary.

The home care record usually includes the following types of documentation:

- Patient identification data and service agreement
- Certification and plan of treatment
- Physician's orders
- Documentation by each discipline involved in home care including treatment plans, summaries, and other progress notes
- Comprehensive assessment (OASIS-C), plan of care, and case conference notes
- Consents and other legal documents
- Referral or transfer information from other facilities
- Discharge summaries

Some parts of home care records may be kept in the patient's home to facilitate communication among multiple caregivers or services. Technology has affected home care documentation through the use of portable computers or devices such as laptops and electronic pads.

Hospice Care Documentation

Hospice care is similar to home care in that most services are provided to patients in their homes. However, hospices also may be located in other healthcare settings such as hospitals, long-term care facilities, or in separate freestanding facilities. Hospice care is unique in that a hospice program provides **palliative care** to terminally ill patients and supportive services to patients and their families. This type of care focuses on symptom management (for example, pain) and patient comfort rather than life-prolonging measures.

When the patient is admitted to a hospice care program, his or her primary caregiver is identified. In addition, basic patient identification information, diagnoses, prognosis, attending physician, and emergency contact information are collected.

An interdisciplinary team establishes a plan of care, which is the foundation for the hospice services to be provided to the patient. The care plan is based on information collected in the physical and psychosocial assessments performed upon admission. The assessments are updated throughout the patient's participation in the program.

Documentation of a care plan review is required every 30 days. The hospice provider must prepare a summary when the patient is transferred between care settings (between hospital and home care, for example). Federal regulations require the hospice provider to follow the patient's care plan even when the patient receives inpatient services.

Federal regulations govern hospice providers, as do accreditation standards established by the same organizations noted under home healthcare documentation. As might be expected, accreditation documentation requirements are based on federal regulations, so the content of all is similar.

There are two basic episodes in hospice care. The first episode begins with the patient's admission to the program and ends when the patient dies, is discharged, or is transferred to another facility. The second begins with the patient's death and follows the family through the bereavement process until the survivors are discharged. Bereavement services can last as long as one year and must be documented.

Behavioral Healthcare Documentation

Behavioral healthcare is delivered in inpatient hospitals, outpatient clinics, physicians' offices, rehabilitation programs, long-term care facilities and community mental health programs. Documentation reflects the type of facility and the level of care and services delivered. For example, an inpatient psychiatric hospital maintains documentation similar to an inpatient hospital in addition to documentation unique to behavioral health.

Following are the common inpatient setting documentation requirements for behavioral health settings as established by the Joint Commission and federal regulations:

- Registration forms and patient identification data
- Referral information
- Patient's legal status
- All appropriate consents for admission, treatment, evaluation, and aftercare
- Admitting psychiatric diagnoses
- Psychiatric history
- Patient assessment, including complaints of others regarding the patient as well as the patient's comments
- Medical history and physical examination
- Medications
- Provisional diagnoses based on assessment that includes other current diseases as well as psychiatric diagnoses
- Individualized treatment plan and updates
- Reports of treatment, evaluations, and examinations
- Multidisciplinary progress notes
- Reports of special treatment procedures
- Multidisciplinary case conferences and consultation notes
- Notes on unusual occurrences such as treatment complications, accidents or injuries to the patient, death of the patient, and procedures that place the patient at risk or cause unusual pain including restraints and seclusion
- Correspondence related to the patient, including letters and notations of telephone conversations
- Discharge or termination summary
- Individualized aftercare or post-treatment plan

CARF, the Council on Quality and Leadership in Support for People with Disabilities, and AOA also have standards for facilities that specialize in mental health, mental disabilities, or developmental disabilities.

Rehabilitation Services Documentation

The focus of services in physical medicine and rehabilitation settings is increasing a patient's ability to function independently within the parameters of the individual's illness or disability. The documentation requirements for rehabilitation facilities vary because facilities range from comprehensive inpatient care to outpatient services or special programs.

Inpatient rehabilitation hospitals and rehabilitation units within hospitals are reimbursed by Medicare under a prospective payment system. A **patient assessment instrument** (PAI) is completed shortly after admission and upon discharge. Based on the patient's condition, services, diagnosis, and medical condition, a payment level is determined for the inpatient rehabilitation stay. Comprehensive outpatient rehabilitation facilities (CORF) have separate Medicare guidelines.

Many rehabilitation facilities are accredited through CARF, although the Joint Commission or AOA also can be chosen. CARF requires a facility to maintain a single case record for any patient it admits. The documentation standard for the health record includes the following requirements:

- Patient identification data
- Pertinent history, including functional history
- Diagnosis of disability/functional diagnosis
- Rehabilitation problems, goals, and prognosis
- Reports of assessments and program plans
- Reports from referring sources and service referrals
- Reports from outside consultations and laboratory, radiology, orthotic, and prosthetic services
- Designation of a manager for the patient's program
- Evidence of the patient's or family's participation in decision making
- Evaluation reports from each service
- Reports of staff conferences
- Progress reports
- Correspondence related to the patient
- Release forms
- Discharge summary
- Follow-up reports

Documentation of Services Provided in Correctional Facilities

Correctional facilities often provide health services to those incarcerated and thus must maintain health records. Prisons, jails, and juvenile detention centers are all examples of correctional facilities. Health records at those sites begin with the collection of certain baseline information obtained during the initial intake process. This information may include a history and physical, a chest x-ray, and laboratory testing as well as a dental examination and a psychological evaluation.

Additional information is added to the inmate's health record when he or she visits health services for treatment of illness or injury, therapy, or medication. Examples include interdisciplinary progress notes and physician's orders. Because inmates may not maintain their own over-the-counter medications, even these types of medications must be received from health services and documented in the health record.

Some inmates are imprisoned for many years, resulting in lengthy records. If the record is in a paper format it may consist of many volumes. Therefore, health information staff must develop and follow procedures that keep the most current and comprehensive information readily available and thin other parts and place them in secured storage areas.

In some states, an inmate's original paper-based health record is transferred with the inmate when he or she moves to a different prison within the system. As a result, HIM professionals in those states must work together to produce standardized policies, procedures, and formats. Federal facilities often have similar practices. Electronic records will certainly have an impact, but the need for coordination among sites remains.

Correctional health services may choose to comply with the general standards of the Joint Commission, the focused basic standards developed by the American Correctional Association, or the more comprehensive standards of the National Commission on Correctional Health Care. All have accreditation programs for correctional facilities.

End-stage Renal Disease Service Documentation

Individuals with severe kidney disease requiring renal dialysis may be treated in outpatient settings of healthcare facilities, in independent dialysis centers, while residents of long-term care settings, or even in their own homes (self-dialysis). Medicare has specific Conditions for Coverage that apply to all these settings. The standards include criteria for record content as well as for record keeping.

Documentation begins with notification of patient rights. A unique component of that notification is the inclusion of information on the facility's policy for hemodialyzer reuse. Treatment record elements include an interdisciplinary patient assessment and a plan of care, with team members commonly consisting of a physician, nurse, social worker, registered dietitian, and the patient. Progress notes, laboratory test results, a discharge summary, and consents also must be found. Special emphasis is placed on recording the patient's nutritional, anemia, vascular access, transplant, and rehabilitation status, as well as social service interventions and dialysis dosages. Patient education and training are important for dialysis success and for continued service. Evidence of both must be documented.

Check Your Understanding 3.3

1. Which type of health record contains information about care provided prior to arrival at a healthcare setting and documentation of care provided to stabilize the patient?

   A. Ambulatory care
   B. Emergency care
   C. Long-term care
   D. Rehabilitative care

2. Patient history questionnaires, problem lists, diagnostic tests results, and immunization records are commonly found in which type of record?

   A. Ambulatory care
   B. Emergency care
   C. Long-term care
   D. Rehabilitative care

3. The ambulatory surgery record contains information most similar to:

   A. Physician's office records
   B. Emergency care records
   C. Hospital operative records
   D. Hospital obstetric records

4. Which standardized tool is used to assess Medicare-certified rehabilitation facilities?

   A. Outcomes and Assessment Information Set (OASIS)
   B. Care area assessment (CAA)
   C. Patient assessment instrument (PAI)
   D. Minimum Data Set (MDS)

5. Interdisciplinary care plans are an important part of which type of health record?

   A. Emergency department
   B. Ambulance
   C. End-stage renal disease
   D. Ambulatory care

6. Portions of a treatment record may be maintained in a patient's home in which two types of settings?

   A. Hospice and behavioral health
   B. Home health and hospice
   C. Obstetric and gynecologic care
   D. Rehabilitation and correctional care

7. A patient's legal status, complaints of others regarding the patient, and reports of restraints or seclusion would be found most frequently in which type of health record?

   A. Rehabilitative care
   B. Ambulatory care
   C. Behavioral health
   D. Personal health

8. Paper records may require thinning in which two settings?

    A. Home health and hospice
    B. Rehabilitation and end-stage renal disease
    C. Ambulatory care and behavioral health
    D. Long-term care and correctional services

9. A growth and development record may be found in what type of record?

    A. Rehabilitative care
    B. Pediatric
    C. Behavioral health
    D. Obstetric

10. The document that indicates current and past medical conditions is:

    A. MDS
    B. CAAs
    C. Problem list
    D. PAI

Principles and Practices of Health Record Documentation

The content of healthcare records not only relates to the types of documents and reports found in the records, but also to practices followed while documenting. Some principles have existed for decades and other practices have evolved as a result of increased emphasis on providing reimbursable evidence of quality care.

Basic Documentation Principles

The basic principles of health record documentation apply to all types of healthcare records. These principles address the uniformity, accuracy, completeness, legibility, authenticity, timeliness, frequency, and format of health record entries. The American Health Information Management Association (AHIMA) has developed the following general documentation guidelines (Smith 2001, 56):

- Every healthcare organization should have policies that ensure the uniformity of both the content and the format of the health record. The policies should be based on all applicable accreditation standards, federal and state regulations, payer requirements, and professional practice standards.

- The health record should be organized systematically in order to facilitate data retrieval and compilation.

- Only individuals authorized by the organization's policies should be allowed to enter documentation in the health record.

- Organizational policy and/or medical staff rules and regulations should specify who may receive and transcribe verbal physician's orders.

- Health record entries should be documented at the time the services they describe are rendered.

- The authors of all entries should be clearly identified in the record.

- Only abbreviations and symbols approved by the organization and/or medical staff rules and regulations should be used in the health record.

- All entries in the health record should be permanent.

- Errors in paper-based records should be corrected according to the following process: Draw a single line in ink through the incorrect entry. Then print the word *error* at the top of the entry along with a legal signature or initials, the date, time, and reason for change, and the title and discipline of the individual making the correction. The correct information is then added to the entry. Errors must never be obliterated. The original entry should remain legible, and the corrections should be entered in chronological order. Any late entries should be labeled as such.

- When errors in the EHR are corrected, the erroneous information should not be displayed; however, there should be a method to view the previous version of the document with the original data (Wiedemann 2010).

- Any corrections or information added to the record by the patient should be inserted as an addendum (a separate note). No changes should be made in the original entries in the record. Any information added to the health record by the patient should be clearly identified as an addendum.

- The HIM department should develop, implement, and evaluate policies and procedures related to the quantitative and qualitative analysis of health records (Quantitative and qualitative analysis are discussed in chapter 7.) Uniform documentation guidelines specific to EHRs have yet to be developed. However, most basic documentation principles apply to every medium. In other cases, the type of medium, paper or electronic, may require that specific details be handled differently to achieve the same documentation goals. For example, the method used to make corrections and amendments in EHRs is often different from the method used for paper-based records noted above. In fact, in 2009 AHIMA published *Amendments, Corrections, and Deletions in the Electronic Health Record Toolkit*. The publication includes definitions of each term, case scenarios, and practice guidelines. Additional resources such as this toolkit will assist practitioners with EHR implementation.

Clinical Documentation Improvement

Because documentation found in health records is crucial as evidence of services provided and the quality of those services, many healthcare settings, particularly acute care hospitals, have initiated clinical documentation improvement (CDI) programs. Increased scrutiny of documentation by third-party payers such as Medicare regarding severity and acuity of a patient's illness, the patient's risk of death or mortality, and the need for detailed clinical data for diagnostic and procedural coding, research, patient safety, and quality scorecards make these programs worthwhile. Documentation by physicians or other qualified healthcare practitioners who can legally determine diagnoses is the focus, but reviews may occur for other healthcare providers' documentation as well.

The AHIMA CDI Toolkit (2010, 6) describes of the goals of CDI as:

- Identify and clarify missing, conflicting, or nonspecific physician documentation related to diagnoses and procedures

- Support accurate diagnostic and procedural coding, DRG assignment, severity of illness, and expected risk of mortality, leading to appropriate reimbursement

- Promote health record completion during the patient's course of care

- Improve communication between physicians and other members of the health-care team

- Provide education

- Improve documentation to reflect quality and outcome scores

- Improve coders' clinical knowledge

CDI health record documentation reviews generally begin the day after a patient's admission and continue regularly, sometimes daily, throughout the entire patient stay (concurrently). Specially trained personnel with coding, disease process, regulatory, and record content knowledge as well as excellent communication skills, review records on the care units for the detail needed to accurately assign codes, receive appropriate reimbursement, and reflect actual treatment. The criteria for these reviews and record content can come from a variety of sources including:

- Facility bylaws, rules, and regulations regarding documentation

- State licensure, federal certification, and voluntary accreditation standards

- Official coding conventions, rules, and guidelines

- Other established regulatory standards (for example, definition of "present on admission")

Reviewers record findings on electronic or paper worksheets noting patient identifying information, working diagnostic group, diagnoses, procedures, and related data. A sample review form can be found in figure 3.18.

Questions for practitioners generated from record reviews are forwarded to the pertinent healthcare provider either in person verbally or via a document (electronic or paper)

Figure 3.18.   Sample CDI Review Form

Clinical Documentation Improvement Review Form

MR #	Account #	Financial Class	Attending Physician

Initial Review

CDS:	Date of review:	LOS:	GLOS:
Working DRG:	Relative weight:	SOI:	ROM:

Principal diagnosis:	Principal procedure:

Relevant secondary diagnoses:	Location in the health record:	Relevance (i.e., CC/MCC, ROM, POA):

Query opportunity/need for additional documentation:

Clinical indicators/medical evidence:	Location in the health record:	Desired outcome/impact:
Physician Response: Yes___ No___	Date of response:	Physician agreed w/ request: Yes___ No___

Revised DRG:	GLOS:	Relative weight:	SOI:	ROM:

Principal diagnosis:	Principal procedure:

Disposition:	Review closed ___	Follow up review required ___	Date of next review:

General comments:

Subsequent Review(s)

CDS:	Date of review:	LOS:

Relevant secondary diagnoses:	Location in the health record:	Relevance (i.e., CC/MCC, ROM, POA):

Query opportunity/need for additional documentation:

Figure 3.18. **Sample CDI Review Form** *(continued)*

Physician Response: Yes___ No___		Date of response:	Physician agreed w/ request: Yes___ No___		
Revised DRG:	GLOS:	Relative weight:	SOI:		ROM:
Principal diagnosis:			Principal procedure:		
Disposition:	Review closed ___		Follow up review required ___		Date of next review:
General comments:					

called a query. Queries draw attention to documentation requiring clarification or additional information. More specifically, the AHIMA Standards for Ethical CDI Professionals describe some of these instances as:

> conflicting, incomplete, or ambiguous information in the health record regarding a significant reportable condition or procedure or other reportable data element dependent on health record documentation (e.g. present on admission indicator). (2010, 1)

Wording of a query is important to allow practitioners to use professional determination of clinical facts rather than leading or directing them to conclusions. Figure 3.19 provides an example of a query or clarification request on a patient who received tissue debridement.

Sometimes the practitioner's response will be documented on the query form itself or at other times directly into the patient's healthcare record. If provided on the query form, facility policy needs to indicate whether it becomes part of the legal medical record. If it does not become part of the legal record, it must still be maintained as evidence in the event of an audit. If a practitioner does not respond to a query within an established time frame, follow-up contacts are made or other actions as determined in facility policies are initiated. These steps continue until the patient leaves the healthcare facility.

The end result should be as complete a record as possible on patient discharge, clarity in assigning final diagnoses and procedure codes, and accurate determination of a reimbursement category. If questions remain at this time, the CDI professional must review the documentation again and obtain resolution.

As the ICD-10 and ICD-10-PCS coding systems are introduced requiring more specificity in diagnostic and procedural information, and as quality measures, present on admission medical information, pay-for-performance initiatives, and both the number and complexity of internal and external record audits increase, a well-designed program can have a significant positive impact financially and legally for the care setting.

Figure 3.19. Sample CDI Query/Clarification Form

Clinical Documentation Improvement Clarification Form—Debridement

Date: _____ Patient Name: _____

CDI Professional: _____Health Record Number: _____

CDI Professional Phone #: _____Account Number: _____

(or place patient sticker)

Attention Medical Staff:

A review of the health record by the clinical documentation team found an opportunity for clarification regarding the debridement performed. Official coding guidelines state **excisional debridement** involves the surgical removal or cutting away of tissue.

The documentation in the record is unclear as to the type of debridement that was performed on this visit. The relevant information is provided below for your expedited review. **Please address these findings in the record by providing a specific procedure description and/or clarification of an existing procedure in the next progress note, dictated report, discharge summary and/or in an addendum.**

A response is requested within 24 hours.

Clinical Indicators/Medical Evidence	Location In The Health Record
1.	1.
2.	2.

Please clarify whether the debridement performed was excisional, nonexcisional, or undetermined AND the depth of the patient's debridement (skin, subcutaneous tissue, fascia, muscle, tendon, and/or bone)

Please note that a lack of response to this request does not reflect disagreement. If no additional documentation is warranted, please check the following box:

☐ I disagree with the need for additional documentation.

Reminder: ALL documentation MUST occur in the health record. This form is NOT part of the health record.

Format of the Health Record

Health records are maintained in two basic formats, paper or electronic. Records are referred to as hybrid if they have some paper and some electronic components. Today, most healthcare facilities are working toward an EHR system. (Chapter 7 covers management of paper-based, hybrid, and electronic health records.)

Paper-based Health Records

The traditional paper-based health record format has several limitations. Because the paper-based record is lengthy and difficult to handle, it most often is kept in a single format that all end users can use. The greater the number of end users, the more important it is to follow a defined format. One format is also supported by accreditation standards and government regulations that require every provider to develop specific guidelines on record content and how the information in health records is to be arranged.

Although the regulatory standards regarding content also apply to electronic records, the foundation of an EHR is defined data elements. In a true EHR, computer screen views can be tailored to the needs of the end user. The paper-based record does not allow for this individual customization. In addition, the EHR allows the system administrator to limit access to information, restructure information, and highlight key information that the end user may need. The paper-based record lacks that flexibility.

As mentioned in chapter 2, three major types of paper-based health records are in use today: the **source-oriented health record,** the **problem-oriented health record,** and the **integrated health record.** It is important to realize, however, that no hard and fast rules exist for arranging the elements of a health record. Healthcare settings are free to select the arrangement that best suits their needs. For example, some organizations arrange the materials in active paper-based records in one way and closed records in another.

Source-oriented Health Records

In the source-oriented health record, documents are grouped together according to their point of origin. That is, laboratory records are grouped together, radiology records are grouped together, clinical notes are grouped together, and so on. Thus, physicians' progress notes for a single episode of patient care would be arranged in either chronological or reverse chronological order and placed together in the patient's health record.

The result is that those individuals charged with filing reports in the paper-based health record can do so easily simply by looking at the source of the document and date of the report. However, the end users of record information do not have as easy a time. To get a full view of the patient's course of treatment, they must search by date of occurrence in each section of the record (that is, laboratory, radiology, and every section of clinical notes). The more types of healthcare professionals contributing to care, the more sections a source-oriented health record can have. It is left to the end user to tie the information from the various sections of the record together to get a picture of the entire course of treatment.

Problem-oriented Health Records

The problem-oriented health record is better suited to serve the patient and the end user of the patient information. The key characteristic of this format is an itemized list of the patient's past and present social, psychological, and medical problems. Each problem is identified by a unique number.

In addition to a problem list, each problem-oriented health record contains a patient database, an initial care plan, and progress notes. The database is formatted much like the source-oriented health record and contains the following information:

- Chief complaint
- Present illness(es)
- Social history
- Medical history
- Physical examination
- Diagnostic test results

The initial plan serves as the guide for addressing each of the patient's problems. The plans are numbered to correspond to the problems they address.

The patient's healthcare provider uses progress notes to document how the patient's problems are being treated and how he or she is responding to treatment. Each progress note is labeled with the unique number assigned to the problem being addressed. Some providers also use a **subjective, objective, assessment plan** (SOAP) format for their problem-oriented progress notes. A subjective (S) entry relates significant information in the patient's words or from the patient's point of view. Objective (O) data includes factual information such as laboratory findings or provider observations. Professional conclusions reached from evaluation of the subjective or objective information make up the assessment (A), and any comments on or changes in plans (P) complete the framework. An example of a SOAP note can be found in figure 3.20. Not all SOAP components must be entered in every note. If the SOAP framework is used, only pertinent parts are documented. This problem-indexing system allows the healthcare provider to easily follow the patient's course of treatment regarding any specific problem. Ideally, other elements of the health record (for example, physician's orders) also would be numbered according to the problems they address.

Integrated Health Records

The third major type of paper-based health record is the integrated health record. The integrated health record is arranged so that the documentation from various sources is intermingled and follows strict chronological (date) order. The advantage of the integrated format is that it is easy to follow the course of the patient's diagnosis and treatment. The disadvantage is that the format makes it difficult to compare information from any one specific type of healthcare professional.

Figure 3.20.   Example of a SOAP progress note

SOAP PROGRESS NOTE		
Identification Number		
Medical Record Number		
Last Name	**First Name**	**Middle Initial**
Date of Birth		

DATE	DEPARTMENT	PROGRESS NOTES
7-28-89	INT MEDICINE	#1 Diabetes Mellitus
		S: Occasionally gets hungry. No insulin reactions. Says she is following diet.
		O: Adequately controlled. FBS 110 mg %, urine sugar, no acetone.
		A: Insulin-dependent diabetes, controlled.
		P: Continue 40 units NPH insulin daily, 1,200 calorie diet, return visit in 2 weeks.
		#6 Hypertension
		S: No headaches, dizziness, etc.
		O: BP 140/90 (RA sitting); pulse 80
		A: BP satisfactory
		P: Continue with Diuril, 500 mg once daily. Return visit in 2 weeks.

Future of Paper-based Health Records

The ultimate goal of every health record is to facilitate communication. A well-designed, well-maintained paper-based health record can significantly improve communication among healthcare providers and other health information end users. Still, the paper-based health record has a number of weaknesses. For example, it has been determined that the average health record is needed by approximately 150 end users. However, the paper-based record can be viewed by only one user at a time and in only one place at a time. Thus, the valuable information recorded in the health record is often unavailable to individuals who need it.

Further, paper-based health records can be difficult to update. An active record of a patient receiving care moves often from provider to provider within the healthcare facility. The individual(s) responsible for updating its content must hand-carry paper documents to wherever the record is located in order to file them or wait until the record is returned. The result is that updates may be delayed.

Finally, paper-based health records are fragile and susceptible to damage from water, fire, and the wear and tear of daily use. They also can easily be misplaced or misfiled. For most organizations, it would be too expensive and difficult to maintain duplicate copies of paper health records as backups.

For all of these reasons and the need to provide better coordinated services, reduce medical errors and duplication of services, and consequently increase the quality of care, national efforts are focused on the adoption of electronic health records.

Electronic Health Records

The EHR can be seen as the natural evolution of the health record. By design, it not only addresses many of the paper-based health record's existing problems but also presents new capabilities. The discussion here focuses on the impact of the EHR on the generation of record content whereas a much broader description and analysis of the EHR is presented in chapters 14 through 17.

Definition of the Electronic Health Record

To address the important task of uniformity in definitions, the Office of the National Coordinator for Health Information Technology charged a workgroup to tackle the topic. NAHIT published its report in April 2008. The report includes proposed definitions for electronic medical records, electronic health records, and personal health records. It differentiates between electronic medical and electronic health records as follows:

> Electronic medical record—an electronic record of health-related information on an individual that can be created, gathered, managed, and consulted by authorized clinicians and staff within one health organization.
>
> Electronic health record—an electronic record of health-related information on an individual that conforms to nationally recognized interoperability standards and that can be created, managed, and consulted by authorized clinicians and staff across more than one health care organization. (NAHIT 2008)

Thus, the suggestion is that the term "electronic health record" be applied to those record systems that support the function of interoperability across healthcare providers. (The definition of a personal health record will be shared later in this chapter.)

Electronic Health Record Core Capabilities

Initial work in developing uniformity in electronic health records came through efforts to identify its functions. The Institute of Medicine (IOM) began that process by identifying eight core functions. "Key Capabilities of an Electronic Health Record System," was released by the IOM's Committee on Data Standards for Patient Safety in 2003. The core functions are:

- Health information and data—patient data using defined data sets and interfaces with related medical treatment and diagnostic reporting systems

- Results management—electronic reporting of tests, consultations, and related patient consents

- Order entry and management—electronic order entry with allergy, interaction, and laboratory report interfaces

- Decision support—reminders, prompts, diagnosis and disease management information, adverse event, disease outbreak, and bioterrorism tracking

- Electronic communication and connectivity—exchange of healthcare data across providers within and outside a care setting to support continuity of care, including telemedicine and telemonitoring options

- Patient support—patient education and home-based telemedicine opportunities

- Administrative processes—electronic scheduling, billing and claims management, and identification of those appropriate for clinical trials or focused disease management

- Reporting and population health management—quality management and regulatory reporting (IOM 2003)

In adopting these capabilities, the Committee agreed that all functions would not be accomplished at one time and that efforts would be ongoing well into the future. In July 2004, using the IOM's work as a foundation, a national standards group called Health Level Seven (HL7) introduced an expanded list of about 130 different functions that would help define an EHR. Although these efforts contributed to the understanding of electronic health records, uniform, consistent content standards still do not exist.

Transitions in Record Practices

There are a number of challenges related to record content and documentation when organizations adopt electronic health records. Adoption changes health information workflow and processes. Sharing of records with other organizations either within a healthcare enterprise or outside requires coordination. Successful adoption has a much higher probability if issues are anticipated and are part of initiation plans.

First, healthcare organizations must maintain legal and regulatory compliance. Applicable record content and documentation standards addressed in this chapter apply to healthcare settings no matter the record format. Complete, accurate, and consistent records must be maintained for each patient. However, new questions are posed as a result of plans for EHR adoption, and policies and procedures must be developed from resulting discussions.

For example, decisions need to be made regarding the timely capture and display of information and when documents become part of a record. The latter is particularly important regarding "preliminary" reports, document versions, or when documents are received as part of health information exchanges. Audit trails to indicate the timing of adding and deleting documents may be important in providing evidence for the chronology of clinical decisions. Guidelines for the correction and editing of information are important, as are policies in the event of purposeful or inadvertent record deletion. A definition of an organization's legal health record will provide guidance when content questions arise and particularly in release of information or potential liability or lawsuit situations.

Content edit checks, evidence of use of decision support information, criteria to evaluate records for completeness, and other support processes must be developed. Role-based guidelines for access to records, including security measures, must be in place. Guidelines for retention of records, determination of backup systems, and procedures for eventual record destruction must be addressed.

Hybrid Records

One method of overcoming some of the EHR hurdles is for the healthcare setting to move in steps from paper-based systems to full EHR adoption. If planned well, this allows the facility to thoroughly investigate the needs of its users and gradually address the weaknesses and challenges of an EHR. A record in this type of system is referred to as a hybrid record. Chapter 7 provides additional information on the management of hybrid record systems.

Definition of Hybrid Record

In a series of practice briefs on hybrid records, an AHIMA e-HIM Work Group used the following description (AHIMA e-HIM Work Group 2003):

> A hybrid health record is a system with functional components that:
> - Include both paper and electronic documents
> - Use both manual and electronic processes

On the basis of this description, a hybrid record has many formats. For example, one facility may have laboratory and other diagnostic reports reported electronically, with the remainder on paper. This facility may take an EHR step by scanning all the paper documents upon patient discharge to make a full record accessible electronically for subsequent users. Another organization may have most record components generated electronically by providers as care is delivered, scan all other documents that are not part of the system, and have alerts and reminders that assist in clinical and care decision support.

Documenting Transitions

Hybrid records are a positive step toward the EHR, but they also create special challenges. Both manual and computer processes must be supported, policies and procedures are needed for both types of systems, and appropriate safeguards must be in place for the privacy and security of both systems. A definition of what constitutes a record in each system must be developed. As the transition occurs, it also is important to regularly update system descriptions, including the location of all care documents, so that patient health information remains readily available to users. The AHIMA e-HIM Work Group (AHIMA e-HIM Work Group 2003, Appendix) suggests a matrix for this step and provides an example (table 3.4).

As the electronic system develops, different versions of documents may exist and these also must be monitored and logged for both legal and practice purposes. Additionally, an AHIMA e-HIM Task Force (AHIMA e-HIM Task Force 2004) describes in detail changes in health information processes and procedures that are required as a record transitions from paper to hybrid to fully electronic formats.

Personal Health Records

A relatively new development, the **personal health record** (PHR) has been defined by a workgroup sponsored by NAHIT as:

> An electronic record of health-related information on an individual that conforms to nationally recognized interoperability standards and that can be drawn from multiple sources while being managed, shared, and controlled by the individual (NAHIT 2008).

The personal health record is unique in that it is maintained and controlled by each individual and is a compilation of information obtained from healthcare providers as well as through personal discovery. It could be found on a personal computer, the Web, desktop and Web, or portable devices. In 2005, an AHIMA e-HIM Personal Health Record Task Force identified minimum common data elements for a PHR as (AHIMA e-HIM Task Force 2005, Appendix B):

- Personal demographic information
- General medical information
- Allergies and drug sensitivities
- Conditions
- Hospitalizations
- Surgeries
- Medications
- Immunizations
- Clinical tests
- Pregnancy history

Table 3.4.   Hybrid health record legal source legend

	Organization's Name HYBRID HEALTH RECORD LEGAL SOURCE LEGEND			
Report/Document Types	LHR Media Type (P)aper/(E)lectronic	Source System Application (nonpaper)	Electronic Storage Start Date	Stop Printing Start Date
Admission History & Physical	P/E	System 1	1/1/2002	1/1/2003
Attending Admission Notes	P			
Physician Orders	E			
Inpatient Progress Notes	P			
Discharge Summary	E	System 1	1/1/2002	4/1/2002
Inpatient Transfer Note	E	System 1	1/1/2002	
Outpatient Progress Notes	P			
Clinical Laboratory Results—(Preliminary/Interim)	E	System 2	1/1/1999	1/1/1999
Clinical Laboratory Results (Final)	E	System 2	1/1/1999	1/1/2000
Radiology Reports	E	System 3	7/1/2003	
Care Flow Sheets	E	System 1	6/1/2003	
Medication Records	E	System 1	7/1/2003	
Clinical Consult Reports	E	System 1	1/1/2002	
Pre-operative, Pre-procedure Notes	P			
Pathology Reports	E	System 2	1/1/1999	1/1/2000
Organ/Tissue Donation or Transplants	P			
Patient Problem List (Summary List)	E	System 1	8/1/2003	
Urgent Care and Emergency Records	P			
Consents[1]	E	System 4	TBD	
Advance Directive				
Correspondence[1]	E	System 4	TBD	
Pre-operative Anesthetic Assessments and Plans	P			
Intra-operative Documentation	P			
Post-Operative Documentation	P			
Brief Post-Operative Note	P			
Surgical Operative Reports	E	System 1	1/1/2002	

[1]Scanned electronic documents

Source: AHIMA 2003.

Because it is a lifelong record, information also could include:

- Information from providers
- Genetic information
- Personal, family, occupational, and environmental history
- Health plans and goals
- Health status of the individual
- Documentation of choices in relation to organ donation, durable power of attorney, and advance directives
- Charges paid for services and products
- Health insurance information
- Provider directory

Although health information professionals may not have direct contact with personal records, they serve as patient advocates and can play important support and educational roles. In addition, in the electronic record environment, patients have portals to communicate with practitioners via such methods as e-mails, their personal health records, patient questionnaires and surveys, and transferring clinical information. This sharing has the potential benefit of providing more comprehensive information to healthcare providers, but it includes challenges such as identification of the original data source and verification of the accuracy of information. Facilities will need policies in place to determine how much and what type of information actually becomes part of the organization's health record. More information on PHRs can be found in chapter 16.

Check Your Understanding 3.4

1. Which type of health record includes both paper and electronic components?
   A. Hybrid
   B. Electronic
   C. Problem-oriented
   D. Source-oriented

2. Which of the following is a disadvantage of an EHR over a paper-based record?
   A. Allows customization to user needs
   B. Permits multiple users at the same time
   C. Enables duplicate copies to be made easily
   D. Requires privacy and security measures

3. In an integrated health record, documentation by health professionals is organized:

    A. In sections by type of professional
    B. In sections by problem number
    C. Intermixed in date sequence
    D. Depends on facility policy

4. The patient indicates that her pain is worse. In which part of a SOAP note would this information be recorded?

    A. Subjective
    B. Objective
    C. Assessment
    D. Plan

5. Which of the following electronic record technological capabilities would allow an x-ray to be sent to a physician in another state?

    A. Database management
    B. Image processing
    C. Text processing
    D. Vocabulary standards

6. Which of the following is true of paper-based records?

    A. They are susceptible to damage from fire or floods.
    B. They lack standardization.
    C. They are easy to access and update.
    D. They require a limited number of personnel to process.

7. A definition of what constitutes a record, recording where each component is located, and noting dates of format changes are particularly important in:

    A. Electronic records
    B. Integrated records
    C. Paper records
    D. Hybrid records

8. In a problem-oriented health record, problems are organized by:

    A. Letter
    B. Number
    C. Patient name
    D. Body system

Real-World Case

When St. James Hospital began developing its electronic record, system designers set out to capture every bit of information available. The unofficial goal of the implementation team was to compile all available health information into a single system and provide the means to deliver the information instantaneously to end users on demand. However, the large volumes of information, overcrowded computer screens, and lack of uniform structure soon proved overwhelming for the system's end users. Their feedback called for useful information formatted in a usable structure.

In response to end-user frustration, designers took a hard look at the information that was being captured. They considered the following questions:

- How is health information formatted and structured?

- How long is health information retained?

- What information is purged from the system?

- What health information is archived?

- How much control should end users have over the information they are allowed to access?

Summary

The records maintained by healthcare providers for patients—no matter the illness or healthcare setting—all contain similar information (for example, chief complaint/reason for visit, history and physical examination or assessment and plan, progress notes, diagnostic test results, and orders). However, some settings and medical specialties have documentation requirements that are unique to their fields.

Accreditation standards, state and federal laws, and facility policies all affect the content of the health record. Although standards and policies must be complied with, facilities should not lose sight of the primary purpose of the health record: to facilitate effective patient healthcare. Facilities must organize and maintain health records in a way that ensures that the information in them is complete and easy to retrieve. The end result is that healthcare providers can use the information effectively to make wise treatment decisions.

HIM professionals are often positioned within their employment settings to significantly influence established documentation practices. Their knowledge of quality coding principles clarifies the impact of documentation on reimbursement. Their experience in performance improvement clarifies the impact of documentation on the quality and continuity of patient care. And their expertise in release-of-information functions clarifies the impact of documentation on liability issues.

Bringing order to chaos is the primary justification for formalizing the content and structure of the health record. Health records that lack structure are of little use to the healthcare providers who use the information in them to make decisions about patient care. Thus, in order for health information to be useful, it must be expressed in a vocabulary that end users understand and it must be organized in a predictable format. It also must provide details specific to the problem being addressed. In addition, the information must be current, legible, and accurate.

The challenge for EHR system designers is to develop computer systems that are flexible, accessible, and portable enough to meet the unique needs of every healthcare provider, administrator, researcher, educator, and policymaker.

References

AHIMA. 2010. CDI toolkit. Chicago: AHIMA.

AHIMA. 2010. Ethical standards for clinical documentation improvement (CDI) professionals. Chicago: AHIMA.

AHIMA e-HIM Task Force. 2004. The strategic importance of electronic health records management. *Journal of AHIMA* 75(9):80C–80E.

AHIMA e-HIM Task Force. 2005. The role of the personal health record in the EHR. *Journal of AHIMA* 76(7):64A–64D.

AHIMA e-HIM Work Group. 2003. The complete medical record in a hybrid EHR environment. Chicago: AHIMA.

Institute of Medicine (IOM) Committee on Data Standards for Patient Safety, Board on Health Care Services. 2003. Key capabilities of an electronic health record system. Washington, DC: The National Academies Press.

National Alliance for Health Information Technology (NAHIT). 2008. Defining key health information technology terms. Washington, DC: ONCHIT.

Smith, C. 2001. Practice brief: Documentation requirements for the acute care inpatient record. *Journal of AHIMA* 72(3):56A–56G.

Wiedemann, Lou Ann. 2010. Deleting errors in the EHR. *Journal of AHIMA* 81(9):52–53.

Additional Resources

AHIMA. 2008. Enterprise content and record management for healthcare. *Journal of AHIMA* 79(10):91–98.

AHIMA. 2008. Managing an effective query process. *Journal of AHIMA* 79(10):83–88.

AHIMA. 2009. Amendments, corrections, and deletions in the electronic health record toolkit. Chicago: AHIMA.

AHIMA. 2009. Recommended regulations and standards for specific healthcare settings (updated). *Journal of AHIMA* 80(1):61–67.

AHIMA. 2010. EHRs as the business and legal records of healthcare organizations (undated). Appendix A: Issues in electronic health record management. Chicago: AHIMA.

AHIMA. 2010. Guidance for clinical documentation improvement programs. *Journal of AHIMA* 81(5): expanded Web version.

AHIMA e-HIM Work Group on Maintaining the Legal EHR. (2005). Update: Maintaining a legally sound health record—paper and electronic. *Journal of AHIMA 76*(10):64A-L.

Dimick, C. 2008. Defining the legal EHR: Simple or complex? *Journal of AHIMA* 79(1):60–61.

Groen, P., and D. Goldstein. 2007. VistA electronic health record (EHR) system: The market today and tomorrow. *Virtual Medical World Monthly.* http://www.hoise.com/vmw/07/articles/vmw/LV-VM-04-07-1.html

Institute of Medicine. 1997. *The Computer-Based Patient Record: An Essential Technology for Health Care*, rev. ed. Washington, DC: National Academy Press.

Odom-Wesley, B., and D. Brown. Edited by C. Meyers. 2009. *Documentation for Medical Records.* Chicago: AHIMA.

Peden, A. 2012. *Comparative Health Information Management*, 3rd ed. Clifton Park, NY: Delmar, Cengage Learning.

U.S. Department of Veterans Affairs. 2011. Healthcare. Medical Centers. http://www.va.gov/health/MedicalCenters.asp

U.S. Department of Veterans Affairs. 2011. Veterans health information systems and technology architecture (VistA)—Description. http://www.virec.research.va.gov/DataSourcesName/VISTA/VISTA.htm

chapter 4

Healthcare Data Sets and Standards

Kathy Giannangelo, MA, RHIA, CCS, CPHIMS, FAHIMA

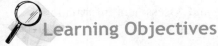

Learning Objectives

- Describe the purpose of healthcare data sets and standards

- Explain the importance of healthcare data sets and standards

- Identify the common health information standardized data sets

- Explain the need for electronic data interchange standards

- Explain the healthcare data needs in an electronic environment

- Discuss how data standards are developed

- Identify well-known standards that support electronic health record (EHR) systems

- Discuss how data standards support the development of EHR systems

- Identify prominent health informatics standards development organizations (SDOs)

- Recognize the impact of the Health Insurance Portability and Accountability Act of 1996 (HIPAA) on the development of health informatics standards

- Explain the relationship of core data elements to healthcare informatics standards in electronic environments

- Describe the role of government agencies, such as the ONC, in healthcare informatics standards development, testing, coordination, and harmonization

Key Terms

American College of Radiology and the National Electrical Manufacturers Association (ACR-NEMA)

American National Standards Institute (ANSI)

ASTM International

Clinical Document Architecture (CDA)

Common Formats Version 1.1

Continuity of Care Document (CCD)

Continuity of Care Record (CCR)

Core data elements

Core measure

Data dictionary

Data element

Data Elements for Emergency Department Systems (DEEDS) 1.0

Data set

Data standard

Department of Health and Human Services (HHS)

Digital Imaging and Communication in Medicine (DICOM)

Electronic data interchange (EDI)

Extensible markup language (XML)

Health Information Technology Expert Panel (HITEP)

Healthcare Effectiveness Data and Information Set (HEDIS)

Healthcare informatics standards

HIT Policy Committee (HITPC)

HIT Standards Committee (HITSC)

Hospital discharge abstract system

Inpatient

Institute of Electrical and Electronics Engineers (IEEE)

Metadata

Minimum Data Set (MDS) Version 3.0

National Center for Health Statistics (NCHS)

National Committee on Vital and Health Statistics (NCVHS)

National Institute for Standards and Technology (NIST)

Nationwide Health Information Network (NHIN)

Office of the National Coordinator of Health Information Technology (ONC)

ORYX initiative

Outcomes and Assessment Information Set (OASIS-C)

Outpatients

Prospective payment system (PPS)

Quality Data Model (QDM)

Standard

Standards and Interoperability (S&I) Framework

Standards development organizations (SDOs)

Structure and content standards

Transaction standards

Uniform Ambulatory Care Data Set (UACDS)

Uniform Hospital Discharge Data Set (UHDDS)

Introduction

Data and information pertaining to individuals who use healthcare services are collected in virtually every setting where healthcare is delivered. As noted in other chapters, data represent basic facts and measurements. In healthcare, these facts usually describe specific characteristics of individual patients. The term *data* is plural. Although the singular form is *datum,* the term that is frequently used to describe a single fact or measurement is

data element. For example, age, gender, insurance company, and blood pressure are all data elements concerning a patient. The term *information* refers to data that have been collected, combined, analyzed, interpreted, and/or converted into a form that can be used for specific purposes. In other words, data represent facts; information represents meaning.

In healthcare settings, data are stored in the individual's health record whether that record is in paper or electronic format. The numerous data elements in the health record are then combined, analyzed, and interpreted by the patient's physician and other clinicians. For example, test results are combined with the physician's observations and the patient's description of his or her symptoms to form information about the disease or condition that is affecting the patient. Physicians use both data and information to diagnose diseases, develop treatment plans, assess the effectiveness of care, and determine the patient's prognosis.

Data about patients can be extracted from individual health records and combined as aggregate data. Aggregate data are used to develop information about groups of patients. For example, data about all of the patients who suffered an acute myocardial infarction during a specific time period could be collected in a database. From the aggregate data, it would be possible to identify common characteristics that might predict the course of the disease or provide information about the most effective way to treat it. Ultimately, research using aggregated data might be used for disease prevention. For example, researchers identified the link between smoking and lung cancer by analyzing aggregate data about patients with a diagnosis of lung cancer; smoking cessation programs grew from the identification of the causal effect of smoking on lung cancer and a variety of other conditions.

History of Healthcare Data Collection

The first known efforts to collect and use healthcare data to produce meaningful statistical profiles date back to the seventeenth century. In the early 1600s, Captain John Graunt gathered data on the common causes of death in London. He called his study the Bills of Mortality. However, few systematic efforts were undertaken to collect statistical data about the incidence and prevalence of disease until the mid-20th century, when technological developments made it possible to collect and analyze large amounts of healthcare data.

Modern efforts at standardizing healthcare data began in the 1960s. At that time, healthcare facilities began to use computers to process larger amounts of data than could be handled manually. The goal was to make comparisons among data from multiple providers. It soon became evident that healthcare organizations needed to use standardized, uniform data definitions in order to arrive at meaningful data comparisons.

The first data standardization efforts focused generally on hospitals and specifically on hospital discharge data. The intent of the efforts was to standardize definitions of key data elements commonly collected in hospitals. Discharge data were collected in **hospital discharge abstract systems.** These systems used databases compiled from aggregate data on all the patients discharged from a particular facility. The need to compare uniform discharge data from one hospital to the next led to the development of **data sets** or lists of recommended data elements with uniform definitions.

Today, hospitals and other healthcare organizations collect more data and develop more information than ever before. Moreover, data and information from the health records of individual patients are used for more purposes than ever before. The demand for information is coming from users within the organizations as well as from external users such as third-party payers, government agencies, accreditation organizations, and others. The extensive use of information within and across organizational boundaries demands standards that promote interoperable electronic interchange of data and information. Information and informatics standards are critical in the migration to electronic health records (EHRs), as described in chapter 16.

Data Sets in the Electronic Environment

The data sets originally developed to support uniform data collection are inadequate for an electronic environment, and many public and private organizations have been actively engaged in the process of developing **healthcare informatics standards** to support EHR development and information interchange. Standards development is a dynamic process as key players in the standards development community negotiate, refine, and revise standards. The critical importance of healthcare information and informatics standards has been recognized in recent federal initiatives including those of the **Office of the National Coordinator of Health Information Technology** (ONC).

According to *Toward a National Health Information Infrastructure* by the **National Committee on Vital and Health Statistics** (NCVHS), "if information in multiple locations is to be searched, shared, and synthesized when needed, we will need agreed-upon information guardians that can exchange data with each other . . . we will need equitable rules of data exchange so that competitors (within or between healthcare provider systems, health information management companies, or health web services) will be willing to connect and share data" (NCVHS 2000).

Developing Standardized Data Sets and Standards

This chapter describes the initial efforts at developing standardized data sets for use in different types of healthcare settings, including acute care, ambulatory care, long-term care, and home care. It explores the recent national initiatives related to interoperability and connectivity of healthcare information systems that will support widespread implementation of EHRs. It also explains the work of developing a **Nationwide Health Information Network** (NHIN) that will improve patient care, increase safety, and assist clinical and administrative decision making.

It is essential that the HIM professional understand the purpose, content, and importance of healthcare data sets and standards. HIM professionals work with many of these data sets and **data standards** on the job. In the years to come, the roles of the HIM professional will be influenced and likely change as standards continue to develop, be adopted, and ultimately implemented.

Theory into Practice

In a large Midwestern health system, the director of health information services leads the system's clinical data standards committee. The committee recently decided to develop a **data dictionary** as a first step toward implementing an EHR system. To assist in this effort, the group used the following guidelines (AHIMA e-HIM Workgroup on EHR Data Content 2006):

- Design a plan
- Develop an enterprise data dictionary
- Ensure collaborative involvement and buy-in
- Develop an approvals process and documentation trail
- Identify and retail details of data versions
- Design for flexibility and growth
- Design room for expansion of field values
- Follow established ISO/International Electrotechnical Commission (IEC) 11179 guidelines or rules for metadata registry
- Adopt nationally recognized standards and normalize field definitions across data sets
- Beware of differing standards for the same concepts
- Use geographic codes and standards that conform to the National Spatial Data Infrastructure and Federal Geographic Data Committee
- Test the information system
- Provide ongoing education and training
- Assess the extent to which the data elements maintain consistency and avoid duplication

Data dictionaries include the following components:

- A list of data elements collected in individual health records
- Definitions of the data elements
- Descriptions of the attributes of each data element
- Specifications for the size of the data field in the information system
- Descriptions of the data views to be accessed by various users
- Location where the data are stored

The committee began the process with what it considered to be a simple data element: patient gender. Committee members reviewed the types of services provided by the health-care system's hospitals and clinics. One of the hospitals offered a gender re-identification program that treated patients who were in the process of transitioning from one gender to the other. Another hospital provided neonatal intensive care services for a large geographical region. Some of the infants treated in the neonatal intensive care unit had been born with congenital defects that made it difficult to determine their gender.

During discussions of the problem, the clinical laboratory representative on the committee stressed the importance of documenting the gender of every patient. She explained that the normal range for most laboratory tests varies by gender. This information was a surprise to many committee members.

After the committee's initial discussion, the health information management director agreed to research data sets and standards for gender. He accessed the United States Health Information Knowledgebase (USHIK) and found gender is defined as administrative sex rather than biological sex. After further review of several options for administrative gender, he noticed the Health Level Seven (HL7) Version 3.0 recommended three values: F, M, UN, with display names of Female, Male, Undifferentiated, and definitions of female and male. When the gender of a person could not be uniquely defined as male or female, such as hermaphrodite, the gender was considered undifferentiated. The HIM director also learned this code system is tied to the **Clinical Document Architecture** (CDA) Release 2 which is one of the content exchange standards for stage 1 meaningful use. The committee decided to adopt the HL7 standard for administrative gender.

The challenges the committee faced in defining this relatively simple data element raised its awareness of how difficult it would be to adequately define every data element to be included in the new EHR system. The committee members gathered information on every available healthcare data set and healthcare informatics standard and carefully compared the data definitions recommended. During their discussions, the HIM manager shared the following from the International Organization for Standardization (ISO 2004):

> The increased use of data processing and electronic data interchange heavily relies on accurate, reliable, controllable, and verifiable data recorded in databases. One of the prerequisites for a correct and proper use and interpretation of data is that both users and owners of data have a common understanding of the meaning and descriptive characteristics (e.g., representation) of that data. To guarantee this shared view, a number of basic attributes has to be defined.

They discovered that implementation of the EHR system would be a huge project. However, they were committed to the process because it would improve the quality of the data collected in the system. The collection of consistent, reliable, and valid data would improve administrative and clinical decision making, make it possible to perform meaningful performance improvement comparisons, and result in the ability to move healthcare information electronically between disparate healthcare information systems.

Data Sets

Without data there is no information. However, because of the vast amounts of data available there needs to be some way to organize them so they can be managed. Creating a data set is a method to capture and arrange certain data elements in order to turn data into information.

Definition of Data Set

A data set is a list of recommended data elements with uniform definitions that are relevant for a particular use. For example, the Medicare Provider Analysis and Review (MEDPAR) File available from the Centers for Medicare and Medicaid Services (CMS) contains data from claims for services provided to beneficiaries admitted to Medicare-certified inpatient hospitals and skilled nursing facilities (SNF). The data set for this file is the data contained in the billing form's fields.

Another example of a data set is the **Quality Data Model** (QDM), formerly known as the Quality Data Set (QDS), published by the National Quality Forum (NQF). The QDM will be discussed later in this chapter.

Importance and Use of Data Sets

The idea of data standardization became widely accepted during the 1960s. Under the leadership of the **National Center for Health Statistics** (NCHS) and the NCVHS in collaboration with other organizations, data sets were developed for a variety of healthcare settings. Data sets for acute care, long-term care, and ambulatory care were the first to be created.

Healthcare data sets have two purposes. The first is to identify the data elements that should be collected for each patient. The second is to provide uniform definitions for common terms. The use of uniform definitions ensures that data collected from a variety of healthcare settings will share a standard definition.

Standardizing data elements and definitions makes it possible to compare the data collected at different facilities. For example, when data are standardized, the term *admission* means the same thing at City Hospital and at University Hospital. Because both hospitals define *admission* in the same way, they can be compared with each other on such things as number of admissions and percentage of occupancy.

The contents of data sets vary by their purpose. However, data sets are not meant to limit the number of data elements that can be collected. Most healthcare organizations collect additional data elements that have meaning for their specific administrative and clinical operations.

Data sets may be formed for such activities as research, clinical trials, quality and safety improvement, reimbursement, accreditation, and exchanging clinical information (Giannangelo 2007). The MEDPAR File, for example, allows researchers to track inpatient history and patterns/outcomes of care over time. Acute care hospitals use the AHRQ **Common Formats Version 1.1** when reporting patient safety events. Contained within Version 1.1 are technical specifications which include a data dictionary. By defining the Common Formats data elements and their attributes, standardization is possible.

Having defined data sets ensures consistent data collection and reporting. Standardized data sets provide information about the effectiveness of interventions and treatments for specific diseases, thereby improving the quality and safety of healthcare, maximizing the effectiveness of health promotions and care, minimizing the burden on those responsible for generating the data, and helping facilitate efficient reuse of data (Giannangelo 2007).

Types of Data Sets

The following are examples of data sets the HIT professional will most likely encounter in his or her daily work.

Data Sets Required or Recommended by the Federal Government

A number of data reporting requirements come from federal initiatives. Some are mandated through published federal regulations, such as the Medicare **prospective payment system** (PPS), while some are only recommendations.

Uniform Hospital Discharge Data Set

In 1969, a conference on hospital discharge abstract systems was sponsored jointly by NCHS, the National Center for Health Services Research and Development, and Johns Hopkins University. Conference participants recommended that all short-term general hospitals in the United States collect a minimum set of patient-specific data elements. They also recommended that these data elements be included in all databases compiled from hospital discharge abstract systems. They called the list of patient-specific data items the **Uniform Hospital Discharge Data Set** (UHDDS).

The purpose of the UHDDS is to list and define a set of common, uniform data elements. The data elements are collected from the health records of every hospital **inpatient** and later abstracted from the health record and included in national databases.

In 1974, the federal government adopted the UHDDS as the standard for collecting data for the Medicare and Medicaid programs. When the Section 1886(d) of the Social Security Act was enacted in 1983, UHDDS definitions were incorporated into the rules and regulations for implementing the inpatient prospective payment system based on diagnosis-related groups (DRGs). A key component of DRGs was the incorporation of the definitions of principal diagnosis, principal procedure, and other significant procedures into the DRG algorithms. As a result, accurate DRG assignment depends on accurate selection and coding of the principal diagnosis and principal procedure and the appropriate sequencing of other significant diagnoses and procedures. NCVHS revised the UHDDS in 1984, and the new UHDDS was adopted for all federal health programs in 1986. Because UHDDS data definitions are a component of DRGs, short-term, general hospitals in the United States generally collect patient-specific data in the format recommended by the UHDDS.

The UHDDS has been revised several times since 1986. The current version includes the recommended data elements shown in figure 4.1.

Figure 4.1.   UHDDS data elements

Data Element	Definition/Descriptor
01. Personal identification	The unique number assigned to each patient within a hospital that distinguishes the patient and his or her hospital record from all others in that institution.
02. Date of birth	Month, day, and year of birth. Capture of the full four-digit year of birth is recommended.
03. Sex	Male or female
04. Race and ethnicity	04a. Race American Indian/Eskimo/Aleut Asian or Pacific Islander Black White Other race Unknown 04b. Ethnicity Spanish origin/Hispanic Non-Spanish origin/Non-Hispanic Unknown
05. Residence	Full address of usual residence Zip code (nine digits, if available) Code for foreign residence
06. Hospital identification	A unique institutional number across data collection systems. The Medicare provider number is the preferred hospital identifier.
07. Admission date	Month, day, and year of admission
08. Type of admission	Scheduled: Arranged with admissions office at least 24 hours prior to admission Unscheduled: All other admissions
09. Discharge date	Month, day, and year of discharge
10 & 11. Physician identification • Attending physician • Operating physician	The Medicare unique physician identification number (UPIN) is the preferred method of identifying the attending physician and operating physician(s) because it is uniform across all data systems.
12. Principal diagnosis	The condition established after study to be chiefly responsible for occasioning the admission of the patient to the hospital for care.
13. Other diagnoses	All conditions that coexist at the time of admission or that develop subsequently or that affect the treatment received and/or the length of stay. Diagnoses that relate to an earlier episode and have no bearing on the current hospital stay are to be excluded.

(continued on next page)

Figure 4.1.   UHDDS data elements *(continued)*

Data Element	Definition/Descriptor
14. Qualifier for other diagnoses	A qualifier is given for each diagnosis coded under "other diagnoses" to indicate whether the onset of the diagnosis preceded or followed admission to the hospital. The option "uncertain" is permitted.
15. External cause-of-injury code	The ICD-9-CM code for the external cause of an injury, poisoning, or adverse effect (commonly referred to as an E code). Hospitals should complete this item whenever there is a diagnosis of an injury, poisoning, or adverse effect.
16. Birth weight of neonate	The specific birth weight of a newborn, preferably recorded in grams
17. Procedures and dates	All significant procedures are to be reported. A significant procedure is one that is: • Surgical in nature, or • Carries a procedural risk, or • Carries an anesthetic risk, or • Requires specialized training. The date of each significant procedure must be reported. When more than one procedure is reported, the principal procedure must be designated. The principal procedure is one that is performed for definitive treatment rather than one performed for diagnostic or exploratory purposes or was necessary to take care of a complication. If there appear to be two procedures that are principal, then the one most closely related to the principal diagnosis should be selected as the principal procedure. The UPIN must be reported for the person performing the principal procedure.
18. Disposition of the patient	• Discharged to home (excludes those patients referred to home health service) • Discharged to acute care hospital • Discharged to nursing facility • Discharged home to be under the care of a home health service (including a hospice) • Discharged to other healthcare facility • Left against medical advice • Alive, other; or alive, not stated • Died
19. Patient's expected source of payment	Primary source Other sources All categories for primary and other sources are: • Blue Cross/Blue Shield • Other health insurance companies • Other liability insurance • Medicare

Figure 4.1.   **UHDDS data elements** *(continued)*

Data Element	Definition/Descriptor
	• Medicaid • Worker's Compensation • Self-insured employer plan • Health maintenance organization (HMO) • CHAMPUS • CHAMPVA • Other government payers • Self-pay • No charge (free, charity, special research, teaching) • Other
20. Total charges	All charges billed by the hospital for this hospitalization. Professional charges for individual patient care by physicians are excluded.

Uniform Ambulatory Care Data Set

Ambulatory care includes medical and surgical care provided to patients who depart from the facility on the same day they receive care. The care is provided in physicians' offices, medical clinics, same-day surgery centers, outpatient hospital clinics and diagnostic departments, emergency treatment centers, and hospital emergency departments. Patients who receive ambulatory care services in hospital-based clinics and departments are referred to as **outpatients**.

Since the 1980s, the number and the length of inpatient hospitalizations have gone down dramatically. At the same time, the number of healthcare procedures performed in ambulatory settings has gone up. There are several reasons for this trend, including:

- Technological improvements in diagnostic and therapeutic procedures and the development of short-acting anesthetics have made it possible to perform many medical and surgical procedures in ambulatory facilities. Surgical procedures that once required inpatient hospitalization and long recovery periods now are being performed in same-day surgery centers.

- Third-party payers have extended coverage to include most procedures performed on an outpatient basis.

- Medicare's acute inpatient hospital prospective payment system limits reimbursement for inpatient care and, in effect, encourages the use of ambulatory and/or outpatient care as an alternative to more costly inpatient services.

Like hospitals, ambulatory care organizations depend on having accurate data and information. A standardized data set to guide the content and structure of ambulatory health records and data collection systems in ambulatory care was needed.

In 1989, NCVHS approved the **Uniform Ambulatory Care Data Set** (UACDS). The committee recommended its use in every facility where ambulatory care is delivered. Several of the data elements that make up the UACDS are similar to those used in the UHDDS. For example, the UACDS data elements that describe the personal identifier, residence, date of birth, gender, and race/ethnicity of the patient are the same as the definitions in the UHDDS. The reason for keeping the same demographic data elements is to make it easier to compare data for inpatients and ambulatory patients in the same facility as well as among different facilities.

The UACDS also includes data elements specific to ambulatory care, such as the reason for the encounter with the healthcare provider. Additionally, it includes optional data elements to describe the patient's living arrangements and marital status. These data elements (shown in figure 4.2) are unique to the UACDS. Ambulatory care practitioners need information about the living conditions of their patients because patients and their families often need to manage at-home nursing care (such as activity restrictions after a surgical procedure). Hospital staff members provide such nursing services in acute care settings.

The goal of the UACDS is to improve data comparison in ambulatory and outpatient care settings. It provides uniform definitions that help providers analyze patterns of care. The data elements in the UACDS are those most likely to be needed by a variety of users. Unlike the UHDDS, the UACDS has not been incorporated into federal regulations. Therefore, it is a recommended, rather than a required, data set. In practical terms, it has been subsumed by other data definition efforts, most notably the **core data elements** recommended as part of the **Standards and Interoperability (S&I) Framework**, described later in this chapter.

Resident Assessment Instrument (RAI) and Minimum Data Set

Uniform data collection is likewise important in the long-term care setting. Long-term care incorporates the healthcare services provided in residential facilities for individuals who are unable to live independently because of a chronic illness or disability. Long-term care facilities also provide dietary and social services as well as housing and nursing care. To participate in the Medicare and Medicaid programs, long-term care facilities must develop a comprehensive functional assessment for every resident. From this assessment, a nursing home resident's plan of care is developed.

The RAI process is a federally mandated standard assessment used to collect demographic and clinical data on residents in a Medicare and/or Medicaid-certified long-term care facility. It consists of three components, the **Minimum Data Set** (**MDS) Version 3.0**, the Care Area Assessment (CAA) process, and the RAI utilization guidelines (CMS 2012). To meet federal requirements, long-term care facilities must complete an assessment for every resident at the time of admission and at designated reassessment points throughout the resident's stay.

The MDS is far more extensive and includes more clinical data than either the UHDDS or the UACDS.

Figure 4.2.   **UACDS data elements**

Data Element	Definition/Descriptor
Provider identification, address, type of practice	Provider identification: Include the full name of the provider as well as the unique physician identification number (UPIN). Address: The complete address of the provider's office. In cases where the provider has multiple offices, the location of the usual or principal place of practice should be given. Profession: • Physician including specialty or field of practice • Other (specify)
Place of encounter	Specify the location of the encounter: • Private office • Clinic or health center • Hospital outpatient department • Hospital emergency department • Other (specify)
Reason for encounter	Includes, but is not limited to, the patient's complaints and symptoms reflecting his or her own perception of needs, provided verbally or in writing by the patient at the point of entry into the healthcare system, or the patient's own words recorded by an intermediary or provider at that time.
Diagnostic services	Includes all diagnostic services of any type.
Problem, diagnosis, or assessment	Describes the provider's level of understanding and the interpretation of the patient's reasons for the encounter and all conditions requiring treatment or management at the time of the encounter.
Therapeutic services	List by name all services done or ordered: • Medical (including drug therapy) • Surgical • Patient education
Preventive services	List by name all preventive services and procedures performed at the time of the encounter.
Disposition	The provider's statement of the next step(s) in the care of the patient. At a minimum, the following classification is suggested: 1. No follow-up planned 2. Follow-up planned • Return when necessary • Return to the current provider at a specified time • Telephone follow-up • Returned to referring provider • Referred to other provider • Admit to hospital • Other

Source: Adapted from Hanken and Water 1994.

The MDS organizes data according to 20 main categories. Each category includes a structured list of choices and responses. The use of structured lists automatically standardizes the data that are collected. The major categories of data collected in the MDS include:

1. Identification information
2. Hearing, speech, and vision
3. Cognitive patterns
4. Mood
5. Behavior
6. Preferences for customary routine and activities
7. Functional status
8. Bladder and bowel
9. Active disease diagnosis
10. Health conditions
11. Swallowing/Nutritional status
12. Oral/Dental status
13. Skin conditions
14. Medications
15. Special treatments and procedures
16. Restraints
17. Participation in assessment and goal setting
18. Care area assessment (CAA) summary
19. Correction request
20. Assessment administration

The data collected by the MDS are used to develop care plans for residents and to document placement at the appropriate level of care. The MDS is also used as a data collection tool to classify Medicare residents into RUGs (Resource Utilization Groups), a system used in the PPS for skilled nursing facilities, hospital swing bed programs, and in many state Medicaid case-mix payment systems. Another use of the MDS assessment data is the monitoring of the quality of care in the nation's nursing homes through MDS-based quality indicators (QIs) and quality measures (QMs).

Because the MDS is used nationwide to collect data about residents in long-term care facilities, the data can and will be used as a basis for identifying and assessing resident safety and quality improvement activities in nursing homes. For example, MDS data can give valuable information about the incidence of falls and their impact on the care of nursing home residents. From those data, prevention measures can be developed and implemented to address a common and significant problem in elderly care.

Outcomes and Assessment Information Set

The **Outcomes and Assessment Information Set** (OASIS-C) is a standardized data set designed to gather and report data about Medicare beneficiaries who are receiving services from a Medicare-certified home health agency. OASIS-C includes a set of core data items that are collected on all adult home health patients whose care is reimbursed by Medicare and Medicaid with the exception of patients receiving pre- or postnatal services only.

The OASIS-C data set became effective January 1, 2010. OASIS-C includes process items that support measurement of evidence-based practices across the post-acute care spectrum that have been shown to prevent exacerbation of serious conditions, can improve care received by individual patients, and can provide guidance to agencies on how to improve care and avoid adverse events. OASIS-C contains more than 30 data elements.

OASIS-C data are grouped into the following categories (CMS 2011):

- Patient Tracking Items
- Clinical Record Items
- Patient History and Diagnoses
- Living Arrangements
- Sensory Status
- Integumentary Status
- Respiratory Status
- Cardiac Status
- Elimination Status
- Neuro/Emotional/Behavioral Status
- Activities of Daily Living (ADLs)/Instrumental Activities of Daily Living (IADLs)
- Medications
- Care Management
- Therapy Need and Plan of Care
- Emergent Care
- Discharge

Data collected through OASIS-C are used to assess the patient's ability to be discharged or transferred from home care services. The data are also used in measuring patient outcomes in order to assess the quality of home healthcare services. Under the prospective payment program for home health, implemented in 2000, data from OASIS-C also form the basis of reimbursement for provided services. In addition, these data are used to create patient case mix profile reports and patient outcome reports that are used by state survey staff in the certification process. Home health agency quality measures that appear on the CMS Home Health Compare website are also based on OASIS-C data.

Healthcare Effectiveness Data and Information Set

The **Healthcare Effectiveness Data and Information Set** (HEDIS) is sponsored by the National Committee for Quality Assurance (NCQA). HEDIS is a set of standard performance measures designed to provide healthcare purchasers and consumers with the information they need to compare the performance of managed healthcare plans.

HEDIS is designed to collect administrative, claims, and health record review data. It collects standardized data about specific health-related conditions or issues so that the success of various treatment plans can be assessed and compared. HEDIS data form the basis of performance improvement (PI) efforts for health plans. They also are used to develop physician profiles. The goal of physician profiling is to positively influence physician practice patterns.

HEDIS contains more than 70 measures related to conditions such as heart disease, cancer, diabetes, asthma, chlamydia infection, osteoporosis, and rheumatoid arthritis. It includes data related to patient outcomes and data about the treatment process used by the clinician in treating the patient.

Standardized HEDIS data elements are abstracted from health records in clinics and hospitals. The health record data are combined with enrollment and claims data and analyzed according to HEDIS specifications.

An example of a HEDIS measure is comprehensive diabetes care. Other examples of HEDIS effectiveness of care measures include:

- Adolescent immunizations
- Medical assistance with smoking and tobacco use cessation
- Antidepressant medication management
- Breast cancer screening
- Cholesterol management for patients with cardiovascular conditions
- Follow-up care for children prescribed ADHD medication

Health plans often release data from HEDIS studies publicly to document substantial positive effects on the health of their clients. Results are compared over time and with data from other sources. From the data, health plans determine opportunities for performance improvement and develop potential interventions.

HEDIS is an example of a population-based data collection tool. It illustrates the need for developing standardized data definitions and uniform collection methods. It also emphasizes the importance of data quality management.

Data Elements for Emergency Departments

Emergency and trauma care in the United States are very sophisticated. Emergency services represent a large part of healthcare delivery. As services increase, it is more and more important to collect relevant aggregate data about emergency and trauma care. Many states require the reporting of trauma cases to state agencies.

In 1997, the Centers for Disease Control and Prevention (CDC) through its National Center for Injury Prevention and Control (NCIPC) published a data set called **Data Elements for Emergency Department Systems** (DEEDS) 1.0. The purpose of this data set is to support the uniform collection of data in hospital-based emergency departments and to reduce incompatibilities in emergency department records.

DEEDS recommends the collection of 156 data elements in hospitals that offer emergency care services. As with the UHDDS and UACDS, this data set contains recommendations on both the content and the structure of the data elements to be collected. The data are organized into the following eight sections:

- Patient identification data

- Facility and practitioner identification data

- Emergency department payment data

- Emergency department arrival and first-assessment data

- Emergency department history and physical examination data

- Emergency department procedure and result data

- Emergency department medication data

- Emergency department disposition and diagnosis data

DEEDS incorporates national standards for **electronic data interchange** (EDI), so its implementation in an EHR system can make possible communication and integration with other information systems (NCIPC 2006).

The Health Level Seven (HL7) Emergency Care Work Group has begun the process of updating and revising DEEDS 1.0 with the intent to expand the scope of DEEDS to harmonize with the prehospital arena, disaster response systems, and the needs of secondary data users such as the CDC and public health agencies (HL7 2011).

Core Measures for ORYX

The Joint Commission (TJC) is one of the largest users of healthcare data and information. Its primary function is the accreditation of hospitals and other healthcare organizations. In 1997, the TJC introduced the **ORYX initiative** to integrate outcomes data and other performance measurement data into its accreditation processes. (The initiative was named ORYX after an African animal that can be thought of as a different kind of zebra.) The goal of the initiative is to promote a comprehensive, continuous, data-driven accreditation process for healthcare facilities (TJC 2012).

The ORYX initiative uses nationally standardized performance measures to improve the safety and quality of healthcare. The ORYX initiative integrates outcomes and other performance measures into the accreditation process through data collection about specific core measures (TJC 2012). The **core measures** are based on selected diagnoses/conditions such as diabetes mellitus, the outcomes of which can be improved by standardizing care. They include the minimum number of data elements needed to provide an accurate and reliable measure of performance. Core measures rely on data elements that are readily available or already collected. The Joint Commission is in the process of reclassifying the core measures as accountability measures.

Data Sets for Interoperable Electronic Information Exchange

ARRA and HITECH provided funding to support the adoption of qualified EHRs. Their subsequent regulations define the meaningful use of HIT systems. To meet the meaningful use requirements, the submission of information on clinical quality measures is necessary. Formed by the National Quality Forum with support from the Agency for Healthcare Research and Quality (AHRQ), the **Health Information Technology Expert Panel** (HITEP) was tasked with creating a better link between current quality measurement and EHR reporting capabilities. The HITEP Quality Data Set (QDS) Workgroup developed a QDS framework, which includes standard elements, quality data elements, and data flow attributes (NQF 2009).

The QDS, now known as the Quality Data Model (QDM), has undergone several revisions. However, its underlying purpose remains. According to NQF (2011), the QDM "clearly defines concepts used in quality measures and clinical care and is intended to enable automation of structured data capture in EHRs, PHRs, and other clinical applications. It provides a grammar to describe clinical concepts in a standardized format so individuals (i.e., providers, researchers, or measure developers) monitoring clinical performance and outcomes can concisely communicate necessary information."

The QDM element, which is defined as an atomic unit of information that has precise meaning to communicate the data required within a quality measure, provides unambiguous definition and enables consistent capture and use of data for quality measurement (NQF 2011).

One of the government's health outcomes policy priorities used to create the framework for meaningful use of EHRs is to improve care coordination. A key to interoperable electronic information exchange is having defined core data sets. **ASTM International** (ASTM) was instrumental in identifying a core data set for a patient's clinical summary with the publication in 2005 of ASTM E2369-05e2 Standard Specification for **Continuity of Care Record** (CCR). The CCR core data set is shown in figure 4.3.

Another organization, Health Level Seven (HL7), developed the CDA. The CDA provides an exchange model for clinical documents (such as discharge summaries and progress notes). It also makes documents machine-readable so that they can be easily processed electronically and makes them human-readable so that they can be retrieved easily and used by the people who need them.

ASTM and HL7 combined their work to create the **Continuity of Care Document** (CCD). The CCD is an implementation guide for sharing CCR patient summary data using the CDA. The CCD was recognized as part of the first set of interoperability standards. The CCR, CDA, and CCD will be discussed later in this chapter.

Continuing the work toward interoperability is the transitions of care (ToC) initiative, one of the projects of the Standards and Interoperability (S&I) Framework. According to the initiative's charter (S&I Framework 2011a para 1), "The exchange of clinical summaries is hampered by ambiguous common definitions of what data elements must at a minimum be exchanged, how they must be encoded, and how those common semantic elements map to MU specified formats (C32/CCD and CCR)." An outcome of the initiative is a clinical information model (CIM) "consisting of unambiguous, clinically-relevant definitions of the core data elements that should be included in care transitions" (ONC 2011a slide 4). The core data element categories are demographics, active medication list, active problem list, and intolerances including allergies. Figure 4.4 lists the core data elements for the active problem list category.

Figure 4.3.   Continuity of Care Record core data set

• Patient administrative and clinical data • Medical devices or equipment needed by the patient

• Patient administrative and clinical data

• Basic information about the patient's payer

• Advance directives

• Patient's sources of support

• Patient's current functional status

• Problems

• Family history

• Social history

• Alerts

• Medications

• Medical devices or equipment needed by the patient

• Immunization history

• Vital signs (as appropriate)

• Results of laboratory, diagnostic, and therapeutic results

• Diagnostic and therapeutic procedures

• Encounters

• Plan of care

• Healthcare providers

Source: Reprinted, with permission, from E2369, copyright ASTM International, 100 Barr Harbor Drive, West Conshohocken, PA 19428. A copy of the complete standard may be obtained from ASTM International, www.astm.org.

Figure 4.4.   Active problem list

• Coded Problem(s) or no known problem(s)

• Start Date (or date of onset) of problem(s)

• Clinician who added it to the problem list (include date/time stamp)

• Reconciled (Yes or No)

• Reconciled by? Date/Time Stamp

• Resolved and/or changed problems in this encounter

Note: What clinician sending the message has determined to be the patient's active problems and/or diagnoses or determination of no known problems—this list may be reconciled at each ToC.

Source: S&I Framework 2011b.

Check Your Understanding 4.1

1. Which of the following is designed to collect a minimum set of data about inpatients?

   A. DRGs
   B. NCHS
   C. UACDS
   D. UHDDS

2. Which of the following is used to collect data about ambulatory care patients?

   A. DRGs
   B. MDS
   C. ORYX
   D. UACDS

3. Which of the following is used to collect data about long-term care residents?

   A. NCHS
   B. MDS
   C. UACDS
   D. UHDDS

4. Which of the following provides a structured way to develop a long-term care resident care plan?

   A. MDS
   B. OASIS-C
   C. UACHD
   D. UHDDS

5. Which of the following is used to gather data about Medicare beneficiaries receiving home care?

   A. MDS
   B. NCHS
   C. OASIS-C
   D. UHDDS

6. Which of the following best describes the DEEDS data set?

   A. Uses data for home health outcomes research
   B. Collects data about hospital emergency encounters
   C. Uses data for inpatient analysis
   D. Collects data for ambulatory care

7. Which of the following is a set of performance measures used to compare the performance of managed healthcare plans?

   A. DEEDS
   B. HEDIS
   C. ORYX
   D. UHDDS

8. Which of the following was developed by the Joint Commission?

    A. HEDIS
    B. MDS
    C. OASIS-C
    D. ORYX

9. Which of the following would be a core data set for a patient's clinical summary?

    A. CDA
    B. CCR
    C. CCD
    D. QDS

10. The Resident Assessment Instrument is triggered by the data collected by the:

    A. Core measures
    B. DEEDS
    C. MDS
    D. HEDIS

Standards for Electronic Data and Electronic Data Interchange

The original uniform data sets such as the UHDDS and the UACDS were created for use in paper-based (manual) health record systems. They were not designed to accommodate the data needs of the current healthcare delivery system or the demands of EHRs and clinical information systems.

Standards are needed in order for data to be easily, accurately, and securely communicated and exchanged electronically among various computer systems. This is referred to as interoperability. Without standards for interoperability, EHRs and the NHIN will not realize their full benefits (Thompson and Brailer 2004).

Many types of standards are being developed to support the EHR and health information exchange. Some involve defining record structure and content, others specify technical approaches for transmitting data, and still others provide rules for protecting the privacy and security of data.

Public and private organizations have been actively engaged in the process of developing healthcare informatics standards to support EHR development, interoperability, and information exchange. The federal government supports this work in a variety of ways. One example is the S&I Framework. According to Fridsma (2010 slide 4), the Framework "is the mechanism by which ONC will manage the implementation of specifications and the harmonization of existing health IT standards to promote interoperability nationwide."

Definition of Data Standard for Electronic Data Exchange

Data standards provide the ability to record a certain data item in accordance with the agreed upon standard (Giannangelo 2007). Data content standards are "clear guidelines for the acceptable values for specified data fields" (Fenton et al. 2007). Data exchange standards are protocols that help ensure that data transmitted from one system to another remain comparable.

One of the purposes of HIPAA's Administrative Simplification rules was to standard-ize information exchange and in August 2000, the **Department of Health and Human Services (HHS)** published regulations for electronic transactions. These regulations apply to transactions that occur among healthcare providers and healthcare plans and payers (Rode 2001). The long-term goal of the **transaction standards** is to allow providers and plans or payers to seamlessly transfer data back and forth with little intervention. To do this, HHS adopted the electronic transaction standards of ASC X12 Insurance Subcom-mittee (Accredited Standards Committee Health Care Task group [X12N]). The standards adopted for EDI are called ANSI ASC X12N.

The HIPAA standards also include code sets standards for the electronic exchange of health-related information. To illustrate how the adoption and utilization of standards for data representation and data exchange facilitates billing functions, consider the codes sets are data standards used to identify specific data elements such as the diagnosis on a claim. The compendium of data elements on the claim form make up a data set. In order to send the diagnosis and other items that make up the data set electronically, the healthcare pro-vider uses the ASC X12N 837 messaging standard. The 837 specifies the format for each data element. For example, one specification for the format of the diagnosis would be that diagnosis codes have a maximum size of seven (7) characters.

A new version of the standard for electronic healthcare transactions (Version 5010 of the X12 standard) was approved in 2009 and implemented in 2012. This new version is essential to the use of ICD-10-CM and ICD-10-PCS codes that are slated for implementa-tion in 2013.

Data Needs in an Electronic Environment

As discussed in chapter 16, healthcare organizations often have several different computer systems operating at the same time. For example, a hospital's laboratory system might be entirely separate from its billing system. In fact, the various departments of large health-care organizations often use different operating systems and are serviced by different ven-dors. In addition to operating multiple systems, it is an ongoing challenge to integrate information from legacy (older) systems operating on old platforms with state-of-the art information systems.

Healthcare organizations must integrate data that originate in various databases within facilities as well as in databases outside the facility. They also must be able to respond to requests to transfer data to other facilities, payers, accrediting and regulating agencies, quality improvement organizations, and other information users. These goals can only be accomplished when every database system is either operating on the same platform or using common standards.

Benefits of Data Exchange Standards

Healthcare informatics standards describe accepted methods for collecting, maintaining, and/or transferring healthcare data among computer systems. These standards are designed to provide a common language that makes it easy to:

- Exchange information
- Share information
- Communicate within and across disciplines and settings
- Integrate disparate data systems
- Compare information at a regional, national, and international level
- Link data in a secure environment

Having the ability to exchange, share, communicate, integrate, compare, and link data is important to healthcare delivery. These activities make possible important activities such as:

- Disease surveillance
- Health and healthcare population monitoring
- Outcomes research
- Decision making and policy development

The long-term vision is to enhance the comparability, quality, integrity, and utility of health information from a wide variety of public sources through uniform data policies and standards (NCVHS 2001). Thompson and Brailer (2004, 13) expressed the federal commitment to standards in their statement that "A key component of progress in interoperable health information is the development of technically sound and robustly specified interoperability standards and policies." In 2010, states, eligible territories, and qualified State Designated Entities received awards from ONC to assist them in facilitating the secure exchange of health information in order to advance state-level health information exchange while moving toward nationwide interoperability. The ONC expects the funding to be used to increase connectivity, enable patient-centric information flow to improve the quality and efficiency of care, and ensure healthcare providers and hospitals meet national standards (ONC 2011b).

Many types of standards are necessary to implement EHRs and a health information technology infrastructure that supports connectivity, interoperability, and seamless data interchange. International, national, state and regional or local standards ensure communication and efficiency and minimization of duplication of effort along the continuum of healthcare. It is especially important to note that healthcare is provided locally and standards must be adopted at the local level to achieve the full benefit of an EHR.

American Recovery and Reinvestment Act

Officially known as the American Recovery and Reinvestment Act (ARRA P.L. 111-5) and Health Information Technology for Economic and Clinical Health Act (HITECH), the "Stimulus Law" was signed on February 17, 2009. ARRA provides $19.2 billion in spending on health IT. Title XIII of ARRA, given a subtitle, "Health Information Technology for Economic and Clinical Health Act (HITECH)," deals with many of the health information communication and technology provisions.

Office of National Coordinator

ARRA includes the statutory authorization of ONC, which makes ONC a permanent office under HHS (Asmonga 2009). Its charge is to help develop a national health IT infrastructure to improve the quality and efficiency of healthcare and the ability of consumers to manage their care and safety. ARRA stipulated $2 billion to ONC for use as follows (Asmonga 2009):

- $20 million: to advance healthcare information enterprise integration through technical standards analysis and establishment of conformance testing infrastructure to be done by the **National Institute of Standards and Technology** (NIST) and coordinated with ONC

- $300 million: to support regional or subnational efforts toward health information exchange

- Remaining funds: to the immediate implementation assistance to support:

  — Health IT architecture

  — Development and adoption of certified electronic health records (EHRs) for categories of healthcare providers not eligible for support under title XVIII or XIX of the Social Security Administration for the adoption of such records

  — Training on best practices to integrate health IT

  — Infrastructure and tools for the promotion of telemedicine

  — Promotion of the interoperability of clinical data repositories or registries

  — Promotion of technologies and best practices

  — Improvement and expansion of the use of health IT by public health departments

The ONC published a final rule establishing standards, implementation specifications, and certification criteria for the certification of EHR technology to support the achievement of meaningful use Stage 1 by eligible professionals and eligible hospitals under the Medicare and Medicaid EHR incentive programs in 2010. Stage 1 standards, which took effect in 2011, fall into three categories: content exchange, vocabulary, and privacy and security (ONC 2010). Transport standards were proposed but removed in the final rule. These standards will be discussed later in this chapter.

Health Information Technology (HIT) Policy Committee and HIT Standards Committee

Two official HHS advisory committees established as a result of ARRA are the **HIT Policy Committee** (HITPC) and the **HIT Standards Committee** (HITSC). The HIT Policy Committee provides recommendations to the National Coordinator on a policy framework for the development and adoption of a nationwide health information technology infrastructure that permits the electronic exchange and use of health information as is consistent with the Federal Health IT Strategic Plan and that includes recommendations on the areas in which standards, implementation specifications, and certification criteria are needed.

The HIT Standards Committee provides recommendations to the National Coordinator on standards, implementation specifications, and certification criteria for the electronic exchange and use of health information for purposes of adoption, consistent with the implementation of the Federal Health IT Strategic Plan, and in accordance with policies developed by the HIT Policy Committee.

Standards Development, Coordination, Testing, and Harmonization

Developing, coordinating, testing, and harmonizing healthcare standards is a complex process in which many organizations are involved. The following definitions provide further information on standards and harmonization (HITSP 2009):

The term **standard** . . . is a well-defined approach that supports a business process and:

- has been agreed upon by a group of experts

- has been publicly vetted

- provides rules, guidelines, or characteristics

- helps to ensure that materials, products, processes, and services are fit for their intended purpose

- is available in an accessible format

- is subject to an ongoing review and revision process.

Harmonization is the name given to the effort by industry to replace the variety of product standards and other regulatory policies adopted by nations, in favor of uniform global standards. Usually used in the context of trade agreements, harmonization has recently been adopted by the United States government to refer to information technology standards.

Most standards are created through a voluntary consensus process that involves identifying the need for a standard, negotiating the content of the standard, and drafting a proposed standard. The final standard is published after undergoing a comment and revision period. This process facilitates wide adoption and improved utility. Figure 4.5 describes the standards value chain.

Figure 4.5.   Standards value chain

Standards typically go through several stages in a process that can take three or more years. It begins with developers, who draft new standards or update existing ones. Profiling organizations select among applicable standards, combine the work of multiple developers, and create use scenarios for how to apply them. Typically, independent, neutral organizations test the standards, and implementers put them to work.

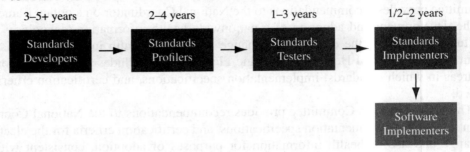

Advocates

Advocacy organizations influence and facilitate the value chain at every step. National governments are prominent standardization advocates, often sponsoring, funding, and staffing standards activities. Private-sector stakeholders include advocacy organizations such as health IT and finance advocates and software vendors, implementers, and users. Consumers also have a stake in standards, although they are underrepresented in standards advocacy.

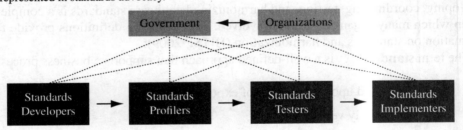

Market Stakeholders

Software vendors, implementers, and users are economic stakeholders. They influence standards development and implementation through participation and funding. Their balance of interest is both strategic and tactical.

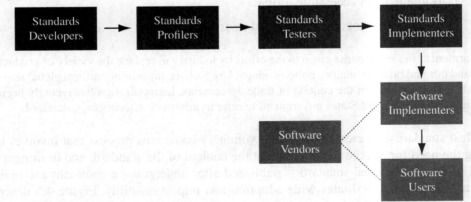

Source: Marshall 2009.

Organizations referred to as **standards development organizations** (SDOs) are involved with the creation or revisions of standards. HL7 and ASTM, for example, are both accredited SDOs. Table 4.1 provides a list of several organizations that are actively involved in developing standards for health-related information management.

Because so many organizations are developing standards, there needs to be coordination. Therefore, some organizations play key roles in coordinating the efforts of other

Table 4.1. Standards development organizations

Private or government organizations involved in the development of healthcare informatics standards at a national or international level.

Resource	Description	Source
AIIM	AIIM is an ANSI (American National Standards Institute) accredited standards development organization. AIIM also holds the Secretariat for the ISO (International Organization for Standardization) committee focused on information management compliance issues, TC171.	http://www.aiim.org
Accredited Standards Committee (ASC) X12	ASC X12 is a designated committee under the Designated Standard Maintenance Organization (DSMO), which develops uniform standards for cross-industry exchange of business transactions through electronic data interchange (EDI) standards. ASC X12 is an ANSI-accredited standards development organization.	http://www.x12.org
American Dental Association (ADA)	The ADA is an ANSI-accredited standards developing organization that develops dental standards that promote safe and effective oral healthcare.	http://www.ada.org/275.aspx
ASTM International	Formerly the American Society for Testing and Materials, ASTM International is an ANSI-accredited standards development organization that develops standards for healthcare data security, standard record content, and protocols for exchange of laboratory data.	http://www.astm.org
European Committee for Standardization (CEN)	CEN contributes to the objectives of the European Union and European Economic Area with voluntary technical standards that promote free trade, the safety of workers and consumers, interoperability of networks, environmental protection, exploitation of research and development programs, and public procurement.	http://www.cenorm.be/cenorm/index.htm
Clinical and Laboratory Standards Institute (CLSI)	A global, nonprofit, standards development organization that promotes the development and use of voluntary consensus standards and guidelines within the healthcare community. Its core business is the development of globally applicable voluntary consensus documents for healthcare testing.	http://www.clsi.org
Clinical Data Interchange Standards Consortium (CDISC)	CDISC is an open, multidisciplinary, nonprofit organization that has established worldwide industry standards to support the electronic acquisition, exchange, submission and archiving of clinical trials data and metadata for medical and biopharmaceutical product development.	http://www.cdisc.org/
Designated Standard Maintenance Organization (DSMO)	The DSMO was established in the final HIPAA rule and is charged with maintaining the standards for electronic transactions, developing or modifying an adopted standard.	http://www.hipaa-dsmo.org
Health Industry Business Communications Council (HIBCC)	HIBCC is an industry-sponsored and supported nonprofit organization. As an ANSI-accredited organization, its primary function is to facilitate electronic communications by developing standards for information exchange among healthcare trading partners.	http://www.hibcc.org/

(continued on next page)

Table 4.1. **Standards development organizations** *(continued)*

Private or government organizations involved in the development of healthcare informatics standards at a national or international level.

Resource	Description	Source
Health Level 7 (HL7)	An ANSI-accredited standards development organization that develops messaging, data content, and document standards to support the exchange of clinical information.	http://www.hl7.org
Institute of Electrical and Electronic Engineers (IEEE)	A national organization that develops standards for hospital system interface transactions, including links between critical care bedside instruments and clinical information systems.	http://www.ieee.org
International Organization for Standardization (ISO)	ISO is a nongovernmental organization and network of national standards institutes from 157 countries.	http://www.iso.org/iso/en/ISOOnline.frontpage
National Council for Prescription Drug Programs (NCPDP)	A designated committee under the Designated Standard Maintenance Organization (DSMO) that specializes in developing standards for exchanging prescription and payment information.	http://www.ncpdp.org
National Information Standards Organization (NISO)	An ANSI-accredited, nonprofit association that identifies, develops, maintains, and publishes technical standards to manage information. NISO standards address areas of retrieval, re-purposing, storage, metadata, and preservation.	http://www.niso.org
National Uniform Billing Committee (NUBC)	A designated committee under the Designated Standard Maintenance Organization (DSMO) that is responsible for identifying data elements and designing the CMS-1500.	http://www.nubc.org
National Uniform Claim Committee (NUCC)	The national group that replaces the Uniform Claim Form Task Force in 1995 and developed a standard data set to be used in the transmission of noninstitutional provider claims to and from third-party payers.	http://www.nucc.org

Source: AHIMA 2007.

SDOs. The **American National Standards Institute** (ANSI) is one example. It coordinates the development of voluntary standards in a variety of industries, including healthcare. Most SDOs in the United States are members of ANSI. ISO coordinates international standards development. ANSI represents the United States at the ISO.

Some other projects that coordinate healthcare standards are the National Library of Medicine's Unified Medical Language System (UMLS) and the USHIK.

The UMLS's Metathesaurus is a centralized vocabulary database that includes more than a hundred vocabularies, classifications, and code sets. Source vocabularies found in the Metathesaurus include those designed for use in patient-record systems such as SNOMED CT as well as those used for healthcare billing such as ICD-9-CM. The code sets mandated for use in electronic administrative transactions in the United States under the provisions of HIPAA are found in the Metathesaurus with the exception of the National Drug Codes (NDC) which are available from the FDA.

The USHIK is a computer-based health metadata registry funded and directed by the AHRQ with CMS and the Veterans Administration as strategic inter-agency partners. It is populated with the data elements and information models of SDO and other healthcare organizations in such a way that public and private organizations can harmonize information formats with healthcare standards. The knowledge base also contains data element information for government initiatives supporting the use and implementation of data standards (for example, HIPAA) and the federal health architecture program.

ARRA called for ONC, in consultation with NIST, to recognize a program for the voluntary certification of health information technology as being in compliance with applicable certification criteria to meet defined meaningful use requirements. In collaboration with ONC, NIST has developed the necessary functional and conformance testing requirements, test cases, and test tools in support of the health IT certification program. The NIST is a non-regulatory agency of the U.S. Department of Commerce.

At present, one of the most challenging aspects of the standards movement is the area of standards harmonization. In 2011, the HITSC Clinical Quality Workgroup and Vocabulary Task Force were tasked with selecting the minimum number of vocabulary standards with the minimum number of values to meet the requirements of meaningful use stages 2 and 3. Content exchange standards are being reviewed as well with the same goal to harmonize HIT standards. It will take the cooperation and collaboration of many, especially the HIM profession, to harmonize HIT standards and implementation guides for the purpose of interoperability and health information exchange HIE.

Types of Standards

Many types of standards are necessary to implement EHRs and a health information technology infrastructure that supports connectivity, interoperability, and seamless data interchange. While progress with standards harmonization and consolidation has occurred, there are still hundreds of standards. Thus, it is impossible to discuss them all in this chapter. Those better-known standards HIM professionals may work with are addressed here. Other chapters, such as chapter 5 Clinical Vocabularies and Classification Systems, provide additional information on specific standards.

Record Structure and Content Standards

Structure and content standards establish and provide clear and uniform definitions of the data elements to be included in EHR systems. They specify the type of data to be collected in each data field and the attributes and values of each data field, all of which are captured in data dictionaries.

ASTM Standard E1384-02a 07

ASTM International is an SDO that develops standards for a variety of industries in the United States. The ASTM Technical Committee on Healthcare Informatics E31 is charged with the responsibility for developing standards related to the EHR. E31 works through subcommittees assigned to various aspects of this endeavor.

The ASTM Subcommittee E31.25 on Healthcare Data Management, Security, Confidentiality, and Privacy developed ASTM Standard E1384-02a 07. This standard identifies the content and structure for EHRs. The scope of this standard covers all types of healthcare services, including acute care hospitals, ambulatory care, skilled nursing facilities, home healthcare, and specialty environments. It applies to short-term contacts such as EDs and emergency medical care services as well as long-term care contacts.

HL7 EHR-S Functional Model and Standards

HL7 provides a comprehensive framework and related standards for the exchange, integration, sharing, and retrieval of electronic health information that supports clinical practice and the management, delivery, and evaluation of health services. It provides a reference list of functions that may be present in an EHR-S (http://www.HL7.org). Figure 4.6 shows the HL7 EHR-S Functional Model. HL7 developed the HL7 EHR-S Functional Model and Standards that address the content and structure of an EHR. The purpose of the functional model is to provide a foundation for common understanding of possible and useful functions of EHR systems.

Content Exchange Standards

Content exchange standards complement record content and structure and vocabulary standards. These standards provide the rules, often called protocols, of how data are actually transmitted from one computer system to another. Content exchange standards supply the specifications for the format of data exchanges, thereby providing the ability to send and receive medical and administrative data in an understandable and usable manner across information systems.

CCR, CDA, and CCD

The CCR standard is a core data set of relevant current and past information about a patient's health status and healthcare treatment. The CCR was created to help

Figure 4.6.   ANSI/HL7 EHR System Functional Model, R1-2007

ANSI/HL7 EHR System Functional Model, R1-2007		
Direct Care	DC.1	Care Management
	DC.2	Clinical Decision Support
	DC.3	Operations Management & Communication
Supportive	S.1	Clinical Support
	S.2	Measurement, Analysis, Research & Reports
	S.3	Administrative & Financial
Information Infrastructure	IN.1	Security
	IN.2	Health Record Information & Management
	IN.3	Registry & Directory Services
	IN.4	Standard Terminologies & Terminology Services
	IN.5	Standards-based Interoperability
	IN.6	Business Rules Management
	IN.7	Workflow Management

communicate that information from one provider to another for referral, transfer, or discharge of the patient or when the patient wishes to create a personal health record. Data from a CCR may also be incorporated into a personal health record. Because it utilizes XML codes, it enhances interoperability and allows its preparation, transmission, and viewing in multiple ways. The CCR is designed to be organized and transportable. It is sponsored by a consortium of healthcare organizations, practitioners, and other stakeholders. The CCR is the other content exchange option available for meeting the requirement for EHR Technology to be certified as being capable of electronically exchanging a patient summary record for stage 1.

HL7 is a SDO that provides standards, guidelines, and methodologies that make data exchange possible among hospitals, physician practices, and other types of provider systems. For example, the standards consist of rules for transmitting demographic data, orders, patient observations, laboratory results, history and physical observations, and findings. They also include message rules for appointment scheduling, referrals, problem list maintenance, and care plans.

The HL7 CDA provides an exchange model for clinical documents (such as discharge summaries and progress notes) and brings the healthcare industry closer to the realization of an EHR. The CDA standard makes documents machine-readable so that they can be easily processed electronically. It also makes documents human-readable so that they can be retrieved easily and used by the people who need them.

ASTM and HL7 negotiated a memorandum of understanding to bring ASTM's CCR initiative into line with HL7's EHR functionality and CDA standards. The CCD was developed as a collaborative effort between ASTM and HL7 to leverage CDA with the CCR specifications. As the use of the CCD increases, it is likely to become the common health information exchange (HIE) methodology between the EHR and PHR systems.

Institute of Electrical and Electronics Engineers 1073

The **Institute of Electrical and Electronics Engineers** (IEEE) 1073 provides for open-systems communications in healthcare applications, primarily between bedside medical devices and patient care information systems, optimized for the acute care setting. The IEEE 1073 series was adopted as a federal health information interoperability standard for electronic data exchange (ONC 2006).

The IEEE 1073 series of standards pertains to connectivity. The standard specifically addresses the requirement for two devices to automatically configure a connection for successful operation, independent of connection type. The standard defines a device-to-device internal messaging system that allows hospitals and other healthcare providers to achieve plug-and-play interoperability between medical instrumentation and electronic healthcare information systems, especially in a manner that is compatible with the acute care environment.

Digital Imaging and Communication in Medicine

Through a cooperative effort between the **American College of Radiology and the National Electrical Manufacturers Association** (ACR-NEMA), **Digital Imaging and**

Communication in Medicine (DICOM) was originally created to permit the interchange of biomedical image wave forms and related information.

DICOM is used by most medical professions that use imaging within the healthcare industry, such as cardiology, dentistry, endoscopy, mammography, ophthalmology, and orthopedics. DICOM was adopted as the federal health information interoperability messaging standard for imaging in March 2003 (ONC 2006).

Vocabulary Standards

Vocabulary standards include vocabularies, code sets, and nomenclatures. These standards go hand in hand with other health informatics standards such as those for information modeling and metadata. Vocabulary standards establish common definitions for medical terms to encourage consistent descriptions of an individual's condition in the health record. Having established standards for clinical data enables consistent definition of data elements. These systems are explored thoroughly in chapter 5.

Privacy and Security Standards

HIPAA mandated the adoption of privacy and security protection for identifiable health information. HIPAA privacy standards have been implemented throughout the healthcare industry to protect personal health information and define appropriate use and disclosure.

Security standards ensure that patient-identifiable health information remains confidential and protected from unauthorized disclosure, alteration, or destruction. Effective security standards are especially important in computer-based environments because patient information is accessible to many users in many locations. Many standards organizations—most notably, the ASTM and HL7—have developed security standards, but no single standard currently addresses all of the HIPAA provisions. Privacy is addressed in chapter 13 and security is addressed in chapter 17.

Check Your Understanding 4.2

1. Which of the following best describes an SDO?

   A. Coordinates standards groups
   B. Develops standards
   C. Develops data sets
   D. Develops best practices

2. Which of the following should be used to communicate information from one provider to another for referral, transfer, or discharge of the patient?

   A. CDA
   B. CCR
   C. HL7
   D. ORYX

3. Which of the following was adopted as the federal health information interoperability messaging standard for imaging?

    A. DEED
    B. DICOM
    C. IEEE
    D. NHIN

4. Which SDO develops messaging, data content, and document standards to support the exchange of clinical information?

    A. IEEE
    B. DSMO
    C. NUBC
    D. HL7

5. Which of these standards is a standard for communication between bedside medical devices and patient care information systems?

    A. ASTM Standard E1384-02a 07
    B. LOINC
    C. HL7 CDA
    D. IEEE 1073

6. One of the two official HHS advisory groups established as a result of ARRA responsible for making recommendations to the National Coordinator is:

    A. Certification Commission for Health Information Technology
    B. HL7
    C. HIT Policy Committee
    D. Accredited Standards Committee Health Care Task group

7. Which standard assists in the sharing of information from one provider to another for patient care?

    A. ASTM CCR
    B. LOINC
    C. HL7 CDA
    D. DICOM

8. What organization coordinates the efforts of other SDOs?

    A. ANSI
    B. HL7
    C. ASTM
    D. ARRA

9. What type of standard establishes common definitions for medical terms?

    A. Content exchange
    B. Interoperability
    C. Record structure and content
    D. Vocabulary

Emerging Health Information Standards

The development of healthcare informatics standards is far from complete. The task is critically important to the development of EHR systems and, ultimately, to implementation of a national health information infrastructure. Leading standards groups are continuously working to reach consensus on a variety of standards, but many issues remain unresolved.

Extensible Markup Language (XML)

A key technology tool for enabling data sharing is called **extensible markup language** (XML). XML was developed as a universal language to facilitate the storage and transmission of data published on the Internet. Markup languages communicate electronic representations of paper documents to computers by inserting additional information into text (Sokolowski 1999).

For example, the CCR standard specifies XML coding that allows users to prepare, transmit, and view the CCR in multiple ways such as in a browser, as an element in a HL7 message, or CDA compliant document, or as a word processing document (ASTM 2009).

Another XML-based standard, the Structured Product Labeling (SPL), is a document markup standard approved by HL7 and adopted by Food and Drug Administration (FDA) as a mechanism for exchanging product information (FDA 2012).

Metadata Standards

AHIMA (2012) defines metadata as "Descriptive data that characterize other data to create a clearer understanding of their meaning and to achieve greater reliability and quality of information. Metadata consist of both indexing terms and attributes. Data about data: for example, creation date, date sent, date received, last access date, last modification date" (221). Metadata standards would be standards that support descriptive data that characterize other data to create a clearer understanding of their meaning and to achieve greater reliability and quality of information.

CDA documents are also encoded in XML. CDA is cited throughout an ONC advance notice of proposed rule making published on August 9, 2011. This notice solicited comments on **metadata** standards to support nationwide electronic health information exchange. Initial categories of metadata under consideration as a minimum set include patient identity, provenance, and privacy in association with a patient obtaining their summary care record from a health care provider (ONC 2011c). Following the notice, the ONC announced the launch of two pilot programs which will test the metadata standards. At the time of publication, a determination had not been made as to whether EHR technology should be capable of applying the metadata standards as part of EHR certification requirements supporting meaningful use under Stage 2 of the Medicare and Medicaid EHR Incentive programs.

Role of HIM Professional

As the domain experts in health record data content, HIM professionals have a large role to play in overseeing healthcare data sets and standards for their organizations. As paper disappears and electronic information environments appear, the HIM professional will be called upon to coordinate and manage the organization's data requirements. HIM professionals have the opportunity to serve as leaders in healthcare organizations and in their professional community to ensure data content standards are identified, understood, implemented and managed. Specific aspects that fall to HIM professionals include (AHIMA 2008):

- Conducting a data content standards requirements analysis

- Developing a local data dictionary to support enterprise-wide interoperability

- Advancing the development of data content standards

- Contributing to domain knowledge by participating in relevant professional association work

- Contributing to the development and harmonization of industry and professional standards

Real-World Case

According to the American Academy of Family Physicians (AAFP), "Continuity of care is the process by which the patient and the physician are cooperatively involved in ongoing health care management toward the goal of high quality, cost-effective medical care" (AAFP 2010, paragraph 1). The CCR, an XML-based health data exchange standard, was created to help communicate summary health information from one provider to another for referral, transfer, or discharge of the patient. Microsoft introduced a personal health record platform that allows sharing of health information.

Microsoft's HealthVault allows the user to gather, store, and share health information online. HealthVault supports the CCR and CCD standards for exchanging patient data. Not only can applications use the CCR standard to exchange data with HealthVault, but a user can extract and reconcile data from a CCR (Microsoft 2009). Microsoft's partners include New York-Presbyterian Hospital, Health Partners, Kaiser Permanente, Aetna, Walgreens, among others.

Summary

According to Brandt (2000), "the vision is clear: a longitudinal, or lifetime, health record for each person that is computer-based, secure, readily accessible when needed, and linked across the continuum of care [is needed]. In reality, we are a long way from that model."

It is impossible to develop a longitudinal EHR that meets Brandt's specifications without standards that guide its development. The complexity of technology, the variations in computer platforms from one system to the next, and the different (and sometimes conflicting) data needs of users demand flexible health data/information systems. The systems must be able to store volumes of data in a standardized format, communicate across vendor-specific systems, and keep data in a secure manner that protects individual privacy and information confidentiality.

The need for standardized data definitions was recognized in the 1960s, and the NCVHS took the lead in developing uniform minimum data sets for various sites of care. As technology has driven the development of the data/information systems, the early data sets have been supplemented with healthcare information standards that focus on EHR systems.

A number of standards-setting organizations have been involved in developing uniform definitions, data fields, and views for health record content and structure. Standards for developing record structure and content, content exchange, vocabulary, and privacy and security are being created and implemented. These standards are dynamic and in constant development by various groups.

Standards development generally takes place as a consensus-driven process among various interested parties. Implementation is often voluntary but may be mandated. However, many groups are involved in standards development and competition exists among those groups. One of the major efforts of the ONC is standards harmonization that consolidates standards into a useful and accepted set of national information technology standards.

Some data sets and standards have been incorporated into federal law and are thus required for use by affected healthcare organizations. For example, in 1983, when Section 1886(d) of the Social Security Act was enacted, UHDDS definitions were incorporated into the rules and regulations for implementing an inpatient prospective payment system based on diagnosis-related groups (DRGs). These definitions are still required for reporting inpatient data for reimbursement under the Medicare program.

HIPAA mandated incorporation of healthcare information standards into all electronic or computer-based health information systems. Of particular importance under HIPAA are transaction/messaging standards for communication of data across systems, privacy standards that protect individual privacy and confidentiality, and security standards that ensure that data are accessed only by those who have a specific right to access them. The rules and regulations for HIPAA are still in development, and, to date, the transaction, privacy, and security standards have been implemented. Other standards are still under development. For example, in 2005 HHS published a proposed rule to adopt of a suite of standards for the electronic health care claim attachment. A final rule was never published. However, the Affordable Care Act requires the final rule defining standards and operating rules for claim attachments be published no later than January 2014 with compliance no later than January 2016.

The selection of health information standards to support EHR adoption gained national support through recent federal initiatives aimed at developing a strategic plan to guide the nation's implementation of interoperable health information technology in both the public and private sectors. The ONC has been given a mandate to advance the development, adoption, and implementation of healthcare information technology nationally through collaboration among public and private interests and to ensure that these standards are consistent with current efforts to set HIT standards for use by the federal government (Thompson and Brailer 2004). As a permanent office under HHS, the ONC oversees implementation plans for the provisions of the HITECH Act within ARRA. In 2010, the ONC published standards, implementation specifications, and certification criteria for the certification of EHR technology to support the achievement of meaningful use Stage 1 by eligible professionals and eligible hospitals under the Medicare and Medicaid EHR incentive programs. The final rule for Stage 2 is expected to be released in third quarter 2012 followed by Stage 3 some years later.

Work will continue on the development of healthcare informatics standards. It is a complex and dynamic task with constant activity in the development, modification, negotiation, and implementation process. The rapid growth of technology and the increasing need for healthcare data/information makes the task a daunting one. According to Fridsma (2011, paragraph 2) "ONC is identifying the vocabularies, the message, and the transport 'building blocks' that will enable interoperability. While vendors should be able to flexibly combine them to support interoperable HIE, these 'building blocks' need to be unambiguous and have very limited (or no) optionality."

References

AHIMA. 2007. Data standards, data quality, and interoperability. Appendix A: Data standards resource. *Journal of AHIMA* 78(2).

AHIMA e-HIM Workgroup on EHR Data Content. 2006. Guidelines for developing a data dictionary. *Journal of AHIMA* 77(2):64A–64D.

AHIMA Leadership Model. 2008. Data content standards. http://library.ahima.org/xpedio/groups/public/documents/ahima/bok1_042568.pdf#page%3D1

American Academy of Family Physicians. 2010. Continuity of care, definition of. http://www.aafp.org/online/en/home/policy/policies/c/continuityofcaredefinition.html

American Recovery and Reinvestment Act of 2009. Public Law 111-5. February 17, 2009. http://www.gpo.gov/fdsys/pkg/PLAW-111publ5/content-detail.html

Asmonga, D. 2009. ARRA Opportunities and omissions: New legislation seeks to jumpstart health IT, but issues remain. *Journal of AHIMA* 80(5):16–18.

ASTM International. 2005. http://www.astm.org/

ASTM International. 2009. http://www.astm.org/Standards/E2369.htm

Brandt, M.D. 2000. Health informatics standards: A user's guide. *Journal of AHIMA* 71(4):39–43.

Centers for Medicare and Medicaid Services. 2011. Outcome and assessment information set: OASIS-C guidance manual. http://www.cms.gov/HomeHealthQualityInits/14_HHQIOASIS UserManual.asp#TopOfPage

Centers for Medicare and Medicaid Services. 2012. Long-term care facility resident assessment instrument user's manual. http://www.cms.gov/NursingHomeQualityInits/45_NHQIMDS30 TrainingMaterials.asp#TopOfPage

Fenton, S., et al. 2007. Data standards, data quality, and interoperability. *Journal of AHIMA* 78(2): Web extra.

Food and Drug Administration. 2012. Structured product labeling resources. http://www.fda.gov/ForIndustry/DataStandards/StructuredProductLabeling/default.htm

Fridsma, D. 2010. ONC S&I framework: Coordination and operations. http://healthit.hhs.gov/portal/server.pt/gateway/PTARGS_0_11673_947553_0_0_18/Fridsma_Harmonization%20Processes%20and%20Governance_v4.pdf

Fridsma, D. 2011. Standards Are Not Optional. HealthIT Buzz. http://www.healthit.gov/buzz-blog/from-the-onc-desk/standards-optional-2/

Giannangelo, K. 2007. Unraveling the data set, an e-HIM essential. *Journal of AHIMA* 78(2):60–61.

Hanken, M.A., and K. Water, eds. 1994. *Glossary of Healthcare Terms.* Chicago: AHIMA.

Health Information Technology Standards Panel. 2009. HITSP glossary. http://wiki.hitsp.org/docs/REF6/REF6-2.html

Health Level Seven (HL7). 2011. Emergency care. http://www.hl7.org/Special/committees/emergencycare/projects.cfm?action=edit&ProjectNumber=820

International Organization for Standardization. 2004. Information technology parts 1–6 (2nd Edition). www.iso.org

The Joint Commission. 2012. Facts about ORYX performance measurement systems. http://www.jointcommission.org/assets/1/18/ORYX_performance_measurement_systems_1_6_11.pdf

Marshall, G.F. 2009. The standards value chain: Where health IT standards come from. *Journal of AHIMA* 80(10):54–55, 60–62.

Microsoft. 2009. Using CCR & CCD with HealthVault. http://www.google.com/url?sa=t&rct=j&q=&esrc=s&source=web&cd=1&ved=0CCcQFjAA&url=http%3A%2F%2Fdownload.microsoft.com%2Fdownload%2F0%2F4%2F9%2F0498cecf-d0b1-4a72-b9b7-17eb7d7ada98%2FUsingCCRandCCRwithHealthVault.pdf&ei=Vz77TvmYEsengwfg4sCLAg&usg=AFQjCNHZ_uUi3Yet0EObUWSz-LuC2So4bw&sig2=Ox4KYSmltpQTWnlC-0Bi7A.

National Center for Injury Prevention and Control. 2006. Data elements for emergency department systems, release 1.0. Atlanta, GA: CDC and HHS. http://www.cdc.gov/ncipc/pub-res/deedspage.htm

National Committee on Vital and Health Statistics. 2000. Toward a health information infrastructure: Interim report. Washington, DC: HHS.

National Committee on Vital and Health Statistics. 2001. Information for health: A strategy for building the national health information infrastructure. Washington, DC: HHS.

National Quality Forum. 2009. Health information technology automation of quality measurement: Quality data set and data flow. Washington, DC: NQF.

National Quality Forum. 2011. Quality data model - Draft October 2011. http://www.qualityforum.org/WorkArea/linkit.aspx?LinkIdentifier=id&ItemID=68545

Office of the National Coordinator for Health Information Technology. 2006. Consolidated health informatics. http://www.hhs.gov/healthit/chiinitiative.html

Office of the National Coordinator for Health Information Technology. 2010. Health information technology: Initial set of standards, implementation specifications, and certification criteria for electronic health record technology. *Federal Register* 75 (144):44649. http://edocket.access.gpo.gov/2010/pdf/2010-17210.pdf

Office of the National Coordinator for Health Information Technology. 2011a. HITSC—Standards and implementation: Update on standards effort. http://healthit.hhs.gov/portal/server.pt/gateway/PTARGS_0_16869_955993_0_0_18/HITSC_StandarddsUpdate102111.pdf

Office of the National Coordinator for Health Information Technology. 2011b. Get the facts about state health information exchange program. http://healthit.hhs.gov/portal/server.pt?open=512&mode=2&objID=1834

Office of the National Coordinator for Health Information Technology. 2011c. Metadata standards to support nationwide electronic health information exchange. *Federal Register* 76(153):48769–48776. http://www.gpo.gov/fdsys/pkg/FR-2011-08-09/pdf/2011-20219.pdf

Rode, D. 2001. Understanding HIPAA transactions and code sets. *Journal of AHIMA* 72(1):26–32.

S&I Framework. 2011a. Transitions of care overview. http://wiki.siframework.org/Transitions+of+Care+Overview

S&I Framework. 2011b. ToC CIM core data elements. http://wiki.siframework.org/ToC+CIM+Core+Data+Elements

Sokolowski, R. 1999. XML makes its mark. *Journal of AHIMA* 70(10):21–24.

Thompson, T.G., and D.J. Brailer. 2004. The decade of health information technology: Delivering consumer-centric and information-rich health care—framework for strategic action. Washington, DC: HHS.

Additional Resources

Health Information and Management Systems Society. 2009. The digital office. http://www.himss.org/digital_office/20091027_DigitalOffice_boldTitle.html

Health Level 7. 2009. http://HL7.org

chapter 5

Clinical Vocabularies and Classification Systems

Karen S. Scott, MEd, RHIA, CCS-P, CPC

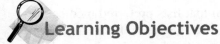

Learning Objectives

- Discuss the history of the development of clinical vocabularies
- Understand the history, uses, and structure of ICD-9-CM, ICD-10-CM, ICD-10-PCS, ICD-O-3, HCPCS, CPT, SNOMED CT, DSM-IV-TR, and nursing vocabularies
- Describe the coding process
- Identify the technology used in the coding process
- Understand the history, elements, policies, and procedures for corporate compliance
- Discuss new directions in clinical vocabularies

Key Terms

Classification system
Clinical vocabulary
Computer-assisted coding (CAC)
Current Procedural Terminology (CPT)
Diagnostic and Statistical Manual of Mental Disorders, Fourth Revision, Text Revision (DSM-IV-TR)
E codes
Encoder

Healthcare Common Procedure Coding System (HCPCS)
Interface
International Classification of Diseases, Ninth Revision, Clinical Modification (ICD-9-CM)
International Classification of Diseases, Tenth Revision, Clinical Modification (ICD-10-CM)

International Classification of Diseases, Tenth Revision, Procedure Coding System (ICD-10-PCS)

International Classification of Diseases for Oncology, Third Edition (ICD-O-3)

Morbidity

Mortality

Natural language processing (NLP)

Nomenclature

Nosology

Nursing vocabularies

Read Codes

Systemized Nomenclature of Medicine Clinical Terminology (SNOMED CT)

V codes

World Health Organization (WHO)

Introduction

Over the years, diseases and medical-surgical procedures have come to be known by different names. For example, Down's syndrome is sometimes referred to as mongolism or trisomy 21. Clearly, the use of more than one term for the same disease makes it difficult to collect and retrieve information. In an effort to organize and standardize medical language, the healthcare industry has developed nomenclatures, classification systems, and clinical vocabularies.

In medicine, a **nomenclature** is a recognized system that lists preferred medical terminology. Nomenclatures, or "naming" systems, such as CPT, also are referred to as *clinical terminology*. **Classification systems** group together similar diseases and procedures. They also organize related entities for easy retrieval. The *International Classification of Diseases, Ninth Revision, Clinical Modification* (ICD-9-CM), is an example of a classification system. **Clinical vocabularies** have been developed to create a list of clinical words or phrases with their meanings.

These systems facilitate the organization, storage, and retrieval of healthcare diagnostic and procedural data. Moreover, they aid in the development and implementation of electronic patient record systems. This chapter discusses the various nomenclatures, classification systems, and clinical vocabularies used in the healthcare industry today.

Theory into Practice

Hillcrest Health Care Clinic is a multispecialty group practice with clinics in five different locations. The offices are implementing an electronic health record system and the office manager is investigating how the current codes are assigned. She noticed that many of the providers do not use codebooks at all but, instead, assign codes by checking off common diagnoses and procedures on superbills and other preprinted forms. Some of the physicians who are using standardized lists provided on software are selecting codes that are not substantiated by the clinical documentation in the patients' health record. The end result is incorrect code assignment, denied reimbursement, and erroneous database entries. Clearly, policies and procedures are needed to control the coding process especially when creating standardization with an electronic health record system.

History and Importance of Clinical Vocabularies

The first medical nomenclature to be universally accepted in the United States was developed by the New York Academy of Medicine and titled the *Standard Nomenclature of Disease and Operations.* In 1937, the American Medical Association (AMA) assumed the copyright and editing responsibility for this work and expanded it to include a nomenclature for procedures as well as diseases. The expanded work was published in one volume titled *Standard Nomenclature of Disease and Standard Nomenclature of Operations.*

ICD-9-CM is the most recognized classification system used today in the United States. It evolved from a classification developed by Dr. Jacques Bertillon. His system was published in 1893 as the *Bertillon Classification of Causes of Death.* In 1898, the American Public Health Association recommended that registrars in the United States, Canada, and Mexico use the Bertillon classification.

This classification system was revised throughout the early 1900s. In 1948, the **World Health Organization** (WHO) published the sixth revision of the system. The sixth revision included a classification for **morbidity** and **mortality** data. Throughout the 1900s, various healthcare associations and public health organizations representing numerous countries worked to create a standardized classification system for healthcare.

In 1975, representatives from numerous countries met in Geneva, Switzerland to develop the *International Classification of Diseases* under the direction of WHO. Today, the ICD classification system is used throughout the world and is undergoing its 11th revision. As noted above a modification of ICD (ICD-9-CM) is used in the United States with a new revision (ICD-10-CM) planned for implementation by October 31, 2013.

Development of these systems has helped to standardize terminology for the collection, processing, and retrieval of medical information. Additional systems of classification and nomenclatures are discussed later in this chapter.

Clinical Vocabularies, Classifications, and Nomenclatures

Users of clinical vocabularies and classifications can be divided into two main groups: clinical and administrative.

Clinical users are providers who use clinical vocabularies and classifications to collect, process, and retrieve data for clinical purposes. They use the vocabularies to support activities such as clinical research, disease prevention, and patient care. An example of a clinical user would be a physician who uses ICD-9-CM codes to track a patient's diagnostic history.

Administrative users include healthcare facilities, professional organizations, and government agencies. These groups use clinical vocabularies and classifications to support administrative, statistical, and reimbursement functions. An example of this is when ***Current Procedural Terminology*** (CPT) codes are used to report physician services to the Medicare program to determine reimbursement. The specific users of clinical vocabularies are discussed in the sections that follow.

The Health Insurance Portability and Accountability Act (HIPAA) required the establishment of electronic transactions and coding standards. In 2000, the Department of Health and Human Services (HHS), in accordance with HIPAA, established official medical coding set standards. To be in compliance with the HIPAA law, all covered entities are required to use the following official medical coding sets:

- *International Classification of Diseases, Ninth Revision, Clinical Modification* (ICD-9-CM), including the Official ICD-9-CM Guidelines for Coding and Reporting: Volumes 1 and 2 are used for reporting all diseases, injuries, impairments, other health problems and causes of such, and Volume 3 is used to report procedures performed on hospital inpatients. (ICD-10-CM and ICD-10-PCS will replace ICD-9-CM in 2013.)

- ***Healthcare Common Procedure Coding System*** (HCPCS), which includes *Current Procedural Terminology* (CPT): This system is used for reporting physician and other healthcare services, including non-inpatient procedures.

- *Current Dental Terminology, Code on Dental Procedures and Nomenclatures* (CDT): This system is used for reporting dental services.

- *National Drug Codes* (NDC): In the original ruling from Medicare, the NDC was designated as the official data set for reporting drugs used by pharmacies. However, this adoption was repealed in 2003. Currently, there is no official standard for reporting medications on pharmacy transactions.

International Classification of Diseases, Ninth Revision, Clinical Modification

The International Classification of Diseases (ICD) is a classification system for reporting medical diagnoses and procedures.

History

ICD-9-CM is one of the most common classification systems used in the United States today. It is an adaptation of the *International Classification of Diseases, Ninth Revision* (ICD-9), published by WHO in Geneva, Switzerland.

In the United States, the federal government, through the National Center for Health Statistics (NCHS), modified ICD-9 to create ICD-9-CM. ICD-9-CM was issued for use in the United States in 1978. The intent of this modification was to provide a classification system for morbidity data.

ICD-9-CM is maintained by four organizations known as the cooperating parties: the National Center for Health Statistics (NCHS), the American Hospital Association (AHA), the American Health Information Management Association (AHIMA), and the Centers for

Medicare and Medicaid Services (CMS). The cooperating parties assume the following responsibilities:

- To serve as a clearinghouse to answer questions on ICD-9-CM
- To develop educational materials and programs on ICD-9-CM
- To work cooperatively in maintaining the integrity of ICD-9-CM
- To recommend revisions and modifications to current and future revisions of ICD

The work of the cooperating parties is supplemented by AHA's Editorial Advisory Board for *Coding Clinic,* which is composed of representatives of hospitals, heath data systems, and the federal government.

NCHS serves as the World Health Organization (WHO) Collaborating Center for the Family of International Classifications for North America and in this capacity is responsible for coordination of all official disease classification activities in the United States relating to the ICD and its use, interpretation, and periodic revision. In regards to their duties in ICD-9-CM and ICD-10-CM, NCHS is responsible for updating the diagnosis classification (Volumes 1 and 2), and CMS is responsible for updating the procedure classification (Volume 3). AHIMA works to help provide training and certification, and the AHA maintains the central office on ICD-9-CM and publishes *Coding Clinic for ICD-9-CM,* which contains the official coding guidelines and official guidance on the usage of ICD-9-CM codes.

In 1985, the ICD-9-CM Coordination and Maintenance Committee was established. Cochaired by representatives of NCHS and CMS, the committee is made up of advisors and representatives of all the cooperating parties. It meets twice a year to provide a public forum for discussing possible revisions and updates to ICD-9-CM. Discussions at these meetings are advisory only as the director of NCHS and the administrator of CMS determine all final revisions. As the U.S. transitions toward ICD-10, the Cooperating Parties are revising draft editions and preparing and updating the resources needed to support the changes.

Purpose and Use

According to the Central Office on ICD-9-CM, ICD-9-CM has the following uses:

- Classifying morbidity and mortality information for statistical purposes
- Indexing hospital records by disease and operations
- Reporting diagnoses by physicians
- Storing and retrieving data
- Reporting national morbidity and mortality data
- Serving as the basis of diagnosis-related group (DRG) assignment for hospital reimbursement

- Reporting and compiling healthcare data to assist in the evaluation of medical care planning for healthcare delivery systems
- Determining patterns of care among healthcare providers
- Analyzing payments for health services
- Conducting epidemiological and clinical research

Overview of Structure

ICD-9-CM is published in three volumes. Volume 1 is known as the Tabular List. It contains the numerical listing of codes that represent diseases and injuries. Volume 2 is the Alphabetic Index. It consists of an alphabetic index for all the codes listed in Volume 1. The Tabular List and Alphabetic Index for Procedures are published as Volume 3. Volume 3 is not part of the international version of ICD-9. It is used only in the United States to report procedures performed on hospital inpatients.

Volume 1

Volume 1 of ICD-9-CM is divided into three subdivisions: classification of diseases and injuries, supplementary classifications, and appendixes.

The classification of diseases and injuries is divided into 17 chapters (figure 5.1). The chapters are organized by type of condition and anatomical system. For example, chapter 5, Mental Disorders, represents a chapter that groups diseases by type of condition. Chapter 6, Diseases of the Nervous System and Sense Organs, represents a chapter that groups diseases by anatomical system. For example, Diseases of the Ear and Mastoid Process are included in categories 380–389.

The chapters are further divided into sections. Sections are groups of three-digit code numbers. An example of a section in chapter 5 is the disease classification for organic psychotic conditions (290–294) (see figure 5.2).

Figure 5.1.   Chapter titles in the *ICD-9-CM Classification of Diseases and Injuries*

1. Infectious and Parasitic Diseases	10. Diseases of the Genitourinary System
2. Neoplasms	11. Complications of Pregnancy, Childbirth, and the Puerperium
3. Endocrine, Nutritional, and Metabolic Diseases and Immunity Disorders	12. Diseases of the Skin and Subcutaneous Tissue
4. Diseases of the Blood and Blood-Forming Organs	13. Diseases of the Musculoskeletal System and Connective Tissue
5. Mental Disorders	14. Congenital Anomalies
6. Diseases of the Nervous System and Sense Organs	15. Certain Conditions Originating in the Perinatal Period
7. Diseases of the Circulatory System	16. Symptoms, Signs, and Ill-Defined Conditions
8. Diseases of the Respiratory System	17. Injury and Poisoning
9. Diseases of the Digestive System	

Figure 5.2. **Example of an ICD-9-CM section**

ORGANIC PSYCHOTIC CONDITIONS (290–294)

Includes: psychotic organic brain syndrome

Excludes: *nonpsychotic syndromes of organic etiology (310.0–310.9)*

psychoses classifiable to 295–298 and without

impairment of orientation, comprehension, calculation, learning capacity, and judgment, but associated with physical disease, injury, or condition affecting the brain [e.g., following childbirth] (295.0–298.8)

290   Senile and presenile organic psychotic conditions

Code first the associated neurological condition

Excludes: *dementia not classified as senile, presenile, or arteriosclerotic (294.10–294.11)*

psychoses classifiable to 295–298 occurring in the senium without dementia or delirium (295.0–298.8)

senility with mental changes of nonpsychotic severity (310.1)

transient organic psychotic conditions (293.0–293.9)

290.0   Senile dementia, uncomplicated

Senile dementia:

NOS

simple type

Excludes: *mild memory disturbances, not amounting to dementia, associated with senile brain disease (310.1)*

senile dementia with:

delirium or confusion (290.3)

delusional [paranoid] features (290.20)

depressive features (290.21)

290.1   Presenile dementia

Brain syndrome with presenile brain disease

Excludes: *arteriosclerotic dementia (290.40–290.43)*

dementia associated with other cerebral conditions (294.10–294.11)

290.10   Presenile dementia, uncomplicated

Presenile dementia:

NOS

simple type

290.11   Presenile dementia with delirium

Presenile dementia with acute confusional state

290.12   Presenile dementia with delusional features

Presenile dementia, paranoid type

290.13   Presenile dementia with depressive features

Presenile dementia, depressed type

Sections are subdivided into categories. Categories represent a group of closely related conditions or a single disease entity. Category 290, Senile and pre-senile organic psychotic conditions, is an example of a category found in chapter 6.

Categories are further divided into subcategories. At this level, four-digit code numbers are used. Figure 5.2 provides an example of a subcategory: code number 290.1, Pre-senile dementia.

The most specific codes in the ICD-9-CM system are found at the sub-classification level. Five-digit code numbers represent this level. In figure 5.2, code 290.10 represents a code at the sub-classification level.

Two supplementary classifications are part of Volume 1: the Supplementary Classification of Factors Influencing Health Status and Contact with Health Services (V codes) and the Supplementary Classification of External Causes of Injury and Poisoning (E codes).

V codes are used to classify occasions when circumstances other than disease or injury are recorded as the reason for the patient's encounter with the healthcare provider. Such circumstances generally occur in one of the following three ways:

- When a person who is not currently sick encounters a health service provider for some specific reason, such as to act as an organ or tissue donor, to receive prophylactic vaccination, or to discuss a problem that in itself is not a disease or injury (for example, when a patient sees a physician for a measles vaccination)

- When a person with a known disease or injury, whether current or resolving, encounters the healthcare system for a specific treatment of that disease or injury (for example, when a patient seeks follow-up care for a previously applied cast)

- When some circumstance or problem influences the person's health status but is not in itself a current injury or illness (for example, when a patient has a personal history of smoking)

V codes are always alphanumeric codes. They are easy to identify because they begin with the alpha character *V* and are followed by numerical digits. An example is V15.04, Allergy to seafood.

E codes provide a means to classify environmental events, circumstances, and conditions as the cause of injury, poisoning, and other adverse effect. These codes must be used in addition to codes from the main chapters of ICD-9-CM. E codes provide additional information used by insurance companies, safety programs, and public health agencies to determine the causes of injuries, poisonings, or other adverse situations. Even though use of many E codes is optional, many facilities use them as secondary codes to identify the cause of accidents and injuries. Some states have mandated reporting of E codes in certain circumstances, such as in reporting head trauma.

E codes begin with the alpha character *E* and are followed by numerical characters. E925.0 represents the code for an accident caused by an electric current in domestic wiring and appliances.

The last subdivision of Volume 1 consists of the appendixes. ICD-9-CM includes two appendixes, however most publishers include references to all five previously existing appendixes:

- Appendix A: Morphology of Neoplasms
- Appendix B: Glossary of Mental Disorders (removed in 2004)
- Appendix C: Classification of Drugs by American Hospital Formulary Service List Number
- Appendix D: Classification of Industrial Accidents According to Agency (removed in 2009)
- Appendix E: List of Three-Digit Categories (removed in 2007)

Volume 2

The Index to Diseases and Injuries is printed as Volume 2 of ICD-9-CM. Main terms appear alphabetically in the index by type of disease, injury, or illness. Subterms are indented under the main term. For example, the main term bradycardia and the subterms for bradycardia appear as shown in figure 5.3.

Volume 3

The third volume of ICD-9-CM contains the tabular and alphabetic lists of procedures. The Tabular List of Procedures contains chapters organized according to anatomical system, except for the last chapter, Miscellaneous Diagnostic and Therapeutic Procedures. Figure 5.4 shows the procedure chapter titles. According to the HIPAA regulations, these codes are to be used only for inpatient hospital billing.

ICD-9-CM procedure codes are organized according to these chapters, and then the chapters are divided into two-, three-, and sometimes four-digit code numbers. All procedure codes are written with two digits to the left of the decimal point. Figure 5.5 provides

Figure 5.3.   Example of index entries for main terms and subterms in ICD-9-CM

Brachycephaly 756.0	sinus 427.89
Brachymorphism and ectopia lentis 759.89	with paroxysmal tachyarrhythmia or tachycardia 427.81
Bradley's disease (epidemic vomiting) 078.82	chronic 427.81
Bradycardia 427.89	persistent 427.81
chronic (sinus) 427.81	severe 427.81
newborn 763.83	tachycardia syndrome 427.81
nodal 427.89	vagal 427.89
postoperative 997.1	**Bradypnea** 786.09
reflex 337.0	**Brailsford's disease** 732.3
sinoatrial 427.89	radial head 732.3
with paroxysmal tachyarrhythmia or tachycardia 427.81	tarsal scaphoid 732.5
chronic 427.81	

Figure 5.4. Chapter titles in the ICD-9-CM Tabular List of Procedures

1. Operations on the Nervous System
2. Operations on the Endocrine System
3. Operations on the Eye
4. Operations on the Ear
5. Operations on the Nose, Mouth, and Pharynx
6. Operations on the Respiratory System
7. Operations on the Cardiovascular System
8. Operations on the Hemic and Lymphatic System

9. Operations on the Digestive System
10. Operations on the Urinary System
11. Operations on the Male Genital Organs
12. Operations on the Female Genital Organs
13. Obstetrical Procedures
14. Operations on the Musculoskeletal System
15. Operations on the Integumentary System
16. Miscellaneous Diagnostic and Therapeutic Procedures

Figure 5.5. Example from the ICD-9-CM Tabular List of Procedures

06   Operations on thyroid and parathyroid glands
Includes: incidental resection of hyoid bone

06.0   Incision of thyroid field
Excludes: *division of isthmus (06.91)*

06.01   Aspiration of thyroid field
Percutaneous or needle drainage of thyroid field
Excludes: *aspiration biopsy of thyroid (06.11)*
drainage by incision (06.09)
postoperative aspiration of field (06.02)

06.02   Reopening of wound of thyroid field
Reopening of wound of thyroid field for:
control of (postoperative) hemorrhage
examination
exploration
removal of hematoma

06.09   Other incision of thyroid field
Drainage of hematoma
Drainage of thyroglossal tract
Exploration:
neck   by incision
thyroid (field)
Removal of foreign body
Thyroidotomy NOS

Excludes: *postoperative exploration (06.02)*
removal of hematoma by aspiration (06.01)

Figure 5.6.   Example of alphabetic entries in the ICD-9-CM index to procedures

Acromioplasty 81.83	**Acupuncture** 99.92
for recurrent dislocation of shoulder 81.82	with smouldering moxa 93.35
partial replacement 81.81	for anesthesia 99.91
total replacement 81.80	**Adams operation**
Actinotherapy 99.82	advancement of round ligament 69.22
Activities of daily living (ADL)	crushing of nasal septum 21.88
therapy 93.83	excision of palmar fascia 82.35
training for the blind 93.78	

an example of a tabular listing from the beginning of chapter 2, Operations on the Endocrine System (06–07).

The Alphabetic Index to Procedures is organized in the same manner as the Alphabetic Index to Diseases. Figure 5.6 shows an example of the alphabetic organization of procedures.

Check Your Understanding 5.1

Instructions: Use the following excerpt from the Alphabetic Index to complete the questions below.

Bacillary—*see* condition
Bacilluria 791.9
    asymptomatic, in pregnancy or puerperium 646.5
    tuberculous (*see also* Tuberculosis) 016.9
Bacillus—*see also* Infection, bacillus
    abortus infection 023.1
    anthracis infection 022.9
    coli
    infection 041.4
        generalized 038.42
        intestinal 008.00
      pyemia 038.42
      septicemia 038.42
    Flexner's 004.1
    fusiformis infestation 101
    mallei infection 024
    Shiga's 004.0
    suipestifer infection (*see also* Infection, Salmonella) 003.9

Back—*see* condition

Backache (postural) 724.5

   psychogenic 307.89

   sacroiliac 724.6

1. List the first four main terms that appear in the excerpt.

   _____ _____ _____ _____

2. List the first four subterms that appear under **Bacillus.**

   _____ _____ _____ _____

3. Indicate whether each of the following codes represents a disease (D) or a procedure (P).

   a. ____ 99.82   d. ____ 73.4
   b. ____ 098.0   e. ____ 844.0
   c. ____ 301.51   f. ____ 45.24

International Classification of Diseases, Tenth Revision, Clinical Modification

Established by WHO, the ICD system was designed to be totally revised at 10-year intervals. In the mid-1990s, WHO published the newest version of ICD: *International Statistical Classification of Diseases and Related Health Problems, Tenth Revision,* known as ICD-10. This revision is currently in use by many countries throughout the world and has been used in the United States to capture mortality statistics since 1999. However, studies in the United States determined that ICD-10 needed to be modified to capture data that would support our reimbursement system prior to implementation.

   ICD-10-CM provides several enhancements that are anticipated to improve coding accuracy. Among these are (Zeisset 2009):

- Including combination codes for conditions and common symptoms or manifestations. A single code may be used to classify two diagnoses, a diagnosis with an associated sign or symptom, or a diagnosis with an associated complication. This allows one code to be assigned, resulting in fewer cases requiring more than one code and reducing sequencing problems.

- Decreasing cross-referencing by writing out the full code title for all codes.

- Providing codes for laterality such as codes for left side, right side, and in some cases bilateral as available in appropriate chapters.

- Providing expanded codes to capture more detail in several sections such as injury, diabetes, postoperative complications, and others. Adding code alpha character extensions (seventh character) in appropriate sections to provide specific information about the characteristics of the encounter such as initial encounter, subsequent encounter, or sequelae.

In addition to the above, ICD-10-CM provides flexibility and expandability, which allow more specificity in the coding of many conditions. This should result in improved usefulness of the data in many areas such as measuring quality of patient care, conducting research, establishing health policy, designing payment systems and processes for reimbursement, tracking public health risks, and monitoring resource utilization to name a few (Zeisset 2009).

Purpose and Use

The Clinical Modification of ICD-10 is known as the *International Classification of Diseases, Tenth Revision, Clinical Modification* (ICD-10-CM). According to NCHS, ICD-10-CM is the planned replacement for ICD-9-CM, Volumes 1 and 2. This revision is considered to be an improvement over both ICD-9-CM and ICD-10, and was developed to contain a great many more codes and allow greater specificity than existing ICD code sets.

Overview of Structure

Although the traditional ICD structure remains, ICD-10-CM is a complete alphanumeric coding scheme. The former supplementary classification information (V and E codes) was incorporated into the main classification system with different letters preceding the numerical portions of the codes. ICD-10 contains new chapters and several categories have been restructured and new features added to maintain consistency with modern medicine. The disease classification has been expanded to provide greater specificity at the sixth-digit level and with a seventh-digit extension.

A draft of ICD-10-CM including a draft of official coding guidelines is available from the NCHS website at http://www.cdc.gov/nchs/icd/icd10cm.htm#10update. Similarities in structure and terms between ICD-10-CM and ICD-9-CM are shown and explained in figure 5.7.

Examples of ICD-10-CM codes include the following:

- Malignant Neoplasm
    - C34.1   Malignant neoplasm of upper lobe, bronchus or lung
    - C34.10 Malignant neoplasm of upper lobe, bronchus or lung, unspecified side
    - C34.11 Malignant neoplasm of upper lobe, right bronchus or lung
    - C34.12 Malignant neoplasm of upper lobe, left bronchus or lung
- Diabetes
    - E10.2   Type 1 diabetes mellitus with kidney complications
    - E10.21 Type 1 diabetes mellitus with diabetic nephropathy
             Type 1 diabetes mellitus with intercapillary glomerulosclerosis
             Type 1 diabetes with intracapillary glomerulonephritis
             Type 1 diabetes mellitus with Kimmelstiel-Wilson disease

Figure 5.7.   Similarities in structure and terms between ICD-10-CM and ICD-9-CM

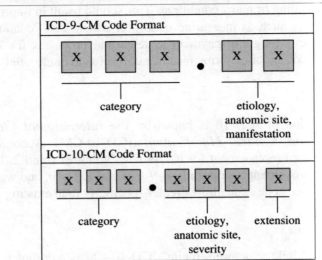

ICD-10-CM:

- Has the same type of hierarchy in its structure as ICD-9-CM. All codes have the same first three digits describing common traits, with each character beyond the first three providing more specificity.

- Has the same organization and use of notes and instructions. When a note appears under a three-character code, it applies to all codes within that category, and notes under a specific code apply to the single code.

- Codes must be at least three characters, with a decimal point used after the third character. The additional characters following the decimal point describe the etiology, anatomic site, or severity.

- Consists of an alphabetic index formatted by main terms listed in alphabetic order with indentations for any applicable qualifiers or descriptors. Familiar punctuation such as brackets, parentheses, colons, and commas are used in ICD-10-CM, as are terms such as Not Elsewhere Classified (NEC), Not Otherwise Specified (NOS), "code first," "Use additional code," and "code also" notes familiar to coding professionals.

- Uses cross-references to provide instructions to reference other or additional terms. The tabular list is present in code number order and used like ICD-9-CM.

— E10.22   Type 1 diabetes mellitus with diabetic chronic kidney disease

   Type 1 diabetes mellitus with chronic kidney disease due to conditions classified to 0.21 and 0.22

   Use additional code to identify stage of chronic kidney disease (N18.1–N18.6)

— E10.29   Type 1 diabetes mellitus with other diabetic kidney complication

   Type 1 diabetes mellitus with renal tubular degeneration

International Classification of Diseases, Tenth Revision, Procedure Coding System

ICD-10-CM does not include a procedure volume. Thus, when the United States began planning to clinically modify WHO's ICD-10, it was determined that creating a separate volume for procedures would be insufficient. As a result, CMS contracted with 3M Health Information Systems to develop a separate procedure code system that would serve as a replacement for ICD-9-CM, Volume 3. This coding system is known as the ***International Classification of Diseases, Tenth Revision, Procedure Coding System,*** or ICD-10-PCS.

Purpose and Use

According to CMS, the agency responsible for updating the procedure section of ICD-9-CM, the design of ICD-10-PCS included the following goals:

- To improve accuracy and efficiency of coding
- To reduce training effort
- To improve communication with physicians

Overview of Structure

ICD-10-PCS has no correlation to the ICD-10-CM structure. It consists of a multiaxial seven-character alphanumeric code structure. The 10 digits 0–9 and the 24 letters A–H, J–N, and P–Z are characters used in ICD-10-PCS. Although this system has the capability and flexibility to replace all existing procedural coding systems, it is only going to replace ICD-9-CM procedure codes. Because of its unique structure, ICD-10-PCS is considered to be both complete and expandable.

Because many different and confusing names of procedures are in use in the medical field, each root procedure has been defined in ICD-10-PCS. This helps to clarify terms that currently have overlapping meaning, such as excision or resection.

Excision:

- Definition: Cutting out or off, without replacement, a portion of a body part
- Examples: Partial nephrectomy, wedge ostectomy, pulmonary segmentectomy

Resection:

- Definition: Cutting out or off, without replacement, all of body part
- Examples: Total nephrectomy, total lobectomy of lung, total mastectomy (Averill et al. nd)

Procedures are divided into 16 sections related to general type of procedure (medical and surgical, imaging, and so on). All procedure codes have seven characters. The first character of the procedure code always specifies the section where the procedure is indexed. The second through seventh characters have a standard meaning within each section. In medical and surgical procedures, the seven characters are defined as follows:

1 = Section of the ICD-10-PCS system where the code resides

2 = The body system

3 = Root operation (such as excision, incision)

4 = Specific body part

5 = Approach used, such as intraluminal or open

6 = Device used to perform the procedure

7 = Qualifier to provide additional information about the procedure (for example, diagnostic versus therapeutic)

An example of an ICD-10-PCS code is 097F7DZ, Dilation Eustachian Tube, Right, Transorifice Intraluminal.

Section	Medical and Surgical	0
Body System	Ear, Nose, Sinus	9
Root Operation	Dilation	7
Body Part	Eustachian tube, right	F
Approach	Via natural or artificial opening	7
Device	Intraluminal	D
Qualifier	No Qualifier	Z

The draft ICD-10-PCS code system and training manual are available online from https://www.cms.gov/ICD10/11b15_2012_ICD10PCS.asp.

Implementation of ICD-10 in the United States

The Department of Health and Human Services published in the *Federal Register* on January 16, 2009 a final rule to establish a timeline for implementation of ICD-10-CM and ICD-10-PCS. These two coding systems will be adopted as the national standards under the HIPAA electronic transactions and coding standards rule to replace the current uses of ICD-9-CM. The effective date for this rule is October 1, 2013. This final rule can be reviewed at http://edocket.access.gpo.gov/2009/pdf/E9-743.pdf. The transition from ICD-9-CM to ICD-10-CM and ICD-10-PCS will be a tremendous effort. Planning for the transition is discussed below. At the time of publication, the Centers for Medicare and Medicaid Services (CMS) has indicated the ICD-10-CM/PCS compliance date of October 1, 2013, but have proposed a one year delay. Providers will not be able to continue to report ICD-9-CM codes for services provided on or after the implementation date. Coders should begin to familiarize themselves with the new systems. The *Journal of American Health Information Management Association* and other publications are publishing preparation articles that will enable coders to stay current and be prepared for the changes as they take effect. Extensive training sessions and coding materials are being developed to assist coders and facilities with this transition.

ICD-9-CM to ICD-10-CM Transition Issues

Historically, change to a new classification system has proven that advance preparation is essential. Organizations should put in place a detailed implementation plan that identifies key tasks to be performed and assigns responsibilities and timelines for completion. An adequate budget needs to be allocated to cover the costs of implementation.

Planning for education at all levels in the organization is important. Training should be tailored to the job performed and ranges from general awareness of ICD-10 to actually learning how to code with the new system. Awareness of ICD-10-CM/PCS would include understanding the general structure of the systems and the potential impact to workflow processes in order to prepare for the systems. Analysis includes trending or providing information that involves coded data but not actual application of codes in daily jobs. Application training for coding professionals includes training on assigning codes on a routine basis and requires a more extensive knowledge of the systems.

Examples of staff that should be included in a training program include coding, billing, quality management, information systems, and researchers to name a few. Different approaches to training should be developed depending on the level and type of training required. For example, coding staff will require different training than, say, billing or quality management staff. Figure 5.8 provides a checklist of training considerations for coding staff.

Figure 5.8.   **ICD-10 training checklist for coding staff**

- Evaluate coding personnel's baseline knowledge in skills to identify knowledge gaps in the areas of medical terminology, anatomy and physiology, pathophysiology, and pharmacology. Measuring coding professionals' baseline knowledge will shorten the learning curve, improve coding accuracy and productivity, prepare for educational needs, and accelerate the realization of benefits of the new coding systems. AHIMA plans to provide self-assessment tools and other resources suitable for skill assessment.

- Review ICD-10-CM coding guidelines, ICD-10-PCS reference manual, and other ICD-10 educational materials to identify areas where increased clinical knowledge will be needed.

- Use information from coding professional knowledge gap assessment to develop individualized education plans for improving clinical knowledge to ensure it meets the requirements of ICD-10-CM and ICD-10-PCS.

- If outsourced staff are used for coding, communicate with the companies that provide these services concerning their plans for ICD-10 related training.

- Consider having the coding personnel practice coding a few records using ICD-10-CM and ICD-10-PCS to increase familiarity with the new coding systems.

   —Download ICD-10-CM information at http://www.cdc.gov/nchs/icd/icd10cm.htm

   —Download ICD-10-PCS information at http://www.cms.gov/ICD10/11b_2011_ICD10PCS.asp

---

Source: Bowman and Zeisset 2007.

Implementation of ICD-10 will also require that changes to be made in the organization's information systems and a detailed plan to handle the transition needs to be developed. For example, it is important to conduct an inventory to identify what databases and applications currently use IC-9-CM codes and how these systems need to be changed to accommodate the new ICD-10 codes. Software changes that may need to be done might include expanding field sizes, accommodating longer code descriptions, making modifications to table structures, and building new system interfaces.

Because the ICD-10 requires a greater level of detail, a medical record documentation assessment should be performed. The assessment should identify documentation deficiencies result in a documentation improvement program. Education of physicians in documentation practices will be key to more precise data capture. Refer to chapter 3 for additional information on documentation improvement.

International Classification of Functioning, Disability, and Health (ICF)

In 2001, the World Health Assembly approved the International Classification of Functioning, Disability, and Health (ICF). The ICF is a classification that was first created in 1980 called the International Classification of Impairments, Disabilities, and Handicaps, or ICIDH, created by the World Health Organization (WHO) to "provide a unifying framework for classifying the consequences of disease." The ICF classification complements WHO's *International Classification of Diseases, Tenth Revision* (ICD), which contains information on diagnosis and health condition, but not on functional status. The ICD and ICF constitute the core classifications in the WHO Family of International Classifications (WHO-FIC).

The ICF is structured around the following broad components:

- Body functions and structure
  - physiological functions of body systems
  - anatomical parts of the body such as organs, limbs, and components
- Activities (related to tasks and actions by an individual) and participation (involvement in a life situation)
  - execution of tasks or actions by an individual
  - involvement in a life situation
- Additional information on severity and environmental factors
  - problems in body function or structure; deviation or loss
  - activity limitations and participation restrictions
  - physical, social, and attitudinal environment in which people live and conduct their lives

Functioning and disability are viewed as a complex interaction between the health condition of the individual and the contextual factors of the environment as well as personal factors. The picture produced by this combination of factors and dimensions is of "the person in his or her world." The classification treats these dimensions as interactive and dynamic rather than linear or static. It allows for an assessment of the degree of disability, although it is not a measurement instrument. It is applicable to all people, whatever their health condition. The language of the ICF is neutral as to etiology, placing the emphasis on function rather than condition or disease. It also is carefully designed to be relevant across cultures as well as age groups and genders, making it highly appropriate for heterogeneous populations. (NCHS)

Revision of the classification in the United States and Canada is performed by the WHO Collaborating Center for the Family of International Classifications for North America (NACC) and is located at the National Center for Health Statistics (NCHS). It promotes the development and use of ICF.

The goals of the NACC are as follows:

- Represents the United States and Canada in international activities related to study and revision of the ICIDH/ICF

- Works with U.S. researchers conducting ICIDH/ICF studies and evaluations

- Collaborates with Canadian researchers through the Canadian Institute for Health Information (CIHI)

International Classification of Diseases for Oncology, Third Edition

The *International Classification of Diseases for Oncology, Third Edition* (ICD-O-3) is a system used for classifying incidences of malignant disease. Hospitals use ICD-O-3 for several purposes, for example, to develop cancer registries. Cancer registries list all the cases of cancer diagnosed and treated in the facility.

History of ICD-O-3

WHO published the first edition of the *International Classification of Diseases for Oncology* (ICD-O) in 1976. It was developed jointly by the United States Cancer Institute and WHO's International Agency for Research on Cancer.

In 1968, the American Cancer Society published *Manual of Tumor Nomenclature and Coding* (MOTNAC). Also in 1968, WHO asked the International Agency for Research on Cancer to develop a chapter on neoplasms for the ninth revision of ICD. WHO decided to publish a supplemental neoplasm classification based on MOTNAC for ICD-9.

ICD-O-3 was published for use in coding cancers diagnosed in the United States after January 1, 2001, and is updated on an annual basis. In 2010, the WHO/IARC ICD-O Update Committee was formed to review proposals for new or revised codes. This committee publishes updates with the effective date of January 1 of the next calendar year.

Purpose and Use

Originally, ICD-O was developed to aid in the collection of information in the field of oncology. (Oncology is the study of neoplasms [new tissue], or tumors.) Its purpose is to provide a detailed classification system for coding the histology (morphology [structure]), topography (site), and behavior of neoplasms (that is, malignant, benign). The current version of ICD-O provides a detailed classification used by pathology departments, cancer registries, and healthcare providers who treat cancer patients.

Overview of Structure

A dual-axis classification is used in ICD-O-3 to code the topography and morphology of the neoplasm. These codes are identical or compatible with other coding classifications and nomenclatures. For example, the topography codes used in ICD-10 for malignant neoplasms are the same codes used in ICD-O-3.

The morphology codes identify the type of tumor found and its behavior. The morphology code numbers consist of the letter *M* followed by five digits. The first four digits identify the histological type of the neoplasm. The fifth digit identifies the behavior of the tumor. The following morphology codes for some leukemias provide an example:

Leukemias

M9891/3	Acute monocytic leukemia
M9895/3	Acute myeloid leukemia with multilineage dysplasia
M9896/3	Acute myeloid leukemia, AML1
M9897/3	Acute myeloid leukemia, MLL

The fifth-digit (behavior) codes that appear after the slash are used to indicate the following:

/0	Benign
/1	Uncertain whether benign or malignant, borderline malignancy
/2	Carcinoma in situ
	Intraepithelial
	Noninfiltrating
	Non-invasive
/3	Malignant, primary site
/6	Malignant, metastatic site
	Secondary site
/9	Malignant, uncertain whether primary or metastatic site

Check Your Understanding 5.2

Instructions: List the type of behavior for the tumors represented by the following codes.

1. _____ M8140/0

2. _____ M8490/6

3. _____ M8331/3

4. _____ M8120/2

Healthcare Common Procedure Coding System

HCPCS (pronounced "Hick Picks") was originally called the HCFA Common Proce-dure Coding System. The name of the system was changed in 2001, when the Health Care Financing Administration (the agency that administered the Medicare and Medicaid programs) changed its name to the Centers for Medicare and Medicaid Services (CMS). HCPCS is used to report physicians' services to Medicare for reimbursement.

History of HCPCS

HCPCS is a collection of codes and descriptors used to represent healthcare procedures, supplies, products, and services. When the Medicare program was first implemented in the early 1980s, the Health Care Financing Administration (HCFA) found it necessary to expand the HCPCS system because not all supplies, procedures, and services could be coded using the CPT system. For example, durable medical equipment (DME) is not found in CPT. Therefore, HCFA developed an additional level of codes to report supplies and services that are not in CPT.

Purpose and Use

In 1983, Medicare introduced HCPCS to promote uniform reporting and statistical data collection of medical procedures, supplies, products, and services. Most state Medicaid programs and other insurance companies recognize portions of the HCPCS coding system. Physicians and providers use HCPCS codes to report the services and procedures they deliver.

Overview of Structure

HCPCS is divided into two code levels or groups: I and II.

Level I

Level I codes are the AMA's CPT codes. These five-digit codes and two-digit modifiers are copyrighted by the AMA. CPT codes primarily cover physicians' services but are used for hospital outpatient coding as well. CPT codes are updated annually, effective January 1. Modifiers are two digit code extenders that are utilizing in both Level I (CPT) and Level II HCPCS to modify or change the code description, such as to indicate a bilateral procedure (modifier 50) or to indicate that a procedure was decreased or limited (modifier 22).

Level II

Level II codes, also called National Codes, are maintained by CMS. With the exception of temporary codes, level II codes are updated annually on January 1. Temporary codes begin with the letters *G, K,* or *Q.* Temporary codes are updated throughout the year. Level II also contains modifiers in the form of letters and alphanumeric characters.

Level II codes were developed to code medical services, equipment, and supplies that are not included in CPT. Today, when people refer to HCPCS codes, they are often referring to level II codes; level I codes are most often referred to merely as CPT. Technically, HCPCS includes both level I (CPT) and level II codes. The codes are alphanumeric and start with an alphabetic character from A to V. The alphabetic character is followed by four numeric characters. The alphabetic character identifies the code section and type of service or supply coded. At times, level II codes were designed to reflect code assignment based on Medicare payment regulations. For example, even though there are colonoscopy codes provided in the CPT book, if a Medicare patient is undergoing a screening colonoscopy Medicare payment policies would require a Level II screening code to be utilized. Figure 5.9 shows the different code choices for patients undergoing a colonoscopy based on their medical necessity.

Figure 5.10 provides a list of the major sections in level II.

Level II also contains modifiers that can be used with all levels of HCPCS codes, including CPT codes. The modifiers permit greater reporting specificity in reference to the main code. Sample level II modifiers appear in figure 5.11.

Figure 5.9.   CPT/HCPCS code choices for colonoscopy

Example:	
Reason for Colonoscopy	**Appropriate code**
Problem, such as bleeding or polyps	CPT codes 45378–45392
Colorectal cancer screening, patient does not meet Medicare definition of high risk	G0121
Colorectal cancer screening, patient meets definition of high risk	G0105

Figure 5.10.   HCPCS Level II section titles

A0000–A0999	Transport Services Including Ambulance
A4000–A4899	Medical and Surgical Supplies
A9000–A9999	Administrative, Miscellaneous, and Investigational
B4000–B9999	Enteral and Parenteral Therapy
D0000–D9999	Dental Procedures
E0100–E9999	Durable Medical Equipment
G0000–G9999	Procedures/Professional Services (Temporary)
J0000–J8999	Drugs Other Than Chemotherapy
J9000–J9999	Chemotherapy Drugs
K0000–K9999	Orthotic Procedures
L5000–L9999	Prosthetic Procedures
M0000–M0009	Medical Services
P2000–P2999	Laboratory Tests
Q0000–Q9999	Temporary Codes
R0000–R5999	Domestic Radiology Services
S0009–S9999	Temporary National Codes
V0000–V2999	Vision Services
V5000–V5299	Hearing Services

Figure 5.11.   Sample HCPCS Level II modifiers

–AA	Anesthesia services performed personally by anesthesiologist
–E1	Upper left eyelid
–E2	Lower left eyelid
–E3	Upper right eyelid
–E4	Lower right eyelid
–NU	New equipment
–QC	Single channel monitoring

Current Procedural Terminology, Version 4

As mentioned earlier, the CPT system is copyrighted and maintained by the AMA. There have been several major updates to the system since the original edition was published in 1966. Code updates are published annually and take effect every January 1.

History of CPT-4

CPT is a comprehensive descriptive listing of terms and codes for reporting diagnostic and therapeutic procedures and medical services. Currently, it is updated annually by the

AMA's CPT Editorial Panel. This panel is composed of physicians and other healthcare professionals who revise, modify, and update the publication.

The Editorial Panel gets advice on revisions from the CPT Advisory Committee. This committee is nominated by the AMA House of Delegates and is composed of representatives from more than 90 medical specialties and healthcare providers. As defined by the AMA, the committee has three objectives:

- To serve as a resource to the Editorial Panel by giving advice on procedure coding and nomenclature as relevant to the member's specialty

- To provide documentation to staff and the Editorial Panel regarding the medical appropriateness of various medical and surgical procedures

- To suggest revisions to CPT

Purpose and Use

The purpose of CPT is to provide a system for standard terminology and coding to report medical procedures and services. CPT is one of the most widely used systems for reporting medical services to health insurance carriers. In addition, it is used for other administrative purposes, such as developing guidelines for medical care review. Organizations that collect data for medical education and research purposes also use CPT.

Today, CMS requires that CPT codes be used to report medical services provided to patients in specific settings. Starting in 1983, HCFA (now called the CMS) required that CPT be used to report services provided to Medicare Part B beneficiaries. In October 1986, HCFA required state Medicaid agencies to use CPT as part of the Medicaid Management Information System. As part of the Omnibus Budget Reconciliation Act, HCFA required in July 1987 that CPT be used for reporting outpatient hospital surgical procedures and ambulatory surgery center procedures. The most recent mandate for CPT use occurred with the final rule of the Health Insurance Portability and Accountability Act (HIPAA). HIPAA mandates that CPT be used as the required code set for physicians' services and other medical services such as physical therapy and most laboratory procedures.

Overview of Structure

The CPT codebook consists of an introduction, eight sections containing the codes, appendixes, and an index. Five digit codes are used—most are numeric, although specific sections include an alpha character. The eight sections include: evaluation and management services, anesthesia, surgery, radiology (including nuclear medicine and diagnostic ultrasound), pathology and laboratory, medicine, Category II and Category III codes.

Introduction

The introduction contains a list of the codebook section numbers and their sequences and instructions for use. Information that appears in the introduction applies to all sections of the codebook. A coder who is unfamiliar with CPT coding should read the introduction.

Symbols and punctuation marks are used to assist coders in correct usage of CPT codes. The symbols used in the CPT codebook are explained in the introduction and are found at the bottom of each page of the coding section of the book. For example, a bullet listed to the left of a code signifies that the code is new for that year's updated book.

Sections

The sections are as follows:

Evaluation and Management	99201–99499
Anesthesia	00100–01999
Surgery	10021–69990
Radiology	70010–79999
Pathology and Laboratory	80047–89398
Medicine	90281–99607
Category II Codes	0001F–7025F
Category III Codes	0016T–0207T

Each of these sections begins with guidelines containing specific instructions and definitions that are unique to the section. Coders must understand the information in the guidelines in order to code correctly from each section.

Category II and III Codes

According to CPT, Category II codes were designed as "supplemental tracking codes that can be used for performance measurement" (AMA 2012). Although these codes are optional, they can be used to provide greater specificity regarding a patient's visit and treatment details.

Category III codes were added to the CPT book to allow for temporary coding assignment for new technology and services that do not meet the rigorous requirements necessary to be added to the main section of the CPT book. The codes are not optional and should be used to report procedures performed. Codes in the Category III section are evaluated and added every six months. As Category I codes (codes ranging from 00100 to 99499) are created to describe new procedures, the corresponding temporary category III codes will be deleted from the CPT system. After approximately five years, if Category III codes have not been utilized, CPT may remove them from the CPT book and archive them.

Appendixes

Appendixes follow the last section of codes. The appendixes provide information to help the coder in the coding process.

- Appendix A provides a complete list of modifiers and their descriptions. Modifiers are written as two-digit codes that follow the main CPT codes. For example, the two-digit modifier for bilateral procedures is modifier 50.

- Appendix B is a summary of the additions, deletions, and revisions that have been implemented for the current CPT edition. This appendix can be used to update information and data that contain CPT codes.

- Appendix C provides clinical examples for codes found in the evaluation and management section (E/M) of the book. These examples can be used as a tool to assist the coder in reporting an E/M code.

- Appendix D is a listing of CPT add-on codes. These codes must be preceded by a primary procedure code and would never be reported alone.

- Appendix E is a summary of CPT codes that are exempt from modifier 51, and appendix F is a summary of CPT codes that are exempt from modifier 63.

- Appendix G contains codes that include conscious/moderate sedation.

- Appendix H is an alphabetic index of performance measures by clinical condition or type but was removed from CPT.

- Appendix I contains genetic testing code modifiers used for reporting with lab procedures related to genetic testing.

- Appendix J includes a listing of sensory, motor, and mixed nerves that are useful for nerve conduction studies.

- Appendix K lists procedures included in the CPT code book that are not yet approved by the FDA.

- Appendix L is a reference of the vascular families including which are considered first-, second-, and third-order vessels.

- Appendix M displays a table of deleted CPT codes and crosswalks to current codes.

- Appendix N is a listing of codes that have been resequenced.

Index

The index of the CPT codebook lists main terms alphabetically. Main term entries are of four types:

- Procedure or service
- Organ or other anatomic site
- Condition
- Synonym, eponym, or abbreviation

Main terms are followed by subterms. The subterms modify the main terms and are indented under them. Coders begin their search for the correct CPT code by checking the alphabetic index in the above order until finding a likely code to describe the procedure

Figure 5.12. **Portion of the CPT index**

Face	
CT Scan	70486–70488
Lesion Destruction	17000–17004, 17280–17286
Magnetic Resonance Imaging (MRI)	70540–70543
Tumor Resection	21015
Face Lift	15824–15828
Facial Asymmetries	
See Hemifacial Microsomia	

performed. The coder should then verify the code(s) selected in the main section of the codebook to be certain the code best describes the procedure(s) performed. Figure 5.12 shows a portion of the CPT index.

Check Your Understanding 5.3

Instructions: List the section of the CPT codebook in which each of the following codes is located.

1. _____ 99311

2. _____ 90807

3. _____ 33470

4. _____ 01200

5. _____ 87551

6. _____ 77295

7. _____ 0071T

Systematized Nomenclature of Medicine

The **Systematized Nomenclature of Medicine Clinical Terminology** (SNOMED CT) is a standardized vocabulary, sometimes referred to as a controlled reference terminology. The American College of Pathologists (ACP) defines SNOMED CT as a systematized, multiaxial, and hierarchically organized nomenclature of medically useful terms.

"SNOMED CT (Systematized Nomenclature of Medicine—Clinical Terms) is a comprehensive clinical terminology, originally created by the College of American Pathologists (CAP) and, as of April 2007, owned, maintained, and distributed by the International Health Terminology Standards Development Organisation (IHTSDO), a not-for-profit association in Denmark. The CAP continues to support SNOMED CT operations under contract to the IHTSDO and provides SNOMED-related products and services as a licensee of the terminology" (NLM 2009). IHTSDO develops and promotes the use of SNOMED CT to support safe and effective health information exchange. SNOMED CT is a clinical terminology and is considered to be the most comprehensive, multilingual healthcare terminology in the world (IHTSDO 2011).

History

ACP published the first edition of SNOMED in 1977. SNOMED is based on the Systematized Nomenclature of Pathology (SNOP), which was published by ACP in 1965 to organize information from surgical pathology reports. Because SNOP was widely used and accepted in the medical community, it was expanded as a nomenclature for other specialties.

Numerous versions of SNOMED have been published since 1977. The current version includes more than 150,000 terms that are used in countries throughout the world. SNOMED CT is the most comprehensive controlled vocabulary developed to date. The updated version of SNOMED is SNOMED CT (clinical terms), which is a "comprehensive multilingual clinical terminology tool providing the information framework for clinical decision making for electronic medical record[s]" (Brouch 2003, 54). This version is an adaptation of earlier versions of SNOMED and also contains the United Kingdom's National Health Service's Clinical Terms (previously known as **Read Codes**). Read Codes users are being migrated over to SNOMED CT.

In 2007, the Health and Human Services (HHS) Secretary announced that the United States would participate in an international effort to encourage more rapid development and worldwide adoption of standard clinical terminology for electronic health records.

> The United States is one of nine charter members of the new International Health Terminology Standards Development Organisation (IHTSDO), which has acquired Systemized Nomenclature of Medicine (SNOMED) Clinical Terms (SNOMED CT) from the College of American Pathologists (CAP). Other charter members are from Australia, Canada, Denmark, Lithuania, the Netherlands, New Zealand, Sweden, and the United Kingdom. Membership is open to all countries.
>
> "International implementation of SNOMED CT is good for everyone engaged in developing electronic health records, and it will open up new opportunities for international collaboration in research and public health surveillance," Secretary Leavitt said. "This use of a standard terminology will enable the use of health information across borders, facilitate public health surveillance and support evidence-based research."

Purpose and Use

In the field of medicine, two physicians may use two different terms for the same medical condition. This makes it difficult to gather and retrieve information. Standardized vocabulary is needed to facilitate the indexing, storage, and retrieval of patient information in an EHR. SNOMED CT creates a standardized vocabulary.

The Computer-based Patient Record Institute (CPRI) has studied the ability of current nomenclatures to capture information for EHRs. The institute has determined that SNOMED CT is the most comprehensive controlled vocabulary for coding the contents of the health record and facilitating the development of electronic records. According to the IHTSDO:

> Each year, avoidable deaths and injuries occur because of poor communication between healthcare practitioners, or because busy practitioners forget or neglect to follow their own criteria for best practices. The delivery of a standard clinical terminology for use across the world's health information systems can therefore make a significant contribution towards improving the quality and safety of healthcare.
>
> SNOMED CT aims to contribute to the improvement of patient care through underpinning the development of systems to accurately record healthcare encounters and to deliver decision support to health care providers. Ultimately, patients will benefit from the use of SNOMED CT to more clearly describe and accurately record their care, in building and facilitating better communication and interoperability in electronic health record exchange, and in creating systems that support healthcare decision making. (IHTSDO 2011)

Overview of Structure

Using SNOMED as a foundation, SNOMED CT presents data in a completely machine-readable format. According to SNOMED International, the main content areas of SNOMED CT include the following tables:

- Concept—A clinical idea to which a unique ConceptID has been assigned in SNOMED CT. Each concept is represented by a row in the concepts table.

- Descriptions—The human-readable phrases or names associated with SNOMED CT concepts. All of the concept descriptions in SNOMED CT are listed in the descriptions table.

- Relationships—An association between two concepts. The nature of the association is indicated by a relationship type. Each relationship is represented by a row in the relationships table.

- History—SNOMED CT includes some information about the history of changes to concepts and descriptions.

SNOMED CT has been mapped to ICD-9-CM and ICD-10 as well as other commonly used vocabularies such as ICD-O-3, ICD-10, and LOINC. Mapping is the comparison of code descriptions used in various coding systems and comparing the two to determine which codes match as closely as possible.

The core tables provide the framework for the organization of the elements within the system. The concepts table lists every concept that appeared in earlier versions of SNOMED CT, starting with version 3. More than 366,000 concepts are organized into 18 hierarchies within the SNOMED CT system. Each concept, or fully-specified name as listed on the table, is given a concept identifier.

Concepts are further identified by various terms or phrases that define them. The combination of a concept and a term is a description. Descriptions are given a Description ID.

Real-world Example

TheraDoc is a medical informatics company that produces software used for clinical decision support. One of its systems, Antibiotic Assistant, was designed to support the appropriate use of antibiotics (TheraDoc 2001). SNOMED CT was integrated into Antibiotic Assistant to allow the system to be integrated with other patient information systems in order to analyze possible drug interactions or adverse reactions to the medications. TheraDoc's Antibiotic Assistant, supported by SNOMED CT, is designed to work within the facility's existing information systems environment. TheraDoc's powerful interface and inference engines can use existing data from ancillary and legacy systems to integrate patient-specific results reporting and monitoring with disease-specific point-of-care decision support. Coupled with existing electronic medical records and order management systems, the Antibiotic Assistant can act as an integrated disease-specific ordering module to address and improve both processes and tasks. Through sophisticated knowledge-based engines, the software considers all possible ways in which an infectious disease can be managed and eliminates those options that are contraindicated due to mitigating factors (for example, allergies, neutropenia) and patient attributes (for example, height, weight, age).

Diagnostic and Statistical Manual of Mental Disorders, Fourth Edition, Text Revision

The American Psychiatric Association (APA) developed the *Diagnostic and Statistical Manual of Mental Disorders* (DSM) as a tool for providing a set of codes that could be used to aid in the collection of clinical data using stand-alone personal computers.

History of DSM-IV

The APA published the first edition of the DSM in 1952. The APA's Committee on Nomenclature and Statistics developed DSM from ICD. DSM-I contained a glossary of descriptions of mental disorders. DSM has been revised three times since 1952 and is now published as the fourth revision, or DSM-IV-TR. The updated text revision (TR) became effective in 2004 to maintain currency with updated clinical terms. There were very few coding changes in the DSM-IV-TR version.

To facilitate ease of use with ICD versions, the APA has worked closely with other organizations to make DSM-IV, ICD-9-CM, and ICD-10 fully compatible. All DSM-IV-TR codes are ICD-9-CM codes. This is even more important because the HIPAA law requires that valid ICD-9-CM codes be used for diagnostic purposes. According to the APA, *"The Diagnostic and Statistical Manual of Mental Disorders* (DSM) is the standard classification of mental disorders used by mental health professionals in the United States. It is intended to be applicable in a wide array of contexts and used by clinicians and researchers of many different orientations (for example, biological, psychodynamic, cognitive, behavioral, interpersonal, family/systems)" (APA 2011).

Purpose and Use

The main purpose of DSM-IV-TR is to provide a means to record data on patients treated for substance abuse and mental disorders. DSM is used as a nomenclature that clinicians can reference to enhance their clinical practices and as a language for communicating diagnostic information. Clinicians use DSM to assign a diagnosis. Mental health professionals use this manual when working with patients in order to better understand their illness and potential treatment and to help third-party payers (e.g., insurance) understand the needs of the patient. The book is typically considered the "bible" for any professional who makes psychiatric diagnoses in the United States and many other countries (Heffner 2011).

DSM contains a listing of the criteria for diagnosing each mental disorder and its key clinical manifestations. Mental conditions are evaluated along five axes.

Overview of Structure

The five axes used in DSM-IV-TR are:

Axis I	Clinical Disorders	diagnoses such as depression or schizophrenia
	Other Conditions That May Be a Focus of Clinical Attention	
Axis II	Personality Disorders	such as paranoia disorders
	Mental Retardation	such as Down's syndrome
Axis III	General Medical Conditions	symptoms or physical conditions such as brain disorders
Axis IV	Psychosocial and Environmental Problems	events such as death of a loved one that impact the patient's condition
Axis V	Global Assessment of Functioning	patient's level of functioning including appropriate to date and time

Use of these axes by clinicians helps to establish a systematic evaluation of patient symptoms which will lead to the establishment of diagnoses for the patient. The diagnoses then are given a code or codes that are the same as ICD-9-CM codes. The newest updated version of DSM, DSM-V, is scheduled to be published in 2013.

The idea is to assemble existing disorders into larger clusters suggested by the scientific evidence and then to encourage researchers, granting agencies, and journal editors to facilitate research within and across clusters. This clustering (which has come to be called a "meta-structure") would be reflected in the *DSM-V* as a new table of contents, but would leave revisions of criteria for individual disorders to the existing *DSM-V* work groups. Ultimately, the goal is to move away from a classification that focused on reliability while inadvertently sacrificing validity toward a classification that is far more clinically useful than that of *DSM-IV* and far more open to validation. (Bernstein 2011)

Nursing Vocabularies

The use of vocabularies is a relatively new concept in the field of nursing. Nursing vocabularies are currently used to classify nursing diagnoses, interventions, and outcomes in various healthcare settings.

History of Nursing Vocabularies

Nursing vocabularies were developed to aid in the collection of data about nursing care. They serve as a way to document nursing care and to facilitate the capture of these data on computer systems. For example, North American Nursing Diagnosis Association-International (NANDA-I) was established to "develop, refine and promote terminology that accurately reflects nurses' clinical judgments. Implementation of nursing diagnosis enhances every aspect of nursing practice, from garnering professional respect to assuring consistent documentation representing nurses' professional clinical judgment, and accurate documentation to enable reimbursement" (NANDA-I 2011).

Purpose and Use

According to NANDA, "A nursing diagnosis is used to determine the appropriate plan of care for the patient. The nursing diagnosis drives interventions and patient outcomes, enabling the nurse to develop the patient care plan. Nursing diagnoses also provide a standard nomenclature for use in the Electronic Health Record, enabling clear communication among care team members and the collection of data for continuous improvement in patient care" (NANDA-I 2011).

The American Nurses Association (ANA) recognizes approximately 13 standardized terminologies. These nursing terminologies are developed by separate agencies for various purposes. These terminologies are described in table 5.1. All the classifications approved by the ANA are included in the Unified Medical Language System (UMLS).

Table 5.1. **Widely used nursing vocabularies and classifications**

Vocabulary or Classification System	Usage	Web Site
North American Nursing Diagnosis Association (NANDA) Taxonomy II	This classification is used to classify nursing diagnoses in all nursing settings. The NANDA multiaxial taxonomy is designed to provide a standardized nursing terminology to define patient responses, document care for reimbursement, and to allow for inclusion of nursing terminology in building clinical EHRs (North American Nursing Diagnosis Association 2005).	http://nanda.org
Nursing Interventions Classifications (NIC)	NIC is used to classify nursing interventions. Nursing interventions are any direct-care treatment that a nurse performs on behalf of the patient. These interventions are used to direct the care of patients.	http://www.nursing.uiowa.edu/excellence/nursing_knowledge/clinical_effectiveness/nic.htm
Nursing Outcomes Classification (NOC)	NOC is used to classify nursing outcomes. Nursing outcomes are the end result of care. They can measure quality of care, cost-efficiency, and progress of treatment.	http://www.nursing.uiowa.edu/excellence/nursing_knowledge/clinical_effectiveness/noc.htm
Home Health Care Classifications (HHCC)	HHCC contains two interrelated vocabularies used for classifying and documenting ambulatory and home health care. The HHCC of Nursing Diagnoses and the HHCC of Nursing Interventions are used.	http://sabacare.com
Nursing Management Minimum Data Set (NMMDS)	NMMDS captures nursing data for the comparison of patient outcomes.	http://www.nursing.umn.edu/ICNP/USANMMDS/home.html
OMAHA System	This classification is used to classify nursing diagnoses, interventions, and outcomes.	http://omahasystem.org/index.htm
SNOMED CT	SNOMED is a reference terminology for healthcare.	http://SNOMED.org
Perioperative Nursing Dataset (PNDS)	This data set is a standardized nursing vocabulary for use when patients undergo surgery. It allows for the capture of data from preadmission care until patient discharge.	http://aorn.org/research/pnds.htm
Clinical Care Classification (CCC)	The CCC is used to classify nursing diagnoses and outcomes, and interventions.	http://sabacare.com
Patient Care Data Set	This terminology is now retired.	http://ncvhs.hhs.gov/990518t3.pdf
International Classification for Nursing Practice (2000) Information (ICNP)	ICNP provides data to influence decision-making, education, and health policy.	http://icn.ch/icnp_about.htm
Alternative Link	Alternative Link's ABC codes represent integrative healthcare products and services (complementary and alternative medicine).	http://alternativelink.com/ali/intro_altlink.html
Logical Observation Identifiers Names & Codes (LOINC)	LOINC is used to pool results—such as blood hemoglobin, serum potassium, or vital signs—for clinical care, outcomes management, and research.	http://regenstrief.org/loinc/

The nursing data sets and classification systems are developed to capture documentation on nursing care. They are designed to capture nursing diagnoses, interventions, and outcomes for acute, surgery, home, and ambulatory care settings.

According to the ANA, "A standardized vocabulary assists nurses to document care while providing a foundation for examining and evaluating the quality and effectiveness of that care. An information infrastructure provides the foundation for benchmarking, measuring and comparing outcome data, and evaluating the quality and effectiveness of care" (ANA 2011). The various ANA-recognized standardized terminologies have different structures. See table 5.1 for a description of each.

Check Your Understanding 5.4

Instructions: Match the following classification systems with their functions.

1. _____ SNOMED CT

2. _____ Nursing vocabularies

3. _____ DSM-IV-TR

a. To document nursing care and to facilitate the capture of nursing information on computer systems
b. To provide a means to record information about patients treated for substance abuse and mental disorders
c. To aid in the collection of clinical data using stand-alone personal computers
d. To provide a system for coding the clinical services provided by physicians and other clinical professionals
e. To provide a controlled vocabulary for coding the contents of the patient record and for facilitating the development of computer-based patient records

The Coding Process

The coding process varies from organization to organization, but some standards, elements, and steps are common to almost all organizations.

Standards of Ethical Coding

In today's healthcare environment, coding plays an important role in the determination of reimbursement for healthcare facilities. Improper coding could result in incorrect reimbursement and potential fraud and/or abuse claims against the provider. AHIMA developed its Standards of Ethical Coding, last updated in 2008. The standards were developed by AHIMA's Coding Policy and Strategy Committee and approved by its Board of Directors. The AHIMA standards are meant to serve as a guide for coding professionals (see figure 5.13).

Elements of Coding Quality

The coding process must be reviewed on an ongoing basis for consistency and accuracy. Audits should occur to review the codes selected by coders and to serve as guides for

Figure 5.13. **AHIMA's Standards of Ethical Coding**

1. Coding professionals are expected to support the importance of accurate, complete, and consistent coding practices for the production of quality healthcare data.

2. Coding professionals in all healthcare settings should adhere to the ICD-9-CM (International Classification of Diseases, 9th revision, Clinical Modification) coding conventions, official coding guidelines approved by the Cooperating Parties,* the CPT (Current Procedural Terminology) rules established by the American Medical Association, and any other official coding rules and guidelines established for use with mandated standard code sets. Selection and sequencing of diagnoses and procedures must meet the definitions of required data sets for applicable healthcare settings.

3. Coding professionals should use their skills, their knowledge of currently mandated coding and classification systems, and official resources to select the appropriate diagnostic and procedural codes.

4. Coding professionals should only assign and report codes that are clearly and consistently supported by physician documentation in the health record.

5. Coding professionals should consult physicians for clarification and additional documentation prior to code assignment when there are conflicting or ambiguous data in the health record.

6. Coding professionals should not change codes or the narratives of codes on the billing abstract so that meanings are misrepresented. Diagnoses or procedures should not be inappropriately included or excluded because payment or insurance policy coverage requirements will be affected. When individual payer policies conflict with official coding rules and guidelines, these policies should be obtained in writing whenever possible. Reasonable efforts should be made to educate the payer on proper coding practices in order to influence a change in the payer's policy.

7. Coding professionals, as members of the healthcare team, should assist and educate physicians and other clinicians by advocating proper documentation practices, further specificity, and resequencing or inclusion of diagnoses or procedures when needed to more accurately reflect the acuity, severity, and the occurrence of events.

8. Coding professionals should participate in the development of institutional coding policies and should ensure that coding policies complement, not conflict with, official coding rules and guidelines.

9. Coding professionals should maintain and continually enhance their coding skills, as they have a professional responsibility to stay abreast of changes in codes, coding guidelines, and regulations.

10. Coding professionals should strive for optimal payment to which the facility is legally entitled, remembering that it is unethical and illegal to maximize payment by means that contradict regulatory guidelines.

*The Cooperating Parties are the American Health Information Management Association, American Hospital Association, Centers for Medicare and Medicaid Services, and National Center for Health Statistics.

further education for the coding professionals. Review of records should be approached as a way to improve quality and not viewed as punitive in nature. Coding processes should be monitored for the following elements of quality:

- *Reliability:* The degree to which the same results are achieved consistently (that is, when different individuals code the same health record, they assign the same codes)

- *Validity:* The degree to which codes accurately reflect the patient's diagnoses and procedures

- *Completeness:* The degree to which the codes capture all the diagnoses and procedures documented in the health record

- *Timeliness:* The time frame in which the health records are coded

Coding Policies and Procedures

Every healthcare facility should establish coding policies and procedures that establish guidelines that coders should follow to ensure coding consistency. Coding consistency can be developed by using the coding guidelines, practice briefs, and sample policies and procedures established by organizations such as the AHA, the AMA, AHIMA, and state health information management association policies. Any areas that are not covered in official policies or guidelines should be covered in the facility's policies/procedures, such as to provide usage guidance regarding optional E codes in diagnosis coding.

The AHA publishes the official guidelines for ICD-9-CM coding in a quarterly newsletter entitled *Coding Clinic.* The AMA publishes information regarding CPT codes in a newsletter entitled *CPT Assistant.* Both publications can be used as a basis for developing facility policies and procedures.

Steps in the Coding Process

For accurate coding, the coder must have a complete health record on the patient. Each facility needs to define what constitutes a complete record. The coder must review the contents of the record to determine the patient's condition and the treatment and care he or she received.

For an inpatient record, the health record should contain the following documents prior to being coded: a face sheet, history and physical, consultations, if applicable, operative and procedural reports, pathology reports, progress notes, and a discharge summary. The coder needs to review these documents to verify diagnoses and procedures.

After the record is reviewed, the coder selects the diagnoses and procedures that need to be coded and assigns appropriate code numbers. Codes then have to be sequenced according to Uniform Hospital Discharge Data Set (UHDDS) guidelines.

After the diagnoses and procedures are coded, the codes are entered into the facility's database. These data then become the foundation for statistical, reimbursement, and clinical information systems.

Quality Assessment for the Coding Process

Assessment of the coding process should occur through regular monitoring of coding accuracy. Monitoring is the ongoing internal review of coding practices conducted by an organization on a regular basis. A monitoring/audit program plan should be a written plan that outlines the objectives and frequency of the audits, the record selection process, the qualifications of auditors, and corrective actions the organization will take as a result of the audit findings.

Initially, a baseline audit should be performed. The audit should be a review of a large sample of the coding completed. It should include a sample of records coded by all coders for all types of services. Moreover, the sample should be representative of all physicians and types of cases treated by the organization. The baseline audit provides an overview of the organization's current coding practices.

The organization should conduct follow-up audits according to the schedule established in the monitoring/audit plan. Follow-up audits will provide ongoing monitoring of the coding process to ensure coding accuracy. The results of the audits also can be used to outline areas in which coder education and training are needed. Figure 5.14 is an example of a coding audit review sheet. Chapter 6 also discusses management of documentation and coding quality and corporate coding compliance programs.

Check Your Understanding 5.5

Instructions: Indicate whether the following statements are true or false (T or F).

1. _____ Coding plays an important role in the determination of reimbursement of healthcare facilities.

2. _____ The coding function must be reviewed on an ongoing basis for coding consistency and accuracy.

3. _____ The AMA publishes the official guidelines for CPT coding in its newsletter, *Coding Clinic*.

4. _____ Codes are sequenced in the patient's health record according to AHIMA's Standards of Ethical Coding.

5. _____ A baseline audit should include a sample of records coded by all coders for all types of services.

Figure 5.14. **Example of a coding audit review sheet**

Coding Audit Review Sheet

Coder _____

Type of Review (IP,OP,ER) _____

Date of Review _____

Medical Record # _____

Discharge Date _____

Initial Codes Assigned	Reviewer's Recommendations

Principal Diagnosis

A. Chosen and coded correctly   _____

B. Chosen correctly, coded incorrectly _____

C. Chosen incorrectly, coded correctly _____

D. Chosen and coded incorrectly   _____

Secondary Diagnoses

A. Chosen and coded correctly   _____

B. Chosen correctly, coded incorrectly _____

C. Chosen incorrectly, coded correctly _____

D. Chosen and coded incorrectly   _____

Principal Procedure

A. Chosen and coded correctly   _____

B. Chosen correctly, coded incorrectly _____

C. Chosen incorrectly, coded correctly _____

D. Chosen and coded incorrectly   _____

Secondary Procedures

A. Chosen and coded correctly   _____

B. Chosen correctly, coded incorrectly _____

C. Chosen incorrectly, coded correctly _____

D. Chosen and coded incorrectly   _____

DRG

A. Chosen and coded correctly   _____

B. Chosen correctly, coded incorrectly _____

C. Chosen incorrectly, coded correctly _____

D. Chosen and coded incorrectly   _____

Note: A review sheet can also be constructed to monitor CPT coding information instead of DRG assignments.

Coding Technology

Technology is changing many aspects of the health information profession. One of the primary areas where it has assisted in making jobs more efficient is in the area of coding. As early as the 1980s, information technology was applied to make the coding process more effective and efficient. The type of tool used to aid in the coding process is commonly referred to as an **encoder.** The development of other technologies, including **natural language processing** (NLP), will likely have an even greater impact on the coding process.

Encoders

Encoders for ICD were developed in the early 1980s. Over the subsequent years, greater sophistication has been built into these technology solutions. An encoder is computer software that helps the coding professional to assign codes. Initially, encoders were developed for assisting coders in assigning ICD-9-CM codes. Today, however, encoders include assistance with other coding systems including CPT, HCPCS, and ICD-10.

The information science and technology behind the encoding software varies from vendor to vendor. Some encoders are built using techniques such as rule-based systems that prompt the coder through a series of questions, commonly known as "logic based" encoders. As the coder answers the questions, the encoder leads the coder to codes for diagnoses and procedures. Alternatively, other encoders, referred to as "knowledge based", utilize more of an electronic code book by automating a look-up function similar to the manual index in ICD or other coding classifications.

Encoders have many different types of interfaces, depending on the vendor. An **interface** can be defined as the total component of screens, navigation, and input mechanisms used to help the end user operate the encoding software. Some encoder systems allow coders to input classification codes directly into the system and then go through a series of edit checks to ensure that only allowable code numbers are entered. In more sophisticated software systems, the encoder also prompts the coder to review the sequencing of the codes that have been selected in order to optimize reimbursement.

Good encoding software should include edit checks to ensure data quality. For example, an inappropriate combination of codes or inconsistent data should be flagged for the coder's attention. Encoding software is frequently linked to other information systems applications. This includes direct links to MS-DRG grouper software and billing systems. The use of encoders has become a predominant tool in the HIM department, particularly in acute care facilities. Today, however, there is even a greater movement toward more complete computerization of the coding function using a supporting technology called **computer-assisted coding** (CAC). As the role of the coding professional changes with more electronically generated records, facilities will need to review their current coding tools including the encoder to determine if they are still appropriate in the CAC environment. The coder will not be assigning codes from "scratch" any longer but will utilize the encoder to verify correct coding and review edits and issues that impact reimbursement. There are several different types of CAC including using software to aid the physician in selecting the correct code with processes such as drop-down boxes or the use of touch screen terminals. One form of CAC is natural language processing, or NLP. In an NLP or artificial intelligence software, digital text from online documents stored in the organization's information system is read directly by the software, which then suggests codes to match the documentation. For example, the digital text in an online emergency department record would be interpreted automatically by the CAC system and, through the use of expert or artificial intelligence software, would automatically suggest appropriate code numbers. The coding professional would then review the selections and verify codes before releasing the case into the billing system. See an example of this in figure 5.15.

The goal of CAC is to become the essential tool for hospital coding by meeting both current and future requirements. While the motivations and goals for CAC are clear, there are significant challenges in the hospital setting. CAC developers must demonstrate the effectiveness of their solutions for hospital inpatient and outpatient services while working with HIM professionals to serve up three important deliverables Since the CAC products work with electronically generated documents, as facilities move closer to a total electronic health record it will prove to be a more usable coding tool.

Figure 5.15. CAC example

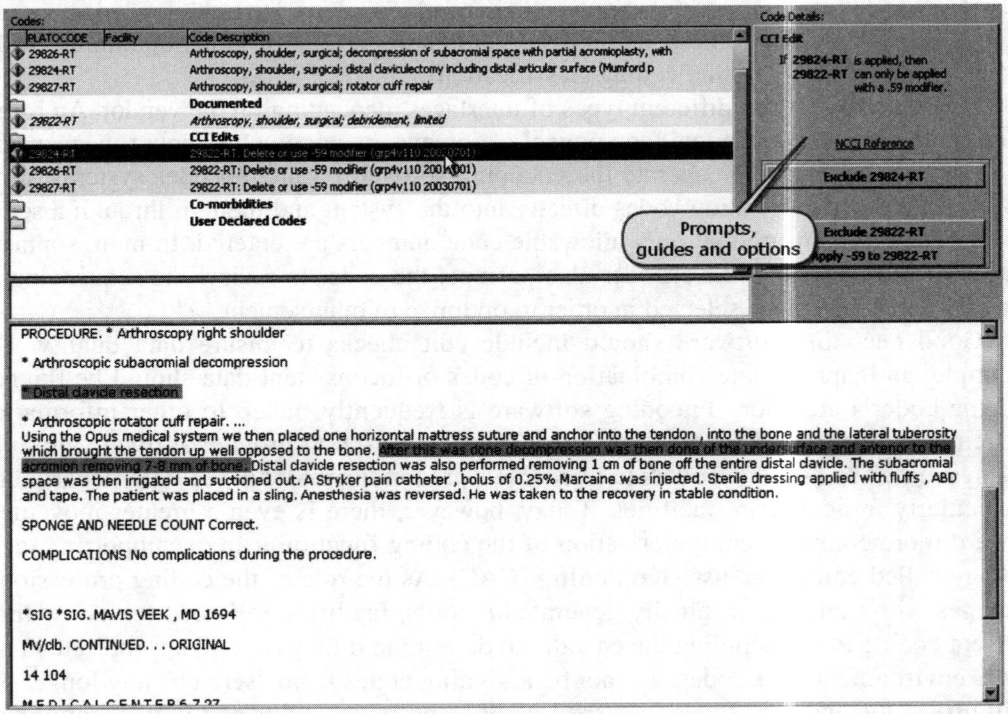

Source: Copyright © PLATOCODE Ltd.

Transitioning to CAC

The Skills and Tools Required to Work with Computer-assisted Coding

The coding world is not immune to technology advancements. Computer-assisted coding (**CAC**) technology is changing how the coding process is accomplished across all healthcare settings. **CAC** technology continues to integrate into a coding professional's daily life. A number of tools are required to facilitate preparation for a successful transition.

The Coder as Editor

Just as word processing did not require individuals to relearn how to spell or create sentences, **CAC** will not require coders to relearn how to code. Rather it allows coders to apply their analytical coding knowledge. The coders's role will transform to editor when working with **CAC** technology.

Generally speaking, an editor reviews content to determine if revisions are necessary. A coding editor determines if the computer-suggested codes are ready for all downstream processes such as billing or public health reporting.

Coders determine the final code selection based upon their knowledge of coding guidelines, clinical concepts, and compliance regulations. They will have the opportunity to agree or disagree with the coding options provided by the software.

This transition from producing the code to editing codes requires critical thinking skills such as knowing why a diagnosis or procedure is or is not coded. **CAC** provides a link between documentation and a suggested code; however, coders need to base their decisions on a combined knowledge of disease processes and coding principles. A common coding example that requires analysis is the determination of coding signs and symptoms.

Each health record is unique and requires coders to decide if the code assignment reflects the patient's clinical story. Having a solid education from a reliable source in clinical foundations related to anatomy, physiology, and pharmacology, as well as a coding education, is important for coders at all levels of their careers and can enhance their analytical skills.

Technology Skills

A qualitative research study revealed coders support automation and technology advancements. In today's healthcare environment individual technology skills are important to assess.

Electronic health record systems are changing the way coders perform the coding function, from accessing records remotely to determining if the documentation necessary for proper code assignment is present in the electronic record.

Working remotely without an on-site IT department requires that coders possess familiarity with technology, such as connecting through a virtual protected network, ensuring information security, and troubleshooting if the technology is not performing at the expected level.

Specifically, coders must understand the logic that supports how the computer generates a list of suggested codes. There is a difference between how systems determine a code. Two common ways are natural language processing and structured text input.

(continued on next page)

Coders should be aware which type of system the organization is investigating, implementing, or maintaining because they will be responsible for validating the output from the system.

Computer-assisted coding technology is most efficient when interfaced with electronic documentation. Just as codes produced by coding professionals are dependent upon documentation, the computer-selected codes are dependent upon the available electronic documentation. The system receives documentation via system interfacing.

CAC systems typically interface with current encoding products, which interface with the organization's financial system. It is important to know which systems are interfacing with each other, as well as what information is part of the interface. Coders thus should assess their interface knowledge.

Next Steps

To prepare for **CAC**, coders should create a continuing education plan based upon individual self-assessment. The plan should include specific actions, such as reviewing **CAC** articles or taking a class in anatomy from a reliable source.

Making a commitment to lifelong learning is important, because guidelines, regulations, and technology change the coding process. Integrating new and prior skills builds a coding professional's confidence in an ever-changing healthcare landscape.

Real World: ICD-10-CM CAC Example

In this example, the **CAC** software assigned the code T15.91A based on documentation in the emergency department record that states the patient had a "foreign body in the right eye." The coder is presented with the decision to accept the code or reject it based on further analysis.

Review of the documentation revealed that the foreign body was located on the edge of the cornea, which changes the fourth character in ICD-10-CM from 9 to 1. The coders replaces the T15.91xA code with T15.01A, Foreign body in cornea, right eye.

Emergency Department Record

A patient is brought to the emergency department due to a foreign body in the right eye. He was working with metal, and a piece flew in his eye. He reports slight irritation to the right eye but no blurred vision.

A slit lamp shows a foreign body approximately 2–3 o'clock on the edge of the cornea. The foreign body appears to be metallic. The iris is intact.

Procedure: Two drops of Alcaine were used in the right eye. Foreign body is removed from the right eye.

Computer-Generated Codes: T15.91xA, Foreign body, external eye, right.

Final Coding Decision: Coder selects the more specific code for foreign body of cornea, T15.01xA.

Article citation: Smith, Gail; Bronnert, June. "Transitioning to CAC: The Skills and Tools Required to Work with Computer-assisted Coding." *Journal of AHIMA* 81, no.7 (July 2010): 60–61.

Check Your Understanding 5.6

Instructions: Indicate whether the following statements are true or false (T or F).

1. ____ An encoder is computer software that assists in determining coding accuracy and reliability.

2. ____ An interface is the total component of screens, navigation, and input mechanisms used to operate encoding software.

3. ____ Good encoding software should include edit checks.

4. ____ The NLP encoding system uses expert or artificial intelligence software to automatically assign code numbers.

5. ____ Good encoding software should include edit checks to ensure data quality.

Unifying Clinical Vocabularies

As the number and sophistication of clinical vocabularies increase, there has been a significant movement toward research in understanding the fundamental elements and structures in both vocabularies and classification systems. One of the most farsighted endeavors toward bringing together the various clinical vocabularies is the Unified Medical Language System (UMLS) project being conducted by the National Library of Medicine (NLM).

National Library of Medicine UMLS Project

The NLM established a research project in 1986. This long-range project is called the Unified Medical Language System (UMLS) project.

The purpose of the UMLS is to aid in the development of systems that help healthcare professionals retrieve and integrate electronic biomedical information from a variety of sources. UMLS uses three knowledge sources to make it easier for users to link separate information systems:

- The *metathesaurus* provides a uniform collection of more than one hundred biomedical/health-related vocabularies, coding systems, and classifications and links the different names used in the various vocabularies and classifications, such as SNOMED CT, LOINC, and RXNorm to a common concept. The UMLS Metathesaurus contains the complete set of SNOMED CT.

- The *specialist lexicon* contains syntactic information for many terms. (For example, it lists the parts of speech, various forms of a word, and spelling variations of the terms within UMLS.)

- The *semantic network* provides a system for categorizing objects and identifying the relationships among various concepts.

The UMLS knowledge sources overcome retrieval problems that occur when different terminology and separate databases are used. They are currently being used in a variety of applications, including patient data creation, natural language processing, and information retrieval. The NLM maintains fact sheets describing the progress of this project on its website, http://www.nlm.nih.gov/pubs/factsheets/umls.html.

Development of the Nosologist Role

Nosology is the branch of medical science that deals with classification systems. A nosologist is a person who works with using and developing classification systems. The AHIMA Coding Futures Task Force envisions that the role of the coder will change dramatically over the next decade. At present, the coder's primary responsibility is the assignment of codes. In the future, the coder will become responsible for the development, maintenance, and management of classification systems and vocabularies.

In today's healthcare environment, HIM professionals, especially those with career paths in clinical coding, are enjoying a wealth of opportunity in the job market. There is a critical need for qualified coding professionals to classify, manage, and maintain clinical information for analysis and transactions. As a result of increased regulation in healthcare, heightened compliance risks, and progressively more complex reimbursement tied to code assignments, coding professionals have a greater array of choices within the profession than ever before (AHIMA Practice Council for Clinical Terminology and Classification 2007).

Along with increased demand for coding professionals is a clear broadening of roles within the HIM profession. Today's work force demands knowledge and job skills that go beyond the basic conventions of standard diagnosis and procedure code assignment from health records. Clinical terminologies are expanding into a broader use of data sets beyond the traditional ICD-9-CM and HCPCS/CPT code sets to include SNOMED-CT, LOINC, specialized terminologies for pharmaceuticals and nursing care, and a host of others to serve an environment hungry for data that is easily digested by computer software and reliable, consistent, and accurate.

Many levels of HIM expertise are needed, and a variety of skills are important for career success. Most employers are seeking a minimum of a bachelor's degree in a healthcare discipline as well as "high-end" knowledge that facilitates integration of data management with a specific business case, software application, or clinical workflow support process. Current employment trends favor master's degree preparation in HIM, health informatics, computer information management, or related fields of study. A solid clinical knowledge base is required for many positions related to clinical terminology use involving clinical coding systems and data analysis.

To complete the picture, there are a number of healthcare professionals managing health information today. HIM roles involve physicians, nurses, technicians, and other allied health professionals in some job settings. Career pathways in HIM frequently merge with an educational foundation or experience in these disciplines. These pathways are helpful for illustrating how selected jobs evolve over time and how entry-level positions lay the foundation for new opportunities with greater responsibility, variety, and compensation potential.

Check Your Understanding 5.7

Instructions: Indicate whether the following statements are true or false (T or F).

1. _____ The UMLS project was initiated to bring together the various medical vocabularies.

2. _____ The metathesaurus, one of the UMLS knowledge sources, contains syntactic information for many terms.

3. _____ The UMLS knowledge sources are currently being used in natural language processing.

4. _____ A nosologist's primary responsibility is the assignment of diagnosis codes.

5. _____ In the future, coders' roles will change.

Real-world Case

Can computer-assisted coding (CAC) be helpful to outpatient coders? CAC is a supporting technology that has reached an exciting stage of development. It holds a great deal of promise for assisting in further automation of the coding process. Although the technology holds great promise, it also faces a huge challenge because of the complexity and variability of human speech. However, promising new CAC products are beginning to emerge in certain medical arenas, such as emergency medicine and radiology. Facilities that have begun to implement CAC report the following benefits (*AHIMA Today* 2009):

- Reduced number of systems requiring review (previously the hybrid record required the review of components in the EHR/scanned documents/paper record)

- Increased productivity and efficiency

- Increased accuracy

- Increase in productivity by 20 percent

- Decrease in overtime by 85 percent
- Decrease in external auditor recommendation changes by 50 percent
- Decrease in external audit fees by 60 percent
- Increase in Medicare Case-Mix Index (CMI) by 0.08 or 4 percent with same patient population

Summary

In recent decades, coding, classification, and vocabulary systems have grown in importance. This is clear in the critical role that coding now plays in the healthcare industry's reimbursement process and its use in research and quality assurance efforts.

Nomenclatures, classification systems, and clinical vocabularies were created to help organize healthcare data. In medicine, a nomenclature is a system that lists preferred medical terminology. A classification system groups together similar diseases and procedures and organizes related entities for easy retrieval.

The purpose and use of clinical classifications today are varied. For example, physicians use classifications such as ICD to classify morbidity and mortality information for statistical purposes, to index hospital records by disease and operations, and to report diagnoses. In addition, clinical classifications are used in the reporting and compilation of healthcare data to assist in evaluating medical care planning for healthcare delivery systems, determining patterns of care among healthcare providers, analyzing payments of healthcare services, and conducting epidemiological and clinical research studies.

Although ICD-9-CM is perhaps the most prominent classification system in use today, health information technicians use many other systems in their daily practice, such as CPT, HCPCS, ICD-O-2, DSM, and nursing vocabularies. The continued development of these and other classification systems and vocabularies reflects the complexity of describing the medical care process. As the healthcare industry prepares for the implementation of ICD-10-CM and ICD-10-PCS, extensive training and educational preparation is underway. This will provide many job opportunities for coding and HIM professionals.

Every healthcare organization must have policies and procedures in place that set guidelines for managing the coding process and ensuring the consistency of the organization's coding output. Further, every organization should establish a monitoring/audit program to review and assess coding accuracy on a regular basis. Moreover, every organization should develop a corporate compliance plan that monitors its billing and coding activities to prevent fraudulent practices.

Finally, technological advances are having a tremendous impact on the coding process today and will likely have an even greater impact in the future. Important projects such as the Unified Medical Language System project conducted by the National Library of Medicine, coupled with the growth and maturity of automated coding and natural language processing systems, will revolutionize the coding function.

References

AHIMA Practice Council for Clinical Terminology and Classification. 2007. Paving the information highway: Career pathways for knowledge workers involved with coded data. Chicago: AHIMA.

AHIMA Today. 2009. Convention daily newsletter: Working smarter with computer-assisted coding. Highlights from 81st Convention and Exhibit.

American Medical Association. 2012. *Current Procedural Terminology.* Chicago: American Medical Association.

American Nurses Association Committee for Nursing Practice Information Infrastructure. 2011. Frequently asked questions: Standardized terminologies. http://users.stargate.net/~lqthede/CNPII/RecognizedTerminologies/ANARecognizedStandardizations.htm

American Psychiatric Association. 2011. http://www.psych.org/MainMenu/Research/DSMIV.aspx

Averill, R., R. Mullin, B. Steinbeck, N. Goldfield, T. Grant, R. Butler. nd. Development of the ICD-10 Procedure Coding System (ICD-10-PCS). https://www.cms.gov/ICD10/Downloads/pcs_final_report2012.pdf

Bernstein, Carol, MD, American Psychiatric Association, *Psychiatric News,* March 2011, "Meta Structure in DSM-V Process." http://www.dsm5.org/Documents/PsychiatryOnline%20_%20Psychiatric%20News%20_%20News%20Article%20Copy.pdf

Bowman, S., and A. Zeisset. 2007. ICD-10 Preparation Checklist. Chicago: AHIMA.

Brouch, K. 2003. AHIMA project offers insights into SNOMED, ICD-9-CM mapping process. *Journal of AHIMA* 74(7):52–55.

Health and Human Services. 2007. News release: HHS joins international partners to promote electronic health records standards. http://www.hhs.gov/news/press/2007pres/04/pr20070426a.html

Heffner, Christopher, MD, Heffner Media Group. 2011. *AllPsych Online, The Virtual Psychology Classroom,* http://allpsych.com/disorders/dsm.html

International Health Terminology Standards Development Organization. 2011. http://www.ihtsdo.org/snomed-ct/

National Center for Health Statistics. 2012. http://www.cdc.gov/nchs/icd.htm

National Library of Medicine. 2009. National Institutes of Health, SNOMED Clinical Terms (SNOMED CT).

North American Nursing Diagnoses Association, NANDA-I, http://www.nanda.org/Portals/0/PDFs/NANDA-I%20Pubs/NANDA_I_Fact_Sheet_Final_07_28_2011.pdf

Office of Inspector General. 1998. Compliance program guidance for hospitals. *Federal Register* 63(35):8987–8998. http://oig.hhs.gov/authorities/docs/cpghosp.pdf

Office of Inspector General. 2005. OIG supplemental compliance program guidance for hospitals. *Federal Register* 70(19):4858–4876. http://oig.hhs.gov/fraud/docs/complianceguidance/012705 hospsupplementalguidance.pdf

TheraDoc. 2001. Antibiotic Assistant. http://www.stochasticaphelion.com/bungee/Build/products/ abx_assist.html

Zeisset, A. 2009. ICD-10-CM enhancements: A look at the features that will improve coding accuracy. *Journal of AHIMA* 80(2):55–58.

Additional Resources

AHIMA Compliance Task Force. 1999. Practice brief: Seven steps to corporate compliance: The HIM role. Chicago: AHIMA.

AHIMA House of Delegates. 2008. AHIMA standards of ethical coding.

Centers for Medicare and Medicaid Services. 2009. HIPAA Information Series: 4. Overview of Electronic Transactions and Code Sets, 1. Baltimore, MD: CMS. http://www.cms.hhs.gov/ educationmaterials/downloads/whateelectronictransactionsandcodesets-4.pdf

Morsch, M., R. Kaul, and S. Briercheck. 2008. Hospital-based computer-assisted coding—A new paradigm. *2008 AHIMA Convention Proceedings*.

chapter 6

Reimbursement Methodologies

Anita C. Hazelwood, MLS, RHIA, FAHIMA
Carol A. Venable, MPH, RHIA, FAHIMA

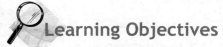

Learning Objectives

- Understand the historical development of healthcare reimbursement in the United States

- Describe current reimbursement processes, forms, and support practices for healthcare reimbursement

- Differentiate between commercial health insurance and employer-based self-insurance

- Describe the purpose and basic benefits of the following government-sponsored health programs: Medicare Part A, Medicare Part B, Medicare Advantage, Medicaid, CHAMPVA, TRICARE, HIS, TANF, PACE, SCHIP, workers' compensation, and FECA

- Understand the concept of managed care and to provide examples of different types of managed care organizations

- Identify and differentiate between the different types of fee-for-service reimbursement methods

- Describe the various Medicare prospective payment systems

- Understand the purpose of the fee schedules, chargemasters, and auditing procedures that support the reimbursement process

- Support accurate billing through chargemaster, claims management, and bill reconciliation processes

- Outline the revenue cycle processes
- Describe the elements of a compliance program
- Explain the relationship between coding practice and corporate compliance

Key Terms

Accept assignment

Accounts receivable

Administrative services only (ASO) contracts

Advance Beneficiary Notice of Noncoverage (ABN)

All patient DRGs (AP-DRGs)

All patient refined DRGs (APR-DRGs)

Ambulatory payment classification (APC) system

Ambulatory surgery center (ASC)

Auditing

Balance billing

Balanced Budget Refinement Act of 1999 (BBRA)

Blue Cross and Blue Shield (BC/BS)

BC/BS Federal Employee Program (FEP)

Bundled payments

Capitation

Case-mix group

Case-mix group (CMG) relative weights

Case-mix index

Categorically needy eligibility groups (Medicaid)

Centers for Medicare and Medicaid Services (CMS)

Chargemaster

Civilian Health and Medical Program of the Uniformed Services (CHAMPUS)

Civilian Health and Medical Program-Veterans Affairs (CHAMPVA)

Claim

CMS-1500

Coinsurance

Comorbidity

Compliance

Compliance program guidance

Complication

Coordination of benefits (COB) transaction

Cost outlier

Cost outlier adjustment

Current Procedural Terminology (CPT)

Department of Health and Human Services (HHS)

Diagnosis-related groups (DRGs)

Discharge planning

Discounting

DRG grouper

Employer-based self-insurance

Episode-of-care (EOC) reimbursement

Exclusive provider organization (EPO)

Explanation of Benefits (EOB)

External reviews (audits)

Federal Employees' Compensation Act (FECA)

Fee schedule

Fee-for-service basis

Fraud and abuse

Geographic practice cost index (GPCI)

Global payment

Global surgery payment

Group health insurance

Group model HMO

Group practice without walls (GPWW)

Hard-coding

Health maintenance organization (HMO)

Healthcare Common Procedure Coding System (HCPCS)

Healthcare Effectiveness Data and Information Set (HEDIS)

Healthcare provider

Home Assessment Validation and Entry (HAVEN)
Home health agency (HHA)
Home health prospective payment system (HH PPS)
Home health resource group (HHRG)
Hospice
Hospital-acquired conditions (HAC)
Hospitalization insurance (HI) (Medicare Part A)
Indemnity plans
Independent practice association (IPA)
Indian Health Service (IHS)
Inpatient psychiatric facility (IPF)
Inpatient rehabilitation facility (IRF)
Inpatient Rehabilitation Validation and Entry (IRVEN)
Insured
Insurer
Integrated delivery system (IDS)
Integrated provider organization (IPO)
Long-term care hospital (LTCH)
Low-utilization payment adjustment (LUPA)
Major diagnostic category (MDC)
Major medical insurance
Managed care
Management service organization (MSO)
Medicaid
Medical foundation
Medically needy option (Medicaid)
Medicare
Medicare Administrative Contractor (MAC)
Medicare Advantage
Medicare carrier
Medicare fee schedule (MFS)
Medicare severity diagnosis-related groups (MS-DRGs)
Medicare Summary Notice (MSN)
Medigap
Minimum Data Set 3.0 (MDS)

National Committee for Quality Assurance (NCQA)
National conversion factor (CF)
National Correct Coding Initiative (NCCI)
National Uniform Billing Committee (NUBC)
Network model HMO
Network provider
Nonparticipating providers
Omnibus Budget Reconciliation Act (OBRA)
Outcomes and Assessment Information Set (OASIS)
Out-of-pocket expenses
Outpatient code editor (OCE)
Outpatient prospective payment system (OPPS)
Packaging
Partial hospitalization
Patient Protection and Affordable Care Act
Payer of last resort (Medicaid)
Payment status indicator (PSI)
Per member per month (PMPM)
Per patient per month (PPPM)
Physician-hospital organization (PHO)
Point-of-service (POS) plan
Policyholder
Precertification
Preferred provider organization (PPO)
Premium
Present on admission (POA)
Primary care physician (PCP)
Principal diagnosis
Principal procedure
Professional component (PC)
Programs of All-Inclusive Care for the Elderly (PACE)
Prospective payment system (PPS)
Public assistance
Relative value unit (RVU)
Remittance advice (RA)
Resident assessment instrument (RAI)

Resident Assessment Validation and Entry (RAVEN)

Resource Utilization Groups, Version IV (RUG-IV)

Resource-based relative value scale (RBRVS)

Respite care

Retrospective payment system

Recovery Audit Contractor (RAC)

Revenue codes

Skilled nursing facility prospective payment system (SNF PPS)

Social Security Act

Staff model HMO

State Children's Health Insurance Program (SCHIP)

State workers' compensation insurance funds

Supplemental medical insurance (SMI) (Medicare Part B)

Tax Equity and Fiscal Responsibility Act of 1982 (TEFRA)

Technical component (TC)

Temporary Assistance for Needy Families (TANF)

Third-party payer

Traditional fee-for-service reimbursement

TRICARE

TRICARE Extra

TRICARE Prime

TRICARE Standard

UB-04 (CMS-1450)

Unbundling

Upcoding

Usual, customary, and reasonable (UCR) charges

Veterans Health Administration

Voluntary Disclosure Program

Workers' compensation

Introduction

In the United States, the systems used to pay healthcare organizations and individual healthcare professionals for the services they provide are very complex. This is due in part to the variety of reimbursement methods as well as to requirements for detailed documentation to support medical **claims.** The government and other third-party payers also are concerned about potential **fraud and abuse** in claims processing. Therefore, ensuring that bills and claims are accurate and correctly presented is an important focus of healthcare **compliance.**

A reimbursement claim is a statement of services submitted by a **healthcare provider** (for example, a physician or a hospital) to a **third-party payer** (for example, an insurance company or **Medicare**). The claim documents the medical and/or surgical services that were provided to a patient during a specific episode of care. Accurate reimbursement is critical to the operational and financial health of healthcare organizations. In most healthcare organizations, health insurance specialists process reimbursement claims. Health information management (HIM) professionals also play an important role in healthcare reimbursement by:

- Ensuring that health record documentation supports services billed

- Assigning diagnostic and procedural codes according to patient record documentation

- Applying coding guidelines and edits when assigning codes or **auditing** for coding quality and accuracy

- Appealing insurance claims denials
- Clarifying ambiguous or missing documentation

This chapter reviews the history of healthcare reimbursement in the United States and explains the different reimbursement systems commonly used since the start of **prospective payment systems** (PPS). A variety of healthcare reimbursement methodologies with a focus on Medicare prospective payment systems are discussed. Reimbursement claims processing and the support processes involved are also explained.

Theory into Practice

It is not uncommon to hear the phrase "if it wasn't documented, it wasn't done" in reference to health record documentation. In the context of reimbursement, this phrase means that when a healthcare provider (for example, a hospital) provides a service to a patient but fails to document the service in the patient's health record, that provider has no evidence to support a claim for the service. As a result, the third-party payer may deny the claim.

For example, a hospital submitted a claim for outpatient services totaling $1,950. When the third-party payer reviewed the claim, it might disallow $200 in charges for which there was no health record documentation. The payer then would recalculate the claim for a total payment of $1,750. The hospital would have lost $200 in revenue on this one case. However, if the hospital was underpaid $200 on every case because of incomplete documentation and there were 36,500 patient encounters per year, the potential revenue loss for one year would be $7,300,000!

History of Healthcare Reimbursement in the United States

Healthcare reimbursement in the United States has a long and complex history. Until the late 1800s, Americans paid their own healthcare expenses. Many people without the means to pay for care received charity care or no care at all. Over the past 100 years, a number of groups have attempted to develop systems that would ensure adequate healthcare for every American. But the development of prepaid insurance plans and third-party reimbursement systems did not follow a straight path. The result is the complicated reimbursement system in place today.

Pre-Medicare/Medicaid Campaigns for National Health Insurance

Campaigns for national health insurance began as early as 1915 with the drafting of health insurance legislation by the American Association of Labor Legislation (AALL). This legislation proposed coverage for the services of physicians, nurses, and hospitals;

sick pay; maternity benefits; and a death benefit of $50 to pay for funeral expenses. Although the plan was supported by the American Medical Association (AMA), it was never passed into law.

Through the 1930s and 1940s similar efforts were attempted, including a plan introduced by President Harry Truman in 1945 for universal comprehensive national health insurance. Truman's plan died in a congressional committee in 1946.

After the Second World War, private insurance systems expanded and union-negotiated healthcare benefits served to protect workers from the impact of unforeseen healthcare expenses. The Hill-Burton Act (formally called the Hospital Survey and Construction Act) was passed in 1946. In return for federal funds for facility construction, healthcare facilities agreed to provide medical services for free or at reduced rates to patients who were unable to pay for their own care.

Congress first introduced a bill to fund coverage of hospital costs for Social Security beneficiaries in 1948, but the concept of federal health insurance programs for the aged and the poor was not accepted until 1965 when President Lyndon Johnson signed the law that created federal healthcare programs for the elderly and poor as part of his Great Society legislation (also called the War on Poverty).

Medicare/Medicaid Programs

Title XVIII of the **Social Security Act,** or Health Insurance for the Aged and Disabled, is commonly known as Medicare. Medicare legislation was enacted as one element of the 1965 amendments to the Social Security Act. Medicare is a health insurance program designed to complement the retirement, survivors, and disability insurance benefits enacted under Title II of the Social Security Act. It covered most Americans over the age of 65 when it was first implemented in 1966.

In 1973, several additional groups became eligible for Medicare benefits, including those entitled to Social Security or Railroad Retirement disability cash benefits for at least 24 months, most persons with end-stage renal disease (ESRD), and certain individuals over 65 who were not eligible for paid coverage but elected to pay for Medicare benefits.

The **Medicaid** program became effective in 1966 under Title XIX of the Social Security Act. It was designed as a cost-sharing program between the federal and state governments. Medicaid pays for the healthcare services provided to many low-income Americans. It allowed states to add health coverage to their **public assistance** programs for low-income groups, families with dependent children, the aged, and the disabled. Because Medicaid eligibility is based on meeting criteria other than income, today the program covers only about 40 percent of the population living in poverty.

The Medicare and Medicaid programs were originally the responsibility of the Department of Health, Education, and Welfare (predecessor to the **Department of Health and Human Services** [HHS]). The **Centers for Medicare and Medicaid Services** (CMS), an administrative agency within HHS, today administers these programs.

The Medicare and Medicaid programs are discussed in more detail later in this chapter.

Cost Management

Since 1983, the prospective payment systems (PPSs) have been used to manage the costs of the Medicare and Medicaid programs. PPS is defined as "A type of reimbursement system that is based on preset payment levels rather than actual charges billed after the service has been provided; specifically, one of several Medicare reimbursement systems based on predetermined payment rates or periods and linked to the anticipated intensity of services delivered as well as the beneficiary's condition" (AHIMA 2012, 283). This was in response to the skyrocketing costs of healthcare, which was depleting the national budget and serving as a drain on the Social Security Administration. The PPS for inpatient acute care was the first to be implemented, followed by numerous others ranging from home health services to outpatient facility services. The most recently implemented system is for inpatient psychiatric facilities. Each of these prospective payment systems is discussed in detail later in this chapter.

Private and self-insured health insurance plans also have implemented a number of cost-containing measures, most notably, managed care delivery and reimbursement systems. Managed care has virtually eliminated **traditional fee-for-service reimbursement** systems in just two decades.

The implementation of managed care systems has had far-reaching effects on healthcare organizations and providers in every setting. However, hospitals have experienced the greatest financial pressure. Managed care is discussed in detail later in this chapter.

Development of Prepaid Health Plans

In 1860, Franklin Health Assurance Company of Massachusetts became the first commercial insurance company in the United States to provide private healthcare coverage for injuries that did not result in death. Within 20 years, 60 other insurance companies offered health insurance policies. By 1900, both accident insurance companies and life insurance companies were offering policies.

Blue Cross/Blue Shield

Modern health insurance was born in 1929 when Baylor University Hospital in Dallas, Texas, agreed to provide healthcare services to Dallas schoolteachers. The hospital agreed to provide room, board, and certain ancillary services to the teachers for a set monthly fee of 50 cents. Payment was made directly to the hospital, not to the patient. This plan is generally considered to be the first Blue Cross plan.

The Blue Cross plans contrasted with standard **indemnity plans.** Indemnity plans were offered by private insurance companies. In these plans, the patient is reimbursed or (indemnified) for covered services up to a specified dollar limit. It was then the responsibility of the hospital to collect the money from the patient. Blue Shield plans were eventually developed by physicians. The plans were similar to Blue Cross plans except that they offered coverage for physicians' services.

Group Health Insurance

Starting in the 1930s and through the Second World War, traditional insurance companies added health insurance coverage for hospital, surgical, and medical expenses to their accident and life insurance plans. During the Second World War, **group health insurance** was offered as a way to attract scarce wartime labor. Group health insurance plans provide healthcare benefits to full-time employees of a company. This trend was strengthened by the favorable tax treatment for fringe benefits. After the war, the Supreme Court ruled that employee benefits, including health insurance, were a legitimate part of the labor–management bargaining process. Health insurance quickly became a popular employee benefit.

Major Medical Insurance

Although early health insurance policies covered expenses associated with common accidents and illnesses, they were inadequate for coverage of extended illnesses and lengthy hospital stays. To correct this deficiency, insurance companies began offering **major medical insurance** coverage for catastrophic illnesses and injuries during the early 1950s. Major medical insurance provides benefits up to a high-dollar limit for most types of medical expenses. However, it usually requires patients to pay large deductibles. It also may place limits on charges (for example, room and board) and require patients to pay a portion of the expenses. **Blue Cross and Blue Shield** (BC/BS) soon followed by offering similar plans.

Typically, the major medical insurance **policyholder** (or **insured**) paid a specified deductible. A deductible is the amount the insured pays before the **insurer** assumes liability for any remaining costs of covered services. After the deductible had been paid, insured and insurer (third-party payer) shared covered losses according to a specified ratio, and the insured paid a **coinsurance** amount. Coinsurance refers to the amount the insured pays as a requirement of the insurance policy.

According to the Washington Insurance Council, by 1955, health insurance coverage continued to expand, and eventually 77 million Americans were covered by either an indemnity plan or a major medical plan. In subsequent years, insurance companies introduced high-benefit-level major medical plans, which limited **out-of-pocket expenses.**

Out-of-pocket expenses are the healthcare expenses that the insured party is responsible for paying. After the insured has paid an amount specified in the insurance plan (that is, the deductible plus any copayments), the plan pays 100 percent of covered expenses. Such health insurance plans are common today and have been expanded to include coverage for advanced medical technology.

Health Insurance Coverage

The U.S. Census Bureau (2010) reported that the percentage of insured decreased to 83.7 percent in 2010, from 83.9 percent in 2009 (table 6.1).

Table 6.1.　**Health insurance coverage status: 1990–2010**

Year	Total U.S. Population (000)	Number Covered (000)	Percentage Covered
2010	306,110	256,206	83.7
2009	304,280	255,295	83.9
2008	301,483	256,702	85.1
2007	299,106	255,018	85.3
2006	296,824	251,610	84.8
2005	293,834	250,799	85.4
2004	291,166	247,669	85.1
2003	288,280	246,332	85.4
2002	285,933	246,157	86.1
2001	282,082	244,059	86.5
2000	279,517	242,932	86.9
1999	274,087	231,533	84.5
1998	271,743	227,462	83.7
1997	269,094	225,646	83.9
1996	266,792	225,077	84.4
1995	264,314	223,733	84.6
1994	262,105	222,387	84.8
1993	259,753	220,040	84.7
1992	256,830	218,189	85.0
1991	251,447	216,003	85.9
1990	248,886	214,167	86.1

Source: Based on U.S. Census Bureau information (http://www.census.gov).

The lack of health insurance for so many Americans continues to be a serious concern. Because of the financial constraints caused by changes in Medicare/Medicaid and managed care reimbursement, many hospitals are no longer able to provide charitable services. As a result, underfunded and overcrowded public hospitals are struggling to provide services to uninsured patients who cannot pay for their own care. In addition, many uninsured patients delay seeking medical treatment until they are extremely ill, with long-term consequences for their own health and for the healthcare system. Thousands of patients with chronic diseases such as diabetes and asthma are brought to hospital emergency departments every day because they do not have access to basic healthcare services nor can they afford the routine medications to treat their diseases. Because of all of the reasons listed above, on March 23, 2010, President Obama signed comprehensive health reform, the **Patient Protection and Affordable Care Act**, into law. Several states and specialty groups nationwide have challenged this law with lawsuits still pending at this time including one in the United States Supreme Court.

Check Your Understanding 6.1

1. The amount of money that the patient is responsible for before the insurance kicks in is called the:

   A. Coinsurance
   B. Deductible
   C. Out-of-pocket expenses
   D. Indemnity

2. Which of the following is a reason why the high percentage of uninsured is a concern?

   A. With so many uninsured insurance companies may not make a profit.
   B. Hospitals cannot afford to provide care to uninsured patients.
   C. Generally speaking, uninsured patients receive medical care at the first sign of a problem.
   D. There are not enough insurance companies available to insure all of the uninsured if they decide to purchase insurance.

3. Prospective payment systems were developed by CMS to:

   A. Increase healthcare access
   B. Manage Medicare and Medicaid costs
   C. Implement managed care programs
   D. Eliminate fee-for-service programs

4. The government agency that administers the Medicaid and Medicare programs is:

   A. HCFA
   B. DHHS
   C. CMS
   D. SSA

5. Major medical insurance covers:

   A. Automobile accidents
   B. Ambulatory care
   C. Catastrophic illnesses
   D. Catastrophic illnesses and injuries

6. Which of the following was the original group of individuals eligible for Medicare?

   A. Americans over the age of 65
   B. Patients with end-stage renal disease
   C. Those eligible for Railroad Retirement disability
   D. Those entitled to Social Security benefits

Healthcare Reimbursement Systems

Before the widespread availability of health insurance coverage, individuals were assured access to healthcare only when they were able to pay for the services themselves. They paid cash for services on a retrospective **fee-for-service basis,** which meant the patient was expected to pay the healthcare provider after a service was rendered. Until managed care, **capitation,** and other PPSs, private insurance plans and government-sponsored programs also reimbursed providers on a retrospective fee-for-service basis.

Fee-for-service reimbursement is now rare for most types of medical services. However, some types of care are not covered by most health insurance plans and are still paid for directly by patients on a fee-for-service basis. Cosmetic surgery is one example of a medical service that is not covered by most insurance plans. Many insurance plans limit coverage for psychiatric services, substance abuse treatment, and the testing and correction of vision and hearing.

Commercial Insurance

Most Americans are covered by private group insurance plans tied to their employment. Typically, employers and employees share the cost of such plans. Two types of commercial insurance are commonly available: private insurance and **employer-based self-insurance.**

Private Health Insurance Plans

Private commercial insurance plans are financed through the payment of **premiums.** Each covered individual or family pays a preestablished amount (usually monthly), and the insurance company sets aside the premiums from all the people covered by the plan in a special fund.

When a claim for medical care is submitted to the insurance company, the claim is paid out of the fund's reserves. Before payment is made, the insurance company reviews every claim to determine whether the services described on the claim are covered by the patient's policy. The company also reviews the diagnosis codes provided on the claim to ensure that the services provided were medically necessary. Payment then is made to either the provider or the policyholder.

When purchasing an insurance policy, the policyholder receives written confirmation from the insurance company when the insurance goes into effect. An insurance policy represents a legal contract for services between the insured and the insurance company.

Most insurance policies include the following information:

- What medical services the company will cover
- When the company will pay for medical services
- How much and for how long the company will pay for covered services
- Which process is to be followed to ensure that covered medical expenses are paid

Employer-Based Self-Insurance Plans

During the 1970s, a number of large companies found that they could save money by self-insuring their employee health plans rather than purchasing coverage from private insurers. Self-insurance costs are lower because additional fees built into premiums by a private insurer can be eliminated. With a large employee group annual medical expenses vary slightly and can be predicted. By budgeting a certain amount to pay its employees' medical claims, the employer retains control over the funds until such time as medical claims need to be paid.

Employer-based self-insurance has become a common form of group health insurance coverage. Many employers enter into **administrative services only** (ASO) **contracts** with private insurers and fund the plans themselves. The private insurers administer self-insurance plans on behalf of the employers.

Not-for-Profit and For-Profit Healthcare Plans

Community-based, noninvestor-owned healthcare plans have existed for decades in the United States. These healthcare plans are referred to as not-for-profit or nonprofit plans.

However, since the 1990s there has been substantial growth of investor or for-profit health plans. In fact, many nonprofit plans have converted to investor-owned plans in recent years.

A primary difference between nonprofit and for-profit entities is where their excess revenues are directed. In a for-profit health plan, like any other stock company, excess revenues are distributed to shareholders. In nonprofit entities, excess revenues are not distributed to shareholders, but are retained for future internal investments. The literature regarding the comparative benefits, quality of care, and performance of nonprofit versus for-profit healthcare entities differs. Some studies indicate that for-profit health plans provide lower quality care and poorer performance than nonprofit plans (Himmelstein et al. 1999; Schneider et al. 2005). Others indicate little or no difference between the two (Kim et al. 2004).

Blue Cross and Blue Shield Plans

Blue Cross and Blue Shield (BC/BS) plans, also known as the Blues, were the first prepaid health plans in the United States. Originally, Blue Cross plans covered hospital care and Blue Shield plans covered physicians' services.

The first Blue Cross plan was created in 1929 and the first Blue Shield Plan was created in 1939. In 1982, the Blue Cross Association and the National Association of Blue Shield Plans merged to create the Blue Cross and Blue Shield Association.

In 2009, the Blue Cross and Blue Shield Association included over 60 independent, locally operated companies with plans in 50 states, the District of Columbia, and Puerto Rico and international plans in Panama and Uruguay. The Blues offer health insurance to individuals, small businesses, seniors, and large employer groups. In addition, federal employees are eligible to enroll in the **BC/BS Federal Employee Program** (FEP) (also called the BC/BS Service Benefit Plan).

Government-Sponsored Healthcare Programs

The federal government administers several healthcare programs. The best known are Medicare and Medicaid. In addition, the federal government offers other health programs to address the needs of military personnel and their dependents, veterans, and Native Americans, which are discussed below.

Medicare

The original Medicare program was implemented on July 1, 1966. The Medicare program pays for the healthcare services provided to Social Security beneficiaries 65 years old and older, people under 65 years old with certain disabilities, and people of all ages with end-stage renal disease.

Medicare has four parts:

1. Medicare Part A Hospital Insurance that helps cover inpatient hospital, skilled nursing, home health, hospice care, and inpatient care in a religious non-medical health care institution.
2. Medicare Part B Medical Insurance that helps cover physician services, outpatient care, and home healthcare
3. Medicare Part C Medicare Advantage Plans (like an HMO or PPO) is a health coverage option that includes Part A and Part B and is operated by private insurance companies that are approved by and under contract with Medicare
4. Medicare Part D Prescription Drug Coverage that helps cover the cost of prescription drugs and is run by private insurance companies that are approved by and under contract with Medicare

Each of these parts is described below in addition to Medigap insurance, which can help pay some of the healthcare costs (gaps) like copayments, coinsurance, and deductibles that Medicare doesn't cover.

Medicare Part A

Medicare Part A provides **hospitalization insurance** (HI) that is generally provided free of charge to individuals age 65 and over who are eligible for Social Security or Railroad Retirement benefits, people under 65 years old with certain disabilities, and people of all ages with end-stage renal disease. In addition, some otherwise-ineligible aged and disabled beneficiaries who voluntarily pay a monthly premium for their coverage are eligible for Medicare Part A.

Healthcare services covered under Medicare Part A include inpatient hospital care, skilled nursing facility (SNF) care, home healthcare, **hospice** care, and inpatient care in a religious non-medical health care institution. Table 6.2 summarizes the benefit periods, deductibles, and copayments according to the healthcare setting.

Table 6.2. **Medicare Part A benefit period, beneficiary deductibles and copayments, and Medicare payment responsibilities according to healthcare setting**

Healthcare Setting	Benefit Period	Patient's Responsibility	Medicare Payments
Hospital (inpatient)	First 60 days	$1,156 deductible	All but $1,156
	Days 61–90	$289 per day	All but $289/day
	Days 91–150 (these reserve days can be used only once in the patient's lifetime)	$578 per day	All but $578/day
	Beyond 150 days	All costs	Nothing
Skilled nursing facility	First 20 days	Nothing	100% approved amount
	Days 21–100	$144.50 per day	All but $144.50 per day
	Beyond 100 days	All costs	Nothing
Home healthcare	For as long as patient meets Medicare medical necessity criteria	Nothing for services, but 20% of approved amount for durable medical equipment (DME)	100% of the approved amount, and 80% of the approved amount for DME
Hospice care	For as long as physician certifies need for care	Limited costs for outpatient drugs and inpatient respite care ($5 per outpatient prescription and 5% for respite care)	All but limited costs for outpatient drugs and inpatient respite care
Blood	Unlimited if medical necessity criteria are met	First three pints unless patient or someone else donates blood to replace what the patient uses	All but first three pints per calendar year

Source: http://www.medicare.gov/costs.

Inpatient Hospital Care: Inpatient hospital care is paid for under Medicare Part A when the care is medically necessary. Medicare Part A coverage is measured in benefit periods. A benefit period begins the day a patient is admitted as an inpatient in a hospital or skilled nursing facility. The benefit period ends when the patient has not received any inpatient hospital care (or skilled care in a SNF) for 60 days in a row. If the patient goes into a hospital or a skilled nursing facility after one benefit period has ended, a new benefit period begins. The patient must pay the inpatient hospital deductible for each benefit period. There is no limit to the number of benefit periods.

In each benefit period there are limits to the number of days Medicare will pay for inpatient care. Inpatient hospital care is usually limited to 90 days during each benefit period. A benefit period begins on the day of admission and ends when the beneficiary has been out of the hospital for 60 days in a row, including the day of discharge. There is no limit to the number of benefit periods. When a beneficiary exhausts the 90 days of inpatient hospital care available during a benefit period, a nonrenewable lifetime reserve of up to a total of 60 additional days of inpatient hospital care can be used.

The beneficiary must pay all inpatient deductibles for each period and copayments for all hospital days following day 60. In 2012, the deductible was $1,156. Additional coinsurance payments ($289 per day in 2012) are required from days 61 through 90. For days 91 to 150 there is a higher copay ($578 per day in 2010). For days past 150 the beneficiary is responsible for all costs. The following is an example of how the benefit period works:

> John goes into the hospital on March 1, 2012 and is discharged on March 5, 2012. The benefit period ends on May 3 and a new benefit period begins. John goes into the hospital again on August 1, 2009 for a 70-day stay. This begins another benefit period. John is responsible for paying the deductible for each benefit period and for paying a copay for each day stay after 60 days.

Skilled Nursing Facility Care: SNF care is covered when a patient requires skilled nursing or rehabilitation services occurring within 30 days of a 3-day-long or longer acute hospitalization and is certified as medically necessary. The number of SNF days provided under Medicare is limited to 100 days per benefit period. Medicare fully covers the first 20 days in a benefit period. For days 21 through 100, a copayment ($144.50 per day in 2012) is required. Medicare benefits expire after the first 100 days of SNF care during a benefit period.

Home Health Care: Care provided by a **home health agency** (HHA) may be furnished part-time in the residence of a homebound beneficiary when intermittent or part-time skilled nursing and/or certain other therapy or rehabilitation care is needed. Certain medical supplies and durable medical equipment (DME) also may be paid for under the Medicare home health benefit.

The Medicare program requires the HHA to develop a treatment plan that is periodically reviewed by a physician. Home healthcare under Medicare Part A has no limitations on duration, no copayments, and no deductibles. For DME, beneficiaries must pay 20 percent coinsurance, as required under Medicare Part B.

Hospice Care: Terminally ill persons, whose life expectancies are certified by their attending physician to be six months or less, may elect to receive hospice services. To qualify for Medicare reimbursement for hospice care, patients must elect to forgo standard Medicare benefits for treatment of their terminal illnesses and agree to receive only hospice care. When a hospice patient requires treatment for a condition that is not related to his or her terminal illness, however, Medicare does pay for all covered services necessary for that condition. The Medicare beneficiary pays no deductible for hospice coverage, but does pay coinsurance amounts for drugs and inpatient **respite care.** (Respite care is any inpatient care provided to the hospice patient for the purpose of providing primary caregivers a break from their care-giving responsibilities.)

Blood: For any Part A service, the beneficiary is responsible for paying fees to cover the first three pints or units of nonreplaced blood per calendar year. The beneficiary has the option of paying the fee or arranging for the blood to be replaced by family and friends.

Medicare Part B

Medicare Part B offers voluntary **supplemental medical insurance** (SMI) to help pay for physicians' services, medical services, and medical–surgical supplies not covered by the hospitalization plan. Most individuals over 65 who are otherwise ineligible for

Medicare Part A coverage can enroll voluntarily by paying a monthly premium when they also enroll in Part B.

Medicare Part B covers the following services and supplies:

- Physicians' and surgeons' services, including some covered services furnished by chiropractors, podiatrists, dentists, and optometrists; and services provided by the following Medicare-approved practitioners who are not physicians: certified registered nurse anesthetists, clinical psychologists, clinical social workers (other than those employed by a hospital or an SNF), physician assistants, and nurse practitioners and clinical nurse specialists working in collaboration with a physician

- Services in an emergency department or outpatient clinic, including same-day surgery and ambulance services

- Home healthcare not covered under Medicare Part A

- Laboratory tests, x-rays, and other diagnostic radiology services, as well as certain preventive care screening tests

- Ambulatory surgery center (ASC) services in Medicare-approved facilities

- Most physical and occupational therapy and speech pathology services

- Comprehensive outpatient rehabilitation facility services and mental healthcare provided as part of a partial hospitalization psychiatric program when a physician certifies that inpatient treatment would be required without the partial hospitalization services. (A **partial hospitalization** program offers intensive psychiatric treatment on an outpatient basis to psychiatric patients, with an expectation that the patient's psychiatric condition and level of functioning will improve and that relapse will be prevented so that re-hospitalization can be avoided.)

- Radiation therapy, renal dialysis and kidney transplants, and heart and liver transplants under certain limited conditions

- DME approved for home use, such as oxygen equipment, wheelchairs, prosthetic devices, surgical dressings, splints, casts, walkers, and hospital beds needed for use in the home

- Drugs and biologicals that cannot be self-administered, such as hepatitis B vaccines and transplant and immunosuppressive drugs (plus certain self-administered anticancer drugs)

- Preventive services such as bone mass measurements, cardiovascular screening blood tests, colorectal cancer screening, diabetes services, glaucoma testing, Pap test and pelvic exam, prostate cancer screening, screening mammograms, and vaccinations (flu, pneumococcal, hepatitis B)

- Inpatient hospitalizations when Part A benefits have been exhausted

Table 6.3.   Medicare Part B benefit deductibles and copayments and Medicare payment responsibilities according to type of service

Type of Service	Benefit	Deductible and Copayment	Medicare Payment
Medical expense	Physician's services, inpatient and outpatient medical and surgical services and supplies, and durable medical equipment (DME)	Annual deductible, plus 20% of approved amount after deductible has been met, except in outpatient setting	80% of approved amount (after patient has paid the deductible)
	Mental healthcare	50% of most outpatient care	50% of most outpatient care
Clinical laboratory services	Blood tests, urinalysis, and more	Nothing	100% of approved amount
Home healthcare	Intermittent skilled care, home health aid services, DME and supplies, and other services	Nothing for home care service; 20% of approved amount for DME	100% of approved amount; 80% of approved amount for DME
Outpatient hospital services	Services for diagnosis and treatment of an illness or injury	A coinsurance amount for *each service* received during an outpatient visit. For *each* outpatient service received, the coinsurance amount cannot be greater than the Medicare Part A inpatient hospital deductible. Charges for items or services that Medicare does not cover	Payment based on ambulatory patient classifications/outpatient prospective payment system
Blood	Unlimited if medical necessity criteria are met	First three pints (if met under Part B, does not have to be met again under Part A)	All but first three pints

Source: Adapted from CMS 2010.

To be covered, all Medicare Part B services must be either documented as medically necessary or covered as one of several prescribed preventive benefits. Part B services also are generally subject to deductibles and coinsurance payments (table 6.3). Certain medical services and related care are subject to special payment rules, for example:

- Deductibles for administration of blood and blood products
- Maximum approved amounts for Medicare-approved physical or occupational therapy services performed in settings other than hospitals
- Higher cost-sharing requirements, such as those for outpatient psychiatric care

Services Not Covered by Part A or Part B

The following healthcare services are usually not covered by Medicare Part A or B and are only covered by private health plans under the Medicare Advantage program:

- Long-term nursing care
- Cosmetic surgery
- Dentures and dental care
- Acupuncture
- Hearing aids and exams for fitting hearing aids

Part C Medicare Advantage (MA Plans)

Medicare Advantage may provide expanded coverage of many healthcare services. Although any Medicare beneficiary may receive benefits through the original fee-for-service program, most beneficiaries enrolled in both Parts A and B can choose to participate in a Medicare Advantage plan instead.

Medicare Advantage Plans may offer extra coverage for such services as vision, hearing, dental, and/or health and wellness programs. Many include Medicare prescription drug coverage. Out-of-pocket costs and rules will vary depending upon the organization offering the plan. Organizations that offer Medicare Advantage plans must meet specific requirements as determined by CMS.

Primary Medicare Advantage products include the following types of plans:

- *Health Maintenance Organization (HMO):* In most HMOs, you can only go to doctors, other healthcare providers, or hospitals on the plan's list of approved providers except in an emergency. You may also need to get a referral from your primary care doctor.

- *PPO plans:* In a PPO plan, patients use doctors, specialists, and hospitals in the plan's network and can go to doctors and hospitals not on the list, usually at an additional cost. Patients do not need referrals to see doctors or go to hospitals that are not part of the plan's network and may pay lower copayments and receive extra benefits.

- *Private fee-for-service plans:* These plans are similar to original Medicare in that you can generally go to any doctor, other healthcare provider, or hospital as long as they agree to treat you. The plan determines how much it will pay doctors, other healthcare providers, and hospitals, and how much you must pay when you receive care.

- *Medicare specialty plans:* These plans provide focused and specialized healthcare for specific groups of people, such as those who have both Medicare and Medicaid, who live in a nursing home, or have certain chronic medical conditions.

Part D Medicare Prescription Drug, Improvement, and Modernization Act

The Medicare Prescription Drug, Improvement, and Modernization Act, also known as the Medicare Reform Bill, was signed into law on December 8, 2003. This legislation provides seniors and individuals with disabilities with a prescription drug benefit, more choices, and better benefits under Medicare. Medicare drug plans are run by insurance companies and other private companies approved by Medicare. Each plan can vary in cost and drugs covered, and beneficiaries select their preferred plan.

Out-of-Pocket Expenses and Medigap Insurance

Medicare beneficiaries who elect the fee-for-service option are responsible for charges not covered by the Medicare program and for various cost-sharing aspects of Parts A and B. These liabilities may be paid by the Medicare beneficiary; by a third party, such as an employer-sponsored health plan or private Medigap insurance; or by Medicaid, when the person is eligible.

Medigap is private health insurance that pays, within limits, most of the healthcare service charges not covered by Medicare Parts A and/or B. These policies must meet federal and state laws.

Check Your Understanding 6.2

Instructions: Select the best answer for the following statements.

1. Medicare Part A provides:

    A. Dental insurance
    B. Hospitalization insurance
    C. Outpatient insurance
    D. All of the above

2. Medicare Part B covers:

    A. Services in an emergency department
    B. Ambulatory surgery center services
    C. Services in an outpatient clinic
    D. All of the above

3. Medicare coverage applies to:

    A. Individuals age 65 and over
    B. Individuals who are disabled
    C. Individuals who undergo chronic kidney dialysis for end-stage renal disease
    D. All of the above

4. These types of plans allow beneficiaries to go to any doctor or hospital that accepts the terms of the plan's payment:

   A. Managed care plans
   B. PPO plans
   C. Private fee-for-service plans
   D. Medicare specialty plans

5. What plans were the first prepaid health plans in the United States?

   A. Blue Cross and Blue Shield Plans
   B. Government-Sponsored Healthcare Programs
   C. Employer-Based Self-Insurance Plans
   D. Private Health Insurance Plans

Medicaid

Title XIX of the Social Security Act enacted Medicaid in 1965. State governments work with the federal Medicaid program to provide healthcare coverage to low-income individuals and families. The Medicaid program pays for medical assistance provided to individuals and families with low incomes and limited financial resources.

Medicaid Eligibility Criteria

Individual states must meet broad national guidelines established by federal statutes, regulations, and policies to qualify for federal matching grants under the Medicaid program. Individual state medical assistance agencies, however, establish the Medicaid eligibility standards for residents of their states. The states also determine the type, amount, duration, and scope of covered services; calculate the rate of payment for covered services; and administer local programs. Medicaid policies on eligibility, services, and payment are complex and vary considerably among states. Therefore, an individual who is eligible for Medicaid in one state may not be eligible in another.

Low income is only one test for Medicaid eligibility. Other financial resources also are compared against eligibility standards. These standards are determined by each state according to federal guidelines.

To be eligible for federal funds, states are required to provide Medicaid coverage to certain individuals. These individuals include recipients of federally assisted income maintenance payments, as well as related groups of individuals who do not receive cash payments. The federal **categorically needy eligibility groups** include:

- Individuals eligible for Medicaid when they meet requirements for **Temporary Assistance for Needy Families** (TANF)

- Children below age six whose family income is at or below 133 percent of the federal poverty level (FPL) (the income threshold established by the federal government)

- Pregnant women whose family income is below 133 percent of the FPL (services are limited to those related to pregnancy-related medical care)

- Supplemental Security Income (SSI) recipients in most states

- Recipients of adoption or foster care assistance under Title IV-E of the Social Security Act

- Specially protected groups (typically individuals who lose their cash assistance due to earnings from work or from increased Social Security benefits, but who may keep Medicaid for a period of time)

- Infants born to Medicaid-eligible pregnant women

- Certain low-income Medicare beneficiaries

States also have the option of providing Medicaid coverage to other categorically related groups. Categorically related groups share the characteristics of the eligible groups (that is, they fall within defined categories), but the eligibility criteria are somewhat more liberally defined. A **medically needy option** also allows states to extend Medicaid eligibility to persons who would be eligible for Medicaid under one of the mandatory or optional groups except that their income and/or resources are above the eligibility level set by their state. Individuals may qualify immediately or may "spend down" by incurring medical expenses that reduce their income to or below their state's income level for the medically needy.

Medicaid Services

To be eligible for federal matching funds, each state's Medicaid program must offer medical assistance for the following basic services:

- Inpatient hospital services

- Outpatient hospital services

- Emergency services

- Prenatal care

- Vaccines for children

- Physicians' services

- SNF services for persons aged 21 or older

- Family planning services and supplies

- Rural health clinic services

- Home healthcare for persons eligible for skilled nursing services

- Laboratory and x-ray services

- Pediatric and family nurse practitioner services
- Nurse-midwife services
- Federally qualified health center (FQHC) services and ambulatory services performed at an FQHC that would be available in other settings
- Early and periodic screening and diagnostic and therapeutic services for children under age 21

States also may receive federal matching funds to provide some of the optional services, the most common being:

- Diagnostic services
- Clinic services
- Prescription drugs and prosthetic devices
- Transportation services
- Rehabilitation and physical therapy services
- Prosthetic devices
- Home care and community-based care services for persons with chronic impairments

The Balanced Budget Act (BBA) of 1997 also called for implementation of a state option called **Programs of All-Inclusive Care for the Elderly** (PACE). PACE provides an alternative to institutional care for individuals 55 years old or older who require a level of care usually provided at nursing facilities. It offers and manages all of the health, medical, and social services needed by a beneficiary and mobilizes other services, as needed, to provide preventive, rehabilitative, curative, and supportive care.

PACE services can be provided in day healthcare centers, homes, hospitals, and nursing homes. The program helps its beneficiaries to maintain their independence, dignity, and quality of life. PACE also functions within the Medicare program. Individuals enrolled in PACE receive benefits solely through the PACE program.

Medicaid-Medicare Relationship

Medicare beneficiaries who have low incomes and limited financial resources also may receive help from the Medicaid program. For persons eligible for full Medicaid coverage, Medicare coverage is supplemented by services that are available under their state's Medicaid program according to their eligibility category. Additional services may include, for example, nursing facility care beyond the 100-day limit covered by Medicare, prescription drugs, eyeglasses, and hearing aids. For those enrolled in both programs, any services covered by Medicare are paid for by the Medicare program before any payments are made by the Medicaid program because Medicaid is always the **payer of last resort.**

Table 6.4.   **Comparison of Medicare and Medicaid programs**

Medicare	Medicaid
Health insurance for people age 65 and older, or people under 65 who are entitled to Medicare because of disability or are receiving dialysis for permanent kidney failure	Health assistance for people of any age
Administered through fiscal intermediaries, insurance companies under contract to the government to process Medicare claims	Administered by the federal government through state and local governments following federal and state guidelines
Medicare regulations are the same in all states	Medicaid regulations vary from state to state
Financed by monthly premiums paid by the beneficiary and by payroll tax deductions	Financed by federal, state, and county tax dollars
For people age 65 and over, eligibility is based on Social Security or Railroad Retirement participation. For people under age 65, eligibility is based on disability. For people who undergo kidney dialysis, eligibility is not dependent on age.	Eligibility based on financial need
Beneficiary responsible for paying deductibles, coinsurance or copayments, and Part B premiums	Medicaid can help pay Medicare deductible, coinsurance or copayment, and premiums
Hospital and medical benefits; preventive care and long-term care benefits are limited	Comprehensive benefits include hospital, preventive care, long-term care, and other services not covered under Medicare such as dental work, prescriptions, transportation, eyeglasses, and hearing aids

This means that Medicaid will not cover anything until after any Medicare coverage has been exhausted (AHIMA 2012, 260). Table 6.4 provides a comparison of the Medicare and Medicaid programs.

State Children's Health Insurance Program

The **State Children's Health Insurance Program** (SCHIP) (Title XXI of the Social Security Act) is a program initiated by the BBA. SCHIP (sometimes referred to as the Children's Health Insurance Program, or CHIP) allows states to expand existing insurance programs to cover children up to age 19. It provides additional federal funds to states so that Medicaid eligibility can be expanded to include a greater number of children.

SCHIP became available on October 1, 1997, and is jointly funded by the federal government and the states. Following broad federal guidelines, states establish eligibility and coverage guidelines and have flexibility in the way they provide services. Recipients in all states must meet three eligibility criteria:

1.   They must come from low-income families
2.   They must be otherwise ineligible for Medicaid
3.   They must be uninsured

States are required to offer the following services:

- Inpatient hospital services
- Outpatient hospital services
- Physicians' surgical and medical services
- Laboratory and x-ray services
- Well-baby/child care services, including age-appropriate immunizations

Check Your Understanding 6.3

1. Title XIX of the Social Security Act Amendment of 1965 is also known as:

   A. Medicare
   B. Medicaid
   C. Medigap
   D. SCHIP

2. Medicaid eligibility standards are established by:

   A. Centers for Medicare and Medicaid Services
   B. Medicare
   C. Individual states
   D. Federal government

3. To be eligible for federal matching funds, each state's Medicaid program must offer medical assistance for:

   A. Inpatient hospital services
   B. Prenatal care
   C. Vaccines for children
   D. All of the above

4. Which program provides additional federal funds to states so that Medicaid eligibility can be expanded to include a greater number of children?

   A. Medicaid
   B. Medigap
   C. SCHIP
   D. PACE

5. Which of the following is *not* a place where PACE services can be provided?

   A. Day healthcare centers
   B. Homes
   C. Hospitals
   D. Hospice

TRICARE

TRICARE, formerly known as **Civilian Health and Medical Program of the Uniformed Services** (CHAMPUS), is a healthcare program for active-duty service members, National Guard and Reserve members, retirees, their families, survivors, and certain former spouses. TRICARE offers three options: **TRICARE Prime, TRICARE Extra,** and **TRICARE Standard.** The plan type depends upon type of eligible individual and where the individual lives.

Veterans Health Administration

The **Veterans Health Administration** is the component of the U.S. Department of Veterans Affairs that implements the medical assistance program of the VA. Veterans of the U.S. armed forces may be eligible for a broad range of programs and services provided by the VA. By federal law, eligibility for benefits is determined by a system of eight Priority Groups. Retirees from military service, veterans with service-connected injuries or conditions rated by VA, and Purple Heart recipients are within the higher priority groups.

VA's healthcare offers a wide variety of services, information, and benefits. The VA is the nation's largest integrated healthcare system and operates more than 1,400 sites of care such as hospitals, community outpatient clinics, community living centers, domicilaries, readjustment counseling centers, and various other types of facilities. Major benefits include Veterans' compensation, Veterans' pension, survivors' benefits, rehabilitation and employment assistance, education assistance, home loan guaranties, and life insurance coverage.

Eligibility for VA dental care and nursing home care are more restricted. VA nursing homes are primarily for veterans needing care for a service-connected condition, or who have service-connected disability ratings of 70 percent or higher. Reservists and National Guardsmen who were called to active duty by a federal executive order qualify for VA healthcare benefits.

CHAMPVA

The **Civilian Health and Medical Program-Veterans Affairs** (CHAMPVA) is a healthcare program for dependents and survivors of permanently and totally disabled veterans, survivors of veterans who died from service-related conditions, and survivors of military personnel who died in the line of duty. CHAMPVA is a voluntary program that allows beneficiaries to be treated for free at participating VA healthcare facilities. Because of the similarity between CHAMPVA and TRICARE (which replaced CHAMPUS), people sometimes confuse the two programs. However, CHAMPVA is separate from TRICARE and there are distinct differences between them.

Indian Health Service

The **Indian Health Service** (IHS) is an agency within the HHS. It is responsible for providing healthcare services to American Indians and Alaska natives. The American Indians and Alaska natives served by the IHS receive preventive healthcare services, primary medical services (hospital and ambulatory care), community health services, substance abuse treatment services, and rehabilitative services. Secondary medical care, highly specialized medical services, and other rehabilitative care are provided by IHS staff or by private healthcare professionals working under contract with the IHS.

A system of acute and ambulatory care facilities operates on Indian reservations and in Indian and Alaska native communities. In locations where the IHS does not have its own facilities or is not equipped to provide a needed service, it contracts with local hospitals, state and local healthcare agencies, tribal health institutions, and individual healthcare providers.

Workers' Compensation

Most employees are eligible for some type of **workers' compensation** insurance. Workers' compensation programs cover healthcare costs and lost income associated with work-related injuries and illnesses. Federal government employees are covered by the **Federal Employees' Compensation Act** (FECA). Individual states pass legislation that addresses workers' compensation coverage for nonfederal government employees. Some states exclude certain workers—for example, business owners, independent contractors, farm workers, and so on. Texas employers are not required to provide workers' compensation coverage.

Federal Workers' Compensation Funds

The Federal Employees' Compensation Act (FECA) provides federal employees injured in the performance of duty with workers' compensation benefits. This includes wage-loss benefits for total or partial disability, monetary benefits for permanent loss of use of a body part, medical benefits, and vocational rehabilitation. FECA also provides survivor benefits to eligible dependents if the injury causes the employee's death.

FECA is administered by the Office of Workers' Compensation Programs (OWCP), within the U.S. Department of Labor's (DOL) Employment Standards Administration (ESA).

State Workers' Compensation Funds

According to the American Association of State Compensation Insurance Funds (AASCIF), state workers' compensation insurance was developed in response to the concerns of employers. Before state workers' compensation programs became widely available, employers faced the possibility of going out of business when insurance companies refused to provide coverage or charged excessive premiums. Legislators in most states have addressed these concerns by establishing **state workers' compensation insurance funds** that provide a stable source of insurance coverage and serve to protect employers from uncertainties about the continuing availability of coverage.

State workers' compensation insurance funds do not operate at taxpayer expense because, by law, the funds support themselves through income derived from premiums and investments. As nonprofit departments of the state or as independent nonprofit companies, they return surplus assets to policyholders as dividends or safety refunds. This system reduces the overall cost of state-level workers' compensation insurance. In states where state funds have not been mandated, employers purchase workers' compensation coverage from private carriers or provide self-insurance coverage.

Check Your Understanding 6.4

1. A healthcare program for active duty members of the military and other qualified family members is called:

    A. HIS
    B. Medicare
    C. Medicaid
    D. TRICARE

2. A healthcare program for dependents and survivors of permanently and totally disabled veterans:

    A. CHAMPUS
    B. CHAMPVA
    C. IHS
    D. TRICARE

3. The agency responsible for providing healthcare services to American Indians and Alaska natives is:

    A. CHAMPUS
    B. CHAMPVA
    C. IHS
    D. TRICARE

4. Insurance that covers healthcare costs and lost income associated with work-related injuries is called:

    A. CHAMPVA
    B. Medicare
    C. Medicaid
    D. Workers' compensation

5. Which agency/program provides federal employees injured in the performance of duty with workers' compensation benefits?

    A. Federal Employees' Compensation Act (FECA)
    B. Center for Medicare and Medicaid Services
    C. Tricare
    D. CHAMPVA

Managed Care
Definition

Managed care is the generic term for prepaid health plans that integrate the financial and delivery aspects of healthcare services. In other words, managed care organizations work to control the cost of, and access to, healthcare services at the same time that they strive to meet high-quality standards. Some of the methods used to control costs inlcude:

- Review of utilization of healthcare services
- Using primary care physicians as gatekeepers to control referrals to specialists
- Limit the providers from which the enrollee can seek treatment
- Use of case managers to monitor and coordinate care of patients with complex problems
- Primary Care Case Management

Managed Care Quality Initiatives

The cost of providing appropriate services also is monitored continuously to determine whether the services are being delivered in the most efficient and cost-effective way possible.

Since 1973, several pieces of federal legislation have been passed with the goal of encouraging the development of managed healthcare systems (table 6.5). The Health Maintenance Organization Assistance Act of 1973 authorized federal grants and loans to private organizations that wished to develop **health maintenance organizations** (HMOs). Another important advancement in managed care was development of the **Healthcare Effectiveness Data and Information Set** (HEDIS) by the **National Committee for Quality Assurance** (NCQA).

The NCQA is a private, not-for-profit organization that accredits, assesses, and reports on the quality of managed care plans in the United States. It worked with public and private healthcare purchasers, health plans, researchers, and consumer advocates to develop HEDIS in 1989. HEDIS is a set of standardized measures used to compare managed care plans in terms of the quality of services they provide. The standards cover areas such as plan membership, utilization of and access to services, and financial indicators. The goals of the program include:

- Helping beneficiaries make informed choices among the numerous managed care plans available
- Improving the quality of care provided by managed care plans
- Helping the government and other third-party payers make informed purchasing decisions

Table 6.5. Federal legislation relevant to managed care

Year	Legislative Title	Legislative Summary
1973	Federal Health Maintenance Organization Assistance Act of 1973 (HMO Act of 1973)	• Authorized grants and loans to develop HMOs under private sponsorship • Defined a federally qualified HMO (certified to provide healthcare services to Medicare and Medicaid enrollees) as one that has applied for and met federal standards established in the HMO Act of 1973 • Required most employers with more than 25 employees to offer HMO coverage when local plans were available
1974	Employee Retirement Income Security Act of 1974 (ERISA)	• Mandated reporting and disclosure requirements for group life and health plans (including managed care plans) • Permitted large employers to self-insure employee healthcare benefits • Exempted large employers from taxes on health insurance premium
1982	Tax Equity and Fiscal Responsibility Act of 1982 (TEFRA)	• Modified the HMO Act of 1973 • Created Medicare risk programs, which allowed federally qualified HMOs and competitive medical plans that met specified Medicare requirements to provide Medicare-covered services under a risk contract • Defined risk contract as an arrangement among providers to provide capitated (fixed, prepaid basis) healthcare services to Medicare beneficiaries • Defined competitive medical plan (CMP) as an HMO that meets federal eligibility requirements for a Medicare risk contract but is not licensed as a federally qualified plan
1981	Omnibus Budget Reconciliation Act of 1981 (OBRA)	• Provided states with flexibility to establish HMOs for Medicare and Medicaid programs • Resulted in increased enrollment
1985	Preferred Provider Health Care Act of 1985	• Eased restrictions on preferred provider organizations • Allowed subscribers to seek healthcare from providers outside the PPO
1985	Consolidated Omnibus Budget Reconciliation Act of 1985 (COBRA)	• Established an employee's right to continue healthcare coverage beyond scheduled benefit termination date (including HMO coverage)
1988	Amendment to the HMO Act of 1973	• Allowed federally qualified HMOs to permit members to occasionally use non-HMO physicians and be partially reimbursed
1989	Healthcare Effectiveness Data and Information Set (HEDIS)—developed by National Committee for Quality Assurance (NCQA)	• Created standards to assess managed care systems in terms of membership, utilization of services, quality, access, health plan management and activities, and financial indicators
1994	HCFA's Office of Managed Care established	• Facilitated innovation and competition among Medicare HMOs
2010	Patient Protection and Affordable Care Act	• Individual mandate requirements, expansion of public programs, Health Insurance Exchanges, changes to private insurance, employer requirements, and cost and coverage estimates are part of this plan

- Several kinds of managed care plans are available in the United States, including:
  - — Health maintenance organizations (HMOs)
  - — Preferred provider organizations (PPOs)
  - — **Point-of-service** (POS) **plans**
  - — **Exclusive provider organizations** (EPOs)
  - — **Integrated delivery systems** (IDSs)

Health Maintenance Organizations

An HMO is a prepaid voluntary health plan that provides healthcare services in return for the payment of a monthly membership premium. HMO premiums are based on a projection of the costs that are likely to be involved in treating the plan's average enrollee over a specified period of time. If the actual cost per enrollee were to exceed the projected cost, the HMO would experience a financial loss. If the actual cost per enrollee turned out to be lower than the projection, the HMO would show a profit. Because most HMOs are for-profit organizations, they emphasize cost control and preventive medicine.

Today, most employers and insurance companies offer enrollees some type of HMO option. The benefit to third-party payers and enrollees alike is cost savings. Most HMO enrollees have significantly lower out-of-pocket expenses than enrollees of traditional fee-for-service and other types of managed care plans. The HMO premiums shared by employers and enrollees also are lower than the premiums for other types of healthcare plans.

HMOs can be organized in several different ways, including the **group model HMO,** the **independent practice association** (IPA), the **network model HMO,** and the **staff model HMO,** or there can also be a combination of the staff, group, and network models.

Group Model HMOs

In the group model HMO, the HMO enters into a contract with an independent multispecialty physician group to provide medical services to members of the plan. The providers usually agree to devote a fixed percentage of their practice time to the HMO. Alternatively, the HMO may own or directly manage the physician group, in which case the physicians and their support staff would be considered its employees.

Group model HMOs are closed-panel arrangements. In other words, the physicians are not allowed to treat patients from other managed care plans. Enrollees of group model HMOs are required to seek services from the designated physician group.

Independent Practice Associations

IPAs are sometimes called individual practice associations. In the IPA model, the HMO enters into a contract with an organized group of physicians who join together for purposes of fulfilling the HMO contract but retain their individual practices. The physicians are not considered employees of the HMO. They work from their own private offices and continue to see other patients. The HMO usually pays the IPA according to a negotiated list of discounted fees. Alternatively, physicians may agree to provide services to HMO members for a set prepaid capitated payment for a specified period of time. Capitation is discussed later in this chapter.

The IPA is an open-panel HMO, which means that the physicians are free to treat patients from other plans. Enrollees of such HMOs are required to seek services from the designated physician group.

Network Model HMOs

Network model HMOs are similar to group model HMOs except that the HMO contracts for services with two or more multispecialty group practices instead of just one practice. Members of network model HMOs receive a list of all the physicians on the approved panel and are required to select providers from the list.

Staff Model HMOs

Staff model HMOs directly employ physicians and other healthcare professionals to provide medical services to members. Members of the salaried medical staff are considered employees of the HMO rather than independent practitioners. Premiums are paid directly to the HMO, and ambulatory care services are usually provided within the HMO's corporate facilities. The staff model HMO is a closed-panel arrangement.

Preferred Provider Organizations

Preferred provider organizations (PPOs) represent contractual agreements between healthcare providers and a self-insured employer or a health insurance carrier. Beneficiaries of PPOs select providers such as physicians or hospitals from a list of participating providers who have agreed to furnish healthcare services to the covered population. Beneficiaries may elect to receive services from nonparticipating providers but must pay a greater portion of the cost (in other words, higher deductibles and copays). Providers are usually reimbursed on a discounted fee-for-service basis.

Point-of-Service Plans

POS plans are similar to HMOs in that subscribers must select a **primary care physician** (PCP) from a network of participating physicians. (The PCP is usually a family or general practice physician or an internal medicine specialist.) The PCP acts as a service gatekeeper to control the patient's access to specialty, surgical, and hospital care as well as expensive diagnostic services.

POS plans are different from HMOs in that subscribers are allowed to seek care from providers outside the network. However, the subscribers must pay a greater share of the charges for out-of-network services. POS plans were created to increase the flexibility of managed care plans and to allow patients more choice in providers.

Exclusive Provider Organizations

EPOs are similar to PPOs except that EPOs provide benefits to enrollees only when the enrollees receive healthcare services from **network providers.** In other words, EPO beneficiaries do not receive reimbursement for services furnished by nonparticipating providers. In addition, healthcare services must be coordinated by a PCP. EPOs are regulated by state insurance departments. In contrast, HMOs are regulated by state departments of commerce or departments of incorporation.

Integrated Delivery Systems

An IDS is a healthcare provider made up of a number of associated medical facilities that furnish coordinated healthcare services. Most IDSs include a number of facilities that provide services along the continuum of care, for example, ambulatory surgery centers, physicians' office practices, outpatient clinics, acute care hospitals, SNFs, and so on.

Integrated delivery systems can be structured according to several different models, including:

- **Group practices without walls** (GPWWs)
- **Integrated provider organizations** (IPOs)
- **Management service organizations** (MSOs)
- **Medical foundations**
- **Physician-hospital organizations** (PHOs)

Group Practices without Walls

A GPWW is an arrangement that allows physicians to maintain their own offices, but to share administrative, management, and marketing services (for example, medical transcription and billing) for the purpose of fulfilling contracts with managed care organizations.

Integrated Provider Organizations

An IPO manages and coordinates the delivery of healthcare services performed by a number of healthcare professionals and facilities. IPOs typically provide acute care (hospital) services, physicians' services, ambulatory care services, and skilled nursing services. The physicians working in an IPO are salaried employees. IPOs are sometimes referred to as delivery systems, horizontally integrated systems, health delivery networks, accountable health plans, integrated service networks (ISNs), vertically integrated plans (VIPs), and vertically integrated systems.

Management Service Organizations

MSOs provide practice management (administrative and support) services to individual physicians' practices. They are usually owned by a group of physicians or a hospital.

Medical Foundations

Medical foundations are nonprofit organizations that enter into contracts with physicians to manage the physicians' practices. The typical medical foundation owns clinical and business resources and makes them available to the participating physicians. Clinical assets include medical equipment and supplies, and treatment facilities. Business assets include billing and administrative support systems.

Physician-Hospital Organizations

PHOs, previously known as medical staff-hospital organizations, provide healthcare services through a contractual arrangement between physicians and hospital(s). PHO arrangements make it possible for the managed care market to view the hospital(s) and physicians as a single entity for the purpose of establishing a contract for services.

Check Your Understanding 6.5

Instructions: Select the best option for the following statements.

1. This model of HMO is created when physicians join together in an organized group for the purposes of fulfilling a contract but retain individual practices:

   A. Group
   B. Independent practice association
   C. Network model
   D. Staff

2. This model of HMO employs physicians and other healthcare professionals to provide healthcare services to members:

   A. Group
   B. Independent practice association
   C. Network
   D. Staff

3. In this model, healthcare services are contracted with two or more multispecialty group practices instead of just one:

   A. Group
   B. Independent practice
   C. Network
   D. Staff

4. In this HMO contract, providers usually agree to devote a fixed percentage of their practice time to the HMO:

   A. Group
   B. Independent practice
   C. Network
   D. Staff

5. Premiums are paid directly to this type of HMO, and services are usually provided within corporate facilities:

   A. Group
   B. Independent practice
   C. Network
   D. Staff

6. This nonprofit organization contracts with physicians to manage their practices and owns clinical/business resources that are made available to participating physicians:

   A. Exclusive provider organization
   B. Group practice without walls
   C. Management service organization
   D. Medical foundation

7. This organization manages and coordinates the delivery of healthcare services performed by a number of healthcare professionals and facilities and its physicians are salaried employees:

   A. Group practice without walls
   B. Integrated delivery system
   C. Integrated provider organization
   D. Management service organization

8. This arrangement makes it possible for the managed care market to view hospitals and physicians as a single entity for the purpose of contracting services:

   A. Management service organization
   B. Medical foundation
   C. Physician-hospital organization
   D. Point-of-service plan

Healthcare Reimbursement Methodologies

As mentioned earlier, about 85 percent of Americans are covered by some type of private prepaid health plan or federal healthcare program. Therefore, third-party payers rather than actual recipients of services pay for most healthcare expenses in the United States. The recipients can be considered the "first parties" and the providers the "second parties." Third-party payers include commercial for-profit insurance companies, nonprofit and for-profit Blue Cross and Blue Shield organizations, self-insured employers, federal programs (Medicare, Medicaid, SCHIP, TRICARE, CHAMPVA, and IHS), and workers' compensation programs.

Providers charge their own determined amounts for services rendered. However, providers are rarely reimbursed this full amount because third-party payers may have a unique reimbursement methodology. For example, commercial insurance plans usually reimburse healthcare providers under some type of **retrospective payment system.** The federal Medicare program uses prospective payment systems (PPSs). In retrospective payment systems, the exact amount of the payment is determined after the service has been delivered. In a PPS, the exact amount of the payment is determined before the service is delivered.

Fee-for-Service Reimbursement Methodologies

Fee-for-service reimbursement methodologies issue payments to healthcare providers on the basis of the charges assigned to each of the separate services that were performed for the patient. **Chargemasters** are used to list the individual charges for every element entailed in providing a service (for example, surgical supplies, surgical equipment, room and board, nursing care, respiratory therapy, pharmaceuticals, medical equipment, and so on). The total bill for an episode of care represents the sum of all the itemized charges for every element of care provided. Independent clinical professionals such as physicians and psychologists who are not employees of the facility issue separate itemized bills to cover their services after the services are completed or on a monthly basis when the services are ongoing.

Before prepaid insurance plans became common in the 1950s and the Medicare and Medicaid programs were developed in the 1960s, healthcare providers sent itemized bills directly to their patients. Patients were held responsible for paying their own medical bills. When prepaid health plans and the Medicare/Medicaid programs were originally developed, they also based reimbursement on itemized fees.

Traditional Fee-for-Service Reimbursement

In traditional fee-for-service (FFS) reimbursement systems, third-party payers and/or patients issue payments to healthcare providers after healthcare services have been provided (for example, after the patient has been discharged from the hospital). Payments are based on the specific services delivered. The fees charged for services vary considerably by the type of services provided, the resources required, and the type and number of healthcare professionals involved.

Payments can be calculated on the basis of actual billed charges, discounted charges, pre-negotiated rate schedules, or the usual or customary charges in a specific community. It is important to remember that the billed charges are not necessarily the actual cost of the services provided.

For example, some third-party payers pay only the maximum allowable charges as determined by the plan. Maximum allowable charges may be significantly lower than the provider's billed charges. Some payers issue payments on the basis of **usual, customary, and reasonable** (UCR) **charges.** UCR is defined as a "Type of retrospective fee-for-service payment method in which the third-party payer pays for fees that are usual, customary, and reasonable, wherein "usual" is usual for the individual provider's practice;

"customary" means customary for the community; and "reasonable" is reasonable for the situation (AHIMA 2012, 352). Commercial insurance and Blue Cross/Blue Shield plans often issue payments based on negotiated discount rates and contractual cost-sharing arrangements with the patient.

For many plans, the health plan and the patient share costs on an 80/20 percent arrangement. The portion of the claim covered by the patient's insurance plan is 80 percent of allowable charges. After the third-party payer transmits its payment to the provider, the provider's billing department issues a final statement to the patient. The statement shows the amount for which the patient is responsible (in this example, 20 percent of allowable charges).

The traditional FFS reimbursement methodology is still used by many commercial insurance companies for visits to physicians' offices.

Managed Fee-for-Service Reimbursement

Managed FFS reimbursement is similar to traditional FFS reimbursement except that managed care plans control costs primarily by managing their members' use of healthcare services. Most managed care plans also negotiate with providers to develop discounted **fee schedules.** A fee schedule is a list of services provided and the charge for that service. Managed FFS reimbursement is common for inpatient hospital care. In some areas of the country, however, it also is applied to outpatient and ambulatory services, surgical procedures, high-cost diagnostic procedures, and physicians' services.

Utilization controls include the prospective and retrospective review of the healthcare services planned for, or provided to, patients. For example, a prospective utilization review of a plan to hospitalize a patient for minor surgery might determine that the surgery could be safely performed less expensively in an outpatient setting or the insurance company could deny the service due to lack of medical necessity or other reason. This prospective utilization review is sometimes called **precertification**.

In a retrospective utilization review, the plan might determine that part or all of the services provided to a patient were not medically necessary or were not covered by the plan. In such cases, the plan would disallow part or all of the provider's charges and the patient would be responsible for paying the provider's outstanding charges.

Discharge planning also can be considered a type of utilization control. The managed care plan may be able to move the patient to a less intensive, and therefore less expensive, care setting as soon as possible by coordinating his or her discharge from inpatient care.

Episode-of-Care Reimbursement Methodologies

Plans that use **episode-of-care** (EOC) **reimbursement** methods issue lump-sum payments to providers to compensate them for all the healthcare services delivered to a patient for a specific illness and/or over a specific period of time. EOC payments also are called **bundled payments.** Bundled payments cover multiple services and also may involve multiple providers of care. EOC reimbursement methods include capitated payments, global payments, global surgery payments, Medicare ambulatory surgery center rates, and Medicare PPSs.

Capitation

Capitation is based on per-person premiums or membership fees rather than on itemized per-procedure or per-service charges. The capitated managed care plan negotiates a contract with an employer or government agency representing a specific group of individuals. According to the contract, the managed care organization agrees to provide all the contracted healthcare services that the covered individuals need over a specified period of time (usually one year). In exchange, the individual enrollee and/or third-party payer agrees to pay a fixed premium for the covered group. Like other insurance plans, a capitated insurance contract stipulates as part of the contract exactly which healthcare services are covered and which ones are not.

Capitated premiums are calculated on the projected cost of providing covered services **per patient per month** or **per member per month** (PPPM or PMPM). The capitated premium for an individual member of a plan includes all the services covered by the plan, regardless of the number of services actually provided during the period or their cost. If the average member of the plan actually used more services than originally assumed in the PPPM calculation, the plan would show a loss for the period. If the average member actually used fewer services, the plan would show a profit.

The purchasers of capitated coverage (usually the member's employer) pay monthly premiums to the managed care plan. The individual enrollees usually pay part of the premium as well. The plan then compensates the providers who actually furnished the services. In some arrangements, the managed care plan accepts all the risk involved in the contract. In others, some of the risk is passed on to the PCPs who agreed to act as gatekeepers for the plan.

The capitated managed care organization may own or operate some or all of the healthcare facilities that provide care to members and directly employ clinical professionals. Staff model HMOs operate in this way. Alternatively, the capitated managed care organization may purchase services from independent physicians and facilities, as do group model HMOs.

Global Payment

Global payment methodology is sometimes applied to radiological and similar types of procedures that involve professional and technical components. Global payments are lump-sum payments distributed among the physicians who perform the procedure or interpret its results and the healthcare facility that provided the equipment, supplies, and technical support required. The procedure's **professional component** is supplied by physicians (for example, radiologists), and its **technical component** (for example, radiological supplies, equipment, and support services) is supplied by a hospital or freestanding diagnostic or surgical center. For example:

Larry underwent a scheduled carotid angiogram as a hospital outpatient. He had complained of ringing in his ears and dizziness, and his physician scheduled the procedure to determine whether there was a blockage in one of Larry's carotid arteries. The procedure required a surgeon to inject radiopaque contrast material through a catheter into Larry's left carotid artery. A radiological technician then took an x-ray of Larry's neck. The technician was supervised by a radiologist, and both were employees of the hospital.

Professional component: Injection of radiopaque contrast material by the surgeon

Technical component: X-ray of the neck region

Global payment: The facility received a lump-sum payment for the procedure and paid for the services of the surgeon from that payment.

Global Surgery Payments

A single **global surgery payment** covers all the healthcare services entailed in planning and completing a specific surgical procedure. In other words, every element of the procedure from the treatment decision through normal postoperative patient care is covered by a single bundled payment. For example:

Tammy received all the prenatal, perinatal, and postnatal care involved in the birth of her daughter from Dr. Michaels. She received one bill from the physician for a total of $2,200. The bill represented the total charges for the obstetrical services associated with her pregnancy. However, the two-day inpatient hospital stay for the normal delivery was not included in the global payment, nor were the laboratory services she received during her hospital stay. Tammy received a separate bill for these services. In addition, if she had suffered a postdelivery complication (for example, a wound infection) or an unrelated medical problem, the physician and hospital services required to treat the complications would not have been covered by the global surgical payment.

Prospective Payment

In 1983, CMS implemented a PPS for inpatient hospital care provided to Medicare beneficiaries. This PPS methodology was called **diagnosis-related groups** (DRGs). The DRG system was implemented as a way to control Medicare spending. It reimburses hospitals a predetermined amount for each Medicare inpatient stay. Payments are determined by the DRG to which each case is assigned according to the patient's **principal diagnosis,** which is defined as the condition, which, after study, is determined to have occasioned the admission of the patient to the hospital for care.

After DRG implementation in 1983, Congress passed the **Omnibus Budget Reconciliation Act** (OBRA) of 1986, which mandated the development of a prospective system for hospital-based outpatient services provided to Medicare beneficiaries. In subsequent years, Congress mandated the development of PPSs for other healthcare providers including care in SNFs, outpatient services and procedures, home healthcare, and rehabilitation care. In addition, the act included a legislative proposal on a PPS for long-term care.

Check Your Understanding 6.6

Instructions: Select the correct term for each of the following statements.

1. The type of payment system where the amount of payment is determined before the service is delivered is called:

    A. Fee-for-service
    B. Per diem
    C. Prospective
    D. Retrospective

2. These payment arrangements are streamlined by the use of chargemasters:

    A. Fee-for-service
    B. Per diem
    C. Prospective
    D. Retrospective

3. The prospective payment system implemented in 1983 is referred to as:

    A. APC
    B. DRG
    C. OPPS
    D. URC

4. Third-party payers and/or patients issue payments to healthcare providers after healthcare services have been provided and payments are based on the specific services delivered refers to _____ reimbursement?

    A. Managed Fee-for-Service
    B. Traditional Fee-for-Service
    C. Episode-of-Care
    D. Fee-for-Service

5. For many plans, the health plan and the patient share costs on a(an) _____ percent arrangement?

    A. 50/50
    B. 80/20
    C. 90/10
    D. 75/25

Medicare Prospective Payment Systems

This section discusses the various Medicare Prospective Payment Systems.

Medicare Acute Inpatient Prospective Payment System (IPPS)

As mentioned previously, prior to 1983, Medicare Part A payments to hospitals were determined on a traditional FFS reimbursement methodology. Payment was based on the cost of services provided, and reasonable cost and/or per-diem costs were used to determine payment. The way payments were made, however, was changed to a prospective payment system after 1982.

Medicare Severity Diagnosis-Related Groups (MS-DRGs)

Congress passed the **Tax Equity and Fiscal Responsibility Act of 1982** (TEFRA). TEFRA mandated implementation of the DRG PPS. Under DRGs, Medicare paid most hospitals for inpatient hospital services according to a predetermined rate for each discharge. Very simply, the DRG system was a way of classifying patients on the basis of diagnosis. Patients within each DRG were said to be "medically meaningful"—that is, patients within a group were expected to evoke a set of clinical responses, which statistically would result in an approximately equal use of hospital resources. On October 1, 2007, the DRG system became the **Medicare severity diagnosis-related groups** (MS-DRGs).

At this time, several types of hospitals are excluded from Medicare acute inpatient PPS because the PPS diagnosis-related groups do not accurately account for the resource costs for the types of patients treated in those facilities. The following facilities are still paid on the basis of reasonable cost, subject to payment limits per discharge or under a separate PPS:

- Psychiatric and rehabilitation hospitals and psychiatric and rehabilitation units within larger medical facilities
- **Long-term care hospitals** (LTCHs), which are defined as hospitals with an average length of stay of 25 days or more
- Children's hospitals
- Cancer hospitals
- Critical access hospitals
- Religious non-medical health care institutions (healthcare furnished under religious tenets that prohibit conventional or unconventional healthcare for a beneficiary)

MS-DRG Assignment

To determine the appropriate MS-DRG, a claim for a healthcare encounter is first classified into one of 25 **major diagnostic categories,** or MDCs. The principal diagnosis determines the MDC assignment. The principal diagnosis is the condition established after study to have resulted in the inpatient admission. Within most MDCs, cases are divided into surgical MS-DRGs (based on a surgical hierarchy that orders individual procedures or groups of procedures by resource intensity) and medical MS-DRGs. Medical MS-DRGs generally are differentiated on the basis of diagnosis and age. Some surgical and medical MS-DRGs are further differentiated on the basis of the presence or absence of **complications** or **comorbidities.**

A complication is a secondary condition that arises during hospitalization and is thought to increase the length of stay by at least one day for approximately 75 percent of patients. A co-morbid condition is a condition that existed at admission and is thought to increase the length of stay at least one day for approximately 75 percent of patients. During the initial years of DRGs there was a standard list of diagnoses that were considered CCs. Each year new CCs are added and others deleted from the CC list.

Prior to the implementation of MS-DRGs, a comprehensive review of the CC list was performed and an important change to the CC concept was made. Each base MS-DRG can be subdivided in one of three possible alternatives:

- MS-DRGs with three subgroups Major Complication/Comorbidity (MCC, CC, and non-CC); referred to as "with MCC," "with CC," and "w/o CC/MCC"

  — MS-DRG 682 Renal Failure w MCC

  — MS-DRG 683 Renal Failure w CC

  — MS-DRG 684 Renal Failure w/o CC/MCC

- MS-DRGs with two subgroups (MCC and CC/non-CC); referred to as "with MCC" and "without MCC"

  — MS-DRG 725 Benign Prostatic Hypertrophy w MCC

  — MS-DRG 726 Benign Prostatic Hypertrophy w/o MCC

- MS-DRGs with two subgroups (non-CC and CC/MCC); referred to as "with CC/MCC" and "without CC/MCC"

  — MS-DRG 294 Deep Vein Thrombophlebitis w CC/MCC

  — MS-DRG 295 Deep Vein Thrombophlebitis w/o CC/MCC

The increased number of classifications is intended to differentiate between the levels of resource consumption within a base MS-DRG group.

Under the acute inpatient prospective payment system (PPS), a predetermined rate based on the MS-DRG (only one is assigned per case) assigned to each case is used to reimburse hospitals for inpatient care provided to Medicare and TRICARE beneficiaries.

Hospitals determine MS-DRGs by assigning ICD-9-CM codes to each patient's principal diagnosis, comorbidities, complications, major complications, **principal procedure,** and secondary procedures. These code numbers and other information on the patient (age, gender, and discharge status) are entered into a grouper. An MS-**DRG grouper** is a computer software program that assigns appropriate MS-DRGs according to the information provided for each episode of care.

Reimbursement for each episode of care is based on the MS-DRG assigned. Different diagnoses require different levels of care and expenditures of resources. Therefore, each MS-DRG is assigned a different level of payment that reflects the average amount of resources required to treat a patient assigned to that MS-DRG. Each MS-DRG is associated with a description, a relative weight, a geometric mean length of stay (LOS), and an arithmetic mean LOS.

The relative weight represents the average resources required to care for cases in that particular MS-DRG relative to the national average of resources used to treat all Medicare patients. An MS-DRG with a relative weight of 2.000, on average, requires twice as many resources as an MS-DRG with a relative weight of 1.000.

The geometric mean LOS is defined as the total days of service, excluding any outliers or transfers, divided by the total number of patients.

The arithmetic mean LOS is defined as the total days of service divided by the total number of patients.

For example, MS-DRG 1, organized within MDC 01, is described as heart transplant or implant of heart assist system with MCC and has a relative weight of 24.2794, a geometric mean LOS of 28.6, and an arithmetic mean LOS of 37.4.

CMS adjusts the Medicare MS-DRG list and reimbursement rates every fiscal year (October 1 through September 30). There are currently 751 MS-DRGs.

In some cases, the MS-DRG payment received by the hospital may be lower than the actual cost of providing Medicare Part A inpatient services. In such cases, the hospital must absorb the loss. In other cases, the cost of providing care is lower than the MS-DRG payment and the hospital may receive a payment for more than its actual cost and, therefore, makes a profit. It is expected that, on average, hospitals will be reimbursed for their total costs in providing services to Medicare patients.

Special circumstances can also apply to inpatient cases and result in an outlier payment to the hospital. An outlier case results in exceptionally high costs when compared with other cases in the same DRG. To qualify for a **cost outlier,** a hospital's charges for a case (adjusted to cost) must exceed the payment rate for the MS-DRG by a fixed amount which changes each year. The additional payment amount is equal to 80 percent of the difference between the hospital's entire cost for the stay and the threshold amount.

There can be further hospital-specific adjustments resulting in add-on payments:

- *Disproportionate share hospital (DSH):* If the hospital treats a high percentage of low-income patients, it receives a percentage add-on payment applied to the MS-DRG-adjusted base payment rate.

- *Indirect medical education (IME):* If the hospital is an approved teaching hospital, it receives a percentage add-on payment for each case paid under MS-DRGs. This percentage varies depending on the ratio of residents to beds.

- *New technologies:* If the hospital can demonstrate the use of a new technology that is a substantial clinical improvement over available existing technologies and the new technology is approved, additional payments are made. Hospitals must submit a formal request to CMS with a significant sample of data to demonstrate that the technology meets the high-cost threshold.

Case-Mix Index

The MS-DRG system creates a hospital's **case-mix index** (types or categories of patients treated by the hospital) based on the relative weights of the MS-DRG. The case-mix index can be figured by multiplying the relative weight of each MS-DRG by the number of discharges within that MS-DRG. This provides the total weight for each MS-DRG. The sum of all total weights divided by the sum of total patient discharges equals the case-mix index. An example follows in table 6.6.

A hospital may relate its case-mix index to the costs incurred for inpatient care. This information allows the hospital to make administrative decisions about services to be offered to its patient population. For example:

> The hospital's case-mix report indicated that a small population of patients was receiving obstetrical services, but that the costs associated with providing such services were disproportionately high. This report along with other data might result in the hospital's administrative decision to discontinue its obstetrical services department.

All Patient DRG

An **all patient DRG** (AP-DRG) system was developed in 1988 by 3M Health Information Systems as the basis for New York's hospital reimbursement program for non-Medicare discharges. AP-DRGs are still used in a number of states as a basis for payment of non-Medicare claims. AP-DRGs use the patient's age, sex, discharge status, and ICD-9-CM diagnoses and procedure codes to determine a DRG that, in turn, determines reimbursement. 3M also has developed **all patient refined DRGs** (APR-DRGs) as an extension of the DRG concept. APR-DRGs adjust patient data for severity of illness and risk of mortality, help to develop clinical pathways, are used as

Table 6.6.   **Calculation of case-mix index**

MS-DRG	Description	Number of Discharges	CMS Relative Weight	Total Relative Weight
280	Heart failure & shock	50	1.8503	92.515
193	Simple pneumonia & pleurisy w CC	42	1.4796	62.1432
377	GI hemorrhage w MCC	23	1.7541	40.3443
190	COPD	18	1.1924	15.0956
483	Major joint & limb reattach upper extreme w CC/MCC	17	2.4019	40.8323
	Total	**150**		**50.9300**

Case-Mix Index (CMI) for the top 5 MS-DRGs above is: 1.67

Total relative weight divided by total discharges = CMI

250.9300 divided by 150 = 1.67 CMI

a basis for quality assurance programs, and are used in comparative profiling and setting capitation rates (Averill et al. 2002).

Hospital-Acquired Conditions and Present on Admission Indicator Reporting

The Deficit Reduction Act of 2005 (DRA) mandated a quality adjustment in the MS-DRG payments for certain hospital-acquired conditions. CMS titled the program "Hospital-Acquired Conditions and Present on Admission Indicator Reporting" (HAC and POA). Inpatient hospitals were required to submit POA information on diagnoses for inpatient discharges on or after October 1, 2007. The following hospitals are exempt from the POA indicator requirement:

- Critical access hospitals
- Long-term care hospitals
- Maryland waiver hospitals
- Cancer hospitals
- Children's inpatient facilities
- Inpatient rehabilitation facilities
- Psychiatric hospitals

Present on admission (POA) is defined as a condition present at the time the order for inpatient admission occurs—conditions that develop during an outpatient encounter, including the emergency department, observation or outpatient surgery, are considered as present on admission. A POA indicator is assigned to principal and secondary diagnoses and the external cause of injury codes. The reporting options that are available are:

Y = Yes, diagnosis was present at the time of inpatient admission.

N = No, diagnosis was not present at the time of inpatient admission.

U = Unknown, documentation is insufficient to determine if condition was present at the time of inpatient admission.

W = Clinically undetermined. The provider is unable to determine whether the condition was present at the time of admission.

Unreported/Not used = Exempt from POA reporting.

Complete guidelines with examples are part of the *ICD-9-CM Official Guidelines for Coding and Reporting* and should be reviewed. The POA indicator guidelines do not provide guidance on when a condition should be coded but, rather, how to apply the POA indicator to the final set of diagnosis codes that have been assigned.

CMS identified **hospital-acquired conditions** (HAC) (not present on admission) as "reasonably preventable," and hospitals do not receive additional payment for cases in which one of the conditions was not present on admission. This is termed the HAC payment provision. The selected conditions include:

- Foreign object retained after surgery

- Air embolism

- Blood incompatibility

- Stage III and IV pressure ulcers

- Falls and trauma

- Catheter-associated urinary tract infection

- Vascular catheter-associated infection

- Surgical site infection—following CABG, bariatric surgery, or orthopedic procedures

- Certain manifestations of poor glycemic control

- Deep vein thrombosis (DVT)/pulmonary embolism (PE) following total knee replacement and hip replacement procedures

The HAC and POA web page at http://www.cms.gov/HospitalAcqCond/ provides up-to-date information on these topics.

Resource-Based Relative Value Scale (RBRVS) System

In 1992, CMS implemented the **resource-based relative value scale** (RBRVS) system for physician's services such as office visits covered under Medicare Part B. The system reimburses physicians according to a fee schedule based on predetermined values assigned to specific services.

The **Medicare fee schedule** (MFS) is the listing of allowed charges that are reimbursable to physicians under Medicare. Each year's MFS is published by CMS in the *Federal Register.*

To calculate fee schedule amounts, Medicare uses a formula that incorporates the following **relative value units** (RVUs) for:

- Physician work (RVUw)

- Practice expenses (RVUpe)

- Malpractice costs (RVUm)

Sample 2011 RVUs for selected HCPCS codes are shown in table 6.7.

Table 6.7.   Sample 2011 RVUs for selected HCPCS codes

HCPCS Code	Description	Work RVU	Facility Practice Expense RVU	Malpractice Expense RVU
99203	Office visit	1.42	.72	.14
99204	Office visit	2.43	1.21	.23
11010	Debridement skin at fracture site	4.19	3.49	.76
45380	Colonoscopy with biopsy	4.43	2.73	.67
52601	TURP, complete	15.26	8.09	1.49

Table 6.8.   Sample GPCIs for selected U.S. cities

City	Work GPCI	Practice Expense GPCI	Malpractice Expense GPCI
St. Louis	.99163	.939923	1.05944
Dallas	1.0113	.99943	.82543311
Spokane	.98989	.932469	1.670886

Payment localities are adjusted according to three **geographic practice cost indices** (GPCIs):

- Physician work (GPCIw)

- Practice expenses (GPCIpe)

- Malpractice costs (GPCIm)

Sample GPCIs for selected U.S. cities are shown in table 6.8.

A geographic practice cost index is a number used to multiply each RVU so that it better reflects a geographical area's relative costs. For example, costs of office rental prices, local taxes, average salaries, and malpractice costs are all affected by geography.

A **national conversion factor** (CF) converts the RVUs into payments. In 2011, the CF was $33.976.

The RBRVS fee schedule uses the following formula:

$$[(RVUw \times GPCIw) + (RVUpe \times GPCIpe) + (RVUm \times GPCIm)] \times CF = Payment$$

As an example, payment for performing a drainage of a repair of a nail bed (code 11760) in Birmingham, Alabama, can be calculated. RVU values include:

- Work RVU (RVUw) = 1.63

- Practice expense RVU (RVUpe) = 1.71

- Malpractice RVU (RVUm) = 0.18

GPCI values include:

- Work GPCI (GPCIw) = .982
- Practice expense GPCI (GPCIpe) = 0.853
- Malpractice GPCI (GPCIm) = 0.496
- National CF = $33.976

The calculation is as follows:

$$(1.63 \times .982) + (1.71 \times 0.853) + (0.18 \times 0.496) \times \$33.9764$$
$$1.60 + 1.458 + 0.089$$
$$3.147 \times \$33.976$$
$$\text{Fee schedule payment} = \$106.92$$

Skilled Nursing Facility Prospective Payment System

The BBA mandated implementation of a **skilled nursing facility prospective payment system** (SNF PPS). The system was to cover all costs (routine, ancillary, and capital) associated with covered SNF services furnished to Medicare Part A beneficiaries. Certain educational activities were exempt from the new system.

The SNF PPS was implemented on July 1, 1998. Under the PPS, SNFs are no longer paid under a system based on reasonable costs. Instead, they are paid according to a perdiem (per day) PPS based on case mix–adjusted payment rates. Per diem rates range from a high of about $737 to a low of about $183.

Medicare Part A covers post-hospital SNF services and all items and services paid under Medicare Part B before July 1, 1998 (other than physician and certain other services specifically excluded under the BBA). Major elements of the SNF PPS include rates, coverage, transition, and consolidated billing.

OBRA required CMS to develop an assessment instrument to standardize the collection of SNF patient data. That instrument is known as the **resident assessment instrument** (RAI) and includes the **Minimum Data Set 3.0** (MDS). The MDS is the minimum core of defined and categorized patient assessment questions that serves as the basis for documentation and reimbursement in an SNF. The MDS form contains a face sheet for documentation of resident identification information, demographic information, and the patient's customary routine. Additional information about MDS is covered in chapter 4.

Resource Utilization Groups

SNF reimbursement rates are paid according to **Resource Utilization Groups, Version IV** (RUG-IV) (a resident classification system) based on the MDS resident assessments.

The RUG-IV classification system uses resident assessment data from the MDS collected by SNFs to assign residents to one of 66 groups.

Resident Assessment Validation and Entry

CMS developed an electronic data-entry system for skilled nursing facilities that offers users the ability to collect MDS assessments in a database and transmit them in CMS-standard format to their state database. The data-entry software is entitled **Resident Assessment Validation and Entry** (RAVEN). RAVEN imports and exports data in standard MDS record format; maintains facility, resident, and employee information; enforces data integrity via rigorous edit checks; and provides comprehensive online help. It includes a data dictionary and a RUG calculator.

Consolidated Billing Provision

The BBA includes a billing provision that requires an SNF to submit consolidated Medicare bills for its residents for services covered under either Part A or Part B except for a limited number of specifically excluded services. For example, when a physician provides a diagnostic radiology service to an SNF patient, the SNF must bill for the technical component of the radiology service because this is included in the SNF consolidated billing payment. The rendering physician must develop a business relationship with the SNF in order to receive payment from the SNF for the services he or she rendered. The professional component of the physician services is excluded from SNF consolidated billing and must be billed separately to the Medicare Administratvie Contractor.

There are, of course, other exclusions to this provision, including physician assistant services, nurse practitioner services, and clinical nurse specialists when these individuals are working under the supervision of, or in collaboration with, a physician, certified midwife services, qualified psychologist services, and certified registered nurse anesthetist services. Other exclusions include hospice care, maintenance dialysis, selected services furnished on an outpatient basis such as cardiac catheterization services, CAT scans and MRIs, radiation therapy, and ambulance services. In addition, SNFs report **Healthcare Common Procedure Coding System** (HCPCS) codes on all Part B bills.

Outpatient Prospective Payment System

The **outpatient prospective payment system** (OPPS) was first implemented for services furnished on or after August 1, 2000. Under the OPPS, the federal government pays for hospital outpatient services on a rate-per-service basis that varies according to the **ambulatory payment classification** (APC) group to which the service is assigned. The Healthcare Common Procedural Coding System (HCPCS) identifies and groups the services within each APC group. Services included under APCs follow:

- Surgical procedures
- Radiology including radiation therapy
- Clinic visits (E/M)
- ER visits

- Partial hospitalization services for the mentally ill
- Chemotherapy
- Preventive services and screening exams
- Dialysis for other than ESRD
- Vaccines, splints, casts, and antigens
- Certain implantable items

The OPPS does not apply to critical access hospitals (CAHs) or hospitals in Maryland that are excluded, IHS hospitals, or hospitals outside the 50 states, the District of Columbia, and Puerto Rico.

Ambulatory Payment Classification Groups (APCs)

The calculation of payment for services under the OPPS is based on the categorization of outpatient services into APC groups according to *Current Procedural Terminology* (CPT)/HCPCS code. ICD-9-CM coding is not utilized in the selection of APCs. The more than 850 APCs are categorized into significant procedure APCs, radiology and other diagnostic APCs, medical visit APCs, and a partial hospitalization APC. Services within an APC are similar, both clinically and with regard to resource consumption, and each APC is assigned a fixed payment rate for the facility fee or technical component of the outpatient visit. Payment rates are also adjusted according to the hospital's wage index. Multiple APCs may be appropriate for a single episode of care as the patient may receive various types of services such as radiology or surgical procedures.

Payment Status Indicators

The OPPS **payment status indicators** (PSIs or SIs) (table 6.9) that are assigned to each HCPCS code and APCs play an important role in determining payment for services under the OPPS. They indicate whether a service represented by an HCPCS code is payable under the OPPS or another payment system and also whether particular OPPS policies apply to the code.

Status indicator N refers to items and services that are packaged into APC rates. **Packaging** means that payment for that service is packaged into payment for other services and, therefore, there is no separate APC payment. Packaged services might include minor ancillary services, inexpensive drugs, medical supplies, and implantable devices.

Discounting applies to multiple surgical procedures furnished during the same operative session. For discounted procedures, the full APC rate is paid for the surgical procedure with the highest rate and other surgical procedures performed at the same time are reimbursed at 50 percent of the APC rate. When a surgical procedure is terminated after a patient is prepared for surgery, but before induction of anesthesia, the facility is reimbursed at 50 percent of the APC rate. Modifier 73 should be appended to the procedure

Table 6.9.   OPPS payment status indicators and description of payment under OPPS

Status Indicator	Description of Payment under OPPS
SI A	Services paid under some other method (such as a fee schedule): • Ambulance services • Clinical diagnostic laboratory services • Nonimplantable prosthetic and orthotic devices • EPO for ESRD patients • Physical, occupational, and speech therapy • Routine dialysis services for ESRD patients provided in a certified dialysis unit of a hospital • Diagnostic mammography • Screening mammography
SI B	Codes that are not recognized by OPPS when submitted on an outpatient hospital Part B bill type
SI C	Inpatient procedures
SI D	Discontinued codes
SI E	Items, codes, and services not covered by Medicare
SI F	Corneal tissue acquisition; certain CRNA services and Hepatitis B vaccines
SI G	Pass-through drugs and biologicals
SI H	Pass-through device categories
SI K	Non-pass-through drugs, nonimplantable biologicals, and therapeutic
SI L	Influenza vaccine; Pneumococcal pneumonia vaccine
SI M	Items and services not billable to the fiscal intermediary/MAC
SI N	Items and services packaged into APC rates
SI P	Partial hospitalization
SI Q	Packaged services subject to separate payment under OPPS payment criteria
SI Q1	STVX-Packaged codes
SI Q2	T-Packaged codes
SI Q3	Codes that may be paid through a composite APC
SI R	Blood and blood products
SI S	Significant procedure, not discounted when multiple
SI T	Significant procedure, multiple reduction applies
SI U	Brachytherapy services
SI V	Clinic or emergency department visit
SI Y	Nonimplantable durable medical equipment
SI X	Ancillary services

code indicating that the procedure was discontinued. Modifier 74 is appended to the procedure code when a procedure is interrupted after its initiation or the administration of anesthesia. The facility receives the full APC payment.

The OPPS does pay outlier payments on a service-by-service basis when the cost of furnishing a service or procedure by a hospital exceeds 1.75 times the APC payment amount and exceeds the APC payment rate plus a fixed-dollar threshold. If a provider meets both of these conditions, the outlier payment is calculated as 50 percent of the amount by which the cost of furnishing the service exceeds 1.75 times the APC payment rate. The fixed-dollar threshold changes each year.

Services that are identified with a status indicator C have been identified as inpatient only services and will not be reimbursed by Medicare when they are provided on an outpatient basis. This inpatient-only list is updated each year.

Special payments are also made for new technology in one of two ways. Transitional pass-through payments are temporary additional payments that are made when certain drugs, biological agents, brachytherapy devices, and other expensive medical devices new to medicine are used. These new technology APCs were created to allow new procedures and services to enter HOPPS quickly even though their complete costs and payment information are not known. New technology APCs house modern procedures and services until enough data is collected to properly place the new procedure in an existing APC or to create a new APC for the service/procedure. Coding for E/M medical visits is difficult under the APC system. CMS states that each facility should develop a system for mapping the provided services furnished to the different levels of effort represented by E/M codes. As long as services furnished are documented and medically necessary and the facility is following its own system, which reasonably relates the intensity of hospital resources to the different levels of codes, CMS assumes that the hospital is in compliance with its reporting requirements.

Ambulatory Surgery Center Prospective Payment System (ASC PPS)

For Medicare purposes, an **ambulatory surgery center** (ASC) is a distinct entity that operates exclusively for the purpose of furnishing outpatient surgical services to patients. An ASC is either independent or operated by a hospital. If it is operated by a hospital, it has the option of being covered under Medicare as an ASC or it can continue to be covered as an outpatient surgery department. To be considered an ASC of a hospital, it has to be a separately identifiable entity physically, administratively, and financially.

The Medicare Modernization Act (MMA) of 2003 extensively revised the ASC payment system with changes going into effect on January 1, 2008. The system is called the ambulatory surgery center prospective payment system (ASC PPS).

ASCs must accept assignment as payment in full. Eighty percent of the payment comes from the government and 20 percent from the beneficiary.

Under the ASC payment system, Medicare will make payments to ASCs only for services on the ASC list of covered procedures. The surgical procedures included in the list are those that have been determined to pose no significant risk to beneficiaries when furnished in an ASC. The ASC payment includes services such as medical and surgical supplies, nursing services, surgical dressings, implanted prosthetic devices not on a pass-through list, and splints and casts. Examples of services not included in the ASC payment are brachytherapy, procurement of corneal tissue, and certain drugs and biologicals.

The payment rates for most covered ASC procedures and covered ancillary services are established prospectively based on a percentage of the OPPS payment rates while a small number of services are contractor-based, such as the pass-through items.

The HCPCS code is used as the basis for payment. Each HCPCS code falls into one of more than 1,500 ASC groups with each group having a unique payment. Medicare pays 80 percent of the wage-adjusted rate and the beneficiary is responsible for the other 20 percent. Similar to the OPPS, each HCPCS has a payment indicator that determines whether the surgical procedure is on the ASC list (A2); device-intensive procedure paid at adjusted rate (J8); or packaged service or item for which no separate payment is made (N1). These are just a few examples of some of the payment indicators.

Again, like the OPPS, there are guidelines for payment of terminated procedures. The following rules apply:

- percent payment for procedures terminated for reasons before the ASC has expended substantial resources
- 50 percent payment for procedures that are terminated due to medical complications prior to anesthesia
- 100 percent payment for procedures that have started but are terminated after anesthesia is induced

Home Health Prospective Payment System (HH PPS)

The BBA called for the development and implementation of a **home health prospective payment system** (HH PPS) for reimbursement of services provided to Medicare beneficiaries. The PPS for home health agencies (HHAs) was implemented on October 1, 2000.

OASIS-C and Home Assessment Validation and Entry (HAVEN)

HHAs use the OASIS-C data set and the Home Assessment Validation and Entry (HAVEN) data-entry software to conduct all patient assessments, not just the assessments for Medicare beneficiaries. OASIS-C stands for **Outcome and Assessment Information Set.** It consists of data elements that (1) represent core items for the comprehensive assessment of an adult home care patient and (2) form the basis for measuring patient outcomes for the purpose of outcome-based quality improvement (OBQI).

OASIS-C is a key component of Medicare's partnership with the home care industry to foster and monitor improved home healthcare outcomes. The Conditions of Participation for HHAs require that HHAs electronically report all OASIS-C data.

CMS also developed the OASIS-C data-entry system called HAVEN (**Home Assessment Validation and Entry**). HAVEN is available to HHAs at no charge through CMS's website or on CD-ROM. HAVEN offers users the ability to collect OASIS-C data in a database and transmit them in a standard format to state databases. The data-entry software imports and exports data in standard OASIS-C record format, maintains agency, patient, and employee information, maintains data integrity through rigorous edit checks, and provides comprehensive on-line help.

Home Health Resource Groups

Home health resource groups (HHRGs) represent the classification system established for the prospective reimbursement of covered home care services to Medicare beneficiaries during a 60-day episode of care. Covered services include skilled nursing visits, home health aide visits, therapy services (for example, physical, occupational, and speech therapy), medical social services, and nonroutine medical supplies. DME is excluded from the episode-of-care payment and is reimbursed under the DME fee schedule.

The classification of a patient into one of 153 HHRGs is based on OASIS-C data, which establish the severity of clinical and functional needs and services utilized. Grouper software is used to establish the appropriate HHRG. The HHRG is a six-character alphanumeric code that represents severity levels in three domains: clinical, functional, and service utilization (table 6.10). For example:

OASIS data collected on a seventy-six-year-old male home care patient resulted in an HHRG of C2, F3, and S2. This HHRG is interpreted as a clinical domain of low severity, a functional domain of moderate severity, and a service utilization domain of low utilization.

Table 6.10. HHRG severity levels in three domains: clinical, functional, and service utilization

Domain	Score	Severity Level
Clinical	C1	Minimum severity
	C2	Low severity
	C3	Moderate severity
Functional	F1	Minimum severity
	F2	Low severity
	F3	Moderate severity
Service utilization	S1	Minimum utilization
	S2	Low severity utilization
	S3	Moderate utilization
	S4	High utilization
	S5	Maximum utilization

The HHRG assigned as well as the type of supplies provided and the number of home health visits comprises the HIPPS code, which is the unit of payment for the episode of care.

Episode of care reimbursements in 2012 varies from $1,700 to almost $7,000 and are affected by treatment level and regional wage differentials. There is no limit to the number of 60-day episodes of care that a patient may receive as long as Medicare coverage criteria are met. The national 60-day episode base payment amount is updated each year.

Low Utilization and Outlier Payments

When a patient receives fewer than four home care visits during a 60-day episode, an alternate (reduced) payment, or **low-utilization payment adjustment** (LUPA), is made instead of the full HHRG reimbursement rate. HHAs are eligible for a **cost outlier adjustment,** which is a payment for certain high-cost home care patients whose costs are in excess of a threshold amount for each HHRG. The threshold is the 60-day episode payment plus a fixed-dollar loss that is constant across the HHRGs.

Ambulance Fee Schedule

A new Medicare payment system for medically necessary transports effective for services provided on or after April 1, 2002, was included as part of the BBA. The final rule established a five-year transition period during which time payment will be based on a blended amount, based in part on the ambulance fee schedule and in part on reasonable cost or reasonable charge. By year five (CY 2006), the fee schedule was fully implemented with 100 percent of payment based on the schedule. The new payment system applies to all ambulance services, including volunteer, municipal, private, independent, and institutional providers (hospitals, critical access hospitals, SNFs, and HHAs).

Ambulance services are reported on claims using HCPCS codes that reflect the seven categories of ground service and two categories of air service. Mandatory assignment is required for all ambulance service providers.

The seven categories of ground (land and water) ambulance services include:

1. Basic life support
2. Advanced life support, level 1
3. Advanced life support, level 2
4. Fixed wing air ambulance
5. Specialty care transport
6. Paramedic intercept
7. Rotary wing air ambulance

The air service categories include fixed-wing air ambulance (airplane) and rotary wing air ambulance (helicopter).

Inpatient Rehabilitation Facility (IRF) Prospective Payment System

The BBA (as amended by the **Balanced Budget Refinement Act of 1999** [BBRA]) authorized implementation of a per-discharge PPS for care provided to Medicare beneficiaries by inpatient rehabilitation hospitals and rehabilitation units, referred to as **inpatient rehabilitation facilities** (IRFs). The PPS for IRFs became effective on January 1, 2002.

IRFs must meet the regulatory requirements to be classified as a rehabilitation hospital or rehabilitation unit that is excluded from the PPS for inpatient acute care services. To meet the criteria, an IRF must operate as a hospital. Requirements state that during the most recent, consecutive, and appropriate 12-month time period, the hospital will have treated an inpatient population of whom at least 60 percent required intensive rehabilitative services for treatment of one or more of 13 medical conditions. Examples of these conditions are listed in figure 6.1.

Patient Assessment Instrument

IRFs are required to complete a patient assessment instrument (PAI) upon each patient's admission and also discharge from the facility. CMS provides facilities with the **Inpatient Rehabilitation Validation and Entry** (IRVEN) system to collect the IRF-PAI in a database that can be transmitted electronically to the IRF-PAI national database. These data are used in assessing clinical characteristics of patients in rehabilitation settings. Ultimately, they can be used to provide survey agencies with a means to objectively measure and compare facility performance and quality and to allow researchers to develop improved standards of care.

The IRF PPS uses information from the IRF-PAI to classify patients into distinct groups on the basis of clinical characteristics and expected resource needs. Data used to construct these groups, called **case-mix groups** (CMGs), include rehabilitation impairment categories (RICs), functional status (both motor and cognitive), age, comorbidities, and other factors. There are currently 92 CMGs into which patients are classified.

Figure 6.1. **Medical conditions that are criteria for classification as inpatient rehabilitation facility**

• Stroke	• Brain injury
• Spinal cord injury	• Neurological disorders including multiple sclerosis, motor neuron diseases, polyneuropathy, muscular dystrophy, and Parkinson's disease
• Congenital deformity	
• Amputation	
• Major multiple trauma	
• Fracture of femur (hip fracture)	• Burns

Source: CMS 2011.

CMG Relative Weight

An appropriate weight, called the **CMG relative weight,** is assigned to each case-mix group and measures the relative difference in facility resource intensity among the various groups. Separate payments are calculated for each group, including the application of case- and facility-level adjustments. Facility-level adjustments include wage-index adjustments, low-income patient adjustments, and rural facility adjustments. Case-level adjustments include transfer adjustments, interrupted-stay adjustments, and cost outlier adjustments.

Long-Term Care Hospital (LTCH) Prospective Payment System

The Balanced Budget Refinement Act of 1999 amended by the Benefits Improvement Act of 2000 mandated the establishment of a per discharge, DRG-based PPS for long-term care hospitals beginning on October 1, 2002.

LTCHs are defined as having an average inpatient LOS greater than 25 days. Typically, patients with the following conditions are treated in LTCHs:

- Chronic cardiac disorders
- Neuromuscular and neurovascular diseases such as after-effects of strokes or Parkinson's disease
- Infectious conditions requiring long-term care such as methicillin-resistant Staphylococcus aureus (MRSA)
- Complex orthopedic conditions such as pelvic fractures or complicated hip fractures
- Wound care complications (traumatic, pressure, diabetic, and venous)
- Multisystem organ failure
- Immunosuppressed conditions
- Respiratory failure and ventilation management and weaning
- Dysphagia management
- Postoperative complications
- Multiple intravenous therapies
- Chemotherapy
- Pre- and postoperative organ transplant care
- Chronic nutritional problems and total parenteral nutrition issues
- Spinal cord injuries
- Burns
- Head injuries

Medicare Severity-LTC-DRGs

Patients are classified into distinct diagnosis groups based on clinical characteristics and expected resource use. These groups are based on the current inpatient MS-DRGs. There are approximately 750 LTC-DRGs. The payment system includes the following three primary elements:

1. Patient classification into an MS-LTC-DRG weight.
2. Relative weight of the MS-LTC-DRG. The weights reflect the variation in cost per discharge as they take into account the utilization for each diagnosis.
3. Federal payment rate. Payment is made at a predetermined per discharge amount for each MS-LTC-DRG.

Adjustments

The PPS does provide for case-level adjustments such as short-stay outlier, interrupted stays, and high-cost outliers. Facility-wide adjustments include area wage index and cost of living adjustments.

A short-stay outlier is an adjustment to the payment rate for stays that are considerably shorter than the average length of stay (ALOS) for a particular MS-LTC-DRG. A case would qualify for short-stay outlier status when the LOS is between one day and up to and including five-sixths of the ALOS for the MS-LTC-DRG. Both the ALOS and the five-sixths of the ALOS periods are published in the *Federal Register.* Payment under the short-stay outlier is made using different payment methodologies. (See table 6.11 for examples of MS-LTC-DRGs and the ALOS for each.)

An interrupted stay occurs when a patient is discharged from the long-term care hospital and then is readmitted to the same facility for further treatment after a specific number of days away from the facility. There are different policies if the patient is readmitted to the facility within three days (called three-day or less interrupted-stay policy) or if the patient is away from the facility more than three days (called the greater than three-day interrupted-stay policy).

A high-cost outlier is an adjustment to the payment rate for a patient when the costs are unusually high and exceed the typical costs associated with an MS-LTC-DRG. High-cost

Table 6.11. **Examples of MS-LTC-DRGs, relative weights, geometric ALOS, and short-stay outlier threshold**

MS-LTC-DRG	Description	Relative Weight	Geometric ALOS	Arithmetic ALOS
28	Spinal procedures w MCC	1.7420	36.0	30.0
114	Orbital procedures w/o CC/MCC	0.7789	23.4	19.5
132	Cranial/facial procedure w/o CC/MCC	0.4607	17.9	14.9
150	Epistaxis w MCC	0.6931	21.9	18.3
163	Major chest procedure w MCC	2.2110	38.5	32.1
181	Respiratory neoplasm w CC	0.5810	17.4	14.5
194	Simple pneumonia and pleurisy w MCC	0.6173	18.9	15.8

outlier payments reduce the facility's potential financial losses that can result from treating patients who require more costly care than is normal. A case qualifies for a high-cost outlier payment when the estimated cost of care exceeds the high-cost outlier threshold, which is published each year.

Inpatient Psychiatric Facilities (IPFs) Prospective Payment System

The Balanced Budget Refinement Act of 1999 mandated the development of a per diem PPS for inpatient psychiatric services furnished in hospitals and exempt units. The PPS became effective on January 1, 2005, establishing a standardized per diem rate to **inpatient psychiatric facilities** (IPFs) based on the national average of operating, ancillary, and capital costs for each patient day of care in the IPF. The system uses the same MS-DRGs as the acute care hospital inpatient system. The payment rate is based on a per diem, which is updated each year.

Adjustments

Patient-level or case-level adjustments are provided for age, specified MS-DRGs, and certain comorbidity categories. Payment adjustments are made for eight age categories beginning with age 45, at which point, statistically, costs are increased as the patient ages.

The IPF receives an MS-DRG payment adjustment for a principal diagnosis that groups to one of 17 psychiatric MS-DRGs. (See table 6.12.) Seventeen comorbidity categories

Table 6.12.   **Psychiatric MS-DRGs**

MS-DRG	MS-DRG Description
056	Degenerative nervous system disorders w MCC
057	Degenerative nervous system disorders w/o MCC
080	Nontraumatic stupor and coma w MCC
081	Nontraumatic stupor and coma w/o MCC
876	OR procedure w principal diagnoses of mental illness
880	Acute adjustment reaction and psychosocial dysfunction
881	Depressive neuroses
882	Neuroses except depressive
883	Disorders of personality and impulse control
884	Organic disturbances and mental retardation
885	Psychoses
886	Behavioral and developmental disorders
887	Other mental disorder diagnoses
894	Alcohol/drug abuse or dependence, left AMA
895	Alcohol/drug abuse or dependence with rehabilitation therapy
896	Alcohol/drug abuse or dependence w/o rehabilitation therapy w MCC
897	Alcohol/drug abuse or dependence w/o rehabilitation therapy w/o MCC

that require comparatively more costly treatment during an inpatient stay also generate a payment adjustment. The list of comorbidity categories and their associated ICD-9-CM diagnosis codes can be found in table 6.13.

The IPF PPS also includes an outlier policy for those patients who require more expensive care than expected in an effort to minimize the financial risk to the IPF. Although the basis of the system is a per diem rate, outlier payments are made on a per case basis rather than on the per diem basis. An IPF receives an additional adjustment for patients who are given electroconvulsive therapy (ECT).

The PPS also includes regulations on payments when there is an interrupted stay, meaning the patient is discharged from an IPF and returns to the same or another facility

Table 6.13.   **Comorbidity categories affecting IPS payments**

Category	ICD-9-CM Diagnosis Codes
Developmental disabilities	317, 318.0, 318.1, 318.2, and 319
Coagulation factor deficit	286.0 through 286.4
Tracheostomy	519.00 through 519.09; V44.0
Renal failure, acute	584.5 through 584.9, 636.30,636.31, 636.32, 637,30, 637.31, 637.32, 638.3, 639.3, 669.32, 669.34, 958.5
Renal failure, chronic	403.01, 403.11, 403.91, 404.02, 404.03, 404.12, 404.13, 404.92, 404.93, 585.3,585.4, 585.5, 585.6, 585.9, 586, V45.1, V56.0, V56.1, V56.2
Oncology treatment	140.0 through 239.9 with either 99.25 or a code from 92.21 through 92.29
Uncontrolled Type I diabetes mellitus w or w/o complications	250.02, 250.03, 250.12, 250.13, 250.22, 250.23, 250.32, 250.33, 250.42, 250.43, 250.52, 250.53, 250.62, 250.63, 250.72,250.73, 250.82, 250.83, 250.92, 250.93
Severe protein calorie malnutrition	260 through 262
Eating and conduct disorders	307.1, 307.50, 312.03, 312.33, 312.34
Infectious diseases	010.00 through 041.10,042,045.00 through 053.19, 054.40 through 054.49,055.0 through 077.0,078.2 through 078.89, 079.50 through 079.59
Drug- or alcohol-induced mental disorders	291.0, 292.0, 292.12, 292.2, 303.00, 304.00
Cardiac conditions	391.0, 391.1, 391.2, 402.01,404.03, 416.0, 421.0, 421.1, 421.9
Gangrene	440.24, 785.4
Chronic obstructive pulmonary disease	491.21, 494.1, 510.0, 518.83, 518.84, V46.11, V46.12, V46.13, V46.14
Artificial openings—digestive and urinary	569.60 through 569.69, 997.5, V44.1 through V44.6
Severe musculoskeletal and connective tissue disorders	696.0, 710.0, 730.00 through 730.09, 730.10 through 730.19, 730.20 through 730.29
Poisoning	965.00 through 965.09, 965.4, 967.0 through 969.9, 977.0, 980.0 through 980.9, 983.0 through 983.9, 986, 989.0 through 989.7
Schwannomatosis	237.73
Other neurofibromatosis	237.79

before midnight on the third consecutive day. The intent of the policy is to prevent a facility from prematurely discharging a patient after the maximum payment is received and subsequently readmitting the patient.

Facility adjustments include a wage-index adjustment, a rural location adjustment, a teaching status adjustment, a cost-of-living adjustment for Alaska and Hawaii, and a qualifying emergency department adjustment.

Check Your Understanding 6.7

1. Which of the following patients qualify for a LUPA?

   A. Patient had 10 visits in the 60-day period.
   B. Patient had 3 visits in the 60-day period.
   C. Patient had 4 visits in the 60-day period.
   D. Patient had 5 visits in the 60-day period.

2. Prior to implementation of the MS-DRG prospective payment system, Medicare Part A payments to hospitals were based on a:

   A. Fee-for-service reimbursement methodology
   B. Level of care and expenditure for resources system
   C. Managed care capitated payment schedule
   D. Predetermined rate for each inpatient discharge

3. The MS-DRG prospected payment system rate is based on what type of diagnosis?

   A. Primary
   B. Principal
   C. Admitting
   D. Additional

4. The computer software program that assigns appropriate MS-DRGs according to information provided for each episode of care is called a:

   A. Classification
   B. Catalog
   C. Register
   D. Grouper

5. Which of the following hospitals are excluded from the Medicare acute care prospective payment system?

   A. Children's
   B. Small community
   C. Tertiary
   D. Trauma

6. MS-diagnostic-related groups are organized into:

    A. Case-mix classifications
    B. Geographic practice cost indices
    C. Major diagnostic categories
    D. Resource-based relative values

7. What reimbursement system utilizes the Medicare fee schedule?

    A. APCs
    B. MS-DRGs
    C. RBRVS
    D. RUG-IV

8. What legislation mandated the implementation of a skilled nursing facility prospective payment system?

    A. BBA
    B. COBRA
    C. OBRA
    D. TEFRA

9. Which of the following is the tool used to collect resident assessment data so that the SNF residents can be assigned to the appropriate resource utilization group?

    A. MDS
    B. RAP
    C. RAVEN
    D. RUG

10. What reimbursement system is associated with the Medicare outpatient prospective payment system?

    A. APCs
    B. MS-DRGs
    C. RBRVS
    D. RUG-IV

11. Which of the following types of organizations is not reimbursed under the outpatient prospective payment system?

    A. Partial hospitalization facilities
    B. Critical access hospitals
    C. Hospital outpatient departments
    D. Outpatient dialysis centers

12. Which of the following concepts is applied when multiple surgical procedures are furnished during the same operative session?

    A. Bundling of services
    B. Outlier adjustment
    C. Pass-through payment
    D. Discounting of procedures

13. What data set is used for patient assessments by the home health prospective payment system?

   A. HEDIS
   B. OASIS-C
   C. RAI
   D. UHDDS

14. The inpatient psychiatric facility prospective reimbursement system is based on:

   A. MS-DRGS
   B. Per diem rate
   C. RUGS-IV
   D. CMGs

15. What tool is used to calculate the CMG?

   A. IRF-PAI
   B. OASIS
   C. MDS
   D. Grouper

Processing of Reimbursement Claims

Understanding payment mechanisms is an important foundation for accurately processing claims forms. However, it is also important to understand how these mechanisms apply to actual claims processing. Many HIM professionals have an active role in various aspects of claims processing support.

A facility's patient accounts department is responsible for billing third-party payers, processing **accounts receivable,** monitoring payments from third-party payers, and verifying insurance coverage. **Medicare Administrative Contractors** (MACs) contract with CMS to serve as the financial agent between providers and the federal government to locally administer Medicare's Parts A and B.

Coordination of Benefits

In many instances, patients have more than one insurance policy and the determination of which policy is primary and which is secondary is necessary so that there is no duplication in payment of benefits. This process is called the coordination of benefits (COB) or the **coordination of benefits transaction.** The monies collected from third-party payers cannot be greater than the amount of the provider's charges.

Submission of Claims

According to the **National Uniform Billing Committee** (NUBC) more than 98 percent of hospital claims are submitted electronically to Medicare. The Administrative

Simplification Compliance Act (ASCA), which was part of HIPAA, mandated the electronic submission of all healthcare claims with a few exceptions.

Healthcare facilities submit claims via the electronic format (screen 837I) which replaces the **UB-04 (CMS-1450)** paper billing form. Physicians submit claims via the electronic format (screen 837P), which takes the place of the **CMS-1500** billing form. For those healthcare facilities with a waiver of the ASCA requirements, UB-04 and CMS-1500 are used.

Explanation of Benefits and Medicare Summary Notice Remittance Advice

An **Explanation of Benefits** (EOB) is a statement sent by a third-party payer to the patient to explain services provided, amounts billed, and payments made by the health plan. Medicare sends a **Medicare Summary Notice** (MSN) to a beneficiary to show how much the provider billed, how much Medicare reimbursed the provider, and what the patient must pay the provider by way of deductible and copayments. (See figure 6.2 for a sample Part B MSN.)

A **remittance advice** (RA) is sent to the provider to explain payments made by third-party payers (figure 6.3). Payments are typically sent in batches with the RA sent to the facility and payments electronically transferred to the provider's bank.

Medicare Administrative Contractors (MACs)

MACs process Part A and Part B claims from hospitals, physicians, and other providers. Currently there are fifteen MAC jurisdictions with an additional four jurisdictions for home health and four for DME. There are plans to decrease this to ten MAC jurisdictions over the next few years.

National Correct Coding Initiative (NCCI)

CMS implemented the **National Correct Coding Initiative** (NCCI) in 1996 to develop correct coding methodologies to improve the appropriate payment of Medicare Part B claims.

NCCI policies are based on:

- Coding conventions defined in the CPT codebooks
- National and local policies and coding edits
- Analysis of standard medical and surgical practice
- Review of current coding practices

The NCCI edits (which most providers have built into their claims software) explain what procedures and services cannot be billed together on the same day of service for a

Figure 6.2. Sample Medicare Summary Notice

CMS CENTERS for MEDICARE & MEDICAID SERVICES

Medicare Summary Notice

Page 1 of 2

July 1, 20XX

BENEFICIARY NAME
STREET ADDRESS
CITY, STATE ZIP CODE

CUSTOMER SERVICE INFORMATION

Your Medicare Number: 111-11-1111A

If you have questions, write or call:
Medicare
555 Medicare Blvd., Suite 200
Medicare Building
Medicare, US XXXXX-XXXX

Local: (XXX) XXX-XXXX
Toll-free: 1-800-XXX-XXXX
TTY for Hearing Impaired: 1-800-XXX-XXXX

BE INFORMED: Beware of "free" medical services or products. If it sounds too good to be true, it probably is.

This is a summary of claims processed from 05/15/20XX through 06/10/20XX.

PART A HOSPITAL INSURANCE – INPATIENT CLAIMS

Dates of Service	Benefit Days Used	Non-Covered Charges	Deductible and Coinsurance	You May Be Billed	See Notes Section
Claim Number: 12435-84956-84556-45621					a
Cure Hospital, 213 Sick Lane, Dallas, TX 75555					
Referred by: Paul Jones, M.D.					
04/25/XX – 05/09/XX	14 days	$0.00	$876.00	$776.00	b, c
Claim Number: 12435-84956-845556-45622					
Continued Care Hospital, 124 Sick Lane, Dallas, TX 75555					
Referred by: Paul Jones, M.D.					
05/09/XX – 06/20/XX	11 days	$0.00	$0.00	$0.00	

PART B MEDICAL INSURANCE – OUTPATIENT FACILITY CLAIMS

Dates of Service	Services Provided	Amount Charged	Non-Covered Charges	Deductible and Coinsurance	You May Be Billed	See Notes Section
Claim Number: 12435-8956-8458						d
Medicare Hospital, 123 Medicare Lane, Dallas, TX 75209						
Referred by: Paul Jones, M.D.						
04/02/XX	I.V. Therapy (Q0081)	$33.00	$0.00	$6.60	$6.60	
	Lab (3810)	1,140.50	0.00	228.10	228.10	
	Operating Room (31628)	786.50	0.00	157.30	157.30	
	Observation Room (99201)	293.00	0.00	58.60	58.60	
	Claim Total	**$2,253.00**	**$0.00**	**$450.60**	**$450.60**	

(continued)

THIS IS NOT A BILL – Keep this notice for your records.

Figure 6.2.   **Sample Medicare Summary Notice** *(continued)*

Your Medicare Number: 111-11-1111A   Page 2 of 2
                                                                       July 1, 20XX

> **Notes Section:**
>
> a   The amount Medicare paid the provider for this claim is $XXXX.XX.
>
> b $776.00 was applied to your inpatient deductible.
>
> c $30.00 was applied to your blood deductible.
>
> d   The amount Medicare paid the provider for this claim is $XXXX.XX.

Deductible Information:

You have met the Part A deductible for this benefit period.

You have met the Part B deductible for 20XX.

You have met the blood deductible for 20XX.

General Information:

You have the right to make a request in writing for an itemized statement which details
each Medicare item or service which you have received from your physician, hospital, or
any other health supplier or health professional. Please contact them directly, in writing, if
you would like an itemized statement.

Compare the services you receive with those that appear on your Medicare Summary
Notice. If you have questions, call your doctor or provider. If you feel further investigation
is needed due to possible fraud and abuse, call the phone number in the Customer Service
Information Box.

Appeals Information—Part A (Inpatient) and Part B (Outpatient)

If you disagree with any claims decision on either Part A or Part B of this notice,
you can request an appeal by November 1, 20XX. Follow the instructions below:

1)   Circle the item(s) you disagree with and explain why you disagree.

2)   Send this notice or a copy, to the address in the "Customer Service Information" box
     on Page 1. (You may also send any additional information you may have about your
     appeal.)

3)   Sign here _____ Phone number _____

Revised 02/XX

Figure 6.3. Sample single-claim remittance advice

```
Medicare National Standard Intermediary Remittance Advice
FPE:                                        07/30/09
PAID:                                       01/25/10
CLM#                                        2
TOB:                                        111

PATIENT:        JOHN DOE                                    PCN:    235617
HIC:            123456              SVC FROM:    01/05/09   MRN:    124767
PAT STAT:    01    CLAIM STAT:    1    THRU:     01/06/10   ICN:    987654

CHARGES:                        PAYMENT DATA: 140=DRG   0.000   =REIM RATE
1939.90      =REPORTED         2741.69   =DRG AMOUNT    0.00    =MSP PRIM PAYER
0.00         =NONCOVERED       2497.26   =DRG/OPER      0.00    =PROF COMPONENT
0.00         =DENIED            244.43   =DRG/CAPITAL   0.00    =ESRD AMOUNT
1939.90      =COVERED             0.00   =OUTLIER       0.00    =HCPCS AMOUNT
DAYS/VISITS:                       0.00   =CAP OUTLIER   0.00    =ALLOWED AMOUNT
1            =COST REPT          768.00   =CASH DEDUCT   0.00    =G/R AMOUNT
1            =COVD/UTIL            0.00   =BLOOD DEDUCT  0.00    =INTEREST
0            =NONCOVERED           0.00   =COINSURANCE  -801.79  =CONTRACT ADJ
0            =COVD VISITS          0.00   =PAT REFUND    675.00  =PER DIEM AMT
0            =NCOV VISITS          0.00   =MSP LIAB MET  1973.69 =NET REIM AMT
ADJ REASON CODES:        CO  A2 -801.79
                         PR      1
                         768
REMARK CODES:            MA02
```

patient. The mutually exclusive edit applies to improbable or impossible combinations of codes. For example, code 58940, Oophorectomy, partial or total, unilateral or bilateral, would never be used with code 58150, Total abdominal hysterectomy (corpus and cervix), with or without removal of tube(s), with or without removal of ovary(s). Modifiers may be used to indicate circumstances in which the NCCI edits should not be applied and payment should be made as requested. Modifier –59, for example, is used when circumstances require that certain procedures or services be reported together even though they usually are not.

Portions of the NCCI are incorporated into the **outpatient code editor** (OCE) against which all ambulatory claims are reviewed. The OCE also applies a set of logical rules to determine whether various combinations of codes are correct and appropriately represent services provided. Billing issues generated from these CCI and OCE edits often result in claim denials.

Physician Query Process

There are instances, however, when it is necessary to query the physician for clarification of data that may influence proper code assignment. This might include instances when there is conflicting or incomplete information in the record. Query forms have proved to be an effective means of communication with physicians. AHIMA cautions coders that these forms are used to improve documentation and understanding of the clinical situation, but not to increase reimbursement. In fact, reimbursement should never be mentioned. The query should contain the following information (AHIMA 2008, 85):

- Patient name
- Admission date and/or date of service
- Health record number
- Account number
- Date query initiated
- Name and contact information of the individual initiating the query
- Statement of the issue in the form of a question along with clinical indicators specified from the chart (e.g., history and physical states urosepsis, lab reports WBC of 14,400. Emergency department report fever of 102)

Queries should be made in writing and should never lead the physician into a specific response. An example of a leading query and a well-written query can be found in table 6.14.

Electronic Data Interchange

Electronic data interchange (EDI) is the electronic transfer of information, such as health claims, in a standard format between trading partners. EDI originated when a number of industries identified cost savings through the electronic transmission of business information. They were convinced that the standardization of formatted information was the most effective means of communicating with multiple trading partners.

Table 6.14. **Leading query**

Leading query
Dr. Smith—Based on your documentation, this patient has anemia and was transfused 2 units of blood. Also, there was a 10 point drop in hematocrit following surgery. Please document "Acute Blood Loss Anemia," as this patient clearly meets the clinical criteria for this diagnosis.
Appropriately written query
Dr. Smith—In your progress note on 6/20, you documented anemia and ordered transfusion of 2 units of whole blood. Also, according to the lab work performed on xx/xx, the patient had a 10 point drop in hematocrit following surgery. Please document in the discharge summary, the type of anemia you were treating.

EDI allows entities within the healthcare system to exchange medical, billing, and other information and to process transactions quickly and cost-effectively. EDI substantially reduces handling and processing time compared to paper and eliminates the risk of lost paper documents. It also can eliminate the inefficiencies of handling paper documents and thus can significantly reduce administrative burden, lower operating costs, and improve overall data quality.

Check Your Understanding 6.8

1. The hospital needs to know how much Medicare paid on a claim so they can bill the secondary insurance. What should they refer to?

   A. Explanation of Benefits
   B. Medicare Summary Notice
   C. Remittance advice
   D. Coordination of benefits

2. Which of the following situations would be identified by the NCCI edits?

   A. Determine the MS-DRG
   B. Billing for two services that are prohibited from being billed on the same day
   C. Whether or not data that were submitted electronically were successfully submitted
   D. Receive the remittance advice

3. The purpose of a physician query is to:

   A. Identify the MS-DRG
   B. Identify the principle diagnosis
   C. Improve documentation
   D. Increase reimbursement

Instructions: Indicate whether the following statements are true or false (T or F).

4. _____ Medicare Administrative Contractors serve as the financial agent between providers and the federal government to locally administer Medicare Part A and Part B.

5. _____ The 837P is submitted to Medicare carriers to process hospital outpatient claims.

6. _____ The 837I is also referred to as the 837P.

7. _____ The abbreviation used to describe the electronic transfer of information such as a claims submission is EDI.

8. _____ The OCE applies a set of logical rules.

Reimbursement Support Processes

Reimbursement support processes are routinely reviewed and revised by third-party payers to control payments to providers. Healthcare facilities also implement reimbursement support processes to make sure that they are receiving the level of reimbursement to which they are entitled. Third-party payers revise fee schedules, and healthcare facilities revise chargemasters, evaluate the quality of documentation and coding, conduct internal audits, and implement compliance programs.

Management of the Fee Schedules

Third-party payers that reimburse providers on a fee-for-service basis generally update fee schedules on an annual basis. A fee schedule is a list of healthcare services and procedures (usually CPT/HCPCS codes) and charges associated with each. (See table 6.15.) The fee schedule (sometimes referred to as a table of allowances) represents the approved payment levels for a given insurance plan (for example, Medicare, Medicaid, and BC/BS).

Physicians, practitioners, and suppliers must notify Medicare by December 31 of each year if they intend to participate in the Medicare program during the coming year. Medicare participation means that the provider or supplier agrees to accept assignment for all covered services provided to Medicare patients. To **accept assignment** means the provider or supplier accepts, as payment in full, the allowed charge (from the fee schedule). The provider or supplier is prohibited from **balance billing,** which means the patient cannot be held responsible for charges in excess of the Medicare fee schedule.

However, participating providers may bill patients for services that are not covered by Medicare. Physicians must notify a patient that the service will not be paid for by giving the patient a Notice of Exclusions from Medicare Benefits.

If a provider believes that a service may be denied by Medicare because it could be considered unnecessary, he must notify the patient before the treatment begins using an **Advance Beneficiary Notice of Noncoverage** (ABN) (figure 6.4). ABNs are provided for various care settings such as home health and SNF facilities.

Table 6.15. **Partial 2011 Medicare physician fee schedule payment amounts for Chicago, Illinois**

Carrier Locality	CPT Code	Nonfacility Fee Schedule Amount	Facility Fee Schedule Amount
95215	10040	109.2	95.93
95215	10060	115.8	98.26
95215	10061	194.89	171.21
95215	10080	1178.50	106.02
95215	10081	277.58	182.86
95215	10120	143.55	97.26
95215	10121	280.42	197.54

Source: CMS 2011.

Figure 6.4.   Advance Beneficiary Notice (ABN)

A. Notifier:

B. Patient Name: **C. Identification Number:**

Advance Beneficiary Notice of Noncoverage (ABN)

<u>NOTE:</u> If Medicare doesn't pay for **D.** ——————— below, you may have to pay.
Medicare does not pay for everything, even some care that you or your health care provider have
good reason to think you need. We expect Medicare may not pay for the **D.** ——————— below.

D.	E. Reason Medicare May Not Pay:	F. Estimated Cost

WHAT YOU NEED TO DO NOW:
- Read this notice, so you can make an informed decision about your care.
- Ask us any questions that you may have after you finish reading.
- Choose an option below about whether to receive the **D.** ——————— listed above.
   Note: If you choose Option 1 or 2, we may help you to use any other insurance
      that you might have, but Medicare cannot require us to do this.

G. OPTIONS: Check only one box. We cannot choose a box for you.

☐ **OPTION 1.** I want the **D.** ——————— listed above. You may ask to be paid now, but I also want Medicare billed for an official decision on payment, which is sent to me on a Medicare Summary Notice (MSN). I understand that if Medicare doesn't pay, I am responsible for payment, but **I can appeal to Medicare** by following the directions on the MSN. If Medicare does pay, you will refund any payments I made to you, less co-pays or deductibles.

☐ **OPTION 2.** I want the **D.** ——————— listed above, but do not bill Medicare. You may ask to be paid now as I am responsible for payment. **I cannot appeal if Medicare is not billed**.

☐ **OPTION 3.** I don't want the **D.** ——————— listed above. I understand with this choice I am **not** responsible for payment, and **I cannot appeal to see if Medicare would pay.**

H. Additional Information:

This notice gives our opinion, not an official Medicare decision. If you have other questions
on this notice or Medicare billing, call **1-800-MEDICARE** (1-800-633-4227/**TTY:** 1-877-486-2048).
Signing below means that you have received and understand this notice. You also receive a copy.

I. Signature:	J. Date:

According to the Paperwork Reduction Act of 1995, no persons are required to respond to a collection of information unless it displays a valid OMB control number. The valid OMB control number for this information collection is 0938-0566. The time required to complete this information collection is estimated to average 7 minutes per response, including the time to review instructions, search existing data resources, gather the data needed, and complete and review the information collection. If you have comments concerning the accuracy of the time estimate or suggestions for improving this form, please write to: CMS, 7500 Security Boulevard, Attn: PRA Reports Clearance Officer, Baltimore, Maryland 21244-1850.

Form CMS-R-131 (03/11)   Form Approved OMB No. 0938-0566

Nonparticipating providers (nonPARs) do not sign a participation agreement with Medicare but may or may not accept assignment. If the nonPAR physician elects to accept assignment, he or she is paid 95 percent (5 percent less than participating physicians) of the MFS. For example, if the MFS amount is $200, the PAR provider receives $160 (80 percent of $200), but the nonPAR provider receives only $152 (95 percent of $160).

NonPAR providers who choose not to accept assignment are subject to Medicare's limiting charge rule, which states that a physician may not charge a patient more than 115 percent of the nonparticipating fee schedule. The provider collects the full amount from the patient, and Medicare reimburses the patient. Figure 6.5 illustrates the various fee schedules by type of provider.

Management of the Chargemaster

The chargemaster (table 6.16), also called the charge description master (CDM), contains information about healthcare services (and transactions) provided to a patient. Its primary purpose is to allow the provider to accurately charge routine services and supplies to the patient. Services, supplies, and procedures included on the chargemaster generate reimbursement for almost 75 percent of UB-92 claims submitted for outpatient services alone.

Figure 6.5. **Fee schedules by provider type**

Participating Provider	
Physician's fee	$180.00
MFS	$105.00
Medicare pays 80% of MFS or	$ 84.00
Patient pays 20% of MFS or	$ 21.00
Physician write-off ($180–$105)	$ 75.00
Nonparticipating provider who accepts assignment	
Physician's fee	$180.00
MFS	$105.00
Medicare nonPAR fee (95% of $105)	$ 99.75
Medicare pays 80% of nonPAR fee	$ 79.80
Patient pays 20% of nonPAR fee	$ 19.95
Physician write-off ($180–$99.75)	$ 80.25
Nonparticipating provider who does not accept assignment	
Physician's normal fee	$180.00
MFS	$105.00
Medicare nonPAR fee (95% of $105)	$ 99.75
Limiting charge (115% of $99.75)	$114.71
Patient billed	$114.71
Medicare pays patient (80% of nonPAR fee)	$ 79.80
Patient out of pocket ($114.71–$79.80)	$ 34.91

Table 6.16.   Sample section from a chargemaster

| Charge Code | Item Description | CPT/HCPCS Code | | | Revenue Code | G/L Key | Activity Date |
		Insurance Code A	Insurance Code B	Insurance Code C			
2110410000	ECHO ENCEPHALOGRAM	76506	76506	Y7030	320	15	12/2/2008
2110410090	F/U ECHO ENCEPHALOGRAM	76506	76506	Y7040	320	15	12/2/2008
2110413000	PORT US ECHO ENCEPHALOGRAM	76506	76506	Y7050	320	15	12/2/2008
2120411000	ULTRASOUND SPINAL CONTENTS	76800	76800	Y7060	320	15	12/2/2008
2130401000	THYROID SONOGRAM	76536	76536	Y7070	320	15	1/1/2010
2151111000	TM JOINTS BILATERAL	70330	70330	Y7080	320	15	8/12/2009
2161111000	NECK LAT ONLY	70360	70360	Y7090	320	15	10/1/2008
2162111000	LARYNX AP & LATERAL	70360	70360	Y7100	320	15	10/1/2008
2201111000	LONG BONE CHLD AP	76061	76061	Y7110	320	15	8/12/2009
2201401000	NON-VASCULAR EXTREM SONO	76880	76880	Y7120	320	15	10/1/2008
2210111000	SKULL 1 VIEW	70250	70250	Y7130	320	15	1/1/2010
2210112000	SKULL 2 VIEWS	70250	70250	Y7140	320	15	8/12/2009
2210114000	SKULL 4 VIEWS	70260	70260	Y7150	320	15	8/12/2009
2211111000	MASTOIDS	70130	70130	Y7160	320	15	1/1/2010
2212111000	MANDIBLE	70110	70110	Y7170	320	15	12/2/2008
2213111000	FACIAL BONES	70140	70140	Y7180	320	15	12/2/2008
2213114000	FACIAL BONES MIN 4	70150	70150	Y7190	320	15	12/2/2008
2214111000	NASAL BONES	70160	70160	Y7200	320	15	1/1/2010
2215111000	ORBITS	70200	70200	Y7210	320	15	1/1/2010
2217111000	PARANASAL SINUSES	70220	70220	Y7220	320	15	1/1/2010

The information that makes up a chargemaster line item may vary from one facility to another. There are, however, some common elements found in a typical chargemaster (Schraffenberger and Kuehn 2011, 223–227). These include:

- *Description of service:* Examples might be the evaluation and management visit, observation, or emergency room visit.
- *CPT/HCPCS code:* This code must correspond to the description of the service.
- ***Revenue code*** *(also called the UB-04 code):* The revenue code is a three-digit code that describes a classification of a product or service provided to the patient. These revenue or UB-04 codes are required by CMS for reporting services.

- *Charge amount:* This is the amount the facility charges for the procedure or service. It is not necessarily what the facility will be reimbursed by the third-party payer.

- *Charge or service code:* The charge or service code is an internally assigned number that is unique to the facility. It identifies each procedure listed on the charge-master and identifies the department or revenue center that initiated the charge. The charge code can be very useful for revenue tracking and budget analysis.

- *General ledger key:* The general ledger key is a two- or three-digit number that assigns a line item to a section of the general ledger in the hospital's accounting system.

- *Activity/status date:* The activity/status date indicates the most recent activity of an item.

Chargemasters may allow more than one CPT/HCPCS code per item to differentiate between payment schedules for different payers.

The CDM also can be used as a tool for collecting workload statistics that can be used to monitor production and compile budgets. Statistics can be used to provide data regarding the use of equipment, personnel, services, and supplies. It is often used as a decision support tool to evaluate costs related to resources and to prepare for contract negotiations with managed care organizations.

The CDM relieves coders from coding repetitive services and supplies that require little, if any, formal documentation analysis. In these circumstances, the patient is billed automatically by linking the service to the appropriate CPT/HCPCS code (referred to as **hard-coding**). The advantage of hard-coding is that the code for the procedure will be reproduced accurately each time that a test, service, or procedure is ordered (Schraffen-berger and Kuehn 2011, 228).

Maintenance of the Chargemaster

The chargemaster must be updated routinely. Maintenance of the chargemaster is best accomplished by representatives from health information management, clinical services, finance, the business office/patient financial services, compliance, and information systems. The HIM professionals are generally consulted regarding the update of CPT codes. The CDM is updated when new CPT codes become available, when departments request a new item, and when the medical fee schedules/PPS rates are updated.

An inaccurate chargemaster adversely affects facility reimbursement, compliance, and data quality. According to a 1999 AHIMA practice brief (Rhodes 1999), negative effects that may result from an inaccurate chargemaster include overpayment, underpayment, undercharging for delivery of healthcare services, claims rejections, and fines/penalties. Chargemaster programs are automated and involve the billing of numerous services for high volumes of patients, often without human intervention. Therefore, it is highly likely that a single error on the chargemaster could result in multiple errors before it is identified and corrected, resulting in a serious financial impact.

Management of the Revenue Cycle

Revenue cycle management involves many different processes and people, all working to make sure that the healthcare facility is properly reimbursed for the services provided. Effectively managing the revenue cycle is paramount to improving the revenues received by the facility. Delays in payment, denied claims, and other lost revenues impact tremendously on the facility's financial health.

The revenue cycle involves many functions in addition to the process of billing. According to an AHIMA practice brief (Youmans 2004), the major functions typically include:

- Admitting, patient access management
- Case management
- Charge capture
- Health information management
- Patient financial services, business office
- Finance
- Compliance
- Information technology

Revenue Cycle Management Committee

An effective method for managing the revenue cycle is through a revenue cycle management committee or team composed of individuals from all the departments involved in the revenue cycle. The HIM professional is an important player on this team. Various team members should analyze the revenue cycle indicators, which include:

- Value and volume of discharged, not final billed encounters
- Number of accounts receivable (AR) days
- Number of bill-hold days
- Percentage and amount of write-offs
- Percentage of clean claims
- Percentage of claims returned to provider
- Percentage of denials
- Percentage of accounts-missing documents
- Number of query forms
- Percentage of late charges

- Percentage of accurate registrations

- Percentage of increased point-of-service collections for elective procedures

- Percentage of increased DRG payments due to improved documentation and coding (Youmans 2004)

The HIM professional's area of expertise is varied and will be extremely useful in denials management, data analysis and presentation, write-off preparation, policy development, response to patient financial services requests, and review of OCEs and groupers.

Management of Documentation and Coding Quality

According to Deborah Elder, manager of inpatient and outpatient coding services, Medical Management Plus, Inc., in Birmingham, Alabama:

> The importance of complete and accurate coding cannot be underestimated. ICD-9-CM and CPT-4 coding drives reimbursement and also presents a mechanism by which external and internal agents evaluate utilization of services, quality of care, and the hospital's patient acuity level. This numerically abbreviated medical information is only as complete as the physician documentation and is only as accurate as the coder's translation. Coders have a monumental impact on the hospital and this impact will broaden as other health care services are converted to a prospective payment method of reimbursement, including Outpatient Services, Extended Care Facilities, and Home Health Agencies. (Elder 2000)

The cornerstone of accurate coding is physician documentation. According to an AHIMA practice brief (Bowman 2008), ensuring the accuracy of coded data is a shared responsibility between coding professionals and physicians. Accurate diagnostic and procedural coded data originate from collaboration between physicians, who have a clinical background, and coding professionals, who have an understanding of classification systems.

Complete, accurate, legible, and timely documentation should:

- Address the clinical significance of abnormal test results

- Support the intensity of patient evaluation and treatment and describe the thought processes and complexity of decision making

- Include all diagnostic and therapeutic procedures, treatments, and tests performed, in addition to their results

- Include any changes in the patient's condition, including psychosocial and physical symptoms

- Include all conditions that coexist at the time of admission, that subsequently develop, or that affect the treatment received and the length of stay. This encompasses all conditions that affect patient care in terms of requiring clinical evaluation, therapeutic treatment, diagnostic procedures, extended length of hospital stay, or increased nursing care and monitoring.

- Be updated as necessary to reflect all diagnoses relevant to the care or services provided

- Be consistent and discuss and reconcile any discrepancies (this reconciliation should be documented in the medical record)

- Be legible and written in ink, typewritten, or electronically signed, stored, and printed (Bowman 2008).

Coding and Corporate Compliance

The federal government has initiated efforts to investigate healthcare fraud and to establish guidelines to ensure corporate compliance with the government guidelines. Part of the initiative involved providing healthcare organizations with guidelines for developing comprehensive compliance programs with specific policies and procedures.

History of Fraud and Abuse and Corporate Compliance in Healthcare

The federal government, specifically the HHS, is the largest purchaser of healthcare in the United States. Because one of the federal government's duties is to use the taxpayers' monies wisely, federal agencies must ensure that the healthcare provided to enrollees in federal healthcare programs is appropriate and is actually provided. Several federal initiatives and pieces of legislation related to investigating, identifying, and preventing healthcare fraud and abuse have been passed. The basis for prosecution of healthcare fraud and abuse is the Federal False Claims Act (FCA). This act was signed into law by Abraham Lincoln in 1863. Its original intent was to encourage private citizens during the Civil War to report fraudulent actions taken against the Union Army. Under this act, the government had to prove that an individual acted with specific intent to defraud the government.

In 1986, the FCA was amended to include provisions that eliminated the requirement that specific intent to defraud be proven. The law now has become the basis for prosecuting healthcare providers who knowingly present a false claim for payment to the government. Therefore, when a healthcare provider shows a pattern or practice of coding that results in overcharges to Medicare and Medicaid, that provider can be prosecuted.

Several government agencies are involved in detecting, prosecuting, and preventing fraud and abuse. Among them are the HHS, the Office of the Inspector General (OIG), the Department of Justice (the attorney general), the Federal Bureau of Investigation (FBI), CMS, the Drug Enforcement Agency (DEA), the Internal Revenue Service (IRS), and state attorneys general.

Many initiatives are joint efforts among the agencies. For example, Operation Restore Trust, which began in 1995, is a joint effort of HHS, OIG, CMS, and the Administration on Aging. Operation Restore Trust spent only $7.9 million in the first two years to identify $188 million in overpayments to providers. It also led to implementation of special fraud alerts notifying providers of current investigative findings and to the **Voluntary Disclosure Program.**

The federal government began to actively investigate fraud in the Medicare program in 1977 with passage of the Anti-Fraud and Abuse Amendments of 1977 to Title XIX of the Social Security Act (SSA). However, detecting, preventing, and prosecuting fraud and abuse did not reach true prominence until the Health Insurance Portability and Accountability Act of 1996 (HIPAA) established Sections 1128C and 1128D of the SSA. These sections authorized the OIG to conduct investigations, audits, and evaluations related to healthcare fraud. The BBA focused on fraud and abuse issues specifically relating to penalties.

The BBA also required that physicians and practitioners provide diagnostic information (to show medical necessity) prior to a facility performing lab or radiology services for a patient.

As previously mentioned, HIPAA expanded the OIG's duties to include:

- Coordination of federal, state, and local enforcement efforts targeting healthcare fraud

- Provision of industry guidance concerning fraudulent healthcare practices

- Establishment of a national data bank for reporting final adverse actions against healthcare providers

Significantly, HIPAA authorizes the OIG to investigate cases of healthcare fraud that involve private healthcare plans as well as federally-funded programs, although, according to information on the OIG website, present policies restrict the OIG's investigative focus to cases of fraud that affect federally funded programs.

A major portion of HIPAA focused on identifying medically unnecessary services, **upcoding,** unbundling, and billing for services not provided. Upcoding is the practice of assigning a diagnosis or procedure code specifically for the purpose of obtaining a higher level of payment. It is most often found when reimbursement-grouping systems are used.

Unbundling is the practice of using multiple codes that describe individual components of a procedure rather than an appropriate single code that describes all steps of the procedure performed. Unbundling is a component of the NCCI.

HIPAA also expanded sanctions related to mandatory exclusion from Medicare, length of exclusion, failure to comply with statutory obligations, and antikickback penalties (Schraffenberger and Kuehn 2011).

From February 1998 until the present, the OIG continues to issue **compliance program guidance** for various types of healthcare organizations. The OIG website (http://www.oig.hhs.gov) posts the documents that most healthcare organizations need to develop fraud and abuse compliance plans. The goal of compliance programs is to prevent accusations of fraud and abuse, make operations run more smoothly, improve services, and contain costs (Anderson 2000).

Elements of Corporate Compliance

In the February 23, 1998, *Federal Register*, the OIG outlined the following seven elements as the minimum necessary for a comprehensive compliance program (p. 8989):

1. The development and distribution of written standards of conduct, as well as written policies and procedures that promote the hospital's commitment to compliance and that address specific areas of potential fraud, such as claims development and submission processes, code gaming, and financial relationships with physicians and other healthcare professionals

2. The designation of a chief compliance officer and appropriate corporate bodies, for example, a corporate compliance committee, charged with the responsibility for operating and monitoring the compliance program, and who report directly to the CEO and the organization's governing body

3. The development and implementation of regular, effective education and training programs for all affected employees

4. The maintenance of a process, such as a hotline, to receive complaints and the adoption of procedures to protect the anonymity of complainants and to protect whistleblowers from retaliation

5. The development of a system to respond to allegations of improper/illegal activities and the enforcement of appropriate disciplinary action against employees who have violated internal compliance policies, applicable statutes, regulations, or federal healthcare program requirements

6. The use of audits and/or other evaluation techniques to monitor compliance and assist in the reduction of identified problem areas

7. The investigation and remediation of identified systemic problems and the development of policies addressing the nonemployment or retention of sanctioned individuals

The OIG believes that a compliance program conforming to these elements will not only "fulfill the organization's legal duty to ensure that it is not submitting false or inaccurate claims to government and private payers," but will also result in additional potential benefits, including, among others (p. 8998):

- Demonstration of the organization's commitment to responsible conduct toward employees and the community

- Provision of a more accurate view of behavior relating to fraud and abuse

- Identification and prevention of criminal and unethical conduct

- Improvements in the quality of patient care

In the January 31, 2005, *Federal Register,* the OIG supplemental compliance program guidance for hospitals was published (pp. 4858–4876). This document supplements

Figure 6.6.   **Online compliance resources**

Department of Health and Human Services, Office of the Inspector General	http://www.oig.hhs.gov
American Health Information Management Association	http://www.ahima.org
Health Care Compliance Association	http://www.hcca-info.org
National Health Care Anti-Fraud Association	http://www.nhcaa.org
Centers for Medicare and Medicaid Services	http://www.cms.hhs.gov
CMS Fraud Page	http://www.medicare.gov

rather than replaces the 1998 compliance program guidance (CPG) document. The supplemental CPG contains new compliance recommendations and an expanded discussion of risk areas, current enforcement priorities, and lessons learned in the area of corporate compliance.

For additional resources on compliance and fraud and abuse, see figure 6.6.

Relationship between Coding Practice and Compliance

Any compliance program must contain references to complete and accurate coding. Many of the documented fraud and abuse convictions have centered on the coding function.

OIG Work Plan

At the beginning of each fiscal year, the OIG publishes an annual Work Plan that describes the specific audits and evaluations that are underway or that the OIG plans to initiate in the coming fiscal year. The Work Plan provides general focus areas for investigative, enforcement, and compliance activities. The current edition and prior editions of the Work Plan are available from the OIG website at http://www.oig.hhs.gov under Reports and Publications.

The HIM Compliance Program

As mentioned previously, one element of the corporate compliance program addresses the coding function. Because the accuracy and completeness of ICD-9-CM and CPT code assignment determine the provider payment, the reference to coding is not surprising. Thus, it is important that healthcare organizations have a strong coding compliance program. This coding compliance plan should be based on the same principles as that of the corporate-wide program. The basic elements of a coding plan should include:

- Code of conduct
- Policies and procedures
- Education and training

- Communication
- Auditing
- Corrective action
- Reporting

Code of Conduct

The HIM department should develop a code of conduct or adopt AHIMA's Standards of Ethical Coding.

Policies and Procedures

Policies and procedures that describe the facility's coding standards and functions should be documented. This should be done through a coding compliance manual. Some of the items that should be included in this manual include policies on the following: ambiguous or incomplete documentation, rebilling of problem claims, use of official coding guidelines, issues where no official guidelines exist, and clarification of new or confusing coding issues.

Education and Training

Periodic and staff-appropriate education of staff is a key factor in a successful coding compliance program. Education for coders should be provided monthly (Schraffenberger and Kuehn 2011).

Areas that could be covered at training sessions include:

- The OIG Work Plan
- Clinical information related to problematic body systems, diagnoses, and procedures
- Changes to the PPSs
- Changes to ICD-9-CM, HCPCS Level II, and CPT codes
- Application of the *ICD-9-CM Official Guidelines for Coding and Reporting*
- Issues in *Coding Clinic for ICD-9-CM*
- Issues in *CPT Assistant*

All newly hired coding personnel should receive extensive training on the facility's and HIM department's compliance programs.

Education of the medical staff on documentation is likewise important to the success of any coding compliance program. Documentation education may be provided monthly, bimonthly, or quarterly depending on the importance of the issues covered (Schraffenberger and Kuehn 2011).

Examples of documentation problems that may need to be addressed with physicians include:

- Inconsistent documentation
- Incomplete progress notes
- Undocumented care
- Test results not addressed in physician documentation
- Historical diagnoses being documented as current diagnoses
- Long-standing, chronic conditions that are not documented
- Lack of documentation of postoperative complications
- Illegibility
- Documentation not completed on time (Bowman 2008)

Communication

Communication between the coding supervisor and the coding professionals is vital to ensure consistency in following coding policies and issues. Simply distributing information on new or revised compliance issues may not be sufficient to convey the importance of these issues. By verbally communicating to the group, possibly through team meetings, the coding supervisor knows that everyone has heard the same message and the coders have had the opportunity to ask questions.

Internal Audits

Ongoing evaluation is critical to successful coding and billing for third-party payer reimbursement. In the past, the goal of internal audit programs was to increase revenues for the provider. Today, the goal is to protect providers from sanctions or fines. Healthcare organizations can implement monitoring programs by conducting regular, periodic audits of (1) ICD-9-CM and CPT/HCPCS coding and (2) claims development and submission. In addition, audits should be conducted to follow up on previous reviews that resulted in the identification of problems (for example, poor coding quality or errors in claims submission).

Auditing involves the performance of internal and/or **external reviews** to identify variations from established baselines (for example, review outpatient coding as compared with CMS outpatient coding guidelines). Internal reviews are conducted by facility-based staff (for example, HIM professionals), and external reviews are conducted by either consultants hired for this purpose (for example, corporations that specialize in such reviews and independent health information consultants) or third-party payers.

The scope and frequency of audits and the size of the sample depend on the size of the organization, available resources, the number of coding professionals, the history of noncompliance, risk factors, case complexity, and the results of initial assessments (Bowman 2008).

One of the elements of the auditing process is identification of risk areas. Some major risk areas include:

- MS-DRG coding accuracy
- Variations in case mix
- Discharge status (transfers versus discharges)
- Services provided under arrangement
- Three-day payment window, formerly called the 72-hour rule (Under this rule, diagnostic services provided within three days of admission should be included [bundled] in the MS-DRG, whether or not they are related to the admission. Non-diagnostic services provided within three days of admission should be included in the MS-DRG only if they are related to the admission. All nondiagnostic services that are unrelated to the admission can be billed separately.)
- Medical necessity
- Evaluation and management services
- Chargemaster description

Selecting types of cases to review also is important. Some examples of various case selection possibilities are found in figure 6.7.

The frequency of audits depends on the individual facility. Daily, weekly, monthly, or quarterly audits may be considered.

The results of the audits must be analyzed to determine the reason(s) for the coding errors. Focused reviews in one particular area may be necessary to review a higher volume

Figure 6.7. Examples of various case selections for auditing

Simple random sample	Unlisted CPT codes
Medical DRGs by high dollar and high volume	"Separate procedure" CPT codes reported in conjunction with related CPT codes
Surgical DRGs by high dollar and high volume	
Medical DRGs without comorbid conditions or complications	Unusual modifier usage patterns
	Not elsewhere classified (NEC) and not otherwise specified (NOS) codes
Surgical DRGs without comorbid conditions or complications	Highest-level evaluation and management (E/M) codes
Major diagnostic category by high dollar and high volume	
Most common diagnosis codes	Consultation E/M codes
Most common procedure codes	Critical Care E/M codes
	Chargemaster review by service
Significant procedure APCs by high dollar and high volume	Superbill, encounter form, and charge sheet review by specialty

of cases in which there were frequent errors. Certainly, focused reviews aimed at OIG target areas would be appropriate. Significant variations from baselines should prompt an investigation to determine cause(s).

Feedback on the results of audits should be presented to interested parties such as coding staff, supervisors, and physicians.

Corrective Action

Certainly, the goal of corrective action activities is the prevention of the same or a similar problem in the future. Typical corrective actions for resolving problems identified during coding audits include:

- Revisions to policies and procedures
- Development of additional policies and procedures
- Process improvements
- Education of coders, physicians, and/or other organizational staff depending on the nature of the identified problem
- Revision or addition of routine monitoring activities
- Additions, deletions, or revisions to systems edits
- Documentation improvement strategies
- Disciplinary action (Bowman 2008)

Reporting

Documentation on coding compliance activities should be maintained and reported as stated in the policies and procedures. Adverse findings should be reviewed with the corporate compliance officer and steps taken as necessary to report these findings.

Recovery Audit Contractor Program

The Medicare Prescription Drug, Improvement, and Modernization Act of 2003 directed the Department of Health and Human Services to conduct a three-year demonstration program using recovery audit contractors (RACs) to detect and correct improper payments in the Medicare Fee for Service (FFS) program. The demonstration proved successful in returning dollars to the Medicare Trust Fund and identifying monies that needed to be returned to providers. The RAC program provided CMS with another tool for detecting improper payments made in the past and has also given CMS a valuable mechanism for preventing future inappropriate payments.

The Tax Relief and Health Care Act of 2006 subsequently made the RAC program a permanent one and required the Secretary of DHHS to expand the program to all 50 states no later than January 1, 2010. RACs are authorized to investigate claims submitted by all physicians, providers, facilities, and supplies. There are four recovery audit contractors (RACs), each one responsible for about a quarter of the country. In 2009, CMS reported that the RAC Pilot Program saved almost $700 million in improper Medicare payments. In FY 2010 over $92 million was recovered.

RACs conduct two types of audits: automated reviews and complex reviews. An automated review occurs when a RAC makes a claim determination at the system level without a human review of the health record, such as data mining. Errors found must be clearly noncovered services or incorrect application of coding rules and must be supported by Medicare policy, approved article, or coding guidance. A complex review occurs when a RAC makes a claim determination utilizing human review of the health record. Records requiring a complex review are those with high probability of noncovered services or when no definitive Medicare policy, Medicare article, or Medicare-sanctioned coding guideline exists.

Check Your Understanding 6.9

Instructions: Select the best term to complete each of the following statements.

1. Fee schedules are updated by third-party payers

   A. Annually
   B. Monthly
   C. Semiannually
   D. Weekly

2. To accept assignment means that the

   A. Patient authorizes payment to be made directly to the provider
   B. Provider accepts as payment in full whatever the payer reimburses
   C. Balance billing is allowed on patient accounts, but at a limited rate
   D. Participating provider always receives a higher rate of reimbursement

3. A fee schedule is

   A. Developed by third-party payers and includes a list of healthcare services and procedures and charges of each
   B. Developed by providers and includes a list of healthcare services provided to a patient
   C. Developed by third-party payers and includes a list of healthcare services provided to a patient
   D. Developed by providers and lists charge codes

4. An inaccurately generated chargemaster affects reimbursement, resulting in

   A. Overpayments
   B. Underpayments
   C. Claims rejections
   D. Any of the above

5. The goal of compliance programs is to prevent:

    A. Accusations of fraud and abuse
    B. Delays in claims processing
    C. Billing errors
    D. Inaccurate code assignments

6. The practice of assigning a diagnosis or procedure code specifically for the purpose of obtaining a higher level of payment is called:

    A. Billing
    B. Unbundling
    C. Upcoding
    D. Unnecessary service

7. The essential elements of a Corporate Compliance Program are defined by:

    A. CMS
    B. HIPAA
    C. Medicare
    D. OIG

Instructions: Indicate whether the following statements are true or false (T or F).

8. _____ The federal Office of the Inspector General established compliance plans for the healthcare industry.

9. _____ The basis for prosecuting healthcare fraud and abuse is the Federal False Compliance Act.

10. _____ A corporate compliance program should include the development and implementation of education and training programs for all affected employees.

11. _____ HIM professionals are not involved in developing policies and procedures for corporate compliance.

Real-World Case

Streamlining the Revenue Cycle Management Process

At Mississippi Baptist Medical Center in Jackson, Mississippi, the organization's revenue cycle is running smoothly. Betsy Hathorn, RHIA, is the director of clinical resource management and oversees a variety of departments, including HIM, social work, case management, utilization review, infection control, and clinical decision support. The confluence of all these departments has worked well for managing the revenue cycle.

Hathorn has elected to oversee revenue cycle management (RCM), with the goal of reducing rework and producing cleaner claims. "It became important because all of the problems were winding up back in our department. Nothing was getting fixed, so we had to sit down and say: This is in our lap. We might as well do what we can to improve the process," Hathorn says.

Mapping the Process

To start, the team developed what it calls a "process map" of the revenue cycle. These maps help them see where problems occur and where improvements could be made. A similar map of the chargemaster management process is also in development.

The team has also developed a comprehensive flow chart of the progress of a claim through the organization. It is a 32-page document that is proving useful as a training tool and as a way to ensure that all the people who work with claims use the same processes and understand how things work.

The team works with small work groups and an executive steering committee to report progress and measure results. The organization has seen a 23 percent increase in advance beneficiary notices and a reduction in failed claims by about 100 a month.

To continue to measure its progress, the team looks at indicators such as discharge not final billed days, OCE edits, local coverage determination reviews, case management numbers, length of stay, and inpatient cases denied, appealed, or overturned. This was an attempt to measure whether what they are doing is making a difference.

Ready for RCM

As RCM increasingly becomes part of the HIM professional's skill portfolio, Hathorn's advice for those interested in this area is simple: find your niche.

"Take your skills and look at a situation and bring something to it," she says. "You need people skills, the ability to collaborate. The ability to bring people together and discuss an issue that everyone feels like they have a part of—that's probably more important than understanding the finance" (Zender 2009).

Summary

From its very beginnings, financial reimbursement for healthcare services has followed several paths. Among these are private pay, commercial insurance, employer self-insurance, and various government programs. The mixture of payment mechanisms has made healthcare reimbursement in the United States very complex.

As a consequence, the processing of medical claims can be complicated. How a claim is processed, what documentation is required, and how much reimbursement will be paid depend on the payer and the type of claim. Many attempts have been made to create a uniform healthcare claim that would accommodate all payment mechanisms. Claims processed for payment under Medicare have been consolidated into a uniform bill.

Healthcare organizations have developed several tools to help manage the billing and reimbursement process, including development of fee schedules and chargemasters. The HIM professional is frequently called on to provide expertise in the development, management, and auditing of these tools. In addition, organizations have recognized that ongoing evaluation of the entire billing process is essential to ensure accurate payment as well as to avoid fraud and abuse sanctions or fines. The HIM professional's work is likely to involve helping to develop such audit programs in addition to conducting the audits themselves.

Over the past two decades, the billing and reimbursement process has become an integral part of the job functions of many HIM professionals. The expertise brought to bear on the process to ensure accurate and timely claims submission is critical to the operations of any healthcare organization.

Payments for the delivery of healthcare services increased from $27 billion in 1960 to more than $3.5 trillion in FY 2010. In response, private insurers introduced managed care programs and the federal government implemented prospective payment systems to replace the costly per diem (or traditional fee-for-service) reimbursement methods. The federal government also incorporated managed care into its healthcare programs.

Health claims reimbursement processing has evolved from the submission of handwritten CMS-1500 and UB-04 forms to specially designed forms to be used for optical scanning purposes to electronic data interchange. EDI was greatly affected by HIPAA legislation passed in 1996. Of recently enacted federal legislation affecting claims reimbursement processing, the NCCI and the OIG coding compliance programs have had the most effect on HIM professionals.

References

AHIMA. 2008. "Managing an Effective Query Process" *Journal of the AHIMA* 79(10):83–88.

AHIMA. 2012. *Pocket Glossary of Health Information Management and Technology.* Chicago: AHIMA.

Anderson, S. 2000. Audit outpatient bills to get all the money you deserve. *Medical Records Briefing* 15(12):6.

Averill, Richard, et al. 2002. "What Are APR-DRGs? An Introduction to Severity of Illness and Risk of Mortality Adjustment Methodology." Salt Lake City: 3M HIS.

Bowman, S. 2008. *Health Information Management Compliance: Guidelines for Preventing Fraud and Abuse.* Chicago: AHIMA.

Centers for Medicare and Medicaid Services. 2012. *Medicare and You.* http://www.cms.hhs.gov

Elder, D. 2000. Coding: The key to compliance. Birmingham, AL: Medical Management Plus.

Himmelstein, D.V., S. Woolhandler, I. Hellander, and S.M. Wolfe. 1999. Quality of care in investor-owned vs. not-for-profit HMOs. *JAMA* 282:159–163.

Kim, C., D.F. Williamson, C.M. Mangione, M.M. Safford, J.V. Selby, D.G. Marrero, J.D. Curb, T.J. Thompson, K.M. Venkat Narayan, and W.H. Herman. 2004. Managed care organizations and the quality of diabetes care: The translating research into action for diabetes (TRIAD) study. *Diabetes Care* 27:1529–1534.

Office of Inspector General. 1998. Program Guidance for Hospitals. *Federal Register* 63(35):8987–8998. http://www.gpo.gov/fdsys/pkg/FR-1998-02-23/pdf/98-4399.pdf

Office of Inspector General. 2005. OIG Supplemental Compliance Program Guidance for Hospitals. *Federal Register* 70(19):4858–4876. http://www.oig.hhs.gov/fraud/docs/complianceguidance/012705HospSupplementalGuidance.pdf

Rhodes, H. 1999. Practice brief: The care and maintenance of charge masters. *Journal of AHIMA* 70(7).

Schraffenberger, L.A., and L. Kuehn. 2011. *Effective Management of Coding Services.* Chicago: AHIMA.

Schneider, E.C., A.M. Zaslaksky, and A.M. Epstein. 2005. Quality of care in for-profit and not-for-profit health plans enrolling Medicare beneficiaries. *American Journal of Medicine* 118(12):1392–1400.

Youmans, K. 2004. Practice brief: An HIM spin on the revenue cycle. *Journal of AHIMA* 75(3):32–36.

Zender, A. 2009. Streamlining the revenue cycle management process. *Journal of AHIMA* 80(3):88.

Additional Resources

American Medical Association. 2011. *Current Procedural Terminology,* 2012 edition. Chicago: American Medical Association.

Averill, R.F. 1999. Honest mistake or fraud? Meeting the coding compliance challenge. *Journal of AHIMA* 70(5):16–21.

Campbell, T. 2003. Opportunities for HIM in revenue cycle management. *Journal of AHIMA* 74(10):62–63.

Coder's Desk Reference. 2011. Salt Lake City: Ingenix.

Hazelwood, A., and C. Venable. 2012. *ICD-9-CM and ICD-10-CM Diagnostic Coding and Reimbursement for Physician Services.* Chicago: AHIMA.

Johnson, S.L. 2000. *Understanding Medical Coding: A Comprehensive Guide.* Albany, NY: Delmar Thomson Learning.

Kuehn, L. 2012. *CPT/HCPCS Coding and Reimbursement for Physician Services.* Chicago: AHIMA.

Palmer, K. 1999. A brief history: Universal health care efforts in the US: late 1800s to Medicare. http://pnhp.org

Schraffenberger, L.A. 2012. *Basic ICD-10-CM/PCS and ICD-9-CM Coding.* Chicago: AHIMA.

Smith, G. 2012. *Basic CPT/HCPCS Coding.* Chicago: AHIMA.

chapter 7

Health Information Functions

Lisa A. Cerrato, MS, RHIA and
Jane Roberts, MS, RHIA

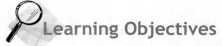

Learning Objectives

- Identify typical health information management functions

- Explain the purpose and techniques used for the maintenance of the master patient index in paper-based and electronic environments

- Identify operational techniques for managing traditional HIM functions in paper-based, hybrid, and electronic record environments

- Discuss techniques used in the processing, storage, retrieval, and maintenance of health records in paper-based, hybrid, and electronic environments

- Explain the use of quality control techniques used for paper-based, hybrid, and electronic health records and for supporting services such as medical transcription, release of information, and coding functions

- Discuss the concept of the legal health record and how it is applied

- Describe practices for authorization and access control of health records in paper-based, hybrid, and electronic formats

- Recognize the interrelationship between the HIM department and other key departments within the healthcare organization

- Describe the purpose, development, and maintenance of registries and indexes such as the master patient index, disease index, and operation index

- Discuss the functions and responsibilities of common HIM support services, including cancer and trauma registries, birth certificate completion, and statistical and research services

- Explain the relationship of accreditation, licensing, and standards requirements to HIM functions and how compliance with these is monitored

- Describe techniques used in the management of the HIM department, such as policy and procedure development and the budgeting process

Key Terms

Abstracting

Access control

Alphabetic filing system

Alphanumeric filing system

APC grouper

Authentication

Authorization

Back-end speech recognition

Certificate of destruction

Clinical coding

Computer-assisted coding (CAC)

Concurrent review

Corrections

Deemed status

Deficiency slip

Delinquent record

Destruction

Digital dictation

Duplicate medical record number

Encoder

Enterprise master person/patient index (EMPI)

Free-text data

Front-end speech recognition

Health information exchange (HIE)

Health record number

Hybrid record

Index

The Joint Commission (TJC)

Legal health record

Master patient index (MPI)

Medical transcription

Middle-digit filing system

MS-DRG grouper

Natural language processing (NLP)

Nonrepudiation

Numeric filing system

Operation index

Outguide

Overlap

Overlay

Patient account number

Policies

Procedures

Purged records

Quantitative analysis

Reassignment

Record completion

Record processing

Record reconciliation

Registry

Release of information (ROI)

Requisition

Resequencing

Retention

Retraction

Retrospective review

Serial numbering system

Serial-unit numbering system

Standard

Storage and retrieval

Straight numeric filing system

Terminal-digit filing system

Transcription

Unit numbering system

Version control

Virtual HIM

Voice recognition technology

Introduction

Health information management (HIM) involves a wide variety of functions that are critical to the operations of the healthcare organization and the healthcare delivery process. This chapter examines the functions of the HIM department and looks at the different management and supervisory processes that HIM professionals assume in the organization. Several chapters in this book are related to this chapter and focus on the purpose and content of patient health records, the different technologies used in obtaining and retrieving patient information, the different information systems used in healthcare organizations, the importance of maintaining data integrity, and ensuring data confidentiality.

HIM functions usually involve ensuring the quality, security, and availability of health information as it follows the patient through the health system. The HIM department also monitors the quality of patient information, ensuring that the information is maintained and protected in accordance with federal, state, and local regulations and the guidelines issued by various accrediting bodies.

Among the HIM department's most important functions is that of storage and retrieval of patient information. The electronic health record (EHR) is rapidly replacing paper-based record and hybrid record systems. Paper-based record systems are transitioning to hybrid record systems. Hybrid record systems are evolving into electronic record systems. As healthcare organizations make the transition to an electronic health record (EHR), paper or hybrid record systems may still be used to store patient information. Regardless of the type of storage system used, patient information must be stored in a manner that ensures its accessibility to authorized users whenever and wherever it is needed.

In most healthcare organizations, the HIM department also manages several critical support services. In addition to the storage and retrieval function, the HIM department also typically manages the following support services:

- Record processing
- Monitoring of record completion
- Transcription
- Release of patient information
- Clinical coding, abstracting, and clinical data analysis

The services managed by the HIM department vary depending on the organization. Besides the typical HIM functions, the HIM department may manage the following functions:

- Research and statistics
- Cancer and/or trauma registries
- Birth certificate completion

An interdepartmental relationship exists between the HIM department and many other departments within a healthcare organization. HIM functions support patient care, quality and resource management, billing, and patient registration. The functions associated with patient care, quality and resource management, billing, and patient registration also affect the processes managed by the HIM department. The information systems department and HIM work together to support the electronic health record environment.

Theory into Practice

A patient arrives at the admitting department of a hospital and is admitted as an inpatient to the medical floor. The registration clerk asks the patient if he has ever been seen or admitted to the hospital before. The patient states that he has never been admitted to this hospital. Upon a search of the registration system (master patient index) by using the patient's name, and date of birth, the clerk finds that the patient had been seen at the hospital previously as an outpatient. The registration clerk updates information in the computer by asking the patient questions. The patient's demographic information and insurance information is updated in the computer. The insurance card is scanned and entered into the computer. The information put into the registration system is automatically sent to the hospital's electronic health record, thus, the patient's health record is created. The patient is transported to the medical unit.

Once in the room, the patient's nurse introduces herself and does an assessment of the patient and carries out the orders received by the patient's physician. While on the unit, the patient has blood drawn for laboratory tests. The patient's physician visits the patient later that afternoon and dictates a history and physical examination. Each clinician and physician that enters the room enters information regarding the patient in the computer located in the patient's room. The history and physical examination report is remotely transcribed by the transcriptionist and the report is electronically transmitted into the electronic health record (EHR). The patient stays in the hospital for four days and is discharged home.

Eighty percent of the health record at this hospital is either captured at point of service via direct input by the clinician, electronically transmitted, or COLD fed into the EHR. The HIM department's record processing clerk checks to make sure the record is received electronically and that any loose sheets are retrieved from the nursing units and scanned into the EHR. The electronic health record is then analyzed for deficiencies and coded. Because a high percentage of the health record is structured data within the EHR, the medical coder checks the codes assigned by the computerized assisted coding (CAC) system to assure that the correct codes were assigned accurately. The medical coder also abstracts any information not found by the CAC system. The physician completes deficiencies found in the health record. The record is completed.

The medical codes and abstracted data from the health record are electronically sent to the business office. The medical coding information, registration information, and charges entered from various departments are used to generate a bill. The bill is sent to the patient's insurance company.

HIM Functions and Services

HIM functions are information-centered. This means that they typically involve ensuring information quality, security, and availability. The medium in which the information is stored will dictate how the specific functions are carried out. The goal of the health record system is to ensure that accurate information is available to authorized users to support quality patient care. For example, storage of information in paper-based records involves different types of tasks than does storage of information in electronic records.

Figure 7.1 provides a description of a fictional HIM department with paper-based, hybrid, and electronic records. The description includes many of the HIM functions discussed in this chapter. It is important to note that these are typical functions. Not all HIM departments are identical in organization or in the functions they perform. Table 7.1 summarizes the some of the typical functions of the HIM department for paper-based and hybrid records and EHRs.

Figure 7.1. HIM functions at Community Hospital Medical Center

Community Hospital Medical Center is located in the suburbs of a large southeastern city. It is a nationally recognized leader in providing specialty and primary healthcare services and in conducting groundbreaking research in the treatment of various health disorders. Located on a fifty-acre campus, the facility includes:

- A 516-licensed-bed facility that includes a Level I trauma center and a 50-bed neonatal intensive care unit, a 16-bed pediatric ICU, and 25 general pediatric beds
- A cancer center with facilities for research, diagnosis, and treatment
- An outpatient center that includes specialized examination and treatment rooms, a clinical laboratory, a diagnostic radiology department, and an ambulatory surgery department

The facility is affiliated with a local medical school and provides education and training for third- and fourth-year medical students as well as internships and residencies for physician training.

The HIM department is responsible for all health records for the entire facility including both inpatient and outpatient records. The medical training aspect of the facility adds another complicated dimension to the management of the health records.

The functions performed within the HIM department include:

- Record processing (concurrent and retrospective analysis and monitoring of health record content)
- Record completion
- Storage and retrieval of health records (including monitoring and tracking of health record location)
- Release of patient information
- Clinical coding of diagnoses and procedures
- Transcription of medical reports (excluding pathology and radiology reports)
- Statistical and internal report generation
- Cancer and trauma registry

The HIM department is staffed with the equivalent of 63 full-time employees and operates 24 hours a day, 7 days a week. The following organizational chart shows how the operations in the department are organized.

```
                              ┌─────────────────┐
                              │  HIM Services   │
                              └─────────────────┘
         ┌──────────────────────────┼──────────────────────────┐
┌────────────────────┐   ┌────────────────────────┐   ┌────────────────────────┐
│  Record Processing │   │  Compliance/Research   │   │ Release of Information  │
│ • Assembly/analysis│   │ • Clinical coding      │   │ • External requests for │
│ • Storage and      │   │ • Research (cancer      │   │   patient information   │
│   retrieval        │   │   registry and trauma  │   │ • Birth certificates    │
│ • Record completion│   │   registry)            │   │                         │
│ • Medical          │   │                        │   │                         │
│   transcription    │   │                        │   │                         │
└────────────────────┘   └────────────────────────┘   └────────────────────────┘
```

Table 7.1.   **Table of common HIM functions**

Function/Service	Description
Storage and retrieval	**Paper-based system:** • Patient care information documented on paper and housed in file folders. • Records retrieved for patient care purposes, quality improvement studies, audits, and other authorized uses. • Records are delivered to the nursing units, outpatient surgery, and the emergency room as the patient is admitted or being treated. **Hybrid system:** **Patient care information documented both on paper and in the computer.** • Record is accessible to patient care areas via the computer by use of an electronic document management system (EDMS). • If hospital is transitioning to the EHR, portions of the health record may be printed for use on the patient care unit. **EHR system:** • Patient care information captured at point of service and/or electronically transmitted to the EHR. • Same electronic components utilized in the hybrid record, but the record resides entirely in electronic format with work processes performed via the computer.
Record processing/ completion	**Paper-based:** • After the patient is discharged from the hospital, the record is retrieved from the nursing unit. The record is then assembled or put in an order prescribed by the facility's policy and procedure manual. For example, the face sheet is usually the first page in the paper record. • Receipt of the health record is checked with a discharge list in a process called record reconciliation. • The postdischarge record order is usually different than the order of the record on the nursing unit. • After the record is assembled, it is analyzed for deficiencies, such as missing reports and signatures. • Physicians visit the HIM department to complete deficiencies in records. • The record is reanalyzed after completion to assure completeness of the process. Deficiencies are cleared from the computer. **Hybrid system:** • Portions of the record can be directly inputted into the EHR through computer interfaces (for example, transcribed reports, laboratory reports, emergency records, etc.). After the patient is discharged from the hospital, the paper record is prepared for imaging (scanning). • Receipt of the health record is checked with a discharge list in a process called record reconciliation. • Physicians complete the record from a computer that may be located remotely from the hospital. • If electronic signatures, computer key, and electronic completion rules are applied, the deficiency system is updated once the physician completes his/her records. • Records are analyzed for deficiencies either manually by the HIM staff and/or by rules built into the computer system. **EHR system:** • Receipt of the health record is checked with a discharge list in a process called record reconciliation. • Entire health record available via the computer for completion. Work queues in the computer are used to route health records to appropriate person or area for completion.

Table 7.1. **Table of common HIM functions** *(continued)*

Function/Service	Description
Transcription	**Paper-based system:** • May be completed in-house or outsourced to an outside service. • Physician dictates reports into a dictation system that records the voice. The transcriptionist types (transcribes) what the physician has dictated. • The transcribed report is placed in the chart. • Reports commonly transcribed include: operative reports, history and physicals, discharge summaries, radiology reports, pathology reports, and consultations. **Hybrid and EHR system:** • The process is basically the same as in the paper-based system, except that the transcribed reports are electronically added to the health record that resides within the computer. Speech recognition technology may be applied to the front-end and back-end of the transcription process to facilitate the process.
Release of information (ROI)	**Paper-based system:** • Reviews requests for health records for validity to assure compliance with federal and state regulations. • Logs and verifies validity of requests for patient information. • May copy the record in response to valid requests or may provide record for an outsourced copy service to process. • May go to court in response to a subpoena or court order. • Must have in-depth knowledge of laws and regulations governing the release of information. **Hybrid and EHR system:** • ROI process is basically the same as in the paper-based environment. • As the EHR evolves there may be opportunities for the HIM professional's role to be expanded.
Clinical coding	**Paper-based system:** • A code number(s) is/are assigned to the diagnoses and procedures documented in the health record. The coder looks the code number up in a coding book or by entering key words into the computer using software called an encoder. • ICD-9-CM and CPT are the two primary coding systems used in a hospital setting. ICD-10-CM and ICD-10-PCS will replace ICD-9-CM. • Other information is abstracted from the record for reporting and reimbursement purposes. • Coding takes place on-site within the HIM department. **Hybrid and EHR system:** • The process is the same as the paper-based system, except that in the EHR environment, the record that is reviewed is the electronic health record. • Coding may be remote to hospital; home-based coding is possible. • Computer-assisted coding may be utilized. • Data abstracting may be reduced or eliminated as automatic data capture is implemented.

The functions (**storage and retrieval, record processing, record completion, transcription, release of information** [ROI], **clinical coding**) discussed here might be considered the most fundamental responsibilities of most HIM departments. (The processes that support these HIM functions are discussed later in this chapter.) As mentioned earlier, in some institutions, HIM functions also include clinical quality performance activities, research and statistics, maintenance of cancer and other registries, support for medical staff committee functions, and responsibility for birth certificate submission to state departments of public health. Even though these functions may not fall within the traditional range of HIM department responsibilities, health information technicians (HITs) sometimes do perform them.

Master Patient Index

Probably the most important index used by the HIM department is the master patient index (MPI). The MPI is the permanent record of every patient ever seen in the healthcare entity. The MPI functions as the primary guide to locating pertinent demographic data about the patient and his or her health record number. Without the information contained in the MPI, it would be almost impossible to locate a patient's health record in most organizations that use a numeric filing system. The demographic information entered in the PMI supplies the patient identifying information for the health record and its supporting databases. Therefore the MPI is the initial point of documentation of the health record. An **enterprise master patient index** (EMPI) references all patients in two or more facilities (e.g. integrated healthcare delivery system or health information exchange [HIE]).

The amount of information contained on each patient in the MPI varies from facility to facility. The recommended core data elements for an EMPI include: (AHIMA 2010b)

- Internal patient identification (medical record number)
- Person name
- Date of birth
- Gender
- Race
- Ethnicity
- Address
- Telephone number
- Alias/previous/maiden names
- Social Security number
- Facility identification
- Universal patient identifier (not yet established)
- Account—visit number
- Admission encounter—visit date

- Discharge departure date

- Encounter—service type

- Encounter—service location

- Encounter—primary physician

- Patient disposition

Figure 7.2 provides an example of an input screen for an electronic MPI system.

Today, it is common practice to have an electronic MPI instead of a manually maintained index. Often the patient registration system, also known at the registration, admission, discharge, transfer (R-ADT) system, functions as the MPI. The benefits of an electronic system include the ability to access data by more than one individual at a time. In addition, edit checks can be applied against specific fields in the database to better ensure data accuracy. An electronic index also can be easily cross-referenced—for example, when a patient has used more than one name during hospital or clinic visits.

An electronic MPI permits the use of several search techniques for locating an existing patient's information. For example, common techniques include: alphabetical or phonetic

Figure 7.2.   Input screen for an electronic MPI system

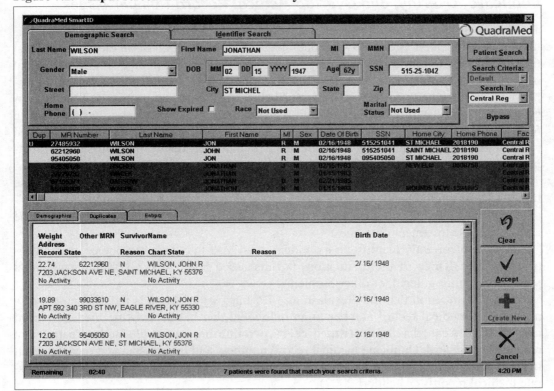

Source: AHIMA Virtual Lab QuadraMed MPI.

searches and searches by specific data elements such as medical record or billing number, date of birth, or Social Security number.

Once the patient's medical record number is identified using the MPI, the health record can be located which facilitates the coordination of care by caregivers and provides the physician and others access to the patient's history of previous encounters.

Maintenance of Master Patient Index

To ensure the integrity of the MPI, several quality control mechanisms are essential. The following section describes some of the quality issues and examines how these can be controlled.

Quality Issues in MPI Systems

MPIs are prone to errors, which adversely affects the integrity of the health record system.

These errors may include misspellings, incorrect demographic data, transposition of numbers, and typographical errors to name a few. When the data integrity of the MPI has been compromised in this way the faulty data are dispersed throughout the organization risking treatment errors and billing problems, and distorting data analysis of the organization's patient population (Dimick 2009).

Duplicate, Overlay, and Overlap Medical Record Number Issues

The most common MPI errors occur at the point of registration when existing MPI information is not located. Frequently an incomplete or rushed search of an electronic MPI at the time of registration can cause creation of a duplicate record number for an individual or match an individual with the wrong health record number. Duplicate, overlay, and overlap medical record number issues, discussed below, are significant problems. To help mitigate these, some facilities have instituted registration improvement programs, which can feature cross-department committees whose purpose is to reduce registration errors and clean up the MPI (Dimick 2009). The cleanup strategies for identifying errors and correcting MPI errors are discussed below.

The MPI is the key to locating specific patient information. Several problems can arise if patient information is not located. For example, as stated earlier, these may include billing errors, performance of unnecessary duplicate tests, and increased legal exposure in the area of adverse treatment outcomes.

Failure to correctly identify an individual in an MPI may result in one or more integrity problems. Three of these situations are discussed below and all result in potential patient care, billing, legal, or other problems.

The first situation that may result in an MPI integrity problem is the assignment of a new patient medical record number to an individual that has an existing medical record number. This is called a **duplicate medical record number** and results in the creation of a new medical record. Duplicate medical record numbers and their associated records result in a patient having duplicate medical record numbers with medical information in disparate medical records (Altendorf 2007).

Another situation arising from the failure to correctly identify an individual in an MPI is called an **overlay.** This is where a patient is assigned another patient's medical record number. The consequence of this situation is that medical information from two or more individuals is comingled or combined, resulting in problems identifying what medical information belongs to which patient.

The third case is called an **overlap.** This is when more than one medical record number exists for the same patient within an enterprise at different facilities or in different databases. Overlaps may occur in organizations that have multiple facilities, such as a multi-hospital system, or can occur in health information exchanges. Frequently this problem arises when there are facility or organization mergers and an enterprise master person/patient index (EMPI) is created.

Strategies for MPI Integrity

With more and more consolidations and mergers occurring among healthcare organizations and the establishment of health information exchanges, tracking patient information is increasingly more difficult. MPI integrity, however, must be maintained in order to avoid patient safety, customer service, risk management, legal, and other issues. "Although no organization expects to have duplicated patient information in the MPI, it is unrealistic to assume that duplicates will never occur. Even though errors may occur at the point of registration, the actual cause of error varies" (AHIMA 2010b). Most integrity issues are caused by human error. Some of these may be input errors by personnel such as misspellings, typographical errors, and transposition of numbers among others. Others may be retrieval errors such as using poor search strategies or reading errors. And still others may be due to inaccurate information being provided by the patient or client.

Initially, the MPI clean-up process is required to fix duplicates, overlay, and overlap errors within the MPI. MPI clean up is generally done by using matching algorithms to identify and fix these problems.

There are three types of matching algorithms that are often part of the MPI application programs used to identify potential duplicate health record numbers.

A deterministic algorithm requires an exact match of combined data elements such as name, birth date, sex, and Social Security number. A probabilistic algorithm is based on complex mathematical formulas that analyze facility-specific MPI data to determine precisely matched weight probabilities for attribute values of various data elements. Probabilistic algorithms are used most often in large databases such as HIEs. A rules-based algorithm assigns weights, for significant values, to particular data elements and later uses these weights in the comparison of one record to another (AHIMA 2010b).

The management of a high-quality, error-free MPI requires constant maintenance that includes oversight, evaluation, and correction of errors. The responsibility for MPI maintenance should be centralized under the direction of a qualified professional. A comprehensive maintenance program should include:

- Ongoing process to identify and address existing errors
- Advanced person search capabilities for minimizing the creation of new errors

- Mechanism for efficiently detecting, reviewing, and resolving potential errors
- Ability to reliably link different medical record numbers and other identifiers for the same person to create an enterprise view of the person
- Consideration of the types of physical merges (files, film, and such) and the interfaces and correction routines to other electronic systems that are populated or updated by the EMPI

MPI maintenance policies and procedures also should be outlined:

- Whether to use the most recent information for each data element or criteria for determining which data elements will be stored as the patient's information
- Identification of duplicate data elements (for example, prior names or aliases)
- Communication of merges to ancillary staff for source system revision
- Regular review of error reports and trending of duplicate percentages (AHIMA 2010b)

Prevention of problems should be the front line of defense. Communication back to the department responsible for the errors is key to providing awareness of the importance of the MPI and identifying opportunities for training and workflow issues.

Patient Identity in a Health Information Exchange Environment

As stated in chapter 16, **health information exchange** (HIE) is frequently used to describe both the sharing of health information electronically among two or more entities and also an organization that provides services to accomplish this information exchange. Regional Health Information Organizations or networks usually cover local or state geographical regions and are the building blocks of the proposed national health information network (NHIN). The purpose of an HIE is to increase the availability of health information to authorized stakeholders in order to improve quality and safety of healthcare delivery across the continuum.

To ensure integrity of patient identity in health information exchange, standardization of health information exchange practices is paramount. The focus on technical exchange of data between systems must ensure the quality of the data exchanged (that is, data validity and integrity, and quality of key data values). A quality health information exchange environment begins with accurate patient identification.

However, mechanisms must be in place to achieve this goal. The challenge of accurately capturing a patient's key demographic data in a single organization and preventing duplicate medical records is difficult. But this challenge becomes even more complicated when attempting to link patient information among a group of different organizations.

There are several competing identification methods that can be used. One common method is probabilistic matching that attempts to match an individual on multiple data elements such as name, date of birth, address, gender, and other items. Probabilistic matching has been used in healthcare and other industries for decades.

Many HIE organizations have formed multidisciplinary data governance steering committees to address how patient identification will be handled in the HIE. These committees determine, for example, what data are used in the matching algorithm, how many potential candidate matches will be presented to the user, and data quality standards.

Health information professionals are taking the lead in ensuring integrity of personal identification in HIEs. They are frequently members of data governance steering committees helping to define how patient identification is performed as well as addressing data security and privacy issues.

Identification Systems

The health record number (also called the medical record number) is a key data element in the MPI. It is used as a unique personal identifier and is also used in paper-based numerical filing systems to locate records and in electronic systems to link records. The health record number is unique to the healthcare facility or enterprise, which assigns it. For example, the same patient is seen at hospital A and Hospital B would have different health record numbers in each facility. Although it is typically assigned at the point of patient registration, the HIM department is usually responsible for the integrity of health record number assignment and for ensuring that no two patients receive the same number. The HIM department also ensures that the identification numbering system is such that all of an individual patient's records are stored together or can be linked together.

The health record number is important because it uniquely identifies not only the patient, but also the patient's record. Patient care documentation generated as part of the patient's episode of care is identified and physically filed or linked in an electronic system. Examples of documentation and medical reports found in health records are the history and physical, the discharge summary, operative notes, pathology reports, laboratory reports, radiology reports, and nursing notes. Thus, having a numbering system is important for efficiently storing and retrieving information about a single patient.

It is generally agreed that Social Security numbers (SSNs) should not be used as patient identifiers. The Social Security Administration is adamant in its opposition to using the SSN for purposes other than those identified by law. The American Health Information Management Association (AHIMA) is in agreement on this issue due to privacy, confidentiality, and security issues related to the use of the SSN.

The type of health record numbering system used varies from facility to facility. Four types of systems used most commonly in association with paper-based record systems are discussed below as is the identification system most frequently used with EHRs. The system used determines the procedure for assigning the health record number and the method for filing the patient record in a paper-based system.

Identification Systems for Paper-based Health Records

Serial Numbering System

In the **serial numbering system,** a patient receives a unique numerical identifier for each encounter or admission to a healthcare facility. The numbering system is called serial because numbers are issued in a series. For example, Mr. Jones is admitted to the hospital at 8:00 a.m. on October 12 and given number 786544. Mrs. Wright, who registered at 8:15 a.m. on the same day, receives the next available number, 786545. Thus, in a serial numbering system each patient receives the next available number in the series.

With this system, a patient admitted to a healthcare facility on three different occasions receives three different health record numbers. The information compiled for each admission is filed with the health record for each encounter. One disadvantage to the serial numbering system is that information about the patient's care and treatment is filed in separate health records and at separate locations. This makes retrieval of all patient information less efficient and storage more costly.

In addition to retrieval inefficiencies and the costs associated with file folders, this numbering system is time-consuming in terms of documentation. Each time a patient returns to the healthcare facility, manual index cards or computer systems must be updated to reflect the addition of a new serial number and each update presents an opportunity for input error.

Unit Numbering System

The **unit numbering system** is most commonly used in large healthcare facilities. Many of the disadvantages to the serial numbering system can be addressed by using a unit number. In the unit numbering system, the patient receives a unique health record number at the time of the first encounter. For all subsequent encounters for a particular patient, the health record number that was assigned for the first encounter is used.

One advantage to this method is that all information, regardless of the number of encounters, can be filed or linked together. Having all the information related to the patient filed in one location facilitates communication among caregivers and improves operational efficiency.

For the unit numbering system to work effectively, patient demographic and health record number information must be available to all areas of the facility that process patient registrations. For example, clerks in the admitting, emergency, and clinical departments must have access to a database of previous patients and their health record numbers. Access to such information is not a problem for organizations that make the information available to the registration areas via a computer network and electronic MPI. However, an incomplete search of an electronic system increases the likelihood that duplicate numbers may be assigned to a patient.

Serial-Unit Numbering System

The **serial-unit numbering system** is an attempt to combine the strengths and minimize the weaknesses of the serial and unit numbering systems. In this system, numbers are assigned in a serial manner, just as they are in the serial numbering system. However, during each new patient encounter, the previous health records are brought forward and filed under the last assigned health record number. This creates a unit record.

The serial-unit numbering system helps alleviate the problem of access to previous patient demographic and health record number information. It also helps in addressing problems associated with retrieval and the cost of the serial system.

Alphabetic Identification and Filing System

Some small facilities and clinics use an alphabetic patient identification and filing system. In this system, the patient's last name is used as the first source of identification and his or her first name and middle initial provide further identification. The disadvantage to this system is that a given community may have several persons with the same or a similar name. In this case, the facility routinely uses date of birth as the next step in the process of identifying a patient.

There are some conveniences to alphabetic identification and filing. It is simple to locate a health record without first accessing an assigned number. However, each entry must be double-checked to verify that the correct patient record is being used.

Identification Systems Used for Electronic Health Records

Unit numbering is the method most commonly used as the unique identifier in the EHR environment. For search and retrieval purposes, identifiers other than the health record number can be used to locate patient records in EHRs. The **patient account number** and patient name are often used to find a patient's health record stored electronically within a computer system.

Because correcting a digital record can be complex, before making entries or using information for care it is very important to confirm the correct patient health record has been accessed by verifying the full name, date of birth, and other factors.

The process for checking patient records should be included in the facility's charting **policies** and **procedures.**

Check Your Understanding 7.1

1. The system in which a health record number is assigned at the first encounter and then used for all subsequent healthcare encounters is the:

    A. Serial numbering system
    B. Unit numbering system
    C. Serial-unit numbering system
    D. Terminal-digit filing system

2. The primary guide to locating a record in a numerical filing system is the:

    A. Master patient index
    B. Admission register
    C. Discharge register
    D. Physician index

3. What type of algorithm(s) may be used to identify duplicate medical record numbers?

    A. Deterministic
    B. Probabilistic
    C. Rules-based
    D. All of the above

4. The health record number is typically assigned by:

   A. Patient registration
   B. Nursing
   C. Billing
   D. HIM staff

5. Which of the following is used to locate an electronic health record?

   A. Health record number
   B. Barcode
   C. Color code
   D. Terminal digit

6. John Smith, treated as a patient at a multi-hospital system, has three medical record numbers. The term used to describe multiple health record numbers is:

   A. Duplicates
   B. Overlay
   C. Overlap
   D. Integrity

7. Which of the following should be part of a comprehensive MPI maintenance program?

   A. Advanced person search
   B. Issuing medical record numbers
   C. Deletion capabilities
   D. Employee training

8. Which of the following is true about the Social Security number?

   A. AHIMA supports using the Social Security number as the health record identifier.
   B. The Social Security Administration supports using the Social Security number as the health record identifier.
   C. Both AHIMA and the Social Security Administration oppose using the Social Security number as the health record identifier.
   D. Both AHIMA and the Social Security Administration support using the Social Security number as the health record identifier.

9. Describes the electronic sharing of Information among two or more entities.

   A. Enterprise group
   B. Health information exchange
   C. Work queues
   D. Overlay organization

10. Which identification system is at a disadvantage when there are two patients with the same name?

   A. Serial numbering
   B. Unit numbering
   C. Serial-unit numbering
   D. Alphabetic

HIM Functions in a Paper-based Environment

Health information management is rapidly changing with the provisions mandated by the American Recovery and Reinvestment Act (ARRA) for the implementation of the electronic health record by 2014. The implementation of the EHR has been long awaited within the HIM profession. The EHR environment requires the HIM professionals expand their knowledge base to include systems and processes needed to support the EHR. Some organizations remain completely paper-based, while others use a combination of paper-based and electronic formats known as a hybrid record. Therefore the HIT professional must be familiar with best practices for all health record environments. The following section describes processes for the creation, storage, and maintenance of paper-based records.

Record Storage and Retrieval Functions

The storage and retrieval of patient information is one of the HIM department's most important functions. The department must ensure that health records are stored safely and that mechanisms are in place to efficiently retrieve them for patient care or other purposes. Moreover, the data contained in patient health records are confidential; thus, mechanisms must be in place to ensure that only authorized individuals have access to them.

Storage of paper-based health records has traditionally been the most common archival medium across healthcare delivery sites. In paper-based storage systems, each health record is contained in a special file folder that is filed either alphabetically or numerically, depending on the size of the organization. A small organization such as a physician's office practice may file its health records alphabetically in open-shelf files. Clinics, hospitals, long-term care facilities, and other larger facilities file their records numerically, using the patient's **health record number** as the primary identifier.

However, the in-house archival of paper-based health records is not the healthcare organization's only storage option. Health records also may be stored off-site, microfilmed, or scanned as digital images. Indeed, large HIM departments may have all these storage mechanisms in place.

Without a good storage and retrieval filing system, it would be impossible to locate and retrieve health records when they are needed. The following subsections discuss these key elements of the storage and retrieval function:

- Identification systems for paper-based health records and EHRs
- Filing systems for paper-based health records
- Storage systems
- Retrieval and tracking systems

Filing Systems for Paper-based Health Records

The filing system used by a healthcare facility maintaining paper-based health records refers to the procedure in which the file folders are placed on shelving units or in filing cabinets. The unique health record number assigned to a patient upon admission to a healthcare facility is the number also used to file the record in a numeric filing system. Likewise, the patient's name is used as the basis for filing in an alphabetical filing system.

Records that cannot be located and retrieved when needed serve no useful function. Thus, the HIM department must carefully consider the types of filing and storage systems it uses to ensure that they meet the needs of the organization. The three major classifications of filing systems are discussed below.

Alphabetic Filing Systems

In **alphabetic filing systems,** records are arranged in alphabetical order. This system is usually satisfactory for a very small volume of records, such as records maintained in small physician practices. The alphabetic filing system is easy to create and use. It is often called a direct filing method because it does not rely on an index or an authority file and the user can find a file by looking directly under the name of the record.

For organizations that have thousands of records, however, alphabetic filing has many disadvantages. First, it does not ensure a unique identifier. For example, a large facility may have several patients named Paula Smith. If it were relying strictly on alphabetical filing by patient last and first name, multiple health records would be labeled Paula Smith on the file shelf.

A second disadvantage is that alphabetic files do not expand evenly. Statistically, almost half the files fall under the letters *B, C, H, M, S,* and *W.* A third disadvantage to the alphabetical filing system is that it is time-consuming to purge or clean out files for inactive storage. With an alphabetical filing system, each individual record needs to be checked for the last patient encounter to determine whether it is inactive (figure 7.3).

Figure 7.3.   Rules for alphabetic filing

---

1. File each record alphabetically by the last name, followed by the first name and middle initial. For example:

   Brown, Michelle L.
   Brown, Michelle S.
   Brown, Robert A.

   When the patient has identical last and first names and middle initial, order the records by date of birth, filing the record with the earliest birth date first.

2. Last names beginning with a prefix or containing an apostrophe are filed in strict alphabetical order, ignoring any apostrophes or spaces. For example, the names Mackel, Mac Bain, and Mc Dougal would be filed as:

   Macbain
   Mackel
   Mcdougal

3. In hyphenated names such as Manasse-O'Brien, the hyphenation is ignored and the record is filed as:

   Manasseobrien

Numeric Filing Systems

In a **numeric filing system,** records are filed by using the health record number. Numeric filing is a type of indirect filing system. To use an indirect filing system, an index or authority file needs to be consulted before the user can identify a record associated with a specific patient. In healthcare, the authority file is usually the **master patient index** (MPI). The filing clerk searches the MPI by patient name. When the correct patient is located in the MPI, the clerk uses the health record number to locate the patient's health record folder within the filing system.

At first glance, the numeric filing system may seem much more work than the alphabetic system. This can be true for organizations that have a very small number of records (hundreds). However, in larger organizations, the numeric filing system actually has many advantages over an alphabetic system. Following are the most common types of numeric filing systems:

- In **straight numeric filing systems,** records are arranged consecutively in ascending numeric order. The number assigned to each file is the health record number.

- The **terminal-digit filing system** is considered by many to be the most efficient. In this system, the last digit or group of last digits (terminal digits) is the primary unit used for filing, followed by the middle unit and the last unit of numbers. For example, 443798 could be broken down as 44-37-98, with 98 as the primary unit for filing, 37 as the secondary (middle) unit, and 44 as the tertiary unit. The record would be filed in the following arrangement: file section, 98; shelf number, 37; and folder number, 44. An example of how health records are filed using terminal-digit filing is shown in figure 7.4.

  The terminal-digit system is excellent for facilities with a heavy record volume. This is because large numbers can be divided into groups of several digits and still be easily managed for filing and retrieval purposes. In addition to ensuring that every record has a unique number, terminal-digit filing allows even file expansion, unlike an alphabetic or straight numerical filing system.

- The **middle-digit filing system** is very similar to the terminal-digit filing system. The primary unit is the middle unit, the secondary unit is the first unit to the left, followed by the last digits. For example, 443798 could be broken down with 37 as the primary unit, 44 as the secondary unit, and 98 as the tertiary unit. The record could be filed in the following arrangement: file section, 37; shelf number, 44; and folder number, 98.

Although the examples provided above for terminal- and middle-digit filing use a six-digit number, the number of digits in the health record number may vary depending on the healthcare facility. The length of any number and how it is divided depends on the organization. For example, one healthcare facility may have a health record number that is six digits in length. The highest number or volume of records that could be accommodated in

Figure 7.4. Example of terminal-digit filing

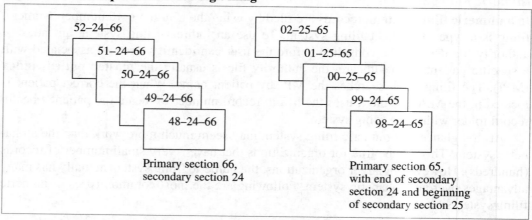

52–24–66
51–24–66
50–24–66
49–24–66
48–24–66

Primary section 66,
secondary section 24

02–25–65
01–25–65
00–25–65
99–24–65
98–24–65

Primary section 65,
with end of secondary
section 24 and beginning
of secondary section 25

Note: Records first are filed by the last two digits, then the middle two digits, and finally in numerical order by the first two digits.

such a numbering scheme would be 999,999 records. Another healthcare organization may have a numbering system containing seven digits. The capacity of this facility is much greater and can accommodate 9,999,999 records. Some facilities may have a three-digit primary unit. However, the method for filing would remain the same. The file section corresponding to the primary unit would be accessed first, followed by the secondary unit, and then the tertiary unit.

Alphanumeric Filing Systems

The **alphanumeric filing system** is the third type of system. This system uses a combination of alpha letters and numbers for identification purposes. The first two letters of the patient's last name are followed by a unique numeric identifier. The alphanumeric filing system is appropriate for small organizations. Although this system may be quicker because file clerks first file the record alphabetically, it still relies on accessing a master index or authority file to identify the unique numerical number.

Centralized Unit Filing Systems

In a centralized unit filing system, individual patient encounters are filed by the same unique identifier and in the same location. The unique identifier can be alphabetic, alphanumeric, or numeric. For example, in a small medical practice all of an individual's encounters may be filed together alphabetically by last name.

Usually, centralized unit filing is associated with the unit numbering system in which file clerks have to look in only one location for the patient's health record. In addition, the supply costs for record folders are reduced because all forms and information are filed together in one folder. Furthermore, computer or index card update issues are lessened using the unit numbering system. The patient retains the same health record number, regardless of the number of admissions or encounters.

Check Your Understanding 7.2

1. Consider the following sequence of numbers: 12-34-55, 13-34-55, and 14-34-55. What filing system is being used if these numbers represent the health record numbers of three records filed together within the filing system?

   A. Straight numerical filing
   B. Terminal-digit filing
   C. Middle-digit filing
   D. Family digit filing

2. The master patient index (MPI) is necessary to locate health records within the paper-based storage system for all the types of filing systems, except:

   A. Straight numerical
   B. Terminal-digit filing
   C. Middle-digit filing
   D. Alphabetical filing

3. The term used to describe a combination of paper-based and electronic health records is:

   A. Flexible
   B. Joint
   C. Mixed
   D. Hybrid

4. Which of the following is an advantage of a centralized unit filing system?

   A. Having the records close to the specialized patient care area
   B. One location in which to look for records
   C. Different file folders for each area of specialty
   D. Having different rules for each area

5. Which filing system is considered to be the most efficient?

   A. Straight numeric
   B. Terminal-digit
   C. Middle-digit
   D. Alphabetic

Storage Systems for Paper-based Records

Many options are available for storing health records. Paper-based records are stored in filing cabinets or shelving units. Other storage options include microfilm, off-site storage, and imaged-based storage. As healthcare facilities transition toward and implement the EHR, imaged-based systems are increasingly utilized. The choice of system depends on the needs of the facility and the amount budgeted within the department for record storage. For organizations with a high record volume, a combination of systems may be the appropriate choice. For organizations that have a very low volume of records, paper storage may be appropriate.

Filing Cabinets or Shelving Units

Paper-based records may be stored in vertical and lateral filing cabinets, open-shelf files, and compressible file systems. Vertical file cabinets are the traditional drawer files and come in sizes that can hold either letter or legal-sized records. The usual configuration is two or four drawers. Vertical file cabinets are appropriate for low-volume record storage. However, this type of filing equipment does not facilitate quick and easy filing and retrieval. Therefore, these file cabinets are rarely used to store health records.

Lateral filing units also have drawers. However, the drawers open laterally rather than vertically. They also include side-to-side rails for hanging files. These filing units range in size from two to five drawers and are usually 30 or 36 inches in width. Although easier for retrieval and filing than vertical cabinets, this type of equipment would only be used in low-volume offices.

The filing equipment of choice for housing health records is usually some configuration of shelf filing. Shelf files resemble open bookshelves. They can either be totally open or have receding doors. Shelf files are ideal for high-volume record storage. Shelving units with six shelves are usually used for record storage purposes. Moreover, shelf files save space. For example, one six-shelf unit offers file capacity equal to eight 30-inch-wide lateral file drawers.

A variation on open-shelf files is the mobile or compact file (figure 7.5). Instead of having aisle space between every row of files, mobile files conserve floor space by providing only one aisle of space. This is accomplished by mounting the file shelves on tracks secured to the floor. The shelves then are moved by hand, with mechanical assistance, or electronically. This type of storage system is ideal in facilities where space is a major concern. In most situations, an organization can double or even triple storage capacity in the same floor space, even when compared to other high-density filing systems such as open shelf.

A type of mobile or compact files is the lateral mobile shelving system. This filing system consists of stationary shelving in the back and file storage shelving that slides side to side in the front. This is an inexpensive way to increase the storage capacity of existing shelving or another record storage system. However, this type of shelving is only appropriate for low-volume record filing and retrieval activity.

Variations on open-shelf files are horizontal and vertical carousel systems. The horizontal carousel contains open-shelf files that revolve around a central spine or track system. Essentially, this type of filing system brings the files to the user, thus avoiding walking through aisles of files. The vertical carousel system brings all files or records to a standing or sitting workstation and can take advantage of vertical ceiling height. Vertical carousel systems are often used to store the manual MPI.

The amount of space, volume of records, and record usage or activity must be considered when determining the type of storage system to use. When space is not sufficient to house the number of shelving units needed to hold the records for the period of time required for patient care and other purposes, older health records are purged or removed from the file area. Generally, files that have been inactive for a certain period of time (for

Figure 7.5. **Mobile file units**

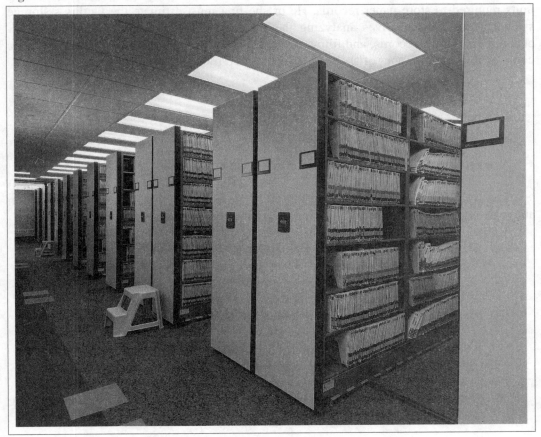

Source: Photo provided by Spacesaver Corporation. Reprinted with permission.

example, three years since the patient's last visit) are removed from the active filing area. **Purged records** are often microfilmed, sent to off-site storage facilities, or scanned. How frequently paper-based records are purged from the storage system is determined by not only space availability, but also the patient readmission rate and the use of patient record data. For example, a research hospital may maintain health records in paper format for a period of time longer than other facilities because researchers may need to access information about patients who have expired or who have not been admitted to the facility for a number of years.

The volume of health records can be enormous in many organizations. For example, when an acute care facility admits 50 patients per day and treats the same number of patients in the emergency department, 100 health records are generated. Over a year, this amounts to 36,500 new records. If approximately one inch is required to store five paper records, the organization would need approximately 7,300 inches, or approximately 608 feet, of filing space.

An HIM professional often has responsibility for planning the file space and shelving units required to store paper records. He or she first must estimate the facility's storage system needs. This involves analyzing the volume indicators, such as number of discharges, size of the records, and filing inch capacity of the storage unit. For example, one could estimate the number of shelving units required by using the following information:

Shelving unit shelf width = 36 inches

Number of shelves per unit = 7 shelves

Average record thickness = ½ inch

Average annual inpatient discharges = 8,500 patients

The following demonstrates how the HIM professional would use the information above to estimate the number of shelving units required to house one year's records:

1. Determine the linear inch capacity of each shelving unit.

    36 inches per shelf × 7 shelves per unit = 252 inches per shelving unit

2. Determine the linear filing inches needed for the volume of records.

    8,500 average annual inpatient discharges × ½ average record thickness
    = 4,250 filing inches required to store one year of inpatient discharge records

3. Determine the number of shelving units required by dividing the required filing space by the shelving unit linear inch capacity.

    4,250 ÷ 252 = 16.8 shelving units

Actually, 17 shelving units would be required to store one year of inpatient records because it is impossible to purchase 16.8 shelving units.

However, most HIM departments store more than inpatient discharge records. Outpatient records also are typically stored in the HIM department, and the storage requirements for the outpatient records must be considered when estimating the record storage needs. Consider the following example:

Hospital XYZ has the following volume statistics:

Average inpatient discharges per year = 10,000

Average inpatient record thickness = 1 inch

Average outpatient visits = 22,500

Average outpatient record thickness = ¼ inch

Each shelving unit has 7 shelves, each 36 inches wide

The following demonstrates how the HIM professional would estimate the number of shelving units required to house one year's records:

1. Determine the linear filing inches required to house inpatient and outpatient records.

10,000 inpatient discharges per year × 1 inch
= 10,000 linear filing inches required

22,500 outpatient visits per year × ¼ inch
= 5,625 linear filing inches required

10,000 + 5,625 = 15,625 linear filing inches
needed for inpatient and outpatient records

2. Determine the linear filing inches per shelving unit.

36 inches per shelf × 7 shelves per unit = 252 inches per shelving unit

3. Divide the required filing space by the shelving unit linear inch capacity.

15,625 inches needed ÷ 252 inches per shelving unit
= 62 shelving units required to store the records

Therefore, for this example 62 shelving units would be required to store one year of records.

In an EHR environment, the HIM professional works with the software vendor and the information technology (IT) department to determine the required computer storage space and medium.

File Folders

Paper-based health records that are stored on shelving units, in compressible filing units, or in filing cabinets are housed in filing folders. During an average inpatient encounter, a health record exceeding 100 pages is common. These various reports and documents must be sorted and stored in their own file folders. File folders come in two standard weights, 11 and 14 point. Higher weights such as 20 point are also available. The higher weight is the most durable and would be the folder of choice for active records that receive heavy filing and retrieval activity. In addition to weight, consideration should be given to the selection of top or side tabs. Top-tab folders are used in vertical or lateral shelving systems. Side-tab folders, which are the usual configuration for health records, are used in all open-shelf filing systems.

Health record folders also should include some type of fastening system to hold the record documents together. Record fasteners are two pronged and can be up to 2 inches long. They can be placed at the top or sides of the file folder. Usually, folders are purchased with fasteners attached, although for low-volume operations self-adhesive fasteners can be

Figure 7.6.   Color-coded file folders

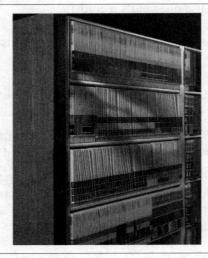

Source: Photo provided by Spacesaver Corporation. Reprinted with permission.

used and installed by office staff. Dividers also may be placed in health records to separate clinical, inpatient, outpatient, and/or administrative documents.

Whether the facility uses an alphabetic or numeric filing system, file folders should be color coded for easy filing and retrieval. For example, in a numeric filing system, each single digit is a specific color. Therefore, one can easily locate misfiles by visually scanning a shelf for disruption of the color pattern of a particular file shelving section. Figure 7.6 demonstrates the use of color coding on file folders. For high-volume systems, color coding of files is done at the factory. For lower-volume systems, color-coded labels can be affixed to the file folders.

Microfilm-based Storage Systems

Storage of paper-based health records consumes an enormous amount of space. There are other options for record storage that significantly reduce space needs. A traditional alternative that has been used over the past three or more decades is micrographics or microfilm. Microfilm is a good storage alternative for inactive or infrequently used health records.

Essentially, the microfilming process converts paper documents to archive-stored images by taking a picture of the original document and storing it as a very small negative. Because the images are so small, a special microfilm viewer or reader that magnifies each image must be used to read them. Microfilm comes in a variety of formats, including:

- *Roll microfilm:* This format stores each document page sequentially in a long roll. One roll of microfilm can potentially hold thousands of images and the health records of hundreds of patients. However, the fact that the roll stores document pages sequentially can be a disadvantage. For example, if the organization is using a serial numbering system, a patient's entire health record covering multiple encounters may be on separate roles of microfilm. This makes retrieval less efficient.

- *Jacket microfilm:* In this format, a roll of microfilm is cut and placed into special four-by-six-inch jackets with several sleeves to hold the images. A benefit of this option is that all the patient's records can be collected together in the same jacket or several jackets can be combined in a small paper folder. Thus, the record becomes a unit record holding all information about the patient. Jackets can be color-coded with the patient's health record number and name. They are usually filed using the same type of filing system (alphabetic, straight numerical, terminal digit) used for paper files.

- *Microfiche:* This format can be a copy of a microfilm jacket or a direct copy of the source health record. It is made on Mylar film and is the same size as the microfilm jacket. When used as a copy from the source health record, the microfiche eliminates the need to cut rolls of film to fit into microfilm jackets. Sometimes organizations store their health records in microfilm jackets. These jackets are never removed from the HIM department. Instead, when the information is needed, a microfiche copy is made using a special duplicator and then provided to the requesting care areas.

One benefit of microfilm is that it is much less costly for backup than digital media. Moreover, microfilm is acceptable as courtroom evidence and provides good security because it is difficult to tamper with.

Off-site Storage Systems

Because space for paper-based records has become limited and/or microfilm has become cost prohibitive, many healthcare facilities use off-site storage companies to house purged records. An off-site storage company is usually a contracted service that stores health records. The company then retrieves and delivers records requested by the healthcare facility's HIM department for a fee.

The healthcare facility should carefully evaluate the off-site storage company's capabilities for storing records securely for the entire retention period. Considerations for off-site storage include climate control, fire protection, pest and dust control, physical protection from burglary or vandalism, and cost.

Image-based Storage Systems

The use of digital document imaging is increasing as healthcare facilities implement EHR or hybrid record systems. Essentially, a document imaging system scans and indexes an original source document to create a digital picture that can be retrieved via the computer. Most document imaging solutions include production scanners that can scan hundreds or thousands of documents a day, plus a workflow or document management application that makes the scanned information available to a department or an entire enterprise. When scanned, the images are stored on electronic media, such as a magnetic or optical disk.

Unlike microfilm rolls, the optical disk is a random-access device and retrieval of documents is much faster. Additionally, document images can be viewed by more than one person at one time and at different locations.

One of the greatest benefits of document imaging is increased efficiency by eliminating the requirement to move and track paper documents through workflow. Document imaging also helps solve the problem of lost or misplaced paper or microfiche documents. Moreover, it saves money by reducing the need for storage space and by decreasing the work of file clerks. Document imaging is discussed in additional detail under hybrid record systems.

Check Your Understanding 7.3

1. What type of paper-based storage system conserves floor space by eliminating all but one or two aisles?

   A. Open-shelf units
   B. Carousel systems
   C. Mobile filing units
   D. Filing cabinets

2. What feature of the filing folder helps locate misfiles within the paper-based filing system?

   A. Fasteners
   B. Folder weight
   C. Color coding
   D. Barcodes

3. In a paper-based system, the HIM department routinely delivers health records to:

   A. Patient registration
   B. Nursing units
   C. Billing department
   D. Administration

4. Which of the following paper weights would be the most durable for the medical record folder?

   A. 11
   B. 14
   C. 20
   D. 8

5. What microfilm format is inefficient when patients have multiple admissions on microfilm?

   A. Roll
   B. Jacket
   C. Microfiche
   D. Both roll and jacket

Retrieval and Tracking Systems for Paper-based Records

Tracking the location of health records removed from a paper-based storage system area is key to ensuring their accessibility to authorized persons. The **outguide** is the most common type of tracking system used to track paper-based health records. An outguide is usually made of strong colored vinyl with two plastic pockets. It is the size of a regular record folder and is placed in the record location when the record is removed from the file. Outguides normally come with either a bottom or a middle tab with the word OUT printed on it to indicate that a health record has been removed from the file shelf.

The larger of the plastic pockets is used to hold loose reports or other documents that come to the HIM department while the original record is charged out. The smaller pocket is used to house information about who checked out the health record, its current location, when it was checked out, and the expected return date. This checkout information may be either a handwritten or computerized requisition slip generated from a tracking system.

A **requisition** is a request from a clinical or other area in the organization to charge out a specific health record. The requisition may be in paper or electronic form. The information contained on a requisition usually includes patient's name, health record number, date of the request, date and time needed, name of the requestor, and location for delivery.

In a paper-based requisition system, the requisition slip has multiple copies. One copy is the routing slip that comes with the health record. Another copy goes in the outguide. A third copy may be used as a transfer notice and sent to the HIM department if the health record is subsequently transferred to another location. For example, if a record were requested from the intensive care unit (ICU), it would be transferred to the medical unit when the patient was transferred from the ICU to the medical floor.

In many institutions, the chart-tracking and requisition systems are built into the automated information system. In this case, paper requisition slips are replaced by automated requisitions sent directly to the HIM department and all pertinent data are retained in a database. Automated systems such as these are similar to a library book checkout system. With an automated system, it is easy to track how many records are charged out of the HIM department at any given time, their location, and whether they have been returned on the due dates indicated. Figure 7.7 provides an example of how the computer screen appears in a chart-tracking system. A barcode representing the health record number is often on the file folder to facilitate data entry into the computer chart-tracking system. The HIM department should create facility-wide policies and procedures for the proper use of tracking systems. Further, an audit for health records not returned in a timely manner should be performed on a regular basis.

In healthcare organizations that use hybrid or EHR systems, tools built into the systems, such as workflow automation and audit trails, can provide tracking information—for example, who accessed which records and for what purpose.

Retention and Destruction of Paper-based Records

An important HIM function is to ensure that there are relevant retention and destruction policies and procedures in place. An organization's duty of care over health information

Figure 7.7.   Chart-tracking computer screen: Location tab

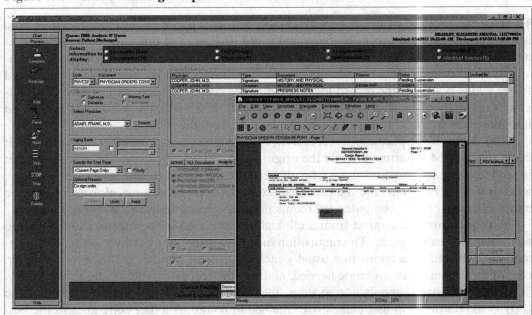

extends from the time of creation to the time of destruction. Therefore, both health information **retention** and **destruction** policies and procedures must be in place. It is recommended good practice that retention and destruction policies be approved by the health information manager, chief executive officer, medical staff, malpractice insurer, and legal counsel.

Retention policies and procedures relate to what information must be retained, for how long, and in what form. Destruction policies and procedures relate to what information may be destroyed, appropriate destruction methods, and required documentation of destruction.

Retention

Established policies and procedures are important to ensure that the healthcare organization is in compliance with appropriate accreditation standards, state statutes, federal regulations, and administrative laws for health information retention. The following are general guidelines recommended for establishing retention policies and procedures (AHIMA 2011e):

- Ensure patient health information is available to meet the needs of continued patient care, legal requirements, research, education, and other legitimate uses of the organization.

- Include guidelines that specify what information is kept, the time period for which it is kept, and the storage medium on which it will be maintained (e.g., paper, microfilm, optical disk, magnet tape).

- Include clear destruction policies and procedures that include appropriate methods of destruction for each medium on which information is maintained.

- Compliance documentation:

  — Compliance programs should establish written policies to address the retention of all types of documentation. This documentation includes clinical and medical records, health records, claims documentation, and compliance documentation. Compliance documentation includes all records necessary to protect the integrity of the compliance process and confirm the effectiveness of the program, including employee training documentation, reports from hotlines, results of internal investigations, results of auditing and monitoring, modifications to the compliance program, and self-disclosures.

  — The documentation should be retained according to applicable federal and state law and regulations and must be maintained for a sufficient length of time to ensure its availability to prove compliance with laws and regulations.

  — The organization's legal counsel should be consulted regarding the retention of compliance documentation.

- The majority of states have specific retention requirements that should be used to establish a facility's retention policy. In the absence of specific state requirements for record retention, providers should keep health information for at least the period specified by the state's statutes of limitations or for a sufficient length of time to prove compliance with laws and regulations. If the patient was a minor, the provider should retain health information until the patient reaches the age of majority (as defined by state law) plus the period of the statute of limitations, unless otherwise provided by state law. A longer retention period is prudent, since the statute may not begin until the potential plaintiff learns of the causal relationship between an injury and the care received. In addition, under the False Claims Act (31 USC 3729), claims may be brought for up to 7 years after the incident; however, on occasion, the time has been extended to 10 years.

- Unless longer periods of time are required by state or federal law, AHIMA recommends that specific patient health information be retained for established minimum time periods (table 7.2).

Table 7.2. **AHIMA's recommended retention standards**

Health Information	Recommended Retention Period
Diagnostic images (such as x-ray film) (adults)	5 years
Diagnostic images (such as x-ray film) (minors)	5 years after the age of majority
Disease index	10 years
Fetal heart monitor records	10 years after the age of majority
Master patient/person index	Permanently
Operative index	10 years
Patient health/medical records (adults)	10 years after the most recent encounter
Patient health/medical records (minors)	Age of majority plus statute of limitations
Physician index	10 years
Register of births	Permanently
Register of deaths	Permanently
Register of surgical procedures	Permanently

Source: AHIMA. "Retention and Destruction of Health Information. Appendix D: AHIMA's Recommended Retention Standards" (updated August 2011).

Destruction

"While ideally records should be kept forever, this is not always practical" (Menke 2009). Record destruction, however, should only be done in accordance with federal and state law and written retention and destruction policies of the organization. Furthermore, records involved in any open investigation, audit, or litigation should not be destroyed.

Some states require creation of an abstract, notification of patients, or specify the method of destruction. In the absence of any state law to the contrary, AHIMA recommends the following guidelines for destruction of health information (AHIMA 2011e):

- Destroy the records so there is no possibility of reconstruction of information.

  — Appropriate methods for destroying paper records include burning, shredding, pulping, and pulverizing.

  — Methods for destroying microfilm or microfiche include recycling and pulverizing.

  — The laser disks used in write once-read many (WORM) document imaging applications cannot be altered or reused, making pulverization an appropriate means of destruction.

  — The preferred method for destroying electronic data is magnetic degaussing. (Data are stored in magnetic media by making very small areas called magnetic domains change their magnetic alignment to be in the direction of an applied magnetic field. Degaussing leaves the domains in random patterns with no preference to orientation, rendering previous data unrecoverable.) Proper degaussing ensures that there is insufficient magnetic remanence to reconstruct the data. Overwriting can also be used to destroy electronic data. (To overwrite, cover the data with a pattern, its complement, and then another pattern—for example, 00110101, followed by 11001010, and then 10010111.) In theory, however, files that have been overwritten as many as six times can be recovered. Total data destruction does not occur until the original data and all backup information have been destroyed.

— Although magnetic tapes can be overwritten, it is time-consuming and there can be areas on a tape that are unresponsive to overwriting. Degaussing is considered preferable.

- Document the destruction, including:

  — Date of destruction

  — Method of destruction

  — Description of the disposed records

  — Inclusive dates covered

  — A statement that the records were destroyed in the normal course of business

  — The signatures of the individuals supervising and witnessing the destruction

- Maintain destruction documents permanently. These are called **certificates of destruction.** Such certificates may be required as evidence to show records were destroyed in the regular course of business. When facilities fail to apply destruction policies uniformly or where destruction is contrary to policy, courts may allow a jury to infer in a negligence suit that if records were available, they would show the facility acted improperly in treating the patient. Figure 7.8 provides an example of a certificate of destruction.

- If destruction services are contracted, the contract must meet the requirements of the Health Insurance Portability and Accountability Act (HIPAA) Privacy Rule. In addition, the contract should:

  — Indemnify the healthcare facility from loss due to unauthorized disclosure

  — Require that the business associate maintain liability insurance in specified amounts, at all times the contract is in effect

  — Provide proof of destruction

  — Specify the method of destruction

  — Specify the time that will elapse between acquisition and destruction of data

The method of destruction should be reassessed annually, based on current technology, accepted practices, and availability of timely and cost-effective destruction services.

Figure 7.8. Sample certificate of destruction

> **Medical Practice Name**
>
> The information described below was destroyed in the normal course of business pursuant to a proper retention schedule and destruction policies and procedures.
>
> Date of destruction: _____
>
> Description of records or record series disposed of: _____
>
> _____
>
> _____
>
> Inclusive dates covered:
>
> _____
>
> _____
>
> Method of destruction:
>
> ☐ Burning   ☐ Shredding   ☐ Pulping
> ☐ Demagnetizing   ☐ Overwriting   ☐ Pulverizing
> ☐ Other: _____
>
> Records destroyed by: _____
>
> Witness signature: _____
>
> Department manager: _____
>
> *Note: This sample form is provided for discussion purposes only. It is not intended for use without advice of legal counsel.*

Source: AHIMA 2011.

Check Your Understanding 7.4

1. Under the False Claims Act, claims may be brought up to how many years?

   A. 10 years
   B. No more than 7 years
   C. Generally 7 years, but could go as high as 10
   D. Depends but is generally 5 to 7 years

2. Record retention should be based on:

   A. Desires of the medical staff only
   B. HIPAA standards
   C. State regulations only
   D. State regulations and AHIMA recommendations

3. Which of the following is the appropriate method for destroying microfilm?

   A. Burning
   B. Shredding
   C. Pulverizing
   D. Degaussing

4. Which of the following is the appropriate method for destroying electronic data?

   A. Burning
   B. Shredding
   C. Pulverizing
   D. Degaussing

5. The tool used to track paper-based health records is:

   A. Compliance documentation
   B. Outguide
   C. Requisition
   D. MPI

Record Processing of Paper-based Records

Record processing refers to the procedures performed that support the maintenance of each individual patient record in an organized and standard manner. This function facilitates efficiency, accuracy, and completeness of the health record. The quality of patient care is adversely affected when complete and correct information is not readily available for delivery of patient care. Moreover, administrative and other functions, such as evaluating clinical quality performance, billing, and research, would be negatively affected without a complete and accurate health record. The following activities are normally considered record processing.

Admission and Discharge Record Reconciliation for Paper-based Records

In a paper-based record environment, when a patient is admitted to the healthcare facility, the HIM professional will search the MPI to see if the patient has had any previous admissions to the facility. If a patient has a previous admission, the health records from the previous admission(s) may be retrieved from the permanent storage area and delivered to the patient care unit for the medical staff to reference the patient's past medical history.

Likewise, once the patient is discharged from the healthcare facility, the health record of each patient discharged is either retrieved by the HIM professional or delivered to the HIM department for record processing. However, before health records can be processed, the HIM professional must assure that all health records for patients discharged on that date have been received. The health records received by the department are compared to a discharge list, which is usually generated from the hospital's registration system. The process of assuring that all the records of discharged patients have been received by the HIM department for processing is called **record reconciliation.**

If the health record of any discharged patient has not been received by the HIM department, the HIM professional must locate the health record. The chart-tracking system is updated to reflect that old records have been returned and filed in the permanent file area. The current records of discharged patients are then sent to the health record processing area.

Record Assembly Functions for Paper-based Records

In a paper-based system, the health record is organized or assembled after the patient is discharged from the hospital or other setting. *Assembly* means that each page in the patient record is organized in a pre-established order. The pre-established record order of the pages varies from facility to facility. Each page in the patient record is reviewed to ensure that it belongs to that record.

Deficiency Analysis for Paper-based Records

After the record is assembled in the correct order, HIM professionals review or analyze it to make sure that there are no missing reports, forms, or required signatures and that all documents contain the patient's name and health record number. This review for deficiencies is an example of **quantitative analysis.**

The quantitative analysis or record content review process can be handled in a number of ways. Some acute care facilities conduct record review on a continuing basis during a patient's hospital stay. Using this method, personnel from the HIM department go to the nursing unit daily (or periodically) to review each patient's record. This type of process is usually referred to as a **concurrent review** because review occurs concurrently with the patient's stay in the hospital. Other acute care facilities perform the quantitative analysis the day following the patient's discharge from the hospital. This type of review is called **retrospective review** because it occurs after the patient has left the facility. In this process, the patient's health record is received in the HIM department, usually the day after discharge, and reviewed by an HIM professional.

Whether done concurrently or retrospectively, the review usually involves checking to ensure that:

- All forms and reports contain correct patient identification (name, health record number, gender, attending physician, and so on).

- All forms and reports are present. For example, when the patient is admitted for a cholecystectomy, a minimum set of operative reports, consents, and forms should be present (operative consent form, anesthesia form, operative report, recovery room report, pathology report, and so on).

- Reports requiring authentication (that is, operative, pathology, discharge summaries, history and physicals, and radiology reports) have signatures or have been appropriately authenticated.

When deficiencies are identified, the HIM professional usually completes a **deficiency slip** that indicates what reports are missing or require authentication and enters this information into a computer system that logs and tracks health record deficiencies or maintains a copy of the deficiency slip in a tickler file. See figure 7.9 for a sample paper deficiency slip. Usually, the deficiency slip is a multipart form, one copy appended to the health record and one or more copies filed by physician name. A record with deficiencies is called an incomplete record.

Automated systems for tracking record deficiencies are commonly used to facilitate the process. An automated health record deficiency tracking system has a computer screen

Figure 7.9. Sample deficiency slip

Physician/Practitioner's Name: _____

Health Record Number: _____

Patient's Name: _____

Discharge Date: _____

Analyzed by: _____

Date: _____

Signatures Required	Dictation Required	Missing Reports
_____ History	_____ History	_____ History
_____ Physical	_____ Physical	_____ Physical
_____ Consultation	_____ Consultation	_____ Consultation
_____ Operative Report	_____ Operative Report	_____ Operative Report
_____ Discharge Summary	_____ Discharge Summary	_____ Discharge Summary
		_____ Radiology Report
Other	Other	_____ Pathology Report
		_____ Progress Notes
_____ _____	_____ _____	
_____ _____	_____ _____	Other
_____ _____	_____ _____	_____ _____
		_____ _____
		_____ _____

Figure 7.10.   Chart deficiency screen

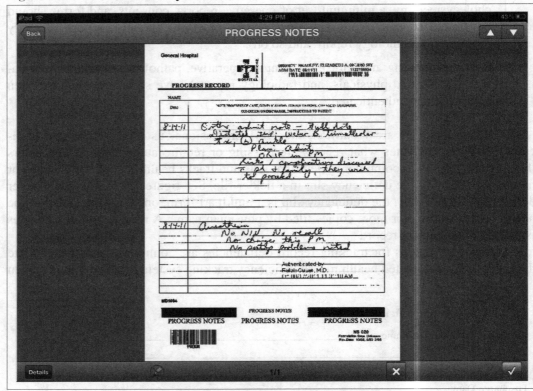

that looks similar to the deficiency slip to allow for data entry (figure 7.10). If an automated deficiency system is utilized, each deficiency for a specific record is entered into the computer as is the name (or identification number) of the physician responsible for completing the deficiencies. This type of system stores the entered data into a database for later retrieval or analysis. Such systems reduce the amount of clerical work, make retrieval of deficiency information faster and easier, and provide for automatic report and statistics generation about deficiencies.

When deficiencies are identified and documented, they must be corrected. When reports or forms are missing, HIM personnel should try to locate them.

The health record content review (its requirements and how extensive it is) depends on the individual organization and its medical staff bylaws, rules, and regulations as well as on licensing and accreditation body requirements. Other inpatient facilities, such as long-term care and rehabilitation institutions, usually follow the same processes as acute care facilities. Outpatient facilities such as clinics or physician office practices usually conduct a quantitative analysis after each patient visit or on a periodic basis.

The HIM department often receives reports belonging to a health record that has already been assembled or scanned. These unprocessed reports are called loose reports or loose filing. In a paper-based system, the medical record must be located and the loose report assembled into the appropriate location within the record.

Monitoring Completion of Paper-based Records

When deficiencies in the health record, such as reports that need to be dictated or signed by a physician or other health professional, are identified through quantitative analysis, the record is filed in a specially designated area of the HIM department, frequently called the incomplete record file. A copy of the deficiency slip is filed in an index box called a tickler file, usually by the name of the responsible healthcare professional. Periodically, the HIM department notifies the appropriate individuals of the incomplete or deficient record status and requests that they come to the department to rectify it. In the EHR environment, or where electronic signatures and electronic authentication of medical records is accepted, the incomplete record file may be eliminated.

After the healthcare professional completes the record deficiencies, the record is reanalyzed to ensure its completeness. If no deficiencies are found, the deficiency slip is removed and/or the deficiency tracking system is updated to reflect that the health record is completed. The health record then is routed to the storage and retrieval area for filing in the permanent file.

When an incomplete record is not rectified within a specific number of days as indicated in the medical staff rules and regulations, the record is considered to be a **delinquent record.** Generally, an incomplete record is considered delinquent after it has been available to the physician for completion for 15 to 30 days. The HIM department monitors the delinquent record rate very closely to ensure compliance with accrediting standards that define performance expectations or processes that must be in place.

Handling Corrections, Errors, and Addendums in Paper-based Records

Health records may occasionally require that entries be amended, corrected, or deleted. Regardless of the media used to store the health record, policies must be in place to assure the integrity of the information contained in the health record as a business record, legal health record, and as a patient care communication tool. The healthcare facility must have written policies that specify who, when, and how amendments, corrections, and deletions may be made to a health record.

Corrections

In a paper-based health record environment, corrections to health record entries are corrected by drawing a single line through the original entry, writing "error" above the entry, and then the practitioner signs, dates, and times the correction. For example:

Error: correction "female" Jane Smith, MD 12/11/11 15:00
The 72-year-old white ~~male~~ presents to the emergency room with a 4-hour history of severe lower right quadrant abdominal pain.

Addendums

Addendums and amendments are a type of correction. An addendum is a supplement to a signed report that provides *additional* health information within the health record. In this type of correction, a previous entry has been made and the addendum provides additional information to address a specific situation or incident. The following guidelines should be followed for making addendums (AHIMA e-HIM Workgroup on Maintaining the Legal EHR 2005):

- Document the current date and time.
- Write "addendum" and state the reason for the addendum, referring back to the original entry.
- Identify any sources of information used to support the addendum.
- When writing an addendum, complete it as soon after the original note as possible.

Amendments

An amendment is a *clarification* made to the health information after the original documentation has been final signed by the provider. An amendment must be dated, timed, signed, and attached to the original document that it is amending (Hall et al. 2009).

Authorization and Access Control for Paper-based Records

"**Access control** is the process that determines who is authorized to access patient information in the health record" (AHIMA Workgroup on Electronic Health Records Management 2004). Access control involves determining which individuals or groups should be granted access, what portions of the health record should be available, and what rights should be granted. For example, HIM professionals responsible for release of information would be granted the right to print the EHR or copy the paper record, whereas a nurse or physician would be granted view-only access to the EHR. Physicians and nurses would be granted the right to enter patient information in the EHR.

For the paper portion of the health record, authentication is the process the HIM staff performs to verify the identity of the person requesting access and determining if that person is authorized to access the record. Checking a photo identification card (for example, employee identification card) is one example of authentication of the person's right to access the paper-based health record. Access cards may also be used to authenticate the user's right to access the record system. Access cards are often used in combination with passwords or personal identification numbers (PINs) as a method of authenticating the person's identity (AHIMA Workgroup on Electronic Health Records Management 2004).

Forms Design, Development, and Control for Paper-based Records

An important part of ensuring adequate health record content is the function of forms design and development. In a paper record system, forms make possible the capture of adequate healthcare documentation. The HIM department often participates in forms design in consultation with a forms vendor. The basic concept behind any form is that it must meet the needs of the end user. This means that the form must fulfill its intended purpose, include all the necessary data, and be easy to use.

Forms Design and Development

One of the first steps in forms design is to identify the purpose, use, and potential users of the form. This basic information will drive the rest of the design process. For example, when the purpose of the form is to meet a licensing requirement, the data elements contained on it must comply with the requirement. When the form is to be used by multiple individuals, a multicopy version might be appropriate. When it is to be completed by hand, it must allow enough space for handwriting.

After the purpose, use, and potential users of the form have been identified, it is important to ensure that the new form does not duplicate one already in place. Organizations often needlessly duplicate forms because they have no mechanism for forms tracking.

Any forms design project should follow a number of guidelines. The following are common design elements for paper forms (AHIMA 1997):

- All forms should contain a unique identifying number for positive identification and easy inventory control.

- Each form should include original and revised dates for the tracking and purging of obsolete forms.

- Each form should have a concise title that clearly identifies the form's purpose.

- The facility's name and logo should appear on each page of the form.

- For clinical forms, patient identification information (name, health record number, billing number, physician name and number, date of birth, admission date, and room number) should appear on every page.

- For clinical forms, a signature line should appear at the bottom, and there should be no question about what has been authenticated. If initials are used, space also should be provided for the full name and title so that each set of initials is identified.

- Data-entry methodology should be considered when the information is to be keyed into a computer. The order of the form should mirror the data-entry order to ensure that information is entered consistently.

- Optical character reader codes and barcodes should be printed in the upper left-hand corner of the form when imaging the health record is a possibility.

- A standard of 8.5 by 11 inches is the best size for a document. Bifold and trifold documents are difficult to handle and copy in a closed chart.

- Form colors should be black ink on white paper. If color coding is desired, a strip of color along one margin is the best option.

- Documents that contain punched holes should have a margin of at least 3/4 inch. All other margins should be at least 3/8-inch wide.

- Vertical and horizontal lines assist the user in completing and reviewing the form. Bold lines should be used to draw the reader's eye to an important field.

- Sufficient space should be provided to complete the entry (for example, 1/16 inch for typed letters and 1/3-inch high for handwritten entries).

- Titles for boxes and fields should be located in the top left-hand corner of the box or field.

- Paper ranging from 20 to 24 pounds in weight is recommended for use in copiers, scanners, and fax machines.

- Type size should be no smaller than 9 points for lowercase letters and 10 points for uppercase letters.

The principles of good design are critical when forms are used in document imaging systems. For example, the use of colored paper or ink other than black should be minimized or eliminated because the color can adversely affect the quality of the scanned images. Also, the use of scanned images requires forms to contain a barcode that identifies the document type, thus enabling the form to be placed in the proper location within the EHR. Forms not containing a barcode must be indexed separately when scanned into the computer.

Clinical Forms Committee

Every healthcare organization should have a forms or design (for EHR systems) committee. The medical records committee also may function in this capacity. This committee should provide oversight for the development, review, and control of all enterprise-wide information capture tools, including paper forms and design of computer screens. The committee should be composed of information users and include representatives from the following:

- Health information management

- Medical staff

- Nursing staff

- Purchasing

- Information services

- Performance improvement

- Support or ancillary departments

- Forms vendor representative

In addition, anyone directly affected by the new form or computer view should be invited to attend the forms committee meeting. For example, when a form is being redesigned for use in the intensive care unit, nurses or physicians from that clinical area should be invited to give their input.

Forms Control, Tracking, and Management

Forms control, tracking, and management are important issues. At a minimum, a good forms control program includes the following activities (Barnett 1996):

- *Establishing standards:* Written standards and guidelines are essential to ensure that good design and production practices are followed. A forms manual should be developed. **Standards** are fixed rules that must be followed for every form (for example, where the form title should be located). A guideline, on the other hand, provides general direction about the design of a form (for example, usual size of the font used).

- *Establishing a numbering and tracking system:* A unique numbering system should be developed to identify all organizational forms. A master form index should be established, and copies of all forms should be maintained for easy retrieval. At a minimum, information in the master form index should include form title, form number, origination date, revision dates, form purpose, and legal requirements. Ideally, the tracking system should be automated.

- *Establishing a testing and evaluation plan:* No new or revised form should be put into production or use without a field test and evaluation. Mechanisms should be in place to ensure appropriate testing of any new or revised form.

- *Checking the quality of new forms:* A mechanism should be in place to check all newly printed forms prior to distribution. This should be a quality check to ensure that the new form conforms to the original procurement order.

- *Systematizing storage, inventory, and distribution:* Processes should be in place to ensure that forms are stored appropriately. Paper forms should be stored in safe and environmentally appropriate environments. Inventory should be maintained at a cost-effective level, and distribution should be timely.

- *Establishing a forms database:* In an electronic system that supports document imaging, a forms database may be used to store and facilitate updating of forms. Such a database can provide information on utilization rates, obsolescence, and replacement of individual forms or documentation templates.

Quality Control Functions in Paper-based Systems

All the HIM functions discussed in this section must be managed appropriately to ensure the quality of health record content as well as the security, accessibility, and timeliness of the information contained in the health record. However, merely having a process for health record review does not totally ensure content quality. Further, having good forms design practices does not necessarily mean that all forms that are developed are necessary. Therefore, the organization must establish systems to help monitor and control the quality of record content and processes. The strategies discussed thus far help ensure quality control over the management of health record content.

In addition to quality monitoring performed to ensure compliance with Joint Commission standards, HIM functions should be monitored for accuracy and timeliness. Below are examples of control measures that may be established to ensure that processes are being performed correctly and that systems are functioning as expected. The department should establish standards and criteria that indicate an acceptable level of performance. After quality control standards are established, it is important to establish a monitoring system to determine whether goals are being met. Corrective action should be implemented when error or accuracy rates are deemed to be at an unacceptable level. Chapter 10 describes specific techniques and quality improvement practices.

Storage and Retrieval

Various standards can be set to monitor the quality of the storage and retrieval process. Filing accuracy can be checked by conducting a random audit of the storage area. To conduct a study, a section of the permanent file room can be checked for misfiles. Any misfiles found are noted, and a filing accuracy rate can be determined and compared against the established standard. For example, if the standard is that 99 percent of the health records will be filed correctly, a sample of filed records can be checked for misfiles. If 550 health records are checked and 7 misfiles are found, the error rate is 1.27 percent (7 divided by 550 multiplied by 100, which would make the accuracy rate 98.7 percent). Some organizations have a rechecking process whereby a record is filed and tagged and another employee follows up and checks the accuracy of the filing. Similarly, in a digital imaging system, indexing and quality should be checked through a defined quality assessment process to ensure the retrievability of health information.

Timeliness of the storage and retrieval processes also can be monitored. Examples of standards that may be established to determine the timeliness of HIM services are:

- An average of 50 records will be filed in an hour.
- Records for the emergency department will be retrieved within 10 minutes of the request.
- Loose materials will be filed in either the record or the outguide pocket within 24 hours of receipt in the HIM department.
- An average of 190 pages of scanned records will be indexed in an hour.
- Scanned records will be available online within 24 hours of discharge.

Record Processing

In a paper-based health record system, physicians come to the incomplete record area to dictate and sign medical records. If records are unavailable when they arrive, the chart completion process is delayed. The availability of records can be monitored by comparing the incomplete chart lists for a sample of physicians against the charts available to the physicians when they come to the HIM department. For example, if seven physicians worked on completing charts on a particular day with a total of 210 incomplete records collectively and a total of 35 charts were not available, the nonavailable chart rate is 16.6, or 17 percent (35 divided by 210 multiplied by 100).

Check Your Understanding 7.5

1. What should be done when the HIM department's error or accuracy rate is deemed unacceptable?

   A. A corrective action should be taken.
   B. The problem should be treated as an isolated incident.
   C. The formula for determining the rate may need to be adjusted.
   D. Re-audit the problem area.

2. The forms design committee:

   A. Provides oversight for the development, review, and control of forms and computer screens
   B. Is responsible for the EHR implementation and maintenance
   C. Is always a subcommittee of the quality improvement committee
   D. Is an optional function for the HIM department

3. Statements that define the performance expectations and/or structures or processes that must be in place are:

   A. Rules
   B. Policies
   C. Outcomes
   D. Standards

4. In a paper-based system, individual health records are organized in a pre-established order. This process is called:

   A. Retrieval
   B. Assembly
   C. Analysis
   D. Reordering

5. Reviewing a health record for missing signatures and missing medical reports is called:

   A. Assembly
   B. Indexing
   C. Analysis
   D. Coding

6. Reviewing the record for deficiencies after the patient is discharged from the hospital is an example of what type of review?

   A. Concurrent
   B. Retrospective
   C. Real-time
   D. Qualitative

7. Incomplete records that are not completed by the physician within the time frame specified in the healthcare facility's policies are called:

   A. Suspended records
   B. Delinquent records
   C. Loose records
   D. Default records

Instructions: Indicate whether the following statements are true or false (T or F).

8. ____ In a paper-based record, errors should be completely obliterated.

9. ____ Addendums should document the date the event actually happened—not the date it was documented.

10. ____ The best practice for forms design is to use white paper with black ink.

HIM Functions in a Hybrid Environment

Many large healthcare organizations are transitioning toward or have implemented electronically stored health records. Facilities transitioning to the EHR sometimes use a **hybrid record.** A hybrid record is a combination of paper-based and electronically stored health data. The hybrid record environment includes a combination of paper-based and EHR systems. Hybrid and electronic records are discussed in more detail in chapter 16 and later in this chapter.

The hybrid record is a transitional health record that at some point becomes an electronic health record. The percentage of paper-based components and electronic components varies from facility to facility. Dictation or transcription, laboratory results, and radiology reports are often the first components to be accessible electronically. Imaging functions that comprise the electronic document management systems are the often utilized as the hybrid record evolves toward becoming an EHR. The Theory into Practice case at the beginning of this chapter is an example of the transition from a paper-based to a hybrid record environment. The following sections describe management of the hybrid record.

The hybrid record comprises individually identifiable data, in any medium, that are collected, processed, stored, displayed, and used by healthcare professionals. For example, dictation, laboratory, and x-ray results might be available electronically, whereas progress notes, ancillary care, provider information, graphic sheets, and doctors' orders remain on paper. Other health information may be maintained on various other media types such as film, video, or an imaging system. This information in the health record is collected and/or directly used to document healthcare delivery or healthcare status (AHIMA e-HIM Workgroup on Health Information in a Hybrid Environment 2003).

Storage, Retrieval, and Retention of Hybrid Records

Although the intent of storage, retrieval, and retention functions for hybrid records is the same as for paper-based systems, how the functions are carried out may differ. This is due in part to the different media and technologies used that require different work functions and workflow patterns.

Use of Electronic Document Management Systems

One commonly used system in the hybrid environment is an electronic document management system (EDMS). An EDMS encompasses a wide range of technologies used to provide portions of an electronic health record and does more than manage documents after they are scanned into the computer. A robust EDMS performs many functions. Among these are scanning a paper document and creating a digital image, using workflow management technologies to schedule and monitor work tasks, multimedia technologies and formats, and technology to move computer-generated content such as a history and physical or discharge summary from a transcription system to an EDMS without creating paper (AHIMA e-HIM Workgroup on Electronic Document Management as a Component of EHR 2003).

In a hybrid record environment, the document imaging component is often used to make paper-based records electronically accessible post-discharge. See figure 7.11 for an example of an EDMS that is used as a chart repository to provide electronic access to the hybrid record.

Some components of the health record may be electronically transmitted to the EDMS via computer interfaces and computer output to laser disk (COLD) fed documentation.

Figure 7.11. EDMS sample screen

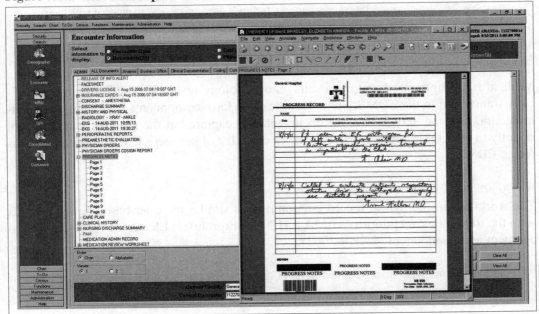

Figure 7.12. Checklist for planning an EDMS

1. **Assembly:** Ensure the record is in the optimal physical order for efficient processing for records to be scanned.

2. **Types of records:** Determine where each of the following is stored and how reconciliation will occur on a daily basis (check in and account for each chart, even outpatients).

3. **Forms inventory/format:** Create inventory with sample of each form.

4. **Loose/late reports:** Determine policy on receipt of loose reports, adding in order or filing in back of chart, and codifying once entered into system.

5. **Physical layout of equipment:** Determine workflow in HIM department.

6. **Analysis, deficiency, and electronic signature process:** Ensure that the medical record is complete and that entries are timely according to established rules and regulations.

7. **Paper storage/filing:** Determine disposition of paper documents after scanning.

8. **Communications:** Ensure that all stakeholders receive critical information about the new system and the impact.

9. **Quality assurance:** Index and perform quality control after documents are scanned. Indexing is performed to assign document names and encounter numbers to each document. Quality control is performed on 100 percent of images to review the quality of the scan. In addition to this initial quality control, ongoing quality monitoring should be performed on a random basis.

10. **Policy and procedures:** Develop new policy and procedures.

11. **Legal considerations:** The information stored is the entity's business record (in healthcare, the legal record). A plan to house this information on media other than paper must be scrutinized by legal counsel to ensure that the technology being considered can comply with federal and state laws, requirements for licensure, and credentialing along with operational needs and that it is consistent with existing policies and procedures. There should also be a risk management component to ensure that there will be no compromise to patient care and that documents required for lawsuits remain available. This latter consideration may impact a facility's decision on how to proceed with their documents once scanned into the imaging system.

Source: AHIMA e-HIM Workgroup on Electronic Document Management as a Component of EHR 2003.

Medical transcription, laboratory results, and radiology results are most often electronically transferred to the EDMS. Some facilities also have components of the nursing documentation and ancillary healthcare documentation captured at the point of care and sent directly to the EDMS. Figure 7.12 provides a checklist of key steps in the planning process for an EDMS.

Workflow Using an EDMS

The workflow in the hybrid record environment is similar to paper-based health records with the following exceptions (AHIMA e-HIM Workgroup on Electronic Document Management as a Component of EHR 2003):

- The permanent storage and retrieval areas are replaced with electronic storage of imaged records.

- The incomplete record area resides in the EDMS.
- Medical coding may be done remotely.

The paper-based record assembly process described earlier is replaced by record preparation and document scanning in the hybrid and EHR environment. Records are prepared for scanning by repairing torn forms, removing staples, and adding header forms to the front of the records. Barcoding is often used to identify the document type for the scanning process. Additionally, checks are made to ensure that all pages are identified accurately as part of the individual patient's record. Depending on the extent to which barcoded forms are used, the record may still need to be assembled to ensure proper order by date and type of report. The record is then scanned using high-speed scanners.

Following is an example of the workflow post-discharge in a hybrid record system where an EDMS is utilized:

1. Paper record is retrieved from the patient care unit.
2. Record receipt is reconciled with the list of patients discharged for that date.
3. Records are prepared by removing staples, clips, and repairing torn pages.
4. Each page of the record is checked to verify that it does indeed belong to that patient.
5. Record is scanned into the EDMS.
6. The quality of the scanned image is reviewed. If the image is not of high quality, the image is enhanced or rescanned.
7. Forms missing a barcode are indexed and placed into the proper location within the health record.
8. Records are analyzed for missing documents (for example, discharge summaries, operative reports, history and physicals, and so forth).
9. Records are analyzed for missing signatures. Deficiencies are electronically tagged.
10. The record is sent to an incomplete work queue for the physician to complete.
11. Records are also placed in a coding queue to await coding.
12. When the record is completed, it is locked to prevent further changes to the health record.
13. Scanned paper records are boxed or sent to storage and kept for the period specified in the record retention policy.

An advantage in using an EDMS is that it can help manage work tasks. Workflow rules built into the system automatically identify the work tasks to be performed, how they should be routed, and sequences and dependencies among tasks. For example, in management of record completion, as the status of dictation changes from dictate to transcribe to sign to signed, the status of the deficiency system is automatically updated without human intervention. At the same time, a request for dictation or review and signature is routed to the physician's in-box.

The use of an EDMS also allows tasks to be performed in secure locations outside the facility. Primary examples include coding and transcription functions (AHIMA e-HIM Workgroup on Electronic Document Management as a Component of EHR 2003).

Record Retention

Retention of health records in a hybrid record environment is similar to that for health records in a paper-based environment. The healthcare facility must consider state and federal regulations, statutes of limitation, research and educational needs, and patient care needs.

Special consideration must be given to how long to keep paper records that have been scanned into the EDMS. Facilities have several quality checks integrated in the record processing function, to assure that the best possible image is included in the electronic portion of the health record. The facility must have a policy on how long the paper portion of the imaged record is maintained after the record is complete. The AHIMA e-HIM Workgroup on Electronic Document Management as a Component of EHR (2003) states, "As a general rule, paper records should be boxed up after all paper is scanned, indexed and released in the EDMS, stored for no longer than six months and then destroyed." Other facilities may decide to maintain the paper records of imaged documents for longer or shorter periods of time. The storage capacity, the cost, and the definition of the facility's legal record will determine how long these paper records are maintained.

When the hybrid records include paper records that are not imaged, this should be indicated in the EDMS. For example, fetal monitoring strips are often cumbersome to scan because they are a continuous feed of paper. The decision may be made by the facility to maintain the fetal monitoring strips and other similar documents on paper and store them within the facility. The location and existence of these paper portions of the record must be noted in EDMS.

Handling Corrections

As noted earlier, health records may occasionally require that entries be amended, corrected, or deleted. Regardless of the media used to store the health record, policies must be in place to assure the integrity of the information contained in the health record as a business record, as a legal health record, and as a patient care communication tool. The healthcare facility must have written policies that specify who, when, and how amendments, corrections, and deletions may be made to a health record.

In a hybrid record environment how corrections are handled will depend upon how the documentation is created. If the record is in paper format then the guidelines discussed earlier under paper-based systems apply. If the record is in an electronic format then the guidelines discussed in the following section under electronic record systems apply. Records stored in EDMSs present unique situations for handling corrections. If the record is stored in an EDMS then the following guidelines should be followed

(AHIMA e-HIM Workgroup on Electronic Document Management as a Component of EHR 2003):

- **Corrections:** Policies and procedures should identify how and by whom corrections are made. Business rules may apply that identify who can access and correct unsigned documents. Facilities should develop guidelines for changes made to signed and unsigned documents. For example, if a document is changed or corrected, typically the copy with the error is removed from view within the EDMS. However, a copy of the original document must be available. This can either be a manual or electronic process. It is important that all staff are aware that these documents are available. Some type of annotation may be made in the EDMS system so that clinical staff will know whom to contact if they feel they may need to see the original document.

- **Retraction** involves removing a document from standard view, removing it from one record, and posting it to another within the electronic document management system. In the record from which the document was removed, the document would not be considered part of the designated record set or visible to anyone. Someone should be designated by the organization to view or print the retracted documents. An annotation should be viewable to the clinical staff so that the retracted document can be consulted if needed.

- **Resequencing** involves moving a document from one place to another within the same episode of care. No annotation of this action is necessary.

- **Reassignment** (synonymous with misfiles) involves moving the document from one episode of care to a different episode of care within the same patient record. As with retractions, someone in the organization should be designated to view or print the reassigned document. An annotation should be viewable to the clinical staff so that the reassigned document can be consulted if needed.

Search, Retrieval, and Manipulation

In a hybrid record environment, health data include both paper and electronic documents and use both manual and electronic processes. The goal of the hybrid record system is to enable retrieval of information to assist healthcare professionals in providing quality patient care and reporting patient outcomes.

As stated earlier, when the hybrid record includes paper records that are not imaged, this should be indicated in the EDMS. In these cases the facility will have to rely on usual paper-based location identification and retrieval processes.

Within the EDMS, documents may be retrieved in various ways and the method used depends upon on how the EDMS has been installed and configured. For example, retrieval could be through the organization's intranet, the Internet, an application on the desktop, or within the clinical system. Access should be integrated so that the end user does not have to move between various systems. To ensure that the right information is delivered to the right person, the system should provide basic and advanced search methods that include filters as well as security measures that track access and limit access on a need-to-know basis.

The facility should have distribution policies in place to safeguard the information. Among the policies that should be established are: online viewing for authorized users, online viewing and printing (usually limited to HIM staff to support release of information functions), and auto fax for authorized users.

For security and privacy reasons retrieval and viewing of information should be in designated work areas throughout the organization. Remote viewing should be provided to authorized individuals and should use customary security processes for remote access. Remote viewing may include viewing documents from physician offices and for remote record completion or remote coding to name a few instances (AHIMA e-HIM Workgroup on Electronic Document Management as a Component of EHR 2003).

Authorization and Access Control for Hybrid Records

As stated earlier, "Access control is the process that determines who is authorized to access patient information in the health record" (AHIMA Workgroup on Electronic Health Records Management 2004). Since the hybrid record is comprised of both paper and electronic components, the healthcare facility must address authorization to access both the paper and electronic portions of the record.

For the electronic portion of the health record, authentication is the process that the computer goes through to assure that the person accessing the system is an authorized user (see chapter 14). The most common method of authentication is the use of user names and passwords (AHIMA Workgroup on Electronic Health Records Management 2004). Access control is strengthened by the use of strong passwords that include numbers, upper- and lowercase letters rather than easily identifiable names or numbers.

As stated earlier, for paper portions of the health record, checking a photo identification card, access cards, or a combination of passwords or personal identifications numbers are methods for authentication.

Nonrepudiation measures "limit an EHR's user's ability to deny (repudiate) the origination, receipt, or authorization of a data exchange by that user" (Dougherty 2008). Nonrepudiate means to accept. An example of a nonrepudiation measure is the use of electronic signatures to assure the authorship of a record entry in which rules built into the EHR will date and time stamp the entry and then lock the notation or report to prevent future changes to the original information documented in the record. Nonrepudiation is also discussed later in the section about electronic health records.

Quality Control Functions for Hybrid Records

Quality control processes are essential for insuring data integrity and availability. In addition to those already discussed, the following are important quality control functions.

Quality Control in Record Processing

The quality control function in the hybrid record should be performed at the time records are processed. Each page of the health record must be checked prior to document scanning to verify that it belongs to that patient's record. After the record is scanned, the images are often reviewed to ensure that a high-quality image has been achieved. If an image is found to be unclear, the document is rescanned after adjustments are made to the computer or scanner.

Record processing is also monitored to assure that records are processed in a timely manner and meet standards set forth by the healthcare facility. For example, a healthcare facility may have a standard that all records for discharged patients are scanned and available in the EDMS for completion within 24 hours of discharge. The HIM professional may monitor the health records processed on a daily basis to determine if this standard is being met.

Reconciliation in the Hybrid Record

Record reconciliation is the process of checking individual data elements, reports, or files against each other to resolve discrepancies in accuracy of data and information. In paper-based systems, reconciliation usually is incorporated into the chart analysis process. In a hybrid record system, reconciliation may be even more challenging because data are being captured from a variety of sources and moving across interfaces. Figure 7.13 provides a comparison of reconciliation quality control tasks across paper-based, hybrid, and electronic health record systems.

Issues and Challenges with Hybrid Records

For many large acute care facilities, the hybrid record environment has been implemented as a transitional state toward the electronic health record. However, with hybrid record environments there are several challenges the facility encounters. Some of the challenges a facility may encounter include:

- Defining the legal record
- Dual work processes
- Legibility of handwritten scanned documents
- Compliance with meaningful use criteria may be difficult to determine

One of the main challenges with the hybrid record is establishing a policy of what comprises the legal health record, discussed later in this chapter. In a hybrid environment the health record includes both paper and electronic elements. Therefore, it is important to document the location of the documentation in the entire health record. The healthcare facility must have the ability to make available disparate documentation sources for patient care and other purposes. Some facilities have addressed this challenge by imaging the paper portion of the health record into an EDMS so that the entire health record is available electronically regardless of the documentation's original source or media type. The

Figure 7.13.   Comparison of reconciliation processes

	Paper Systems	Hybrid or Transitional Systems	Fully Electronic Systems
Inpatient visits	Verify that a record exists for each discharge. Verify correct patient type registered (for example, inpatient, short stay, observation status) to ensure accurate billing.	Same with addition of monitoring canceled admits.	Same
Emergency department, outpatient, and clinic visits	Verify that record exists for every registration. Verify correct registration of multiple visits in one day according to APC regulations.	Same with addition of monitoring canceled admits.	Same
Interface engine	No	Monitor at least daily interface engine logs for failed reports. Research and correct documents that fail to cross an interface between disparate computer systems (for example, stand-alone transcription system to an EHR). Ensure that documents are posted to the correct encounter and are in the correct location. Verify that content remains constant when moved from one system or database to another. The extent of reconciliation increases with the number of disparate computer systems.	Same
MPI and EMPI	Correction of duplicate patient name and number entries by accurately matching patients to paper records. Ensure match to all computer systems (for example, lab, radiology, pharmacy, billing). Correct other or duplicate names in system (for example, legal guardian names) through verification of secondary matched data elements.	Same issues as in the paper-based record.	Same issues as paper-based and hybrid records. The EHR may be able to automatically identify components of records in other electronic systems and provide notification of changes.
In-box maintenance	None	Monitor unopened mail and incomplete documentation (for example, unsigned dictations, unreviewed results, and documents copied to others that have failed).	Same

Figure 7.13.   Comparison of reconciliation processes *(continued)*

	Paper Systems	Hybrid or Transitional Systems	Fully Electronic Systems
Auto-faxing files and automatic data transfers	Monitor transcription systems for failures of sent documents. Periodically validate fax numbers and that remote fax machines are located in secure locations.	Expanded monitoring including voice recognition and direct charting.	Expanded to include transfer of EHR files for ROI, download of EHR data to patient personal health records, and community-based health records or databases
Work queues	Primarily focused on HIM department systems such as coding and incomplete chart tracking	Expanded to include scanning system	Extended to entire EHR
Downtime processes	None except for HIM functions	Ensure online data are captured following downtime through direct entry or scanning.	In addition to more detailed and lengthy post-downtime data capture, ensure that data flow to data warehouse or other repository in a timely manner and in the correct sequence. Track legal EHR variations from policy on individual records for all downtimes as well as historically for lengthy downtimes.
Patient/legal guardian amendments Living wills and durable powers of attorney for healthcare decision making	Ensure documentation is filed in paper record.	Ensure documentation is scanned into EHR or post a flag that indicates such documents exist and how to access them.	Ensure documentation is either scanned into EHR or ensure amendment made online adheres to the agreed upon amendment process.

Source: AHIMA Workgroup on Electronic Health Records Management 2004.

policies defining the legal health record must be updated as the paper-based component and functions transition into electronic formats.

A useful tool for planning and managing the transition is a grid or matrix that describes where and how to find specific document types that constitute the hybrid health record. The grid can be used as a planning tool to ensure each major document type is addressed during the document's transition from paper to electronic media. It is important to maintain the grid in real time so that users will be able to see the paper-to-electronic status of all documents. Over time, the grid will serve as a monitoring tool and as a dynamic source that can be used to help define the legal status of each document (for example, the point at which an electronic document stored in a system replaces its former paper document as the legal document). (AHIMA 2010c)

Figure 7.14 shows a sample grid or matrix called a Legal Source Legend that may be used to help define the legal health record and monitor the transition to the electronic health record.

Figure 7.14. **Sample legal source legend**

	[Organization's Name] Hybrid Health Record Legal Source Legend

Report/Document Types	Media Type (P)aper/ (E)lectronic	Source System Application (non-paper)	Currently Printed	Currently Scanned	Date Stored Electronically	Stop Printing Start Date
Admission History and Physical	P/E	System 1 (e.g., laboratory system)			1/1/2002	1/1/2003
Attending Admission Notes	P					
Physician Orders	E					
Inpatient Progress Notes	P					
Discharge Summary	E	System 2 (e.g., transcription system)			1/1/2002	4/1/2002
Inpatient Transfer Notes	E	System 1			1/1/2002	
Outpatient Progress Notes	P					
Clinical Laboratory Results (Preliminary/Interim)	E	System 2			1/1/1999	1/1/1999
Clinical Laboratory Results (Final)	E	System 2			1/1/1999	1/1/2000
Radiology Reports	E	System 3 (e.g., radiology system)			7/1/2003	
Care Flow Sheets	E	System 1			6/1/2003	
Medication Records	E	System 1			7/1/2003	
Clinical Consult Reports	E	System 1			1/1/2002	
Preoperative, Preprocedure Notes	P					
Pathology Reports	E	System 2			1/1/1999	1/1/2000
Organ or Tissue Donation or Transplants	P					
Patient Problem List (Summary List)	E	System 1			8/1/2003	
Urgent Care and Emergency Records	P					
Consents*	E	System 4 (e.g., document imaging system)			TBD	
Advance Directive						
Correspondence*	E	System 4			TBD	
Preoperative Anesthetic Assessments and Plans	P					
Intraoperative Documentation	P					
Postoperative Documentation	P					
Brief Postoperative Notes	P					
Surgical Operative Reports	E	System 1			1/1/2002	

*Scanned electronic documents.

The policies must clearly identify what components will be disclosed upon request.

Dual work processes often exist with a hybrid record. Dual work processes refer to coexisting paper and electronic processes used in the hybrid health record environment. The management of the health record may be challenging as paper and electronic work processes coexist. Health records may still need to be assembled to some degree before scanning and imaging can be done. Additionally, when scanning and imaging are part of the hybrid record process, there is a cost associated with the existence of paper records and the cost of imaging equipment to provide an electronic view of the health record. Paper records still need to be retrieved from patient care units and then reconciled with discharged patient lists to assure that all health records are received in preparation for the scanning process.

Handwritten paper documents of hybrid health records also present challenges of legibility. In addition to the issue of legibility of the handwritten documents, these scanned documents are sources of unstructured data. Although electronically available through the imaging process, these unstructured data sources reduce the ability of the electronic system to data mine or search the health records for specific information.

As part of the incentive program for use of the electronic health records set forth by ARRA, eligible healthcare professionals and hospitals must demonstrate that they are meaningfully using the data stored within the EHR they adopt. Depending on the functionality and the extent of the use of an EDMS, the user of a hybrid health record may have difficulty demonstrating that they have met some of the meaningful use criteria. For example, several of the stage one meaningful use criteria for eligible hospitals require structured data. If a large portion of the health record is imaged, data capture would be unstructured, thus making retrieving the information from the EDMS difficult. Another key issue in implementing an EHR is the varying levels of computer experience of the clinicians who will use the system. Some clinicians will embrace the use of the EHR as a tool that has been long overdue in adoption, while other clinicians will be reluctant to use the technology because of their unease with the use of computer technology. The HIM professional must be a change agent in the process and recognize that the transition to an electronic health record will be easier for some than others. Not all clinicians embrace the use of technology and some may be reluctant to use the new technology.

Check Your Understanding 7.6

1. Which of the following chart-processing activities is eliminated with an EDMS that uses scanned images of barcoded forms?

   A. Chart preparation
   B. Scanning
   C. Assembly
   D. Quality review

2. One of the advantages of an EDMS is that it can:

   A. Help manage work tasks
   B. Decrease the time records should be retained
   C. Improve communications with physicians
   D. Eliminate all of the problems encountered with the paper record

3. Which term indicates that a document has been removed from standard view?

   A. Correction
   B. Resequencing
   C. Reassignment
   D. Retraction

4. Which term is the process of checking individual data elements, reports, or files against each other to resolve discrepancies?

   A. Nonrepudiation
   B. Reconciliation
   C. Reassignment
   D. Resequencing

5. Which of the following could be used to determine if someone has the right to view a health record?

   A. Photo identification
   B. Signature
   C. Verbal request for record
   D. Phone call prior to arrival

HIM Functions in an Electronic Environment

An electronic health record (EHR) is an organization-wide health record that is stored and accessible via the computer. The EHR is comprised of many of the same electronic components utilized in the hybrid record, but is a record that resides entirely in electronic format with work processes performed via the computer. The EHR provides for clinical decision support through the availability of references, interoperability to promote health information exchange (HIE), and standardized terminology that supports data mining for data use. The Healthcare Information and Management Systems Society defines the EHR as (HIMSS 2012):

> A longitudinal electronic record of patient health information generated by one or more encounters in any care delivery setting. Included in this information are patient demographics, progress notes, problems, medications, vital signs, past medical history, immunizations, laboratory data and radiology reports. The EHR automates and streamlines the clinician's workflow. The EHR has the ability to generate a complete record of a clinical patient encounter—as well as supporting other care-related activities directly or indirectly via interface—including evidence-based decision support, quality management, and outcomes reporting.

With the signing of the American Recovery and Reinvestment Act (ARRA) in February 2009, the federal government further defined a qualified electronic health record as including "patient demographics and clinical health information, such as medical history and problem lists and has the capacity." "The Medicare and Medicaid EHR Incentive Programs require the use of certified EHR technology. Standards, implementation specifications, and certification criteria for EHR technology have been adopted by the Secretary of the Department of Health and Human Services. EHR technology must be tested and certified by an Office of the National Coordinator (ONC) Authorized Testing and Certification Body (ATCB) in order for a provider to qualify for EHR incentive payments" (CMS November 2011).

The following is a list of the ONC certification criteria.

- Computerized provider order entry
- Drug-drug, drug-allergy interaction checks
- Maintenance of up-to-date problem list
- Maintenance of active medication list
- Maintenance of active medication allergy list
- Record demographics
- Record and chart vital signs
- Smoking status
- Calculation and submittal of clinical quality measures
- Clinical decision support
- Electronic copy of health information
- Electronic copy of discharge instructions
- Exchange of clinical information and patient summary record
- Access control
- Emergency access
- Automatic log-off
- Audit log
- Integrity
- Authentication
- General encryption
- Encryption and decryption of electronic health information
- Accounting of disclosures
- Drug-formulary checks

- Advance directives
- Incorporation of laboratory test results
- Generation of patient lists
- Patient-specific education resources
- Medication reconciliation
- Submission to immunization registries
- Electronic submission of lab results to public health agencies
- Public health surveillance
- Automated measure calculation

The EHR has evolved into more than an imaged record residing within an electronic document management system. Chapter 16 provides a full description of the EHR and its capabilities.

Transition Functions to an EHR

The hybrid record as discussed earlier is a transitional health record that exists as the paper-based record evolves to an electronic health record. Both paper and electronic components comprise the hybrid record.

> Yes, the EHR promises to streamline information handling and ultimately reduce costs and improve care, but it's important to remember that the EHR is really just automation, not a magic bullet. If a hospital has poor workflow processes, migrating to electronic records will simply automate those poor processes, not solve them. Therefore, re-engineering manual systems and processes represents a major opportunity for reducing costs, improving service and establishing the correct infrastructure to transition to the automated hospital record. (Santangelo 2009)

The planning process must include key clinical and administrative departments that contribute to the health record. The following steps must be considered and are key throughout the planning process to move to a totally electronic environment (Reino 2005):

- Workflow analysis
- Defining the facility's legal record
- Standardization of forms and processes
- Development of a forms catalog or inventory
- Barcoding of forms
- Criteria development for hardware, software, and vendors

- Vendor selection (certified vendors)
- IT plan
- Privacy and security procedure establishment
- Change management
- Training of staff and medical staff

A complete discussion of transition to the EHR is provided in chapter 16. Issues related to the planning, design, development, implementation, and maintenance of information systems including vendor selection processes are explained in chapter 14.

Record Filing and Tracking of EHRs

Record filing is a function that is either eliminated or reduced in an electronic health record environment. As data are increasingly captured and entered into the computer at the point of care, paper documentation is greatly reduced and therefore the need to file the record is either reduced or eliminated. As discussed earlier, for portions of a record that are stored in an EDMS, there may be some stored paper records awaiting destruction based on the facility's retention policies.

The traditional tracking of record access and the locations of charts removed from the paper-record system is replaced by the monitoring for access of the electronic health record by the use of an audit trail. The Center for Medicare and Medicaid Services EHR certification criteria require an audit trail. The CMS certification criteria state, "Generate audit log. Enable a user to generate an audit log for a specific time period and to sort entries in the audit log according to any of the elements specified in the standard" (45 CFR §170.302(r)). The function and content of audit trails are discussed in chapter 14.

Record Processing of EHRs

In an EHR, the loose report is indexed. Indexing is similar to filing in the paper record and ensures that documents are placed in the right location within the right record to allow future retrieval.

Record completion in the electronic health record environment is done via the computer. Healthcare professionals can access, complete, and authenticate records using an electronic in-box, work list, or other tool. Management reports related to record completion can be generated by the system. Work queues allow the record to be routed to multiple locations within the EHR to allow simultaneous completion of the record by multiple users. Health records with deficiencies assigned to multiple physicians for completion are completed in a more timely manner in the EHR environment because more than one person can access the record at a time. Health records can be routed to the medical coding queues at the same time the records are available for completion in the record completion queues, thus facilitating the medical coding and billing process.

As with record filing discussed earlier, the traditional tracking of the locations of charts removed from the paper-record system is replaced by monitoring access to the electronic health record by the use of an audit trail.

Version Control of EHRs

Paper-based, hybrid, and electronic health records may have different versions of a document within the health record. One example where multiple versions could exist is in an electronic health record where there is a medical report that is unsigned and then the physician signs the report. This represents two versions of the same document, one signed and the other unsigned. Similarly, when a physician makes changes to a health record or amends it, multiple versions of the document exist. Each healthcare facility must have policies and procedures for **version control** stating which versions of the document will be viewable within the health record. Documents must be flagged when an earlier version of a document exists and the date and time of the availability of each version of the document must be clearly documented (AHIMA Workgroup on Electronic Health Records Management 2004).

Management of Free Text in EHRs

Free-text data is the unstructured narrative data that is the result of a person typing data into a word-processing system. The nature of free text is that it is undefined, unlimited, and unstructured. For these reasons, it is more difficult for a search engine to find, retrieve, and manipulate data than structured text.

The use of free text should be limited in an electronic health record environment. Transcribed medical reports are an example of documents comprised of free text data (AHIMA Workgroup on Electronic Health Records Management 2004). Many of the advantages of manipulation of data that the EHR offers are lost when the health record is comprised of large amounts of unstructured data.

Pointing and clicking to select structured text is one option that may be utilized by users of the electronic health record. The use of voice recognition software also provides for structured data capture.

Some EHR users prefer to copy and paste text from existing documents in order to speed up the documentation process. Allowing this practice should be assessed carefully as certain risks are inherent in the use of copy functionality. These tools, if used inappropriately, may undermine the clinical decision-making process. For example, copying information into the wrong patient health record could adversely impact patient care. And overuse of disk space, from redundant copied information, can affect overall system response time. Specific risks to documentation integrity of using copy functionality include (Gelzer et al. 2008, 6):

- Inaccurate or outdated information that may adversely impact patient care
- Inability to identify the author or what they thought

- Inability to identify when the documentation was created

- Inability to accurately support or defend E/M codes for professional or technical billing notes

- Propagation of false information

- Internally inconsistent progress notes

Because of these issues, the healthcare facility should have in place policies and procedures related to the copying and pasting of free text in the electronic health record. Similar to documentation in paper-based records, individuals who document in the EHR must be held accountable for their entries.

Management and Integration of Digital Dictation, Transcription, and Voice Recognition

The most common method to capture dictation in the EHR is the use of **digital dictation.** With digital dictation, the physician dictates a medical report and the transcriptionist transcribes the dictation into a structured medical report. The transcribed reports are electronically transmitted to the EHR. The EDMS attaches an auto-signature deficiency and the transcribed report is then electronically routed to a physician work queue for signature.

Voice recognition technology is another method used to capture dictated reports in the EHR. With voice recognition technology the computer software captures the dictation and converts the dictation to text. Back-end voice recognition software or voice recognition at the point of transcription is most commonly used for routine transcription of reports. As the practice of medical transcription evolves and voice recognition software is utilized, emphasis is placed on medical language editing, data quality control, and text/document management.

The HIM professional must establish a monitoring system and implement productivity standards to access the accurate capture of dictation and transmission to the EHR. The implementation of quality and productivity standards reduces turnaround time and improves the quality of information for workflow processes and regional health data exchange.

Reconciliation Processes for EHRs

As with the reconciliation process for the paper-based and hybrid records, electronic health records require that the HIM professional verify that there is an electronic health record present in the system for every discharged patient and verification of reports. Figure 7.15 provides a comparison of these processes for the paper-based, hybrid, and electronic systems.

Figure 7.15.   Comparison of reconciliation processes

	Paper Systems	Hybrid or Transitional Systems	Fully Electronic Systems
Inpatient visits	Verify that a record exists for each discharge. Verify correct patient type registered (for example, inpatient, short stay, observation status) to ensure accurate billing.	Same with addition of monitoring canceled admits.	Same
Emergency department, outpatient, and clinic visits	Verify that record exists for every registration. Verify correct registration of multiple visits in one day according to APC regulations.	Same with addition of monitoring canceled admits.	Same
Interface engine	No	Monitor at least daily interface engine logs for failed reports. Research and correct documents that fail to cross an interface between disparate computer systems (for example, stand-alone transcription system to an EHR). Ensure that documents are posted to the correct encounter and are in the correct location. Verify that content remains constant when moved from one system or database to another. The extent of reconciliation increases with the number of disparate computer systems.	Same
MPI and EMPI	Correction of duplicate patient name and number entries by accurately matching patients to paper records. Ensure match to all computer systems (for example, lab, radiology, pharmacy, billing). Correct other or duplicate names in system (for example, legal guardian names) through verification of secondary matched data elements.	Same issues as in the paper-based record.	Same issues as paper-based and hybrid records. The EHR may be able to automatically identify components of records in other electronic systems and provide notification of changes.
In-box maintenance	None	Monitor unopened mail and incomplete documentation (for example, unsigned dictations, unreviewed results, and documents copied to others that have failed).	Same

Figure 7.15.   **Comparison of reconciliation processes** (*continued*)

	Paper Systems	Hybrid or Transitional Systems	Fully Electronic Systems
Auto-faxing files and automatic data transfers	Monitor transcription systems for failures of sent documents. Periodically validate fax numbers and that remote fax machines are located in secure locations.	Expanded monitoring including voice recognition and direct charting.	Expanded to include transfer of EHR files for ROI, download of EHR data to patient personal health records, and community-based health records or databases
Work queues	Primarily focused on HIM department systems such as coding and incomplete chart tracking	Expanded to include scanning system	Extended to entire EHR
Downtime processes	None except for HIM functions	Ensure online data are captured following downtime through direct entry or scanning.	In addition to more detailed and lengthy post-downtime data capture, ensure that data flow to data warehouse or other repository in a timely manner and in the correct sequence. Track legal EHR variations from policy on individual records for all downtimes as well as historically for lengthy downtimes.
Patient/legal guardian amendments Living wills and durable powers of attorney for healthcare decision making	Ensure documentation is filed in paper record.	Ensure documentation is scanned into EHR or post a flag that indicates such documents exist and how to access them.	Ensure documentation is either scanned into EHR or ensure amendment made online adheres to the agreed upon amendment process.

Source: AHIMA Workgroup on Electronic Health Records Management 2004.

Managing Other Electronic Documentation

New information technologies are producing patient health information and documentation that was unknown even a decade ago. For example, e-mail and voice mail records and audio and video data could be part of an EHR. Consequently, policies and procedures should be in place for the management of all electronic information that is generated about patients in healthcare organizations, regardless of the record type and medium (AHIMA Workgroup on Electronic Health Records Management 2004). The following section discusses some of these media and associated issues.

E-mail

In today's healthcare setting, e-mail is often used as a main form of communication. Often e-mail is used to communicate patient-specific information. The organization should have in place policies and procedures that address the creation, storage, and maintenance of e-mail messages. When patient-identifying information is communicated via e-mail, an e-mail management system should be used for inclusion of the data in the electronic health record. An e-mail management system should consist of a centralized archive capable of enforcing archiving policies. The e-mail management system should also allow e-mails to be classified by type (that is, patient e-mail) and apply rules for archiving, retention, and integration of e-mails into the electronic health record. The management system can also be set up to automatically encrypt patient e-mails to provide a level of security (AHIMA Workgroup on Electronic Health Records Management 2004).

The patient portal is a functionality of the electronic health record that allows patients to access information from protected health information (e.g., lab results), educational information, etc. The patient portal may also include an e-mail communication component for patient–provider communication. If a patient portal is utilized, providers must have policies to address the inclusion of patient–provider communication in the EHR.

Voice Mail

Voice mail containing patient-specific information regarding the patient condition and/or treatment should also be included in the electronic record. In paper-based systems, this is usually handled by transcribed notes placed into the medical record. In an EHR environment, voice mail messages and telephone conversations should be documented. The messages should include provider and patient identification, date and time of actual conversation or message, and the date and time of entry into the EHR. Each of these messages should also be indexed so that they can be searched, retrieved, routed, or purged (AHIMA Workgroup on Electronic Health Records Management 2004).

Handling Materials from Other Facilities

Materials in the form of hardcopy records, diagnostic images, cine films (non-static imaging), or compact discs (CDs) may be received from other facilities that have provided an individual with care. In paper-based systems, the disposition of hardcopy materials is handled according to the organization's written policies and procedures. Usually the material is incorporated into the medical record.

> Some state laws address how to classify external records; however, in the absence of state law, the organization must determine if external records will be a part of the health record. . . . The organization's legal counsel should be consulted prior to determining policy regarding the inclusion of external records as part of the legal health record. (AHIMA 2011b)

Search, Retrieval, and Manipulation Functions of EHRs

In an electronic record environment, large volumes of data are entered into the EHR in structured and unstructured formats. For additional information on structured and unstructured formats, see chapter 16. The goal of the electronic health record system is to enable retrieval of information to assist healthcare professionals in providing quality patient care and reporting patient outcomes. The higher degree of structure in the data entered into the EHR provides for the retrieval of meaningful data and ease of manipulation of that data.

Data mining is the process of analyzing data from different perspectives and summarizing it into useful information. Data mining software is one of a number of analytical tools for analyzing large amounts of data. It allows users to analyze data from many different dimensions, categorize it, and summarize the relationships identified (Palace 1996).

Data mining is "the process of extracting information from a database and then quantifying and filtering discrete, structured data" (AHIMA, Health Data Analysis Tool Kit, 2011, 32). Chapter 14 provides additional information on data mining.

Access Control for EHRs

One of the main advantages of the EHR is that the health record can be viewed by multiple users and from multiple locations and at anytime. This advantage also has the potential for abuse and security risks. Therefore, organizations must have in place appropriate security access control measures to ensure the safety of data. The Center of Medicare and Medicaid Services EHR certification criteria requires access control of the EHR. The certification criteria states, "Assign a unique name and/or number for identifying and tracking user identity and establish controls that permit only authorized users to access electronic health information" (45 CFR §170.302(o)). Chapter 14 provides a full discussion of the methods summarized below.

The foundation on which access control is based includes identification, authentication, and authorization.

Identification

The basic building block of access control is identification of an individual. Usually identification is performed through the user name or user number.

Authentication

The second element of access control is **authentication.** Authentication is the act of verifying a claim of identity. The Center of Medicare and Medicaid Services EHR certification criteria requires authentication. The certification criteria states, "Verify that a person or entity seeking access to electronic health information is the one claimed and is authorized to access such information" (45 CFR 170.302 §170.302(t)).

There are three different types of information that can be used for authentication: something you know, something you have, or something you are. The most common method of authentication is the use of user names and passwords (AHIMA Workgroup on Electronic Health Records Management 2004). As discussed earlier, access control is strengthened by the use of strong passwords that include numbers and upper- and lower-case letters and that are not easily identifiable names or numbers.

A higher level of authentication may also be accomplished with the use of biometrics identification. Biometrics are individual-specific identifiers such as fingerprints, retinal scans, and voice recognition that uniquely identifies the person. Biometric identifiers are sometimes found on desktop computers, laptops, and other access devices (AHIMA Workgroup on Electronic Health Records Management 2004).

Access cards may also be used to authenticate the user's right to access the record system. Access cards are often used in combination with passwords or personal identification numbers (PINs) as a method of authenticating the person's identity (AHIMA Workgroup on Electronic Health Records Management 2004).

Authorization

The third element of access control is authorization. **Authorization** is a right or permission given to an individual to use a computer resource or to use specific applications and access specific data. It is also a set of actions that gives permission to an individual to perform specific functions such as view, write, edit, delete, or execute tasks.

Authorization for using a computer system is usually addressed through identification and authentication described previously. Authorization to use specific applications (that is, order entry, coding, and registration) and specific data would be different among individuals in an organization. For example, employees in the admitting and registration department would not be given the same authorization to use computers, programs, and data as nursing care employees.

Usually authorization is managed through special authorization software that uses various criteria to determine if an individual has authorization for access, sometimes referred to as an access control matrix. For example, authorization may be based on not only the individual's identity but also the individual's role (called role-based authorization), physical location of the resource (that is, access to only certain computers), and time of day.

Nonrepudiation

As stated earlier, nonrepudiation measures "limit an EHR's user's ability to deny (repudiate) the origination, receipt, or authorization of a data exchange by that user" (Dougherty 2008). Nonrepudiate means to accept. An example of a nonrepudiation measure in the electronic environment is the use of electronic signatures. Electronic signatures assure the authorship of a record entry by using rules built into the EHR that date and time stamp the entry and then lock the notation or report to prevent future changes to the original information documented in the record. The use of nonrepudiation reduces the likelihood that an individual can deny making an entry or the timing of an entry.

Handling Amendments and Corrections in EHRs

As stated earlier, health records may occasionally require that entries be amended, corrected, or deleted. Regardless of the media used to store the health record, policies must be in place to assure the integrity of the information contained in the health record as a business record, as a legal health record, and as a patient care communication tool. The healthcare facility must have written policies that specify who, when, and how amendments, corrections, and deletions may be made to a health record.

In the electronic health record the same premise applies to making changes to a health record as it does to a paper-based record. However, with the functionality of the EHR and increased accessibility of the health record, policies must specifically address who may make changes to the health record, within what time frame corrections can be made, and how these changes will be documented.

The functionality of the EHR varies depending on the system used. Functionality refers to features in the EHR that allow the user to maintain different versions of a document, track changes made to a document, lock a document from changes, and create user profiles that limit who may edit entries and so forth. The ability to unlock a record should be given to only a few individuals and typically this would be the health information manager. The HIM professional must track changes to the health record and assure appropriate follow-up in any source systems or other data repositories. Source systems refer to other computer systems that feed information into the EHR, which would also need to be corrected according to policy when corrections are made in the EHR.

Examples of policies that may be written regarding amending, correcting, or deleting health record entries are (Hall et al. 2009):

- After a document or entry in a health record has a final signature on it, the only way to correct it is to add an addendum to the record. The addendum must have a separate signature, date, and time from the original entry.

- The original version of the document in a corrected health record must be maintained. The version should be clearly indicated on the document. For example, reports should indicate, "final copy," "preliminary copy," or "final copy with corrections."

- A health record should be locked from editing once the final signature has been applied.

- The appearance of information added to the record to amend or correct it should be different than the original entry (that is, it may be a different color, italic, or bolded).

Purge and Destruction of EHRs

Retention of electronic health records is similar to health records in paper-based and hybrid environments. The healthcare facility must consider state and federal regulations, statutes of limitation, research and educational needs, and patient care needs. Many healthcare facilities maintain health records indefinitely or for a period that exceeds the statutes of limitations. Retention periods for records vary from state to state and by patient populations. For example, retention requirements or guidelines are typically longer for the records of minors than adult health records. Regardless of the media used to store records, at some point the healthcare facility will need to address when and how health records will be purged and/or destroyed.

In the EHR environment the facility must also have a policy for destruction of computer equipment and computer storage media when it is no longer functioning properly or has become obsolete. The EHR equipment may have patient health information stored on it. Policies must specifically address how health information will be removed from servers, workstations, laptop computers, and other storage media once this hardware will no longer be used for the EHR. The removal of information from computer equipment requires more than simply deleting files. The healthcare facility must run utility software to remove data or neutralize the data by applying magnetic erasers. If these methods of destroying the data are not possible, the hard drive must be removed from the computer and physically destroyed. CDs used for storing data may be destroyed by shredding or pulverizing and then disposal (AHIMA Workgroup on Electronic Health Records Management 2004).

Quality Control Functions for EHRs

Data quality begins at the point of creation (Johns 2002). In the electronic environment, managing data input through good design of end-user interfaces increases the probability of quality data. As noted earlier in this chapter, in the EHR data are captured by:

- Data are entered directly into the computer at the point of care
- Paper documents are scanned and imaged
- Other computer systems are interfaced with the EHR (for example, laboratory results, radiology)
- Transcribed reports are electronically transmitted to the EHR

Input masks, lookup values, and validation rules can provide for quality discrete, structured data that are more easily manipulated and analyzed (AHIMA 2008). Validation rules are applied to data fields to determine the validity of data entered into the EHR. Specifically, these features include drop-down menus, built-in data values, and checkboxes. Although these features provide for consistent entry of data for routine data, they are limited in allowing the practitioner to document complex cases.

More complex cases may require the physician to use free text to adequately document a patient's condition. Free text is unstructured data and limits the facility's ability to report data. Dictation templates may be utilized to structure or prompt the physician for needed documentation, thus improving the quality of dictated reports. Additionally, illegibility is also a quality issue when scanned images are used in the EHR. Therefore, the decision as to how much structured data may be required and when to allow unstructured data should be collaboratively decided by all stakeholders.

Another step to managing the quality data in the EHR is to monitor errors that occur. Most EHRs generate error reports or utilize error queues when there are mismatches between the EHR and the other computer systems that feed information into the EHR. When errors are identified, there must be a process in place for correction.

When selecting an EHR, the screen design should be evaluated for features that will contribute to the capturing of quality health data. Similar to good forms design in the paper-based environment, well-designed EHR screens will provide ease of use, which in turn helps to provide quality data. Screen design or system features that should be evaluated when assessing a computer system are (Williams 2006):

- Clear navigational buttons that direct the user to the next step in the documentation process and buttons to view the previous screen are imperative to assuring the user can use the system with ease.

- Clear labeling of buttons and data fields

- Limiting the use of abbreviations on buttons and data fields

- Consistent location on the screen of navigation buttons

- Built-in alerts to notify the user of possible errors

- Availability of references at the appropriate data field

- Prompt for more information where appropriate

- Checks for warning signs or errors

Additional considerations that should be followed when developing user views or screens include the following:

Navigation design

- All controls should be clear and placed in an intuitive location on the screen.

- Use neutral colors and limit highlighting, flashing, and so forth to reduce eye fatigue.

- Limit choices and label commands.

- Provide undo buttons to make mistakes easy to override.

- Use consistent grammar and terminology.

- Provide a confirmation message for any critical function (such as deleting a file).

Input design

- Simplify data collection.

- Sequence data input to follow workflow.

- Provide a title for each screen.

- Minimize keystrokes by using pop-up menus.

- Use text boxes to enter text.
- Use a number box to enter numbers.
- Use a selection box to allow the user to select a value from a predefined list:
  — Check boxes (used for multiple selections)
  — Radio buttons (used for single selections)
  — On-screen list boxes
    ▪ Drop-down list boxes
    ▪ Combo boxes

Data validation

- Perform a completeness check to ensure that all required data have been entered.
- Perform a format check to ensure that data are the right type (numeric, alphabetic, and so on).
- Perform a range check to ensure that numeric data are in the correct range.
- Perform a consistency check to ensure that combinations of data are correct.
- Perform a database check to compare data against a database or file to ensure data are correct as entered.

Output design

- Minimize the number of clicks needed to reach data or a specific screen.
- Combine data into a single, organized menu to eliminate layers of screens.

The system should also mark required data fields so that the EHR user cannot proceed to the next screen without completing required information. The system may highlight the field or mark it with an asterisk to indicate that the user must complete that field.

As discussed in chapter 16, the quality of patient care is also improved through a well-designed user interface and decision support features. For example, quality patient care is enhanced when there are built-in alerts that check for possible medication interactions and allergy information when medication orders are documented. "However, in too many systems, too little attention is being paid to ensure the judicious use of alerts and to work on the problem of contextual relevancy for the alert the systems generates during actual use" (Ash et al. 2004). If the EHR contains too many alerts that are not relevant to the user, the clinician may click past the alert because he has become desensitized to the use of alerts.

Another valuable feature of clinical decision support systems is the availability of references. The availability of references allows the physician to easily look up information, without having to rely on memory in prescribing medications or considering a course of treatment. For example, treatment options for specific diagnoses such as diabetes are available for the physician in determining the best treatment for the patient.

Check Your Understanding 7.7

1. Version control of documents in the EHR requires:

   A. The deletion of old versions and the retention of the most recent
   B. Policies and procedures to control which version(s) is displayed
   C. Signed and unsigned documents not to be considered two versions
   D. Previous versions to be accessible to administration only

2. Which of the following is a risk of copying and pasting?

   A. Reduction in the time required to document
   B. System may not save data
   C. Copying the note in the wrong patient's record
   D. System thinking that the the information belongs to the patient from whom the content is being copied.

3. How are materials from other facilities documented in the EHR?

   A. They are still filed in the paper medical record.
   B. They are scanned and filed in the EHR.
   C. They are destroyed—not documented in the EHR.
   D. They are returned to the originating organization.

4. Which term verifies claim of identity?

   A. Identification
   B. Authentication
   C. Authorization
   D. Nonrepudiation

5. How are amendments handled in the EHR?

   A. Automatically appended to the original note. No additional signature is required.
   B. Amendments must be entered by the same person as the original note.
   C. Amendments cannot be entered if after 24 hours of the event.
   D. The amendment must have a separate signature, date, and time.

Instructions: Indicate whether the following statements are true or false (T or F).

6. ____ EHR data are captured by scanning and direct entry.

7. ____ Data validation includes an undo button.

8. ____ Policies should address how the patient information will be removed from computers at the end of their useful life.

9. ____ Data quality begins at the point of creation.

10. ____ Authorization is identifying a patient through the use of a user name.

Medical Transcription

The **medical transcription** function is often included among the HIM department's responsibilities. Physicians and other clinicians use automated computer medical dictation (sometimes referred to as voice capture) systems for dictating reports. Medical reports commonly dictated (recorded) include the clinical history, physical examination, consultation report, operative report, discharge summary, pathology reports, and radiology reports. The dictation is stored in either tape or disk format in the dictation system. Medical transcriptionists retrieve the dictated reports and type them using word-processing systems. The final typed report can be printed in paper format or stored electronically in an EHR.

Management of Medical Transcription

Historically, the HIM department has provided medical transcription services. More recently, however, these services have been subsumed by other departments or have been centralized in a separate department. In other cases, the entire medical transcription function has been outsourced (contracted out to a vendor). In many instances, outsourcing part or all of the transcription function can provide substantial benefits, including cost reductions and relief from staffing issues that sometimes result in transcription delays.

More recently, large in-house transcription areas and outsourcing agencies have begun using speech recognition technology to transcribe recorded dictation. Speech recognition technology may be applied on the front-end (at the point of dictation) or back-end (after dictation has taken place). When the speech recognition is applied at the front-end of the process, the physcian must train the system to recognize speech patterns unique to the individual physician. The disadvantage to **front-end speech recognition** is the time required for the physician to train the system. The advantage of front-end speech recognition is that the transcription is completed at the point of dictation. When speech recognition is applied at the back-end or the point of transcription, the transcriptionist must edit the transcribed report to assure that the system correctly reflects the physician's dictation. Since the physician is not required to train the system when using **back-end speech recognition**, it saves the physician time. It enables the dictator's digitized voice recording to be processed through a computer that converts it into text. Templates or standardized documents can be used to reduce the number of errors.

When speech recognition technology is used, the role of the medical transcriptionist is that of a medical language editor. The medical language editor reviews the reports created by the system from the physician's dictation and assures that the system correctly transcribed what was dictated.

Quality Control

Like the other HIM functions discussed in this chapter, it is important to monitor the quality and timeliness of medical transcription. The following are examples of the quality of the medical transcription service that can be monitored:

- To monitor transcription accuracy, a sample of the transcriptionists' reports can be checked for wrong terms, misspelled words, incorrect format, and/or grammatical errors. The number of errors found is noted, and an error or accuracy rate is determined and compared against an established standard.

- Transcription turnaround time also can also be monitored to determine whether reports are being transcribed within the expected time frame set in a standard. Most dictation/transcription computer management systems track the date and time reports are dictated and transcribed. A report indicating dictation and transcription time and date can be used to determine turnaround time.

Release of Information (ROI)

As discussed in other chapters, protecting the security and privacy of patient information is one of the healthcare institution's top priorities. The HIM department usually has responsibility for determining appropriate access to and release of information from patient health records. For example, release of information (ROI) may take the form of a patient's request to mail copies of his or her records to a healthcare provider.

The management of the release of information function includes the following steps:

1. Enter the request in the ROI database: Generally, information such as patient name, date of birth, health record number, name of requester, address of requester, telephone number of requester, purpose of the request, and specific health record information requested is entered in the computer. Figure 7.16 is an example of the computer screens used for entering ROI data.

2. Validity of the authorization is determined: The HIM professional will compare the authorization form signed by the patient with the facility's requirements for authorization to determine the validity of the authorization form. The facility's requirements are based on federal and state regulations. Certain types of information such as substance-abuse treatment records, behavioral records, and HIV records require specific components be included in the authorization form per state (varies per state) and federal regulations. If the authorization is determined to be invalid, the request is returned to the requester with an explanation as to why the request has been returned. If the request is valid, the HIM professional proceeds to the next step.

3. Verify the patient's identity: The HIM professional must first verify that the patient has been a patient at the facility. Verification is done by comparing the information on the authorization with information in the master patient index. The patient's name, date of birth, Social Security number, address, and phone number are used to verify the identity of the patient whose record is requested. The patient's signature in the health record is compared with the patient's signature on the authorization for release of information form.

4. Process the request: The record is retrieved and the only information authorized for the release is copied and released.

Figure 7.16.   **Computer screen of ROI data**

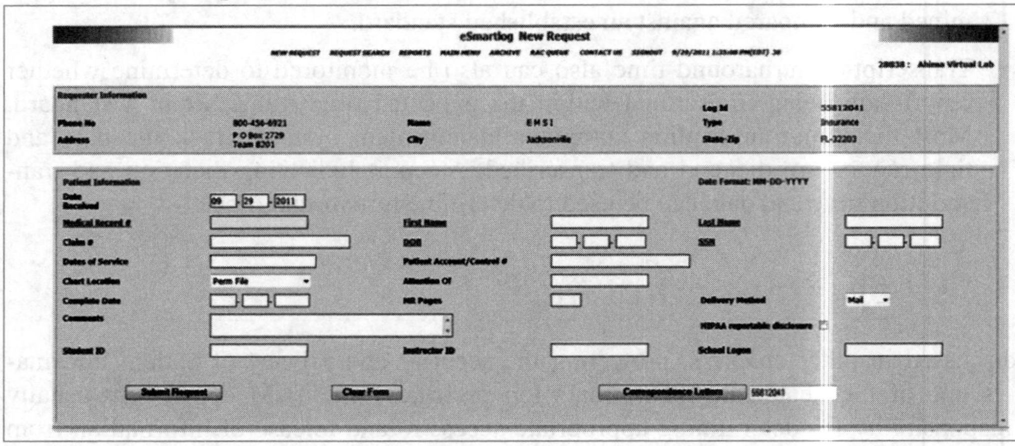

Source: AHIMA Virtual Lab HealthPort eSmart.

Because federal regulations such as Health Insurance Portability and Accountability Act (HIPAA) and state laws govern the release of health record information, HIM department personnel must know what information needs to be included on the authorization for it to be considered valid. If the written request or authorization is valid, the specific information is copied and sent. If the authorization is invalid, the problem with the authorization is noted in the computer and the request is returned to the sender. To comply with HIPAA standards, a healthcare facility must maintain a record that accounts for all disclosures from the health record.

In another case, ROI may take the form of a response to a subpoena duces tecum in a legal case. (A subpoena duces tecum is a judicial request for certain information or evidence. Refer to chapter 13 for further information on subpoenas.) In this instance, the HIM department verifies that the subpoena is valid and that the requested information can be released to the court in compliance with state or federal law or regulations. In such instances, a representative from the HIM department may appear in person in court or at a deposition and give sworn testimony as to the health record's authenticity.

The ROI function has grown immensely in the past decade, in part due to the HIPAA privacy standards. As a result, some HIM departments outsource this function to companies that specialize in release of medical information. Even though it has outsourced the function, the HIM department is ultimately responsible for ensuring that proper practices are followed and that all laws and regulations are adhered to.

ROI Quality Control

The HIM department receives a high volume of requests and must prioritize the processing of release of information. Continuity of care requests are processed before other types of requests. Standards for turnaround time for requests are established by the department. With standards for turnaround times established, the average turnaround times for release of information may be tracked and delays in responding to requests for information addressed. The following two examples illustrate how the timeliness and quality of the release of information can be monitored.

ROI Turnaround Time Monitoring

The turnaround time for the ROI function is monitored. The date a request is received and the date the record copies are sent are entered into a computer database. This information can be used to generate a report that will determine whether the records are being sent in a timely manner.

The accuracy of the ROI function can be monitored by checking a sample of authorization forms that have been sent or that are ready to be sent to verify the validity of the authorization and to ensure compliance with federal and state regulations. The error rate or accuracy rate can be determined and compared against a set standard.

Productivity and Backlog Management

Productivity standards must be established in order to meet the expected turnaround time for the various types of requests.

> While productivity information may be collected manually, electronic systems offer more tools for data manipulation and can provide individual production statistics, departmental request volumes, and information regarding request turnaround times. Timely fulfillment of requests that ensure continuity of care aligns with the overall mission of most healthcare organizations. Thus these types of requests frequently take precedence over other categories of requestors. Monitoring the volume of backlog requests with the available resources and making appropriate staffing adjustments ensures the patient's needs are being met. (Bock et al. 2008)

When the volume of requests reaches beyond the workload capacity of staff meeting productivity and quality standards, the facility may decide to contract with a release of information service to process the backlog.

Legal Health Record

Regardless of the media used to store the health record, the legal health record must be clearly defined by each facility. The **legal health record** refers to the health record that is maintained as the business record and is the health record that may be disclosed to authorized users and for evidentiary purposes. Healthcare facilities must have a policy that clearly identifies the legal health record. Figure 7.17 is an example of a legal health record policy from the AHIMA EHR Practice Council (2007). As noted in the policy template in figure 7.17, "The determining factor in whether a document is considered part of the legal health record is not where the information resides or its format, but rather how the

Figure 7.17.   Sample legal health record policy template

Policy Name: The Health Record for Legal and Business Purposes

Effective Date:

Departments Affected: HIM, Information Systems, Legal Services, *[any additional departments affected]*

Purpose: This policy identifies the health record of *[organization]* for business and legal purposes and to ensure that the integrity of the health record is maintained so that it can support business and legal needs.

Scope: This policy applies to all uses and disclosures of the health record for administrative, business, or evidentiary purposes. It encompasses records that may be kept in a variety of media including, but not limited to, electronic, paper, digital images, video, and audio. It excludes those health records not normally made and kept in the regular course of the business of *[organization]*.

Note: The determining factor in whether a document is considered part of the legal health record is not where the information resides or its format, but rather how the information is used and whether it is reasonable to expect the information to be routinely released when a request for a complete health record is received. The legal health record excludes health records that are not official business records of a healthcare provider. Organizations should seek legal counsel when deciding what constitutes the organization's legal health record.

Policy: It is the policy of *[organization]* to create and maintain health records that, in addition to their primary intended purpose of clinical and patient care use, will also serve the business and legal needs of *[organization]*.

It is the policy of *[organization]* to maintain health records that will not be compromised and will support the business and legal needs of *[organization]*.

Responsibilities

It is the responsibility of *[the health records manager or other designated position]* to:

• Work in conjunction with information services, legal services, and *[other stakeholders]* to create and maintain a matrix or other document that tracks the source, location, and media of each component of the health record. *[Reference an addendum or other source where the health record information is found.]*

• Identify any content that may be used in decision making and care of the patient that may be external to the organization (outside records and reports, PHRs, e-mail, etc.) that is not included as part of the legal record because it was not made or kept in the regular course of business.

• Develop, coordinate, and administer a plan that manages all information content, regardless of location or form that comprises the legal health record of *[organization]*.

• Develop, coordinate, and administer the process of disclosure of health information.

• Devise and administer a health record retention schedule that complies with applicable regulatory and business needs.

• *[Other responsibilities]*

It is the responsibility of the information services department *[or other appropriate department(s)]* to:

• Ensure appropriate access to information systems containing components of the health record.

• Execute the archiving and retention schedule pursuant to the established retention schedule.

• *[Other responsibilities]*

[Additional responsibilities for other individuals or departments]

Source: AHIMA EHR Practice Council 2007.

information is used and whether it is reasonable to expect the information to be routinely released when a request for a complete health record is received" (AHIMA EHR Practice Council 2007). As the healthcare facility transitions to the EHR, consideration must be given to all media (for example, paper, CD, video, images, films, reference materials, downtime documents) and documentation sources. "Legal health records must meet accepted standards as defined by applicable Centers for Medicare and Medicaid Services (CMS), federal regulations, state laws, and standards of accrediting agencies such as the Joint Comission, as well as, the policies of the healthcare providers" (AHIMA 2010c). Many of the EHR quality management components that assure the integrity of the data contained with the health record are key to defining the health record, including version control, authentication, lockdown procedures, and amendment and correction policies. Chapter 13 provides additional discussion about the legal health record.

Tracking and Reporting of Disclosures

HIPAA requires that healthcare facilities maintain an account of each required disclosure type of protected health information (PHI). The following disclosures must be accounted for (Stuard 2003):

- Government mandated reporting
- Research
- Disclosures by business associates that are not for treatment, payment, and healthcare operations

The facility must be able to provide upon request, the date, name of person receiving the information, the address of the recipient, a description of the PHI disclosed, and a statement of the purpose of the disclosure (Stuard 2003). These types of disclosures may reach beyond the requests and disclosures that are under the auspices of the HIM department. Therefore, there must be an organization-wide policy on how compliance with the accounting for disclosure regulation of HIPAA will be accomplished. Examples of departments that are involved with disclosures that fall under the realms of the HIPAA accounting of disclosures regulations might be cancer and trauma registries, institutional review boards, social work departments, and so forth. The enactment of the American Recovery and Reinvestment Act (ARRA) changed HIPAA requirements. Additional information about HIPAA and reporting disclosures is covered in chapter 13.

Clinical Coding

Clinical coding is another important function usually performed by the HIM department. (The specifics of clinical coding are described in chapter 5.) Using a classification or nomenclature system such as ICD-9-CM and/or CPT, clinical coding is a method for categorizing diagnoses and procedures. (Adoption of a new coding system called ICD-10-CM and ICD-10-PCS is planned to replace ICD-9-CM on October 1, 2013.) This categorization is used subsequently for billing and payment purposes as well as for research and clinical quality performance reviews.

The clinical coding function includes the processes of **abstracting** and assigning ICD-9-CM and/or CPT codes to an encounter or hospital stay. The coding professional reviews the health record and enters specific data from it into a computer database. The process of extracting data from the health record and entering them into a computer database is called abstracting. Figure 7.18 is an example, but not an exhaustive list, of data that may be abstracted and entered into the computer database.

The data items included in figure 7.18 are only a partial listing of data abstracted from the health record. A hospital may abstract more than 200 data items from each record. In addition to abstracting, the coding professional is responsible for translating healthcare providers' diagnostic and procedural documentation into coded form using code sets such

Figure 7.18.   Examples of abstracted data fields

Admit source:
- Physician referral
- Clinic referral
- HMO referral
- Transfer from a hospital
- Transfer from a skilled nursing facility
- Transfer from another healthcare facility
- Emergency room
- Court/law enforcement
- Information not available

Transfer facility

Hospital service
- Hospice inpatient
- Psychiatric and alcohol

Inpatients/outpatients
- Skilled nursing inpatients
- Surgical inpatients
- Oncology inpatients
- Obstetrics
- Trauma
- Newborn
- Cardiology
- Medicine

Discharge disposition
- Self-care (home)
- Skilled nursing facility
- Rehabilitation facility

Against medical advice
Psychiatric facility
Long-term care facility
Intermediate care facility
Assisted living
Hospice
Home health
Acute care facility
Expired
Unknown

Discharge facility

Anesthesia type
- Conscious sedation
- General
- Monitored anesthesia care
- Regional

ASA classification

Gestation

C-section
- No previous C-section
- Previous C-section
- C-section performed for complications

VBAC (vaginal birth after cesarean section)

Apgar score (0–10)

Birth weight

Note: This is not an exhaustive list of data items collected.

Source: Adapted from materials provided by OhioHealth, Columbus, OH.

as ICD-9-CM, CPT, and HCPCS Level II. The coding function may be done manually by finding the correct codes in a coding book or done by using a computer program called an **encoder.** Encoders are software programs that help guide the coder through the various coding conventions and rules to arrive at a correct diagnosis, procedural, or service code (figure 7.19). Other programs that are usually part of an encoding system are called MS-DRG and APC groupers for acute care hospitals. **MS-DRG groupers** are software programs that help coders determine the appropriate Medicare severity diagnosis-related group (MS-DRG) assignment based on the logic of the system for hospital inpatients. **APC groupers** are software programs that help coders determine the appropriate ambulatory payment classification for an outpatient encounter.

In an EHR environment, **computer-assisted coding** (CAC) software may be used to generate ICD-9-CM (or ICD-10-CM/PCS) and CPT codes for each episode of care. The technology commonly behind a CAC engine is known as **natural language processing** (NLP). NLP is a computer process that analyzes text and extracts implied facts as coded data (AHIMA 2011). The codes assigned by the CAC software are then reviewed by a

Figure 7.19.   Screen from encoder system

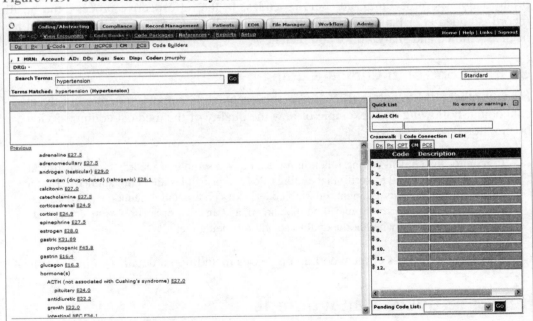

Source: AHIMA Virtual Lab QuadraMed Encoder.

medical coding professional to assure the accuracy of the CAC assigned code(s) based on the documentation and application of coding principals.

> NLP results typically have a confidence factor associated with them. The confidence factor is a rating on how likely the produced NLP code is considered accurate by a coding professional given similar documentation. The higher the confidence factor, the more likely a coding professional will determine the code is accurate. The lower the confidence factor, the less likely the code will be deemed accurate. (Bronnert July 2011)

In today's environment, codes for diagnoses, procedures, and services are usually entered directly into a computer system along with pertinent patient information and other demographics. Data abstracted and the clinical code(s) assigned to a health record make it possible to create automated disease, operation, and physician indexes (discussed later in this chapter). Such indexes are essential in order to retrieve data or specific health records to conduct research or clinical quality performance studies.

Like quantitative analysis, clinical coding can be either concurrent or retrospective. In some acute care and long-term care facilities, the coding of diagnoses, procedures, and services occurs during the patient's hospital stay. In this method, the HIM professional goes to the nursing unit daily or periodically reviews the health record and assigns appropriate diagnosis, procedural, and service codes. In the retrospective process, the health record is coded after patient discharge. Coding usually occurs after the health record has been assembled and analyzed for completeness.

Quality Control in Clinical Coding

Like the other HIM functions discussed in this chapter, it is important to monitor the medical coding. Following is an example of how the quality of the medical coding service can be monitored:

> To monitor the clinical coding function for accuracy, a sample of records for each clinical coder can be reviewed to verify that coding rules and principles are being applied. Criteria such as correct code assignment, missing codes, extra codes, and sequencing of codes can be established. Any errors found should be noted, and an error or accuracy rate can be calculated to determine whether the quality standard is being met.

Chapters 5 and 6 discuss clinical coding processes in additional detail.

Revenue Cycle Management

Revenue cycle management is a system that involves several processes working together to ensure that the healthcare facility is properly reimbursed for the services provided. Major functions of revenue cycle management include: admitting/access management, case management, charge capture, HIM, patient financial services/business office, finance, compliance, and information technology (Amatayakul 2005). Chapter 6 discusses the specifics of revenue cycle management.

Other HIM Functions

Research, statistical reporting, cancer registries, trauma registries, and birth certificate functions require data contained in the health record. Therefore, the HIM department often manages these functions.

Data Reporting and Interpretation

Many HIM departments include a research division. The type of research assistance provided to clinicians, medical staff committees, and clinical administrative decision support varies from organization to organization. Some HIM research sections are responsible for identifying candidate health records for research projects that clinicians are conducting. An example might be that of a physician doing a study on patients diagnosed with hypertension and diabetes who are being given a specific type of medication. In this case, the research section would use disease and procedure indexes to identify and retrieve the appropriate health records. In some cases, the HIM research professionals might not only identify and retrieve the health records, but also actually review the selected records and abstract or collect data from them for the physician researchers.

In addition to research functions, many HIM departments are responsible for collecting and calculating various statistics about the operation of the healthcare facility. (See chapter 9.) Among these are ratios and percentages such as the percentage of occupancy, death and autopsy rates, and hospital census reports. Where the institution has integrated computer information systems, many of these types of statistics are generated automatically. This is particularly the case with daily hospital census reports and percentage of occupancy. However, data entry and other errors often produce incorrect results, so it is still usually the function of the HIM department to verify the accuracy of many of the statistics calculated about institutional operations.

Maintenance of Indexes and Registries

HIM departments often also have responsibility for maintaining indexes and registries. An **index** is a guide that serves as a pointer or indicator to locate something. For example, the index at the back of this book lists key terms. The page number(s) by each term indicates where in the book the reader can find information about that particular term.

The following is a brief overview of indexes and registries. More detailed information is provided in chapter 8.

Disease and Operation Indexes

Compiling and maintaining disease and **operation indexes** has always been an important function of the HIM department. In these indexes, diagnoses, and operative codes, like those used in a classification system such as ICD-9-CM, are used as guides or pointers to the health records of patients who have had a specific disease or operation. Disease and operation indexes are essential for locating health records to conduct quality improvement and research studies, as well as for monitoring quality of care.

The minimal amount of data required for a disease or operation index usually includes:

- The principal diagnosis and relevant secondary diagnoses
- Associated procedures
- Patient's health record number
- Patient's gender, age, and race
- Attending physician's code or name
- The hospital service
- The end result of hospitalization
- Dates of encounter (including admission and discharge for inpatients)

Given this type of information, the index can be used as a guide for retrieving health records for research or other studies. For example, if the clinical quality committee wanted to see the health records for all male patients who had been diagnosed with myocardial infarction, were 50 years old or less, had been treated in the past 6 months, and had been discharged alive, the records could be easily identified and subsequently retrieved using the information in the index.

Today, most indexes are automated except for those in very, very small facilities. The automated disease and operation index usually is accomplished by generating standard or ad hoc reports of data already existing in the computer. Ad hoc reporting capabilities enable the user to select the field items he or she wants in the reports. Standard reports are preexisting reports that have been programmed into the computer to include predefined data fields.

In many institutions, much of the information needed for disease and operation indexes is entered into the computer system concurrently with the diagnosis coding process. In other facilities, the data may be entered during a separate function of abstracting data from the health record and entering them into the computer system. In some cases, pertinent demographic patient information is exchanged from the automated R-ADT system and passed to the coding system. This type of data exchange helps to reduce work and data-entry redundancy and to increase data integrity and consistency.

Physician Index

Like the disease and operation indexes, the physician index is a guide to identifying medical cases associated with a specific physician. Often the information gathered for disease and operation indexes is sufficient for the physician index. Essentially, the data required in such an index include the physician's name or code; the health record number, diagnosis, operations, and disposition of the patients the physician treated; the dates of the patient's admission and discharge; and the patient's gender and age. In addition, certain other patient demographic information may be useful.

Registries

A **registry** or register is a chronological listing of data. With regard to HIM functions, traditional registries include the patient admission and discharge register, operating room register, and birth and death registers. Most information collected today for registries is a byproduct of other automated systems. A more complete discussion of registries is provided in chapter 10.

Cancer and Trauma Registries

The HIM department also may manage the cancer and trauma registry functions. Cancer registries use information from patient records to collect data for the study and treatment of cancer. Likewise, trauma registries use information from the patient record to collect data for the study and treatment of trauma patients. Both registries maintain large computer databases to store patient data.

Birth Certificates

Sometimes the HIM department is responsible for submitting an accurate birth certificate to the health department. A birth certificate must be completed for each newborn before the infant is discharged from the hospital. Information is gathered from the mother's and baby's medical record for completion of the birth certificate. Chapter 9 discusses birth certificate requirements and functions in additional detail.

HIM Interdepartmental Relationships

Performing HIM functions efficiently and effectively involves the interface and cooperation with many clinical and administrative departments in the organization. Good working relationships and communication among all of these departments are essential. These interdepartmental relationships are described below.

Patient Registration

As discussed earlier in the section on the MPI, typically, the first point of data collection in any healthcare organization is patient registration. During the registration process, the patient provides the registration or admitting clerk with personal information. The patient's information is needed for the identification, treatment, and payment of healthcare services. For example, the patient provides demographic information such as name, address, telephone number, and emergency contact information. He or she also provides information about how payment should be handled (for example, insurance company name and insurance group number). For inpatient or same-day surgery admissions, other information, including attending physician, provisional diagnosis, and planned treatment, is provided by the patient's attending physician and integrated into the registration data collection and processing. For a laboratory or radiology referral, an order for a test or treatment must be accompanied by a tentative diagnosis or a reason for the order. The patient registration function essentially begins the process of documenting the patient's care and treatment.

Thus, patient registration is the area where the health record begins. Additionally, it is the area where the health record number is assigned. The accuracy of the information entered into the computer by the patient registration area has a significant impact on the HIM department, patient care areas, and billing department.

Data quality always begins at the source of the data. When data are recorded or obtained incorrectly at the start of the process, the errors follow the data throughout their use in the healthcare organization's business and patient care processes. For example, an error made in entering a patient's health insurance number in the computer system will likely cause serious problems for the billing office. An error made in recording a patient's provisional diagnosis may have adverse effects on the delivery of patient care. An error in assigning a new health record number to a patient who has previously been a patient at the facility and already has a number can cause filing and MPI problems if a unit numbering system is used. As explained earlier in the section about the MPI, two numbers assigned to a single patient are often referred to as duplicate numbers. Because the health record is located using the health record number, duplicate numbers result in the record having two separate locations and compromise the integrity of the MPI. Thus, the importance of getting information correct the first time and at the point where it is initially collected, entered, or recorded cannot be overstated.

Figure 7.20 shows the various areas where patient registration can occur in a large healthcare organization. In some organizations, responsibility for patient registration or admitting falls to the director of HIM services. In others, the admitting department reports to nursing or some other unit or is a separate department.

In smaller organizations such as freestanding clinics or long-term care facilities, patient registration usually occurs in, and is the responsibility of, only one area. In larger facilities, it can occur in various areas. For example, when the patient is being admitted to

Figure 7.20.   Points of patient registration in a large healthcare facility

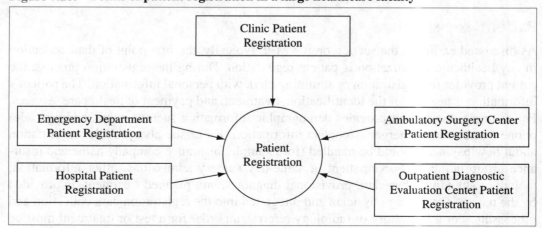

an acute care hospital, registration usually occurs in the patient registration or admitting department. However, when the patient comes to the emergency department for diagnosis or treatment, registration can occur in that department. Still another scenario is that the patient is being seen for the first time in one of the healthcare facility's clinics. In this case, patient registration occurs in the clinic office.

Documentation of information gathered during patient registration is handled either electronically or in paper format. Most acute care facilities now process all patient registration data using computer systems. Although patients may complete a paper form, the registration clerk usually enters their information into a computer system. In a smaller healthcare delivery unit such as a physician's office, however, registration data may still be collected and stored in a paper file.

Billing Department

The billing department uses health record information that is entered into the computer by the HIM department. The HIM department assigns clinical codes and abstracts information from the patient's health record that is required on the patient's bill. Therefore, the patient's bill cannot be submitted for payment until the HIM department enters the required health record information into the computer.

The HIM department also affects the healthcare facility's reimbursement cycle by tracking health records where coding has been delayed and the bill has not been sent for payment. In many facilities, a report is generated weekly that identifies patient accounts that have not been billed because of missing ICD-9-CM codes and/or CPT codes. It is HIM personnel who locate the records to determine why there has been a delay in coding and initiate completion of the coding process so the bill can be submitted to the party responsible for payment of services.

The ROI function in the HIM department also can affect the billing process. Third-party payers often request additional information from the health record before payment (reimbursement for services provided) is sent to the healthcare facility. The information requested from the payer varies from a request for the entire health record for a single episode of care to a single operative report or discharge summary.

Patient Care Departments

The HIM department also works closely with patient care departments such as nursing, laboratory, radiology, physical and occupational therapy, and so on. All patient care departments document the services they provide to patients in the health record. Therefore, they are contributors to health record content.

In a paper-based record system, the HIM department also delivers health records from previous admissions to the nursing units when the patient is readmitted to the hospital. In other healthcare settings, the HIM department pulls and delivers charts of established patients to clinics or other patient care areas. When the patient is discharged from the hospital or leaves a clinic, the HIM department retrieves records from previous admissions or visits in addition to records of the patient's recent admission/visit. The health record then is routed to the record-processing area of the HIM department.

Information Systems

As the EHR is implemented, the relationship between the HIM and IT departments becomes complex. It takes the expertise of both the HIM department and IT department to have a successful EHR.

The HIM professionals are the experts in health record content and provide knowledge of regulations to assure that records comply with federal, state, and accreditation standards. The HIM professional also provides input to the efficient and effective health record information flow. The HIM professional also understands privacy standards and protects health record content from unauthorized access. The HIM professional is the resource person for the health record data needs of the facility.

The IT department provides the experts to assure that the computer equipment and software are working properly. The IT professional assures that the infrastructure needed to support the computer needs is in place. The IT professional is responsible to assure that interfaces between computer systems work properly, system backups are completed in order to protect from the loss of data, software is installed and working properly, and computer equipment is maintained.

With the transition to the EHR, the HIM department and IT department have partnered to assure that the EHR functionality is realized to the fullest. The HIM professional is the administrative EHR expert and the IT professional is the technical expert for a successful EHR.

Quality Management

Quality management includes three fundamental tasks: measurement, assessment, and improvement (Spath 2009). These activities, when included in a formal quality improvement program, can positively impact the cost and quality of healthcare by improving the efficiency and effectiveness of how healthcare is delivered to patients. HIM professionals may assist in collecting data used to measure healthcare performance and assess quality management activities.

Participation on Medical Staff and Organizational Committees

HIM professionals frequently serve as liaisons or support personnel on various medical staff committees. For example, the HIT may be a member of the health record, quality management, or some other medical staff committee. In a support capacity, the HIT may be responsible for taking minutes of the committee meeting, distributing the meeting agenda to committee members, and providing statistics or other required information. As a liaison, the HIT's expertise is frequently required. For example, serving on the organization's health record committee, the HIT may be asked to clarify policies, procedures, and accreditation requirements.

Managing Documentation Requirements

As explained in chapter 2, the health record is the principal repository for data and information about the healthcare services provided to individual patients. Traditionally, the HIM department has been responsible for a variety of content issues. In fulfilling this role, the HIM department has worked with appropriate medical staff committees, clinical departments, and administration.

With regard to a paper-based health record, HIM usually sets standards for record content, chart order, and forms design and development to ensure that content meets accrediting, licensing, and other best practices for documentation. HIM performs many of the same functions when working with an EHR. The department helps ensure that record content and authentication (signatures) in the EHR meet accreditation and licensing requirements and also participates in user-interface design for electronic data input.

Virtual HIM

Virtual HIM refers to a HIM department that is not contained within the walls of a traditional facility. Virtual HIM refers to the HIM functions traditionally performed within the walls of the healthcare facility being done remotely. For the past several decades, many medical transcriptionists have worked from home. Digital dictation technology has allowed the medical transcriptionist to access dictation via phone lines or computer WAV files. With the implementation of hybrid and electronic health records some facilities have permitted medical coders to work from home.

As the full EHR is implemented, it is possible for more of the HIM departmental functions to move to a remote location or to home-based work environments. As paper-based functions are eliminated from the HIM workflow, it becomes possible to perform HIM functions from remote locations. Additionally, virtual HIM also provides opportunities for HIM functions to be outsourced.

Accreditation and Licensing Documentation Requirements

Accrediting bodies such as **The Joint Commission** (TJC) and state licensing bodies are among the groups that have established standards for health record documentation. The Joint Commission is a not-for-profit organization that offers an accreditation program for hospitals and other healthcare organizations based on pre-established accreditation standards.

In addition to TJC, other entities that have established documentation standards include:

- Medicare Conditions of Participation
- National Committee for Quality Assurance (NCQA)

- American Accreditation Health Care Commission/Utilization Review Accreditation Commission (AAHCC/URAC)
- American Osteopathic Association (AOA)
- Commission on Accreditation of Rehabilitation Facilities (CARF)
- Health Accreditation Program of the National League of Nursing
- College of American Pathologists (CAP)
- American Association of Blood Banks (AABB)
- American College of Surgeons (ACS)
- Accreditation Association for Ambulatory Health Care (AAAHC)
- American Medical Accreditation Program (AMAP)

U.S. hospitals, as well as the majority of other healthcare organizations, seek Joint Commission accreditation. Joint Commission accreditation has been an indicator that the accredited hospital or healthcare facility provides high-quality care. As part of the accreditation process, the healthcare facility undergoes an on-site evaluation by a team of Joint Commission surveyors. It is during the survey that TJC evaluates the quality of care provided to patients, the systems in place for ensuring caregiver and medical staff competence, and the performance of important patient functions.

In the past, the on-site survey was a scheduled event. TJC also conducts unannounced surveys.

The on-site survey follows a Tracer Methodology, which follows a sample of patients through their experiences of care in the organization, to evaluate individual components of care and systems of care. The survey follows actual patient records through the facility and includes interviews with key personnel, observation of the organization's administrative and clinical activity, assessment of the physical facilities and equipment and review of documentation. (TJC 2011)

The accreditation process includes a periodic performance review (PPR) and a priority focus process (PFP) that facilitates the newer continual standards compliance process. Midpoint in the accreditation process, the hospital must submit the PPR to the Joint Commission. The PPR is a hospital's review of standards, compliance with standards, action plans implemented to address noncompliance with standards, and measures to follow up on the success of the action plans. The PFP uses information from the PPR and other data sources to identify priority focus areas that are used to guide the survey process. TJC survey, the PPR, and the PFP are used to indicate that the healthcare facility is in compliance with Joint Commission standards.

Healthcare organizations accredited by TJC are also deemed to be in compliance with the Medicare Conditions of Participation. This is referred to as **deemed status.** Medicare randomly selects hospitals recently surveyed by TJC and conducts another survey to validate TJC survey results.

It is essential that HIM professionals become familiar with TJC and Medicare standards and documentation requirements.

It is important to note that each accrediting and licensing agency has its own standards, which must be followed by the healthcare facilities under their auspices.

Monitoring of Accreditation, Licensure, and Standards Requirements

No program for ensuring the quality of health record content would be complete without a process for monitoring accreditation, licensure, and other federal or state agency requirements. Good documentation practices require organizations to be in compliance with regulations and standards from a variety of groups. The HIM department director should establish a mechanism that targets specific regulatory or standards groups and monitors for compliance with these standards. New standards and changes to regulations must be monitored and HIM functions revised if necessary.

Because the HIM department's functions include review and analysis of the health record, several processes are typically in place to monitor the healthcare facility's compliance with Joint Commission standards. The following are examples of such processes.

- Record completion process

  — *Monitoring delinquency rates:* As part of its record completion processes, the HIM department monitors the number of delinquent records. Many facilities determine the number of delinquent records each month and notify their medical staff members of their incomplete and delinquent records. The HIM professional determines the quarterly medical record delinquency rate for the facility and determines whether the hospital is in compliance with Joint Commission standards. If the hospital is not in compliance with TJC, the medical records committee, administration, and other appropriate parties are notified and corrective action is taken. There may be various consequences for physicians when they have not completed delinquent charts within a specified period of time. TJC's Hospital Medical Record Statistics form used by hospitals to monitor compliance with TJC's standard for record completion can be found on the Joint Commission's website (TJC 2011). http://www.jointcommission.org/Hospital_Medical_Record_Statistics_Form/

  — *Monitoring timely completion of medical reports:* Other Joint Commission standards specify time frames within which various medical reports (history and physicals, operative reports, autopsy reports, and so on) must be completed. The HIM department's transcription area may monitor compliance in this area. The transcriptionist can compare the date a report was dictated against the date of service or admission to determine whether the report has been completed within the time frame specified by the standards.

— *Monitoring health record completion:* The quantitative analysis function of the HIM department monitors whether health record documents have been authenticated. Unauthenticated parts of the health record are identified for completion by either handwritten or electronic signature. If the physician does not complete the record within a timely manner, the record is counted in the delinquent record rate.

- Documentation

— *Monitoring the use of abbreviations, acronyms, and symbols:* Transcriptionists can assist with monitoring the use of abbreviations, acronyms, and symbols as they transcribe dictation. Clinical coding personnel also can identify the use of unauthorized abbreviations, acronyms, and symbols as they abstract information from health records. This is an example of the HIM professional's role in monitoring hospital compliance with TJC's standard on abbreviation usage in the health record.

- Confidentiality of information

— *Monitoring access to protected health information:* The HIM department's daily ROI activities can help ensure and monitor access to patient-specific information after discharge. HIM personnel are knowledgeable in the laws and regulations governing the release of patient information. Thus, the department's ROI function is instrumental in monitoring compliance with Joint Commission standards regarding access to protected health information.

- Access to patient records

— *Storage and retrieval processes:* The storage and retrieval processes are managed to ensure that health information is accessible for patient care. These processes are pivotal for compliance with the Joint Commission standards.

There are many additional Joint Commission standards that help healthcare organizations improve quality of care and patient safety. For example, TJC also has a list of abbreviations that may not be used in the healthcare facility, because these abbreviations may be misinterpreted. The HIM professional must consult the *Comprehensive Accreditation Manual for Hospitals* published by TJC for a complete listing of standards and elements of performance. TJC also publishes accreditation manuals for specialty areas, such as long-term care and behavioral healthcare facilities. In addition to monitoring performed as part of daily HIM functions, health record reviews are often done periodically to ensure facility compliance with other standards. The health records review process is a multidisciplinary process coordinated by the HIM department.

Management and Supervisory Processes

Regardless of size, all HIM departments involve a great deal of organization, management, and supervision of personnel. This section provides an overview of some of the more common supervisory responsibilities associated with the management of the HIM functions. Chapter 18 also provides a detailed discussion on management and supervisory issues.

Policy and Procedure Development

Policies and procedures serve as the foundation for the management and supervision of employees of any department or unit. Policies are statements that describe general guidelines that direct behavior or direct and constrain decision making in the organization. Some policies apply to the entire organization; departmental policies apply only to specific business units.

Policies follow a specific format. For example, the policy statement from the University of Houston shown in figure 7.21 provides a specific format that includes a policy title, description of the scope of the policy, the expected standard, and guidelines to achieve the expected standard (University of Houston 2001). Figure 7.21 is an example of a policy that provides guidance for the assignment of overtime within the HIM department. Every policy must be dated, and if there has been a revision, the date of the revision also

Figure 7.21. Sample policy on computer terminal controls

Purpose:	To prevent unauthorized access to University Hospital data by providing terminal controls
Scope:	University Hospital's terminals
Standard:	Proper physical and software control mechanisms shall be in place to control access to and use of devices connected to University Hospital's computer systems

Guidelines:

1. Hardware Terminal Locking: In areas that are not physically secured, terminals should be equipped with locking devices to prevent their use during unattended periods. The locks should be installed in addition to programmed restrictions, such as automatic disconnect after a given period of inactivity.

2. Operating System Identification of Terminal: All terminal activity should be controlled by the operating system, which should be able to identify terminals, whether they are hardwired or connected through communications lines. The operating system should inspect log-on requests to determine which application the terminal user desires. The user should identify an existing application and supply a valid user ID and password combination. If the log-on request is valid, the operating system should make a logical connection between the user and the application.

3. Limitation of Log-On Attempts: Limit system log-on attempts from remote terminal devices. More than three unsuccessful attempts should result in termination of the session, generation of a real-time security violation message to the operator and/or the ISO (and log of said message in an audit file), and purging of the input queue of messages from the terminal.

4. Time-Out Feature: Ensure that the operating system provides the timing services required to support a secure operational environment. Inactive processes or terminals (in an interactive environment) should be terminated after a predetermined period.

5. Dial-Up Control: The communications software should ensure a clean end of connection in all cases, especially in the event of abnormal disconnection.

should appear on the policy. The format of a policy statement varies from organization to organization.

The success of policy relies on procedures. Unlike broad statements included in a policy, procedures are specific statements about how work is to be carried out. Essentially, they are specific instructions to help employees carry out a function or activity. An example of a policy can be seen in figure 7.22. Procedures provide step-by-step instructions on

Figure 7.22. Sample departmental policy: Overtime

HEALTH INFORMATION SERVICES STANDARD POLICY		
Title: OVERTIME		Issued:
Prepared by:		Effective:
Approved		Revised:

PURPOSE: To provide a fair, consistent guideline for assignment of overtime.

POLICY

Overtime will be assigned at the discretion of the manager/supervisor when it is deemed necessary.

- Volume of work exceeds staffing hours present
- Backlog
- Vacancy/extended absences

An Overtime Approval Form must be completed and returned to the Operations Manager/Coding Manager to obtain advanced approval of any necessary overtime.

The assignment will be based on

- past performance
- knowledge of the work area
- productivity
- availability

When overtime is deemed necessary the manager/supervisor(s) will utilize a rotating schedule of individuals trained in the area. If an individual declines an offer they will go to the end of the rotation. If the designated individual for OT fails to complete the assigned OT, it will count as an unexcused absence for the individual.

The manager/supervisor reserves the right to make the final determination in assignment of overtime based on the needs of the department.

Source: OhioHealth, Columbus, OH. Reprinted with permission.

how to complete a specific task. Written procedures are beneficial as a training tool for new employees. They also are beneficial for providing staff with a consistent method of completing tasks.

The format of procedures varies from facility to facility. Figure 7.23 is an example of a procedure that explains the process of collecting scanning records from the nursing unit. This procedure demonstrates the detail that should be included in a written procedure. This procedure also demonstrates the interrelationship of the HIM department

Figure 7.23. Sample departmental procedure: Scanning

POLICY: The HIM Department is committed to ensuring that every record is scanned into the document-imaging system within 24 hours of discharge. HIM Associates (Scanners) retrieve records from the "To Scan" area for capture in the document imaging system on a daily basis. Records are scanned according to discharge date with the oldest date being scanned first.

Emergency Department records are scanned immediately after prepping by ED personnel. All inpatient, outpatient surgery and observation discharges are scanned into the imaging system within 24 hours of discharge. Outpatient encounters and loose reports are scanned on a daily basis according to established scanning priorities.

PURPOSE: To ensure that all medical record information is scanned into the document imaging system with a 95% accuracy rate thereby expediting release of images for availability to system users within 24 hours of date chart made available for retrieval by HIM Dept.

PROCEDURE:
  I. Select prepped batch for scanning from 'To Scan" shelf according to the following priority:
   A. Emergency Department—decentralized to ED.
   B. Late: Inpatient, Observation, Outpatient Surgery, Outpatient Ancillary
   C. Routine: Inpatient, Observation, Outpatient Surgery, Outpatient Ancillary
   D. Loose Reports—different Imaging employee responsible for scanning these.
   Always select batch with the oldest discharge date to scan first.
 II. Scan all documents on the high volume scanner except the following:
   Insert list of additional documents that must be scanned on flatbed scanner.
   • EKGs
   • NB ID
   • Photographs
   • Telemetry strips
III. Turn on scanner (scanner will conduct a "health check").
IV. Login to system:
   A. Enter **User Name**.
   B. Enter **Password** ———— .
   C. Select **Login** button or press **Enter** on keyboard.

(continued on next page)

Figure 7.23. **Sample departmental procedure: Scanning** *(continued)*

V. First time Login

  A. Load index form.

    a. Click Forms on Quickbar.

VI. Create A New Batch: Batch = Chart

  A. Place pages to be scanned in scanner tray.

  B. Enter batch label name (up to 32 characters)

    Recommended Batch Label Name Formats:

    Inpatient/Observation/Outpatient Surgery Encounter Batches: Discharge Date/Patient Last Name/Encounter Number—032503 Jones 1234567

    Multiple Encounter Batches (emergency department, outpatient ancillary, loose): Scanning Date/Batch Type/Batch Number—032503 ED 123

  C. Select appropriate batch type—Move the batchcover sheet to the back of the chart before scanning.

  D. Click **OK** or **Enter**.

  E. Press Green run button on high volume scanner.

  F. Once scanning is complete, press red **Stop** button on high volume scanner.

    (*Skip this step for flatbed scanner.)

VII. Write batch (batch must be associated with batch type that has been assigned Batch Routing Rules):

  A. Automatically:

    1. Click on **Write Next** button on toolbar.

      OR

    Select **Batch/Auto Write to next Queue** on menu. Use **Alt BQ** instead.

  B. Manually:

    1. Click on **Batch/Write Batch**

      OR

    Select **Write** from Quickbar.

    2. Select queue to receive batch from drop-down list (i.e., qcindexq)

      OR

    Click queue icon on Quickbar.

VIII. Enter date, batch i.d. # and name on Batch Cover Sheet in "Scanned" area.

IX. Place rubber band around batch and place on "To Index" shelf in discharge date order.

X. Select next batch to be scanned and return to Step VI for further scanning.

XI. Exit system upon completion of scanning.

Source: Adapted from material provided by OhioHealth, Columbus, OH.

with the nursing units and the intra-relationship among the different functions of the HIM department.

Health information technicians have to follow both policies and procedures in their job functions. In some instances, the HIT will be involved in the development of policies and procedures as they pertain to the HIM department or information management in the organization. Figure 7.24 provides a listing of common HIM policies and procedures.

Figure 7.24. Common HIM department policies and procedures

The following list provides an example of the types of policies and procedures that may be included in a manual for health information services. The titles and content of the policies and procedures may vary by facility or corporation. Some of the policies and procedures are listed more than once for cross-referencing purposes.

Abbreviations
Access to Automated/Computerized Records
Access to Records (Release of Information) by
　　　Resident and by Staff
Admission/Discharge Register
Admission Procedures
　　Facility Procedures—Establishing/Closing the
　　　Record
　　Preparing the Medical Record
　　Preparing the Master Patient Index Card
　　Readmission—Continued Use of Previous
　　　Record
　　Readmission—New Record
Amendment of Clinical Records
Audit Schedule
Audit and Monitoring System
　　Audit/Monitoring Schedule
　　Admission/Readmission Audit
　　Concurrent Audit
　　Discharge Audit
　　Specialized Audits (examples)
　　Change in Condition
　　MDS
　　Nursing Assistant Flow Sheet
　　Psychotropic Drug Documentation
　　Pressure Sore
　　Restrictive Device/Restraint
　　Therapy
Certification, Medicare
Chart Removal and Chart Locator Log
Clinical Records, Definition of Records,
　　　and Record Service
　　General Policies
　　　Access to Records
　　　Automation of Records (See also
　　　　Computerization)
　　　Availability
　　　Change in Ownership
　　　Coding from home
　　　Completion and Correction of Records
　　　Confidentiality
　　　Definition of the legal record
　　　Indexes
　　　Ownership of Records

　　　Permanent and Capable of Being
　　　　Photocopied
　　　Retention
　　　Storage of Records
　　　Subpoena
　　　Unit Record
　　　Willful Falsification/Willful Omission
Closing the Record
Coding and Indexing, Disease Index
Committee Minutes Guidelines
Computerization and Security of Automated Data/
　　　Records
Confidentiality (See Release of Information)
Consulting Services for Clinical Records and Plan
　　　of Service
Content, Record *(the list provided is not all-
　　　inclusive and should be tailored to the
　　　facility/corporation)*
　　General
　　Advanced Directives
　　Transfer Form/Discharge Plan of Care
　　Discharge against Medical Advice
　　Physician Consultant Reports
　　Medicare Certification/Recertification
　　Physician Orders/Telephone Orders
　　Physician Services Guidelines and Progress
　　　Notes
　　Physician History and Physical Exam
　　Discharge Summary
　　Interdisciplinary Progress Notes
Copying/Release of Records—General
Correcting Clinical Records
Data Collection/Monitoring
Definition of Clinical Records/Health Information
　　　Service
Delinquent Physician Visit
Denial Letters, Medicare
Destruction of Records, Log
Disaster Planning for Health Information
Discharge Procedures
　　Assembly of Discharge Record
　　Chart Order on Discharge

(continued on next page)

Figure 7.24. Common HIM department policies and procedures *(continued)*

Completing and Filing Master Patient Index Card
Discharge Chart Audit
Notification of Deficiencies
Incomplete Record File
Closure of Incomplete Clinical Record
Preparation of the record, imaging of records, quality review
Emergency Disaster Evacuation
Establishing/Closing Record
Falsification of Records, Willful
Fax/Facsimile, Faxing
Filing Order, Discharge (Chart Order)
Filing Order, In-house (Chart Order)
Filing System
Filing System, Unit Record
Forms Management
Forms, Release of Information
Forms, Subpoena
Guide to Location of Items in the Health Information Department
Guidelines, Committee Minutes
Incomplete Record File
Indexes
  Disease Index and Forms for Indexing
  Master Patient Index
  Release of Information Index/Log
In-service Training Minutes/Record
Job Descriptions
  Health Information Coordinator
  Health Unit Coordinator
  Other Health Information Staff (if applicable)
Late Entries
Lost Record—Reconstruction
Master Patient Index
Medicare Documentation
  Certification and Recertification
  Medicare Denial Procedure and Letter
  Medicare Log
Numbering System
Ombudsman, Review/Access to Records
Omission, Willful
Order of Filing, Discharge
Order of Filing, In-house
Organizational Chart for Health Information Department
Orientation/Training of Health Information Department
Outguides

Physician Visit Schedule, Letters, and Monitoring
Physician Visits, Delinquent Visit Follow-up
Quality Assurance
  Health Information Participation
  QA Studies and Reporting
Readmission—Continued Use of Previous Record
Readmission—New Record
Recertification or Certification (Medicare)
Reconstruction of Lost Record
Refusal of Treatment
Release of Information
  Confidentiality
  Confidentiality Statement by Staff
  Copying/Release of Records—General
  Faxing Medical Information
  Procedure for Release—Sample Letters and Authorizations
  Redisclosure of Clinical Information
  Resident Access to Records
  Retrieval of Records (sign-out system)
  Subpoena
  Uses and disclosures of protected health information, uses and disclosures of de-identified documentation, business-associated contracts, audit trails
  Witnessing Legal Documents
Requesting Information
  From Hospitals and Other Healthcare Providers
  Request for Information Form
Retention of Records and Destruction after Retention Period
  Example Statement for Destruction
  Retention Guidelines
Retrieval of Records
Security of Automated Data/Electronic Medical Records
  General Procedures
  Back-up Procedures
  Passwords
Sign-out Logs
Storage of Records
Telephone Orders
Thinning
  In-house Records
  Maintaining Overflow Record
Unit Record System

Source: Adapted from Amatayakul 2003 and AHIMA nd.

Future Directions in Health Information Management Technology

The role of the HIM professional continues to evolve as healthcare and technology evolve. Some of the factors influencing the evolution of the role of HIM professionals are as follows:

- Political initiatives

- Expansion of network capabilities

- Emergence of new technologies such as EHRs, natural language processing, and computer-assisted coding

- Move toward ICD-10-CM and ICD-10-PCS

- Societal and regulatory requirements for information privacy and security

- Greater demand and accountability for improved healthcare quality and patient safety that can be facilitated through the use of information technology

- Increased consumer knowledge of personal healthcare decisions and increased focus on personal health records

Hospitals in the United States spend billions of dollars annually to store and manage both paper and electronic health records. The ever-expanding wealth of patient information increasingly strains the U.S. economy. President Obama has made electronic record-keeping a key feature of his healthcare reform effort (Brown 2009). The ARRA of 2009 provides funds to promote the use of interoperable, certified health information technologies including EHR adoption. ARRA provides financial assistance and incentives necessary for the transition to electronic health records. The Office of the National Coordinator for Health Information Technology (ONC), a federal entity located within the Office of the Secretary for the U.S. Department of Health and Human Services (HHS), is responsible for the coordination of the national initiative that all providers adopt an EHR by 2014. The ONC was established in 2004 and in February 2009 the ARRA expanded the role of this office to further support the EHR initiative through funding and the establishment of standards (ONC 2009).

It has been said that we are currently in the information age. In part, this means that information is recognized as a commodity with value. As part of the information age, an explosion of information technology (IT) is transforming the workplace. Many healthcare facilities have either implemented an EHR or are in the transitional stages of implementing one; however, many of the EHRs today use a large amount of imaged documents. As EHRs evolve, the expanded use of database technology and direct data input will be necessary to meet industry standards and demands for information.

The Internet and the IT explosion have transformed HIM functions and will continue to contribute to the evolution of the HIM professional's role. In addition to making EHRs possible, technology is transforming specific work tasks. The IT explosion continues to break down the brick and mortar of the HIM department, making virtual HIM a viable option as HIM departments restructure and adopt the EHR. As the EHR is implemented, more and more facilities are allowing staff to code from remote locations. As the EHR continues to evolve and data are structured within these systems, natural language processing (NLP) will be used for computer-assisted coding (CAC). NLP is the process in which digital text stored on computer can be read by software and automatically coded. As more healthcare settings utilize CAC, the clinical coder's role will be for quality control of the automated process.

Perhaps a more immediate influence likely to affect the role of the clinical coding professional is implementation of ICD-10-CM and ICD-10-PCS. The ICD-10-CM and ICD-10-PCS coding systems will replace ICD-9-CM for coding diagnoses and procedures. Implementation of the revised or new coding systems will require that clinical coders be retrained to use them. Moreover, it will require software vendors to provide new products, which could expand opportunities for HIM professionals.

Because information transcends boundaries, the HIM department may not be a department at all in the future. Instead, it may become a function that is integrated throughout the organization and exists in many departments. Thus, the HIT may be working in information functions managed by departments other than health information management.

Evidence suggests that this phenomenon is already occurring as HIM professionals move into roles in data security, organizational compliance, health data analysis, medical staff services, and so on. The AHIMA Vision 2016 prioritizes the need to revamp the associate degree–level HIM professional from a "generalist to a technical specialist by 2016" (AHIMA Vision 2016 2007). Vision 2016 also discusses the need to provide a pathway for advanced practice role for HIM professionals through the development of graduate degree programs. AHIMA outlined the following roles as those most likely to evolve:

- The *health information manager* (a line or staff manager) would have enterprise- or facility-wide responsibility for health information management. The position includes working with the chief information executive and system users to advance systems, methods, and application support and to improve data quality, access, privacy, security, and usability.

- The *clinical data specialist* would perform data management functions in a variety of application areas, including clinical coding, outcomes management, specialty registries, and research databases.

- The *patient information coordinator* would perform new service roles that help consumers manage their personal health information, including personal health history management, ROI, managed care services, and information resources.

- The *data quality manager* would perform functions involving formalized continuous quality improvement for data integrity throughout the enterprise, beginning with data dictionary and policy development and including quality monitoring and audits.

- The *data resource administrator* would be responsible for the next generation of records and data management using media such as the CPR, the data repository, and electronic warehousing for meeting current and future care needs across the continuum, providing access to the needed information, and ensuring long-term integrity and access.

- The *research and decision support analyst* would support senior management with information for decision making and strategy development using a variety of analytical tools and databases. The position would work with product and policy organizations on high-level analysis projects such as clinical trials and outcomes research.

- The *security officer* would manage the security of all electronically maintained information, including the promulgation of security requirements, policies and privilege systems, and performance audits.

In 2011, the AHIMA Board of Directors undertook the challenge of developing a new view of Health Information Management (HIM)—one that addressed changing practice roles, settings, and functions emerging from increased automation, changing regulations, and dissemination of data (AHIMA's Draft Core Model 2011 "A New View of HIM: Introducing the Core Model"). According to AHIMA's Draft Core Model 2011 ("A New View of HIM: Introducing the Core Model"), there are six functional components in the Core Model. The six functional components are:

- Data Capture, Validation, and Maintenance
- Data/Information, Analysis, Transformation, and Decision Support
- Information Dissemination and Liaison
- Health Information Resource Management and Innovation
- Information Governance and Stewardship
- Quality and Patient Safety

See figure 7.25.

Figure 7.25.   **Functional Components of HIM Core Model**

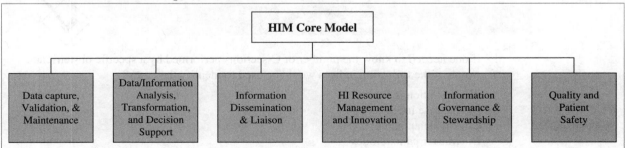

Source: AHIMA's Draft Core Model 2011 "A New View of HIM: Introducing the Core Model."

Some HIM professionals have taken the role of security officer as the healthcare facility implements measures to comply with HIPAA. Others have assumed the role of facility- or enterprise-wide health information managers as healthcare facilities are transitioning toward the EHR. As AHIMA Vision 2016 predictions continue to become a reality, new roles for the HIM professional will continue to emerge. The Draft Core Model expands upon the AHIMA Vision 2016 Roles. "New roles may include business change manager, EHR system manager, IT training specialist, business process engineer, clinical vocabulary manager, workflow and data analyst, consumer advocate, clinical alerts and reminder manager, clinical research coordinator, privacy coordinator, enterprise application specialist, and many more" (Cassidy and Hanson 2005).

Many of these positions will fall outside traditional roles and workplaces. Most will call for additional skills and education. Yet, with their unique mixture of clinical and information skills, HITs are poised for success.

Further evidence of the changing role of the HIM professional is noted in the HITECH provision of the ARRA. The HITECH component of the ARRA provides funding to community colleges to train individuals in the following roles:

- Practice workflow and information management redesign specialists
- Clinician/practitioner consultants
- Implementation support specialists
- Implementation managers
- Technical/software support staff
- Trainers

As a result of the expected change in job functions, the conclusion drawn from AHIMA was that trend data indicate that employers in the twenty-first century will require flexible and multi-skilled workers. Employers also will demand that employees continually add to their skill sets to meet changing needs. That is why another fundamental principle of AHIMA is the need for lifelong learning. HIM professionals must be committed to ongoing education and professional development.

Check Your Understanding 7.8

1. If one needed to know the number of C-sections performed by a specific obstetrician, which of the following indices would be used to identify the cases?

    A. Operation index
    B. Disease index
    C. Physician index
    D. Master patient index

2. The computer system that may serve as the MPI function is the:

   A. Patient registration system
   B. Abstract system
   C. Encoder
   D. Chart-tracking system

3. A chronological listing of data is called a/an:

   A. Index
   B. Registry
   C. Abstract
   D. Record

4. What department within the hospital uses the information abstracted and coded by the HIM department to send for payment from third-party payers?

   A. Patient registration
   B. Nursing unit
   C. Billing department
   D. Administration

5. The function within the HIM department responsible for listening to dictated reports and typing them into a medical report format is called:

   A. Clinical coding
   B. Medical transcription
   C. Clerical services
   D. Release of information

6. Reviewing requests for health record copies and determining if they are valid is part of what function within the HIM department?

   A. Analysis function
   B. Clinical coding
   C. Storage and retrieval function
   D. Release of information function

7. Where does the health record begin?

   A. Patient registration
   B. Nursing unit
   C. Billing department
   D. HIM department

8. One of the most sought after accreditation distinction by healthcare facilities is offered by the:

   A. American Medical Association
   B. American Hospital Association
   C. The Joint Commission
   D. American Health Information Management Association

9. Statements that describe general guidelines that direct behavior or direct or constrain decision making are called:

   A. Policies
   B. Procedures
   C. Standards
   D. Criteria

10. Step-by-step instructions on how to complete a specific task are called:

   A. Policies
   B. Procedures
   C. Standards
   D. Criteria

11. Assigning ICD-9-CM and CPT codes to the diagnoses and procedures documented in the medical record is called:

   A. Clinical coding
   B. Release of information
   C. Billing
   D. Medical transcription

12. Which of the following is an example of how the HIM professional interacts with the medical staff?

   A. Serve on medical staff committees
   B. Provide security for information systems
   C. Retain the health record
   D. Support research

Real-World Case

This case study presents a healthcare facility's journey toward implementation of an electronic health record. It demonstrates the complexity of the process and similarities that exist between paper-based, hybrid, and electronic health records.

Background

Central Community Medical Center (CCMC) is a 600-bed urban hospital located in the downtown of a major metropolitan area. The medical center is one of five hospitals belonging to the Midwest Healthcare systems. The medical center is a full-service teaching hospital with services ranging from medical, surgical, obstetrics, pediatrics, wound care, trauma care, and heart care, to outpatient clinics and services. CCMC has an average of 15,000 inpatient discharges each year and approximately 90,000 outpatient visits per year. Up until two years ago, Central Community Medical Center's HIM department operated as a traditional paper-based health records department. An administrative decision was made to implement an electronic health record. CCMC is the second hospital within the Midwest Healthcare system to implement the EHR; therefore, the vendor selection was already established. The Healthcare system decided that all hospitals would use the same vendor to facilitate the interoperability and consistency of the EHR between facilities.

The Planning Process

Establishment of a Steering Committee

The first step in planning for the various components of implementing an EHR was to establish a steering committee. Key players needed to be identified and included in the planning process. The steering committee consisted of a project manager and approximately 20 individuals from the health information management team and information systems team. Appropriate representatives from administration, medical staff, nursing, and other ancillary departments were included on the steering committee, along with vendor representatives. The steering committee was charged with determining how the vendor product would be implemented at the CCMC facility. Workgroups were developed. The HIM workgroup activities are discussed in this case study.

Forms Redesign and Documentation Analysis

The HIM workgroup completed the task of identifying all forms utilized in the health record, as well as other sources of documentation that comprised the health record. This process took approximately one year to complete and included the creation of a forms catalog, development of a documentation matrix, forms redesign/standardization, and bar-code application.

The forms catalog included a copy of every form used by the healthcare facility to document patient care in the paper-based record. Duplicate forms or forms with similar data were reviewed to determine if a common form could be used across departments.

The next step was to develop a documentation matrix. The forms included in the forms catalog, as well as other sources of health record documentation, were included in the matrix. For example, health record documentation generated and printed from the computer for inclusion in the health record (for example, printed laboratory results) was also identified and included in the documentation matrix. The following information was included in the documentation matrix:

- Name of form or documentation (for example, history and physical, progress notes, physician orders, graphic nursing forms, laboratory results, medication administration form, and so forth)

- Source of the documentation (for example, internal, external)

- Documenter of the information (for example, nursing, physician, physical therapist, radiology, surgical department, laboratory, and so forth)

- Data capture methodology (for example, paper form, printed results, voice recognition, transcription, electronic forms, and so forth)

- Health record location (for example, physician section, nursing section, laboratory section, radiology section, and so forth)

- Name of computer systems used to provide electronic documentation

The documentation matrix was then used to determine what documentation would be scanned and imaged in the electronic document management system (EDMS), what documentation would be electronically transmitted into the EDMS, and what departments or individuals would need to assist with the integration of health record documentation into the EDMS.

Once each form was identified, a barcode was applied to paper forms that would be scanned into the EDMS. The barcode on the forms was needed so forms could be automatically indexed and routed to the correct location within the EDMS. Indexing rules were applied to scanned images and electronically fed documentation. The rules allowed the documentation to be auto-indexed to the correct location within the EDMS. Another task in form redesign was to standardize the location of the barcode on paper forms to be scanned.

The information systems (IS) workgroup used the documentation matrix to assist with the identification of computer interfaces that needed to be in place in order for electronic transmission of the documentation to work properly.

Workflow Analysis

Workflow analysis was also performed on the paper-based HIM procedures to see what processes in the current workflow could be eliminated and what new processes would need to be implemented with the adoption of the electronic health record components. The current workflow was graphically demonstrated in a process flow chart. Several work processes that existed in the paper-based environment were replaced or revised in transitioning to a high-functioning hybrid record. New productivity standards were established to reflect the work processes of the hybrid record.

Work queues were established in the EDMS to mirror the many processes and uses of the electronic health record. A sample of work queues established to accomplish the electronic work processes were:

Internal HIM work queues:

- Record deficiency analysis queues

- Quality review of imaged documents

- Indexing documents for proper placement in the health record

- Loose sheet queues

- Birth certificate queues

- Release of information queues

- Physician decline queues

- Medical coding queues

Physician work queues:

- Records needing dictation
- Records needing signature
- Records requiring text editing
- Medical coding queries
  - Outpatient surgeries
  - Inpatient
  - Emergency department records
  - Ancillary coding

Management work queues:

- Medical coding questions

Supervisor monitoring:

- Questions regarding records from HIM personnel
- Productivity
- Quality review

Review work queues:

- Quality outcome review
- Cancer chart reviews
- External review (temporary queues)
  - Medicare
  - Other payers
  - Auditor review
  - Accreditation review
  - Department of health reviews

Through the documentation matrix and workflow analysis, it was determined that 60 percent of the health record could be captured in the EDMS through electronic transmission of data and 40 percent of the health record would require the paper record be prepped and scanned as images into the EDMS. It was determined that fetal monitoring strips would be maintained on paper because of the inability to capture the monitoring information electronically and the time required to scan the continuous feed of monitoring strip paper after discharge.

After the documentation matrix and workflow analysis were completed, the healthcare facility formally defined the legal health record in a formal policy.

Implementation

Prior to implementation, the EDMS was tested in a test environment to assure that scanned images and electronically transmitted documentation were routed correctly. As the facility approached the implementation date, focus shifted to training. Key clinical staff were trained in the train-the-trainer style. Online training modules were available for staff unable to attend live training sessions. Most of the physician training was accomplished on an individual basis.

Change Management

The implementation of a high-functioning hybrid record and the planned evolution of the paper health record to an electronic health record was a significant culture change for the health facility. It is natural to experience apprehension and resistance as part of the change process. Central Community Medical Center included change management in the planning process. Because of the significant change in work processes, HIM employees needed to be retrained for the new processes of prepping/scanning, indexing, quality review, and electronic chart analysis. Some employees feared that with the automation of the health record there might be job loss. The employee assistance program was utilized to help manage the fears associated with the change. Although the new processes did allow the facility to eliminate 2.0 FTE, the reduction of staff was handled through the process of not replacing employees who resigned from their jobs during the 18-month planning and implementation period.

Ongoing Plan

Central Community Medical Center transitioned to the high-functioning hybrid record with the ultimate goal being to evolve to an electronic health record with minimal paper. With 40 percent of the health record being scanned and imaged for inclusion into the EDMS, the long-term plan is to eliminate as much as possible of the scanned paper portions of the health record and increase the amount of documentation electronically transmitted. As computer systems that are not interfaced with the EDMS are replaced or updated, the IS department will work with vendors to assure the inclusion of the data in the EDMS via electronic transmission. In the future, there will be more emphasis on point-of-care documentation being entered directly into the computer via the use of databases or automated online forms. Improvements to interoperability will be the focus of future enhancements of the electronic health record, which will support the health information exchange initiatives of the healthcare system and regional and national initiatives.

Summary

The health information management department performs a variety of functions within the healthcare institution. These functions include health records storage and retrieval, monitoring record completion, clinical coding, medical transcription, and release of medical information. The department also may manage research and statistics, the cancer and trauma registries, and birth certificate completion. The HIM functions vary from facility to facility. In fact, in any given HIM department, many more functions may be performed in paper, hybrid, and electronic environments.

Probably one of the most fundamental functions of any HIM department is storage and maintenance of health data. The goal of any health record system is to enable retrieval of meaningful data that assists healthcare professionals in providing quality patient care. Paper systems require storage space, equipment, and a system of record identification. Most record systems use a numerical filing system. However, small organizations such as physician offices may use an alphabetic filing system. Although filing systems have been used traditionally for storage of paper records, document-imaging technologies are making it possible to scan records digitally and store them electronically. Keeping track of health records and being able to locate and retrieve them when and where they are needed is an essential HIM function. To provide high-quality retrieval services, the HIM department must have good tracking systems in place and continuously audit its filing and retrieval practices.

The record processing function performed by the HIM department is key to monitoring health record content. It includes conducting quantitative analysis of the record by checking the record content against accreditation standards, rules, and regulations internal to the organization and best practices of information handling.

Clinical coding for purposes of research, claims submission, and quality of care studies has been another foundational aspect of HIM practice. Today, various automated systems support the clinical coder, resulting in increased productivity and improved coding quality.

The HIM department has usually been the custodian of the master patient index, the key to identifying and locating any health record in a numerical filing system. Although the patient registration area assigns the health record number (the primary identifier), the HIM department is responsible for the integrity of this important index. The functions performed by the HIM department also have an impact on the billing and patient care departments and the medical staff.

Forms design and management is another critical HIM function both in the paper and electronic environment. Accurate health information can only be developed through effective data capture methods. Thus, the role of developing good forms, whether in paper or electronic form, continues to be an important part of ensuring high-quality health record content. Associated with forms development is the entire process of tracking and managing forms. This entails development of a forms committee, establishment of forms standards, and implementation of forms numbering and tracking systems.

HIM practice will continue its evolution as discussed in this chapter's section Future Directions in Health Information Management Technology. HIM functions are being transformed as a result of the explosion of information technologies and incentives brought about by ARRA for the transition to electronic health records. AHIMA's initiatives provide a picture of how functions are likely to change in the future. One thing for certain is that the HIT must become increasingly technologically savvy and remain committed to learning throughout his or her professional career.

References

AHIMA. 1997. Practice brief: Developing information capture tools. *Journal of AHIMA* 68(3): Supplement.

AHIMA. 2002. Practice brief: Destruction of patient health information. *Journal of AHIMA*: Web extra.

AHIMA. 2008. Quality data and documentation for EHRs in physician practice. *Journal of AHIMA* 79(8):43–48.

AHIMA. 2010a. Fundamentals for Building a Master Patient Index/ Enterprise Master Patient Index (Updated, Practice brief: Building an enterprise master person index. 2004).

AHIMA. 2010b. "Fundamentals for Building a Master Patient Index/Enterprise Master Patient Index (Updated). Appendix A: Recommended Core Data Elements for EMPIs." *Journal of AHIMA*.

AHIMA. 2010c. "Managing the Transition from Paper to EHRs. (Updated November 2010)" AHIMA. "Managing the Transition from Paper to EHRs. Appendix A: Legal Source Legend." http://library.ahima.org/xpedio/idcplg?IdcService=GET_HIGHLIGHT_INFO&QueryText= %28Managing+the+Transition+from+Paper+to+EHRs%0D%0A%29++%3CAND% 3E++%28xPublishSite%3Csubstring%3E%60BoK%60%29&SortField=xPubDate&SortOrder= Desc&dDocName=bok1_048419&HighlightType=HtmlHighlight&dWebExtension=hcsp

AHIMA. 2011a. "CAC 2010–11 Industry Outlook and Resources Report." Available in the AHIMA Body of Knowledge at http://library.ahima.org/xpedio/groups/public/documents/ahima/ bok1_048947.pdf#xml=http://library.ahima.org/xpedio/idcplg?IdcService=GET_XML_HIGHLIGHT_ INFO&QueryText=%28cac%29%3cand%3e%28xPublishSite%3csubstring%3e%60BoK%60% 29&SortField=xPubDate&SortOrder=Desc&dDocName=bok1_048947&HighlightType=Pdf Highlight

AHIMA. 2011b. "Fundamentals of the Legal Health Record and Designated Record Set." *Journal of AHIMA* 82(2) (February 2011): available at http://library.ahima.org/xpedio/ idcplg?IdcService=GET_HIGHLIGHT_INFO&QueryText=%28Fundamentals+of+the+Legal+ Health+Record+and+Designated+Record+Set%0d%0a%29++%3cAND%3e++%28xPublish Site%3csubstring%3e%60BoK%60%29&SortField=xPubDate&SortOrder=Desc&dDocName= bok1_048604&HighlightType=HtmlHighlight&dWebExtension=hcsp

AHIMA. 2011c. "Health Data Analysis Tool Kit": 32. Available in AHIMA Body of Knowledge at http://library.ahima.org/xpedio/groups/public/documents/ahima/bok1_048618.pdf

AHIMA. 2011d. A New View of HIM: Introducing the Core Model Review Draft Review. Available at http://library.ahima.org/xpedio/groups/public/documents/ahima/bok1_049283.pdf

AHIMA. 2011e. "Retention and Destruction of Health Information." (Updated August 2011). http://library.ahima.org/xpedio/idcplg?IdcService=GET_HIGHLIGHT_INFO&QueryText=%28retention+and+destruction+of++health+information%29%3Cand%3E%28xPublishSite%3Csubstring%3E%60BoK%60%29&SortField=xPubDate&SortOrder=Desc&dDocName=bok1_049252&HighlightType=HtmlHighlight&dWebExtension=hcsp

AHIMA e-HIM Workgroup on Electronic Document Management as a Component of EHR. 2003. Practice brief: Electronic Document Management as a Component of the Electronic Health Record. *Journal of AHIMA*: Web extra.

AHIMA e-HIM Workgroup on Health Information in a Hybrid Environment. 2003. Practice brief: Complete medical record in a hybrid EHR environment: Part I: Managing the transition. *Journal of AHIMA*: Web extra.

AHIMA e-HIM Workgroup on Maintaining the Legal EHR. 2005. Update: Maintaining a legally sound health record—paper and electronic. *Journal of AHIMA* 76(10):64A–L.

AHIMA EHR Practice Council. 2007. Developing a legal health record policy. *Journal of AHIMA* 78(9):93–97.

AHIMA Vision 2016. 2007. A blueprint for quality education in health information management. Chicago: AHIMA.

AHIMA Workgroup on Electronic Health Records Management. 2004. The strategic importance of electronic health records management. Appendix A: Issues in electronic health records management. *Journal of AHIMA* 75(9):80A–80B.

Altendorf, R.L. 2007. Establishment of a quality program for the master patient index. *AHIMA's 79th National Convention and Exhibit Proceedings*.

Amatayakul, M. 2003. Practical advice for effective policies, procedures. *Journal of AHIMA* 74(4):16A–16D.

Amatayakul, M. 2005. *Best Practices in Revenue Cycle Management*. Chicago: AHIMA.

American Reinvestment and Recovery Act. 2009. Sec. 3000. Definitions (13). http://www.bsa.ca.gov/pdfs/stimulus/arra.pdf

Ash, J.S., M. Berg, and E. Coiera. March/April 2004. Some unintended consequences of information technology in health care: The nature of patient care information system-related errors. *Journal of the American Medical Informatics Association* 11(2):104–111.

Barnett, R. 1996. *Managing Business Forms*. Canberra, Australia: Robert Narnett and Associates.

Bock, L.J., B. Demster, A.K. Dinh, E.R. Gorton, and J.R. Lantis, Jr. 2008. Management practices for the release of information. *Journal of AHIMA* 79(11):77–80.

Bronnert, June. (July 2011). "Preparing for the CAC Transition." *Journal of AHIMA* 82(7):60–61.

Brown, D. 2009 (April 4). Obama pledges new data system for veterans. *Washington Post*.

Cassidy, B., and S.P. Hanson. 2005. HIM practice transformation. *Journal of AHIMA* 76(5):56A–56B.

Center for Medicare and Medicaid Service. 2011. http://healthit.hhs.gov/media/MU/n508/MU-%28EH-CAH%29_SCC-InpatientOnlyGrid.pdf

Center for Medicare and Medicaid Service. 2012. "EHR Incentive Programs." https://www.cms.gov/EHRIncentivePrograms/25_Certification.asp#TopOfPage

Dimick, C. 2009. Exposing double identity at patient registration. *Journal of AHIMA* 80(11): Web extra.

Dougherty, M. 2008. How legal is your EHR?: Identifying key functions that support a legal record. *Journal of AHIMA* 79(2):24–30.

Gelzer, R., T. Hall, E. Liette, M.G. Reeves, J. Sundby, A. Tegen, D. Warner, and L.A. Wiedemann. 2008. Copy functionality toolkit. Chicago: AHIMA.

Grant Medical Center. nd. http://www.ohiohealth.com/facilities/grant/

Hall, T., K. Olenik, A. Tegen, D. Warner, L.A. Wiedemann, and T. Wiseman-Kuhlman. 2009. Amendments, corrections, and deletions in the electronic health record: An AHIMA toolkit. Appendix B.

Healthcare Information and Management Systems Society. 2012. Overview of health information exchange. http://www.himss.org/asp/topics_ehr.asp

Johns, M.L. 2002. *Information Management for Health Professions,* 2nd edition. Albany, NY: Thomson Learning/Delmar.

The Joint Commission. 2011. *Accreditation Guide for Hospitals.* Page 14 (viewed November 27. 2011). http://www.jointcommission.org/assets/1/6/Accreditation_Guide_Hospitals_2011.pdf

The Joint Commission. 2011. Hospital Medical Record Statistics Form. (viewed November 27, 2011). http://www.jointcommission.org/Hospital_Medical_Record_Statistics_Form/

Menke, A.M. 2009. Record retention and destruction. American Academy of Ophthalmology, YO Info Newsletter. http://www.aao.org/yo/newsletter/200901/article01.cfm

Office of the National Coordinator for Health Information Technology. 2009. http://healthit.hhs.gov/portal/server.pt?open=512&objID=1200&parentname=CommunityPage&parentid=1&mode=2&in_hi_userid=10741&cached=true

Palace, B. 1996. *Technology Note prepared for Management 274A.* Anderson Graduate School of Management at UCLA. http://www.anderson.ucla.edu/faculty/jason.frand/teacher/technologies/palace/datamining.htm.

Reino, L. 2005. Leading the transition to e-HIM: Strategies for success through collaboration. *AHIMA's 77th National Convention and Exhibit Proceedings.*

Santangelo, E. 2009. Iron Mountain White Paper: Best practices: A self-funding transition plan to electronic health records.

Spath, P.L. 2009. *Fundamentals of Health Care Quality Management, 3rd edition.* Forest Grove, OR: Brown-Spath & Associates, p. 15.

Stuard, S. 2003. Developing a plan of action—How to conduct an accounting of disclosures. *In Confidence* 11(7):4–5.

University of Houston. 2001. *Information Security Manual.*

Williams, A. 2006. Design for better data: How software and users interact on screen matters to data quality. *Journal of AHIMA* 77(2):56–60.

Additional Resources

AHIMA. 2004. Your guide to implementing the EHR: AHIMA Workgroups deliver best practices. *Journal of AHIMA* 75(1):26–31.

AHIMA e-HIM Workgroup on Health Information Management in Health Information Exchange. 2007. Practice brief: HIM principles in health information exchange: Appendix: Use case scenarios. *Journal of AHIMA* 78(8):69–74.

Tegan, A., et al. 2005. The EHR's impact on HIM functions. *Journal of AHIMA* 76(5):56C–56H.

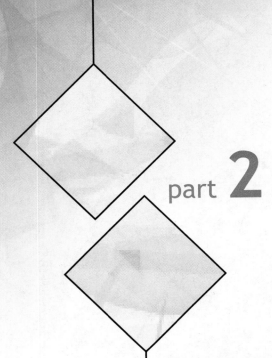

part **2**

Health Statistics, Biomedical Research, and Quality Management

chapter 8

Secondary Data Sources

Marcia Sharp, EdD, RHIA

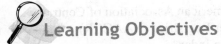

Learning Objectives

- Distinguish between primary and secondary data and between patient-identifiable and aggregate data

- Identify the internal and external users of secondary data

- Compare the facility-specific indexes commonly found in hospitals

- Describe the registries used in hospitals according to purpose, methods of case definition and case finding, data collection methods, reporting and follow-up, and pertinent laws and regulations affecting registry operations

- Define the terms pertinent to each type of secondary record or database

- Discuss the agencies for approval, education, and certification for cancer, immunization, and trauma registries

- Distinguish among healthcare databases in terms of purpose and content

- Compare manual and automated methods of data collection and vendor systems with facility-specific systems

- Describe data stewardship concepts as they relate to secondary data including data quality, security, and confidentiality, as well as data definitions and standards, rights of stakeholders, and data exchange and interoperability

- Identify the role of the health information management professional in data stewardship of primary and secondary health data

Key Terms

Abbreviated Injury Scale (AIS)
Abstracting
Accession number
Accession registry
Activities of daily living (ADL)
Agency for Healthcare Research and
    Quality (AHRQ)
American College of Surgeons (ACS)
    Commission on Cancer
Autodialing system
Case definition
Case finding
Centers for Disease Control and
    Prevention (CDC)
Certified Tumor Registrar (CTR)
Claim
Clinical trial
Collaborative Stage Data Set
Credentialing
Data confidentiality
Data stewardship
Data timeliness
Database
Demographic information
Disease index
Disease registry
Edit
Facility-based registry
Facility-specific system
Food and Drug Administration (FDA)
Health Services Research
Healthcare Cost and Utilization Project
    (HCUP)
Healthcare Integrity and Protection Data
    Bank (HIPDB)

Histocompatibility
Incidence
Index
Injury Severity Score (ISS)
Interrater reliability
Medical Literature, Analysis, and
    Retrieval System Online (MEDLINE)
Medicare Provider Analysis and Review
    (MEDPAR) File
National Cancer Registrars Association
    (NCRA)
National Center for Health Statistics
National Library of Medicine
National Practitioner Data Bank (NPDB)
National Vaccine Advisory Committee
    (NVAC)
North American Association of Central
    Cancer Registries (NAACCR)
Operation index
Patient-specific/identifiable data
Physician index
Population-based registry
Primary data source
Protocol
Public health
Secondary data source
Stage of the neoplasm
Stakeholder
Transparency
Traumatic injury
Unified Medical Language System
    (UMLS)
Vendor system
Vital statistics

Introduction

As a rich source of data about an individual patient, the health record's primary purpose
is in patient care and reimbursement for individual encounters (see chapter 2). However,
it is not easy to see trends in a population of patients by looking at individual records. For

this purpose, data must be extracted from individual records and entered into **databases.** These data may be used in a facility-specific or population-based registry for research and improvement in patient care. In addition, the data may be reported to the state and become part of state- and federal-level databases used to set health policy and improve healthcare. With the electronic health record, it is possible for data to be collected once in the EHR and used many times for a variety of purposes as outlined in this chapter.

The health information management (HIM) professional can play a variety of roles in managing secondary records and databases. He or she plays a key role in helping to set up databases. This task includes determining the content of the database and ensuring compliance with the laws, regulations, and accreditation standards that affect its content and use. All data elements included in the database or registry must be defined in a data dictionary. The HIM professional may serve as a **data steward** to oversee the completeness and accuracy of the data abstracted for inclusion in the database or registry.

This chapter explains the difference between primary and secondary data and their users. It also offers an in-depth look at the types of secondary databases, including indexes and registries, and their functions. Finally, this chapter discusses how secondary databases are processed and maintained.

Theory into Practice

A hospital with a level I trauma center serving a tristate area had an ongoing problem. It was required to provide care to all major trauma cases from the three states within its service area regardless of the patients' ability to pay. However, one of the states (state X) was unwilling to pay for the care provided to its indigent patients. Because trauma care can be extremely intensive and costly, the hospital was losing a lot of money.

The American College of Surgeons requires certified trauma centers to maintain a trauma registry. To demonstrate the extent of the problem, the hospital administrator asked the trauma registrar to gather data on patients from state X. The trauma registrar easily identified the patients and provided information by zip code on their location and the type and severity of their injuries. After the patients had been identified, the business office was able to calculate the cost to the hospital of providing their care. The administrator then presented this information to state X's legislature to obtain the money to pay for the care the trauma center provided to the state's indigent patients.

Differences between Primary and Secondary Data Sources and Databases

The health record is considered a **primary data source** because it contains information about a patient that has been documented by the professionals who provided care or services to that patient. Data contained in registries and similar databases are considered a **secondary data source.**

Data also are categorized as either **patient-specific/identified data, patient identifiable data,** or aggregate data. With patient-identified data, the patient is identified within the data. The health record consists entirely of patient-identified data. In other words, every fact recorded in the record relates to a particular patient identified by name. Secondary data also may be patient identified. In some instances, data are entered into a database along with information such as the patient's name maintained in an identified form. Registries are an example of patient-identified data on groups of patients. Data are patient-identifiable if the identity of the patient can be derived or inferred from the data, with or without the assistance of computers and artificial intelligence (Mon 2007). For example, if an individual can be identified by using a combination of elements such as date of birth, zip code, gender, marital status, and phone number, this would be considered patient-identifiable data.

More often, however, secondary data are considered aggregate data. Aggregate data include data on groups of people or patients without identifying any particular patient individually. Examples of aggregate data are statistics on the average length of stay (ALOS) for patients discharged within a particular diagnosis-related group (DRG).

Purposes and Users of Secondary Data Sources

There are four major purposes for collecting secondary data (figure 8.1). The first is for quality, performance, and patient safety. Healthcare facilities, for example, collect core measures information from the health record for the Centers for Medicare and Medicaid Services to evaluate the quality of care within the facility.

The second area of secondary data use is research. Data taken from health records and entered into disease-oriented databases can help researchers determine the effectiveness of alternate treatment methods. They also can quickly demonstrate survival rates at different stages of diseases.

Figure 8.1.   **Four purposes for collecting secondary data**

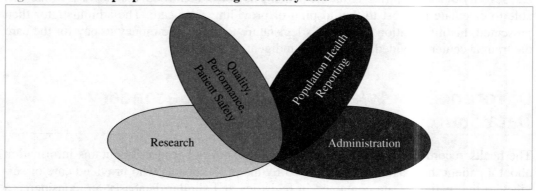

Source: Mon 2007, 11.

The third major use is for population health. States, for example, require that information be reported to them on certain diseases so that the extent of the disease can be determined and measures to prevent its spread can be initiated.

The final use of secondary data is for administration. In credentialing physicians, for example, facilities are required to access a national database for information on previous malpractice or other adverse decisions against a physician (Mon 2007).

Internal Users

Internal users of secondary data are individuals located within the healthcare facility. For example, internal users include medical staff and administrative and management staff. Secondary data enable these users to identify patterns and trends that are helpful in patient care, long-range planning, budgeting, and benchmarking with other facilities.

External Users

External users of patient data are individuals and institutions outside the facility. Examples of external users are state data banks and federal agencies. States have laws that cases of patients with diseases such as tuberculosis and AIDS must be reported to the state department of health. Moreover, the federal government collects data from the states on vital events such as births and deaths.

The secondary data provided to external users are generally aggregate data and not patient-identifiable data. Thus, these data can be used as needed without risking breaches of confidentiality.

Check Your Understanding 8.1

1. Bob Smith is a 56-year-old white male. This is an example of what type of data?

    A. Patient-specific
    B. Primary
    C. Aggregate
    D. Secondary

2. Which of the following is an example of how an internal user utilizes secondary data?

    A. State infectious disease reporting
    B. Birth certificates
    C. Death certificates
    D. Benchmarking with other facilities

3. Secondary data is used for multiple reasons including:

    A. Assisting researchers in determining effectiveness of treatments
    B. Assisting physicians and other healthcare providers in providing patient care
    C. Billing for services provided to the patient
    D. Coding diagnoses and procedures treated

Instructions: Indicate whether the following statements are true or false (T or F).

4. ＿＿＿ A registry is a secondary data source.

5. ＿＿＿ A patient health record contains aggregate data.

6. ＿＿＿ Administrative and management staff members are internal users of secondary data.

7. ＿＿＿ Medical staff members are external users of secondary data.

Types of Secondary Data Sources

Secondary data sources consist of facility-specific indexes; registries, either facility or population based; or other healthcare databases.

Facility-Specific Indexes

The most long-standing secondary data sources are those that have been developed within facilities to meet their individual needs. These **indexes** enable health records to be located by diagnosis, procedure, or physician. Prior to extensive computerization in healthcare, these indexes were kept on cards. Today, most indexes are maintained as computerized reports based on data from databases routinely developed in the healthcare facility. (Facility-specific indexes are discussed more fully in chapter 7.)

Master Population/Patient Index

The master population/patient index (MPI), which is sometimes called the master person index, contains patient-identifiable data such as name, address, date of birth, dates of hospitalizations or encounters, name of attending physician, and health record number. Because paper-based health records are filed numerically in most facilities, the MPI is an important source of patient health record numbers. These numbers enable the facility to quickly retrieve health information for specific patients.

Hospitals with unit numbering systems also depend on the MPI to determine whether a patient has been seen in the facility before and has an existing health record number. Having this information in the MPI avoids the duplication of record numbers. Most of the information in the MPI is entered into the facility database at the time of admission/ preadmission or registration.

Disease and Operation Indexes

The **disease index** is a listing in diagnosis code number order of patients discharged from the facility during a particular time period. Each patient's diagnoses are converted from a verbal description to a numerical code, usually using the *International Classification of*

Diseases. The patient's diagnosis codes are entered into the facility's health information system as part of the discharge processing of the patient's health record. The index always includes the patient's health record number as well as the diagnosis codes so that records can be retrieved by diagnosis. Because each patient is listed with the health record number, which may be linked back to the patient's name, the disease index is considered patient-identifiable data. The disease index also may include information such as the attending physician's name and the date of discharge.

The **operation index** is similar to the disease index except that it is arranged in numerical order by the patient's procedure code(s) using *International Classification of Diseases* or *Current Procedural Terminology* (CPT) codes. The other information listed in the operation index is generally the same as that listed in the disease index except that the surgeon may be listed in addition to, or instead of, the attending physician. For additional information, please see chapter 7.

Physician Index

The **physician index** is a listing of cases in order by physician name or physician identification number. It also includes the patient's health record number and may include other information, such as date of discharge. The physician index enables users to retrieve information about a particular physician, including the number of cases seen during a particular time period.

Registries

Disease registries are collections of secondary data related to patients with a specific diagnosis, condition, or procedure. Registries are different from indexes in that they contain more extensive data. Index reports can usually be produced using data from the facility's existing databases. Registries often require more extensive entry of data from the patient record. Each registry must define the cases that are to be included in it. This process is called **case definition.** In a trauma registry, for example, the case definition might be all patients admitted with a diagnosis falling into the *International Classification of Diseases* trauma diagnosis codes.

After the cases to be included have been determined, the next step in data acquisition is usually **case finding.** Case finding is a method used to identify the patients who have been seen and/or treated in the facility for the particular disease or condition of interest to the registry. After cases have been identified, extensive information is abstracted from the patients' paper-based health records into the registry database or extracted from other databases and automatically entered into the registry database.

The sole purpose of some registries is to collect data from health records and to make them available for users. Other registries take further steps to enter additional information in the registry database, such as routine follow-up of patients at specified intervals. Follow-up information might include rate and duration of survival and quality of life over time.

Cancer Registries

Cancer registries have a long history in healthcare. According to the National Cancer Registrars Association (NCRA), the first hospital cancer registry was founded in 1926 at Yale-New Haven Hospital. It has long been recognized that information is needed to improve the diagnosis and treatment of cancer. Cancer registries were developed as an organized method to collect these data. The data may be facility based (for example, within a hospital or clinic) or population based (for example, from more than one facility within a state or region).

The data from **facility-based registries** are used to provide information for the improved understanding of cancer, including its causes and methods of diagnosis and treatment. The data collected also may provide comparisons in survival rates and quality of life for patients with different treatments and at different stages of cancer at the time of diagnosis. In **population-based registries,** emphasis is on identifying trends and changes in the **incidence** (new cases) of cancer within the area covered by the registry.

The Cancer Registries Amendment Act of 1992 provided funding for a national program of cancer registries with population-based registries in each state. According to the law, these registries were mandated to collect data such as:

- Demographic information about each case of cancer

- Information on the industrial or occupational history of the individuals with the cancers (to the extent such information is available from the same record)

- Administrative information, including date of diagnosis and source of information

- Pathological data characterizing the cancer, including site, **stage of the neoplasm,** incidence, and type of treatment

Case Definition and Case Finding in the Cancer Registry

As defined previously, case definition is the process of deciding which cases should be entered in the registry. In a cancer registry, for example, all cancer cases except skin cancer might meet the definition for the cases to be included. In addition to information on malignant neoplasms, data on benign and borderline brain/central nervous system tumors must be collected by the National Program of Cancer Registries (CDC nd).

In the facility-based cancer registry, the first step is case finding. One way to find cases is through the discharge process in the HIM department. During the discharge procedure, coders and/or discharge analysts can easily earmark cases of patients with cancer for inclusion in the registry. Another case-finding method is to use the facility-specific disease indexes to identify patients with diagnoses of cancer. Additional methods may include reviews of pathology reports and lists of patients receiving radiation therapy or other cancer treatments to determine cases that have not been found by other methods.

Population-based registries usually depend on hospitals, physician offices, radiation facilities, ambulatory surgery centers (ASCs), and pathology laboratories to identify and report cases to the central registry. The administrators of a population-based registry have a responsibility to ensure that all cases of cancer have been identified and reported to the central registry.

Data Collection for the Cancer Registry

Data collection methods vary between facility-based registries and population-based registries. When a case is first entered in the registry, an **accession number** is assigned. This number consists of the first digits of the year the patient was first seen at the facility, and the remaining digits are assigned sequentially throughout the year. The first case in the year, for example, might be 10-0001. The accession number may be assigned manually or by the automated cancer database used by the organization. An **accession registry** of all cases can be kept manually or provided as a report by the database software. This listing of patients in accession number order provides a way to ensure that all cases have been entered into the registry.

In a facility-based registry, data are initially obtained by reviewing and collecting them from the patient's health record. In addition to **demographic information** (such as name, health record number, and address), data in the registry about the patient include:

- Type and site of the cancer
- Diagnostic methodologies
- Treatment methodologies
- Stage at the time of diagnosis

The stage provides information on the size and extent of spread of the tumor throughout the body. There are currently several staging systems. The American Joint Committee on Cancer (AJCC) has worked through its Collaborative Stage Task Force with other organizations with staging systems to develop a new standardized staging system, the **Collaborative Stage Data Set.** This system uses computer algorithms to describe how far a cancer has spread (AJCC 2009). After the initial information is collected at the patient's first encounter, information in the registry is updated periodically through the follow-up process discussed below.

Frequently, the population-based registry only collects information when the patient is diagnosed. Sometimes, however, it receives follow-up information from its reporting entities. These entities usually submit information to the central registry electronically.

Reporting and Follow-up for Cancer Registry Data

Formal reporting of cancer registry data is done through an annual report. The annual report includes aggregate data on the number of cases in the past year by site and type of cancer. It also may include information on patients by gender, age, and ethnic group. Often a particular site or type of cancer is featured with more in-depth data provided.

Other reports are provided as needed. Data from the cancer registry are frequently used in the quality assessment process for a facility as well as in research. Data on survival rates by site of cancer and methods of treatment, for example, would be helpful in researching the most effective treatment for a type of cancer.

Another activity of the cancer registry is patient follow-up. On an annual basis, the registry attempts to obtain information about each patient in the registry, including whether he or she is still alive, status of the cancer, and treatment received during the period. Various methods are used to obtain this information. For a facility-based registry, the facility's patient health records may be checked for return hospitalizations or visits for treatment. Additionally, the patient's physician may be contacted to determine whether the patient is still living and to obtain information about the cancer.

When patient status cannot be determined through these methods, an attempt may be made to contact the patient directly using information in the registry such as the patient's address and telephone number. In addition, contact information from the patient's health record may be used to request information from the patient's relatives. Other methods used include reading newspaper obituaries for deaths and using the Internet to locate patients through sites such as the Social Security Death Index and online telephone books. The information obtained through follow-up is important to allow the registry to develop statistics on survival rates for particular cancers and different treatment methodologies.

Population-based registries do not always include follow-up information on the patients in their databases. However, those who do follow up usually receive the information from the reporting entities such as hospitals, physician offices, and other organizations providing follow-up care.

Standards and Approval Processes for Cancer Registries

Several organizations have developed standards or approval processes for cancer programs. The **American College of Surgeons** (ACS) **Commission on Cancer** has an approval process for cancer programs. One of the requirements of this process is the existence of a cancer registry as part of the program. The ACS standards are published in the Cancer Program Standards (ACS COC 2011). When the ACS surveys the cancer program, part of the survey process is a review of cancer registry activities.

The **North American Association of Central Cancer Registries** (NAACCR) has a certification program for state population-based registries. Certification is based on the quality of data collected and reported by the state registry. NAACCR has developed standards for data quality and format and works with other cancer organizations to align their various standards sets.

The **Centers for Disease Control and Prevention** (CDC) also has national standards regarding the completeness, timeliness, and quality of cancer registry data from state registries through the National Program of Cancer Registries (NPCR). NPCR was developed as a result of the Cancer Registries Amendment Act of 1992. The CDC collects data from the NPCR state registries.

Education and Certification for Cancer Registrars

Traditionally, cancer registrars have been trained through on-the-job training and professional workshops and seminars. The **National Cancer Registrars Association** (NCRA) has worked with colleges to develop formal educational programs for cancer registrars. A cancer registrar may become credentialed as a **Certified Tumor Registrar** (CTR) by passing an examination provided by the National Board for Certification of Registrars (NBCR). Eligibility requirements for the certification examination include a combination of experience and education (NCRA 2009).

Trauma Registries

Trauma registries maintain databases on patients with severe traumatic injuries. A **traumatic injury** is a wound or other injury caused by an external physical force such as an automobile accident, a shooting, a stabbing, or a fall. Information collected by the trauma registry may be used for performance improvement and research in the area of trauma care. Trauma registries may be facility based or may include data for a region or state.

Case Definition and Case Finding for Trauma Registries

The case definition for the trauma registry varies from registry to registry but frequently involves inclusion of cases with diagnoses from the trauma diagnosis codes from the *International Classification of Diseases*. To find cases with trauma diagnoses, the trauma registrar can access the disease indexes looking for cases with codes from this section of *International Classification of Diseases*. In addition, the registrar may look at deaths in services with frequent trauma diagnoses—such as trauma, neurosurgery, orthopedics, and plastic surgery—to find additional cases.

Data Collection for Trauma Registries

After the cases have been identified, information is abstracted from the health records of the injured patients and entered into the trauma registry database. The data elements collected in the **abstracting** process vary from registry to registry but usually include:

- Demographic information on the patient

- Information on the injury

- Care the patient received before hospitalization (such as care at another transferring hospital or care from an emergency medical technician who provided care at the scene of the accident and/or in transport from the accident site to the hospital)

- Status of the patient at the time of admission

- Patient's course in the hospital

- Diagnosis and procedure codes

- **Abbreviated Injury Scale** (AIS)
- **Injury Severity Score** (ISS)

The AIS reflects the nature of the injury and the threat to life of the injury by body system. It may be assigned manually by the registrar or generated as part of the database from data entered by the registrar. The ISS is an overall severity measurement calculated from the AIS scores for patients with multiple injuries (Trauma.org 2012).

Reporting and Follow-up for Trauma Registries

Reporting varies among trauma registries. An annual report is often developed to show the activity of the trauma registry. Other reports may be generated as part of the performance improvement process, such as self-extubation (patients removing their own tubes) and delays in abdominal surgery or patient complications. Some hospitals report data to the National Trauma Data Bank (ACS 2011).

Trauma registries may or may not do follow-up on the patients entered in the registry. When follow-up is done, emphasis is frequently on the patient's quality of life after a period of time. Unlike cancer, where physician follow-up is crucial to detect recurrence, many traumatic injuries do not require continued patient care over time. Thus, follow-up is often not given the emphasis it receives in cancer registries.

Standards and Approval Process for Trauma Registries

The ACS verifies levels I, II, III, and IV trauma centers. As part of its requirements, the ACS states that the level I trauma center must have a trauma registry (ACS Trauma Programs 2012).

Education and Certification of Trauma Registrars

Trauma registrars may be Registered Health Information Technicians (RHITs), Registered Health Information Administrators (RHIAs), Registered Nurses (RNs), Licensed Practical Nurses (LPNs), Emergency Medical Technicians (EMTs), or other health professionals. Training for trauma registrars is through workshops and on-the-job training. The American Trauma Society (ATS), for example, provides core and advanced workshops for trauma registrars. It also provides a certification examination for trauma registrars who meet their education and experience requirements through its Registrar Certification Board. Certified trauma registrars have earned the credential CSTR (certified specialist in trauma registry).

Birth Defects Registries

Birth defects registries collect information on newborns with birth defects. Often population based, these registries serve a variety of purposes. For example, they provide information on the incidence of birth defects to study causes and prevention of birth defects, to monitor trends in birth defects, to improve medical care for children with birth defects, and to target interventions for preventable birth defects, such as folic acid to prevent neural tube defects.

In some cases, registries have been developed after specific events have put a spotlight on birth defects. After the initial Persian Gulf War, for example, some feared an increased incidence of birth defects among the children of Gulf War veterans. The Department of Defense subsequently started a birth defects registry to collect data on the children of these veterans to determine whether any pattern could be detected.

Case Definition and Case Finding for Birth Defects Registries

Birth defects registries use a variety of criteria to determine which cases to include in the registry. Some registries limit cases to those with defects found within the first year of life. Others include those children with a major defect that occurred in the first year of life and was discovered within the first five years of life. Still other registries include only children who were live born or stillborn babies with discernible birth defects.

Cases may be detected in a variety of ways, including review of disease indexes, labor and delivery logs, pathology and autopsy reports, ultrasound reports, and cytogenetic reports. In addition to information from hospitals and physicians, cases may be identified from rehabilitation centers and children's hospitals and from vital records such as birth, death, and fetal death certificates.

Data Collection for Birth Defects Registries

A variety of information is abstracted for the birth defects registry, including:

- Demographic information
- Codes for diagnoses
- Birth weight
- Status at birth, including live born, stillborn, aborted
- Autopsy
- Cytogenetics results
- Whether the infant was a single birth or one in a multiple birth
- Mother's use of alcohol, tobacco, or illicit drugs
- Father's use of drugs and alcohol
- Family history of birth defects

Diabetes Registries

Diabetes registries include cases of patients with diabetes for the purpose of assistance in managing care as well as for research. Patients whose diabetes is not kept under good control frequently have numerous complications. The diabetes registry can keep up with whether the patient has been seen by a physician in an effort to prevent complications.

Case Definition and Case Finding for Diabetes Registries

There are two types of diabetes mellitus: type 1 and type 2 diabetes. Registries sometimes limit their cases by type of diabetes. In some instances, there may be further definition by age. Some diabetes registries, for example, only include children with diabetes.

Case finding includes the review of health records of patients with diabetes. Other case-finding methods include review of the following types of information:

- Diagnostic codes
- Billing data
- Medication lists
- Physician identification
- Health plans

Although facility-based registries for cancer and trauma are usually hospital based, facility-based diabetes registries are often found in physician offices or clinics. The office or clinic is the main location for diabetes care. Thus, data about the patient to be entered into the registry are available at these sites rather than at the hospital. The health records of diabetes patients treated in physician practices may be identified through diagnosis code numbers for diabetes, billing data for diabetes-related services, medication lists for patients on diabetic medications, or identification of patients as the physician sees them.

Health plans also are interested in optimal care for their enrollees because diabetes can have serious complications when not managed correctly. The plans can provide information to the office or clinic on enrollees who are diabetics.

Data Collection for Diabetes Registries

In addition to demographic information about the cases, other data collected may include laboratory values such as glycated hemoglobin also known as HBA1c. This test is used to determine the patient's blood glucose for a period of approximately 60 days prior to the time of the test. Moreover, facility registries may track patient visits to follow up with patients who have not been seen in the past year.

Reporting and Follow-up for Diabetes Registries

A variety of reports can be developed from the diabetes registry. For facility-based registries, one report might keep up with laboratory monitoring of the patient's diabetes to allow intensive intervention with patients whose diabetes is not well controlled. Another report might concern patients who have not been tested within a year or have not had a primary care provider visit within a year.

Population-based diabetes registries might provide reporting on the incidence of diabetes for the geographic area covered by the registry. Registry data also might be used to investigate risk factors for diabetes.

Follow-up is aimed primarily at ensuring that the diabetic is seen by the physician at appropriate intervals to prevent complications.

Implant Registries

An implant is a material or substance inserted into the body, such as breast implants, heart valves, and pacemakers. Implant registries have been developed for the purpose of tracking the performance of implants, including complications, deaths, and defects resulting from implants, as well as implant longevity. In the recent past, the safety of implants has been questioned in a number of highly publicized cases. In Texas, a woman who had a partial mastectomy after her breast implant ruptured was awarded $25 million dollars. Implant manufacturers Corning, Baxter, Bristol-Myers Squibb/MEC, and 3M settled a class action lawsuit after women claimed to suffer autoimmune disease from their silicone breast implants. In some cases, implant registries have been developed in response to such events. For example, there have been questions about the safety of silicone breast implants and temporomandibular joint implants. When such cases arise, it has often been difficult to ensure that all patients with the implants have been notified of safety concerns. A number of federal laws have been enacted to regulate medical devices, including implants. These devices were first covered under Section 15 of the Food, Drug, and Cosmetic Act. The Safe Medical Devices Act of 1990 was passed and then amended through the Medical Device Amendments of 1992. These acts required a sample of facilities to report deaths and severe complications thought to be due to a device to the manufacturer and the **Food and Drug Administration** (FDA) through its MedWatch reporting system. The MedWatch reporting system alerts health professionals and the public of safety alerts and medical device recalls (FDA 2009). Implant registries may help to assure compliance with legal reporting requirements for device related deaths and complications.

Case Definition and Case Finding for Implant Registries

Implant registries sometimes include all types of implants but often are restricted to a specific type of implant such as cochlear, saline breast, or temporomandibular joint.

Data Collection for Implant Registries

Demographic data on patients receiving implants are included in the registry. The FDA requires that all reportable events involving medical devices include the following information (FDA 2011):

- User facility report number
- Name and address of the device manufacturer
- Device brand name and common name
- Product model, catalog, serial, and lot numbers
- Brief description of the event reported to the manufacturer and/or the FDA
- Where the report was submitted (for example, to the FDA, manufacturer, or distributor)

Thus, these data items also should be included in the implant registry to facilitate reporting.

Reporting and Follow-up for Implant Registries

Data from the implant registry may be used to report to the FDA and the manufacturer when devices cause death or serious illness or injury.

Follow-up is important to track the performance of the implant. When patients are tracked, they can be easily notified of product failures, recalls, or upgrades.

Transplant Registries

Transplant registries may have varied purposes. Some organ transplant registries maintain databases of patients who need organs. When an organ becomes available, a fair way then may be used to allocate the organ to the patient with the highest priority. In other cases, the purpose of the registry is to provide a database of potential donors for transplants using live donors, such as bone marrow transplants. Post-transplant information also is kept on organ recipients and donors.

Because transplant registries are used to try to match donor organs with recipients, they are often national or even international in scope. Examples of national registries include the UNet of the United Network for Organ Sharing (UNOS) and the registry of the National Marrow Donor Program (NMDP).

Data collected in the transplant registry also may be used for research, policy analysis, and quality control.

Case Definition and Case Finding for Transplant Registries

Physicians identify patients needing transplants. Information about the patient is provided to the registry. When an organ becomes available, information about it is matched with potential donors. For donor registries, donors are solicited through community information efforts similar to those carried out by blood banks to encourage blood donations.

Data Collection for Transplant Registries

The type of information collected varies according to the type of registry. Pre-transplant data about the recipient include:

- Demographic data
- Patient's diagnosis
- Patient's status codes regarding medical urgency
- Patient's functional status
- Whether the patient is on life support
- Previous transplantations
- **Histocompatibility** (compatibility of donor and recipient tissues)

Information on donors varies according to whether the donor is living. For organs harvested from patients who have died, information is collected on:

- Cause and circumstances of the death
- Organ procurement and consent process
- Medications the donor was taking
- Other donor history

For a living donor, information includes:

- Relationship of the donor to the recipient (if any)
- Clinical information
- Information on organ recovery
- Histocompatibility

Reporting and Follow-up for Transplant Registries

Reporting includes information on donors and recipients as well as survival rates, length of time on the waiting list for an organ, and death rates.

Follow-up information is collected for recipients as well as living donors. For living donors, the information collected might include complications of the procedure and length of stay in the hospital. Follow-up on recipients includes information on status at the time of follow-up (for example, living, expired, lost to follow-up), functional status, graft status, and treatment, such as immunosuppressive drugs. Follow-up is carried out at intervals throughout the first year after the transplant and then annually after that.

Immunization Registries

Children are supposed to receive a large number of immunizations during the first six years of life. These immunizations are so important that the federal government has set several objectives related to immunizations in Healthy People 2020, a set of health goals for the nation. These include increasing the proportion of children and adolescents that are fully immunized (objectives 7–12) and increasing the proportion of children in population-based immunization registries (objectives 18–20) (Healthy People 2012).

Immunization registries usually have the purpose of increasing the number of infants and children who receive the required immunizations at the proper intervals. To accomplish this goal, registries collect information within a particular geographic area on children and their immunization status. They also help by maintaining a central source of information for a particular child's immunization history, even when the child has received immunizations from a variety of providers. This central location for immunization data also relieves parents of the responsibility of maintaining immunization records for their children.

Case Definition and Case Finding for Immunization Registries

All children in the population area served by the registry should be included in the registry. Some registries limit their inclusion of patients to those seen at public clinics, excluding those seen exclusively by private practitioners. Although children are usually targeted in immunization registries, some registries do include information on adults for influenza and pneumonia vaccines.

Children are often entered in the registry at birth. Registry personnel may review birth and death certificates and adoption records to determine which children to include and which children to exclude because they died after birth. In some cases, children are entered electronically through a connection with an electronic birth record system.

Data Collection for Immunization Registries

The National Immunization Program at the CDC has worked with the **National Vaccine Advisory Committee** (NVAC) to develop a core set of immunization data elements to be included in all immunization registries. These data elements include (CDC 2011b):

- Patient name (first, middle, and last)
- Patient birth date
- Patient sex
- Patient race
- Patient ethnicity
- Patient birth order
- Patient birth state/country
- Mother's name (first, middle, last, and maiden)
- Vaccine type
- Vaccine manufacturer
- Vaccination date
- Vaccine lot number

Other items may be included as needed by the individual registry.

Reporting and Follow-up for Immunization Registries

Because the purpose of the immunization registry is to increase the number of children who receive immunizations in a timely manner, reporting should emphasize immunization rates, especially changes in rates in target areas. Immunization registries also can provide automatic reporting of children's immunization to schools to check the immunization status of their students.

Follow-up is directed toward reminding parents that it is time for immunizations as well as seeing whether parents fail to bring the child in for the immunization after a reminder. Reminders may include a letter or postcard or telephone calls. **Autodialing systems** may be used to call parents and deliver a prerecorded reminder. Moreover, registries must decide how frequently to follow up with parents who do not bring their children in for immunization. Maintaining up-to-date addresses and telephone numbers is an important factor in providing follow-up. Registries may allow parents to opt out of the registry if they prefer not to be reminded.

Standards and Approval Processes for Immunization Registries

The CDC, through its National Immunization Program, provides funding for some population-based immunization registries. It has identified 12 minimum functional standards for immunization registries (CDC 2011b), including:

- Electronically store data on all NVAC-approved core data elements.

- Establish a registry record within six weeks of birth for each newborn child born in the catchment area.

- Enable access to and retrieval of immunization information in the registry at the time of the encounter.

- Receive and process immunization information within one month of vaccine administration.

- Protect the confidentiality of healthcare information.

- Ensure the security of healthcare information.

- Exchange immunization records using Health Level Seven (HL7) standards.

- Automatically determine the routine childhood immunization(s) needed, in compliance with current ACIP (Advisory Committee on Immunization Practices) recommendations, when an individual presents for a scheduled immunization.

- Automatically identify individuals due/late for immunization(s) to enable the production of reminder/recall notifications.

- Automatically produce immunization coverage reports by providers, age groups, and geographic areas.

- Produce official immunization records.

- Promote the accuracy and completeness of registry data.

The CDC provides funding for population-based immunization registries.

Other Registries

Registries may be developed for any type of disease or condition. Other commonly kept types of registries are HIV/AIDS and cardiac registries. In 2007 the state of Nebraska initiated a partnership within the state called the Nebraska Registry Partnership (NRP) to introduce, sustain and gradually expand a registry for chronic disease management for cardiovascular diseases and diabetes care improvement for patients seen in rural health clinics (Smith 2007).

In addition, the American Gastroenterological Association (AGA) sponsors the AGA Digestive Health Outcomes Registry. The AGA Registry is the only gastroenterology registry sponsored by the Centers for Medicare and Medicaid Services (CMS), enabling practices to directly submit data for the CMS Physician Quality Reporting System. It is a national outcomes-driven registry that allows clinicians to monitor and improve patient care, while generating data to compare the efficacy of treatments (GMed 2011).

Registries may be developed for administrative purposes also. The National Provider Identifier Registry is an example of an administrative registry. The NPI Registry enables users to search for a provider's national plan and provider enumeration system information, including the national provider identification number. The NPI number is a 10-digit unique identification number assigned to healthcare providers in the United States (CMS 2011). There is no charge to use the registry and it is updated daily (National Plan and Provider Enumeration System 2012). Data collected for healthcare administrative purposes are discussed in the next subsection.

Healthcare Databases

Databases also may be developed for a variety of purposes. For example, the federal government has developed a variety of databases to enable it to carry out surveillance, improvement, and prevention duties. HIM managers may provide information for these databases through data abstraction or from data reported by a facility to state and local entities. They also may use these data to do research or work with other researchers on issues related to reimbursement and health status.

National and State Administrative Databases

Some databases are established for administrative rather than disease-oriented reasons. Data banks are developed, for example, for **claims** data submitted on Medicare claims. Other administrative databases assist in the **credentialing** and privileging of health practitioners.

Medicare Provider Analysis and Review File

The **Medicare Provider Analysis and Review** (MEDPAR) **File** is made up of acute care hospital and skilled nursing facility (SNF) claims data for all Medicare claims. It consists of the following types of data:

- Demographic data on the patient
- Data on the provider

- Information on Medicare coverage for the claim
- Total charges
- Charges broken down by specific type of service, such as operating room, physical therapy, and pharmacy charges
- International Classification of Diseases diagnosis and procedure codes
- MS-DRGs

The MEDPAR file is frequently used for research on topics such as charges for particular types of care and MS-DRGs. The limitation of the MEDPAR data for research purposes is that the file contains only Medicare patients.

National Practitioner Data Bank

The **National Practitioner Data Bank** (NPDB) was mandated under the Health Care Quality Improvement Act of 1986 to provide a database of medical malpractice payments, adverse licensure actions, and certain professional review actions (such as denial of medical staff privileges) taken by healthcare entities such as hospitals against physicians, dentists, and other healthcare providers as well as private accrediting organizations and peer review organizations (NPDB 2010). The NPDB was developed to alleviate the lack of information about malpractice decisions, denial of medical staff privileges, or loss of medical license. Because these data were not widely available, physicians who lost their license to practice in one state or facility could move to another state or another facility and begin practicing again with the current state and/or facility unaware of previous actions against the physician.

Information in the NPDB is provided through a required reporting mechanism. Entities making malpractice payments, including insurance companies, boards of medical examiners, and entities such as hospitals and professional societies, must report to the NPDB. The information to be reported includes information about the practitioner, the reporting entity, and the judgment or settlement. Information about physicians and other healthcare providers must be provided (NPDB 2010). A recent change to the law now requires entities such as private accrediting organizations and peer review organizations to report adverse actions to the data bank. In addition, adverse licensure and other actions against any health care entity must be reported, not just physicians and dentists. Adverse actions may include reporting incidents of license suspensions or revocations. It may also include issues related to professional competence, and malpractice payments. Monetary penalties may be assessed for failure to report.

The law requires healthcare facilities to query the NPDB as part of the credentialing process when a physician initially applies for medical staff privileges and every two years thereafter.

Healthcare Integrity and Protection Data Bank

Part of the Health Insurance Portability and Accountability Act of 1996 (HIPAA) mandated the collection of information on healthcare fraud and abuse because there was no central place to obtain this information. As a result, the national **Healthcare Integrity and Protection Data Bank** (HIPDB) was developed. The types of items that must be reported to the data bank include reportable final adverse actions such as (HHS 2010):

- Federal or state licensing and certification actions, including revocation, reprimands, censures, probations, suspensions, and any other loss of license, or the right to apply for or renew a license, whether by voluntary surrender, non-renewability, or otherwise

- Exclusions from participation in federal or state healthcare programs

- Any other adjudicated actions or decisions defined in the HIPDB regulations

There may be some overlap with the NPDB, so a single report is made and then sorted to the appropriate data bank.

Information to be reported includes information about the healthcare provider, supplier, or practitioner that is the subject of the final adverse action, the nature of the act, and a description of the actions on which the decision was based. Only federal and state government agencies and health plans are required to report, and access to the data bank is limited to these organizations and to practitioners, providers, and suppliers who may only query about themselves.

State Administrative Data Banks

States also frequently have health-related administrative databases. For example, many states collect either UHDDS or UB-04/837 Institutional data on patients discharged from hospitals located within their area. The Statewide Planning and Research Cooperative System (SPARCS) in New York is an example of this type of administrative database. It combines UB-04/837 Institutional data with data required by the state of New York.

National, State, and County Public Health Databases

Public health is the area of healthcare dealing with the health of populations in geographic areas such as states or counties. Publicly reported healthcare data vary from quality and patient safety measurement data to patient satisfaction results. The aggregated data range from a local to national perspective, such as state-specific public health conditions to national morbidity and mortality statistics. In addition, consumers are becoming more actively involved in their healthcare. Publicly reported data may be presented for consumer use through various star ratings on different quality measures via organizations such as The Leapfrog Group, HealthGrades, or Hospital Compare. The Leapfrog Group and Hospital Compare allow users to select various hospitals to compare data such as specific medical conditions, surgical procedures, or overall patient safety ratings. Based on the selections made, data is compared to the hospitals selected as well as to state and national averages. One of the duties of public health agencies is surveillance of the health status of the population within their jurisdiction.

The databases developed by public health departments provide information on the incidence and prevalence of diseases, possible high-risk populations, survival statistics, and trends over time. Data for the databases may be collected using a variety of methods, including interviews, physical examinations of individuals, and reviews of health records. Thus, the HIM manager may have input in these databases through data provided from health records. At the national level, the **National Center for Health Statistics** has responsibility for these databases.

National Health Care Survey

One of the major national public health surveys is the National Health Care Survey. To a large extent, it relies on data from patients' health records. It consists of a number of parts, including:

- The National Hospital Care Survey
- The National Ambulatory Medical Care Survey
- The National Survey of Ambulatory Surgery
- The National Nursing Home Survey
- The National Home and Hospice Care Survey

Data in the National Hospital Care Survey are either abstracted manually from a sample of acute care discharged inpatient records or obtained from state or other discharge databases. Items collected follow the Uniform Hospital Discharge Data Set (UHDDS), including demographic data, admission and discharge dates, and final diagnoses and procedures.

The National Ambulatory Medical Care Survey includes data collected by a sample of office-based physicians and their staffs from the health records of patients seen in a one-week reporting period. Data included are demographic data, the patients' reasons for visit, the diagnoses, diagnostic/screening services, therapeutic and preventive services, ambulatory surgical procedures, and medications/injections, in addition to information on the visit disposition and time spent with the physician.

Data for the National Survey of Ambulatory Surgery are collected on a representative sample of hospital-based and freestanding ambulatory surgery centers. Data include patient demographic characteristics, source of payment, and information on anesthesia given, the diagnoses, and the surgical and nonsurgical procedures on patient visits of hospital-based and freestanding ambulatory surgery centers. The survey consists of a mailed survey about the facility and abstracts of patient data.

The National Nursing Home Survey provides data on each facility, current residents, and discharged residents. Information is gathered through an interview process. The administrator or designee provides information about the facility being surveyed. For information on the residents, the nursing staff member most familiar with the resident's care is interviewed. The staff member uses the resident's health record for reference during the interview. Data collected on the facility include information on ownership, size, certification status, admissions, services, full-time equivalent employees, and basic charges. Interviews about both current and discharged residents provide demographic information on the resident as well as length of stay, diagnoses, level of care received, **activities of daily living** (ADL), and charges.

For the National Home and Hospice Care Survey, data are collected on the home health or hospice agency as well as on their current and discharged patients. Data include referral and length of service, diagnoses, number of visits, patient charges, health status, reason for discharge, and types of services provided. Facility data are provided through an interview with the administrator or designee. Patient information is obtained from the caregiver most familiar with the patient's care. The caregiver may use the patient's health record in answering the interview questions.

Because of the bioterrorism scares in recent years, the CDC has developed the National Electronic Disease Surveillance System (NEDSS) that serves as a major part of the Public Health Information Network (PHIN). This system provides a national surveillance system by connecting the CDC with local and state public health partners. It allows the CDC to monitor trends from disease reporting at the local and state levels to look for possible bioterrorism incidents.

Other national public health databases include the National Health Interview Survey, which is used to monitor the health status of the population of the United States, and the National Immunization Survey, which collects data on the immunization status of children between the ages of 19 months and 35 months living in the United States. Table 8.1 summarizes the national databases.

State and local public health departments also develop databases, as needed, to perform their duties of health surveillance, disease prevention, and research. An example of state databases is infectious/notifiable disease databases. Each state has a list of diseases that must be reported to the state, such as AIDS, measles, and syphilis, so that containment and prevention measures can be taken to avoid large outbreaks of these diseases. As mentioned above, state and local reporting systems connect with the CDC through NEDSS to evaluate trends in disease outbreaks. There also may be statewide databases/registries that collect extensive information on particular diseases and conditions such as birth defects, immunizations, and cancer.

The National Center for Health Statistics, Centers for Disease Control began the National Hospital Care Survey (NHCS) in 2011. This survey combines the National Hospital Discharge Survey (NHDS) and the National Hospital Ambulatory Medical Care Survey (NHAMCS). In 2013, in addition to inpatient data, the hospitals will be asked to provide data on the utilization of healthcare services provided in their emergency, outpatient departments, and ambulatory surgery centers, thus integrating the NHDS and NHAMCS into NHCS. NHCS replaced NHDS and NHAMCS but continues to provide nationally representative data on utilization of hospital care and general purpose healthcare statistics on inpatient care as well as care delivered in emergency, outpatient departments, and ambulatory surgery centers (CDC 2011a).

Table 8.1.   **National heathcare databases**

Database	Type of Setting	Content	Data Source	Method of Data Collection
National Ambulatory Medical Care Survey	Office-based physician practice	Data on the patient and the visit	State discharge databases Office-based physician records	Abstract
National Nursing Home Survey	Nursing home	Data on the facility, current and discharged residents	Administrator Nurse caregiver	Interview
National Hospital Ambulatory Medical Care Survey	Hospital emergency departments and outpatient clinics	Data on the patient, the visit, and the method of payment	Emergency department and outpatient clinic records	Abstract
National Home and Hospice Care Survey	Home health and hospice	Facility data and patient data	Administrator Caregiver	Interview
National Electronic Disease Surveillance System (NEDSS)	Public health departments	Possible bioterrorism incidents	Local and state public health departments	Electronic surveillance

Vital Statistics

Vital statistics include data on births, deaths, fetal deaths, marriages, and divorces. Responsibility for the collection of vital statistics rests with the states. The states share information with the National Center for Health Statistics (NCHS). The actual collection of the information is carried out at the local level. For example, birth certificates are completed at the facility where the birth occurred and then are sent to the state. The state serves as the official repository for the certificate and provides vital statistics information to the NCHS. From the vital statistics collected, states and the national government develop a variety of databases.

One vital statistics database at the national level is the Linked Birth and Infant Death Data Set. In this database, the information from birth certificates is compared to death certificates for infants under one year of age. This database provides data to conduct analyses for patterns of infant death. Other national programs that use vital statistics data include the National Mortality Followback Survey, the National Survey of Family Growth, and the National Death Index (CDC 2012). In some of these databases, such as the National Maternal and Infant Health Survey and the National Mortality Followback Survey, additional information is collected on deaths originally identified through the vital statistics system.

Similar databases using vital statistics data as a basis are found at the state level. Birth defects registries, for example, frequently use vital records data with information on the birth defect as part of their data collection process. For additional information on vital statistics, see chapter 9.

Clinical Trials

A **clinical trial** is a research project in which new treatments and tests are investigated to determine whether they are safe and effective. The trial proceeds according to a **protocol,** which is the list of rules and procedures to be followed. Clinical trials databases have been developed to allow physicians and patients to find clinical trials. A patient with cancer or AIDS, for example, might be interested in participating in a clinical trial but not know how to locate one applicable to his or her type of disease. Clinical trials databases provide the data to enable patients and practitioners to determine what clinical trials are available and applicable to the patient.

The Food and Drug Administration Modernization Act of 1997 mandated that a clinical trials database be developed. The **National Library of Medicine** has developed the database, which is available on the Internet for use by both patients and practitioners at http://www.clinicaltrials.gov. Information in the database includes:

- Abstracts of study protocols
  - Brief summary of the purpose of the study
  - Recruiting status
  - Criteria for patient participation
  - Location of the trial and specific contact information
- Additional information (may help a patient decide whether to consider a particular trial)
  - Research study design
  - Phase of the trial
  - Disease or condition and drug or therapy under study

Each data element has been defined. For example, a brief summary gives an overview of the treatments being studied and types of patients to be included. Recruiting status indicates whether subjects are currently being entered in the trial or will be in the future or whether the trial is closed to new subjects. Criteria for patient participation include information on the type of condition to be studied (in some cases, the stage of the disease) and what other treatments are allowed during the trial or must be completed before entering the trial. Age is a frequent eligibility criterion (Clinicaltrials.gov 2009). Study design includes the research design being followed.

A clinical trial consists of four study phases. Phase I studies research the safety of the treatment in a small group of people. In phase II studies, emphasis is on determining the treatment's effectiveness and further investigating safety. Phase III studies look at effectiveness and side effects and make comparisons to other available treatments in larger populations. Phase IV studies look at the treatment after it has entered the market.

Some clinical trials databases concentrate on a particular disease. The Department of Health and Human Services, for example, has developed ACTIS, the AIDS Clinical Trials Information Service. The National Cancer Institute sponsors PDQ (Physician Data Query), a database for cancer clinical trials. These databases contain information similar to Clinicaltrials.gov. Although Clinicaltrials.gov has been set up for use by both patients and health practitioners, some databases are more oriented toward practitioners.

Health Services Research Databases

Health services research is research concerning healthcare delivery systems, including organization and delivery and care effectiveness and efficiency. Within the federal government, the organization most involved in health services research is the **Agency for Healthcare Research and Quality** (AHRQ). AHRQ looks at issues related to the efficiency and effectiveness of the healthcare delivery system, disease protocols, and guidelines for improved disease outcomes.

A major initiative for AHRQ has been the **Healthcare Cost and Utilization Project** (HCUP). HCUP uses data collected at the state level from either claims data or discharge-abstracted data, including the UHDDS items reported by individual hospitals and, in some cases, by freestanding ambulatory care centers. Which data are reported depends on the individual state. Data may be reported by the facilities to a state agency or to the state hospital association, depending on state regulations. The data then are reported from the state to AHRQ, where they become part of the HCUP databases (AHRQ 2012)

HCUP consists of a set of databases, including:

- The Nationwide Inpatient Sample (NIS), which consists of inpatient discharge data from a sample of hospitals in 35 states throughout the United States

- The State Inpatient Database (SID), which includes data collected by states on hospital discharges

- The State Ambulatory Surgery Database (SASD), which includes information from a sample of states on hospital-affiliated ASCs and, from some states, data from freestanding surgery centers

- State Emergency Department Databases include data from hospital-affiliation emergency departments (EDs) for visits that do not result in a hospitalization

- The Kids Inpatient Database (KID) is made up of inpatient discharge data on children younger than 19 years old (Healthcare Costs and Utilization Project 2009)

These databases are unique because they include data on inpatients whose care is paid for by all types of payers, including Medicare, Medicaid, private insurance, self-paying, and uninsured patients. Data elements include demographic information, information on diagnoses and procedures, admission and discharge status, payment sources, total charges, length of stay, and information on the hospital or freestanding ambulatory surgery center. Researchers may use these databases to look at issues such as those related to the costs of treating particular diseases, the extent to which treatments are used, and differences in outcomes and cost for alternative treatments.

National Library of Medicine

The National Library of Medicine (NLM) produces two databases of special interest to the HIM manager: MEDLINE and UMLS.

1) **Medical Literature, Analysis, and Retrieval System Online** (MEDLINE) is the best-known database from the NLM. It includes bibliographic listings for publications in the areas of medicine, dentistry, nursing, pharmacy, allied health, and veterinary medicine. HIM managers use MEDLINE to locate articles on HIM issues as well as articles on medical topics necessary to carry out quality improvement and medical research activities.

2) The **Unified Medical Language System** (UMLS) provides a way to integrate biomedical concepts from a variety of sources to show their relationships. This process allows links to be made between different information systems for purposes such as electronic health record systems. UMLS is of particular interest to the HIM manager because medical vocabularies such as the *International Classification of Diseases, Ninth Revision, Clinical Modification* (ICD-9-CM), *Current Procedural Terminology* (CPT), and the *Healthcare Common Procedure Coding System* (HCPCS) are among the items included.

Health Information Exchange

Health information exchange (HIE) initiatives have been developed in an effort to move toward a longitudinal patient record with complete information about the patient available at the point of care. This is patient-specific rather than aggregate data and is used primarily for patient care. Some researchers have looked at the amount of data available through the health information exchanges as a possible source of data to aggregate for research. Since HIE is a fairly new concept, it is important that HIEs take the time to develop policies and procedures covering the use of data collected for patient care for other purposes. Special attention needs to be paid to whether patients included in the HIE need to provide individual consent to be included when the data is aggregated for research and other purposes. Aggregated data can be deidentified to add another layer of protection for the patient's identity. For additional information on HIE, see chapter 16.

Data for Performance Measurement

The Joint Commission, the Centers for Medicare and Medicaid Services, and some health plans require healthcare facilities to collect data on core performance measures. These measures are secondary data because they are taken from patient medical records. Facilities must determine how to collect these measures and how to aggregate the data for reporting purposes. Whether a facility reports such measures will be used as a basis for pay for performance systems. It is, therefore, extremely important that the data accurately reflect the quality of care provided by the facility.

Check Your Understanding 8.2

1. Which of the following indexes is an important source of patient health record numbers?

   A. Physician index
   B. Master patient index
   C. Operation index
   D. Disease index

2. After the types of cases to be included in a registry have been determined, what is the next step in data acquisition?

   A. Case registration
   B. Case definition
   C. Case abstracting
   D. Case finding

3. What number is assigned to a case when it is first entered in a cancer registry?

   A. Accession number
   B. Patient number
   C. Health record number
   D. Medical record number

4. What are the patient data such as name, age, address, and so on called?

   A. Demographic data
   B. Secondary data
   C. Aggregate data
   D. Identification data

5. What type of registry maintains a database on patients injured by an external physical force?

   A. Implant registry
   B. Birth defects registry
   C. Trauma registry
   D. Transplant registry

6. Why is the MEDPAR File limited in terms of being used for research purposes?

   A. It only provides demographic data about patients.
   B. It only contains Medicare patients.
   C. It uses ICD-9-CM diagnoses and procedure codes.
   D. It breaks charges down by specific type of service.

7. Which of the following acts mandated establishment of the National Practitioner Data Bank?

    A. Health Care Quality Improvement Act of 1986

    B. Health Insurance Portability and Accountability Act of 1996

    C. Safe Medical Devices Act of 1990

    D. Food and Drug Administration Modernization Act of 1997

8. I started work today on a clinical trial. I need to familiarize myself with the rules and procedures to be followed. This information is called the:

    A. Protocol

    B. MEDPAR

    C. UMLS

    D. HCUP

9. An advantage of HCUP is that it:

    A. Contains only Medicare data

    B. Is used to determine pay for performance

    C. Contains data on all payer types

    D. Contains bibliographic listings from medical journals

Processing and Maintenance of Secondary Databases

Several issues surround the processing and maintenance of secondary databases. HIM managers are often involved in decisions concerning these issues.

Manual versus Automated Methods of Data Collection

Although registries and databases are almost universally electronic, data collection is commonly done manually. The most frequent method is abstracting. Abstracting is the process of reviewing the patient health record and entering the required data elements into the database. In some cases, the abstracting may be done initially on an abstract form. The data then would be entered into the database from the form. In many cases, it is done directly from the primary patient health record into a data collection screen in the electronic database system.

However, not all data collection is done manually. In some cases, data can be downloaded directly from other electronic systems. Birth defects registries, for example, often download information on births and birth defects from the vital records system. In some cases, providers such as hospitals and physicians send information in electronic format to the registry or database. The National Hospital Care Survey, formerly known as the National Hospital Discharge Survey, from the National Center for Health Statistics uses information in electronic format from state databases. As the electronic health record (EHR) develops further, less and less data will need to be manually abstracted since they will be available electronically through the EHR.

Vendor Systems versus Facility-Specific Systems

Each facility must determine what information technology solution best meets its needs.

A **vendor system** is an information system developed by an outside company and sold to a variety of organizations. A **facility-specific system** is an information system developed within the facility for its own use. It may be part of the facility health information system (HIS). It is important that either type of product is able to incorporate demographic and other pertinent information from the facility HIS system. In this way, time is saved and data integrity between the registry information and the HIS system is maintained.

Data Stewardship Issues Associated with Secondary Data Collection and Use

With the increased availability of secondary data in electronic format, there are concerns about collecting healthcare data in an environment without clear guidance about ownership of secondary data, unauthorized reuse of data, and spotty confidentiality and security regulations. Patients have concerns that secondary data collected about them may adversely affect their employment or ability to obtain health insurance. It is much more difficult for patients to determine what information about them is maintained in secondary databases than it is to view their primary health records. Such concerns have led to increasing emphasis on data stewardship.

According to the National Center for Vital and Health Statistics, **data stewardship** is ". . . a responsibility, guided by principles and practices, to ensure the knowledgeable and appropriate use of data derived from individuals' personal health information. These uses include (but are not limited to) data collection, viewing, storage, exchange, aggregation, and analysis" (NCVHS 2009). Data stewardship encompasses the concepts of data quality, security, confidentiality, and uniformity. Issues involve the rights of stakeholders to access, use, and control the data maintained about their care.

Many of these data stewardship issues have been the domain of health information managers since the profession began. It is important for HIM professionals to migrate these skills from the paper to the electronic environment to maintain their leadership in this area.

Data Quality Issues

Indexes, registries, and databases are only helpful when the data they contain are accurate. Decisions concerning new treatment methods, healthcare policy, and physician credentialing and privileging are based on these databases. Incorrect data will likely result in serious errors in decision making.

An important tenet in quality of secondary data is the quality of the primary data source. The patient health record often contains inconsistencies and errors that can lead to data quality issues in secondary data sources. It is important that facilities and providers pursue clinical documentation improvement to ensure the quality of the primary data source necessary for quality secondary data.

Several factors must be addressed when assessing data quality. These include data accuracy, consistency, completeness, and timeliness. (Elements of data quality are also discussed in chapter 2.)

Accuracy of the Data

Data accuracy, also referred to as data *validity* means that data are correct. For example, in a cancer registry, the stage of the neoplasm must be recorded accurately because statistical information on survival rates by stage is commonly reported.

Several methods may be used to ensure validity. One method is to incorporate **edits** in the database. An edit is a check on the accuracy of the data, such as setting data types. If a particular data element, such as admission date, is set up with a data type of date, the computer will not allow other types of data, such as name, to be entered in that field. Other edits may use comparisons between fields to ensure accuracy. For example, an edit might check to see that all patients with the diagnosis of prostate cancer are listed as males in the database.

Consistency of the Data

Another factor to be considered in looking at data quality is consistency, sometimes referred to as data *reliability*. For example, all patients in a trauma registry with the same level, severity, and site of injury should have the same score on the Abbreviated Injury Scale. Reliability is frequently checked by having more than one person abstract data for the same case. The results are then compared to identify any discrepancies. This is called an **interrater reliability** method of checking. Several different people may be used to do the checking. In a cancer registry, for example, physician members of the cancer committee may be called on to check the reliability of the data.

Comprehensiveness of the Data

Comprehensiveness, also referred to as completeness is another factor to be considered in data quality. Missing data may prevent the database from being useful for research or clinical decision making. To avoid missing data, some databases will not allow the user to move to the next field without making an entry in the current one, especially for fields considered crucial. Looking at a variety of sources in case findings is a way to avoid missing patients who should be included in a registry.

Timeliness of the Data

Another concept important in data quality is timeliness. **Data timeliness** means that healthcare data should be up-to-date. Data must also be available within a time frame helpful to the user. Factors that influence decisions may change over time, so it is important that the data reflect up-to-date information.

Data Confidentiality

Data confidentiality usually refers to efforts to guarantee the privacy of personal health information.

HIPAA-Covered Entities

When looking at confidentiality issues, it is important to consider the HIPAA regulations for privacy. For HIPAA covered entities, the data collection done by registries is considered part of "healthcare operations." Therefore, the patient does not have to sign an authorization for release of protected health information (PHI) to be included in the registry. Reporting of notifiable diseases to the state also comes under "healthcare operations" and does not require patient authorization for release (Anonymous 2003). Release of information to requestors other than the state will depend on the requestor. Data may be released to internal users, such as physicians for research, without the patient's consent as well because research also comes under "healthcare operations." External users, such as the American College of Surgeons, collect aggregate data from facilities, so individual patient authorization is not required. Information about patients that may be included in registries or other secondary data sources and reported to outside entities must be included in the facility's Notice of Privacy Practices given to patients on their initial encounters. Through this mechanism, patients are made aware that data about them may be reported to outside entities. (More information about HIPAA privacy regulations may be found in chapter 13.)

Entities Not Covered by HIPAA

Not all registries and databases are covered under HIPAA if the organization maintaining them does not bill for patient care services. Central registries would be an example of registries that are not covered under HIPAA. In such cases, the general norms for data confidentiality should be followed.

Data Definitions and Standards

The use of uniform terminology is an important way to improve data reliability. This has been evident in case definition for registries. The criteria for including a patient in a registry must have a clear definition. Definitions for terms such as race, for example, must include the categories to be used in determining race. If uniform terms are not used, the data will not be consistent. Also, it will be impossible to make comparisons between systems if uniform terms have not been used for all data. A data dictionary in which all data elements are defined helps ensure that uniform data definitions are being followed.

Rights of Stakeholders to Rights of Access, Use, and Control

In the past, a great deal of emphasis has been placed on who owned the data—both primary and secondary. With the primary data source—the patient health record—the consensus was that the facility owned the patient record while the patient controlled its use.

This consensus has broken down, however, with extensive use of data from the primary data source in secondary data banks that were unknown to patients, much less under their control.

Emphasis has switched to the rights of stakeholders regarding access, use, and control of both primary and secondary data. A **stakeholder** is someone who is affected by an issue. In the field of health data, the main stakeholders are patients and providers. In looking back at the four main purposes of collecting secondary data, it is evident that researchers and governments are also stakeholders in this arena.

Patients must be informed that they do not have exclusive ownership of their information but have the right to know what is collected about them and what uses are made of the data. **Transparency** refers to the degree to which patients included in secondary data sets are aware of their inclusion. In its report, *Toward a National Framework for the Secondary Use of Health Data*, the American Medical Informatics Association (2006) has recommended that full disclosure be the policy for all secondary uses of data.

Providers must be aware that patients have rights regarding their patient records to access what is collected about them as well as to amend or correct erroneous information. Patients have a limited right to determine who has access to their primary data. This right is limited by laws and regulations allowing access to data by governments, researchers, and other legitimate users of the data (Burrington-Brown et al. 2007).

Check Your Understanding 8.3

1. Using uniform terminology is a way to improve:

    A. Validity
    B. Data timeliness
    C. Audit trails
    D. Data reliability

2. Which of the following is a true statement about data stewardship?

    A. HIM professionals are not qualified to address data stewardship issues.
    B. Data stewardship addresses the needs of the healthcare organization but not the patient.
    C. HIM professionals have worked with many data stewardship issues for years.
    D. Data stewardship excludes privacy issues.

3. What is used to check the quality of data entered into an information system?

    A. Edits
    B. Interrater reliability
    C. Audit trail
    D. Validity

Instructions: Indicate whether the following statements are true or false (T or F).

4. _____ Now that registries and databases are almost universally electronic, data collection is done manually.

5. _____ One advantage to a vendor system is that purchasers can find out about the system's performance from other users.

6. _____ With regard to data quality, validity refers to the consistency of the data.

7. _____ Among the HIM professional's traditional roles is that of maintaining the confidentiality of health data.

Real-World Case

Hundreds of hospitals, clinics, and health departments automatically report certain symptoms and diagnoses to the government each day. This practice of biosurveillance helps officials track the spread of flu, detect outbreaks, and watch for odd symptoms that might signal a brand new disease or bioterrorism. Although information is reported each day, doctors rarely know what their colleagues nearby are diagnosing. Instead they often call the health department to ask if anyone's heard of any outbreak of certain cases. Work is being done to create a mechanism to track diseases before they become outbreaks (*USA Today* 2011).

Researchers are now working on technology that will link local biosurveillance to electronic health records, and even mobile applications. Providing data on the amount of disease or infection that is spreading locally can improve diagnosis and treatment methods.

Federal health officials are working to create an easy-to-use web tool that will allow doctors to search for local surveillance information. Websites such as Google Flu Trends and HealthMap offer a free web service that tracks the number of influenza and other cases in an area (Guth 2008).

Summary

Health records contain extensive information about individual patients but are difficult to use when attempting to perceive trends in care or quality. With the advent of greater use of the EHR, it is possible to collect data once and use them many times for a variety of purposes. Secondary data are used for quality, performance, and patient safety; research; and population health and administration.

One type of secondary record is the index. An index is a report from the hospital database that provides information on patients and allows retrieval by diagnosis, procedure, or physician. Health information management departments routinely produce indexes.

Disease registries are developed when extensive information is needed about specific diagnoses, procedures, or conditions. They are commonly used for research and to improve patient care and health status. From the database created through the data collection process, reports can be developed to answer questions regarding patient care or issues such as rates of immunization and birth defects. In some cases, patient follow-up is done to assess survival rates and quality of life after a disease or accident.

HIM professionals perform a variety of roles in relation to registries. In some cases, they work on setting up the registry. Moreover, they may work in data collection and management of registry functions. HIM professionals are well suited to such positions because of their background and training in management, patient health record content, regulatory and legal compliance, and medical science and terminology.

Today, organizations and institutions of all types commonly maintain databases pertaining to healthcare. At the federal level, some administrative databases provide data and information for decisions regarding claims and practitioner credentialing. Other databases focus on the public health area, using data collected at the local level and shared with states and the federal government. These databases assist in government surveillance of health status in the United States. Some databases, such as the clinical trials database, are mandated by law and help patients and providers to locate clinical trials regardless of source or location.

Registries and databases raise a number of managerial issues. Data collection is often time-consuming, so some databases now use automated entry methods. In addition, decisions must be made between vendor and facility-specific products. Data use and reuse raises issues related to data stewardship including the quality, confidentiality, and security of the data. Issues concerning the access, use, and control of secondary data have become more pressing. Health information managers must embrace a leadership role as data stewards.

References

Agency for Healthcare Research and Quality. 2012. Healthcare Cost & Utilization Project (HCUP). http://www.ahrq.gov/data/hcup/

American College of Surgeons Commission on Cancer. 2011. Commission on Cancer. http://www.facs.org/cancer/

American College of Surgeons National Trauma Data Bank. 2011. http://www.facs.org/trauma/ntdb/index.html

American College of Surgeons Trauma Programs. 2012. http://www.facs.org/trauma/index.html

American Joint Committee on Cancer. 2009. AJCC home page. http://www.cancerstaging.org

American Medical Informatics Association. 2006. *Toward a National Framework for the Secondary Use of Health Data*. Bethesda, MD: AMIA.

Anonymous. 2003. Handling cancer registry requests for information. *In Confidence* 11(8):7.

Burrington-Brown, J., B. Hjort, and L. Washington. 2007. Health data access, use, and control. *Journal of AHIMA* 78:63–66.

Centers for Disease Control. nd. *Program Manual: National Program of Cancer Registries*, version 1.0. http://www.cdc.gov/cancer/npcr/pdf/program_manual.pdf

Centers for Disease Control. 2011a. National Center for Health Statistics. http://www.cdc.gov/nchs/nhds/about_nhds.htm

Centers for Disease Control. 2011b. National Immunization Program. http://www.cdc.gov/vaccines/programs/iis/default.htm

Centers for Disease Control. 2012. National Center for Health Statistics. http://www.cdc.gov/nchs/nvss.htm

Centers for Medicare and Medicaid Services. 2011. https://www.cms.gov/NationalProvIdentStand/

Clinicaltrials.gov. 2009. Home page. http://www.clinicaltrials.gov

CNBC. 2012. http://www.cnbc.com/id/35988343/Top_10_Class_Action_Lawsuits?slide=6

Department of Health and Human Services. 2010. Fact Sheet on the Healthcare Protection and Integrity Data Bank. http://www.npdb-hipdb.hrsa.gov/resources/brochures/FactSheet-Section1921.pdf

Food and Drug Administration. 2009. Reporting by Health Professionals. http://www.fda.gov/Safety/MedWatch/HowToReport/ucm085568.htm

Food and Drug Administration. 2011. http://www.fda.gov/Safety/MedWatch/default.htm

GMed. 2011. gMed Users Can Now Submit Data Directly to the AGA Registry. http://www.gmed.com/gMed%20Users%20Can%20Now%20Submit%20Data%20Directly%20to%20the%20AGA%20Registry.html

Guth, R.A. 2008 (November 12). Sniffling surfing: Google unveils flu-bug tracker. *Wall Street Journal*.

Healthcare Costs and Utilization Project. 2009. http://www.hcup-us.ahrq.gov/overview.jsp

Healthy People. 2012. Immunizations and Infectious Diseases. http://healthypeople.gov/2020/topicsobjectives2020/overview.aspx?topicid=23

Mon, D. 2007. Development of a national health data stewardship entity: Response to request for information. Chicago: AHIMA. http://library.ahima.org/xpedio/groups/public/documents/ahima/bok1_044422.pdf

National Cancer Registrars Association. 2009. NCRA home page. http://www.ncra-usa.org

National Center for Vital and Health Statistics. 2009. Health data stewardship: What, why, who, how, An NCVHS primer. http://www.ncvhs.hhs.gov/090930lt.pdf

National Plan and Provider Enumeration System. 2012. https://nppes.cms.hhs.gov/NPPES/NPIRegistryHome.do

National Practitioner Data Bank for Adverse Information on Physicians and Other Health Care Practitioners: Reporting on Adverse and Negative Actions. 2010 (Jan. 28) *Federal Register* 75.

Smith, J. 2007. Health Information Technology Initiatives in Nebraska. http://www.nitc.ne.gov/eHc/clearing/HITUpdateJSmith.pdf

Trauma.org. 2012. Injury Severity Score. http://www.trauma.org/index.php/main/article/383/

USA Today. 2011.Tracking diseases before they become outbreaks. http://yourlife.usatoday.com/health/healthcare/prevention/story/2011-09-20/Tracking-diseases-before-they-become-outbreaks/50475608/1

Additional Resources

American Gastroenterological Association. 2011. AGA digestive health outcomes registry. http://www.gastro.org/practice/digestive-health-outcomes-registry

Department of Health and Human Services. 2010. The national hospital care survey. Federal Register 75(226).

chapter 9

Healthcare Statistics and Productivity

Loretta A. Horton, MEd, RHIA

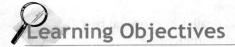

Learning Objectives

- Define measurement
- Differentiate among nominal-level, ordinal-level, interval-level, and ratio-level data
- Identify various ways in which statistics are used in healthcare
- Differentiate between descriptive and inferential statistics
- Define hospital-related statistical terms
- Calculate hospital-related inpatient and outpatient statistics
- Define community-based morbidity and mortality rates
- Calculate community-based morbidity and mortality rates
- Define and calculate measures of central tendency and variability
- Describe the characteristics of the normal distribution
- Identify the relationships of measures of central tendency and variation to the normal distribution
- Display healthcare data using tables, charts, and graphs, as appropriate
- Calculate the case-mix index
- Locate healthcare-related state and federal databases on the Internet
- Use healthcare data collected from online databases in comparative statistical reports

Key Terms

Acute care
Ambulatory surgery center (ASC)
Average daily census
Average length of stay (ALOS)
Bar chart
Bed count
Bed count day
Bed turnover rate
Boxplot
Bubble charts
Case fatality rate
Case mix
Case-mix index (CMI)
Cause-specific mortality rate
Census
Clinic outpatient
Consultation rate
Continuous variables
Crude birth rate
Crude death/mortality rate
Daily inpatient census
Descriptive statistics
Discrete variables
Emergency patient
Encounter
Fetal autopsy rate
Fetal death (stillborn)
Fetal death rate
Frequency distribution
Frequency polygon
Full-time equivalent employee (FTE)
Gross autopsy rate
Gross death rate
Histogram
Hospital-acquired (nosocomial) infection
    rate
Hospital ambulatory care
Hospital autopsy
Hospital autopsy rate
Hospital death rate

Hospital inpatient
Hospital inpatient autopsy
Hospital newborn inpatient
Hospital outpatient
Incidence rate
Infant mortality rate
Inferential statistics
Inpatient admission
Inpatient bed occupancy rate (percentage
    of occupancy)
Inpatient discharge
Inpatient hospitalization
Inpatient service day (IPSD)
Interval-level data
Length of stay (LOS)
Line graph
Maternal death rate (hospital based)
Maternal mortality rate
    (community-based)
Mean
Measures of central tendency
Median
Mode
National Vital Statistics System (NVSS)
Neonatal mortality rate
Net autopsy rate
Net death rate
Newborn (NB)
Newborn autopsy rate
Newborn death rate
Nominal-level data
Normal distribution
Nosocomial (hospital-acquired) infection
Notifiable disease
Occasion of service
Ordinal-level data
Outpatient
Outpatient visit
Pie chart
Population-based statistics

Postneonatal mortality rate
Postoperative infection rate
Prevalence rate
Productivity
Proportion
Proportionate mortality rate (PMR)
Range
Rate
Ratio
Ratio-level data
Referred outpatient

Scales of measurement
Scatter plot
Staffing level
Standard deviation
Stem and leaf plots
Surgical operation
Surgical procedure
Total length of stay (discharge days)
Variability
Variance
Vital statistics

Introduction to Measurement

Complete and accurate information is at the heart of good decision making. The health information management (HIM) professional has responsibility for ensuring that the data collected are accurate and organized into information that is useful to healthcare decision makers.

The primary source of clinical data in a healthcare facility is the health record. To be useful in decision making, data taken from the health record must be as complete and accurate as possible. Data are compiled in various ways to help in making decisions about patient care, the facility's financial status, and facility planning, to name a few.

This chapter discusses common statistical measures and types of data used by organizations in different healthcare settings and data collection and reporting on a community, regional, and national basis. Methods and tools for graphically displaying data are then presented along with a discussion of normal distribution and descriptive statistics.

Before discussing statistical measures used in healthcare, it is important to understand what measurement is and how the data collected are classified. Measurement simply refers to measuring an "attribute or property of a person, object, or event according to a particular set of rules" (Osborn 2005, 66). The result of the measurement will be numbers. And, the "particular set of rules" refers to what will be collected and how it will be collected so that the resulting numbers "will be meaningful, accurate, and informative" (Osborn 2005, 66). In other words, the process of collecting the data must be consistent in order to ensure the results are the same no matter who is collecting the data. If there is consistency in the data collection, we will be able to make comparisons in our own facilities and across facilities.

Data collected falls on one of four **scales of measurement:** nominal, ordinal, interval, or ratio. Furthermore, the data collected is described as either continuous or discrete. These characteristics influence the type of graphic technique that can be used to display the data and the types of statistical analyses that can be performed.

Nominal-level data fall into groups or categories. This is a scale that measures data by name only. The groups or categories are mutually exclusive, that is, a data element cannot be classified to more than one group. Some examples of nominal data collected in healthcare are related to patient demographics such as third-party payer, race, and sex. There is no order to the data collected within these categories.

Data that fall on the ordinal scale have some inherent order, and higher numbers are usually associated with higher values. In **ordinal-level data,** the order of the numbers is meaningful, not the number itself. Staging of a pressure ulcer is an example of a variable that has order. A pressure ulcer has four stages, with stage I being the least severe ulcer and stage IV being the most severe. In this example, the higher number is associated with the most severe type of pressure ulcer; however, we cannot measure the difference between the levels in exact numerical terms.

The most important characteristic of **interval-level data** is that the intervals between successive values are equal. On the Fahrenheit scale, for example, the interval between 20°F and 21°F is the same as between 21°F and 22°F. But because there is no true zero on this scale, we cannot say that 40°F is twice as warm as 20°F.

The **ratio-level data** is the highest level of measurement. On the ratio scale there is a defined unit of measure, a real zero point, and the intervals between successive values are equal. A real zero point means that there is an absolute zero. Only when a zero on a scale truly means the total absence of a property being assessed can that scale be described as ratio-level. For example, consider the variable length of stay. **Length of stay** (LOS) has a defined unit of measurement, day, and a real zero point—0 days. Because there is a real zero point, we can state that an LOS of six days is twice as long as an LOS of three days. Multiplication on the ratio scale by a constant does not change its ratio character, but addition of a constant to a ratio measure does. For example, if we add two days to each LOS so that the stays are 8 and 5 days respectively, the ratio of their stays is no longer 2:1. However, if we multiply the respective lengths of stay by 2 (for example, 6×2 and 3×2), the ratio between the two lengths of stay remains 2:1.

The difference between the ratio and interval scales of measurement is that there is no true zero point on the interval scale.

This four-fold structure is a useful classification for data and the four levels are hierarchically arranged so that higher levels include the key properties of the levels so that ratio level data include the three key properties found in nominal-, ordinal-, and interval-level data. Table 9.1 below lists the scales of measurement and examples.

Table 9.1.   **Scales of measurement**

Scale of measurement	Examples
Nominal	Name, gender, race
Ordinal	Likert scale, anything that is ordered
Interval	Temperature
Ratio	Age, height, length of stay

Discrete versus Continuous Data

Another way to classify data involves categorizing them as either being discrete or continuous. Data that are nominal or ordinal are also considered discrete. **Discrete variables** are those that fall into categories. For example, the variable "gender" has two categories: male and female. The variable "third-party payer" has a number of categories, depending on the healthcare facility. Examples include Medicare, Medicaid, commercial insurance, and private insurance or self-pay.

Discrete variables can only take on a limited number of values and have gaps between successive values. In the pressure ulcer example, the ulcer can be a stage I, II, III, or IV (limited number of values). It cannot be staged as 2.5 or 3.2 because the stages cannot be subdivided into smaller units. This is an example of a discrete variable that has order to its categories.

Continuous variables are either interval or ratio-level, but some ratio-level variables are discrete. For example, if you wanted to compare the number of patients on two different nursing units you could count 5 on one unit and 10 on another. This data are discrete. But you could also say that there are twice as many patients on one unit as there are on the other. And, there could be zero patients on one unit; this would be a true zero because it absolutely corresponds to the total absence of the variable you are assessing—the number of patients on each unit. With **continuous variables** measurements can be subdivided into smaller values. For example, an individual's weight may be 120 or 121 or any weight between 120 and 121. Continuous variables include fractions. Arithmetic operations—addition, subtraction, multiplication, and division—may be performed on continuous variables.

Check Your Understanding 9.1

Instructions: On a separate piece of paper, identify the scale of measurement for each of the following variables and indicate whether each variable is discrete or continuous.

1. _____ Zip code

2. _____ Blood pressure

3. _____ Heart Failure Classification I, II, III, IV

4. _____ Age

5. _____ Ethnicity

6. _____ Marital status

7. _____ Length of stay

8. ____ Discharge disposition (home, SNF, and so on)

9. ____ Weight

10. ____ Level of education

11. ____ Race

12. ____ Temperature in degrees Fahrenheit

13. ____ Types of third-party payers

14. ____ Gender

15. ____ Height

Common Statistical Measures Used in Healthcare

Healthcare data are collected to describe the health status of groups or populations. The data reported about healthcare facilities and communities describe the occurrence of illnesses, births, and deaths for specific periods of time. Data that are collected may be either facility based or population based. The sources of facility-based statistics are **acute care** facilities, long-term care facilities, and other types of healthcare organizations. The population-based statistics are gathered from cities, counties, states, or specific groups within the population, such as individuals affected by diabetes.

Reporting statistics for a healthcare facility is similar to reporting statistics for a community. Rates for healthcare facilities are reported as per 100 cases or percent; a community rate is reported as per 1,000, 10,000, or 100,000 people. For example, if a hospital experienced 2 deaths in a given month and 100 patients were discharged in the same month, the death rate would be 2 percent ([2 × 100]/100). If there were 200 deaths in a community of 80,000 for a given period of time, the death rate would be reported as 25 deaths per 10,000 population ([200 × 10,000]/80,000) for the same period of time.

Ratios, Proportions, and Rates: Three Common Examples of Ratio-Level Data Worth Knowing

Many healthcare statistics are reported in the form of a ratio, proportion, or rate. These measures are used to report morbidity (illness), mortality (death), and natality (birth) at the local, state, and national levels. Basically, these measures indicate the number of times something happened relative to the number of times it could have happened. All three measures are based on formula 9.1. In this formula, x and y are the quantities being compared and x is divided by y. Further, 10^n is 10 to the nth power. The size of 10^n may equal 10, 100, 1,000, 10,000, and so on, depending on the value of n:

$$10^0 = 1$$
$$10^1 = 10$$
$$10^2 = 10 \times 10 = 100$$
$$10^3 = 10 \times 10 \times 10 = 1,000$$

Ratios

In a **ratio,** the quantities being compared, such as patient discharge status (x = alive, y = dead), may be expressed so that x and y are completely independent of each other, or x may be included in y. For example, the outcome of patients discharged from Community Hospital could be compared in one of two ways:

$$\text{Alive/dead, or } x/y$$
$$\text{Alive/(alive + dead), or } x/(x + y)$$

In the first example, x is completely independent of y. The ratio represents the number of patients discharged alive compared to the number of patients who died. In the second example, x is part of the whole ($x + y$). The ratio represents the number of patients discharged alive compared to all patients discharged. Both expressions are considered ratios.

Proportions

A **proportion** is a particular type of ratio in which x is a portion of the whole ($x + y$). In a proportion, the numerator is always included in the denominator. Figures 9.1 and 9.2 describe the procedures for calculating ratios and proportions.

Formula 9.1.   General formula for calculating rates, proportions, and ratios

Ratio, proportion, rate = $x/y \times 10^n$

Rates

Rates are often used to measure events over a period of time. Sometimes they also are used in performance improvement studies. Like ratios and proportions, rates may be reported daily, weekly, monthly, or yearly. This allows for trend analysis and comparisons over time. The basic formula for calculating a rate is shown in formula 9.1.

Figure 9.1.   Calculation of a ratio; discharge status of patients discharged in a month

1. Define x and y:

   x = number of patients discharged alive

   y = number of patients who died

2. Identify x and y:

   $x = 235$

   $y = 22$

3. Set up the ratio x/y:

   235/22

4. Reduce the fraction so that either x or y equals 1:

   10.68/1

There were 10.68 live discharges for every patient who died.

Figure 9.2.   Calculation of a proportion; discharge status of patients discharged in a month

1. Define x and y:

   x = number of patients discharged alive

   y = number of patients who died

2. Identify x and y:

   $x = 235$

   $y = 22$

3. Set up the ratio $x/(x + y)$:

   $235/(235 + 22) = 235/257$

4. Reduce the fraction so that either x or y equals 1:

   0.91/1

The proportion of patients discharged alive was 0.91.

Healthcare facilities calculate many types of morbidity and mortality rates. For example, the C-section rate is a measure of the proportion, or percentage, of C-sections performed during a given period of time. C-section rates are closely monitored because they present more risk to the mother and baby and because they are more expensive than vaginal deliveries. In calculating the C-section rate, the number of C-sections performed during the specified period of time is counted and this value is placed in the numerator. The number of cases, or the population at risk, is the number of women who delivered during the same time period. This number is placed in the denominator. By convention, inpatient hospital rates are reported as the rate per 100 cases ($10^n = 10^2 = 10 \times 10 = 100$) and are expressed as percentages.

Formula 9.2. Calculating risk for contracting a disease

$$\text{Risk rate} = \frac{\text{Number of cases occurring during a given time period}}{\text{Total number of cases or population at risk during the same time period}}$$

Figure 9.3 shows the procedure for calculating a rate. In the example, 30 of the 263 deliveries at Community Hospital during the month of May were C-sections. In the formula, the numerator is the number of C-sections performed in May (given period of time) and the denominator is the total number of deliveries including C-sections (the population at risk) performed within the same time frame. In calculating the rate, the numerator is always included in the denominator. Also, when calculating a facility-based rate, the numerator is first multiplied by 100, and then divided by the denominator.

Because hospital rates rarely result in a whole number, they usually must be rounded. The hospital should set a policy on whether rates are to be reported to one or two decimal places. The division should be carried out to at least one more decimal place than desired.

When rounding, if the last number is five or greater, the preceding number should be increased one digit. In contrast, if the last number is less than five, the preceding number remains the same. For example, when rounding 25.56 percent to one decimal place, the rate becomes 25.6 percent because the last number is greater than five. When rounding 1.563 percent to two places, the rate becomes 1.56 percent because the last digit is less than five. Rates of less than 1 percent are usually carried out to three decimal places and

Figure 9.3. Calculation of a rate; C-section rate for May 20XX

During May, 263 women delivered; of these, 30 deliveries were by C-section. What is the C-section rate for May?

1. Define the numerator (number of times an event occurred) and the denominator (number of times an event could have occurred):

    Numerator = total number of C-sections performed during the time period

    Denominator = total number of deliveries, including C-sections, in the same time period

2. Identify the numerator and the denominator:

    Numerator = 30

    Denominator = 263

3. Set up the rate:

    30/263

4. Multiply the numerator by 100 and then divide by the denominator:

    $([30 \times 100]/263) = 11.4\%$

The C-section rate for May is 11.4 percent.

rounded to two. For rates less than 1 percent, a zero should precede the decimal to emphasize that the rate is less than 1 percent, for example, 0.56 percent.

Check Your Understanding 9.2

Instructions: on a separate piece of paper, identify the following statements as a rate, a ratio, or a proportion.

1. Medicare admissions outnumber commercial insurance admissions 3 to 2.

2. At the annual state HIM meeting, 85 of the registrants were female and 35 were male. Therefore 0.71 percent of the registrants were female.

3. Of the 250 patients admitted in the last six months, 36 percent had Type II diabetes mellitus.

Statistical Data Used in Healthcare Facilities

Acute Care Statistical Data

In the daily operations of any organization, whether in business, manufacturing, or healthcare, data are collected for decision making. To be effective, the decision makers must have confidence in the data collected. Confidence requires that the data collected be accurate, reliable, and timely. The types of data collected in the acute care setting are discussed in the following section.

Administrative Statistical Data

Hospitals collect data on both inpatients and outpatients on a daily basis. They use these statistics to monitor the volume of patients treated daily, weekly, monthly, or within some other specified time frame. The statistics give healthcare decision makers the information they need to plan facilities and services and to monitor inpatient and outpatient revenue streams. For these reasons, the HIM professional must be well versed in data collection, reporting, and analysis methods.

Standard definitions have been developed to ensure that all healthcare providers collect and report data in a consistent manner. The *Pocket Glossary of Health Information Management and Technology* (2012), developed by the American Health Information Management Association (AHIMA), is a resource commonly used to describe the types of healthcare events for which data are collected. It includes definitions of terms related to healthcare organizations, health maintenance organizations (HMOs), and other health-related programs and facilities. Some basic terms that HIM professionals should be familiar with include:

- **Hospital inpatient:** A patient who is provided with room, board, and continuous general nursing service in an area of an acute care facility where patients generally stay overnight at a minimum

- **Hospital newborn inpatient:** A patient born in the hospital at the beginning of the current inpatient hospitalization

  — Newborns are usually counted separately because their care is so different from that of other inpatients

  — Infants born on the way to the hospital or at home are considered hospital inpatients, not hospital newborn inpatients

- **Inpatient hospitalization:** The period during an individual's life when he or she is a patient in a single hospital without interruption except by possible intervening leaves of absence

- **Inpatient admission:** An acute care facility's formal acceptance of a patient who is to be provided with room, board, and continuous nursing service in an area of the facility where patients generally stay overnight

- **Inpatient discharge:** The termination of hospitalization through the formal release of an inpatient by the hospital

  — The term includes patients who are discharged alive (by physician's order), who are discharged against medical advice (AMA), or who died while hospitalized

  — Unless otherwise indicated, inpatient discharges include deaths

- **Hospital outpatient:** A hospital patient who receives services in one or more of the hospital's facilities when he or she is not currently an inpatient or home care patient

  — An outpatient may be classified as either an emergency outpatient or a clinic outpatient

    - An emergency outpatient is admitted to the emergency department of a hospital for diagnosis and treatment of a condition that requires immediate medical, dental, or other emergency services

    - A clinic outpatient is admitted to a clinical service of the clinic or hospital for diagnosis and treatment on an ambulatory basis

Inpatient Census Data

Even though much of the data collection process has been automated, an ongoing responsibility of the HIM professional is to verify the **census** data that are collected daily. The census reports patient activity for a 24-hour reporting period. Included in the census report is the number of inpatients admitted and discharged for the previous 24-hour period as well as the number of intra-hospital transfers. An intra-hospital transfer is a patient who is moved from one patient care unit to another (for example, a patient may be transferred from the intensive care unit [ICU] to the medicine unit). The usual 24-hour reporting period begins at 12:01 a.m. and ends at 12:00 midnight. In the census count, adults and children (A&C) are reported separately from newborns.

Before compiling census data, however, it is important to understand related terminology. The census is the number of hospital inpatients present at any one time. For example, the census in a 300-bed hospital may be 250 patients at 2:00 p.m. on May 1, but 245 an hour later. Because the census may change throughout the day as admissions and discharges occur, hospitals designate an official census-taking time. In most facilities, the official count takes place at midnight. The census-reporting time can be any other time, but it must be consistent throughout the healthcare facility and occur at the same time each day.

The result of the official count taken at midnight is called the **daily inpatient census.** This is the number of inpatients present at the official census-taking time each day. Also included in the daily inpatient census are any patients who were admitted and discharged that same day. For example, if a patient was admitted to the cardiac care unit (CCU) at 1:00 p.m. on May 1 and died at 4:00 p.m. on May 1, he would be counted as a patient who was both admitted and discharged the same day.

Because patients admitted and discharged the same day may not be present at the census-taking time, the hospital must account for them separately. If it did not, credit for the services provided these patients would be lost. The daily inpatient census reflects the total number of patients treated during the 24-hour period. Figure 9.4 displays a sample daily inpatient census report.

Figure 9.4.   Daily inpatient census report—adults and children

May 2	
Number of patients in hospital at midnight, May 1	230
+ Number of patients admitted May 2	+35
− Number of patients discharged, including deaths, May 2	−40
Number of patients in hospital at midnight, May 2	225
+ Number of patients both admitted and discharged, including deaths	+5
Daily inpatient census at midnight, May 2	230
Total inpatient service days, May 2	230

Table 9.2.   **Number of IPSDs**

Day	Census	Same Day Admissions and Discharges	Inpatient Service Days
Day 1	240	0	240
Day 2	253	0	253
Day 3	235	2	237
		Total	**730**

A unit of measure that reflects the services received by one inpatient during a 24-hour period is called an **inpatient service day** (IPSD). The number of IPSDs for a 24-hour period is equal to the daily inpatient census, that is, one service day for each patient treated. In figure 9.4, the total number of inpatient service days for May 2 is 230.

IPSDs are compiled daily, weekly, monthly, and annually. They reflect the volume of services provided by the healthcare facility: the greater the volume of services, the greater the revenues to the facility. Daily reporting of the number of IPSDs is an indicator of the hospital's financial condition.

As mentioned, the daily inpatient census is equal to the number of IPSDs provided for that day as shown in Table 9.2.

The total number of IPSDs for a week, a month, and so on can be divided by the total number of days in the period of interest to obtain the **average daily census.** In the example above, 730 IPSDs is divided by three days to obtain an average daily census of 243.3. The average daily census is the average number of inpatients treated during a given period of time. The general formula for calculating the average daily census is shown in formula 9.3.

In calculating the average daily census, adults and children (A&C) and **newborns** (NB) are reported separately. This is because the intensity of services provided to adults and children is greater than it is for newborns. To calculate the A&C average daily census, the general formula is modified as shown in formula 9.4. Many facilities use a whole number when calculating the census.

Formula 9.3. Calculating the average daily census

$$\text{Average daily census} = \frac{\text{Total number of inpatient service days for a given period}}{\text{Total number of days in the same period}}$$

Formula 9.4. Calculating the average daily census for adults and children

$$\text{Average daily census for A\&C} = \frac{\text{Total number of inpatient service days for A\&C for a given period}}{\text{Total number of days for the same period}}$$

Table 9.3.   Calculation of census statistics

Indicator	Numerator	Denominator
Average daily inpatient census	Total number of inpatient service days for a given period	Total number of days for the same period
Average daily inpatient census for adults and children (A&C)	Total number of inpatient service days for A&C for a given period	Total number of days for the same period
Average daily inpatient census for newborns (NBs)	Total number of inpatient service days for NBs for a given period	Total number of days for the same period

The formula for the average daily census for newborns is shown in formula 9.5. For example, the total number of IPSDs provided to adults and children for the week of May 1 is 1,729, and the total for newborns is 119. Using the formulas, the average daily census for adults and children is 247 (1,729/7) and for newborns it is 17 (119/7). The average daily census for all hospital inpatients for the week of May 1 is 264 ([1,729 + 119]/7). Table 9.3 compares the various formulas for calculating the average daily census.

Formula 9.5. Calculating the average daily census for newborns

$$\text{Average daily census for NBs} = \frac{\text{Total number of inpatient service days for NBs for a given period}}{\text{Total number of days for the same period}}$$

Check Your Understanding 9.3

Instructions: Answer the following questions on a separate piece of paper.

1. Community Hospital reported the following statistics for adults and children at 12:01 a.m. April 1: Census 150; Admissions 20; Discharges 15; 1 patient admitted and died the same day; 1 patient admitted and discharged alive the same day. Calculate the following for April 2:

   a. Inpatient census
   b. Daily inpatient census
   c. Inpatient service days

2. Community Hospital reported the following statistics for their newborn unit at 12:01 a.m. April 1: Census 14: Births 5; Discharges 3; 1 Newborn born and transferred to the state University Hospital. Calculate the following for April 2:

   a. Inpatient census
   b. Daily inpatient census

3. Community Hospital reported the following statistics for their intensive care unit at 12:01 a.m. April 1: Census 10; 1 patient admitted directly from the ESD; 1 patient transferred from Surgery unit; 1 patient transferred from the Medicine unit; 1 patient transferred to the Medicine unit; 1 patient admitted and died the same day. Calculate the following for April 2:

   a. Inpatient census
   b. Daily inpatient census

Inpatient Bed Occupancy Rate

Another indicator of the hospital's financial position is the **inpatient bed occupancy rate,** also called the percentage of occupancy. The inpatient bed occupancy rate is the percentage of official beds occupied by hospital inpatients for a given period of time. In general, the greater the occupancy rate, the greater the revenues for the hospital. For a bed to be included in the official count, it must be set up, staffed, equipped, and available for patient care. The total number of inpatient service days is used in the numerator because it is equal to the daily inpatient census or the number of patients treated daily. The occupancy rate compares the number of patients treated over a given period of time to the total number of beds available for the same period of time.

For example, if 200 patients occupied 280 beds on May 2, the inpatient bed occupancy rate would be 71.4 percent ($[200/\{280 \times 1\}] \times 100$). If the rate were for more than one day, the number of beds would be multiplied by the number of days within that particular time frame. For example, if 1,729 IPSDs were provided during the week of May 1, the inpatient bed occupancy rate for that week would be 88.2 percent ($[1,729/\{280 \times 7\}] \times 100$).

The denominator in this formula is actually the total possible number of inpatient service days. That is, if every available bed in the hospital were occupied every single day, this would be the maximum number of IPSDs that could be provided. This is an important concept, especially when the official **bed count** changes for a given reporting period. For example, if the bed count changed from 280 beds to 300, the bed occupancy rate would reflect the change. The total number of inpatient beds times the total number of days in the period is called the total number of **bed count days.** The general formula for the inpatient bed occupancy rate is shown in formula 9.6.

Formula 9.6. Calculating the inpatient bed occupancy rate

$$\text{Inpatient bed occupancy rate} = \frac{\text{Total number of inpatient service days for a given period}}{\text{Total number of inpatient bed count days for the same period}} \times 100$$

For example, in May the total number of inpatient service days provided was 7,582. The bed count for the month of May changed from 280 beds to 300 on May 20. To calculate the inpatient bed occupancy rate for May, the total number of bed count days must be determined. There are 31 days in May; therefore, the total number of bed count days is calculated as:

Number of beds, May 1–May 19 = 280 × 19 days = 5,320 bed count days
Number of beds, May 20–May 31 = 300 × 12 days = 3,600 bed count days
5,320 + 3,600 = 8,920 bed count days

The inpatient bed occupancy rate for the month of May is 85.0 percent ([7,582/8,920] × 100).

As with the average daily census, the inpatient bed occupancy rate for adults and children is reported separately from that of newborns. To calculate the total number of bed count days for newborns, the official count for newborn bassinets is used. Table 9.4 reviews the formulas for calculating inpatient bed occupancy rates.

It is possible for the inpatient bed occupancy rate to be greater than 100 percent. This occurs when the hospital faces an epidemic or disaster. In this type of situation, hospitals set up temporary beds that usually are not included in the official bed count. As an example, Community Hospital experienced an excessive number of admissions in January because of an outbreak of influenza. In January, the official bed count was 150 beds. On January 5, the daily inpatient census was 156. Therefore, the inpatient bed occupancy rate for January 5 was 104 percent ([156/150] × 100).

Bed Turnover Rate

The **bed turnover rate** is a measure of hospital utilization. It includes the number of times each hospital bed changed occupants. The formula for the bed turnover rate is shown in formula 9.7. For example, Community Hospital had 2,060 discharges and deaths for the month of May. Its bed count for May averaged 677. The bed turnover rate is 3.0 (2,060/677). This simply means that on average, each hospital bed had three occupants during May.

Formula 9.7. Calculating the bed turnover rate
$$\text{Bed turnover rate} = \frac{\text{Total number of discharges, including deaths, for a given period}}{\text{Average bed count for the same time period}}$$

Table 9.4.   **Calculation of inpatient bed occupancy rates**

Rate	Numerator	Denominator
Inpatient bed occupancy rate	Total number of inpatient service days for a given period × 100	Total number of inpatient bed count days for the same period
Inpatient bed occupancy rate for adults and children (A&C)	Total number of inpatient service days for A&C for a given period × 100	Total number of inpatient bed count days for A&C for the same period
Newborn (NB) bed occupancy rate	Total number of NB inpatient service days for a given period × 100	Total number of bassinet bed count days for the same period

Check Your Understanding 9.4

Instructions: Answer the following questions on a separate piece of paper.

1. What is the inpatient bed occupancy rate for each of the following patient care units at Community Hospital for the month of June? (Calculate to one decimal point.)

Table 9.5. **Check Your Understanding 9.4**

Inpatient Unit	Service Days	Bed Count	Occupancy Rate
Medicine	580	36	_____
Surgery	689	42	_____
Pediatric	232	18	_____
Psychiatry	889	35	_____
Obstetrics	222	10	_____
Newborn	222	15	_____

2. Use the preceding information to determine the Occupancy Rate for Community Hospital—all Adults and Children (exclude newborns). Calculate to one decimal point.

3. On July 1, Community Hospital expanded the number of patient beds from 156 to 200. Use the following information to determine the Occupancy Rate for January to June; July to December; and the total for the year (non-leap year).

Table 9.6. **Check Your Understanding 9.4**

Months	Service Days	Bed Count
January–June	15672	156
July–December	25876	200

Length of Stay Data

Length of stay (LOS) data is calculated for each patient after he or she is discharged from the hospital. It is the number of calendar days from the day of patient admission to the day of patient discharge. When the patient is admitted and discharged in the same month, the LOS is determined by simply subtracting the date of admission from the date of discharge. For example, the LOS for a patient admitted on May 12 and discharged on May 17 is five days (17 – 12 = 5)

When the patient is admitted in one month and discharged in another, the calculations must be adjusted. One way to calculate the LOS in this case is to subtract the date of admission from the total number of days in the month the patient was admitted and then add the total number of hospitalized days for the month in which the patient was discharged. For example, the LOS for a patient admitted on May 28 and discharged on June 6 is nine days ([May 31–May 28 = 3 days] + [June 1–June 6 = 6 days]; LOS = 9 days).

When a patient is admitted and discharged on the same day, the LOS is one day. A partial day's stay is never reported as a fraction of a day. The LOS for a patient discharged the day after admission also is one day. Thus, the LOS for a patient who was admitted to the ICU on May 10 at 9:00 a.m. and died at 3:00 p.m. on the same day is one day. Likewise, the LOS for a patient admitted on May 12 and discharged on May 13 is one day.

When the LOS for all patients discharged for a given period of time is summed, the result is the **total length of stay (discharge days)**. As an example, five patients were discharged from the pediatric unit on May 9. The LOS for each patient was as follows:

Table 9.7.   **Length of stay for five patients discharged May 9**

Patient	LOS
1	5
2	3
3	1
4	8
5	10
Total	**27**

In the preceding example, the total LOS is 27 days (5 + 3 + 1 + 8 + 10). The total LOS is also referred to as the number of days of care provided to patients who were discharged or died (discharge days) during a given period of time.

The **average length of stay** (ALOS) is calculated from the total LOS. The total LOS divided by the number of patients discharged is the ALOS. Using the data in the preceding example, the ALOS for the five patients discharged from the pediatric unit on May 9 is 5.4 days (27/5)

The general formula for calculating ALOS is shown in formula 9.8. As with the measures already discussed, the ALOS for adults and children is reported separately from the ALOS for newborns. Table 9.8 reviews the formulas for ALOS. Table 9.9 displays an example of a hospital statistical summary prepared by the HIM department using census and discharge data.

Formula 9.8. Calculating the average length of stay

$$\text{Average length of stay} = \frac{\text{Total length of stay for a given period}}{\text{Total number of discharges, including deaths, for the same period}}$$

Table 9.8.   **Calculation of LOS statistics**

Indicator	Numerator	Denominator
Average LOS	Total length of stay (discharge days) for a given period	Total number of discharges, including deaths, for the same period
Average LOS for adults and children (A&C)	Total length of stay for A&C (discharge days) for a given period	Total number of discharges, including deaths, for A&C for the same period
Average LOS for newborns (NB)	Total length of stay for all NB (discharge days) for a given period	Total number of NB discharges, including deaths, for the same period

Table 9.9. **Statistical summary, Community Hospital, for the period ending July 20XX**

Admissions	July 20XX		Year-to-Date 20XX	
	Actual	Budget	Actual	Budget
Medical	728	769	5,075	5,082
Surgical	578	583	3,964	3,964
OB/GYN	402	440	2,839	3,027
Psychiatry	113	99	818	711
Physical Medicine & Rehab	48	57	380	384
Other Adult	191	178	1,209	1,212
Total Adult	2,060	2,126	14,285	14,380
Newborn	294	312	2,143	2,195
Total Admissions	**2,354**	**2,438**	**16,428**	**16,575**

Average Length of Stay	July 20XX		Year-to-Date 20XX	
	Actual	Budget	Actual	Budget
Medical	6.1	6.4	6.0	6.1
Surgical	7.0	7.2	7.7	7.7
OB/GYN	2.9	3.2	3.5	3.1
Psychiatry	10.8	11.6	10.4	11.6
Physical Medicine & Rehab	27.5	23.0	28.1	24.3
Other Adult	3.6	3.9	4.0	4.1
Total Adult	6.3	6.4	6.7	6.5
Newborn	5.6	5.0	5.6	5.0
Total ALOS	**6.2**	**6.3**	**6.5**	**6.3**

Patient Days	July 20XX		Year-to-Date 20XX	
	Actual	Budget	Actual	Budget
Medical	4,436	4,915	30,654	30,762
Surgical	4,036	4,215	30,381	30,331
OB/GYN	1,170	1,417	10,051	9,442
Psychiatry	1,223	1,144	8,524	8,242
Physical Medicine & Rehab	1,318	1,310	10,672	9,338
Other Adult	688	699	4,858	4,921
Total Adult	12,871	13,700	95,140	93,036
Newborn	1,633	1,552	12,015	10,963
Total Patient Days	**14,504**	**15,252**	**107,155**	**103,999**

Other Key Statistics	July 20XX		Year-to-Date 20XX	
	Actual	Budget	Actual	Budget
Average Daily Census	485	482	498	486
Average Beds Available	677	660	677	660
Clinic Visits	21,621	18,975	144,271	136,513
Emergency Visits	3,822	3,688	26,262	25,604
Inpatient Surgery Patients	657	583	4,546	4,093
Outpatient Surgery Patients	603	554	4,457	3,987

Check Your Understanding 9.5

Instructions: Complete the following exercise on a separate piece of paper.

Table 9.10.　**Check Your Understanding 9.5**

Day	Number of Patients Discharged	Discharge Days
August 1	12	72
August 2	10	70
August 3	12	72
August 4	17	136
August 5	8	32
August 6	9	81
August 7	11	68
August 8	10	80
August 9	14	63
August 10	12	84

1. Calculate the total length of stay for the patient discharges and the average length of stay. Calculate to one decimal point.

    a. Total length of stay _____
    b. Number of patients discharged _____
    c. Average length of stay _____

Patient Care and Clinical Statistical Data

Thus far, this chapter has discussed statistical measures that are indicators of volume of services and utilization of services. The collection of data related to morbidity and mortality is also an important aspect of evaluating the quality of hospital services. Morbidity and mortality rates are reported for all patient discharges within a certain time frame. They also may be reported by service or by physician or other variable of interest in order to identify trends, issues or opportunities for improvement that may require corrective action. The most frequently collected morbidity and mortality rates are presented in this section.

Hospital Death (Mortality) Rates

The **hospital death rate** is based on the number of patients discharged, alive and dead, from the hospital. Deaths are considered discharges because they are the end point of a period of hospitalization. In contrast to the rates discussed in the preceding section, newborns are not counted separately from adults and children.

Gross Death Rate

The **gross death rate** is the proportion of all hospital discharges that ended in death. It is the basic indicator of mortality in a healthcare facility. The gross death rate is calculated by dividing the total number of deaths occurring in a given time period by the total number of discharges, including deaths, for the same time period. The formula for calculating the gross death rate is shown in formula 9.9.

As an example, Community Hospital experienced 21 deaths (A&C and NBs) during the month of May. There were 633 total discharges, including deaths. The gross death rate is 3.3 percent ([21/633] × 100).

Formula 9.9. Calculating the gross death rate

$$\text{Gross death rate} = \frac{\text{Total number of inpatient deaths (including NBs) for a given period}}{\text{Total number of discharges, including A\&C and NB deaths, for the same period}} \times 100$$

Net Death Rate

The **net death rate** is an adjusted death rate. It is calculated with the assumption that certain deaths should not count against the hospital. The net death rate is an adjusted rate because it does not include patients who die within 48 hours of admission. The reason for excluding these deaths is that 48 hours is not enough time to positively affect patient outcome. In other words, the patient was not admitted to the hospital in a manner timely enough for treatment to have an effect on his or her outcome. The formula for calculating the net death rate is shown in formula 9.10.

Continuing with the preceding example of the 21 patients who died at Community Hospital, three died within 48 hours of admission. Therefore, the net death rate is 2.9 percent ([{21 − 3}/{633 − 3}] × 100). The fact that the net death rate is less than the gross death rate is favorable to Community Hospital because lower death rates may be an indicator of better care.

Formula 9.10. Calculating the net death rate

$$\text{Net death rate} = \frac{\text{Total number of inpatient deaths (including NBs) minus deaths} < 48 \text{ hours for a given period}}{\text{Total number of discharges, (including A\&C and NB deaths) minus deaths} < 48 \text{ hours for the same period}} \times 100$$

Newborn Death Rate

Even though newborn deaths are included in the hospital's gross and net death rates, the **newborn death rate** is often calculated separately. Newborns include only infants born alive in the hospital. The newborn death rate is the number of newborns who died in comparison to the total number of newborns discharged, alive and dead. To qualify as a newborn death, the newborn must have been delivered alive. A stillborn infant is not included in either the newborn death rate or the gross or net death rate. The formula for calculating the newborn death rate is shown in formula 9.11.

For example, Community Hospital experienced two newborn deaths during the month of May. There were 53 newborn discharges (including these two deaths). The newborn death rate is 3.8 percent ([2/53] × 100).

Formula 9.11. Calculating the newborn death rate

$$\text{Newborn death rate} = \frac{\text{Total number of NB deaths for a given period}}{\substack{\text{Total number of NB discharges (including deaths)} \\ \text{for the same period}}} \times 100$$

Fetal Death Rate

In healthcare terminology, the death of a stillborn baby is called a **fetal death (stillborn).** A fetal death is a death prior to the fetus's complete expulsion or extraction from the mother in a hospital facility, regardless of the length of the pregnancy. Thus, stillborns are neither admitted nor discharged from the hospital. A fetal death occurs when the fetus fails to breathe or show any other evidence of life, such as a heartbeat, a pulsation of the umbilical cord, or a movement of the voluntary muscles.

Fetal deaths also are classified into categories based on length of gestation or weight. (See table 9.11.) To calculate the **fetal death rate,** divide the total number of intermediate and late fetal deaths for the period by the total number of live births and intermediate and late fetal deaths for the same period. The formula for calculating the fetal death rate is shown in formula 9.12. For example, during the month of May, Community Hospital experienced 269 live births and 7 intermediate and 6 late fetal deaths. The fetal death rate is 4.6 percent ([7 + 6/{269 + 7 + 6}] × 100).

Formula 9.12. Calculating the fetal death rate

$$\text{Fetal death rate} = \frac{\substack{\text{Total number of intermediate and late fetal deaths} \\ \text{for a given period}}}{\substack{\text{Total number of live births plus total number of} \\ \text{intermediate and late fetal deaths for the same period}}} \times 100$$

Table 9.11. **Classifications of fetal death**

Classification	Length of Gestation	Weight
Early fetal death	Less than 20 weeks' gestation	500 g or less
Intermediate fetal death	20 weeks' completed gestation, but less than 28 weeks	501 to 1,000 g
Late fetal death	28 weeks' completed gestation	Over 1,000 g

Maternal Death Rate

Hospitals are also interested in calculating their **maternal death rates (hospital based).** A maternal death is the death of any woman from any cause related to, or aggravated by, pregnancy or its management, regardless of the duration or site of the pregnancy. Maternal deaths that result from accidental or incidental causes are not included in the maternal death rate.

Maternal deaths are classified as either direct or indirect. A direct maternal death is the death of a woman resulting from obstetrical (OB) complications of the pregnancy, labor, or puerperium (the period including the six weeks after delivery). Direct maternal deaths are included in the maternal death rate. An indirect maternal death is the death of a woman from a previously existing disease or a disease that developed during pregnancy, labor, or the puerperium that was not due to obstetric causes, although the physiologic effects of pregnancy were partially responsible.

The maternal death rate may be an indicator of the availability of prenatal care in a community. The hospital also may use it to help identify conditions that could lead to a maternal death. The formula for calculating the maternal death rate is shown in formula 9.13. For example, during the month of May, Community Hospital experienced 275 maternal discharges. Two of these patients died. The maternal death rate for May is 0.73 percent ([2/275] × 100). Table 9.12 summarizes hospital-based mortality rates.

Formula 9.13. Calculating the maternal death rate

$$\text{Maternal death rate} = \frac{\text{Total number of direct maternal deaths for a given period}}{\begin{array}{c}\text{Total number of maternal (OB) discharges,}\\\text{including deaths, for the same period}\end{array}} \times 100$$

Table 9.12.   Calculation of hospital-based mortality rates

Rate	Numerator (x)	Denominator (y)
Gross death rate	Total number of inpatient deaths, including NBs, for a given period × 100	Total number of discharges, including A&C and NB deaths, for the same period
Net death rate (institutional death rate)	Total number of inpatient deaths, including NBs, minus deaths <48 hours for a given period × 100	Total number of discharges, including A&C and NB deaths, minus deaths <48 hours for the same period
Newborn death rate	Total number of NB deaths for a given period × 100	Total number of NB discharges, including deaths, for the same period
Fetal death rate	Total number of intermediate and late fetal deaths for a given period × 100	Total number of live births plus total number of intermediate and late fetal deaths for the same period
Maternal death rate	Total number of direct maternal deaths for a given period × 100	Total number of maternal (obstetric) discharges, including deaths, for the same period
Infant death rate	Number of deaths under 1 year of age during a given time period	Number of live births during the same time period

Check Your Understanding 9.6

Instructions: Using the data provided on deaths and discharges at Community Hospital for the past calendar year, answer the following questions on a separate sheet of paper. Calculate to two decimal points.

Table 9.13.   Check Your Understanding 9.6

Type of Death or Discharge	Total
Total discharges, including deaths (A&C)	1,250
Total deaths (A&C)	20
Deaths less than 48 hours after admission (A&C)	3
Fetal deaths (intermediate and late)	4
Live births	155
Newborn deaths	2
Newborn discharges, including deaths	155
Maternal deaths (direct)	1
OB discharges, including deaths	155

1. _____ What is the gross death rate for adults and children?

2. _____ What is the net death rate for adults and children?

3. _____ What is the fetal death rate?

4. _____ What is the newborn death rate?

5. _____ What is the gross death rate for adults and children and newborns combined?

6. _____ What is the maternal death rate (direct)?

Autopsy Rates

An autopsy is an examination of a dead body to determine the cause of death. Another name that may be used is a post-mortem examination. Autopsies are very useful in the education of medical students and residents. In addition, they can alert family members to conditions or diseases for which they may be at risk.

Two categories of hospital autopsies are conducted in acute care facilities: hospital inpatient autopsies and hospital autopsies. A **hospital inpatient autopsy** is an examination of the body of a patient who died while being treated in the hospital. The patient's death marked the end of his or her stay in the hospital. A pathologist or some other physician on the medical staff performs this type of autopsy in the facility.

A **hospital autopsy** is an examination of the body of an individual who at some time in the past had been a hospital patient and was not a hospital inpatient at the time of death. A pathologist or some other physician on the medical staff performs this type of autopsy as well. The following sections describe the different types of autopsy rates calculated by acute care hospitals.

Gross Autopsy Rates

A **gross autopsy rate** is the proportion or percentage of deaths that are followed by the performance of autopsy. The formula for calculating the gross autopsy rate is shown in formula 9.14. For example, during the month of May, Community Hospital experienced 21 deaths. Autopsies were performed on four of these patients. The gross autopsy rate is 19.0 percent ([4/21] × 100).

Formula 9.14. Calculating the gross autopsy rate

$$\text{Gross autopsy rate} = \frac{\text{Total inpatient autopsies for a given period}}{\text{Total number of inpatient deaths for the same period}} \times 100$$

Net Autopsy Rates

The bodies of patients who have died are not always available for autopsy. For example, a coroner or medical examiner may claim a body for an autopsy for legal reasons. In these situations, the hospital calculates a **net autopsy rate.** In calculating the net autopsy rate, bodies that have been removed by the coroner or medical examiner are excluded from the denominator. The formula for calculating the net autopsy rate is shown in formula 9.15. Continuing with the example in the preceding section, the medical examiner claimed three of the patients for autopsy. The numerator remains the same because four autopsies were performed by the hospital pathologist. However, because three of the deaths were identified as medical examiner's cases and removed from the hospital, 3 is subtracted from 21. The net autopsy rate is 22.2 percent ([4/{21 − 3}] × 100).

Formula 9.15. Calculating the net autopsy rate

$$\text{Net autopsy rate} = \frac{\text{Total number of autopsies on inpatient deaths for a period}}{\substack{\text{Total number of inpatient deaths minus unautopsied} \\ \text{coroners' or medical examiners' cases for the same period}}} \times 100$$

Hospital Autopsy Rates

A third type of autopsy rate is called the **hospital autopsy rate.** This is an adjusted rate that includes autopsies on anyone who may have at one time been a hospital patient. The formula for calculating the hospital autopsy rate is shown in formula 9.16. The hospital autopsy rate includes autopsies performed on any of the following:

- Bodies of inpatients, except those removed by the coroner or medical examiner. When the hospital pathologist or other designated physician acts as an agent in the performance of an autopsy on an inpatient, the death and the autopsy are included in the percentage.

- Bodies of other hospital patients, including ambulatory care patients, hospital home care patients, and former hospital patients who died elsewhere, but whose bodies have been made available for autopsy to be performed by the hospital pathologist or other designated physician. These autopsies and deaths are included in computations of the percentage.

Generally, it is difficult to determine the number of bodies of former hospital patients who may have died in a given time period. In the formula, the phrase available for hospital autopsy involves several conditions, including:

- The autopsy must be performed by the hospital pathologist or a designated physician on the body of a patient treated at some time at the hospital.

- The report of the autopsy must be filed in the patient's health record and in the hospital laboratory or pathology department.

- The tissue specimens must be maintained in the hospital laboratory.

Figure 9.5 explains how to calculate the hospital autopsy rate.

Formula 9.16. Calculating the hospital autopsy rate

$$\text{Hospital autopsy rate} = \frac{\text{Total number of hospital autopsies for a given period}}{\begin{array}{c}\text{Total number of deaths of hospital patients whose}\\ \text{bodies were available for autopsy for the same period}\end{array}} \times 100$$

Figure 9.5.   **Calculation of hospital autopsy rate**

In May, 33 inpatient deaths occurred at Community Hospital. Three of these were medical examiner's cases. Two of the bodies were removed from the hospital and so were not available for hospital autopsy. One of the medical examiner's cases was autopsied by the hospital pathologist. Fourteen other autopsies were performed on hospital inpatients who died during the month of May. In addition, autopsies were performed in the hospital on:

- A child with congenital heart disease who died in the emergency department
- A former hospital inpatient who died in an extended care facility and whose body was brought to the hospital for autopsy
- A former hospital inpatient who died at home and whose body was brought to the hospital for autopsy
- A hospital outpatient who died while receiving chemotherapy for cancer
- A hospital home care patient whose body was brought to the hospital for autopsy
- A former hospital inpatient who died in an emergency vehicle on the way to the hospital

Calculation of total hospital autopsies:

$$\begin{array}{r}
1 \text{ autopsy on medical examiner's case}\\
+14 \text{ autopsies on hospital inpatients}\\
\underline{+6 \text{ autopsies on hospital patients whose bodies were available for autopsy}}\\
21 \text{ autopsies performed by the hospital pathologist}
\end{array}$$

Calculation of number of deaths of hospital patients whose bodies were available for autopsy:

$$\begin{array}{r}
33 \text{ inpatient deaths}\\
-2 \text{ medical examiner's cases}\\
\underline{+6 \text{ deaths of hospital patients}}\\
37 \text{ bodies available for autopsy}
\end{array}$$

Calculation of hospital autopsy rate:

$$\frac{\text{Total number of hospital autopsies for the period} \times 100}{\begin{array}{c}\text{Total number of deaths of hospital patients with bodies available}\\ \text{for hospital autopsy for the period}\end{array}}$$

$$(21 \times 100)/37 = 56.8\%$$

Newborn Autopsy Rates

Autopsy rates usually include autopsies performed on newborn infants unless a separate rate is requested. The formula for calculating the **newborn autopsy rate** is shown in formula 9.17.

In our previous example of two newborn deaths at Community Hospital in May, one of the deaths was autopsied. This represents 50 percent ([1/2] × 100).

> **Formula 9.17. Calculating the newborn autopsy rate**
>
> $$\text{Newborn autopsy rate} = \frac{\text{Total number of autopsies on NB deaths for a given time period}}{\text{Total number of NB deaths for the same period}} \times 100$$

Fetal Autopsy Rates

Hospitals sometimes also calculate the **fetal autopsy rate.** Fetal autopsies are important for the clinician to determine the cause of the fetal loss and to the parents to determine if they need genetic counseling or other types of prenatal care in the future. Fetal autopsies are performed on stillborn infants who have been classified as either intermediate or late fetal deaths. This is the proportion or percentage of autopsies done on intermediate or late fetal deaths out of the total number of intermediate or late fetal deaths. The formula for calculating the fetal autopsy rate is shown in formula 9.18.

In our previous example there were 13 intermediate and late fetal deaths at Community Hospital in May. Three of those deaths were autopsied. The fetal autopsy rate is 23.1 percent ([3/13] × 100).

Table 9.14 summarizes the different hospital autopsy rates.

> **Formula 9.18. Calculating the fetal autopsy rate**
>
> $$\text{Fetal autopsy rate} = \frac{\text{Total number of autopsies on intermediate and late fetal deaths for a given period}}{\text{Total number of intermediate and late fetal deaths for the same period}} \times 100$$

Table 9.14.   Calculation of hospital autopsy rates

Rate	Numerator	Denominator
Gross autopsy rate	Total number of autopsies on inpatient deaths for a given period × 100	Total number of inpatient deaths for the same period
Net autopsy rate	Total number of autopsies on inpatient deaths for a given period × 100	Total number of inpatient deaths minus unautopsied coroner or medical examiner cases for the same period
Hospital autopsy rate	Total number of hospital autopsies for a given period × 100	Total number of deaths of hospital patients whose bodies are available for hospital autopsy for the same period
Newborn (NB) autopsy rate	Total number of autopsies on NB deaths for a given period × 100	Total number of NB deaths for the same period
Fetal autopsy rate	Total number of autopsies on intermediate and late fetal deaths for a given period × 100	Total number of intermediate and late fetal deaths for the same period

Check Your Understanding 9.7

Instructions: Read the following scenario and answer the questions on a separate sheet of paper.

In April, Community Hospital experienced 25 inpatient deaths. Two of these were coroner's cases. One additional death was a former hospital patient who died in hospice and was autopsied by the hospital pathologist. Twelve autopsies were performed on the remaining deaths. Calculate to one decimal point.

    1. ____ What is the gross autopsy rate for this month?

    2. ____ What is the net autopsy rate for this month?

    3. ____ What is the hospital autopsy rate?

Hospital Infection Rates

The most common morbidity rates calculated for hospitals are related to hospital-acquired infections, called **nosocomial (hospital-acquired) infections.** The hospital must continuously monitor the number of infections that occur in its various patient care units because infection can adversely affect the course of a patient's treatment and possibly result in death. The Joint Commission requires hospitals to follow written guidelines for reporting all types of infections. Examples of the different types of infections are respiratory, gastrointestinal, surgical wound, skin, urinary tract, septicemias, and infections related to intravascular catheters.

Hospital-Acquired Infection Rates

Hospital-acquired (nosocomial) infection rates may be calculated for the entire hospital or for a specific unit in the hospital. They also may be calculated for the specific types of infections. Ideally, the hospital should strive for an infection rate of zero. The formula for calculating the hospital-acquired or nosocomial infection rate is shown in formula 9.19. For example, Community Hospital discharged 725 patients during the month of May. Thirty-two of these patients experienced hospital-acquired infections. The hospital-acquired infection rate is 4.4 percent ([32/725] × 100).

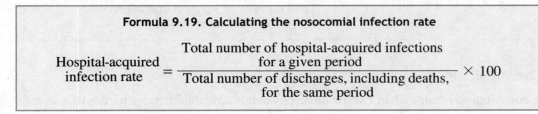

Formula 9.19. Calculating the nosocomial infection rate

$$\text{Hospital-acquired infection rate} = \frac{\text{Total number of hospital-acquired infections for a given period}}{\text{Total number of discharges, including deaths, for the same period}} \times 100$$

Postoperative Infection Rates

Hospitals often track their **postoperative infection rate.** The postoperative infection rate is the proportion or percentage of infections in clean surgical cases out of the total number of surgical operations performed. A clean surgical case is one in which no infection existed prior to surgery. The postoperative infection rate may be an indicator of a problem in the hospital environment or of some type of surgical contamination.

The individual calculating the postoperative infection rate must know the difference between a surgical procedure and a surgical operation. A **surgical procedure** is any single, separate, systematic process on or within the body that can be complete in itself. A physician, dentist, or some other licensed practitioner performs a surgical procedure, with or without instruments, to:

- Restore disunited or deficient parts
- Remove diseased or injured tissues
- Extract foreign matter
- Assist in obstetrical delivery
- Aid in diagnosis

A **surgical operation** involves one or more surgical procedures that are performed on one patient at one time using one approach to achieve a common purpose. An example of a surgical operation is the resection of a portion of both the intestine and the liver in a cancer patient. This involves two procedures, removal of a portion of the liver and removal of a portion of the colon; but it is considered only one operation because there is only one operative approach or incision. In contrast, an esophagogastroduodenoscopy (EGD) and a colonoscopy performed at the same time are two procedures with two different approaches. In the former, the approach is the upper gastrointestinal tract; in the latter, the approach is the lower gastrointestinal tract. In this case, the two procedures do not have a common approach or purpose. The formula for calculating the postoperative infection rate is shown in formula 9.20.

Formula 9.20. Calculating the postoperative infection rate

$$\text{Postoperative infection rate} = \frac{\substack{\text{Number of infections in clean surgical cases} \\ \text{for a given period}}}{\substack{\text{Total number of surgical operations} \\ \text{for the same period}}} \times 100$$

Consultation Rates

A consultation occurs when two or more physicians collaborate on a particular patient's diagnosis or treatment. The attending physician requests the consultation and explains his or her reason for doing so. The consultant then examines the patient and the patient's health record and makes recommendations in a written report. The formula for calculating the **consultation rate** is shown in formula 9.21.

During May, Community Hospital had 725 discharges and deaths. Fifty-seven patients received consultations. The consultation rate for May is 7.9 percent ([57/725] × 100).

Formula 9.21. Calculating the consultation rate

$$\text{Consultation rate} = \frac{\begin{array}{c}\text{Total number of patients receiving}\\\text{consultations for a given period}\end{array}}{\begin{array}{c}\text{Total number of discharges}\\\text{and deaths for the same period}\end{array}} \times 100$$

Case-Mix Statistical Data

Case mix is a method of grouping patients according to a predefined set of characteristics. Medicare severity diagnosis-related groups (MS-DRGs) are often used to determine case mix in hospitals. When calculating case mix using MS-DRGs, the **case-mix index** (CMI) is the average relative weight of all cases treated at a given facility or by a given physician, which reflects the resource intensity or clinical severity of a specific group in relation to the other groups in the classification system.

The CMI is a measure of the resources used in treating the patients in each hospital or group of hospitals. It may be calculated for all patients discharged, discharges by payer (table 9.15), or the discharges by particular physicians (table 9.16).

Table 9.17 provides an example of a case-mix calculation for the top ten MS-DRGs at Community Hospital. The CMI is calculated by multiplying the number of cases for each MS-DRG by the relative weight of the MS-DRG, summing the result (687.8310) and dividing by the total number of cases (484). By convention, the CMI is calculated to five decimal points and rounded to four.

The CMI can be used to indicate the average reimbursement for the hospital. From table 9.14, the reimbursement is approximately 1.5670 multiplied by the hospital's base rate. It also is a measure of the severity of illness of Medicare patients. In table 9.15, you can see that Medicare patients, as expected, have the highest CMI at 2.0059.

Other data analyzed by MS-DRG include LOS and mortality rates. LOS and mortality data are benchmarked against the hospital's peer group and national data. The process of benchmarking involves comparing the hospital's performance against an external standard or benchmark. An excellent source of information for benchmarking purposes is the Healthcare Cost Utilization Project database (HCUPnet), which is available online. Table 9.16 shows the case mix by physician and table 9.17 shows the case mix for the top ten MS-DRGs. A comparison of hospital and national data for MS-DRG 293 appears in table 9.18.

Gross analysis of the data indicates that Community Hospital's mortality rate and ALOS are slightly better than the national average. But, at the same time, the hospital's average charges are higher than the national average.

Table 9.15.   Case-mix index by payer, Community Hospital, 20XX

Payer	CMI	N
Commercial	1.8830	283
Government managed care	0.9880	470
Managed care	1.4703	2,326
Medicaid	1.3400	962
Medicare	2.0059	1,776
Other	1.3251	148
Self-pay	1.3462	528
Average Case Mix by Payer	**1.5670**	**6,503**

Table 9.16.   Case mix of physicians, 20XX

Physician	CMI	N
A	1.0235	71
B	1.6397	71
C	1.1114	86
Average Case Mix by Physician	**1.2501**	**228**

Table 9.17.   Calculation of case-mix index for the top ten MS-DRGs, Community Hospital, 20XX

MS-DRG	Number (N)	MS-DRG Weight	N × MS-DRG Weight
286	84	1.9634	164.9256
293	62	0.6940	43.0280
982	61	2.8954	176.6194
986	51	1.1079	56.5029
434	45	0.6489	29.2005
391	43	1.0958	47.1194
378	41	0.9873	40.4793
287	40	1.0321	41.2840
871	31	1.8437	57.1547
689	26	1.2122	31.5172
Total	**484**		**687.8310**
CMI			**1.4211**

Table 9.18.   Benchmark data, Community Hospital vs. national average for MS-DRG 293, Heart failure and shock w/o CC/MCC

	ALOS	Mortality Rate	Average Charges
Community Hospital	3.1	0.9%	$18,042
National average	3.2	1.1%	$15,900

Check Your Understanding 9.8

Instructions: Using the following table, answer the following questions on a separate piece of paper. Calculate to one decimal point.

Table 9.19.   **Check Your Understanding 9.8**

MS-DRG	MS-DRG Title	Rel. Wt.	No. of Pts.	Total Wt. ANSWERS:
179	Respiratory infections and inflammations w/o CC/MCC	1.0088	5	5.0440
187	Pleural effusion w/ CC	1.0620	2	2.1240
189	Pulmonary edema and respiratory failure	1.3455	3	4.0365
194	Simple pneumonia and pleurisy w/ CC	0.9976	1	0.9976
208	Respiratory system diagnosis w/ ventilator support <96 hours	2.2358	1	2.2358
280	Acute myocardial infarction, discharged alive w/ MCC	1.8313	3	5.4939
299	Peripheral vascular disorders w/ MCC	1.4045	2	2.809
313	Chest pain	0.5404	4	2.1616
377	G.I. hemorrhage w/ MCC	1.6149	1	1.6149
391	Esophagitis, gastroent. and misc. digest. disorders w/ MCC	1.0958	1	1.0958
547	Connective tissue disorders w/o CC/MCC	0.7475	1	0.7475
552	Medical back problems w/o MCC	0.7937	1	0.7937
684	Renal failure w/o CC/MCC	0.6746	1	0.6746
812	Red blood cell disorders w/o MCC	0.7751	2	1.5502
872	Septicemia w/o MV 96+ hours w/o MCC	1.1155	1	1.1155
918	Poisoning and toxic effects of drugs w/o MCC	0.5839	1	0.5839
Total			30	33.0785

Case-mix index = 33/0785 / 30 = 1.1026

1. _____ Last month, Community Hospital had 57 discharges from its Medicine unit. Six patients developed a urinary tract infection while in the hospital. Calculate the nosocomial infection rate for the last month.

2. _____ During June, Community Hospital had 149 patients discharged. Fifty-seven patients had consultations from specialty physicians. What was the consultation rate for June?

3. _____ Dr. Green discharged 30 patients from Medicine Service during the month of August. The table above presents the number of patients discharged by MS-DRG. Calculate the total weight for each MS-DRG and the CMI for Dr. Green.

4. A name given to describe an infection acquired in a healthcare facility is _____.

Ambulatory Care Statistical Data

Ambulatory care includes healthcare services provided to patients who are not hospitalized (that is, who are not considered inpatients or residents and do not stay in the healthcare facility overnight). Such patients are referred to as outpatients. Most ambulatory care services today are provided in freestanding physicians' offices, emergency care centers, and ambulatory surgery centers that are not owned or operated by acute care organizations. Hospitals do, however, provide many hospital-based healthcare services to outpatients. Hospital outpatients may receive services in one or more areas within the hospital, including clinics, same-day surgery departments, diagnostic departments, and emergency departments.

Outpatient statistics include records of the number of patient visits and the types of services provided. Many different terms are used to describe outpatients and ambulatory care services, including:

- **Hospital ambulatory care:** All hospital-directed preventive, therapeutic, and rehabilitative services provided by physicians and their surrogates to patients who are not hospital inpatients

- **Outpatient:** A patient who receives ambulatory care services in a hospital-based clinic or department

- **Hospital outpatient:** A hospital patient who receives services in one or more of a hospital's facilities when he or she is not currently an inpatient or a home care patient

- **Emergency patient:** A patient who is admitted to the emergency department of a hospital for diagnosis and treatment of a condition that requires immediate medical, dental, or allied health services in order to sustain life or to prevent critical consequences

- **Clinic outpatient:** A patient who is admitted to a clinical service of a clinic or hospital for diagnosis or treatment on an ambulatory basis

- **Referred outpatient:** An outpatient who is provided special diagnostic or therapeutic services by a hospital on an ambulatory basis but whose medical care remains the responsibility of the referring physician

- **Outpatient visit:** A patient's visit to one or more units or facilities located in the ambulatory services area (clinic or physician's office) of an acute care hospital in which an overnight stay does not occur

- **Encounter:** The professional, direct personal contact between a patient and a physician or other person who is authorized by state licensure law and, if applicable, by medical staff bylaws, to order or furnish healthcare services for the diagnosis or treatment of the patient; face-to-face contact between a patient and a provider who has primary responsibility for assessing and treating the condition of the patient at a given contact and exercise

- **Occasion of service:** A specified, identifiable service involved in the care of a patient that is not an encounter (for example, a lab test ordered during an encounter)

- **Ambulatory surgery center or ambulatory surgical center (ASC):** Under Medicare, an outpatient surgical facility that has its own national identifier; is a separate entity with respect to its licensure, accreditation, governance, professional supervision, administrative functions, clinical services, recordkeeping, and financial and accounting systems; has as its sole purpose the provision of services in connection with surgical procedures that do not require inpatient hospitalization; and meets the conditions and requirements set forth in the Medicare Conditions of Participation

  — May be referred to as short-stay surgery, one-day surgery, same-day surgery, or come-and-go surgery services

Check Your Understanding 9.9

Match the definitions with the choices on the right:

1. _____ A patient's visit to one or more units or facilities located in the ambulatory services area (clinic or physician's office) of an acute care hospital in which an overnight stay does not occur

2. _____ A specified, identifiable service involved in the care of a patient that is not an encounter (for example, a lab test ordered during an encounter)

3. _____ All hospital-directed preventive, therapeutic, and rehabilitative services provided by physicians and their surrogates to patients who are not hospital inpatients

4. _____ A patient who receives ambulatory care services in a hospital-based clinic or department

5. _____ An outpatient who is provided special diagnostic or therapeutic services by a hospital on an ambulatory basis but whose medical care remains the responsibility of the referring physician

6. _____ The professional, direct personal contact between a patient and a physician or other person who is authorized by state licensure law, and if application, by medical staff bylaws to order or furnish healthcare services for the diagnosis or treatment of the patient; face-to-face contact between a patient and a provider who has primary responsibility for assessing and treating the condition of the patient at a given contact and exercise

a. Ambulatory surgery center

b. Outpatient visit

c. Encounter

d. Occasion of service

e. Referred outpatient

f. Clinic outpatient

g. Emergency outpatient

h. Hospital outpatient

i. Hospital ambulatory care

j. Outpatient

7. ____ A patient who is admitted to a clinical service of a clinic or hospital for diagnosis or treatment on an ambulatory basis

8. ____ A hospital patient who receives services in one or more of a hospital's facilities when he or she is not currently an inpatient or a home care patient

9. ____ A patient who is admitted to the emergency department of a hospital for diagnosis and treatment of a condition that requires immediate medical, dental, or allied health services in order to sustain life or to prevent critical consequences

10. ____ An outpatient surgical facility that has its own national identifier; is a separate entity with respect to its licensure, accreditation, governance, professional supervision, administrative functions, clinical services, recordkeeping, and financial and accounting systems

Public Health Statistics and Epidemiological Information

Just as statistics are collected in the healthcare organizational setting, they also are collected on a community, regional, and national basis. **Vital statistics** are an example of data collected and reported at these levels. The term *vital statistics* refers to the collection and analysis of data related to the crucial events in life: birth, death, marriage, divorce, fetal death, and induced terminations of pregnancy. These statistics are used to identify trends. For example, a higher-than-expected death rate among newborns may be an indication of the lack of prenatal services in a community. A number of deaths in a region due to the same cause may indicate an environmental problem.

These types of data are used as part of the effort to preserve and improve the health of a defined population—the public health. The study of factors that influence the health status of a population is called epidemiology.

National Vital Statistics System

The **National Vital Statistics System** (NVSS) is responsible for maintaining the official vital statistics of the United States. These statistics are provided to the federal government by state-operated registration systems. The NVSS is housed in the National Center for Health Statistics (NCHS) of the Centers for Disease Control and Prevention (CDC).

To facilitate data collection, standard forms and model procedures for the uniform registration of events are developed and recommended for state use through cooperative activities of the individual states and the NCHS. The standard certificates represent the minimum basic data set necessary for the collection and publication of comparable national, state, and local vital statistics data. The standard forms are revised about every

10 years, with the last revision completed in 2003. To effectively implement these new certificates, the NCHS collaborates with its state partners to improve the timeliness, quality, and sustainability of the vital statistics system, along with collection of the revised and new content of the 2003 certificates (CDC 2011).

The certificate of live birth is used for registration purposes and is composed of two parts. The first part contains the information related to the child and the parents. The second part is used to collect data about the mother's pregnancy. This information is used for the collection of aggregate data only. No identification information appears on this portion of the certificate nor does it ever appear on the official certificate of birth. Pregnancy-related information includes complications of pregnancy, concurrent illnesses or conditions affecting pregnancy, and abnormal conditions and/or congenital anomalies of the newborn. Lifestyle factors such as use of alcohol and tobacco also are collected. Thus, the birth certificate is the major source of maternal and natality statistics. A listing of pregnancy-related information appears in figure 9.6.

Data collected from death certificates are used to compile causes of death in the United States. The certificate of death contains decedent information, place of death information, medical certification, and disposition information. Data on causes of death are classified and coded using the International Classification of Diseases (ICD). Beginning in 1999, the United States implemented ICD-10 for the coding of causes of death. Examples of the content of death certificates appear in figure 9.7.

A report of fetal death is completed when a pregnancy results in a stillbirth. This report contains information on the parents, the history of the pregnancy, and the cause of the fetal death. Information collected on the pregnancy is the same as that recorded on the birth certificate. To assess the effects of environmental exposures on the fetus, the parents' occupational data are collected. A listing of the content of the fetal death certificate appears in figure 9.8

The report of induced termination of pregnancy records information on the place of the induced termination of pregnancy, the type of termination procedure, and the patient. (See figure 9.9.)

A tool for monitoring and exploring the interrelationships between infant death and risk factors at birth is the linked birth and infant death data set. This is a service provided by the NCHS. In this data set, the information from the death certificate (such as age and underlying or multiple causes of death) is linked to the information in the birth certificate (such as age, race, birth weight, prenatal care, maternal education, and so on) for each infant who dies in the United States, Puerto Rico, the Virgin Islands, and Guam. The purpose of the data set is to use the many additional variables available from the birth certificate to conduct a detailed analysis of infant mortality patterns.

Birth, death, fetal death, and termination of pregnancy certificates provide vital information for use in medical research, epidemiological studies, and other public health programs. In addition, they are the source of data for compiling morbidity, birth, and mortality rates that describe the health of a given population at the local, state, or national level. Because of their many uses, the data on these certificates must be complete and accurate.

Figure 9.6.   Content of US certificate of live birth, 2003

Child's Information	**Pregnancy History**
Child's name	Date of first prenatal care visit
Time of birth	Date of last prenatal care visit
Sex	Total number of prenatal visits for this pregnancy
Date of birth	Mother's height
Facility (hospital) name (if not an institution, give	Mother's prepregnancy weight
street address)	Mother's weight at delivery
City, town, or location of birth	Did mother get WIC food for herself during this
County of birth	pregnancy?
	Number of previous live births
Mother's Information	Number now living
Current legal name	Number now dead
Date of birth	Date of last live birth
Mother's name prior to first marriage	Number of other pregnancy outcomes
Birthplace	Other outcomes
Residence (state)	Date of last other pregnancy outcomes
County	Cigarette smoking before and during pregnancy
City, town, or location	Principal source of payment for this delivery
Street number	Date last normal menses began
Apartment number	Mother's medical record number
Zip code	Risk factors in this pregnancy
Inside city limits?	Infections present and/or treated during this
Mother's mailing address	pregnancy
Mother married?	Obstetric procedures
If no, has paternity acknowledgment been signed in	Onset of labor
the hospital?	Characteristics of labor and delivery
Social Security number (SSN) requested for child?	Method of delivery
Mother's SSN	Maternal mortality
Education	
Hispanic origin?	**Newborn Information**
Race	Newborn medical record number
Place where birth occurred	Birth weight
Attendant's name, title, and NPI	Obstetric estimate of gestation
Mother transferred for maternal, medical, or fetal	Apgar score (1 and 5 minutes)
indications for delivery?	Plurality
	If not born first (born first, second, third, etc.)
Father's Information	Abnormal conditions of newborn
Current legal name	Congenital anomalies of the newborn
Date of birth	Was infant transferred within 24 hours of delivery?
Birthplace	Is infant living at time of report?
Education	Is infant being breastfed at discharge?
Hispanic origin?	
Race	
Father's SSN	

Source: NVSS 2005.

Figure 9.7. Content of US certificate of death, 2003

Decedent Information	Medical Certification
Name	Date pronounced dead
Sex	Time pronounced dead
Social Security number	Signature of person pronouncing death
Age	Date signed
Under 1 year—month; days	Actual or presumed date of death
Under 1 day—hours; minutes	Actual or presumed time of death
Date of birth	Was medical examiner contacted?
Birthplace	Immediate cause of death
Residence (state)	Due to _____
County	Due to _____
City or town	Due to _____
Street and number	Other significant conditions contributing to death
Apartment number	Was an autopsy performed?
Zip code	Were autopsy findings available to complete the
Inside city limits?	cause of death?
Ever in U.S. armed forces?	Did tobacco use contribute to death?
Marital status at time of death	If female, indicate pregnancy status
Surviving spouse's name (if wife, give name prior	Manner of death
to first marriage)	For deaths due to injury:
Father's name	Date of injury
Mother's name (prior to first marriage)	Time of injury
Informant's name	Place of injury
Relationship to decedent	Injury at work?
Mailing address	Location of injury
Decedent's education	Describe how injury occurred
Hispanic origin?	If transportation injury, specify if driver/operator,
Race	passenger, pedestrian, other
Disposition Information	**Certifier Information**
Method of disposition	Certifier
Place of disposition (cemetery, crematory, other)	Name, address, and zip code of person completing
Location—city, town, and state	Cause of Death
Name and complete address of funeral facility	Title of certifier
Signature of Funeral Service Licensee or other agent	License number
License number	Date certified
Place of Death Information	
Place of death	
If hospital, indicate inpatient, emergency room/	
outpatient, dead on arrival	
If somewhere other than hospital, indicate hospice,	
nursing home/long-term care facility, decedent's	
home, other	
Facility name	
City or town, state, zip code	
County	

Source: NVSS 2011.

Figure 9.8. **Content of US standard report of fetal death, 2003**

Mother's Information	Number of other pregnancy outcomes
Name of fetus (optional—at the discretion of the parents)	Other outcomes
	Date of last other pregnancy outcomes
Time of delivery	Cigarette smoking before and during pregnancy
Sex	Date last normal menses began
Date of delivery	Plurality
City, town, or location of delivery	If not born first (born second, third, etc.)
Zip code of delivery	Mother transferred for maternal, medical, or fetal indications for delivery?
County of delivery	
Place where delivery occurred	**Medical and Health Information**
Facility name	Risk factors in this pregnancy
Facility ID	Infections present and/or treated during this pregnancy
Mother's current legal name	
Date of birth	Method of delivery
Mother's name prior to first marriage	Maternal mortality
Birthplace	Congenital anomalies of the newborn
Residence of mother (state)	
County	**Father's Information**
City, town, or location	Current legal name
Street number	Date of birth
Apartment number	Birthplace
Zip code	
Inside city limits?	**Disposition**
Education	Method of Disposition
Hispanic origin?	
Race	**Attendant and Registrant Information**
Mother married at delivery, conception, or any time between?	Attendant's name, title, and NPI
	Name of person completing report
Date of first prenatal care visit	Date report completed
Date of last prenatal care visit	Date received by registrar
Total number of prenatal visits for this pregnancy	
Mother's height	**Cause of Fetal Death**
Mother's prepregnancy weight	Initiating cause/condition
Mother's weight at delivery	Other significant causes or conditions
Did mother get WIC food for herself during this pregnancy?	Weight of fetus
	Obstetric estimate of gestation at delivery
Number of previous live births	Estimated time of fetal death
Number now living	Was an autopsy performed?
Number now dead	Was a histological placental examination performed?
Date of last live birth	Were autopsy or histological placental examination results used in determining the cause of fetal death?

Figure 9.9.   Content of US standard report of induced termination of pregnancy, 1997

Place of Induced Termination	Hispanic origin?
Facility name	Race
City, town, or location of pregnancy termination	Education
County of pregnancy termination	Elementary/secondary
	College
Patient Information	Date last normal menses began
Patient identification	Clinical estimate of gestation
Age at last birthday	Previous pregnancies
Marital status	Live births
Date or pregnancy termination	Other terminations
Residence (state)	Type of termination procedure
County	**Other Information**
City, town, or location	Name of attending physician
Inside city limits?	Name of person completing report
Zip code	

Source: NVSS 2011.

Population-Based Statistics

Population-based statistics are based on the mortality and morbidity rates from which the health of a population can be inferred. The entire defined population is used in the collection and reporting of these statistics. The size of the defined population serves as the denominator in the calculation of these rates.

Birth Rates and Measures of Infant Mortality

Two community-based rates that are commonly used to describe a community's health are the crude birth rate and measures of infant mortality. The World Health Organization's definition of a live birth is the complete expulsion or extraction from its mother of a product of conception, irrespective of the duration of the pregnancy, which after such separation, breathes or shows other evidence of life, such as beating of the heart, pulsation of the umbilical cord, or definite movement of voluntary muscles, whether or not the umbilical cord has been cut or the placenta is attached.

Rates that describe infant mortality are based on age. Therefore, the definitions for the various age groups must be strictly followed. Table 9.20 summarizes the calculations for community-based birth and infant mortality rates. These mortality or death rates are broken down as follows:

- **Crude birth rate:** As shown in table 9.20, the crude birth rate is the number of live births divided by the population at risk. Community rates are calculated using the multiplier 1,000, 10,000, or 100,000. The purpose is to bring the rate to a whole number, as discussed earlier in the chapter. The result of the formula would be stated as the number of live births per 1,000 population. The formula for calculating the crude birth rate is:

> **Formula 9.22. Calculating the crude birth rate**
>
> $$\text{Crude birth rate} = \frac{\text{Number of live births for a given community for a specified time period}}{\text{Estimated population for the same community and the same time period}} \times 1{,}000$$

For example, if there were 7,532 live births in a community of 600,000 in 2011, the crude birth rate for that year would be 13 per 1,000 population ([7,532/600,000] × 1,000).

- **Neonatal mortality rate:** The neonatal mortality rate can be used as an indirect measure of the quality of prenatal care and/or the mother's prenatal behavior (for example, alcohol, drug, or tobacco use). The neonatal period is the period from birth up to, but not including, 28 days of age. In the formula for calculating the neonatal mortality rate, the numerator is the number of deaths of infants from birth up to but not including 28 days of age during a given time period and the denominator is the total number of live births during the same time period.

> **Formula 9.23. Calculating the neonatal mortality rate**
>
> $$\text{Neonatal mortality rate} = \frac{\text{Number of deaths of infants from birth up to, but not including, 28 days of age during a given time period}}{\text{Number of live births during the same time period}} \times 1{,}000$$

For example, in your community there were 7,532 live births in 20XX and 21 infants under age 28 days who died in that year. The neonatal mortality rate is 3 per 1,000 live births for the period ([21/7,532] × 1,000).

- **Postneonatal mortality rate:** The postneonatal mortality rate is often used as an indicator of the quality of the home or community environment of infants. The postneonatal period is from 28 days of age up to, but not including, one year of age. In the formula for calculating the postneonatal mortality rate, the numerator is the number of deaths among infants from 28 days of age up to, but not including, one year of age during a given time period and the denominator is the total number of live births minus the number of neonatal deaths during the same time period.

Formula 9.24. Calculating the postneonatal mortality rate

$$\text{Postneonatal mortality rate} = \frac{\substack{\text{Number of deaths of infants from 28 days of age} \\ \text{up to, but not including, one year of age} \\ \text{during a given time period}}}{\substack{\text{Number of live births minus neonatal deaths} \\ \text{during the same time period}}} \times 1,000$$

For example, in your community there were 7,532 live births, 21 neonatal deaths and 17 postneonatal deaths during 20XX. The postneonatal mortality rate is 2 per 1,000 live births minus neonatal deaths for the period ($17/[7,532 - 21] \times 1,000$).

- **Infant mortality rate:** The infant mortality rate is the summary of the neonatal and postneonatal mortality rates. In the formula for calculating the infant mortality rate, the numerator is the number of deaths among infants under one year of age and the denominator is the number of live births during the same period. The infant mortality rate is the most commonly used measure for comparing health status among nations. All the rates are expressed in terms of the number of deaths per 1,000 live births.

Formula 9.25. Calculating the infant mortality rate

$$\text{Infant mortality rate} = \frac{\substack{\text{Number of deaths of infants under} \\ \text{one year of age during a given time period}}}{\text{Number of live births during the same time period}} \times 1,000$$

For example, in your community there were 21 neonatal deaths, 17 postneonatal deaths and 7,532 live births in 20XX. The infant mortality rate is 5 per 1,000 live births in that year ($[17 + 21]/7,532 \times 1,000$).

Table 9.20.   Calculation of community-based birth and infant death (mortality) rates

Measure	Numerator (x)	Denominator (y)	10^n
Crude birth rate	Number of live births for a given community for a specified time period	Estimated population for the same community and the same time period	1,000
Neonatal mortality rate	Number of deaths of infants from birth up to, but not including, 28 days of age during a given time period	Number of live births during the same time period	1,000
Postneonatal mortality rate	Number of deaths of infants from 28 days of age up to, but not including, one year of age during a given time period	Number of live births minus neonatal deaths during the same time period	1,000
Infant mortality rate	Number of deaths of infants under one year of age during a given time period	Number of live births during the same time period	1,000

Death (Mortality) Rates

Other measures of mortality with which the HIM professional should be familiar include the following:

- **Crude death/mortality rate:** The crude death rate is a measure of the actual or observed mortality in a given population. Crude death rates apply to a population without regard to characteristics such as age, race, and sex. They measure the proportion of the population that has died during a given period of time (usually one year) or the number of deaths in a community per 1,000 for a given period of time. In the formula, the numerator is the total number of deaths in a population for a specified time period and the denominator is the estimated population for the same time period.

Formula 9.26. Calculating the crude death/mortality rate

$$\text{Crude death rate} = \frac{\begin{array}{c}\text{Total number of deaths for a population}\\\text{during a specified time period}\end{array}}{\text{Estimated population for the same time period}} \times 1,000$$

For example, in our previous examples, we used a community population of 600,000. There were 1,498 deaths in 20XX. Dividing 1,498 by 600,000 equals 0.024966. Using a multiplier of 1,000 gives a crude death rate of 2.5 deaths per 1,000 population for 20XX ([1,498/600,000] × 1,000).

- **Cause-specific mortality rate:** As its name indicates, the cause-specific mortality rate is the rate of death due to a specified cause. It may be calculated for an entire population or for any age, sex, or race. In the formula, the numerator is the number of deaths due to a specified cause for a given time period and the denominator is the estimated population for the same time period. Table 9.21 displays cause-specific mortality rates for men and women due to influenza and pneumonia for the year 2007. The cause-specific death rates for each age group are consistently higher for men than for women. This information could lead to an investigation of why men are more susceptible to death from influenza and pneumonia than women.

Formula 9.27. Calculating the cause-specific mortality rate

$$\begin{array}{c}\text{Cause-specific}\\\text{mortality rate}\end{array} = \frac{\begin{array}{c}\text{Total number of deaths due to a specific cause}\\\text{during a specified time period}\end{array}}{\text{Estimated population for the same time period}} \times 100,000$$

Table 9.21. **Cause-specific mortality rates, by sex, due to influenza and pneumonia (ICD-10 codes J10–J18.9), age 45+, in the United States, 2007**

Age Group	Women			Men		
	Population	Deaths	Rate/100,000	Population	Deaths	Rate/100,000
45–54	22,279,847	783	3.5	21,594,913	1,126	5.2
55–64	16,936,988	1,271	7.5	15,775,088	1,881	11.9
65–74	10,465,176	2,503	23.9	8,888,973	3,044	34.3
75–84	7,710,838	7,447	96.6	5,312,673	7,412	139.5
85+	3,735,499	15,893	425.5	1,776,799	9,642	542.7
Total	**61,128,348**	**27,897**	**45.6**	**53,346,446**	**23,105**	**43.3**

Source: CDC Wonder 2012.

- **Case fatality rate:** The case fatality rate measures the total number of deaths among the diagnosed cases of a specific disease, most often acute illness. In the formula for calculating the case fatality rate, the numerator is the number of deaths due to a specific disease that occurred during a specific time period and the denominator is the number of diagnosed cases during the same time period. The higher the case fatality rate, the more virulent the infection.

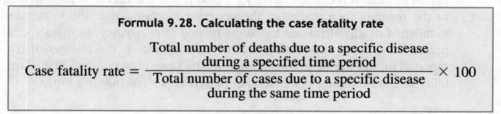

Formula 9.28. Calculating the case fatality rate

$$\text{Case fatality rate} = \frac{\text{Total number of deaths due to a specific disease during a specified time period}}{\text{Total number of cases due to a specific disease during the same time period}} \times 100$$

For example, in our community there were fifteen cases of meningitis resulting in two deaths. The case fatality rate of meningitis is 13.3 percent ([2/15] × 100).

- **Proportionate mortality rate:** The proportionate mortality rate (PMR) is a measure of mortality due to a specific cause for a specific time period. In the formula for calculating the PMR, the numerator is the number of deaths due to a specific disease for a specific time period and the denominator is the number of deaths from all causes for the same time period. Table 9.22 displays the PMRs for influenza and pneumonia in the United States in 2007 by age groups.

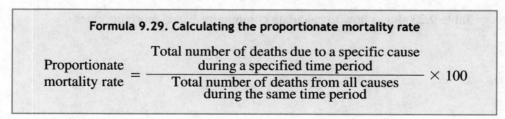

Formula 9.29. Calculating the proportionate mortality rate

$$\text{Proportionate mortality rate} = \frac{\text{Total number of deaths due to a specific cause during a specified time period}}{\text{Total number of deaths from all causes during the same time period}} \times 100$$

Table 9.22.   **Proportionate mortality rates for influenza and pneumonia (ICD-10 codes J10–J18.9), all ages, in the United States, 2007**

Age Group	Influenza and Pneumonia Deaths	Total Deaths	PMR/100
0–4	331	33,841	0.98
5–14	103	6,147	1.68
15–24	163	33,982	0.48
25–34	331	42,572	0.78
35–44	784	79,606	0.98
45–54	1,909	184,686	1.03
55–64	3,152	287,110	1.10
65–74	5,547	389,238	1.43
75–84	14,859	652,682	2.28
85+	25,535	713,647	3.58

Source: CDC 2012.

- **Maternal mortality rate (community based):** The maternal mortality rate measures the deaths associated with pregnancy for a specific community for a specific period of time. It is calculated only for deaths that are directly related to pregnancy. In the formula for calculating the maternal mortality rate, the numerator is the number of deaths attributed to causes related to pregnancy during a specific time period for a given community and the denominator is the number of live births reported during the same time period for the same community. The maternal mortality rate is expressed as the number of deaths per 100,000 live births.

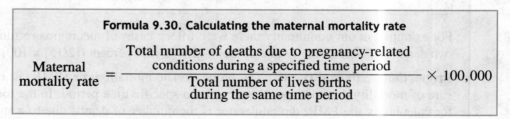

Formula 9.30. Calculating the maternal mortality rate

$$\text{Maternal mortality rate} = \frac{\text{Total number of deaths due to pregnancy-related conditions during a specified time period}}{\text{Total number of lives births during the same time period}} \times 100,000$$

For example, in the United States in 2007 there were 4,317,119 live births and 548 maternal deaths. This is a maternal mortality rate of 13 maternal deaths per 100,000 live births ([548/4,317,119] × 100,000).

Table 9.23 shows how to calculate community-based mortality rates.

Table 9.23.   **Calculation of community-based mortality rates**

Measure	Numerator (x)	Denominator (y)	10^n
Crude death/ mortality rate	Total number of deaths for a population during a specified time period	Estimated population for the same time period	1,000 or 10,000 or 100,000
Cause-specific mortality rate	Total number of deaths due to a specific cause during a specified time period	Estimated population for the same time period	100,000
Case fatality rate	Total number of deaths due to a specific disease during a specified time period	Total number of cases due to a specific disease during the same time period	100
Proportionate mortality rate	Total number of deaths due to a specific cause during a specified time period	Total number of deaths from all causes during the same time period	NA
Maternal mortality rate	Total number of deaths due to pregnancy-related conditions during a specified time period	Total number of live births during the same time period	100,000

Check Your Understanding 9.10

Instructions: Review the mortality data in the following and then answer the following questions on a separate piece of paper.

Table 9.24.   **Check Your Understanding 9.10**

	Mortality Rates, United States, 2007			
	Female		Male	
Age Group	Population	Deaths	Population	Deaths
Less than 1 year	2,078,212	12,845	2,178,808	16,293
1–4 years	8,043,056	2,069	8,424,049	2,634
5–9	9,701,050	1,192	10,148,578	1,519
10–14	9,914,382	1,370	10,399,927	2,066
15–19	10,466,821	3,741	11,006,869	9,558
20–24	10,179,459	4,925	10,852,937	15,758
25–34	19,908,376	12,780	20,682,550	29,792
35–44	21,542,555	29,501	21,618,734	50,105
45–54	22,279,847	70,230	21,594,913	114,456
55–64	16,936,988	113,492	15,775,088	173,618
65–74	10,465,176	170,894	8,888,973	218,344
75–84	7,710,838	331,879	5,312,673	320,803
85 +	3,735,499	464,781	1,776,799	248,866
Total	152,962,259	1,219,699	148,660,898	1,203,812

Source: CDC Wonder 2012.

1. ____ What is the crude death rate per 10,000 for men?

2. ____ What is the crude death rate per 10,000 for women?

3. ____ What is the crude death rate per 10,000 for the entire group?

4. ____ What is the crude death rate per 10,000 for men ages 35–44?

5. ____ What is the crude death rate per 10,000 for women ages 35–55?

Measures of Morbidity

Two measures are commonly used to describe the presence of disease in a community or specific location (for example, a nursing home): incidence and prevalence rates. Disease is defined as any illness, injury, or disability. Incidence and prevalence measures can be broken down by race, sex, age, or other characteristics of a population.

An **incidence rate** is used to compare the frequency of new cases of disease in populations. Populations are compared using rates instead of raw numbers because rates adjust for differences in population size. The incidence rate is the probability or risk of illness in a population over a period of time. The formula for calculating the incidence rate is shown in formula 9.31. The denominator represents the population from which the case in the numerator arose, such as a nursing home, school, or organization. For 10^n, a value is selected so that the smallest rate calculated results in a whole number. For example in a small population such as a nursing home you might select 100, in studying a larger population you might select 1,000. For example, in a local nursing home of 110 patients, two new cases of H1N1 (a strain of Influenza A virus) occurred during November. Using this formula, the incidence rate is 2 percent ([2/110] × 100).

The **prevalence rate** is the proportion of persons in a population who have a particular disease at a specific point in time or over a specified period of time. The formula for calculating the prevalence rate is shown in formula 9.32. The prevalence rate describes the magnitude of an epidemic and can be an indicator of the medical resources needed in a community for the duration of the epidemic. For example, in a community of 600,000 individuals, there were 2,486 individuals identified as having AIDS and an additional 309 cases identified in 20XX. The prevalence rate is 4.66 cases per 1,000 population ([2,486 + 309]/600,000 × 1,000).

It is easy to confuse incidence and prevalence rates. The distinction is in the numerators of their formulas. The numerator in the formula for the incidence rate is the number of new cases occurring in a given time period. The numerator in the formula for the prevalence rate is all cases present during a given time period. In addition, the incidence rate includes only patients whose illness began during a specified time period whereas the prevalence rate includes all patients from a specified cause regardless of when the illness began. Moreover, the prevalence rate includes a patient until he or she recovers.

Formula 9.31. Calculating the incidence rate

$$\text{Incidence rate} = \frac{\begin{array}{c}\text{Total number of new cases of a specific disease}\\\text{during a given time period}\end{array}}{\text{Total population at risk during the same time period}} \times 10^n$$

Formula 9.32. Calculating the prevalence rate

$$\text{Prevelence rate} = \frac{\begin{array}{c}\text{All new and preexisting cases of a specific disease}\\\text{during a given time period}\end{array}}{\text{Total population during the same time period}} \times 10^n$$

National Notifiable Diseases Surveillance System

In 1878, Congress authorized the US Marine Hospital Service, the precursor to the Public Health Service, to collect morbidity reports on cholera, smallpox, plague, and yellow fever from US consuls overseas. This information was used to implement quarantine measures to prevent the spread of these diseases to the United States. In 1879, Congress provided for the weekly collection and publication of reports of these diseases. In 1893, Congress expanded the scope to include weekly reporting from states and municipalities. To provide for more uniformity in data collection, Congress enacted a law in 1902 that directed the surgeon general to provide standard forms for the collection, compilation, and publication of reports at the national level. In 1912, the states and U.S. territories recommended that infectious disease be immediately reported by telegraph. By 1928, all states, the District of Columbia, Hawaii, and Puerto Rico were participating in the national reporting of 29 specified diseases. In 1961, the CDC assumed responsibility for the collection and publication of data concerning nationally notifiable diseases.

A **notifiable disease** is one for which regular, frequent, and timely information on individual cases is considered necessary to prevent and control disease. The list of notifiable diseases varies over time and by state. The Council of State and Territorial Epidemiologists (CSTE) collaborates with the CDC to determine which diseases should be reported. State reporting to the CDC is voluntary. However, all states generally report the internationally quarantinable diseases in accordance with the World Health Organization's International Health Regulations. Completeness of reporting varies by state and type of disease and may be influenced by any of the following factors:

- Type and severity of the illness
- Whether treatment in a healthcare facility was sought
- Diagnosis of an illness
- Availability of diagnostic services

- Disease-control measures in effect
- Public awareness of the disease
- Resources, priorities, and interests of state and local public health officials

Information that is reported includes date, county, age, sex, race and ethnicity, and disease-specific epidemiologic information; personal identifiers are not included. A strict CSTE Data Release Policy regulates dissemination of the data. A list of nationally notifiable infectious diseases appears in figure 9.10. The list is updated annually.

National morbidity data are reported weekly. Public health managers and providers use the reports to rapidly identify disease epidemics and to understand patterns of disease occurrence. Case-specific information is included in the reports. Changes in age, sex, race and ethnicity, and geographic distributions can be monitored and investigated as necessary.

Check Your Understanding 9.11

Instructions: Answer the following questions on a separate piece of paper.

1. Define incidence rate and prevalence rate.

2. What is a notifiable disease?

3. Calculate the incidence rate, per 100,000, for the following hypothetical data: In 20XX, 189,000 new cases of coronary artery disease were reported in the United States. The estimated population for 20XX was 301,623,157.

Presentation of Statistical Data

Collected data are often more meaningful when presented in graphic form (consider any of the acute or ambulatory care data previously described). How one presents such data will be governed by whether they are nominal, ordinal, interval or ratio.

Tables, charts, and graphs offer the opportunity to analyze data sets and to explore, understand, and present frequency distributions, trends, and relationships in the data. The purpose of tables, charts, and graphs is to communicate information about the data to the user of the data.

Whatever type of graphic form is used, it should:

- Display the data
- Allow the user to think about the meaning of the data
- Avoid distortion of the data

Figure 9.10. Nationally notifiable infectious diseases in the United States, 2012

Anthrax
Arboviral neuroinvasive and non-
neuroinvasive diseases
- California serogroup virus disease
- Eastern equine encephalitis virus
disease
- Powassan virus disease
- St. Louis encephalitis virus
disease
- West Nile virus disease
- Western equine encephalitis virus
disease
Babesiosis
Botulism
- Botulism, foodborne
- Botulism, infant
- Botulism, other (wound and
unspecified)
Brucellosis
Chancroid
Chlamydia trachomatis, infections
Cholera
Coccidioidomycosis
Cryptosporidiosis
Cyclosporiasis
Dengue
- Dengue fever
- Dengue hemorrhagic fever
- Dengue shock syndrome
Diphtheria
Ehrlichiosis/Anaplasmosis
- *Ehrlichia chaffeensis*
- *Ehrlichia ewingii*
- *Anaplasma phagocytophilum*
- Undetermined
Giardiasis
Gonorrhea
Haemophilus influenzae, invasive
disease
Hansen disease (leprosy)
Hantavirus pulmonary syndrome
Hemolytic uremic syndrome,
post-diarrheal

Hepatitis
- Hepatitis A, acute
- Hepatitis B, acute
- Hepatitis B, chronic
- Hepatitis B, virus, perinatal
infection
- Hepatitis C, acute
- Hepatitis C, past or present
HIV infection (AIDS has been
reclassified as HIV stage III)
- HIV infection, adult/adolescent
(age ≥ 13 years)
- HIV infection, child (age ≥ 18
months and < 13 years)
- HIV infection, pediatric (age < 18
months)
Influenza-associated pediatric mortality
Legionellosis
Listeriosis
Lyme disease
Malaria
Measles
Meningococcal disease
Mumps
Novel influenza A virus infections
Pertussis
Plague
Poliomyelitis, paralytic
Poliovirus infection, nonparalytic
Psittacosis
Q fever
- Acute
- Chronic
Rabies
- Rabies, animal
- Rabies, human
Rubella (German Measles)
Rubella, congenital syndrome
Salmonellosis
Severe Acute Respiratory Syndrome–
associated Coronavirus (SARS–
CoV) disease
Shiga toxin-producing *Escherichia coli*
(STEC)

Shigellosis
Smallpox
Spotted fever rickettsiosis
Streptococcal toxic-shock syndrome
Streptococcus pneumoniae, invasive
disease
Syphilis
- Primary
- Secondary
- Latent
- Early latent
- Late latent
- Latent, unknown duration
- Neurosyphilis
- Late, non-neurological
- Stillbirth
- Congenital
Tetanus
Toxic-shock syndrome (other than
Streptococcal)
Trichinellosis (Trichinosis)
Tuberculosis
Tularemia
Typhoid fever
Vancomycin-intermediate
Staphylococcus aureus (VISA)
Vancomycin-resistant *Staphylococcus
aureus* (VRSA)
Varicella (morbidity)
Varicella (deaths only)
Vibriosis
Viral hemorrhagic fevers, due to
- Ebola virus
- Marburg virus
- Crimean-Congo hemorrhagic
fever virus
- Lassa virus
- Lujo virus
- New World arenaviruses
(Gunarito, Machupo, Junin and
Sabia viruses)
Yellow fever

Source: CDC 2012.

- Encourage the user to make comparisons

- Reveal data at several levels, from a broad overview to the fine detail

Methods of displaying the data in graphic form are discussed in the following subsections.

Tables

A table is an orderly arrangement of values that groups data into rows and columns. Almost any type of quantitative information can be organized into a table. Tables are useful for demonstrating patterns and other kinds of relationships. In addition, they may serve as the basis for more visual displays of data, such as charts and graphs, where some of the detail may be lost. However, because tables are not very interesting, they should be used sparingly.

A useful first step is to prepare a table shell that shows how the data will be organized and displayed. A *table shell* is the outline of a table with everything in place except for the data. (See table 9.25.) A table should contain all the information the reader needs to understand the data in it. It should have the following characteristics:

- It is a logical unit.

- It is self-explanatory and can stand on its own when photocopied or removed from its context.

- All sources are specified.

- Specific, understandable headings are provided for every column and row.

- Row and column totals are checked for accuracy.

- Blank cells are not left empty. When no information is available for a particular cell, the cell should contain a zero or a dash.

- Categories are mutually exclusive and exhaustive.

The data contained in tables should be aligned. Guidelines for aligning text and numbers include:

- Text in the table should be aligned at left.

- Text that serves as a column label may be centered.

- Numeric values should be aligned at right.

- When numeric values contain decimals, the decimals should be aligned.

The essential components of a table are summarized in figure 9.11.

Tables may contain information on one, two, or three variables. Tables 9.26 and 9.27 are examples of one- and two-variable tables, respectively.

Table 9.25.   **Table shell**

				TITLE					
		Sex						Total	
		Male		Female					
Box Head	Age	Number	%	Number	%			Number	%
Stub	Row Variable	→→→	→→→	→→→	→→→			→→→	→→→
	<45			Column Variable					
↓	45–54			↓					
↓	55–64			↓					
↓	65–74			↓					
↓	75+			↓					

Source: HHS 1994.

Figure 9.11.   **Essential components of a table**

Title	The title should be as complete as possible and should clearly relate to the content of the table. It should answer the following questions: • What are the data (e.g., counts, percentages)? • Who (e.g., white females with breast cancer; black males with lung cancer)? • Where are the data from (e.g., hospital, state, community)? • When (e.g., year, month)? A sample title might be: Site Distribution by Age and Sex of Cancer Patients upon First Admission to Community Hospital, 2010–2012
Box Head	The box head contains the captions or column headings. The heading of each column should contain as few words as possible but should explain exactly what the data in the column represent.
Stub	The row captions are known as the stub. Items in the stub should be grouped to make it easy to interpret the data (e.g., ages grouped into five-year intervals).
Cell	The cell is the box formed by the intersection of a column and a row.
Optional Items:	
Note	Notes are used to explain anything in the table that the reader cannot understand from the title, box head, or stub. They contain numbers, preliminary or revised numbers, or explanations of any unusual numbers. Definitions, abbreviations, and/or qualifications for captions or cell names should be footnoted. A note usually applies to a specific cell(s) within the table, and a symbol (e.g., ** or #) may be used to key the cell to the note. If several notes are used, it is better to use small letters than symbols or numbers. Note any numbers that may be confused with the numbers within the table.
Source	If data are used from a source outside your research, the exact reference to the source should be given. The source lends authenticity to the data and allows the reader to locate the original information if he or she needs it.

Source: HHS 1994.

Table 9.26.   One-variable table, Community Hospital admissions by gender, 20XX

Gender	Number	Percentage
Male	3,141	46.0
Female	3,683	54.0
Total	**6,824**	**100.0**

Table 9.27.   Two-variable table, Community Hospital admissions by race and gender, 20XX

Race	Gender		Total
	Male	Female	
White	2,607	2,946	**5,553**
Non-white	534	737	**1,271**
Total	**3,141**	**3,683**	**6,824**

Charts and Graphs

Charts and graphs of various types are the best means for presenting data for quick visualization of relationships. They emphasize the main points and analyze and clarify relationships among variables.

Several principles are involved in the construction of charts and graphs. When constructing charts and graphs, the following points should be considered:

- *Distortion:* To avoid distorting the data, the representation of the numbers should be proportional to the numerical quantities represented.

- *Proportion and scale:* Graphs should emphasize the horizontal. It is easier for the eye to read along the horizontal axis from left to right. Also, graphs should be greater in length than height. A useful guideline is to follow the three-quarter-high rule. This rule states that the height (*y*-axis) of the graph should be three-fourths the length (*x*-axis) of the graph.

- *Abbreviations:* Any abbreviations should be spelled out in notes.

- *Color:* Color may be used to highlight groupings that appear in the graph.

- *Print:* Both upper- and lowercase letters should be used in titles; the use of all capital letters can be difficult to read.

Bar Charts

Bar charts are used to display data from one or more variables. The bars may be drawn vertically or horizontally. The simplest bar chart is the one-variable bar chart. In this type of chart, a bar represents each category of the variable. For example, if the data figure 9.19 were displayed in a bar chart, "gender" would be the variable and "male and female" would be the variable categories. Bar charts are used for nominal or ordinal variables. Sometimes ratio data that is discrete tend to be represented with bar charts rather than histograms because they are not continuous. Figure 9.12 displays the data from table 9.26 as a bar chart. The length or height of each bar is proportional to the number of males and females admitted. Presentation of the data in a bar chart makes it easy to see that more females than males were admitted to Community Hospital.

Figure 9.13 displays the two-variable data from table 9.27 as a two-variable chart. Computer software makes it easy to create bar graphs. Be careful, though, if you choose to present data in a three-dimensional format. The reader may not always be able to estimate the true height of the bar. In a three-dimensional bar chart, the back edges of the bar appear higher than the front edge. To make sure the reader correctly interprets the chart, the bars should include the actual values for each category.

Figure 9.14 presents guidelines for constructing bar charts.

When constructing a bar chart, keep the following points in mind:

- Arrange the bar categories in a natural order, such as alphabetical order, order by increasing age, or an order that will produce increasing or decreasing bar lengths.

- The bars may be positioned vertically or horizontally.

- The length of the bars should be proportional to the frequency of the event.

Figure 9.12.   One-variable bar chart, Community Hospital admissions by gender, 20XX

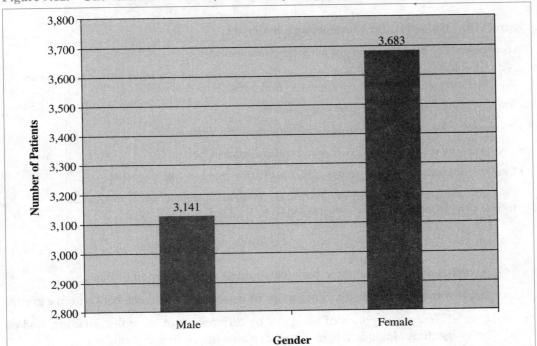

Figure 9.13. **Two-variable bar chart, Community Hospital admissions by race and gender, 20XX**

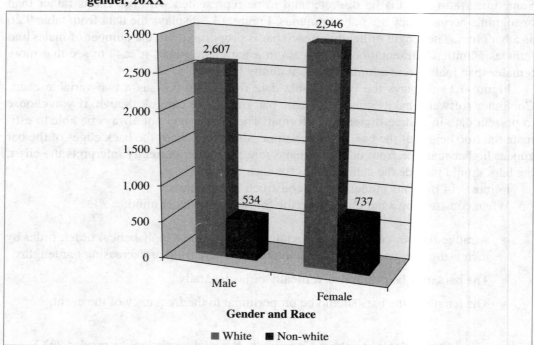

Figure 9.14. **Guidelines for constructing a bar chart**

When constructing a bar chart, keep the following points in mind:

• Arrange the bar categories in a natural order, such as alphabetical order, order by increasing age, or an order that will produce increasing or decreasing bar lengths.

• The bars may be positioned vertically or horizontally.

• The length of the bars should be proportional to the frequency of the event.

• Avoid using more than three bars (categories) within a group of bars.

• Leave a space between adjacent groups of bars, but not between bars within a group.

• Code different categories of variables by differences in bar color, shading, and/or cross-hatching. Include a legend that explains the coding system.

• Avoid using more than three bars (categories) within a group of bars.

• Leave a space between adjacent groups of bars, but not between bars within a group.

• Code different categories of variables by differences in bar color, shading, and/or cross-hatching. Include a legend that explains the coding system.

Pie Charts

A **pie chart** is an easily understood chart in which the sizes of the slices of the pie show the proportional contribution of each part. Pie charts can be used to show the component parts of a single group or variable. Pie charts are intended for interval or ratio data.

To calculate the size of each slice of the pie, first determine the proportion that each slice is to represent. Multiplying the proportion by 360 (the total number of degrees in a circle) will give the size of each slice of the pie in degrees.

Figure 9.15 shows payer data collected on admissions to Community Hospital. The summary data for one year show that managed care was the payer for 39 percent of the patients, Medicare was the payer for 30 percent, Medicaid was the payer for 18 percent, government-managed care was the payer for 8 percent of the patients, and 5 percent of the patients had commercial insurance.

With 39 percent of the pie chart, the managed care category equals approximately 140° (360° × 0.39 = 140°). The Medicare category equals 108° (360° × 0.30 = 108°). The Medicaid category equals 65° (360° × 0.18 = 65°). The government-managed care category equals approximately 29° (360° × 0.08 = 29°). And commercial insurance equals 18° (360° × 0.05 = 18°). Taken together, the slices equal 360° (140° + 108° + 65° + 29° + 18° = 360°).

The slices of the pie should be arranged in some logical order. By convention, the largest slices begin at twelve o'clock. Computer software is available to make the construction of pie charts easy. The pie chart in figure 9.15 was prepared using Excel software.

Line Graphs

A **line graph** may be used to display time trends. A line graph can show trends or patterns of quantitative data over time. The *x*-axis shows the unit of time from left to right, and the *y*-axis measures the values of the variable being plotted. A line graph does not represent a **frequency distribution**.

Figure 9.15.   Pie chart, Community Hospital admissions by payer, 20XX

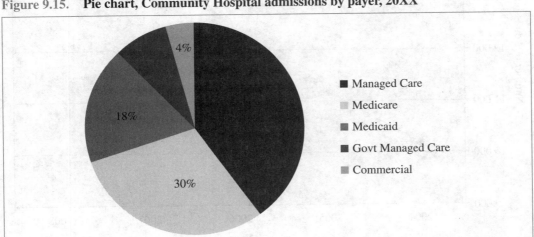

A line graph consists of a line connecting a series of points. Like all graphs, a line graph should be constructed so that it is easy to read. Selection of the proper scale, a complete and accurate title, and an informative legend is important. When a graph is too long and narrow, either vertically or horizontally, it has an awkward appearance and may exaggerate one aspect of the data.

A line graph is especially useful for plotting a large number of observations. It also allows several sets of data to be presented on one graph.

Either actual numbers or percentages may be used on the *y*-axis of the graph. Percentages should be used on the *y*-axis when more than one distribution is to be shown. A percentage distribution allows comparisons among groups where the actual totals are different.

When two or more sets of data are plotted on the same graph, the lines should be made different—solid or broken—for each set. However, the number of lines should be kept to a minimum to avoid confusion. Each line then should be identified in a legend located on the graph.

There are two kinds of time-trend data: point data and period data. Point data reflect an instant in time. Figure 9.16 displays point data—the total number of admissions for each year represented in the graph. Period data are averages or totals over a specified period of time, such as a five-year time frame. Table 9.28 summarizes period data for survival rates of patients diagnosed with kidney cancer at Community Hospital. Figure 9.16 displays these period data in a line graph.

Figure 9.16.   Line graph with point data, Community Hospital admissions, 2004–2008

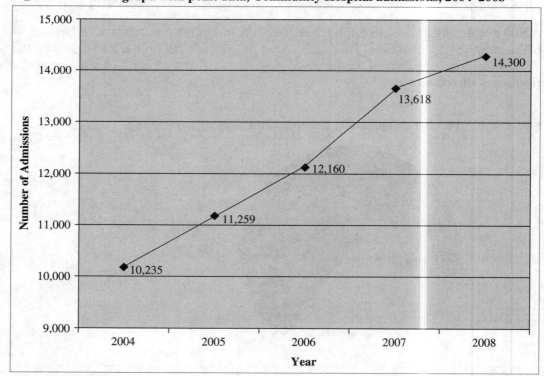

Table 9.28.   **Sample five-year survival rates for kidney cancer by stage, for patients diagnosed between 2003 and 2011**

Year of Diagnosis	Midpoint of Interval	Survival Rate (%)		
		Localized	Regional	Distant
2003–2005	2004	80	71	28
2006–2008	2007	84	74	29
2009–2011	2010	85	74	31

Figure 9.17.   **Period data trend line: survival rates for kidney cancer by stage for patients diagnosed from 2000–2008**

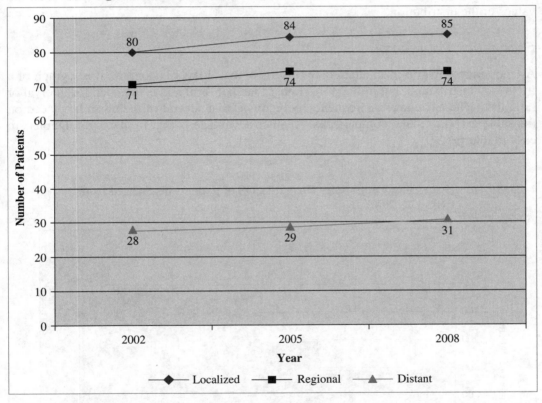

Histograms

A **histogram** is used to display a frequency distribution. It is different from a bar graph in that a bar graph is used to display data that fall into groups or categories (nominal or ordinal data). The categories are noncontinuous, or discrete. In a bar chart, the bars representing the different categories are separated. (Refer to figures 9.12 and 9.13.) On the other hand, histograms are used to illustrate frequency distributions of continuous variables, such as age or LOS. A continuous variable can take on a fractional value (for example,

75.345°F). With continuous variables, there are no gaps between values because the values progress fractionally. Histograms are used for interval or ratio variables.

In a histogram, the frequency distribution may be displayed as a number or a percentage. The histogram consists of a series of bars. Each bar has one class interval as its base and the number (frequency) or percentage of cases in that class interval as its height. A class interval is a type of category. It can represent one value in a frequency distribution (for example, three years of age) or a group of values (for example, ages three to five).

In histograms, there are no spaces between the bars. (See figure 9.18.) The lack of spaces between bars depicts the continuous nature of the distribution. The sum of the heights of the bars represents the total number, or 100 percent, of the cases. Histograms should be used when the distribution of the data needs to be emphasized more than the values of the distribution.

Frequency Polygons

A **frequency polygon** is an alternative to a histogram. Like a histogram, it is a graph of a frequency distribution, but in line form rather than bar form and is intended for interval or ratio data. The advantage of frequency polygons is that several of them can be placed on the same graph to make comparisons. Another advantage is that frequency polygons are easy to interpret.

Figure 9.18.   Histogram, Community Hospital LOS of patients discharged from DRG 127, 20XX

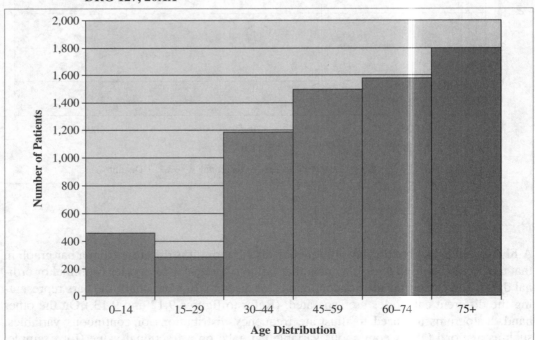

When constructing a frequency polygon, the *x*-axis should be made longer than the *y*-axis to avoid distorting the data. The frequency of observations is always placed on the *y*-axis and the scale of the variable on the *x*-axis. The frequency polygon in figure 9.19 plots the same data that appear in the histogram in figure 9.18. Because the *x*-axis represents the entire frequency distribution, the line starts at zero cases and ends with zero cases.

Scatter Charts

Scatter charts, also called scatter plots or scatter diagrams, are used when one wants to determine if there is a relationship between two variables, such as charges and LOS. Data collected for scatter charts must be at the interval or ratio level of measurement. The data for the two variables are arranged in pairs; one of the two variables is plotted on the *x*-axis and the other variable is plotted on the *y*-axis. The closer the data points come to making a straight line, the stronger the relationship between the two variables. If the data points form a straight line from the lower left of the *x*-axis to the upper right on the *y*-axis, the relationship is positive. (See figure 9.20.) If the line begins at a high value on the *y*-axis and descends to a low value, the relationship is negative. (See figure 9.21.) If the data points are widely scattered, there is no relationship between the two variables. (See figure 9.22.)

Bubble Charts

A **bubble chart** is a type of scatter plot with circular symbols used to compare three variables; the size of the symbol indicates the value of a third variable. In developing the chart,

Figure 9.19.   Frequency polygon, Community Hospital LOS of patients discharged from DRG 127, 20XX

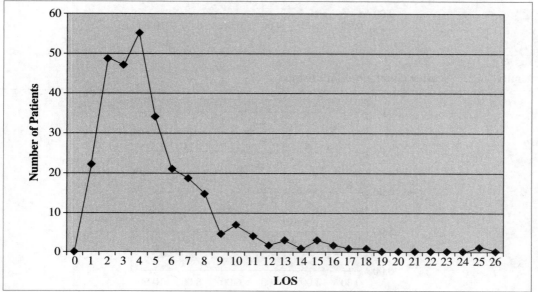

Figure 9.20.   **Scatter chart, positive relationship**

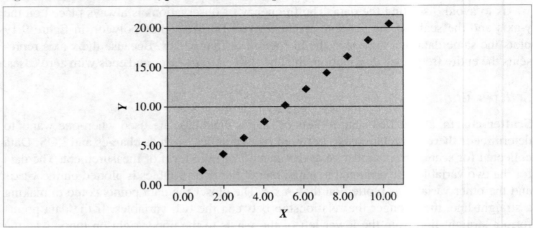

Figure 9.21.   **Scatter chart, negative relationship**

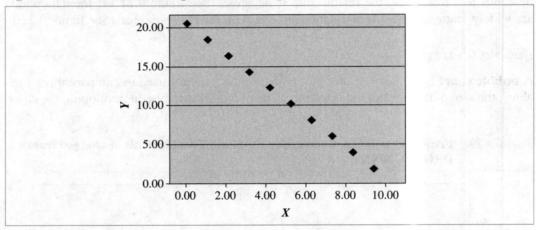

Figure 9.22.   **Scatter chart, no relationship**

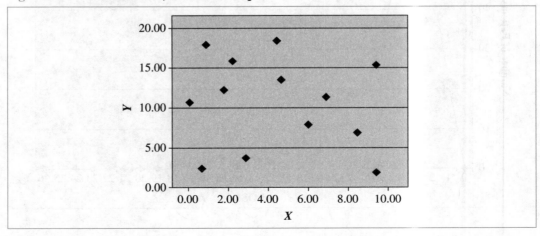

one variable is displayed on the vertical or *y*-axis and on the horizontal or *x*-axis. The size of the bubble is determined by the value of the third variable. Data must be at the interval or ratio-level of measurement.

As an example, an Administrator at Community Hospital is interested in displaying the average charges for the five highest volume MS-DRGs in the organization. The number of discharges will be displayed on the *x*-axis, and average charges will be displayed on the *y*-axis. The size of the bubble indicates the percentage of total discharges for each MS-DRG. The data are displayed in table 9.29, and the corresponding bubble chart is displayed in figure 9.23. It can easily be seen that MS-DRG 795, Normal Newborn, has the highest proportion of overall discharges and the lowest average charges among the top-volume MS-DRGs.

Table 9.29. **Top five high-volume discharges, average charges, and percent of total discharges, Community Hospital, 20XX**

MS-DRG	Number of Discharges	Average Charges	Percent of Total Discharges
795—Normal Newborn	637	$1,239	9.8%
946—Rehabilitation w/o CC/MCC	542	$21,517	8.4%
775—Vaginal Delivery w/o Complicating Diagnoses	505	$5,576	7.8%
293—Heart Failure and Shock w/o CC/MCC	287	$12,043	4.4%
766—Cesarean Section w/o CC/MCC	189	$7,626	2.9%

Figure 9.23. **Bubble chart, top five high-volume discharges, average charges, and percent of total discharges, Community Hospital, 20XX**

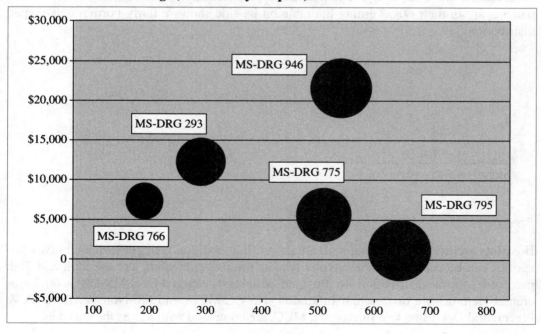

Stem and Leaf Plots

In **stem and leaf plots,** data can be organized so that the shape of a frequency distribution is revealed. As an example, a stem and leaf plot will be constructed on the age of 12 patients discharged from MS-DRG 68, Nonspecific CVA and Precerebral Occlusion w/o Infarct w/o MCC. The ages are ranked in order from lowest to highest:

44   51   52   52   62   65   65   66   68   72   76   82

To develop the plot, break each number into two parts. The last number is called the leaf and the rest of the number is called the stem. Thus, for the number 51, 1 is the leaf and 5 is the stem, and for the number 125, 5 is the leaf and 12 is the stem. The data are then arranged in a table that looks somewhat like a T, with the stem portion in the first column and the leaf portion in the second column. For our data set, the stems are 4, 5, 6, 7 and 8. The leaf portion is then filled in with the last digits that correspond to each stem as shown here:

Stem	Leaf
4	4
5	122
6	25568
7	26
8	2

The completed plot reveals the distribution of the data set. It can immediately be seen that the lowest value in the distribution is 44 and the highest is 82 and that there are five observations in the 60s age group. With this type of display you can quickly see that most patients are in their 60s. Turning the table on its side shows a fairly normal bell-shaped distribution.

```
                8
  L             8
  e             6
  a         2   5
  f         2   5   6
        4   1   2   2   2
  Stem  4   5   6   7   8
```

Boxplots

Boxplots are useful in summarizing a data set. In a boxplot, a single variable in two categories can be compared. The boxplot reveals the range, median, and the 25th and 75th percentiles for the distribution. To illustrate, patients discharged from MS-DRGs 66, Intracranial Hemorrhage or Cerebral Infarction w/o CC/MCC, and 68, Nonspecific CVA & Precerebral Occlusion w/o Infarct w/o MCC, are compared with age as the variable.

The frequency distributions appear in figures 9.24 and 9.25. Twelve patients were discharged from MS-DRG 68 ranging in age from 44 to 82; 38 patients were discharged from MS-DRG 66 ranging in age from 22 to 86. The boxplot, shown in figure 9.26, displays these data side by side. Even though there are more discharges from MS-DRG 66 with a wider range in age, the median age for both MS-DRGs is similar, 62 and 65 respectively. The interquartile range (25th to 75th quartile) for both groups is age 52 to 72 for MS-DRG 66 and age 51 to 73 for MS-DRG 68.

Spreadsheets and Statistical Packages

Electronic spreadsheets, such as Microsoft Excel, and statistical packages, such as SPSS or SAS, can be used to facilitate the data collection and analysis processes. The advantage of using one of these tools is that charts and graphs can be formulated at the time the data are being analyzed. Instruction on the use of these tools is beyond the scope of this chapter; however, they are available on the market and readers are encouraged to learn how to use them.

Figure 9.24. **Frequency distribution for age, MS-DRG 68 Nonspecific CVA and Precerebral Occlusion without Infarct without MCC**

Age		
N	Valid	12
	Missing	0
Median		65.00
Percentiles	25	52.00
	50	65.00
	75	71.00

Age		Frequency	Percent	Valid Percent	Cumulative Percent
Valid	44	1	8.3*	8.3*	8.3*
	51	1	8.3*	8.3*	16.7*
	52	2	16.7*	16.7*	33.3*
	62	1	8.3*	8.3*	41.7*
	65	2	16.7*	16.7*	58.3*
	66	1	8.3*	8.3*	66.7*
	68	1	8.3*	8.3*	75.0*
	72	1	8.3*	8.3*	83.3*
	76	1	8.3*	8.3*	91.7*
	82	1	8.3*	8.3*	100.0*
	Total	12	100.0*	100.0*	

*rounded

Figure 9.25.   Frequency distribution for age, MS-DRG 66 Intracranial Hemorrhage or Cerebral Infarction without CC/MCC

Age			
N	Valid		38
	Missing		0
Median			62.00
Percentiles	25		51.50
	50		62.00
	75		73.50

Age		Frequency	Percent	Valid Percent	Cumulative Percent
Valid	22	1	2.6	2.6	2.6
	23	1	2.6	2.6	5.3
	26	1	2.6	2.6	7.9
	39	1	2.6	2.6	10.5
	44	1	2.6	2.6	13.2
	46	1	2.6	2.6	15.8
	47	1	2.6	2.6	18.4
	49	1	2.6	2.6	21.1
	50	1	2.6	2.6	23.7
	52	1	2.6	2.6	26.3
	55	1	2.6	2.6	28.9
	56	1	2.6	2.6	31.6
	57	3	7.9	7.9	39.5
	58	2	5.3	5.3	44.7
	60	2	5.3	5.3	50.0
	64	1	2.6	2.6	52.6
	68	2	5.3	5.3	57.9
	70	2	5.3	5.3	63.2
	71	2	5.3	5.3	68.4
	72	2	5.3	5.3	73.7
	73	1	2.6	2.6	76.3
	75	1	2.6	2.6	78.9
	76	1	2.6	2.6	81.6
	77	2	5.3	5.3	86.8
	78	1	2.6	2.6	89.5
	83	1	2.6	2.6	92.1
	84	1	2.6	2.6	94.7
	86	2	5.3	5.3	100.0*
	Total	38	100.0*	100.0*	

*rounded

Figure 9.26.   Boxplot of age, MS-DRGs 66 and 68

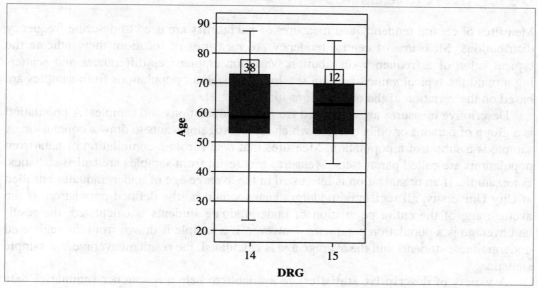

Check Your Understanding 9.12

Instructions: Complete the following sentences on a separate sheet of paper.

1. A presentation of data in rows and columns is a _____.

2. A graphic display technique used to display parts of a whole is a _____.

3. A graphic display technique used to show trends over time is a _____.

4. A graphic display technique used to display categories of a variable is a _____.

5. A graphic display technique that may be used to show the age distribution of a population is a _____.

6. A graphic technique that can visually compare the range of a variable between two categories is a _____.

7. A graphic display that can help one determine if there is a relationship between two variables is a _____.

Descriptive Statistics

Measures of central tendency and measures of **variability** are used to describe frequency distributions. Measures of central tendency are measures of location; they indicate the typical value of a frequency distribution. Variation emphasizes differences and scattering around the typical value of a data set. Inferences about populations from samples are based on the variation of the observations in the data set.

Descriptive measures are computed from both populations and samples. A population is a group of persons or objects about which an investigator wants to draw a conclusion. A sample is a subset of a population. Measures that result from a compilation of data from populations are called parameters. Measures that result from samples are called statistics. For example, if an organization is interested in the average age of undergraduates enrolled at City University, all registered undergraduates would be the defined population. If the average age of the entire population of undergraduate students is calculated, the resultant average is a population parameter. However, if a sample is drawn from the registered undergraduate students and the average age is calculated, the resultant average is a sample statistic.

A variety of **descriptive statistics** are available to help a researcher summarize data for a variable in a frequency distribution. The choice of which descriptive statistics to use is determined, for the most part, by a variable's scale of measurement. Later, the shape of a variable's frequency distribution will be identified as another relevant factor.

Measures of Central Tendency—The Center of a Variable's Values

Measures of central tendency and variability also can be used to describe populations. Measures of central tendency discussed in this subsection are the mean, median, and mode. There are three measures of the center of a distribution of values. The most appropriate center to use can often be determined on the basis of the scale of measurement of the variable considered. Modes are used for nominal-level variables; medians for ordinal-level variables; and means are used for interval and ratio-level variables.

A frequency distribution shows the values that a variable can take and the number of observations associated with each value. For example, using LOS as the variable, five patients were discharged with the following lengths of stay:

Patient	LOS
1	2 days
2	3 days
3	4 days
4	2 days
5	3 days

The data displayed in the table above are referred to as a frequency distribution. A frequency distribution displays the number of times a particular observation occurs for the variable being measured. In this example, the number of times a certain LOS occurs is the variable of interest. The frequency distribution for LOS, in ascending order, is 2, 2, 3, 3, and 4 days.

Frequency distributions may be constructed for both discrete and continuous data. As an example, Community Hospital wants to construct a frequency distribution showing the LOS of patients who were discharged on May 10. LOS is a continuous variable falling on the ratio scale of measurement. The hospital wants to see how many of these patients were in the hospital for a particular LOS (for example, four days). The variable is the LOS, and the frequency is the number of times a particular LOS occurred among the patients discharged on May 10.

To construct the frequency distribution, list all the values that the particular LOS can take, from the lowest observed value to the highest. Then enter the number of times a discharged patient had that particular LOS. Table 9.30 shows a frequency distribution for LOS on May 10. Notice that the frequency distribution lists all the values for LOS between the lowest and the highest, even when there are no observations for some of the values. For

Table 9.30. Calculation of the variance, LOS data

LOS	LOS – Mean (5.8) $(X - \bar{X})$	$(LOS – Mean)^2$ $(X - \bar{X})^2$	LOS	LOS – Mean (5.8) $(X - \bar{X})$	$(LOS – Mean)^2$ $(X - \bar{X})^2$
1	24.8	23.04	6	0.2	0.04
1	24.8	23.04	6	0.2	0.04
2	23.8	14.44	6	0.2	0.04
2	23.8	14.44	6	0.2	0.04
4	21.8	3.24	6	0.2	0.04
4	21.8	3.24	7	1.2	1.44
4	21.8	3.24	7	1.2	1.44
4	21.8	3.24	7	1.2	1.44
4	21.8	3.24	7	1.2	1.44
4	21.8	3.24	7	1.2	1.44
5	20.8	0.64	7	1.2	1.44
5	20.8	0.64	8	2.2	4.84
5	20.8	0.64	8	2.2	4.84
5	20.8	0.64	8	2.2	4.84
5	20.8	0.64	8	2.2	4.84
5	20.8	0.64	8	2.2	4.84
6	0.2	0.04	9	3.2	10.24
6	0.2	0.04	9	3.2	10.24
6	0.2	0.04	9	3.2	10.24
6	0.2	0.04	10	4.2	17.64
6	0.2	0.04	**Total**	**0***	**179.88**
6	0.2	0.04			

*rounded

example, there are no observations of patients spending three days in the hospital. Six patients have LOS of four days. The data in table 9.30 can be used to calculate measures of both central tendency and variability.

Mean

The **mean** is the arithmetic average of a frequency distribution. To calculate a mean, the data must fall on the interval or ratio scales of measurement. The mean is the sum of all scores in a frequency distribution divided by the number of scores. The symbol for the mean is $\overline{X}_i$ (pronounced x-bar). The formula for calculating the mean in a frequency distribution is:

$$\overline{X} = \sum_i^n X_i / N$$

where $\sum$ is summation, $\overline{X}_i$ is each successive observation from the first one in the frequency distribution, $i = 1$, to the last observation (n), and N is the total number of observations.

To calculate the ALOS for the data in table 9.30, substitute the appropriate figures into the following formula:

$$\overline{X} = 5 \sum_i^n X_i / N$$

$$\overline{X} = 1 + 1 + 2 + 2 + 4 + 4 + 4 + 4 + 4 + 4 + 5 + 5 + 5 + 5 + 5 + 5 +$$
$$\frac{6 + 6 + 6 + 6 + 6 + 6 + 6 + 6 + 6 + 6 + 6 + 7 + 7 + 7 + 7 + 7 + 7 +}{8 + 8 + 8 + 8 + 8 + 9 + 9 + 9 + 10}$$
$$42$$

$$\overline{X} = 245/42$$

$$\overline{X} = 5.8$$

The ALOS for patients discharged from Community Hospital on May 10 is 5.8 days (rounded).

Two disadvantages are associated with using the mean as the most typical value in a frequency distribution. First, in this example, the LOS for the 42 patients are integers (whole numbers). However, the ALOS is fractional (5.8), even though there is no fractional LOS. Fractional values are considered more a problem of interpretation than a result that is not meaningful. In this case, the ALOS is interpreted as, "On average, the length of stay for the patients discharged from the Community Hospital on May 10 is between 5 and 6 days."

Second, the mean is sensitive to extreme measures. That is, it is strongly influenced by outliers. For example, if the 10-day LOS were actually a 25-day LOS, the ALOS would increase to 6.2 days.

Thus, the average or arithmetic mean may not always be the most appropriate way to summarize the most typical value of a frequency distribution. The measure of central tendency selected to describe the typical value of a frequency distribution should be based on the characteristics of that particular frequency distribution.

Median

The **median** is the midpoint of a frequency distribution and falls in the ordinal scale of measurement. It is the point at which 50 percent of the observations fall above and 50 percent fall below. If an odd number of observations is in the frequency distribution, the median is the middle number. In the following frequency distribution, the median is 13. Three observations fall above the value of 13, and three fall below it:

10 11 12 **13** 14 15 16

If an even number of observations is in the frequency distribution, the median is the midpoint between the two middle observations. It is found by averaging the two middle scores ($[x + y]/2$). In the following example, the median is 13.5 ($[13 + 14]/2$):

10 11 12 **13** **14** 15 16 17

If the two middle observations take on the same value, the median is that value. When determining the median, it does not matter whether there are duplicate observations in the frequency distribution. Consider the following frequency distribution:

10 11 11 12 **13** **13** 14 15 16 17

In this frequency distribution, the median falls between the fifth and sixth observations. Therefore, the median is 13 ($[13 + 13]/2$).

Table 9.30 records LOS data for 42 patients. In this example, the median falls between the 21st and 22nd observations. Placed in order from lowest to highest, the distribution is as follows:

1 1 2 2 4 4 4 4 4 4 5 5 5 5 5 5 6 6 6 6 6 **6**
6 6 6 6 6 7 7 7 7 7 7 8 8 8 8 8 9 9 9 9 10

The median is 6 ($[6 + 6]/2$).

The median offers the following three advantages:

- Relatively easy to calculate
- Based on the whole distribution and not just a portion of it, as is the case with the mode
- Unlike the mean, it is not influenced by extreme values or unusual outliers in the frequency distribution

Mode

The **mode** is the simplest measure of central tendency. It is used to indicate the most frequent observation in a frequency distribution. The mode offers several advantages, including:

- Easy to obtain and interpret
- Not sensitive to extreme observations in the frequency distribution
- Is easy to communicate and explain to others
- Can be used with nominal-level data

However, there are also disadvantages, including:

- It may not be descriptive of the distribution when the most frequent observation does not occur very often, especially when the number of observations is large.
- It may not be unique. That is, more than one mode may be in a distribution. A frequency distribution may be unimodal, bimodal, or multimodal. When each observation occurs an equal number of times, the distribution does not have a mode.
- It does not provide information about the entire distribution, only the observation that occurs most frequently.

In table 9.30, the mode is 6 because 11 patients had a length of stay of 6 days. To summarize, for the LOS data in table 9.30, the measures of central tendency are similar. The mean is 5.8 days, the median is 6 days, and the mode is 6 days. These statistics are summarized in table 9.31.

Measures of Variability—Spread of a Variable's Values

In addition to measures of central tendency, the hospital can use measures of variability to describe frequency distributions. These measures indicate how widely the observations are spread out around the measures of central tendency. The measures of spread increase with

Table 9.31.   Descriptive statistics for LOS data

N	Valid	42
	Missing	0
Mean		5.8333
Median		6.0000
Mode		6.00
Standard deviation		2.09432
Variance		4.386
Range		9.00
Minimum		1.00
Maximum		10.00

greater variation in the frequency distribution. The spread is equal to zero when there is no variation. The spread of a nominal-level's variable can only be depicted by frequency data. Ordinal-level data may also be displayed as frequencies, but sometimes it may help to calculate a range. Standard deviations and their squared values are used to represent interval and ratio-level data so long as such data are normally distributed; otherwise ranges are used for these kinds of data. This subsection discusses the following measures of spread: the range, the variance, and the standard deviation.

Range

The **range** is the simplest measure of spread. It is the difference between the smallest and largest values in a frequency distribution:

$$Range = X_{max} - X_{min}$$

The range for the LOS data in table 9.30 is 9 (10 − 1 = 9).

One disadvantage of the range is that it can be affected by extreme values, or outliers, in the distribution. Also, the range varies widely from sample to sample. Only the two most extreme observations affect its value, so it is not sensitive to other observations in the distribution.

Two frequency distributions may have the same range but differ greatly in variation. For example, the range for the following frequency distributions is 9 (10 − 1 = 9):

| Distribution 1: | 1 | 2 | 3 | 4 | 5 | 6 | 7 | 8 | 9 | 10 |
| Distribution 2: | 1 | 1.5 | 3 | 3.5 | 3.7 | 7 | 8 | 8.26 | 10 | 10 |

However, when the two distributions are compared, the second distribution has more variation than the first distribution. This is demonstrated when the variance is calculated. The variance for the first distribution is 9.1, and the variance for the second distribution is 11.8.

Variance

The **variance** of a frequency distribution is the average of the squared deviations from the mean. The variance of a sample is symbolized by s^2. The variance of a distribution is larger when the observations are widely spread. The formula for calculating the variance is:

$$s^2 = \frac{\sum (X - \overline{X})^2}{N - 1}$$

The squared deviations of the mean are calculated by subtracting the mean of the frequency distribution from each value in the distribution. The difference between the two values is squared $(X - \overline{X})^2$. The squared differences are summed and divided by $N - 1$. The calculations for the variance for the LOS data are shown in table 9.30.

In the calculations for the variance, the sum of $(X - \overline{X})$ is equal to zero. This is because the mean is the balance point in the distribution. When a value is less than the mean, the difference is negative ($1 - 5.8 = -4.8$); when the value is greater than the mean, the difference is positive ($6 - 5.8 = 0.2$). Therefore, the sum of the differences from the mean is equal to zero. In this example, the sum approximates zero because the actual mean of 5.8333 was rounded to 5.8 for ease in calculation.

The concept of variance is meaningful in more advanced procedures, but in the case of describing the distribution of a single variable, the standard deviation is preferred.

Standard Deviation

The variance for the LOS data in table 9.30 is 4.39, but what does this mean? The interpretation of the variance is not meaningful at the descriptive level because the original units of measure—the lengths of stay—are squared to arrive at the variance. By calculating the square root of the variance, the data are returned to the original units of measurement. This is called the **standard deviation**, which is symbolized by s. The formula for the standard deviation is:

$$s = \sqrt{\frac{\sum (X - \overline{X})}{N - 1}}$$

The standard deviation for the LOS data is 2.1.

The standard deviation is the most widely used measure of variability in descriptive statistics. Because it is easy to interpret, it is the preferred measure of dispersion for frequency distributions. Most handheld calculators include features for calculating the variance and the standard deviation.

The measures of central tendency and variation may be calculated using a handheld calculator. Also, statistical packages such as SPSS are available for performing these and other descriptive and **inferential statistics.** The histograms were prepared using SPSS. The SPSS output for the LOS data appears in table 9.31. The slight differences between the handheld calculator results and the SPSS results in the mean, variance, and standard deviation are because of rounding.

Check Your Understanding 9.13

Instructions: Fifteen infants were born at Community Hospital during the week of December 1. Using a handheld calculator, determine the measures of central tendency and variability for the following infant birth weights (in grams):

2,450	2,750	2,600
2,540	2,815	2,540
2,300	1,735	1,720
2,715	1,800	2,780
2,400	2,485	2,640

1. ____ Mean

2. ____ Median

3. ____ Mode

4. ____ Range

5. ____ Variance

6. ____ Standard deviation

Table 9.32.   Check Your Understanding 9.13

A	B	C	C^2
Weight	Mean	Weight – Mean	
2,450	2,418	32	1024
2,540	2,418	122	14,884
2,300	2,418	–118	13,924
2,715	2,418	297	88,209
2,400	2,418	–18	324
2,750	2,418	332	110,224
2,815	2,418	397	157,609
1,735	2,418	–683	466,489
1,800	2,418	–618	381,924
2,485	2,418	67	4,489
2,600	2,418	182	33,124
2,540	2,418	122	14,884
1,720	2,418	–698	487,204
2,780	2,418	362	131,044
2,640	2,418	222	49,284

Sum of C^2 = 1,954,640

1,954,640/14 = 139,617.1

Use your calculator ($\sqrt{}$ key) or function key if students complete this in a spreadsheet to determine the standard deviation.

$\sqrt{}$ = 373.65371

Normal Distribution

The **normal distribution** is actually a theoretical family of distributions that may have any mean or any standard deviation. It is bell-shaped and symmetrical about the mean. Because it is symmetrical, 50 percent of the observations fall above the mean and 50 percent fall below it. In a normal distribution, the mean, median, and mode are equal.

In the normal distribution, the standard deviation indicates how many observations fall within a certain range of the mean. The areas under the curve corresponding to one, two, and three standard deviations are 68.3 percent, 95.4 percent, and 99.7 percent.

Figure 9.27 shows an example of a normal distribution superimposed on a histogram. The center of the distribution, or mean, is 6. (The median and the mode also are 6.) The standard deviation is 2.45. This means that 68 percent of the observations in the frequency distribution fall within 2.45 standard deviations of 6 (6 ± 2.45). Thus, 68 percent fall between 3.55 and 8.45; 95 percent fall between 1.1 and 10.9; and 99.7 percent fall between 21.35 and 13.35.

As shown in figure 9.27, a characteristic of the normal distribution is that each tail of the curve approaches the *x*-axis but never touches it, no matter how far from center the line is.

A histogram of the frequency distribution for the LOS data in table 9.31 is shown in figure 9.28. The distribution is more peaked than the normal distribution and so is considered kurtotic. *Kurtosis* is the vertical stretching of a distribution.

Figure 9.27.   Histogram of normal distribution

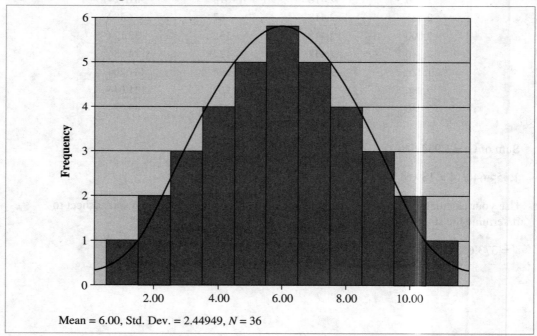

Mean = 6.00, Std. Dev. = 2.44949, *N* = 36

Figure 9.28.   **Histogram of LOS with superimposed normal curve**

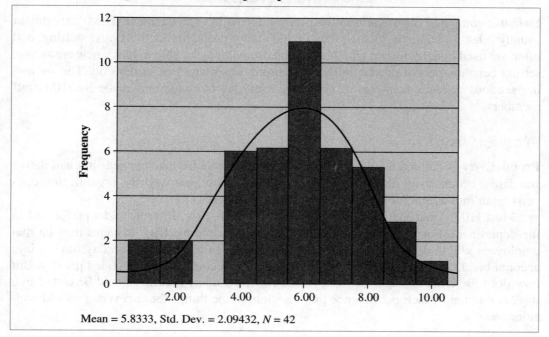

Mean = 5.8333, Std. Dev. = 2.09432, *N* = 42

A skewed distribution is asymmetrical. Skewness is the horizontal stretching of a frequency distribution to one side or the other so that one tail is longer than the other. The longer tail has more observations. Because the mean is sensitive to extreme observations, it moves in the direction of the long tail when a distribution is skewed. When the direction of the tail is off to the right, the distribution is positively skewed, or skewed to the right. When the direction of the tail is off to the left, the distribution is negatively skewed, or skewed to the left. When the mean and the median approximate one another (as with the LOS data), the distribution is not significantly skewed. A perfect normal distribution has a zero skew. If an interval or ratio-level distribution is skewed, the median may be more appropriate than the mean in representing the center of such a distribution.

Check Your Understanding 9.14

Instructions: Answer the following questions on a separate piece of paper.

1. What are the characteristics of a normal distribution?

2. What is the definition of the term *skewness*?

3. What is kurtosis?

Health Information Management Statistics

Statistics computed for use within the health information management (HIM) department usually relate to budgeting which may include labor costs, productivity, and staffing, and often are used in determining whether the department may be able to hire a new employee, setting benchmarks for productivity, determining absentee rates, and so on. The following sections provide examples of common, everyday computations made by HIM staff members.

Productivity

Productivity is defined as a unit of performance defined by management in quantitative standards. Productivity allows organizations to measure how well the organization converts input into output, or labor into a product or service.

Most HIM departments have productivity standards for different tasks performed in the department. For example, in the coding section, a productivity standard may be that employees will code four inpatient records per hour. In a 7.5 hour workday (taking into account breaks the employee will take), 30 inpatient records would be coded per day. But how does the HIM manager or supervisor know how many records should be coded in a day? A number of factors influence this decision. Some things the supervisor should consider are:

- Does the coder do anything in addition to coding, such as abstracting, answering the phone, or obtaining additional information about the diagnoses and procedures?
- What kinds of records is the coder coding? Are they long lengths of stay or short? Are they complex cases or relatively simple cases to code?

There are two simple formulas that accurately calculate labor productivity (Miller and Waterstraat 2004) shown here as formulas 9.33 and 9.34:

Formula 9.33. Calculation of completed work

Completed work = Total work output − Defective work

---

and

Formula 9.34. Calculation of labor productivity

$$\text{Labor productivity} = \frac{\text{Completed work}}{\text{Hours worked to produce total work output}}$$

Determining the total work output and the hours worked is clear; however, determining the defective work involves auditing the work to determine if any work is defective.

Three ways are described to audit employees' work output. First, the manager could perform a review of all the work performed; second, the manager could perform a review of work chosen through a random sample; or third, the manager could use a fixed-percent random sample audit. The last suggestion is the easiest. This method requires the manager to select a fixed percent of total work for each employee to review. The manager also has a predetermined quality standard in mind and then reviews the work and classifies it as completed work or defective work. Additional work could be reviewed if more information is needed to determine the type of defect or until all the work has been reviewed.

Table 9.33 shows the calculation for determining inpatient coding productivity for one month.

Notice in table 9.33 that Coder D's average work output is 4.69 records per hour (work output/total hours worked = 375/80 = 4.69. However, after auditing the work, it was determined that 240 of those records were coded accurately (completed work output). Coder D's completed work is really 3.00 (240/80 = 3.00).

Staffing Levels

Healthcare organizations use a variety of methods to determine appropriate **staffing levels.** For example, many outpatient facilities use patient encounters per **full-time equivalent employee** (FTE) per month. A patient encounter is any personal contact between a patient and a physician or other person authorized to furnish healthcare services for the diagnosis or treatment of the patient. These may include laboratory services, x-ray services, physical therapy, and other ancillary services.

Table 9.33.   Inpatient coding productivity calculation for one month

Coder	Work Output (all records coded)	Total Hours Worked	Average Work Output per Hour	Completed Work Percentage	Completed Work Output (records coded accurately)	Completed Work per Hours Worked
A	500	140	3.57	91%	455	3.25
B	475	140	3.39	96%	456	3.26
C	300	80	3.75	96%	240	3.00
D	375	80	4.69	64%	240	3.00
Department Average			**3.69**			**3.13**

Work Output: number of work units as recorded by the employee or the process
Total Hours Worked: number of hours worked by the employee to produce work, which does not include time on meals, breaks, and meetings
Average Work Output per Hour: work output divided by total hours worked
Completed Work Percentage: percentage of completed work from audit
Completed Work Output: work output multiplied by completed work percentage
Completed Work per Hours Worked: completed work output divided by total hours worked

The staffing level is determined by dividing the number of patient encounters by the expected productivity. An FTE is the total number of workers, including part-time, in an area as the equivalent of full-time positions. The number of FTEs does not always equal the actual number of employees because two or more part-time employees might equal one FTE.

Formula 9.35. Calculating the staffing level

$$\text{Number of FTEs needed} = \frac{\text{Patient encounters}}{\text{Productivity}}$$

For example, the ten physicians in a physician clinic see 250 patient encounters per day. A coder is expected to code 100 records per day. To determine the number of coders needed, divide 250 by 100. Thus, two and a half coders are needed to perform the coding for the physician clinic each day (250/100 = 2.5 FTEs). When computing the FTE, managers are ordinarily instructed to not round up or down. The reason is that managers must justify the need for any employees. For example, in our example above, the administration may only want to approve a person working 50 percent time (0.5 FTE) if a full-time employee is not needed to perform the work.

Hospital HIM departments often use discharges as their method to determine staff levels. For example, to determine the number of employees needed in a coding section, the health information manager first multiplies the average number of inpatient records coded per hour (let us use the example of six records per hour) by the number of productive hours in the workday (7.5), which amounts to 45 records coded per day. If Community Hospital discharges numbered approximately 50 inpatients per day, the manager would then calculate that she needed 1.1 FTEs to accomplish the coding task (50/45 = 1.1 FTEs). In this example, the manager would need one full-time employee plus one 0.1 FTE, which is computed as 40 hours per week multiplied by 0.1. Thus, she would need another employee to work four hours per week to handle the workload. In this example we also determined the productive hours in the workday to be 7.5, taking into consideration any breaks that the employee would take.

Here is another way to determine the number of employees needed. Determine how many minutes and hours it would take to perform all the work, then divide by the number of productive hours. For example, an HIM Director would like to know how many FTEs are needed to analyze the weekly discharges in her facility. There are 275 discharges per week. Timing the records analysts, she determines that it takes one employee 15 minutes to analyze one record, and using a productive week as 37.5 (7.5 x 5 days in the work week) hours, the Director determines that she will need 1.8 FTEs to analyze the weekly discharges (15 minutes x 275 records = 4,125 minutes; 4,125 minutes / 60 minutes (in one hour) = 68.75 hours; 68.75 hours / 37.5 productive hours = 1.8 FTEs).

Check Your Understanding 9.15

1. An HIM manager must determine the number of FTEs needed to code 400 discharges per week. It has been determined that it takes 25 minutes to code each record. Each coder works 37.5 productive hours per week. Round to one digit after the decimal.

2. A full-time scanning specialist was just hired in your HIM department at $10.23 per hour. What is the employee's annual salary?

How to Analyze Information

As health information management professionals we are able to access much patient information. The information in a health care facility is vital to the health and future of that facility. Because of the quantity of the information, we need to know how to use the information to our best advantage. It is not the amount of information that will help administrators make decisions but the knowledge within that information that is important.

We make decisions everyday based on the information we have. For example, if you receive a failing grade on a test, you know you must study harder to receive a passing grade in a class. Personal decisions we make have a powerful effect on our lives. If you receive that failing grade and do not study harder, you may not pass your classes and be forced to leave school thereby not fulfilling your dreams. Just as personal decisions have an impact on us, professional decisions can affect a health care facility. If a hospital Board of Directors decides not to take into consideration changes in payment methodologies for its patients, there could be widespread ramifications. So, just how can we analyze information?

In his book *How to Analyze Information* (2010), Herbert Meyer suggests that there is a seven-step process that will help someone do the best he or she can with the information available:

- First, figure out where you are. You will need to know where your business is currently in order to make decisions about it. You do not need all the detail in this step, but having a good idea how your business is doing will allow you to move forward.

- Second, be sure you are seeing clearly. You need to have a generally accurate idea of the issues at hand.

- Third, decide what you need to decide. In this step you need to be certain that you are asking the right questions. What is it you are really trying to accomplish?

- Next, determine what you need to know. Make a list of the information you need in order to make a decision. Take your time; list everything and if you miss something you discover later on, just go back to this step and add it to the list.

- Fifth, collect the information. But, first ask yourself, what is the most reliable source for the information? Go to the best source you know. This may include checking all your indices, or interviewing individuals. Get all the information you can.

- Next, turn the information into knowledge. After you have collected the information, turn it into facts and keep an eye out for any patterns that may occur. When facts and patterns are determined, the information becomes knowledge.

- Finally, add your own judgment. Your judgment is made up of the knowledge you gleaned from the information you gathered and you—your character, your personality, and your instincts. You can see from this last step that faced with the same knowledge, two people may make entirely different decisions.

The effect of the decisions made through the analysis of data is enormous and can affect the viability of the facility.

Real-World Case

The Performance Improvement Committee of Community Regional Medical Center wanted to study MS-DRG 689 kidney and urinary tract infections w/MCC, because of wide variations in LOS and total charges. The committee asked the HIM director to prepare a profile of patients discharged from MS-DRG 689. A summary of the patients discharged from MS-DRG 689 at Community Hospital was prepared using information found in the hospital's online database.

Real-World Case Discussion Questions

Instructions: Answer the questions using the following information.

A summary of the patients discharged from MS-DRG 689 at Community Hospital is presented in Table 9.34.

The committee also had specific questions regarding DRG MS-689, as follows.

1. What was the average length of stay?

2. What was the modal length of stay?

3. What was the median length of stay?

4. What were the variance and the standard deviation?

Table 9.34.   **Data for real-world case discussion**

Case	Principal Diagnosis	Principal Procedure	Age	LOS	Discharge Destination	Charges	Payer
1	599.0	38.93	53.5	4	HOMEIV	$8,851	MEDICAID
2	599.0	45.13	28.2	7	HOMEHEALTH	$18,966	MEDICARE
3	590.8		45.5	3	HOME	$4,370	MANAGED CARE
4	590.8	86.27	27.9	3	HOMEHEALTH	$7,121	GOV MNGD CARE
5	590.8		38.8	3	HOME	$13,350	MEDICAID
6	590.8	45.23	67.1	4	HOME	$15,854	MANAGED CARE
7	599.0	39.95	88.5	6	SNF	$22,373	MEDICARE
8	599.0		27.8	6	HOMEHEALTH	$11,381	GOV MNGD CARE
9	590.1		52.6	2	HOME	$4,082	MEDICAID
10	599.0		81.9	6	HOMEHEALTH	$17,025	MEDICARE
11	590.8		23.3	3	HOME	$5,039	MEDICAID
12	599.0	43.11	90.1	5	HOMEHEALTH	$17,411	MEDICARE
13	599.0	99.6	91.3	1	UNKNOWN	$5,302	MEDICARE
14	599.0	88.72	73.1	4	HOME	$11,091	MEDICARE
15	599.0		81.3	12	SNF	$23,341	MEDICARE
16	590.8	45.16	74.7	4	HOMEHEALTH	$16,277	MEDICARE
17	599.0		71.2	5	HOMEHEALTH	$9,239	MEDICARE
18	599.0		79.3	7	SNF	$21,050	MEDICARE
19	590.1		31.3	4	HOME	$7,085	GOV MNGD CARE
20	590.8	38.93	74.1	13	ACUTECARE	$49,487	MEDICAID
21	599.0		65.7	2	HOMEHEALTH	$8,980	MEDICARE
22	599.0	86.27	83.1	5	SNF	$11,651	MEDICARE
23	599.0		77.0	5	SNF	$12,295	MEDICARE
24	599.0	99.04	81.2	7	HOMEHEALTH	$23,745	MEDICARE
25	599.0		43.3	10	HOMEHEALTH	$25,130	MEDICARE
26	599.0		81.5	3	SNF	$10,092	MEDICARE
27	599.0	38.93	25.6	3	HOMEIV	$8,722	MEDICAID
28	599.0		61.4	2	SNF	$6,670	MEDICAID
29	599.0	45.13	76.0	8	SNF	$17,741	GOV MNGD CARE
30	590.1		44.4	4	HOME	$10,800	MANAGED CARE
31	590.8		44.8	2	HOME	$10,916	MEDICAID
32	599.0	45.13	61.2	8	SNF	$32,796	MEDICARE

5. What was the average gross charge?

6. What was the average age?

7. What was the average age of patients discharged to skilled nursing facilities?

8. What was the average age of patients discharged home?

Table 9.35.   Variance and the standard deviation

N	Valid	32
	Missing	0
Mean		5.03
Median		4.00
Mode		3(a)
Standard deviation		2.857
Variance		8.160

Multiple modes exist. The smallest value is shown.

Table 9.36.   Average gross charge

N	Valid	32
	Missing	0
Mean		$14,632.16
Median		$11,516.02
Mode		$4,082(a)
Standard deviation		$9,420.543
Variance		88746626.260

Multiple modes exist. The smallest value is shown.

Table 9.37.   Average age of patients discharged home

Discharge Destination	Mean	N	Std. Deviation
ACUTECARE	74.120	1	.
HOME	46.744	9	15.8207
HOMEHEALTH	59.200	10	24.8415
HOMEIV	39.545	2	19.7071
SNF	76.577	9	9.3806
UNKNOWN	91.250	1	.
Total	**60.823**	**32**	**21.7763**

9. Prepare two boxplots comparing:
   a. Charges by payer
   b. LOS by payer

Table 9.38.   **Charges by payer**

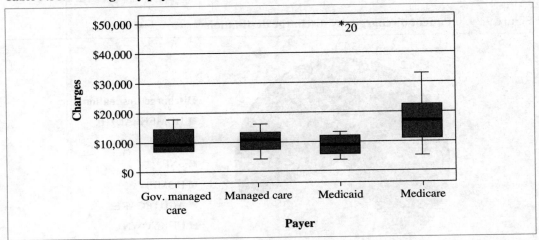

Table 9.39.   **Length by stay of payer**

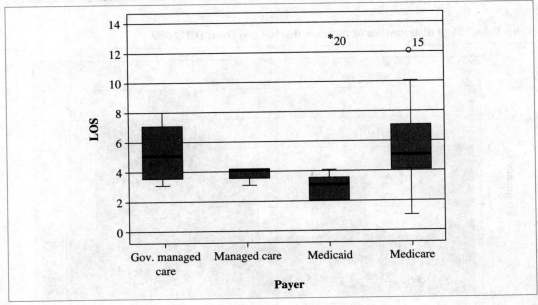

10. Calculate the statistics requested by the Performance Improvement Committee.

   a. Prepare a pie chart showing patient discharges by discharge destination.
   b. Prepare a histogram of the age distribution of patients discharged from DRG 689.
   c. Prepare a bar graph of the principal diagnosis codes.
   d. Discuss the results of your analysis with classmates.

Figure 9.29.   Patient discharges by discharge destination

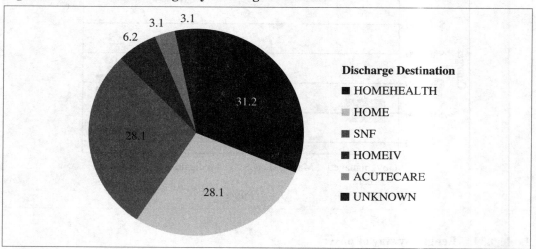

Table 9.40.   Age distribution of patients discharged from DRG 689

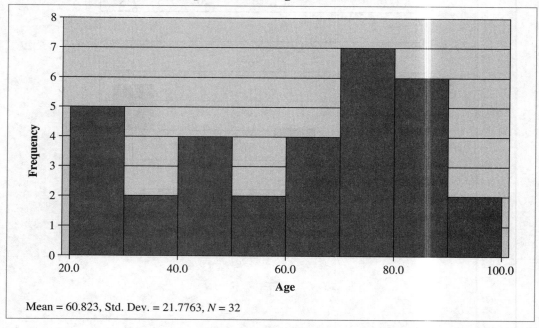

Mean = 60.823, Std. Dev. = 21.7763, *N* = 32

Table 9.41.   Patients by principle diagnosis codes

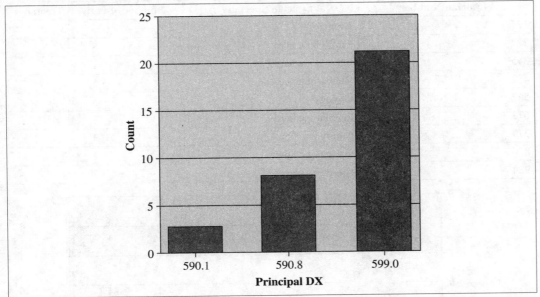

11. After the committee meeting, the members also wanted to know information about the
     physicians treating these patients (see table 9.42).

     a. Using the additional information prepared by the Performance Improvement
         Department prepare a bar graph of the physicians.
     b. Prepare a pie chart showing the specialties of these physicians.

Summary

The nominal, ordinal, interval, and ratio scales of measurement are discussed in this chapter. In nominal measures, names are given to objects or categories. Nominal data's measure of central tendency is the mode. Examples of nominal data include gender, marital status, health insurance type, race, and place of residence. In ordinal data the numbers given to categories represent rank order. The central tendency of ordinal data can be represented by its mode or its median. Examples of ordinal data include patient health status (that is, critical, stable, good) or opinion scales (strongly agree to strongly disagree). The most important characteristic of interval-level data is that the intervals between successive values are equal. Examples include temperature or years. The central tendency of a variable measured at the interval level can be represented by its mode, median, or mean. Ratio-level data is the highest level of measurement. On the ratio scale there is a defined unit of measure, a real zero point, and the intervals between successive values are equal.

Table 9.42. **Information about physicians treating these patients**

Physician Number	Physician Specialty	Number of Patients Treated
127	Urology	3
222	Family practice	8
345	Internal medicine	2
452	Family practice	5
567	Urology	3
673	Internal medicine	3
779	Family practice	3
856	Internal medicine	2
984	Urology	3

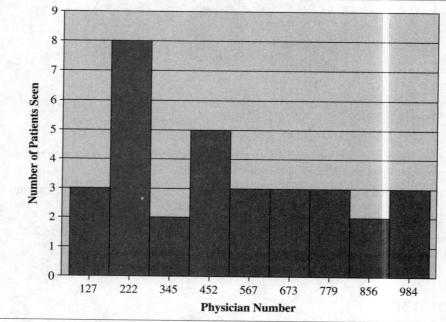

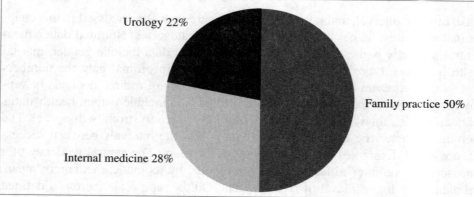

Rates, ratios, proportions, and statistics are commonly used to describe community and hospital populations. They are considered to be descriptive statistics because they portray the characteristics of a group or population. Public health officials use community-based rates, ratios, and proportions to evaluate the general health status of a community. Morbidity and mortality rates are used as indicators of the accessibility and availability of healthcare services in a community.

Hospital-based rates are used for a variety of purposes. First, they describe the general characteristics of the patients treated at the facility. Hospital administrators use the data to monitor the volume of patients treated monthly, weekly, or within some other specified time frame. The statistics give healthcare decision makers the information they need to plan facilities and to monitor inpatient and outpatient revenue streams.

Graphic techniques are often used to summarize and clarify data. Data may be displayed in a variety of ways, for example, as charts, graphs, and tables. Graphic forms are effective ways to present large quantities of information.

Health information management professionals are often in management or supervisory positions, and, as such, must be familiar with methods to determine the statistics having to do with budgets including productivity, staffing, salary, payback period, and return on investment.

Analysis of data is a seven-step process that can assist health information professionals in learning how to think about the data presented and allow them to help the facility's administration in their decision-making processes.

The health information management professional is in a position to serve as a data broker for the healthcare organization. To do this, he or she must fully understand the clinical data that are collected and their application to the decision-making process. In addition, he or she must know what information is needed and how to provide it in a timely manner. With this knowledge, the HIM professional can become an invaluable member of the healthcare team.

References

Agency for Health Care Policy and Research. 2000. HCUPnet: Healthcare cost and utilization project. Rockville, MD: AHRQ. http://www.hcup-us.ahrq.gov/overview.jsp

American Health Information Management Association. 2012. *Pocket Glossary of Health Information Management and Technology,* 3rd ed. Chicago: AHIMA.

Centers for Disease Control and Prevention. 2011. National Center for Health Statistics. 2003 Revisions of the U.S. Standard Certificates of Live Birth and Death and the Fetal Death Report. http://www.cdc.gov/nchs/nvss/vital_certificate_revisions.htm

Centers for Disease Control and Prevention. 2012. CDC Wonder Data Base. http://wonder.cdc.gov

Department of Health and Human Services, Public Health Service. 1994. *Self-Instructional Manual for Tumor Registrars, Book 7: Statistics and Epidemiology for Cancer Registries.* NIH Publication No. 94-3766. Washington, DC: HHS. http://seer.cancer.gov/training/manuals/Book7.pdf

Meyer, H.E. 2010. *How to Analyze Information.* Friday Harbor, WA: Storm King Press.

Miller, P.J., and F.L. Waterstraat. 2004. Apples to apples: Using autobenchmarking to measure productivity. *Journal of AHIMA* 75(1):44–49.

National Vital Statistics System. 2011. Revisions of the U.S. Standard Certificates of Live Birth and Death and the Fetal Death Report. http://www.cdc.gov/nchs/nvss/vital_certificate_revisions.htm

Osborn, C.E. 2005. *Statistical Applications for Health Information Management.* Sudbury, MA: Jones and Bartlett.

Additional Resources

Agency for Healthcare Research and Quality. 2010. AHRQ Profile: Quality research for quality healthcare. AHRQ publication no. 00-P005. Rockville, MD: AHRQ. http://ahrq.gov/about/profile.htm

Centers for Disease Control and Prevention. 2010. National Vital Statistics Report. Deaths: Final Data for 2007. Volume 58. No.19.

Centers for Disease Control and Prevention. 2011. National Center for Health Statistics. Handbook on the Reporting of Induced Termination of Pregnancy. www.cdc.gov/nchs/data/misc/hb_itop.pdf

Centers for Disease Control and Prevention. 2012. Division of Public Health Surveillance and Informatics. Nationally notifiable infectious diseases. United States,. http://www.cdc.gov/osels/ph_surveillance/nndss/phs/infdis.htm

chapter 10

Clinical Quality Performance Improvement and Management

Chris R. Elliott, MS, RHIA

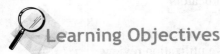

Learning Objectives

- Explain performance improvement (PI) principles
- Discuss various PI tools and techniques used to facilitate communication, identify root causes, and collect, analyze, and report data
- Describe team-based performance improvement processes
- Summarize the concept of quality and its importance in healthcare
- Summarize the importance of patient safety and national patient safety goals
- Define and differentiate between the terms clinical quality assessment, infection control, utilization management, case management, and risk management
- Explain the elements of a quality assessment (QA) program
- Identify major organizations that publish clinical quality standards and guidelines
- Explain common ways that healthcare organizations manage the prevention and occurrence of infections
- Understand the Medicare requirements for utilization management (UM)
- List the basic procedures in the utilization review (UR) process
- Explain the clinical and administrative use of UM information
- Understand the use of severity-of-illness and intensity-of-service screening criteria

Key Terms

Accountable Care Organization (ACO)
Admission utilization review
Affinity grouping
Agency for Healthcare Research and
    Quality (AHRQ)
Bar graph
Benchmark
Brainstorming
Case management
Cause-and-effect diagram
Checksheet
Claims management
Clinical practice guidelines
Clinical protocols
Common-cause variation
Continued-stay (or concurrent) utilization
    review
Continuous improvement
Customer
Dashboards
Data abstracts
Discharge abstract system
Discharge planning
Discharge utilization review
External customers
Financial indicators
Fishbone diagram
Flowcharts
Force-field analysis
Ground rules
Health Care Quality Improvement
    Program (HCQIP)
Histogram
Incident/occurrence report
Inputs
Intensity-of-service screening criteria
Internal customers
ISO 9000 certification

The Joint Commission
Mission
Multivoting technique
National patient safety goals (NPSGs)
Nominal group technique
Opportunity for improvement
Outcome indicators
Outcome measures
Outputs
Pareto chart
Patient advocacy
Performance improvement (PI)
Performance indicators
Potentially compensable event
Preadmission utilization review
Process indicators
Processes
Productivity indicators
Prospective utilization review
Quality indicators
Retrospective utilization review
Risk
Risk management program
Root-cause analysis
Run chart
Scatter diagrams
Scorecards
Severity-of-illness screening criteria
Six Sigma
Special-cause variation
Standard
Statistical process control chart
Structure indicators
Structured brainstorming
Time ladders
Unstructured brainstorming method
Utilization review (UR)
Virtuoso teams

Introduction

The concept of "better" is a mainstay of American life. American people expect that the quality of their lives and the lives of their offspring will become better, that is, improve, over the course of their lifetimes. And it is the pursuit of the better life that has driven the development of most everything we Americans involve ourselves in as a society: development of our educational systems, the conformation of our political processes, our personal and family habits of product consumption, our innovation of new products and services to send out to the world, and, most importantly for this text, our expectations of our interactions with the US healthcare delivery system. If we go to a doctor we expect to get better. If we receive services from one of the myriad of healthcare organizations available in this country today, we expect the experience to be as comfortable as possible and the end results of the services to be beneficial. Are our expectations always fulfilled? We all know that is not the case. Especially today, we know from the recent and continuing public debate about healthcare access, eligibility, and economics that that is not the case. However, all members of our society still have huge expectations that we and those close to us will be better off with respect to our personal and collective health in the future. We have huge expectations that the quality of the services provided by our healthcare system will be the best that they can possibly be.

Those who provide healthcare services in the United States also have expectations of themselves and by and large always have had. Caregivers were concerned about the quality of care they provided to people even in ancient times. Around the 5th century BCE, for example, the Greek physician Hippocrates advised young physicians to "First, do no harm." That directive is still part of the physician's oath today. Throughout the history of medicine, providers have had benefit to their patients and clients at the heart of their desire to practice and by and large still do so today. As scientific inquiry advanced in its process, healthcare providers were interested in improving the outcomes of patient care. Florence Nightingale, for instance, is considered to have been the founder of modern nursing in the mid-19th century. She advocated the use of a uniform scientific method of collecting and evaluating statistics that compared mortality rates among hospitals. The results of her measurement efforts showed wide variation among hospitals in their respective rates. So, she implemented sanitary procedures such as simple hand-washing that greatly improved the results or outcomes of hospital care. Over and over in this history we can find individuals involved in the provision of healthcare services making minor as well as major improvements in the way the services are provided including those involved in the healthcare delivery system today. But today, everyone involved must be willing to help.

Debate regarding issues apparent in our healthcare delivery system from the access, eligibility, and economic perspectives has made us recognize the webs of complexity of the system. Even before this recent debate, the healthcare system had recognized in the late 20th century that it had significant issues around the quality of its processes and results. It also recognized that everyone who worked in the system potentially affected that quality. Obviously, individuals who actually interact with and assist patients can affect healthcare quality. But because of the complexity of the system, individuals who basically have little to no contact with the patient can impact the perceptions of patients regarding their healthcare and whether the experience was better or worse than expectations. This recognition now becomes the reason why this chapter must be undertaken in this textbook. You, the developing health information technician, along with all of your colleagues in health professions programs and practicing nurses, doctors, and therapists in healthcare organizations in the country, make contributions to the perceptions of the quality of healthcare services with which patients come away from the healthcare system every day.

The principal concepts that you will be exploring in this chapter are that patients and clients (also known as *customers*) have perceptions and expectations (also known as *values*) with respect to the healthcare services (also known as the *product*) that they receive from the healthcare system in all its complexity (also known as the ***processes***). The results of their use of the products and processes are known as *outcomes*. The level at which healthcare products, processes, and outcomes meet the values of customers when measured scientifically is the basic definition of *quality* in the United States today.

Theory into Practice

Physicians and surgeons as well as nurses and quality managers continuously assess the quality of the clinical services they provide in healthcare organizations. They also continuously search for ways to improve it. The data collected during the process of providing patient services are the best source of information on the effectiveness of care.

One cardiovascular surgery department at a large Midwestern university hospital identified a potential problem with its program. The department's medical staff noted that many of the patients who had undergone percutaneous transluminal coronary angioplasty (PTCA) in the facility subsequently needed emergency open-heart surgery. Over a period of five years, the hospital's rate of post-PTCA coronary artery bypass graft (CABG) surgery was significantly higher than the national average.

An interdisciplinary team was convened to study the problem. Its members searched the clinical literature on the subject. Based on their research, the team decided to investigate the following factors in relation to the long-term success rate for PTCAs:

- Whether a stent had been placed during the original PTCA procedure

- The patient's age, gender, and comorbidities (unstable angina, severe angina, past myocardial infarction, left ventricular function, number of vessels involved, and diabetes)

- The surgeon's age and gender

- The number of PTCAs performed each year by each surgeon

The study team wanted to perform a statistical analysis of these key factors to determine the root causes of the facility's high rate of emergency surgery after PTCA procedures. The team's leader contacted the director of the health information management (HIM) department and asked for information from the department's databases and the health records of former patients. In addition, the team leader asked the hospital's risk manager to compile information on the surgeons who had performed PTCAs in the facility over the past five years.

The study team was able to answer some of its questions by looking at relevant coded data abstracted from the patients' medical records and input into the hospital's **discharge abstract system.** The team also obtained some interesting insights by analyzing the documentation in the health records of all the patients who had undergone a PTCA in the facility over the past five years or had undergone a PTCA and subsequent emergency CABG surgery. In addition, the HIM director was able to direct the study team to additional sources of clinical guidelines and protocols for PTCA and CABG procedures.

By analyzing and comparing all this information, the study team determined that most of the variance from national success rates was based on a higher-than-average level of comorbidity in the hospital's patient base. However, the team also found that the PTCA success rate was affected by the surgeon's level of experience. The surgeons who performed the most PTCA procedures had the highest success rates.

Performance Measurement and Quality Improvement

Probably the most important concept in the introductory discussion of quality is that of measurement. Over the decades of attempting to deal with the issues involved in healthcare quality, healthcare professionals have struggled with where to put the focus of their resources. Ultimately, they recognized—with the assistance of the theoretical writings of general industry quality masters—that the key to improvement lay in the measurement of the important characteristics of their practice (figure 10.1). This practice could be that of a physician, nurse, or therapist, or it could be the practice of an organization. The important thing to notice is that the model fits for most all individuals, groups, and levels of a healthcare organization.

Definition of Performance

Ultimately, it was recognized that what they were discussing was the performance of various components of organizations. The word *performance* has been defined as "the execution of an activity or pattern of behavior; the application of inherent or learned capabilities to complete a process according to prescribed specifications or standards" (Meisenheimer 1997). Performance is measured using one or more **performance indicators.** For example, performance can be measured against **financial indicators,** such as the average cost per laboratory test, or **productivity indicators,** such as the number of patients seen per physician per day. What is important is to measure the aspects of performance that really reflect quality and that point conclusively to the aspects of performance that require improvement.

Figure 10.1.   Quality masters

A number of individuals have contributed to the theoretical underpinnings of continuous performance improvement. Over the decades, various aspects of their writings have been integrated into the current philosophy of improving quality in the healthcare arena. Go online and see what you can find about two or three of these theoreticians.

Walter A. Shewhart

Walter Shewhart was a statistician and research engineer for Bell Telephone Laboratories from 1925 until 1956. During that time, he pioneered the use of a quality control mechanism called statistical process control. Its purpose was to reduce variation in processes. Shewhart was the first person to suggest that two types of variation could be at work in a process: variation that was the result of chance, and variation that was the result of a definable cause. He used this method to improve the stability of processes.

He also was the first to develop what he called the "act of control." This concept evolved into the plan–do–check–act cycle. W. Edwards Deming built on Shewhart's work.

W. Edwards Deming

W. Edwards Deming was an American statistician. He is often credited with revitalizing the Japanese economy after the Second World War. He wrote the book *Out of the Crisis* in 1983. In his book, he described his methods for improving quality. Like Shewhart, Deming discussed variation and identified two types: common-cause variation (variation caused by chance) and special-cause variation (variation assigned a cause).

Deming believed that quality must be built into the product. He made a number of controversial statements about standard management techniques. For example, he declared that he did not believe in performance appraisals, management by objectives, or work standards.

Deming also developed a 14-point plan to help executives lead their organizations. Several of his points can be recognized in the principles of performance improvement. He believed that senior administrators need to communicate a constancy of purpose in which the vision and mission statements are made known. He proposed focusing on the process and not the results. Another of the 14 points was that organizations must not rely on inspection for defects but, rather, continually work to improve production and service.

According to Deming, the organization's leadership also must provide training, education, and self-improvement opportunities for employees and work to help employees achieve excellence in their jobs. Fear must be driven out of the organization because it impedes self-actualization. Barriers among departments and staff must be broken because barriers prevent people from communicating effectively and processes from being improved.

Joseph M. Juran

Joseph Juran also consulted with the Japanese in the 1950s and wrote several books on quality control. In the 1980s, he claimed that management could control over 80 percent of quality defects by using the three central principles of quality: planning, control, and improvement. He believed that training and hands-on management are basic requirements for meeting the needs of customers.

Armand F. Feigenbaum

Armand Feigenbaum built on Deming's statistical approach. In the early 1980s, he emphasized the necessity of integrating the functions of total quality control. Feigenbaum stated that the planning, design, and setup of the product or service must be integrated with its production and distribution. In turn, the product's production and distribution must be integrated with training, data analysis, and user feedback. Thus, customers and suppliers are all incorporated into the total quality concept. The goal is to meet the expectations and requirements of the organizations' customers.

Figure 10.1. **Quality masters** *(continued)*

Philip B. Crosby

Philip Crosby was a quality consultant working in the 1980s. He did not agree with his predecessors' focus on statistics. Instead, he proposed the concepts of zero defects and conformance to requirements. Crosby also proposed four absolutes of quality:

- Do it right the first time.
- Defect prevention is the only acceptable approach.
- Zero defects is the only performance standard.
- The cost of quality is the only measure of quality. This means that it is less costly to produce a high-quality product the first time than to manage the losses that result from producing a low-quality product.

Brian Joiner

Brian Joiner, also consulting in the 1980s, maintained that quality begins at the top and funnels down through the organization. He developed the Joiner triangle. This concept has three basic elements:

- Quality to ensure customer satisfaction and loyalty
- A scientific approach to root out underlying causes of problems
- The all-one-team method that encourages and empowers employees to work together to break down departmental barriers and creates buy-in to improvement, ownership in the process, and commitment to quality

---

Performance Improvement

The term **performance improvement** (PI) in healthcare is a "process for involving personnel in planning and executing a continuous flow of improvements to provide quality health care that meets or exceeds expectations" (McLaughlin and Kaluzny 2006). Although a number of terms and acronyms are frequently used to represent this PI concept (for example, continuous quality improvement [CQI] and total quality management [TQM]), this chapter uses performance improvement. Numerous improvement models and quality philosophies have been developed over the years. The key feature of performance improvement as implemented in today's healthcare organizations is that it is a continuous cycle of measurement, analysis, monitoring, planning, designing, and evaluating.

Performance monitoring is data driven. Monitoring performance based on internal and external data is the foundation of all PI activities. Each healthcare organization must identify and prioritize which processes and outcomes (in other words, which types of data) are important to monitor based on its mission and the scope of care and services it provides. A logical starting point in identifying areas to monitor performance includes important organization functions, particularly those that are high-risk, high-volume, or problem-prone. Outcomes of care, customer feedback, and the requirements of regulatory agencies are additional areas that organizations consider when prioritizing performance measures. Once the scope and focus of performance monitoring are determined, the leaders define the data collection requirements for each performance measure (Shaw and Elliott 2012).

As shown in figure 10.2, measuring performance depends on the identification of performance measures for each service, process, or outcome determined important to track. A performance measure is a quantitative tool (for example, a rate, ratio, index, percentage) that provides an indication of an organization's performance in relation to a specified process or outcome. Monitoring selected performance measures can help an organization determine process stability or can identify improvement opportunities. Specific criteria are used to define the organization's performance measures. Components of a good performance measure include a documented numerator statement, a denominator statement, and a description of the population to which the measure is applicable. In addition, the measurement period, baseline goal, data collection method, and frequency of data collection, analysis, and reporting must be identified (Shaw and Elliott 2012). The sum total of the performance measures selected as applicable to a healthcare organization make up the Performance Measurement System required by the Joint Commission for use in accreditation processes (Joint Commission 2009a).

For example, one indicator of quality might be that a physician sees patients within 30 minutes after their arrival at the facility. The organization could measure the minutes that it took from the time the patient stated his or her name to the time the physician first

Figure 10.2.   Organization-wide performance improvement process

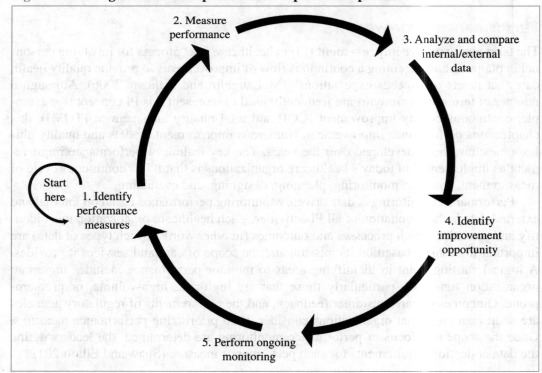

Source: Shaw and Elliot 2012, 5.

saw the patient. As long as patients were seen within that 30-minute time frame, the organization could assume that it was providing high-quality care. No attempts would be made to analyze the process or take corrective action unless the number of minutes increased beyond the 30-minute threshold. In this traditional approach, organizations actively address quality and performance issues only when they fail to meet the level of quality they had defined for themselves in performance measures (Shaw and Elliot 2012).

One important outcome that hospitals are required to continuously monitor is the monthly delinquent health record rate. The criteria used to establish this performance measure include:

$$\frac{\text{Number of incomplete health records that exceed the}}{\text{Medical staff-established time frame for record completion}}$$
$$\text{Average monthly discharges}$$

The populations included in this performance measure are the medical staff and inpatient health records. Tracking this outcome allows the hospital to continuously monitor its rate or percentage of delinquent health records. If the health record delinquency rate exceeds the hospital's established performance standards (an internal comparison) or nationally established performance standards (external comparison), an **opportunity for improvement** has been identified. Following this, a team-based performance improvement process may be initiated.

When an organization compares its current performance to its own internal historical data, or uses data from similar external organizations across the country, it helps establish a *benchmark*, also known as a standard of performance or best practice, for a particular process or outcome. Establishing a benchmark for each monitored performance measure assists the healthcare organization in setting performance baselines, describing process performance or stability, or identifying areas for more focused data collection. **The Joint Commission** (until 2007, known as the Joint Commission on Accreditation of Healthcare Organizations) is one available external resource that can be used to establish the performance measure of the average monthly health record delinquency rate for a hospital. The Joint Commission will cite the healthcare organization with a requirement for improvement if the total average health record delinquency exceeds 50 percent of the average monthly discharges in any one quarter. Hospitals commonly set the benchmark for their health record delinquency rate at less than 50 percent.

Many people advocate that every department in a healthcare organization today should be continuously monitoring its key performance indicators on a regular basis. Some of the decisions for key performance indicators used to monitor HIM functions are:

- Collecting information that is neither too specific nor too general
- Monitoring the overall performance of the department, not simply one or two aspects but, on the other hand, not hundreds of little work processes

- Breaking the department into the units where specialized work is performed, such as a filing unit, report sorting unit, or record pulling unit

- Finding the measures that describe the unit's performance over time, recording on a daily basis but reporting on a weekly basis

- Designing a report that can track data over time, including percentage measures to identify problem areas

Quality Dimensions

Donabedian (1988) contributed significantly to our understanding of measuring quality. He recognized that quality had multiple dimensions that needed to be measured using various types of indicators. He proposed three types of **quality indicators**:

- **Structure indicators** measure the attributes of the setting, such as number and qualifications of the staff, adequacy of equipment and facilities, and adequacy of organizational policies and procedures.

- **Process indicators** measure the actions by which services are provided, the things people or devices do, from conducting appropriate tests, to making a diagnosis, to actually carrying out a treatment.

- **Outcome indicators** measure the actual results of care for patients and populations, including patient and family satisfaction.

In addition to identifying types of quality indicators, Donabedian introduced the idea that quality has both a technical and an interpersonal dimension. The *technical* dimension recognizes that caregivers must have the knowledge and judgment to arrive at an appropriate strategy for providing service and the technical skills to carry it out. The *interpersonal* aspect recognizes that caregivers must have the communication skills and social attributes necessary to serve patients appropriately. The interpersonal aspect of quality recognizes the importance of empathy, honesty, respectfulness, tactfulness, and sensitivity to others. Donabedian acknowledged that it was far easier to measure quality's technical dimension than its interpersonal dimension.

Contemporary Approach to PI

The contemporary approach to PI is much more proactive than the traditional quality management approach. Although PI uses several traditional quality management techniques such as quality indicators, most often its primary focus is on continually making small, targeted changes for improvement, which over time lead to significant overall improvement. Performance improvement is not a philosophy that is satisfied with the status quo; it is not based on the if it ain't broke, don't fix it assumption. Nor does PI operate on the theory of identifying bad apples, where one conducts inspections to identify defects. PI does not attempt to assign individual blame and punish lapses in quality. Instead, PI is based on the assumption that organizations should continuously and systematically identify and test small, planned changes in processes and systems. Over time, the theory proposes, these changes will improve the quality of care provided to patients (Berwick 1989). Opportunities for improvement are identified by gathering and analyzing data on an ongoing basis.

The Focus Is on the Customer

It becomes apparent relatively quickly as one works through the definition of an organization's quality monitors that many cannot be measured without the input of the individuals who are the consumers of the product or service or the receiver of a process's output. Many also cannot be evaluated as to their effectiveness without that input. So, as performance improvement practices evolved, an important focus has developed on the opinions of customers. Many organizations and quality experts define *quality* as meeting or exceeding customer expectations. The term **customer** is used frequently in performance management activities. **External customers** are those people outside the organization for whom it provides services. For example, the external customers of a hospital would include patients, physicians, and third-party payers. Organizations also have **internal customers.** Employees are internal customers. They receive services from other areas in the organization that make it possible for them to do their jobs. For example, a nurse on an intensive care unit would be an internal customer of the hospital pharmacy. The nurse depends on the pharmacy to provide the medications needed to fill the physicians' orders for his or her patients.

Employees in one system or subsystem use the outputs from other systems or subsystems of the organization as inputs to their own system or subsystem. The employees then produce new outputs, which in turn may become inputs for still another system or subsystem. In this way, the performance of one system can affect the performance of many others.

To measure the requirements and perceptions of external customers today, many healthcare organizations utilize polling consultancies to canvass the opinions of their patients and clients following an episode of care. The Centers for Medicare and Medicaid Services also publishes quality information that it gleans from data reported during the reimbursement cycle regarding hospitals that provide services to its beneficiaries (see table 10.1).

Another means by which customers can see how a healthcare organization performs is through the publication of dashboards and scorecards. As discussed earlier, quality has many dimensions. Healthcare leaders cannot just focus on one aspect of quality (such as financial measures) without also considering other aspects (such as patient satisfaction or clinical quality) or they miss the whole picture. **Dashboards** and **scorecards** are tools that present metrics from a variety of quality aspects in one concise report. They may present measures of clinical quality (such as infection rates), financial quality, volume, and patient satisfaction. The indicators provide snapshots of all areas of quality to give leaders and communities of interest an overall perspective of the service the organization is providing.

Table 10.1. **A sample of patient satisfaction survey vendors**

NRC+Picker 1245 Q Street Lincoln, NE 68508 http://www.nationalresearch.com	California Institute for Health Systems Performance 1215 K Street Sacramento, CA 95814 http://www.cihsp.org	CAMC Institute 3200 MacCorkie Avenue, SE Charleston, WV 25304 http://www.camcinstitute.org
Deyta, Inc. 7400 New LaGrange Road, Suite 200 Louisville, KY 40222 http://www.deyta.com	Alexandria Marketing Research Group, Inc. 212 1/2 West 5th Street, Suite 209 Joplin, MO 64801 http://www.alexandriamarketing.com	HealthStream Research 209 10th Avenue South, Suite 536 Nashville, TN 37203 http://www.healthstream.com
Press Ganey Associates 404 Columbia Place South Bend, IN 46601 http://www.pressganey.com	Center for the Study of Services 1625 K Street, NW, 8th Floor Washington, DC 20006 http://cssresearch.org	Minnesota Rural Health Cooperative 190 East 4th Street North, PO Box 155 Cottonwood, MN 56229 http://www.mrhc.net
LSUS Institute for Human Services and Public Policy One University Place Bronson Hall 123 Shreveport, LA 71115 http://www.lsus.edu	Gallup 1001 Gallup Drive Omaha, NE 68102 http://www.gallup.com	Quality Data Management, Inc. 4015 East Royalton Broadview Heights, OH 44147 http://www.qdmnet.com
Professional Research Consultants, Inc. 11326 P Street Omaha, NE 68137 http://www.prconline.com	J. D. Power and Associates 5435 Corporate Drive Ste. 300 Troy, MI 48098 http://www.jdpower.com	WestGroup Research 2702 North 44th Street, Suite 100a Phoenix, AZ 85008 http://westgroupresearch.com
Sullivan/Luallin, Inc. 3760 Fourth Avenue, Suite 1 San Diego, CA 92103 http://www.sullivan-luallin.com	Regenstrief Institute, Inc. 1050 Wishard Blvd RG6 Indianapolis, IN 46202-2872 http://www.regenstrief.org	RAND Health Communications 1776 Main St. Santa Monica, CA 90407 http://www.rand.org/health

Source: HCAHPS Approved Vendor List, http://www.hcahpsonline.org/app_vendor.aspx.

The terms *dashboard* and *scorecard* are often used interchangeably, but technically, dashboards (like dashboards on a car) are reports of process measures that help leaders know what is currently going on so that they can plan strategically where they want to go next, and scorecards (like baseball scorecards) are reports of outcomes measures to help leaders know what they have accomplished. These concise reports help leaders "align organizational effort to achieve higher levels of organizational performance" (Pugh 2005).

The primary focus of PI efforts must be on the customer. The expectations and needs of both external and internal customers must be kept in mind throughout the PI process. Those involved in PI projects must know and understand their customers and involve them in the process so they can express their needs.

Check Your Understanding 10.1

1. Which of the following provide process measure metrics in a precise format?

    A. Dashboard
    B. Scoreboard
    C. Structured indicator
    D. Outcome indicator

2. The focus of performance improvement should be on:

    A. Employees
    B. Financial stability of the organization
    C. Customers
    D. Interpersonal skills

3. Fifty percent of our HIM staff have a nationally recognized credential. This is an example of what type of indicator:

    A. Structured
    B. Process
    C. Outcome
    D. Internal

Instructions: Indicate whether the statements below are true or false (T or F).

4. ____ Performance monitoring is outcomes driven.

5. ____ Performance improvement is something that is done periodically.

6. ____ An outcome indicator measures results of care provided to the patient.

Fundamental Principles of Continuous Performance Improvement

Performance improvement is based on several fundamental principles, including:

- The structure of a system determines its performance. Therefore, problems are more often within systems than within individual people.

- All systems demonstrate variation. Some variation occurs because of common causes and some because of special causes.

- Improvements rely on the collection and analysis of data that increase knowledge.

- PI requires the commitment and support of top administration.

- PI works best when leaders and employees know and share the organization's mission, vision, and values.

- PI efforts take time and require a big investment in people.

- Excellent teamwork is essential.

- Communication must be open, honest, and multidirectional.

- Success must be celebrated to encourage more success.

The Problem Is Usually the System

Problems in patient care and other areas of the healthcare organization are usually symptoms of shortcomings inherent in a system or a process. Kelly defines a system as "a collection of parts that interact with each other to form an interdependent whole" (Kelly 2003). Practically everything one can think of (both entities and processes) can be viewed as systems. Human beings are systems (very complicated systems made up of a lot of subsystems). Families are systems. Shopping for the family's weekly groceries can be viewed as a system. Healthcare organizations are very large systems. Each department in a healthcare facility is a system with numerous subsystems.

Every system has **inputs.** The system **processes** the inputs and eventually produces **outputs.** One system's outputs may then become inputs for another system.

The hospital's admitting department is an example of a system. When a patient enters the hospital, he or she presents to the admitting clerk. The clerk uses a computer to collect data for the admitting system. The patient with knowledge of his or her condition, the admitting clerk with knowledge of the admitting process, and the computer with its admitting template can all be considered inputs for the admitting system. When the clerk begins asking for the patient's address, insurance coverage, and reason for admission and the patient begins responding, the admitting process is under way. The output of the process is the patient's admission to the hospital and a completed face sheet for his or her medical record. These outputs can then be viewed as inputs into the next system in the hospital, the patient care system.

Systems thinking is a vital part of performance improvement. Systems thinking requires individuals to think about patterns and interrelationships between work units in the organization. Performance problems often occur because sources of problems were actually built into the interunit system (Batalden and Stoltz 1993). More recently, the National Academy of Engineering and the Institute of Medicine jointly published *Building a Better Delivery System* (2005) in which means of utilizing systems engineering concepts to improve the healthcare system are demonstrated. *Improvements* must address the system's shortcomings. For example, if the admitting clerk had to follow a series of cumbersome procedures to obtain data about referring physicians in order to enter them into the admitting template, this could seriously affect the clerk's performance and produce a less-than-desirable output. Examples of poor-quality output might be inaccurate information or long delays in admissions or additional work for other departments who must research the demographic data on the physician themselves. The problems in the admitting department may create problems for other departments in the hospital. Using systems thinking as a principle, information on all physicians with privileges at a facility can be maintained in the patient registration system and continuously and automatically updated by the medical staff office credentialing system, thereby preventing such negative occurrences and additional work for others in the organization.

Variation Is Constant

Every system has some degree of variation built into it. No system produces the exact same output every time. It would be desirable to reduce variation within systems as much as possible so that system output could be more predictable and better controlled. However, there will always be some variation, albeit sometimes minor (Omachonu 1999). Variation that is inherent within the system is known as **common-cause variation.** For example, when a nurse takes a patient's blood pressure, she may believe that she is performing the procedure in exactly the same way every time, but she will get slightly different readings each time. Although the blood pressure cuff, the patient, and the nurse are all the same inputs into the system, variations can occur. For example, the cuff may be applied to a different place on the patient's arm. The patient may have a slightly different emotional or physiological status at the time of the measurement. The nurse may have a different level of focus or concentration. Any one of these factors, plus countless others, can affect the values obtained. However, they are potentially present in every single episode of blood pressure measurement in every single patient. It is important to recognize that not every variation is a defect. The variation may just be an example of common-cause variation found inherently in the process.

Some variations are caused by factors outside the system. This type of variation is known as **special-cause variation.** If the special cause produces a negative effect, we will want to identify the special cause and eliminate it. If the special cause produces a positive effect, we will want to reinforce it so the good effect will continue and perhaps be expanded into the processes of others in the organization. An example of this type of variation occurs when a patient is taking blood pressure medication and there is a substantial drop in the measurement. The medication has caused the decrease in blood pressure values and can clearly be considered a special cause. In this situation, the variation is intentional and desired. In other situations, the variation may produce an undesirable and unintentional effect. For example, if a patient is upset about a phone call he received just before the nurse came in to take his vitals, his blood pressure could be exceptionally high. The change in values occurred due to a special cause (the phone call) and resulted in a blood pressure reading much higher than normally expected.

Similar examples of special-cause variation can be identified in our hospital systems. In the health information management (HIM) department, for example, there is always some common-cause variation in the number of records that can be coded each day. On a day when one of the regular coders is out sick, however, the number of records coded might drop significantly. This would be an example of special-cause variation. As much as is possible, the goal should be to remove special causes if they are creating an undesirable effect.

Data Must Support PI Activities and Decisions

Data drive performance improvement. Omachonu states that "the ability to collect, analyze, and use data is a vital component of a successful performance improvement process. Healthcare organizations that do not devote sufficient attention to data collection may be able to speak of only marginal success in their process improvement journey" (Omachonu 1999).

In the past, healthcare organizations relied on unsupported assumptions about which processes were functioning well and which ones were not. Without real data, however, no objective and accurate assessment can take place. Collecting data provides information about the current level of customer satisfaction, potential areas for improvement efforts, and the effectiveness of changes already implemented.

A number of methods can be used in data collection. PI activities must plan the best method for obtaining timely, accurate, and relevant data. Examples of data collection methods and instruments include retrospective record review with specific quality criteria, written surveys, direct observation, and individual or focus group interviews.

After adequate data have been collected, they must be carefully analyzed. Improvement efforts must be built on knowledge, and knowledge is gained through data analysis.

Support Must Come from the Top Down

PI as a vital, continuous process must be built into the organization's culture. The executive leaders of the organization must believe in its value in order for it to permeate the entire organization. Moreover, they must ensure that their management teams are well versed in the principles and techniques of continuous performance improvement.

Training for managers and supervisors can be provided by outside consultants or through in-service training. Managers and supervisors then can train their own employees and model the **continuous improvement** philosophy. Every employee must understand the importance of continually improving processes so as to provide better service to the organization's customers.

The Organization Must Have a Shared Vision

The organization's executive leaders and board of directors are responsible for developing and communicating a clear vision of the organization's future. The organization's vision, mission, and values set its direction and support the norms it considers important.

For a description of an organization's vision, mission, and values, please see chapter 18. They communicate a constancy of purpose. Vision, mission, and values statements help employees to understand the vision and embrace it as their own. The statements also guide employees as they make their own contributions to the organization by fulfilling their professional responsibilities.

Staff and Management Must Be Involved in the Process

As mentioned earlier, executive leaders must be committed to the philosophy of continuous improvement and work to ensure that every manager and every employee is committed to its value. This commitment demands an investment in people and requires substantial time and training. PI depends on everyone in the organization actively seeking to meet internal and external customers' spoken or anticipated needs.

This is particularly important for employees who have direct contact with external customers. These employees are perhaps in the best position to recognize which needs of the customer are not being met. They often offer helpful ideas for improvement. It works to the organization's benefit when staff are empowered to make a difference for their fellow workers and the patients they serve.

Setting Goals Is Crucial

All PI programs must have established goals. Goals are essentially targets that the organization strives to achieve in a given PI program year. They should be specific and define measurable end results. An example of an organizational goal might be "To provide high-quality patient care that is cost-effective."

After goals are established, it is important to identify specific, measurable objectives that can be completed within a certain time frame. An objective associated with the above goal might be "By the end of the year, a high-quality, cost-effective care program will be designed for the management of diabetes patients."

Effective Communication Is Important

Effective communication is absolutely essential for the PI process to work. It must exist at all levels of the organization and in all directions. Managers must hear from staff how the organization is functioning. Staff must feel comfortable in telling management when things are going well and when there are problems. This level of communication requires trust and respect for all individuals and the recognition that everyone wants to do the best job possible.

Obviously, openly identifying and discussing problems is not always comfortable or easy. However, an organization that is committed to serving its customers must view problems as opportunities for improvement. The Japanese call it *kaizen:* the continuous search for opportunities for all processes to get better (Imai 1986). Defects are looked on as treasures because a chance for improvement lies in the discovery of imperfection (Berwick 1989). None of this can happen without effective communication.

Effective communication is two-way communication. It requires clear, articulate, and tactful speaking. Even more important, it requires careful, attentive listening and understanding. Organizations must take the time to listen to their customers, both internal and external, so they can hear information about where services need improvement.

Success Should Be Celebrated

Although PI demands that organizations focus on identifying and addressing problems, it also must celebrate the organization's successes. A celebration of success communicates to everyone that the participants' efforts are applauded, that success can occur from such efforts, and that others should be encouraged to participate in PI initiatives. Those people involved in improving the process need to be recognized and appreciated. One of the reasons organizations collect and analyze data is to let them know when they have reasons to celebrate. Achieving service excellence is certainly a great reason to celebrate.

Formal Performance Improvement Activities

Performance improvement is always some combination of everyday managerial improvements and more formal performance improvement activities. The mix may at times conform with the types of activities discussed thus far in this chapter, which can be undertaken by managers and staff in a more informal manner, and at other times the issues at hand may require a more formal approach due to the significance of the issues, the multidepartment effects, or the complexity of the processes involved in the identified issues. At that point, a formal performance improvement team can be convened to examine the issues and make recommendations utilizing the classic techniques of continuous quality and performance improvement.

Formal performance improvement activities tend to be cyclical in nature. They are based on the kinds of monitoring of internal and external data, or performance measures, discussed above in this chapter.

When an organization compares its current performance to its own internal historical data, or uses data from similar external organizations, it helps establish an organizational **benchmark.** A benchmark is a systematic comparison of one organization's measured characteristics with those of another similar organization or with regional or national standards. Once a benchmark for a performance measure is determined, analyzing data collection results becomes more meaningful. Often, further study or more focused data collection on a performance measure is triggered when data collection results fall outside the established benchmark. This is cycle #1 of the common performance improvement model discussed by Shaw and Elliot as graphically depicted in figure 10.3. When variation is discovered through continuous monitoring or when unexpected events suggest performance problems, the organization may decide that there is an opportunity for improvement and initiate a team performance improvement process. This is cycle #2 of the common performance improvement model discussed by Shaw and Elliot as graphically depicted in figure 10.4 (2012).

Figure 10.3. Monitoring and improving customer satisfaction

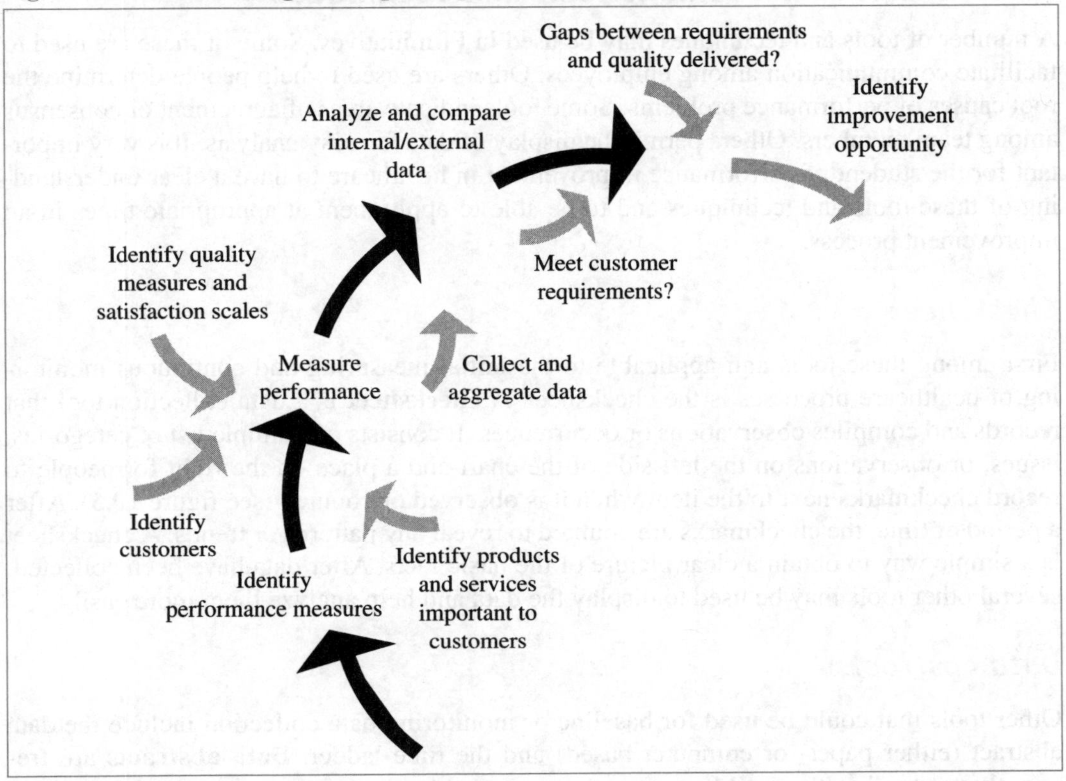

Gaps between requirements
and quality delivered?

Identify
improvement
opportunity

Analyze and compare
internal/external
data

Meet customer
requirements?

Identify quality
measures and
satisfaction scales

Measure
performance

Collect and
aggregate data

Identify
customers

Identify
performance measures

Identify products
and services
important to
customers

Source: Shaw and Elliot 2012, 89.

Figure 10.4. Team-based performance improvement process

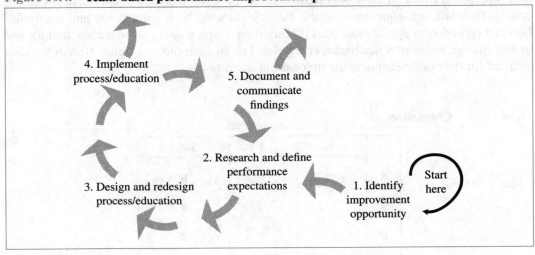

4. Implement
process/education

5. Document and
communicate
findings

2. Research and define
performance
expectations

3. Design and redesign
process/education

1. Identify
improvement
opportunity

Start
here

Source: Shaw and Elliot 2012, 5.

Performance Improvement Tools and Techniques

A number of tools and techniques may be used in PI initiatives. Some of these are used to facilitate communication among employees. Others are used to help people determine the root causes of performance problems. Some tools indicate areas of agreement or consensus among team members. Others permit the display of data for easy analysis. It is very important for the student of performance improvement in healthcare to have a clear understanding of these tools and techniques and to be able to apply them at appropriate times in an improvement process.

Checksheet

First among these tools and applicable to the initial measuring and continuous monitoring of healthcare processes is the checksheet. A **checksheet** is a data collection tool that records and compiles observations or occurrences. It consists of a simple list of categories, issues, or observations on the left side of the chart and a place on the right for people to record checkmarks next to the item when it is observed or counted (see figure 10.5). After a period of time, the checkmarks are counted to reveal any patterns or trends. A checksheet is a simple way to obtain a clear picture of the basic facts. After data have been collected, several other tools may be used to display the data and help analyze them more easily.

Data Abstracts

Other tools that could be used for baseline or monitoring data collection include the data abstract (either paper- or computer-based) and the time ladder. **Data abstracts** are frequently used in healthcare. Most often they are used in clinical process monitoring where data points are retrieved patient by patient from clinical data stored in the health record and recorded in the specified fields of an abstract on paper or in a relatively simple database application like Microsoft Access. Using the computer-based application can, of course, facilitate subsequent use of the data by allowing their summation and manipulation in a spreadsheet application. And if housed on a laptop data can be transported for use in multiple locations of a healthcare enterprise. For an example, see figure 10.6 of the data abstract for the core measure acute myocardial infarction.

Figure 10.5.   **Checksheet**

	1	2	Total
A	╫╫	/ / /	8
B	/ / / /	/ / / /	8
C	/ /	/	3

Figure 10.6.   Acute myocardial infarction (AMI) core measure set

UHC®   *University HealthSystem Consortium*

Acute Myocardial Infarction Core Measures Data Collection (Qtr 4 Yr 2009)
Institution Name: _____

Patient Encounter Number	Patient ID	Admission Date	Discharge Date	Admission Type	Sex

MS-DRG   Race

Name change *Provider ID# changed* to   Zip Code
Certification Number ("6" values)

Primary Payer   **Secondary Payer**   **Attesting Physician Code**   **Attesting Physician Specialty Code**

Payment Source Values   HIC value not linked to
Medicare "1. Yes 2. No"   payment source

Principal Diagnosis   **Principal Procedure**   **Principal Procedure Date**   **Principal Procedure Physician Code**

Present on Admission Diagnosis

Other Diagnosis Codes   Other Procedure Codes

    A. Hispanic ethnicity or Latino: ☐ Yes   ☐ No

    B. What is the date the patient was admitted to   Calendar   Mm/dd/yyyy   CDB Value
        <u>acute</u> inpatient care (Admit Date):
                        Please note the initially pre-populated value is the CDB value
        (Priority order: Verify date of physician admit to
        inpatient order)

1. Point of Origin for Admission or Visit: ☐ 1-Non-Health Care Facility Point of Origin
    (replaced "Admission Source")   ☐ 2-Clinic
              ☐ 3-(discontinued value effective Q4 2007)
    (If Point of Origin is 4 or D, **questions 3 and 7**   ☐ 4-Transfer from a hospital (Different facility)
    through 19 are not required)   ☐ 5-Transfer from Skilled Nursing Facility (SNF) or Intermediate Care
                    Facility (ICF)
    (AMI-1, AMI-7, AMI-7a, AMI-8, AMI-8a, AMI-9)   ☐ 6-Transfer from another Health Care Facility
              ☐ 7-Emergency room
              ☐ 8-Court/law enforcement
              ☐ 9-Information not available
              ☐ A-(discontinued value effective Q4 2007)

              ☐ D-Transfer from One Distinct Unit of the Hospital to another Distinct
                    Unit of the Same Hospital Resulting in a Separate Claim to the Payer

              ☐ E-Transfer from Ambulatory Surgery Center*

              ☐ F-Transfer from Hospice and is Under a Hospice Plan of Care or
                    Enrolled in a Hospice Program*

(continued on next page)

Figure 10.6.   Acute myocardial infarction (AMI) core measure set *(continued)*

2.   Discharge Status:

   (If Discharge Status is 2, 7, 20, 43, 50, 51, or 66, questions 20 through 40 are not required)

   (If Discharge Status is 02,07,20, 43 and 66, and length of stay =1 day then questions 8 and 9 are not required)

   (AMI-1, AMI-2, AMI-3, AMI-4, AMI-5, AMI-9, AMI-T1, AMI-T2)

   Refer to Appendix H, Table 2.5 Discharge Status Disposition

   ❑ 01-Discharged to home care or self care (routine discharge)
   ❑ 02-Discharged/transferred to another short term general hospital for inpatient care
   ❑ 03-Discharged/transferred to skilled nursing facility (SNF) with Medicare certification **in anticipation of covered skilled care****
   ❑ 04-Discharged/transferred to a facility that provides custodial or supportive case
   ❑ 05- Discharged/transferred to a Designated Cancer Center or Children's Hospital
   Usage Note: Transfers to non-designated cancer hospitals should use Code 02. A list of (National Cancer Institute) Designated Cancer Centers can be found at http://www3.cancer.gov/cancercenters/centerslist.html
   ❑ 06-Discharged/transferred to home **under care of organized home health service organization in anticipation of covered skilled care**** with a written plan of care for home care services.
   ❑ 07-Left against medical advice or discontinued care
   ❑ 20-Expired
   ❑ 21- Discharged/transferred to court/law enforcement
   ❑ 43-Discharged/transferred to a federal hospital
   ❑ 50-Hospice – home
   ❑ 51-Hospice – medical facility (certified) providing hospice level of care
   ❑ 61-Discharged/transferred to hospital-based Medicare approved swing bed within the hospital's approved swing bed arrangements.
   ❑ 62-Discharged/transferred to an inpatient rehabilitation facility including rehabilitation distinct part units of a hospital
   ❑ 63-Discharged/transferred to Medicare certified long term care hospital (LTCH)
   ❑ 64-Discharged/transferred to a nursing facility certified under Medicaid but not certified under Medicare
   ❑ 65-Discharged/transferred to a psychiatric hospital or psychiatric distinct part unit of a hospital
   ❑ 66- Discharged to a Critical Access Hospital (CAH)
   ❑ 70- *Discharged/transferred to another Type of Health Care Institution not defined elsewhere in this code list (see Code 05)

3.   Was the patient <u>received as a transfer</u> from an emergency department of **another** hospital: (AMI-1, AMI-7, Ami-7a, AMI-8, AMI-8a)

   ❑ Yes   ❑ No/unable to determine

   (If Yes, questions 7 through 19 are not required)

4.   Patient's Birthdate: (mm-dd-yyyy)

   ____/____/_____   ❑ Not Available
   YYYY (1880 – current year)

   Age: **year/s   month/s   day/s** (if age < 18 years, skip all)

Time Ladders

Time ladders support the collection of data that must be oriented by time. Very simply, they are usually paper-based with the intervals of time necessary to address the problem under consideration listed down the right side of one, two, or three columns on a sheet of paper. Then, as the data collector makes her observations she records them next to the time of occurrence. Frequently, first-line employees are asked to use time ladders since the nature of their work is highly specific and oriented to the processing of single occurrences. For example, a receptionist might be asked to record on a time ladder when a patient arrives at her workstation and then record again on the same time ladder when the patient is called to an exam room. If we wanted to get a picture of how the receptionist's work is broken up by other considerations, we might also ask her to record timing of phone calls, provider requests for assistance, and the like to see how other duties had an impact on her interactions with patients. Time ladders of this type are usually collected for at least a week so a fairly detailed, clear picture can be developed of the flow of work or a process over time. Another example of a time ladder is that derived from computer-based data. If one needed to, for instance, evaluate the times at which patients without appointments arrived to seek treatment in a clinic, one could request reporting again oriented by time over a substantial period like a month of the initial registration times in the clinic of those types of patients.

Statistics-Based Modeling Techniques

In some areas of a healthcare organization where the data generated are predominantly numerical, staff may want to regularly maintain one of two statistics-based modeling techniques: run charts or process control charts. They can help to make it patently obvious when a system that generates a lot of data is out of control.

A **run chart** displays data points over a period of time to provide information about performance (see figure 10.7). The measured points of a process are plotted on a graph at regular time intervals to help team members see whether there are substantial changes in the numbers over time. For example, suppose a health information technician wished to reduce the number of incomplete records in the HIM department. He might first plot the number of incomplete records each month for the past six months. Based on an analysis of the records process, he then might enact a change in the process designed to improve it. Following the improvement effort, he would continue to collect data on the number of incomplete records and plot the data on the graph. If the run chart showed that the number of incomplete charts had decreased, the health information technician could attribute the decrease to the improvement effort. A run chart is an excellent tool for providing visual verification of how a process is performing and whether an improvement effort has worked.

A **statistical process control chart** looks very much like a run chart except that it has lines drawn at the top and bottom. The upper line represents the upper control limit (UCL), and the lower line represents the lower control limit (LCL) (see figure 10.8). These lines

Figure 10.7.   Run chart

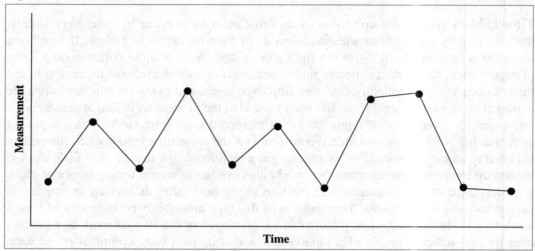

represent two or three standard deviations above and below the mean that have been statistically calculated from the data generated in the process. Remember that two standard deviations from the mean statistically include 95 percent of the observations of a process and three standard deviations include 99 percent. Like the run chart, the statistical process control chart plots points over time to show how a process is performing. However, the two control limit lines permit the evaluator to use the rules of probability to interpret whether the process is stable (in other words, predictable and within the bounds of probability) or out of control (many points of data outside the second or third standard deviations).

As mentioned earlier, Deming and Shewhart talked about systems and how some variation always occurs within a system. The statistical process control chart makes it possible to see whether the variation within a process is the result of a common cause or a special cause. It lets the PI team know whether the team needs to try to reduce the ordinary

Figure 10.8.   Statistical process control chart

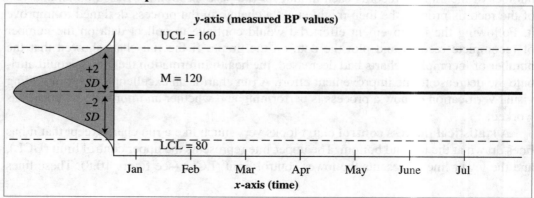

variation occurring through common cause or to seek out a special cause of the variation and try to eliminate it. Removing the variation will bring the upper and lower control limit lines closer together.

Check Your Understanding 10.2

1. Which tool is used to display performance data over time?

   A. Status process control chart
   B. Run chart
   C. Benchmark
   D. Time ladder

2. The nosocomial infection rate for our hospital is 0.2% while the rate at a similar hospital across town is 0.3%. This is an example of:

   A. Checksheet
   B. Data abstract
   C. Run chart
   D. Benchmark

3. The type of variation that is caused by factors outside a system is called:

   A. Input/output
   B. Processes
   C. Common-cause variation
   D. Special-cause variation

Instructions: Indicate whether the statements below are true or false (T or F).

4. _____ Goals should be measurable.

5. _____ Effective communication is the responsibility of administration only.

6. _____ A checksheet is used to record and complete observations and occurrences.

Team-Based Performance Improvement Processes

The first step in a formal process improvement is to assemble the team. If a performance improvement is to be undertaken, staff with knowledge and background in the process under examination should be involved. Because staff have fundamental knowledge of the process, they are vital to the success of process redesign activities. It is important to empower staff members to change processes and then to recognize them for their part in the improvements. In addition, staff members accept change much more easily when they have been part of the decision-making process. By being part of the process redesign team, staff also will have an easier time going through the early phases of the transition period. The team's success depends on the following seven elements:

- Establishing ground rules
- Stating the team's purpose or mission
- Identifying customers and their requirements
- Documenting current processes and identifying barriers
- Collecting and analyzing data
- Identifying possible solutions by brainstorming or using other PI techniques
- Making recommendations for changes in the process

Establishing Ground Rules

Ground rules must be agreed upon at the very beginning of the process improvement team work. All members of the team should have input into the ground rules. They should agree to abide by them for the sake of the team's success. Some ground rules that team members should consider are:

- To arrive on time for meetings
- To complete and present the results of assignments from the previous meeting
- To respect the opinions of all team members
- To listen to other team members' points of view without criticism
- To abide by decisions made by the team

Stating the Team's Purpose or Mission

The team must answer this question: Why has this team been formed? The team must define its **mission** in order to create a map or plan of the means by which it will examine the issues and plan its activities.

Identifying Customers and Their Requirements

The performance improvement team must identify the customers associated with the processes under discussion. Customers are both internal (for example, the facility's business office) and external (for example, third-party payers). The process improvement team identifies these customers and what their requirements are. Having identified its customers, the team works toward modifying the process to meet the customers' requirements.

Documenting Current Processes and Identifying Barriers

The process improvement team members work together to discuss and document current processes. For this step, the team's knowledge is vital because members must answer the following questions:

- What is the current process?
- Where are the start and end points of the process?
- What are the barriers to the process?

Collecting Current Process Data

Once an improvement opportunity has been identified through performance monitoring, and a team that consists of staff involved in the process under study has been assembled, the first task is to research and define performance expectations for the process targeted. Performance improvement teams have a variety of tools that they can use to accomplish their goals. The tools make it easier to gather and analyze information, and they help team members stay focused on PI activities and move the process along efficiently. If the organization has already been routinely monitoring the process as discussed above, it is important to remember that that information is available for use by the assembled PI team as well.

The first steps may include the following and may use additional PI tools and techniques.

FlowChart Current Process

Create a flowchart of the current process. Whenever a team examines a process with the intention of making improvements, it must first understand the process thoroughly. Each team member has a unique perspective on and significant insight into how a portion of the process works. **Flowcharts** help all the team members understand the process in the same way (see figure 10.9).

The work involved in developing the flowchart allows the team to thoroughly understand every step in the process as well as the sequence of steps. The flowchart provides a visual picture of each decision point and each event that must be completed. It readily points out places where there are redundancies and complex and problematic areas.

Brainstorm Problem Areas

Brainstorm problem areas within the current process. **Brainstorming** is a technique used to generate a large number of creative ideas from a group. It encourages PI team members to think out of the box and offer original ideas. There are a number of approaches to brainstorming. Teams can use an unstructured or a structured method.

Figure 10.9.   Flowchart

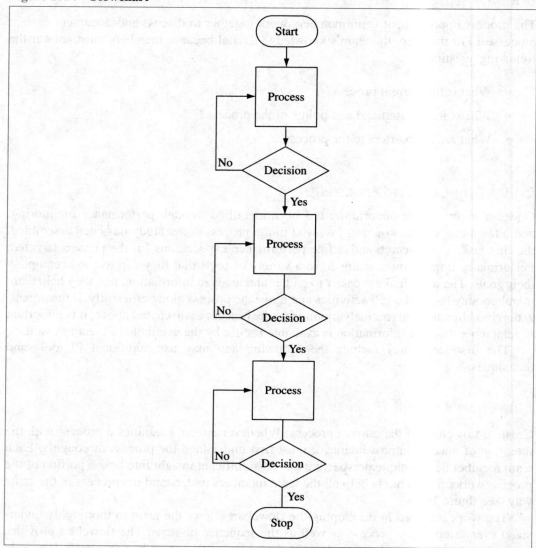

Unstructured Brainstorming Method

The **unstructured brainstorming method** results in a free flow of ideas. The team leader or facilitator writes the ideas on a flip chart as they are offered so that everyone can see the list as it forms. There should be no discussion or evaluation of the ideas at this point. The goal of brainstorming is to encourage creativity and to come up with a lot of ideas. Most brainstorming sessions are short (perhaps five minutes long). The ideas then are used as the basis for later discussions of the subject.

Structured Brainstorming Method

In **structured brainstorming,** the team leader or facilitator asks team members to generate their own list of ideas. Team members can work by themselves or in small groups. Again, the sessions are usually timed. Then, one by one, the team elicits a new idea from each member in turn. The process may take several rounds. As team members run out of new ideas, they pass. The next person then offers an idea until no team member can produce a fresh idea.

Brainstorming is highly effective for identifying a number of potential process steps that may benefit from improvement efforts and for generating solutions to specific problems. It helps people to begin thinking in new ways and gets them involved in the process. It is an excellent method for facilitating open communication.

Cause and Effect Diagram

One of the common quality improvement tools used for risk management purposes is the cause and effect diagram. A **cause-and-effect diagram** facilitates **root-cause analysis.** The diagram is sometimes called a **fishbone diagram** because of its characteristic shape (see figure 10.10). The problem is placed in a box on the right side of the diagram. A horizontal line is drawn and diagonal lines resembling ribs are added to connect the boxes above and below the main horizontal line (or backbone). Each box contains a different category of information.

The categories may represent broad classifications of problem areas. For example, possible categories include people, methods, equipment, materials, policies, procedures, environment, measurement, and others. The team determines how many categories it needs to classify all the possible sources of the problem. Usually, there are four categories.

After constructing the diagram, the team brainstorms the possible root causes of the problem. These are then placed on horizontal lines extending from the diagonal category line. Brainstorming continues until all the team's ideas about causes are exhausted. The purpose of this tool is to permit the team to explore, identify, and graphically display all of the root causes of a problem.

Figure 10.10.   Fishbone diagram

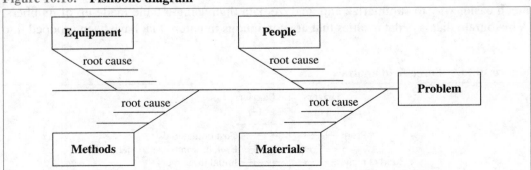

Force-Field Analysis

Force-field analysis is another tool used to visually display data generated through brainstorming. The team leader draws a large T shape on a board (figure 10.11). The word *drivers* is written above the crossbar and on the left side of the T. The word *barriers* is written above the bar and on the right side of the T. Team members then brainstorm the reasons or factors that would encourage a change for improvement and those that might create barriers. The team leader places the factors in the appropriate column on the chart.

Force-field analysis enables team members to identify factors that support or work against a proposed solution. Often the next step after force-field analysis is to work on ways that would eliminate barriers or reinforce drivers.

In addition, the team may need to undertake the following:

- Research any regulatory requirements related to the current process.

- Benchmark the organization's current process against performance standards and/ or nationally recognized standards.

- Conduct a survey to gather customer input on their needs and expectations.

Analyzing Process Data

Following the collection of data, it is important for the team to be able to consider it in a meaningful way. Obviously if the team is handed reams and reams of check sheets, time ladders, or abstracts and asked to prioritize problem areas for focused improvement, there will be no meaningful decisions made. Again, the PI tools and techniques can be of some assistance in providing the team with meaningful documents from which it can draw some conclusions. Consider the following techniques:

A **bar graph,** sometimes referred to as a bar chart, is used to display discrete categories, such as the gender of respondents or the type of health insurance respondents have. Such categories are shown on the horizontal (or *x*) axis of the graph. The vertical (or *y*) axis, shows the number of frequency of responses. The vertical scale always begins with zero (0) (figure 10.12).

A **histogram** can be used to display frequencies of responses (figure 10.13). It is a much easier way to summarize and analyze data than using a table made up of numbers. A histogram displays data values that are continuous in nature that have been grouped into

Figure 10.11.   **Force-field analysis**

Drivers (+)	Barriers (−)
$ Profit ⟶	⟵ Cost of materials
⟶	⟵ Lack of trained personnel
Market niche ⟶	⟵ Initial investment

Figure 10.12.   **Bar graph**

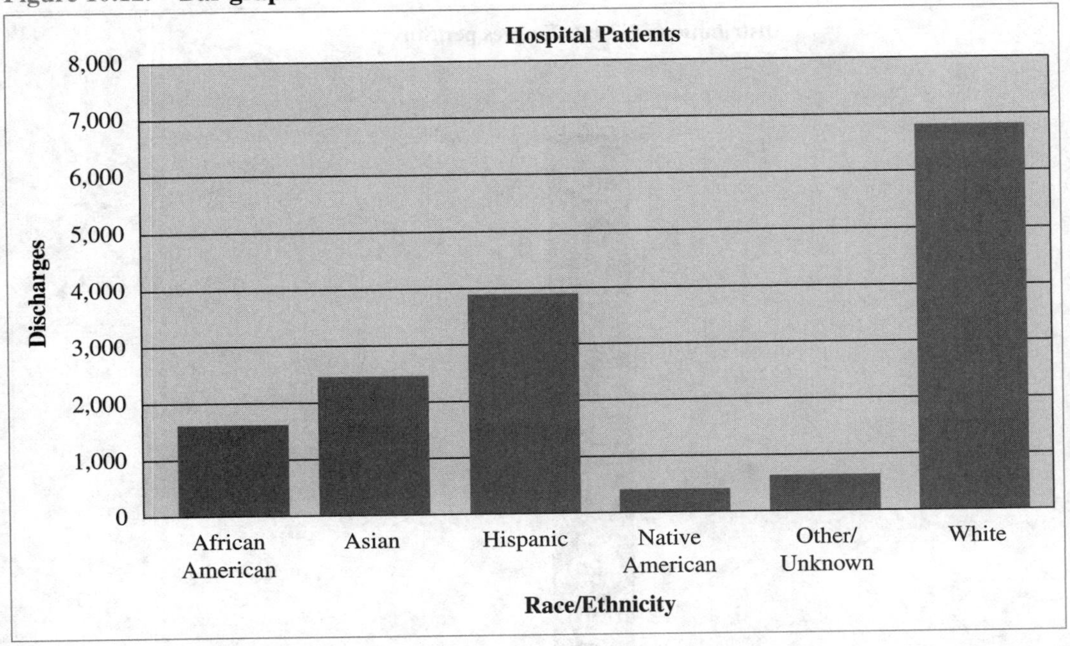

Hospital Patients

Source: Shaw and Elliot 2012, 49.

categories. For example, the data from the time ladder could be displayed on a histogram grouping the individual patient wait times in categories of 0–5 mins, 6–10 mins, 11–15 mins, 16–20 mins, and so forth. The bars on the histogram reveal how the data frequencies were distributed in each category.

The histogram is plotted with the frequencies shown on the *y*-axis and the minute intervals shown on the *x*-axis. The graph would indicate the different intervals that patients had to wait before being called. It can give PI teams an excellent idea of how well their process is performing. It is also possible to calculate the percentages that each bar is representing of the whole and display the percentage scale on the right *y*-axis. Thus, a histogram can show how frequently data values occur among the various intervals, how centered or skewed the distribution of data is, and what the likelihood of future occurrences will be. (Bar graphs and histograms are also covered in chapter 9.)

Scatter diagrams are used to plot the points for two continuous variables that may be related to each other in some way. For example, one might want to look at whether age and blood pressure are related. One variable, age, would be plotted on the horizontal axis of the graph, and the other variable, blood pressure, would be plotted on the vertical axis (figure 10.14). After a number of blood pressures and patients' ages were plotted, a pattern might emerge. If the diagram indicated that blood pressure increased with age, it would reveal a positive relationship between these variables. In some cases, a negative relationship might exist, such as with the variables of age and flexibility or the number of hours of training and the number of mistakes made.

Figure 10.13. **Histogram**

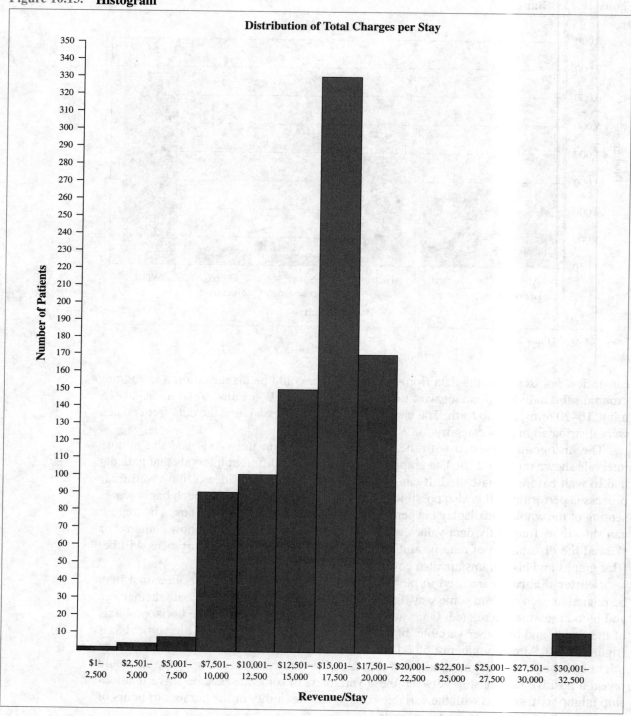

Distribution of Total Charges per Stay

Figure 10.14.   **Scatter diagram**

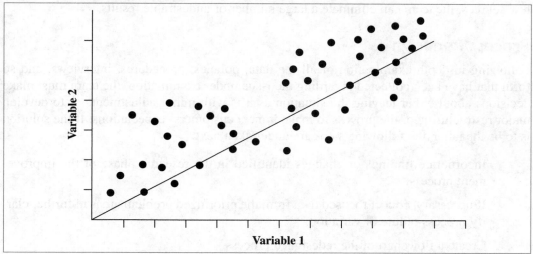

Whenever a scatter diagram indicates that the points are moving together in one direction or another, conclusions about the variables' relationship, either positive or negative, become evident. In other cases, however, the scatter diagram may indicate that there is no linear relationship between the variables because the points are scattered randomly and no pattern emerges. In this case, there would be no linear relationship between the two variables.

The ranking of various categories can be displayed visually using a **Pareto chart** (see figure 10.15). A Pareto chart looks very much like a bar chart except that the highest-ranking item is listed first, followed by the second highest, down to the lowest-ranked item. Its purpose is to display how the team ranked the problems and to allow the team to focus on those problems that may have the biggest potential for improving the process. The chart is based on the Pareto principle. According to the Pareto principle, 20 percent of a problem's

Figure 10.15.   **Pareto chart**

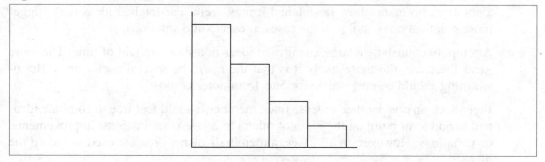

sources are responsible for 80 percent of its actual effects. By concentrating on the vital few sources, the team can eliminate a large number of undesirable results.

Process Redesign

Following in-depth examination of all the data, policies, procedures, interviews, and so forth that have been collected regarding the issue under examination, the team must make decisions about either leaving the situation as it is with minor adjustments or to develop major restructuring of the process to make it meet customers' expectations. If the solution is to be the latter, the following steps are undertaken next:

- Incorporate findings or changes identified in the research phase of the improvement process.

- If necessary, collect focused data from the prioritized problem areas to further clarify process failure or variation.

- Create a flowchart of the redesigned process.

- Develop policies and procedures that support the redesigned process.

- Educate involved staff about the new process.

Brainstorming

Brainstorming can again be a useful QI toolbox technique at this point in the process, one that promotes creative thinking as team members identify possible solutions for process improvement. During solution brainstorming, the team generates new, potentially useful ideas that can help to elaborate the solution. Creative solution brainstorming requires team members to follow four basic ground rules:

- Welcome all ideas. During brainstorming, no judgments are made about ideas presented—there are no wrong or ridiculous proposals.

- Be creative in contributions. Think out of the box! Because change involves risk taking, it is important to be open to new ideas. Every person's point of view is valuable. Team members should be encouraged to say whatever occurs to them as a solution, no matter how far-fetched it may seem. Far-fetched ideas may trigger more practical ones and, in some cases, present valid solutions.

- Attempt to contribute a large quantity of ideas in a short amount of time. The more ideas there are, the more likely it is that there will be several useful ones. Brainstorming should be undertaken for 5 to 15 minutes at most.

- Piggyback on one another's ideas. Team members should feel free to combine ideas and to add to or build on the ideas of others to create combinations, improvements, or variations. However, in all cases, a member's own words are used to record the ideas.

After a lot of ideas have been generated, a team often must find a logical way of reducing them to a set that is manageable and most effective for the problem. The following techniques can be of assistance in this phase of the team's work.

Affinity Grouping

Affinity grouping allows the team to organize similar ideas into logical groupings. Ideas that are generated in a brainstorming session may be written on sticky notes and arranged on a table or posted on a board. Without talking to each other, each team member is asked to walk around the table or board, look at the ideas, and place them in natural groupings that seem related or connected to each other. Each member is empowered to move the ideas in a way that makes the most sense.

As team members move the ideas back or place them in other groupings, the other team members consider the merits of the placements and decide whether further action is needed. The goal is to have the team become comfortable with the arrangement. Finally, the natural groupings that emerge are labeled with a category. The intent in using this tool is to bring focus to the new ideas (see figure 10.16).

Nominal Group Technique

Nominal group technique is a process used to develop agreement about an issue or an idea that the team considers most important. It helps the team reach consensus. Each team member ranks each idea according to importance. For example, if there were six ideas, the idea that is most important would be given the number six. The second most important

Figure 10.16.   **Affinity diagram**

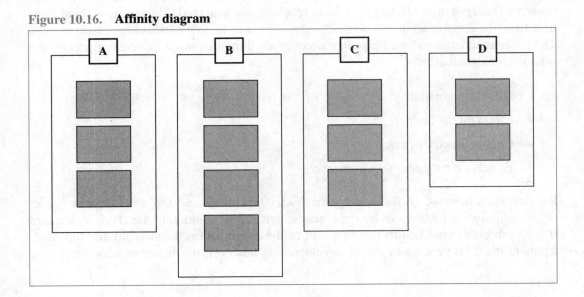

idea would be given the number five, and so on. After each individual team member has had a chance to rank the list of ideas, the numbers are totaled. The ideas ranked most important are clearly visible to all. Those ideas that people did not think were as important also become obvious owing to their low scores. The nominal group technique demonstrates where the team's priorities lie.

Multivoting Technique

The **multivoting technique** is a variation of the nominal group technique and serves the same purpose. Instead of ranking each issue or idea, team members are asked to rate issues by marking them with a distribution of points. In weighted multivoting, a team member is asked to distribute his or her allotment of points among as few or as many issues as he or she wants. For example, the team member might give 13 out of 25 points to one issue of particular importance, 3 points each to four other issues, and no points to the remaining issues. After the voting, the numbers are added. Thus, the team will be able to see which issue emerged as particularly important to the team as a whole.

This technique also can be done using colored dots. For example, if eight items are on a chart, the team members might be given four dots each to distribute among the four items that are most important to them. This method provides a visual demonstration of where the consensus lies and what issue has been ranked most important by the team as a whole.

Recommendations for Process Change

The process improvement team is responsible for putting the outcome of its work in a report format, along with recommendations for improving the process. The recommendations are finalized after all data have been received and analyzed. These data include findings from the benchmarking studies as well as from productivity and other measurements. The recommendations should take into account anything that might have an impact on the organization, such as:

- Utilization of staff
- Effect on the budget
- Change in productivity
- Effects on customer requirements

Recommendations are considered by the leadership group and top management for an organization-wide problem or by the management group heading up the HIM department if the problem is confined to just that unit of the organization. Leadership and top management must be kept aware of all developments however, no matter at what level they are occurring. Implementation resources and timing must be supported and committed by them.

After implementing a new process, the team continues to measure performance against customers' expectations and established performance standards. The team may then need to redesign the process or product if measurements indicate that there is room for further improvement. When measurement data indicate that the improvement is effective, ongoing monitoring of the process is resumed (as in figure 10.3). The team documents and communicates its findings to the leadership group and other interested parties in the organization. Results also may be communicated to interested groups in the community.

The team is usually disbanded at this point in the cycle, and routine organizational monitoring of the performance measures is resumed. If another opportunity for improvement arises, the team-based improvement process may be reinstituted. The relationship between organization-wide performance monitoring and team-based PI processes is illustrated in figure 10.17.

Figure 10.17. **Organization-wide and team-based performance improvement model**

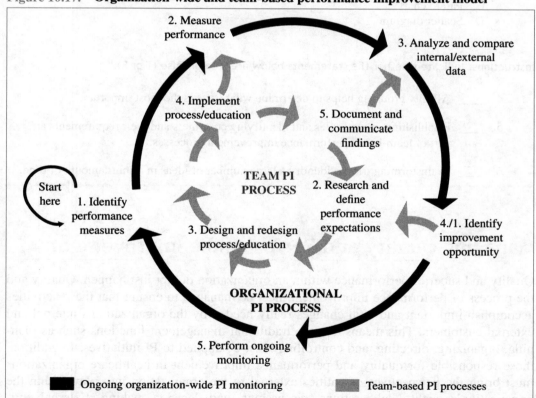

Source: Shaw and Elliot 2012, 6.

Check Your Understanding 10.3

1. Staff members adapt to change more readily when:

   A. Change is mandated by the administration.
   B. They have been part of the decision.
   C. Change is the result of change in accreditation or legislation.
   D. They have seen the value of the desired outcome.

2. Which of the following documents the current process?

   A. Flowchart
   B. Force field analysis
   C. Unstructured brainstorming
   D. Structured brainstorming

3. What technique would be the best to display rankings?

   A. Histogram
   B. Bar graph
   C. Pareto chart
   D. Scatter diagram

Instructions: Indicate whether the statements below are true or false (T or F).

4. ____ Affinity grouping helps to determine what issue is the most important.

5. ____ Establishing ground rules and identifying customers and their requirements are part of team-based performance improvement processes.

6. ____ Brainstorming tries to identify a large number of ideas in a short amount of time.

Managing Quality and Performance Improvement

Quality and superior performance within an organization do not just happen. Quality and the process of performance improvement must be managed to ensure that these activities accomplish important and vital changes really needed by the organization's internal and external customers. This means that the traditional management functions such as planning, organizing, directing, and controlling must be applied to PI initiatives. In addition, those responsible for quality and performance improvement in healthcare organizations must bring the perspectives of entities external to the organization into play within the organization's quality deliberations, discussions, and decision making. External entities that must be considered include agencies offering voluntary accreditation services, agencies involved in the reimbursement cycle, agencies administering licensure services, and agencies offering national quality policy and direction. All must be considered and reflected in an organization's approach to improving its quality and professional performance in order for the quality program to be considered an effective asset to the attaining of the organization's mission and goals as a healthcare organization of superior quality.

Organizational Components of Performance Improvement

To be successful in implementing PI programs, healthcare organizations may have to restructure and create a new culture to accommodate the enormous changes and competition that exist in today's healthcare environment. Changes in customer expectations and the way that healthcare is financed may demand organizational restructuring. Traditional, hierarchical management methods do not necessarily meet the needs of today's customers, the organization's employees, or the organization's operations.

PI must be encompassed in an environment of cooperation. It is most successful in organizations that have an interdisciplinary and participative management approach. As discussed previously, shared vision is one of the cornerstones of a successful PI program. A shared vision puts everyone, including the governing board, upper management, and employees on the same path to organizational success. Changing to a shared leadership environment can create a new organizational culture of shared vision, responsibility, and accountability. Because every employee is a vital part of this shared leadership, this type of environment helps to increase employee motivation and empowerment.

In addition to an enterprise-wide vision, a shared leadership framework is essential for implementing PI. Shared leadership essentially means that organizations ensure that all employees participate in an integrated, continuous PI program. Various organizational frameworks or structures can be developed that encourage shared leadership. One suggested framework includes the following components:

- *Governing board of directors (GBOD):* A GBOD has overall responsibility and accountability for the successful operation of the organization's quality and PI activities and should include membership from the communities of interest, the medical staff, and top organizational administration. The governing board should regularly review current status of quality and PI initiatives and approve all strategic decisions and organizational expenditures of resources concerning them.

- *Quality management board (QMB)*: A QMB has responsibility for the PI program across all subunits of the organization and should include membership from top administration, medical staff officers, top clinical operations staff, and top quality management staff. It should be facilitating all proposals for quality and PI initiatives, making recommendations to the governing board regarding strategic quality direction. It should monitor the progress of all initiatives, providing assistance and advisement as necessary to keep initiatives moving along to completion.

- *Quality management liaison group (QMLG):* A QMLG has responsibility for disseminating information about the organization's quality and PI initiatives throughout the middle management of the organization, for educating managers regarding their roles and the roles of their organizational units in quality and PI initiatives, and for developing cross-functional coordination and communication across organizational units in order to accomplish quality and PI initiatives. In many organizations this type of group is also responsible for maintaining the organization in continuous readiness for accreditation and/or licensure survey.

The organizational structures and processes that constitute a quality management program must be integrated across the entire healthcare organization. To be effective, the organizational unit responsible for quality management must be able to communicate with all areas of the organization and foster interdisciplinary cooperation. Many organizations have actually created a quality management department to help the organization pursue its quality and performance improvement efforts.

The basic responsibilities of the quality management department include:

- Helping departments or groups of departments with similar issues to identify potential quality problems

- Assisting determination of the best methods for studying potential problems (for example, survey, chart review, or interview with staff)

- Participating in regular meetings across the organization, as appropriate, and training organization members on quality and performance improvement methodology, tools, and techniques.

In addition, the quality management department tracks progress on specific quality studies; distributes study results and recommendations to the appropriate bodies (departments, committees, administration, board of directors or trustees); facilitates implementation of educational or structural changes that flow from the recommendations; and ensures that follow-up studies are performed in a timely manner (Longo 1990). Recently, many quality management departments began to assume leadership in the assessing and tracking of organizational compliance with accreditation standards, focus areas, and national patient safety goals.

In hospitals and other large healthcare organizations, the board of directors has ultimate responsibility for ensuring the quality of the medical care provided by the organization. In addition, the board is responsible for the organization's fiscal (financial) stability. If the board is to perform its role, it must be provided regular updates on the organization's clinical quality assessment processes and special projects.

Quality management is best implemented as a cross-functional program. Staff training is critical to success, and new employee orientation should include training in quality management. A permanent multidisciplinary committee should be created to coordinate the program and ensure the consistency of clinical quality assessment processes throughout the organization. The committee should include representatives of the medical staff, nursing staff, and infection control team. Depending on the issue under study, representatives from other areas may be consulted and/or included on a particular assessment. For example, maintenance personnel, safety committee representatives, or departmental supervisors may be included on an issue concerning physical security. In some organizations, specific teams are brought together under the auspices of the quality assessment committee to study a specific issue.

Standards of Organizational Quality in Healthcare

A number of private and government entities develop and maintain standards of organizational quality for healthcare. These entities include agencies and departments of the federal government, accreditation organizations, private for-profit organizations, and not-for-profit organizations such as medical societies and organizations dedicated to research on a specific disease or condition. Standards of quality include descriptive statements called by a number of names, including standards of care, quality of care standards, performance standards, accreditation standards, and practice standards.

A **standard** is a written description of the expected features, characteristics, or outcomes of a healthcare-related service. Standards are generally based on a minimum level of performance. In other words, standards represent the level of performance expected of every healthcare provider and/or providing organization.

Four types of standards are relevant within the context of clinical quality assessment:

- *Clinical practice guidelines* and *clinical protocols:* Detailed step-by-step guides used by healthcare practitioners to make knowledge-based clinical decisions directly related to patient care

- *Accreditation standards:* Predefined statements of the criteria against which the performance of participating healthcare organizations will be assessed during the voluntary accreditation process

- *Government regulations:* Detailed descriptions of the compulsory requirements for participation in the federal Medicare and Medicaid programs

- *Licensure requirements:* Detailed descriptions of the criteria healthcare organizations must fulfill in order to obtain and maintain state licenses to provide specific healthcare services

Clinical Practice Guidelines and Protocols

Standards of clinical quality include both clinical practice guidelines and clinical protocols. According to the Agency for Healthcare Research and Quality, clinical practice guidelines are "systematically developed statements used to assist provider and patient decisions about appropriate health care for specific clinical circumstances" (AHRQ 2005).

The **Agency for Healthcare Research and Quality** (AHRQ) is an agency within the Department of Health and Human Services (HHS). AHRQ's mission is to improve the quality, safety, efficiency, and effectiveness of healthcare for all Americans. Clinical practice guidelines are developed with the goal of standardizing clinical decision making. As the word *guideline* suggests, clinical practice guidelines are not meant to be inflexible and do not apply in every case. Guidelines are updated periodically to reflect the results of recent research studies (figure 10.18).

In contrast to clinical practice guidelines, clinical protocols are treatment recommendations that are often based on guidelines. They describe "generally accepted procedure[s] with clinical steps explicitly recommended by an authoritative body, such as the medical staff" (Larsen-Denning et al. 1997, 575). One example of a clinical protocol is the step-by-step description of the accepted procedure for preparing intravenous solutions at a specific acute care hospital. Another example is described in figure 10.19.

Accreditation Standards

In the United States today, many different organizations monitor the quality of healthcare services and offer accreditation programs for healthcare organizations. All the programs base accreditation on a data collection and submission process followed by a comprehensive survey process. The survey involves measurement of a healthcare facility's performance in comparison to preestablished accreditation standards. Participation in accreditation programs is voluntary. Most accreditation standards are provided to participating healthcare organizations in the form of manuals, such as the Joint Commission's *Comprehensive Accreditation Manual for Hospitals*. (See chapters 7 and 11 for a discussion of accreditation standards.)

The Joint Commission

Since its beginning in 1952, the Joint Commission has continually evolved to meet the changing needs of healthcare organizations. Today, the Joint Commission is the largest healthcare standards-setting body in the world. It conducts accreditation surveys in healthcare organizations and programs in the United States, including hospitals and home care organizations and other healthcare organizations that provide long-term care, assisted living, behavioral healthcare, and laboratory and ambulatory care services (Joint Commission 2010, 2).

In the late 1990s, the Joint Commission moved away from traditional quality assessment processes and began emphasizing performance improvement. Today, the Commission's standards give organizations substantial leeway in selecting performance measures and improvement projects. Required since 1998, all hospitals and long-term care facilities must report outcome measures on at least 20 percent of their patients. **Outcome measures** document the results of care for individual patients as well as for specific types of patients grouped by diagnostic category. For example, an acute care hospital's overall rate of post-surgical infection would be considered an outcome measure. The outcome measures must

Figure 10.18. **Clinical guidelines**

GUIDELINES FOR SCREENING DIABETES IN PREGNANCY
SAN FRANCISCO COMMUNITY HEALTH NETWORK

First prenatal visit: Screen and test clients who present with one or more of the following risk factors:

• Obesity (BMI >30, pre-pregnancy weight)

• Diabetes Mellitus in 1st degree relative

• Prior history of

  • Gestational diabetes or glucose intolerance or use of metformin

  • Macrosomia (>4.0 kg or 8lbs 8oz) or large for gestational age infant (90th percentile)

  • Unexplained stillbirth

  • Malformed infant

• Current glucosuria (100 mg/dl or greater)

24–28 weeks: Screen and test all clients not as yet identified as having gestational diabetes. If initial screening was normal, repeat evaluation.

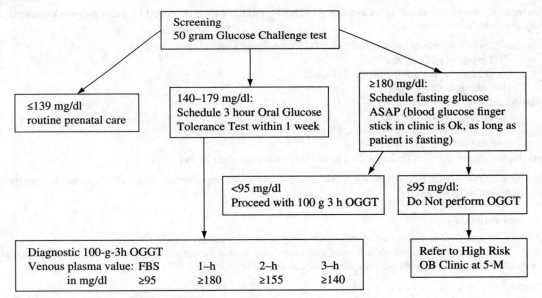

*If two or more values are elevated: treat as gestational diabetes
**If one value is elevated: refer for nutritional counseling. No further testing is necessary. No treatment needed. Re-testing is not necessary if test was done ≥24 weeks.

(continued on next page)

Figure 10.18.   Clinical guidelines *(continued)*

Screening Test for Gestational Diabetes:
50 Gram Oral Glucose Challenge Test (50-g OGCT)

No fasting or dietary restriction required.
Administered during office hours, without respect to time of the day or last meal.
50 grams of glucose, consumed in less than 5 minutes
No smoking
Venous plasma level is drawn one hour from the start of glucose ingestion.

Diagnostic (Confirmatory) Test for Gestational Diabetes:
100 Gram Oral Glucose Tolerance Test (100-g OGTT)

a. Pre-test instructions:
   • Fast for at least 8 hours and no more than 14 hours (water is OK)
   • Instruct clients to eat "normally" (without dietary restrictions) for at least 3 days before the test.
b. Fasting venous plasma drawn
c. 100 grams of glucose, consumed in less than 5 minutes
d. No smoking
e. Venous plasma level is drawn at 1, 2, and 3 hours from start of ingestion of the glucose load.

Postpartum: all clients diagnosed with Gestational Diabetes need to be tested for overt Diabetes 6–8 weeks postpartum and annually thereafter with either:

a. 75 gram 2 hour Glucose Tolerance Test (75-g GTT) (preferred test)
   ≥200 mg/dl overt Diabetes*
   140–199 mg/dl Impaired Glucose Tolerance
   <140 mg/dl normoglycemia
b. fasting glucose (if declines the 75-g GTT)
   ≥126 mg/dl overt Diabetes*
   ≥110 < 126 mg/dl Impaired Fasting Glucose
   <100 mg/dl normoglycemia
Patients that are diagnosed with Diabetes need to be referred back to their PCPs!

*In the absence of unequivocal hyperglycemia and acute metabolic decompensation, these criteria should be confirmed by repeat testing on a different day.

Late-to-care patients:

a. <36 weeks apply same strategy as universal screening at 24–28 weeks.
b. >36 weeks or impending labor regardless of gestational age: obtain fasting glucose (best) >105 mg/dl manage as if GDM, or random glucose (2nd best) >200 mg/dl manage as if GDM.

References:

1. Carr SR. Screening for gestational diabetes mellitus. A perspective in 1998. Diabetes Care. 1998 Aug:21 Suppl 2:B14–8.

2. Brody SC, Harris R, Lohr K. Screening for gestational diabetes: a summary of the evidence for the U.S. Preventive Services Task Force. Obstet Gynecol. 2003 Feb:101(2):380–92. Review.

3. Kjos SL, Buchanan TA. Current Concepts: Gestational Diabetes Mellitus. N Engl J Med 1999:341:1749–1756.

Figure 10.19.   Example of a clinical protocol

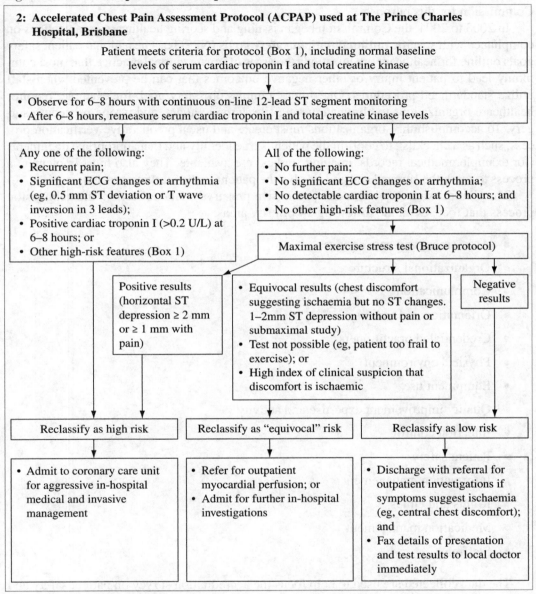

2: Accelerated Chest Pain Assessment Protocol (ACPAP) used at The Prince Charles Hospital, Brisbane

Patient meets criteria for protocol (Box 1), including normal baseline levels of serum cardiac troponin I and total creatine kinase

- Observe for 6–8 hours with continuous on-line 12-lead ST segment monitoring
- After 6–8 hours, remeasure serum cardiac troponin I and total creatine kinase levels

Any one of the following:
- Recurrent pain;
- Significant ECG changes or arrhythmia (eg, 0.5 mm ST deviation or T wave inversion in 3 leads);
- Positive cardiac troponin I (>0.2 U/L) at 6–8 hours; or
- Other high-risk features (Box 1)

All of the following:
- No further pain;
- No significant ECG changes or arrhythmia;
- No detectable cardiac troponin I at 6–8 hours; and
- No other high-risk features (Box 1)

Maximal exercise stress test (Bruce protocol)

Positive results (horizontal ST depression ≥ 2 mm or ≥ 1 mm with pain)

- Equivocal results (chest discomfort suggesting ischaemia but no ST changes. 1–2mm ST depression without pain or submaximal study)
- Test not possible (eg, patient too frail to exercise); or
- High index of clinical suspicion that discomfort is ischaemic

Negative results

Reclassify as high risk

Reclassify as "equivocal" risk

Reclassify as low risk

- Admit to coronary care unit for aggressive in-hospital medical and invasive management

- Refer for outpatient myocardial perfusion; or
- Admit for further in-hospital investigations

- Discharge with referral for outpatient investigations if symptoms suggest ischaemia (eg, central chest discomfort); and
- Fax details of presentation and test results to local doctor immediately

Source: The Prince Charles Hospital, Brisbane

be reported to the Commission via software from vendors that have been approved by the Commission for this purpose.

In 2003 to 2004, the Commission began issuing and scoring healthcare organizations on compliance with specific **national patient safety goals** (NPSGs). The national patient safety goals outline for healthcare organizations the areas of organizational practice that most commonly lead to patient injury or other negative outcomes that can be prevented when staff utilize standardized procedures. One Joint Commission safety goal, for example, requires healthcare organizations to eliminate wrong-site, wrong-patient, and wrong-procedure surgery. To accomplish this, organizations must create and use a preoperative verification process, such as a checklist, to confirm the patient's true identity and that appropriate documents (for example, medical records, imaging studies) are available. They also must implement a process to mark the surgical site and involve the patient in the marking process.

The Commission requires a comprehensive presurvey data collection and submission process that focuses on the following 14 priority areas:

- Assessment and care services
- Organizational structure
- Communication
- Orientation and training
- Credentialed practitioners
- Physical environment
- Equipment use
- Quality improvement expertise and activity
- Infection control
- Patient safety
- Information management
- Rights and ethics
- Medication management
- Staffing

The data collected are used to help focus the accreditation survey on patient safety and high-quality patient care and to select specific patients to "trace" during the on-site survey. This approach, known as tracer methodology, consists of following (tracing) at the time of on-site survey a few patients through their entire stay at the hospital in order to identify quality and patient safety issues that might indicate quality problems and/or patterns of less than optimum care. According to the Commission, "tracer methodology is an evaluation method in which surveyors select a patient, resident or client and use that individual's record as a roadmap to move through an organization to assess and evaluate the organization's compliance with selected standards and the organization's systems of providing care and services" (Joint Commission 2009b). A trace of a surgical patient, for example, might reveal a missing updated history and physical (H&P) on the patient's medical record within 24 hours before surgery. Following this lead, the surveyor might discover that the organization is having an ongoing problem with H&Ps in general, a problem with obtaining the required updated H&P within 24 hours before surgery, or perhaps a problem with just one particular physician.

Other Voluntary Accreditation Organizations

Other voluntary accreditation organizations include the National Committee on Quality Assurance, which focuses its accreditation activities on health plans and outpatient provider organizations, and the Commission on the Accreditation or Rehabilitation Facilities, which focuses on long-term and mental health rehabilitation facilities. Both maintain Internet websites where more information regarding them can be found.

Government Regulations and Licensure Requirements

Various agencies and departments of the federal, state, and local governments also review the quality of services provided in healthcare organizations. However, government regulations and licensure requirements are compulsory rather than voluntary.

Medicare Conditions of Participation

To participate in the Medicare program, healthcare providers must comply with federal regulations known as the Conditions of Participation. The Conditions of Participation are distributed by the Centers for Medicare and Medicaid Services (CMS). CMS administers the Medicare program as well as the federal portion of the Medicaid program. Participation in the Medicare program is critical to the success of many healthcare organizations because a high percentage of healthcare services are delivered to elderly Medicare beneficiaries.

Health Care Quality Improvement Program

In 1992, CMS and peer review organizations (PROs) working under contract with CMS instituted the **Health Care Quality Improvement Program** (HCQIP). Originally, the mission of HCQIP was to promote the quality, effectiveness, and efficiency of services to Medicare beneficiaries by strengthening the community of those committed to improving quality. HCQIP was to monitor and improve quality of care; communicate with beneficiaries, healthcare providers, and practitioners; promote informed health choices; and protect beneficiaries from poor care. Today, HCQIP's approach to improving the health of Medicare beneficiaries involves the analysis of patterns of care to promote changes in the healthcare delivery system.

In 2002, CMS changed the name of the PROs to quality improvement organizations (QIOs). CMS and the QIOs collaborate with practitioners, beneficiaries, providers, plans, and other purchasers of healthcare services to achieve the following goals:

- Develop **quality indicators** that are firmly based in science
- Identify opportunities for healthcare improvements through careful measurement of patterns of care
- Communicate with professional and provider communities about patterns of care
- Intervene to foster quality improvement through system improvements
- Conduct follow-up studies to evaluate success and redirect efforts

HCQIP began work in 1992 with a national quality improvement (QI) project on acute myocardial infarction, the Cooperative Cardiovascular Project. Since then, CMS has expanded its national QI activities and now focuses on six clinical priority areas:

- Acute myocardial infarction
- Breast cancer
- Diabetes
- Heart failure
- Pneumonia
- Stroke

Table 10.2 presents the quality indicators and data sources for each of these clinical topics. CMS selected these priorities because of their importance to public health. In addition, performance in these areas was measurable and there appeared to be a real possibility of improving quality. All are important causes of morbidity and mortality in the US population as a whole and account for large numbers of hospitalizations as well as healthcare expenditures.

CMS's seventh national priority is the reduction of disparities in the healthcare services provided to Medicare beneficiaries. For example, compared to the population overall, African-American Medicare beneficiaries receive fewer preventive services, such as influenza vaccinations. Under CMS's direction, the QIOs are analyzing these disparities in order to implement programs aimed at narrowing the gaps in service.

QIOs use medical peer review, data analysis, and other tools to identify patterns of care and outcomes that need improvement. They then work cooperatively with facilities and individual physicians to improve care. CMS established a comprehensive program in which QIOs use a data-driven approach to monitoring care and outcomes and a shared approach to working with the healthcare community to improve care. In this effort, QIOs also will pursue other types of HCQIP projects, such as important state or local issues, care provided in nonacute hospital settings, and managed care.

Table 10.2. Quality indicators: Medicare's Health Care Quality Improvement Program

Clinical Topic	Quality Indicators	Data Sources
Acute myocardial infarction	1. Early administration of aspirin 2. Early administration of beta blocker 3. Timely reperfusion 4. Aspirin at discharge 5. Beta blocker at discharge 6. Angiotensin-converting enzyme inhibitor (ACEI) at discharge for low left ventricular ejection fraction 7. Smoking cessation counseling during hospitalization	Hospital health records for acute myocardial infarction patients
Breast cancer	1. Biennial mammography screening	Medicare claims (bills) for all female beneficiaries
Diabetes	1. Biennial retinal exam by an eye professional 2. Annual hemoglobin (HbA1c) testing 3. Biennial lipid profile	Medicare claims (bills) for all diabetic beneficiaries
Heart failure	1. Appropriate use/nonuse of ACEI at discharge [excluding discharges on angiotensin-II receptor blocker (ARB)]	Hospital health records for heart failure patients
Pneumonia	1. Influenza vaccinations 2. Pneumococcal vaccinations 3. Blood culture before antibiotics are administered 4. Appropriate initial empiric antibiotic selection 5. Initial antibiotic dose within 8 hours of hospital arrival 6. Influenza vaccination or appropriate screening 7. Pneumococcal vaccination or appropriate screening	1–2: Centers for Disease Control and Prevention Behavioral Risk Factor Surveillance System data 3–7: Hospital health records for pneumonia patients
Stroke	1. Discharged on antithrombotic [acute stroke or transient ischemic attack (TIA)] 2. Discharged on warfarin (atrial fibrillation) 3. Avoidance of sublingual nifedipine (acute stroke)	Hospital health records for stroke, TIA, and chronic atrial fibrillation patients

Source: Originally published as part of CMS publication number 10156.

CMS requires QIOs to offer technical assistance and collaboration on QI projects to every Medicare+Choice plan in their state. QIOs can provide clinical and biostatistical expertise. Further, they can design and conduct quality projects, review and analyze project findings, recommend interventions, and provide advice on data collection (CMS 2005).

State and Local Licensure Requirements

Every state government has required the licensure of hospitals and other types of healthcare organizations since the early 20th century. Some city and county governments also regulate healthcare facilities that operate within local boundaries. The individual states issue licenses that permit facilities to operate within a defined scope of operation. For example, a long-term care organization would be licensed to perform long-term care services, but not acute care services.

To maintain its licensed status, each facility must adhere to the state regulations that govern issues related to staffing, physical facilities, services, documentation requirements, and quality of care. Each facility's performance is usually evaluated annually by survey teams from the state department of health. Healthcare facilities that lose their licenses are no longer allowed to operate in the state.

Check Your Understanding 10.4

1. QIOs use peer review, data analysis, and other tools to:

   A. Evaluate whether or not a healthcare facility is meeting standards for accreditation and licensing
   B. Calculate reimbursement
   C. Penalize healthcare organizations
   D. Identify areas that need improvement

2. Shared leadership means:

   A. Employees are participants in the performance improvement program.
   B. All vice presidents and above are involved in the performance improvement program.
   C. Union leadership and administration lead the performance improvement program.
   D. Board of directors and organizational leadership are responsible for the performance improvement program.

3. The NPSG scores organizations on areas that:

   A. Affect finance stability of the organization
   B. Affect customers
   C. Affect compliance with state law
   D. Commonly lead to patient injury

Instructions: Indicate whether the statements below are true or false (T or F).

4. _____ Accreditation standards were developed to standardize clinical decision making.

5. _____ The Conditions of Participation are used to monitor hospitals and other healthcare organizations in becoming licensed by the state.

6. _____ The mission of AHRQ is to improve quality, safety, efficiency, and effectiveness for all Americans.

Utilization Management

Utilization management (UM) is composed of a set of processes used to determine the appropriateness of medical services provided during specific episodes of care. Whether the services are determined to be appropriate is based on the patient's diagnosis, the site of care, the length of stay (LOS), and other clinical factors. UM processes evaluate the level of care each patient requires. At the same time, they move patients to the most appropriate healthcare setting, evaluate alternative healthcare options, monitor over- and underutilization of services, and attempt to coordinate inefficient scheduling of services.

Basically, UM provides information on how efficiently and cost-effectively the healthcare organization provides the services its customers need. Medicare Conditions of Participation and Joint Commission accreditation standards require acute care hospitals to institute UM programs. In addition, managed care plans such as health maintenance organizations usually conduct rigorous UM processes to control the use of expensive diagnostic, specialty, and hospital care.

Many hospitals have established alternative services to meet the cost-control demands of government payers and managed care plans. Observation beds, same-day surgery services, skilled nursing services, swing beds, and home care services all have decreased inpatient hospital care.

Hospitals can use UM information during contract negotiations with managed care plans to ensure that they are adequately reimbursed for the services they provide. UM information also can be used to evaluate the performance of individual members of the medical staff during the credentialing process.

Functions of Utilization Management

In most hospitals, UM programs perform three important functions: utilization review, case management, and discharge planning.

Utilization Review

Utilization review (UR) is the process of determining whether the medical care provided to a specific patient is necessary. Pre-established objective screening criteria are used as the basis of UR, which is performed according to time frames specified in the organization's UM plan and according to the requirements of the payer guaranteeing the patient's bill.

During the UR process, information about the patient and his or her condition is provided by the patient's physician(s). That information is compared to the organization's screening criteria to determine whether an inpatient admission and/or a clinical service is appropriate and medically necessary. At this point, the payer is usually contacted to approve the findings of the UR process. UR can be performed *prospectively,* before care is provided; *concurrently,* while care is being provided; or *retrospectively,* after the episode of care is complete.

Screening Criteria

UR is based on pre-established screening criteria for inpatient care. **Intensity-of-service screening criteria** determine whether the patient's needed services could be fulfilled most efficiently in an inpatient hospital setting or safely provided on an outpatient basis. For example, if the patient requires invasive surgery that involves a long recovery period, inpatient care would be appropriate. If, however, the procedure could be performed in an ambulatory surgery center, inpatient care would be inappropriate. **Severity-of-illness screening criteria** determine whether the patient's level of physical impairment requires inpatient care.

The hospital may choose whether to develop its own criteria for utilization review or to use criteria established by other sources. Hospital UR may be required to use the criteria established by the payer. Regardless of the criteria selected or developed, the hospital's medical staff should review them periodically and document their formal approval. Screening criteria also are developed and applied by CMS's quality improvement organizations as well as by other third-party payers to establish medical necessity.

Timing

For hospital services, UR is usually performed before the patient is admitted for inpatient care or at the time of admission. Most health insurance and managed care plans require preadmission certification at or before admission to a hospital. Precertification is the process of collecting information to be used for advance eligibility verification, determination of insurance coverage, communication with the physician and/or insured, and initiation of preservice discharge planning and specialized programs such as disease or case management.

Preadmission Utilization Review

Preadmission utilization review is conducted to determine whether the planned service (intensity of service) or the patient's condition (severity of illness) warrants care in an inpatient setting. The purpose of preadmission (or **prospective utilization review**) is to identify patients who do not qualify for inpatient benefits before they are actually admitted. In this way, patients can be referred to the appropriate healthcare setting in a timely manner.

UR also can be conducted at the time of admission, for example, when a patient is admitted to a hospital through its emergency department. The purpose of **admission utilization review** is the same as the purpose of preadmission UR, that is, to identify patients who do not require inpatient care and to direct them to the appropriate healthcare provider.

Continued-Stay Utilization Review

Continued-stay (or **concurrent**) **utilization review** is conducted to determine whether the patient continues to require inpatient care. The purpose of continued-stay review is to ensure that the patient's LOS is not being unnecessarily prolonged and that the hospital's resources are being used efficiently. Some third-party payers require continued-stay UR at specified points during an inpatient stay.

Similar to continued-stay review, **discharge utilization review** is performed to determine whether the patient meets discharge screening criteria and no longer requires services available only in an acute care setting.

Retrospective Utilization Review

Retrospective utilization review is conducted after the patient has been discharged. Retrospective review examines the medical necessity of the services provided to the patient. It may be conducted by a peer review organization or a hospital committee. The purpose of retrospective review is to evaluate quality issues, cost issues, and LOS factors, as well as the appropriateness of the patient's admission and the utilization of hospital resources.

Utilization Review Process

Most hospitals follow a two-step UR process. Nonphysician staff members perform the initial review using information provided by the admitting physician(s). The documentation provided by the physician(s) is compared to the predetermined screening criteria for inpatient admission or continued inpatient stay. When the staff reviewer finds that the screening criteria have not been met, he or she may ask the attending physician(s) to provide additional information. Alternatively, the staff reviewer may refer the case to a member of the medical staff for peer review.

When the reviewing physician determines that the case does not meet the criteria for admission or continued stay, a written notification of denial is prepared. The notification is sent to the attending physician(s), the patient, the business office, and the peer review organization. The patient and the attending physician(s) have the right to request that the decision be reconsidered.

Case Management

A process used in some hospitals, **case management** is the ongoing review of clinical care to ensure the necessity and effectiveness of the services being provided to the patient. It is conducted concurrently with the patient's stay and is performed by clinical professionals (usually registered nurses) employed by acute care hospitals.

The primary role of the case manager is to coordinate and facilitate care. The care-planning process extends beyond the acute care setting to ensure that the patient receives appropriate follow-up services. Many healthcare insurers and managed care organizations also employ case managers to coordinate medical care and ensure the medical necessity of the services provided to beneficiaries.

According to the Center for Case Management (nd), the process of case management is performed to meet the following goals:

- To coordinate multidisciplinary and/or multisetting patient care
- To ensure positive outcomes of care
- To manage the patient's LOS in the acute care facility
- To ensure that the healthcare organization's resources are used efficiently

The need for case management is illustrated by a June 2005 report issued by the Office of Inspector General (OIG). According to the report, which studied patients with three or more stays at an inpatient facility where the admission date for each stay was within one day of the discharge date for the previous stay, 20 percent of the consecutive inpatient stays involved poor-quality care and/or unnecessary fragmentation of care. The report states that the 20 percent was the result of failure to treat patients in a timely manner, inadequate monitoring and treatment of patients, and inadequate care planning (OIG 2005).

Discharge Planning

The purpose of **discharge planning** is to ensure that patients are released from acute care hospitals when they no longer need inpatient care and that if services at a lower level of care are necessary, the patient is referred to that level. Discharge planning is usually managed by the patient's case manager or nurse or by a clinical professional who coordinates discharge planning for the facility. The discharge planner works with the patient and his or her physician(s) and family and/or caregivers to ensure that arrangements have been made to address his or her needs after discharge from the hospital.

Careful discharge planning ensures that the patient can leave the hospital safely and receive the follow-up medical and nursing care he or she needs. For example, a stroke patient who suffered residual hemiplegia might no longer require acute care services and yet still be unable to care for herself at home. She might need continued inpatient care at a rehabilitation facility. Early discharge planning and careful assessment of her medical stability would ensure that she could be transferred safely to the other facility and that the rehabilitation facility would have a room for her after she was discharged from the acute care hospital.

Risk Management

In healthcare, **risk** can be defined as any occurrence or circumstance that might result in a loss. Losses include any damage to an entity's person, property, or rights, including physical injury, cognitive injury, emotional injury, wrongful death, and financial loss. Risk management, therefore, can be defined as a set of policies, processes, and procedures that identify potential operational and financial losses, prevent losses whenever possible, and lessen the effects of losses that cannot be prevented.

The purpose of the **risk management program** should be to link risk management functions to the related processes of quality assessment and performance improvement. The aims of the program are to (1) help provide high-quality patient care while also enhancing a safe environment for patients, employees, and visitors and (2) minimize financial loss by reducing risk through prevention and evaluation.

The basic functions of healthcare risk management programs are similar for most organizations and include:

- Risk identification and analysis
- Loss prevention and reduction
- Claims management

Risk Identification and Analysis

The role of the risk manager is to collect and analyze information on actual losses and potential risks and to design systems that lessen potential losses in the future. Risk managers use information from a variety of sources to identify areas of risk exposure within the organization. Sources of risk management information include:

- Incident reports (sometimes called occurrence reports or occurrence screens)
- Current and past liability claims against the organization
- Performance improvement reports
- Internal inspections of the organization's physical plant and medical equipment
- Reviews conducted by the organization's insurance carriers
- Survey reports from state and local licensing agencies
- Survey reports from accreditation organizations
- Reports of complaints from patients, visitors, medical staff, and employees
- Results of patient satisfaction surveys

An **incident/occurrence report** is a structured tool used to collect data and information about any event *not* consistent with routine operational procedures. In the language of risk management, the documentation of these events is undertaken to identify **potentially compensable events.** A potentially compensable event is an occurrence, such as an accident or medical error, that may result in personal injury or loss of property to patients, staff, visitors, or the healthcare organization.

Incident/occurrence reports are prepared to help healthcare facilities identify and correct problem areas and prepare for legal defense. They are considered extremely confidential documents that are never filed in the patient record and should not be photocopied or prepared in duplicate.

Loss Prevention and Reduction

The risk manager is responsible for developing systems to prevent injuries and other losses within the organization. Performance improvement actions are often initiated in response to suggestions offered by the risk manager. Education also is an invaluable tool in risk management and sometimes is the only activity required to prevent potential safety problems.

Risk managers in many healthcare organizations also are responsible for developing policies and procedures aimed at preventing accidents and injuries and reducing the organization's risk exposure.

Figure 10.20.   Incident or occurrence report

Med Rec #: *00-0545*
Name: *Jackson, Julia*
Date of Birth: *06-22-23*
Street: *6401 Fremont Ave*
City: *Western City, CA*

Risk Management use only: _____   Patient ID/Name of individual involved.
                                                 Use addressograph for patient.

INSTRUCTIONS: (1) Fill out the first page of the Incident Report Form. (2) Select the type of incident from the bottom of page 2. (3) Fill out all appropriate sections as directed. The report must be dated and filled out by the end of the shift in which the incident occurred or was discovered. **DO NOT COPY THIS FORM.** Please print; this report must be legible. **Please fill out all applicable parts of this form.** Upon completion of this form, route it to your Nurse Manager or Supervisor. Do not leave this form in the patient's chart.

Date of incident: *05/29/03*   Time (2400 Clock): *1645*   Hospital Unit: *Med/Surg*

What day of the week
did it occur?   Did the incident occur during: Employee involved worked a(n):
Sun   [√]   Thurs [ ]   Day 0701–1500   [ ]   8 Hour shift   [√]
Mon   [ ]   Fri   [ ]   Evening 1501–2300   [√]   10 Hour shift   [ ]
Tues [ ]   Sat   [ ]   Night 2301–0700   [ ]   12 Hour shift   [ ]
Wed   [ ]   Double shift   [ ]
                                                                        Other _____

Where did the incident occur? *patient room*

Description of incident. Include follow-up care given (i.e., vital signs, x-ray, laboratory tests, etc.).
Pt. developed a macular rash over trunk and extremities after 10 mg

dose of Compazine given for postop nausea. Compazine stopped

and Benadryl given IM.

IMMEDIATE EFFECT OF THE INCIDENT: *Severe macular rash over trunk*

Involved Person Data

Date of Admission: *05/29/03*   Inpatient   [√]
What sex is the person?   Outpatient   [ ]
Male   [ ]   Student   [ ]
Female   [√]   Employee   [ ]
                                        Visitor   [ ]
What is the person's age? _____   Volunteer   [ ]
                                        Other: _____

Current Diagnosis/Reason for visit: *Bowel Obstruction*

Is the involved person aware of the incident?   Yes   [√]   No   [ ]
Is the family aware of incident?   Yes   [ ]   No   [√]

Figure 10.20.   Incident or occurrence report *(continued)*

DO NOT COPY

****   PLEASE PRINT   ****

Person preparing report (Signature): _Gwen Nelson, R.N._   Print: _Gwen Nelson, R.N._

Name of individual witnessing incident (Print): _Bob Patterson, R.N._

Dept/Address: _Med/Surg Team Leader_

Name of employee involved in incident: _Gwen Nelson, R.N._ Dept/Address: _Med/Surg_

Name of employee discovering incident: _Gwen Nelson, R.N._ Dept/Address: _Med/Surg_

**** STAFF TO NOTIFY ATTENDING PHYSICIAN AND/OR DESIGNATED RESIDENT/NURSE PRACTITIONER OF INCIDENT ****

I notified Dr./NP: _Jeff Cook_   at: _1650_   (time).

M.D./NP responded   ☐ in person   ☑ by phone at: _1705_   (time).

Was the attending physician notified?

Yes   [√]   Date: _05 / 29 / 03_ Time: _1650_

No   [ ]   Why not? _____

Examining Physician/Nurse Practitioner statement regarding condition/outcome of person involved:

Pt. was examined by me at 1700 hours. Trunk and extremities
show a macular rash on them. One dose of Benadryl given IM to pt.
and rash began to subside. Compazine stopped.

Examining MD/NP signature: _Tom Lander, M.D. House Staff_

Examining MD/NP name (print): _Tom Lander, M.D._

Date: _05 / 29 / 03_ Time: _1700_   Clinical Service: _Medicine_

CHOOSE THE TYPE OF INCIDENT YOU ARE REPORTING. Use the index below to locate the type of incident you are reporting, go to that section and mark the appropriate box(es). THERE MAY BE MORE THAN ONE ITEM APPLICABLE IN A SECTION. CHECK BOX(ES) IN APPROPRIATE SECTIONS.

Medication/IV Incident	Page 3, Section 1	Patient Behavioral Incident	Page 5, Section 6
Blood/Blood incident	Page 3, Section 2	Safety Incident	Page 5, Section 9
Burn	Page 5, Section 7	Security Incident	Page 5, Section 8
Equipment Incident	Page 5, Section 10	Surgery Incident	Page 5, Section 4
Fall	Page 4, Section 3	Treatment/Procedure Incident	Page 5, Section 5
Fire Incident	Page 5, Section 11		

CONFIDENTIAL: This material is prepared pursuant to Code Annotated, §26-25-1, et seq., and 58-12-43(7, 8, and 9), for the purpose of evaluating healthcare rendered by hospitals or physicians and is NOT PART of the medical record.

(continued on next page)

Figure 10.20.   Incident or occurrence report *(continued)*

SECTION 1 MEDICATION/IV INCIDENT

1A. TYPE OF MEDICATION

Fill in specific medication/solution on the adjacent line.

Analgesic _____
Anesthetic agent _____
Antibiotic _____
Anticoagulant _____
Anticonvulsant _____
Antidepressant _____
Antiemetic___ *Compazine* _____
Antihistamine _____
Antineoplastic _____
Bronchodilator _____
Cardiovascular _____
Contrast media _____
Diuretic _____
Immunizations _____
Immunosuppressive _____
Insulin _____
Intralipids _____
Investigational drug _____
IV solution _____
Laxative_____
Narcotic _____
Oxytocics _____
Psychotherapeutic _____
Radionuclides _____
Sedative/tranquilizer _____
TPN _____
Vasodilator _____
Vasopressor _____
Vitamin _____
Other _____

1B. TYPE OF MEDICATION OR IV INCIDENT

Adverse reaction . . . . [ ] 1B01
Allergic/contraindication. . . . . [ ] 1B02
Delayed stat order . . . . [ ] 1B03
Improper order (MD/NP) . . . . [ ] 1B04
Incompatible additive . . . . [ ] 1B05
Incorrect additive . . . . [ ] 1B06
Incorrect dosage . . . . [ ] 1B07
Incorrect drug . . . . [ ] 1B08
Incorrect narcotic count . . . . [ ] 1B09
Incorrect patient . . . . [ ] 1B10
Incorrect rate of flow . . . . [ ] 1B11
Incorrect route. . . . . [ ] 1B12
Incorrect schedule . . . . [ ] 1B13
Incorrect solution/type . . . . [ ] 1B14
Incorrect time . . . . [ ] 1B15
Incorrect volume. . . . . [ ] 1B16
Infiltration . . . . [ ] 1B17
Given before culture taken . . . . [ ] 1B18
Medication given before lab
  results returned . . . . [ ] 1B19
Medication missing from cart. . . . . [ ] 1B20

Not documented . . . . [ ] 1B21
Not prescribed. . . . . [ ] 1B22
Omitted . . . . [ ] 1B23
Outdated . . . . [ ] 1B24
Out-of-sequence . . . . [ ] 1B25
Patient took unprescribed medication. . . . . . . [ ] 1B26
Repeat administration . . . . [ ] 1B27
Transcription error . . . . [ ] 1B28
Other_____ 1B29

1C. ROUTE OF MEDICATION ORDERED:

IM . . . . [ ] 1C01
IV . . . . [ ] 1C02
PO . . . . [ ] 1C03
Other___ *Suppository* _____ 1C04

1D. MEDICATION DISPENSING INCIDENT

Meds not sent/delayed from pharmacy. . . . . . . [ ] 1D01
Incorrectly labeled . . . . [ ] 1D02
Incorrect dose . . . . [ ] 1D03
Incorrect drug sent . . . . [ ] 1D04
Incorrect IV additive . . . . [ ] 1D05
Incorrect IV fluid . . . . [ ] 1D06
Incorrect route (IV, PO, IM, PR) . . . . [ ] 1D07
Mislabeled. . . . . [ ] 1D08
Other_____ 1D09

SECTION 2
BLOOD/BLOOD COMPONENT INCIDENT

2A. BLOOD/BLOOD COMPONENT TYPE

Albumin. . . . . [ ] 2A01
Cryoprecipitate . . . . [ ] 2A02
Factor VIII (AHF). . . . . [ ] 2A03
Factor IX (Konyne). . . . . [ ] 2A04
Fresh frozen plasma. . . . . [ ] 2A05
Packed red blood cells (PRBC) . . . . [ ] 2A06
Plasmanate®. . . . . [ ] 2A07
Platelets. . . . . [ ] 2A08
RhoGAM®. . . . . [ ] 2A09
Washed red blood cells (WRBC) . . . . [ ] 2A10
Whole blood . . . . [ ] 2A11
Other_____ 2A12

2B. TYPE OF BLOOD/BLOOD COMPONENT
INCIDENT

Crossmatch problem . . . . [ ] 2B01
Improper unit verification. . . . . [ ] 2B02
Inappropriate IV fluids administered
  with blood components. . . . . [ ] 2B03
Inappropriate documentation . . . . [ ] 2B04
Inappropriate storage. [ ] 2B05
Incomplete patient ID . . . . [ ] 2B06
Incorrect patient . . . . [ ] 2B07
Incorrect rate. . . . . [ ] 2B08
Incorrect type . . . . [ ] 2B09
Incorrect volume. . . . . [ ] 2B10
Patient refused . . . . [ ] 2B11
Other_____ 2B12

CONFIDENTIAL: This material is prepared pursuant to Code Annotated, §26-25-1, et seq., and 58-12-43(7, 8. and 9), for the purpose of evaluating healthcare rendered by hospitals or physicians and is NOT PART of the medical record.

Figure 10.20.   Incident or occurrence report *(continued)*

SECTION 3
FALLS

3A. FALL CODE STATUS OF PATIENT
Attended.............................. [ ] 3A01
Unattended .... [ ] 3A02

3B. LOCATION OF FALL
Bathroom in patient's room .... [ ] 3B01
Bathroom (other location)................ [ ] 3B02
Elevator .... [ ] 3B03
Examining/treatment room .... [ ] 3B04
Hallway/corridor .... [ ] 3B05
Nursing station .... [ ] 3B06
Parking lot........................... [ ] 3B07
Patient's room .... [ ] 3B08
Recreation area .... [ ] 3B09
Shower/tub room....................... [ ] 3B10
Stairs .... [ ] 3B11
Waiting room......................... [ ] 3B12
Walkway/sidewalk...................... [ ] 3B13
Other_____   3B14

3C. FALL OCCURRED IN CONJUNCTION WITH:
Bedside commode....................... [ ] 3C01
Chair .... [ ] 3C02
Due to toy .... [ ] 3C03
During transfer .... [ ] 3C04
Exam table........................... [ ] 3C05
Fainting/dizzy .... [ ] 3C06
Fall/slip .... [ ] 3C07
From bed............................. [ ] 3C08
Improperly locked device .... [ ] 3C09
Recreational activity .... [ ] 3C10
Scales .... [ ] 3C11
Stretcher .... [ ] 3C12
Table .... [ ] 3C13
Tripped .... [ ] 3C14
While ambulating unattended .... [ ] 3C15
While ambulating with assist .... [ ] 3C16
While entering or leaving bed............. [ ] 3C17
While using ambulatory device .... [ ] 3C18
Other_____   3C19

3D. PATIENT ACTIVITY PRIVILEGES
(As per medical order)
Ambulate with assistance................. [ ] 3D01
Ambulate with walker.................... [ ] 3D02
Ambulate without assistance.............. [ ] 3D03
Bathroom privileges with assistance .... [ ] 3D04
Bathroom privileges without assistance ...... [ ] 3D05
Bedrest .... [ ] 3D06
Up Ad lib............................ [ ] 3D07
Up in chair/wheelchair .... [ ] 3D08
Other_____   3D09

3E. PATIENT MENTAL CONDITION AT THE
TIME OF THE FALL
Confused/poor judgment.................. [ ] 3E01
Language barrier .... [ ] 3E02
Oriented............................. [ ] 3E03
Unconscious .... [ ] 3E04
Uncooperative .... [ ] 3E05
Unresponsive/medicated .... [ ] 3E06
Other_____

3F. PATIENT'S CALL LIGHT WAS:
On................................. [ ] 3F01
Off................................. [ ] 3F02
Not within reach .... [ ] 3F03
Patient unable to use .... [ ] 3F04
Not applicable .... [ ] 3F05

3G. POSITION OF BED
High................................ [ ] 3G01
Low................................. [ ] 3G02
Intermediate .... [ ] 3G03
Not applicable........................ [ ] 3G04

3H. BED ALARM
On .... [ ] 3H01
Off .... [ ] 3H02
Not applicable........................ [ ] 3H03

3I. POSITION OF SIDE RAILS
(At the time of the fall)

Half Rails   [ ] 3I01   Full Rails   [ ] 3I06
    1 Up   [ ] 3I02   1 Up   [ ] 3I07
    2 Up   [ ] 3I03   2 Up   [ ] 3I08
    3 Up   [ ] 3I04
    4 Up   [ ] 3I05

Not applicable   [ ] 3I09

3J. PATIENT RESTRAINTS
Removed by patient .... [ ] 3J01
Restraints intact .... [ ] 3J02
Not applicable........................ [ ] 3J03
Other_____   3J04

3K. CONDITION OF AREA WHERE FALL
OCCURRED
Normal/dry .... [ ] 3K01
Wet floor............................ [ ] 3K02
Ice condition .... [ ] 3K03
Other_____   3K04

3L. FALLS IN CONJUNCTION
WITH MEDICATION
Narcotic or sedative received by patient
in the past 12 hours?.................... [ ] 3L01
When was the last dose? _____ 3L02
What was the drug? _____ 3L03
What was the route of administration?_____ 3L04

(continued on next page)

Figure 10.20. **Incident or occurrence report** *(continued)*

DO NOT COPY

SECTION 4
SURGERY INCIDENT

Anesthesia occurrence . . . . [ ] 0401
Contamination . . . . [ ] 0402
Incorrect needle count . . . . [ ] 0403
Incorrect sponge count . . . . [ ] 0404
Informed consent absent . . . . [ ] 0405
Informed consent incorrect . . . . [ ] 0406
Instrument lost/broken . . . . [ ] 0407
Retained foreign body . . . . [ ] 0408
Other_____ 0409

SECTION 5
TREATMENT/PROCEDURE INCIDENT

Adverse reaction . . . . [ ] 0501
Allergic response . . . . [ ] 0502
Application/removal of cast/splint . . . . [ ] 0503
Cancellation of procedures . . . . [ ] 0504
Catheter or tube related . . . . [ ] 0505
Delay . . . . [ ] 0506
Dietary problem . . . . [ ] 0507
Dressing/wound occurrence . . . . [ ] 0508
Informed consent absent . . . . [ ] 0509
Informed consent incorrect . . . . [ ] 0510
Injection site . . . . [ ] 0511
Invasive procedure/placement . . . . [ ] 0512
Mislabeled specimen . . . . [ ] 0513
Missing specimen . . . . [ ] 0514
Not documented . . . . [ ] 0515
Omitted . . . . [ ] 0516
Patient/site identification . . . . [ ] 0517
Positioning . . . . [ ] 0518
Prep problem . . . . [ ] 0519
Repeat procedure . . . . [ ] 0520
Reporting of test results . . . . [ ] 0521
Thermoregulation problem . . . . [ ] 0522
Transcription error . . . . [ ] 0523
Transfer/moving of patient . . . . [ ] 0524
Other_____ 0525

SECTION 6
PATIENT BEHAVIORAL INCIDENT

Attempted AWOL . . . . [ ] 0601
AWOL . . . . [ ] 0602
Inappropriate sexual behavior . . . . [ ] 0603
Injured by other patient . . . . [ ] 0604
Patient altercation . . . . [ ] 0605
Self-inflicted injury . . . . [ ] 0606
Suicide gesture . . . . [ ] 0607
Other_____ 0608

SECTION 7
BURNS

Chemical . . . . [ ] 0701
Electrical . . . . [ ] 0702
Inhalation . . . . [ ] 0703
Radioactive . . . . [ ] 0704
Thermal . . . . [ ] 0705

SECTION 8
SECURITY INCIDENTS

Bomb threat . . . . [ ] 0801
Breaking and entering . . . . [ ] 0802
Drug theft . . . . [ ] 0803
Secure area key loss/missing . . . . [ ] 0804
Major theft (over $250) . . . . [ ] 0805
   Amount:_____
Minor theft . . . . [ ] 0806
   Amount:_____
Personal property damage/loss . . . . [ ] 0807
   Amount:_____
Hospital property damage . . . . [ ] 0808
   Amount:_____
Other_____

SECTION 9
SAFETY INCIDENTS (patients and visitors only)

Body fluid exposure . . . . [ ] 0901
Chemical exposure . . . . [ ] 0902
Chemotherapy spill . . . . [ ] 0903
Drug exposure . . . . [ ] 0904
Hazardous material spill . . . . [ ] 0905
Needlestick . . . . [ ] 0906
Other_____ 0907

SECTION 10
EQUIPMENT INCIDENT

Disconnected . . . . [ ] 1001
Electrical problem . . . . [ ] 1002
Improper use . . . . [ ] 1003
Malfunction/defect . . . . [ ] 1004
Mechanical problem . . . . [ ] 1005
Not available . . . . [ ] 1006
Electrical shock . . . . [ ] 1007
Electrical spark . . . . [ ] 1008
Struck by . . . . [ ] 1009
Wrong equipment . . . . [ ] 1010
Tampered with
   By patient . . . . [ ] 1011
   Non-patient . . . . [ ] 1012
Other_____ 1013

SECTION 11
FIRE INCIDENT

Equipment caused . . . . [ ] 1101
Cigarette caused . . . . [ ] 1102
Laser caused . . . . [ ] 1103
Other_____ 1104

CONFIDENTIAL: This material is prepared pursuant to Code Annotated, §26-25-1, et seq., and 58-12-43(7, 8, and 9), for the purpose of evaluating healthcare rendered by hospitals or physicians and is NOT PART of the medical record.

Figure 10.20.   Incident or occurrence report *(continued)*

DO NOT COPY

**EMPLOYEES DO NOT COMPLETE BELOW,
FOR NURSE MANAGER/SUPERVISOR USE ONLY.**

Recommendations and/or corrective actions based on review of report and discussion with employee:

NURSE MANAGER/SUPERVISOR Follow-Up [Check appropriate box(es)/Corrective action]

Policy/Procedure:

Evaluate .... [ ] 1201	**Discussed with:**	
Recommend change................ [ ] 1202	Physician....................... [ ] 1209	
Changed .... [ ] 1203	Staff .... [ ] 1210	
No action taken .... [ ] 1204	Patient......................... [ ] 1211	
Non-compliance .... [ ] 1205	Other........................... [ ] 1212	
Inadequate .... [ ] 1206		
Needs enforcement .... [ ] 1207	Date: _____	
Review with involved individual(s).... [ ] 1208	Time: _____	

Describe specific follow-up actions taken (if applicable include names of depts). _____
_____
_____

SIGN AND DATE: (Indicates review of report)

1. Quality Management/Risk Management_____ ___/___/___

2. Nurse Manager/Supervisor (as applicable) _____ ___/___/___

3. Department Head/DON (as applicable) _____ ___/___/___

4. QM Coordinator (as applicable)_____ ___/___/___

5. Other: Title_____ Name _____ ___/___/___

BIOENGINEERING USE ONLY

Manufacturer contacted	[ ] 1301
Manufacturer instructions followed....................................	[ ] 1302
Needs enforcement of policy/procedure................................	[ ] 1303
Include instructions in staff education and training	[ ] 1304
Preventative maintenance or biomedical evaluation of equipment ordered ...	[ ] 1305
Recommend repair or replacement....................................	[ ] 1306
Removed from service	[ ] 1307
Other _____	[ ] 1308

RISK MANAGEMENT USE ONLY

IMMEDIATE EFFECT OF THE INCIDENT

Alteration in skin integrity .... [ ] 1401	Patient discomfort/inconvenience...... [ ] 1411	
Birth related injury .... [ ] 1402	Psycho/social trauma .... [ ] 1412	
Breach of confidentiality .... [ ] 1403	Reproductive injury or loss .... [ ] 1413	
Death........................... [ ] 1404	Sensory impairment .... [ ] 1414	
Disability .... [ ] 1405	Severe internal injuries.............. [ ] 1415	
Disfigurement.................... [ ] 1406	Substantial disability .... [ ] 1416	
Drug/blood reaction............... [ ] 1407	Unanticipated neuro deficit........... [ ] 1417	
Fluid imbalance .... [ ] 1408	Unanticipated systemic deficit .... [ ] 1418	
Neuro deficit .... [ ] 1409	Indeterminate .... [ ] 1419	
Orthopedic injury .... [ ] 1410	None .... [ ] 1420	
	Other_____ [ ] 1421	

Description_____

CONFIDENTIAL: This material is prepared pursuant to Code Annotated, §26-25-1, et seq., and 58-12-43(7, 8, and 9), for the purpose of evaluating healthcare rendered by hospitals or physicians and is NOT PART of the medical record.

Source: Shaw and Elliot 2012, 190–196.

Claims Management

Claims management is the process of managing the legal and administrative aspects of the healthcare organization's response to injury claims. It is handled differently by different sizes and types of organizations. Accordingly, the role of the risk manager in managing claims varies. Many organizations place the entire process in the hands of their liability insurance vendors. In such cases, the risk manager may act as the organization's liaison with the insurance company. However, some organizations are self-insured, meaning that they establish a dedicated fund for financing future liability settlements. In such cases, the risk manager may manage the entire claims management process.

In most healthcare organizations, the claims management process involves the following general steps (Barton 1997):

1. *Reporting of claims:* Written claims for damages and/or formal legal notifications of the intent to seek compensation for injuries are given to the person responsible for risk management in the organization. The risk manager then notifies the organization's administration and its insurance vendor and/or corporate counsel. The risk manager also reports and investigates potentially compensable events for which no claims have been filed.

2. *Initial investigation of claims:* The risk manager gathers all the information relevant to the claim or the potentially compensable event, including information about the injured parties or claimants; information about the departments and/or caregivers involved in the incident; information about the individuals named as defendants in lawsuits; dates; insurance information; extent of injuries; current status of the case; summary of the claimant's allegations; summary of health record information; summaries of interviews with witnesses and participants; and copies of relevant policies, procedures, clinical protocols, practice standards, and equipment maintenance records.

3. *Protection of primary and secondary health records:* The health records of patients involved in potentially compensable events and claims should be completed as soon as possible after the patients are discharged. The primary and secondary records should then be secured in a locked storage place. Any written incident reports, investigative reports, peer review records, and credentialing files relevant to the case also should be protected.

4. *Negotiation of settlements:* Many claims for compensatory damages are settled out of court. After the healthcare organization has determined whether it is at fault in a case, the organization's risk manager, insurance representative, administration, and/or legal counsel decide whether to offer a monetary settlement. If the organization and the injured party agree on a settlement, the case is brought to a close before judicial proceedings are undertaken.

Patient Advocacy

Many large healthcare organizations such as acute care hospitals have instituted **patient advocacy** programs. In such programs, a patient representative (sometimes called an ombudsperson) responds personally to complaints from patients and their families. Many times, patients and their families are looking for nothing more than an explanation of an adverse occurrence or an apology for a mistake or misunderstanding. Patient representatives are trained to handle minor complaints and to seek remedies on behalf of patients. They also are trained to recognize serious problems that need to be forwarded to performance improvement and/or risk management personnel.

According to the healthcare ombudsperson model, all parties benefit because the ombudsperson (Houk 2003):

- Intervenes at the earliest possible opportunity at the lowest possible level
- Maintains informality, confidentiality, and independence
- Resolves potentially compensable events through timely communication
- Is a professional trained in communicating adverse outcomes and mediation skills
- Has the time built into his or her job to spend with patients and providers
- Is sanctioned by top leadership to move fluidly horizontally and vertically within the existing organizational structure

Regulatory and Accreditation Requirements for Risk Management in Acute Care Hospitals

Anything that undermines patient safety is a risk issue. According to the Joint Commission, all hospital activities must be evaluated as to the potential risk to the patient or to the organization. Leadership is responsible for ensuring adequate resources for patient safety.

Sentinel Events

The Joint Commission requires healthcare organizations to conduct in-depth investigations of occurrences that resulted—or could have resulted—in life-threatening injuries to patients, medical staff, visitors, or employees. The Joint Commission uses the term *sentinel event* for such occurrences.

A sentinel event, therefore, describes an occurrence with an undesirable outcome usually occurring only once. The occurrence, however, points to serious issues involved in care processes that must be resolved in order not to suffer the occurrence again. According to the Joint Commission, it is:

- An unexpected occurrence involving death or serious physical or psychological injury, or the risk thereof. Serious injury specifically includes loss of limb or function. The phrase "or the risk thereof" includes any process variation for which a recurrence would carry a significant chance of a serious adverse outcome.

- An outcome of such magnitude that each event requires an investigation and response.

Examples of sentinel events include medical errors, explosions and fires, and acts of violence. When these occur, the healthcare organization is required to prepare a detailed report of its investigation to explain the root cause of the event so that similar events can be averted in the future. The Joint Commission issues sentinel event alerts when it detects a pattern of similar events reported by the healthcare organizations it accredits. The Joint Commission uses its sentinel events data as a basis for its National Patient Safety Goals.

Check Your Understanding 10.5

1. A group of processes that determine the appropriateness of medical services is:
   A. Utilization management
   B. Utilization review
   C. Case management
   D. Risk management

2. A patient has been discharged prior to an administrative utilization review being conducted. Which of the following should be performed?
   A. Continued stay utilization review
   B. Discharge plan
   C. Retrospective utilization review
   D. Case management

3. A patient fell out of the bed. What should be done?
   A. Case management
   B. Conduct a continued stay utilization review
   C. Perform claims management functions
   D. Complete an incident occurrence report

4. A patient is dissatisfied with his or her care. Who should the patient contact at the hospital?
   A. Utilization review coordinator
   B. Risk manager
   C. Patient representative/advocate
   D. Discharge planner

5. A woman dies in labor and delivery. The Joint Commission would call this type of outcome a(n):

    A. Sentinel event

    B. Potentially compensable event

    C. Incident

    D. Occurrence screens

Recent Clinical Quality Management Initiatives

New initiatives and processes that seek to ensure high-quality care and patient safety characterize the beginning of the 21st century. Stemming from the IOM 1999 and 2001 reports on the quality of healthcare in America, a consensus developed around the need to use information technology as both a methodology and a pathway for managing and improving healthcare quality.

The beginning of the 21st century also has witnessed attempts to link clinical quality to reimbursement for health services. Recent pay-for-performance initiatives by the federal government, the Joint Commmission, and private payers are rewarding organizations for quality outcomes. It is hoped that these funds will encourage healthcare providers to invest in technology that will improve patient care and safety.

In recent years, CMS has become an advocate for pay for performance within the Medicare program. One of its efforts requires hospitals participating in the Medicare program to collect and report on 10 proven hospital quality measures in 3 clinical areas to qualify for full inpatient prospective payment. Those that do not report their data on acute myocardial infarction, heart failure, and pneumonia face a 4 percent penalty per case. Medicare expects hospitals to compare their own data to national and regional averages in order to identify areas for quality improvement (see figure 10.21).

Finally, the early part of the 21st century has witnessed new and creative efforts to encourage medical error reporting. Federal legislation enacted in 2005 allows for the voluntary reporting of medical errors, serious adverse events, and their underlying causes. According to then Joint Commission President Dennis O'Leary, the Patient Safety and Quality Improvement Act "was a breakthrough in the blame and punishment culture that has literally held a death grip on health care. When caregivers feel safe to report errors, patients will be safer because we can learn from these events and put proven solutions into place" (Joint Commission 2005). Subsequent emphasis by the Joint Commission on patient safety issues has resulted in voluminous research and new programs sponsored by the Commission to assist its accreditation customers in improving this all-important area of healthcare organization functioning.

Figure 10.21.   Ten clinical quality measures

To receive full reimbursement from Medicare under the inpatient prospective payment system (IPPS), hospitals must report data for the following 10 quality measures to CMS:

Acute myocardial infarction

1. Acute myocardial infarction (AMI) patients without aspirin contraindications who received aspirin within 24 hours before or after hospital arrival

2. AMI patients without aspirin contraindications who are prescribed aspirin at hospital discharge

3. AMI patients with left ventricular systolic dysfunction (LVSD) and without angiotensin converting enzyme inhibitor (ACEI) contraindications who are prescribed ACEI at hospital discharge

4. AMI patients without beta blocker contraindications who received a beta blocker within 24 hours after hospital arrival

5. AMI patients without beta blocker contraindications who are prescribed a beta blocker at hospital discharge

Heart failure

6. Heart failure patients with documentation in the hospital record that left ventricular function was assessed before arrival, during hospitalization, or is planned for after discharge

7. Heart failure patients with LVSD and without ACEI contraindications who are prescribed an ACEI at hospital discharge

Pneumonia

8. Pneumonia patients who receive their first dose of antibiotics within four hours after arrival at the hospital

9. Pneumonia patients age 65 and older who were screened for pneumococcal vaccine status and were administered the vaccine prior to discharge, if indicated

10. Pneumonia patients who had an assessment of arterial oxygenation by arterial blood gas measurement or pulse oximetry within 24 hours prior to or after arrival at the hospital

Source: Adapted from CMS 2005.

Accountable Care Organizations

Proposed in the Affordable Care Act of 2010, an **Accountable Care Organization** (ACO) is a network of doctors and hospitals that shares responsibility for providing care to patients. An ACO would agree to manage all of the healthcare needs of a minimum of 5,000 Medicare beneficiaries for at least three years. "By focusing on the needs of patients and linking payment rewards to outcomes, this delivery system reform will help improve the health of individuals and communities while saving as much as $960 million over three years for the Medicare program. Under the proposal, ACOs—teams of doctors, hospitals, and other health care providers and suppliers working together—would coordinate and improve care for patients with Original Medicare (that is, those who are not in Medicare Advantage private health plans). To share in savings, ACOs would meet quality standards in five key areas:

- Care coordination
- Patient/caregiver care experiences
- Patient safety
- Preventive health
- At-risk population/frail elderly health

The proposed rules also include strong protections to ensure patients do not have their care choices limited by an ACO" (HHS 2011).

Six Sigma

Benchmarking has been long practiced within the domain of the healthcare system. However, some healthcare organizations have begun to benchmark against other industries and are selecting models that may be adapted to the healthcare industry. For example, some healthcare organizations have begun applying the Six Sigma philosophy to their PI programs. **Six Sigma** is practiced widely in business sectors outside healthcare, and this philosophy is gaining acceptance in the healthcare industry (Shortell and Selberg 2002).

Six Sigma uses statistics for measuring variation in a process with the intent of producing error-free results. Sigma refers to the standard deviation used in descriptive statistics to determine how much an event or observation varies from the estimated average of the population sample. For example, a student who scores 130 on an IQ test would be considered to have a higher IQ than 97.5 percent of the population. The average IQ is considered to be 100, and the standard deviation for IQ is 15 points. Thus, a score of 130 is a variation of two standard deviations above the average. Only 2.5 percent of the population is estimated to have scores above two standard deviations.

Six Sigma was chosen as a target statistic because even two or three standard deviations would not be acceptable in certain scenarios. A 2.5 percent error rate for making correct change at a movie theater may be acceptable, but that error rate for airlines avoiding fatal crashes is completely unacceptable, because airlines have hundreds of flights in the air on any given day. Even if there were only 100 flights per day, two to three fatal crashes per day would be devastating to the airline industry, not to mention the population as a whole. Therefore, it is important to keep this PI approach in proper perspective when it is applied to healthcare.

The Six Sigma measure indicates no more than 3.4 errors per 1 million encounters. Consider the challenge of achieving no more than 3.4 errors per 1 million prescriptions, surgeries, or diagnoses. In certain areas, this standard may seem unattainable, and in others, it may not be rigorous enough. However, incorporating Six Sigma into PI requires considerable organizational change.

Actually deploying Six Sigma in healthcare requires the identification of elements of a product line that are "critical to quality" or CTQs. Focus groups or interviews can be used to elicit the CTQs from the customers for the product. Typically in healthcare, the customers will be the patients/consumers and the providers/physicians. All others involved—the corporations, the payers, the accreditors/licensers—are identified as stakeholders, entities with an important interest in the product that do not have consumer relationships to it. Underpinning the CTQs are elements "critical to process" (CTPs). These also can be identified by such techniques as focus groups or interviews and represent those aspects of the process that make the accomplishment of CTQs possible.

For example, the American Diabetes Association (ADA) and the National Committee on Quality Assurance (NCQA) have joined together to promote a CTQ (http://www.ncqa.org/tabid/139/Default.aspx), "to provide physicians with tools to support the delivery of high quality diabetes mellitus care" and to recognize those providers who are able to maintain the CTQ in their practices. The CTPs supporting this CTQ include the first 10 evidence-based measures of the diabetes care seen in Table 10.3. In addition, the program offered by the ADA/NCQA provides a computer application in which the provider can record the findings for each patient on a regular basis. The output of the application is forwarded to the ADA/NCQA on a regular basis, and when validated by them, the provider is placed on a public recognition list as meeting these evidence-based criteria and thus offering superior care for diabetes mellitus. Patients win as customers. Providers win as customers. ADA wins as a stakeholder in promoting better diabetes mellitus care. Payers win as stakeholders in identifying providers who use best practices in the management of diabetes mellitus.

Table 10.3.   Diabetes care CTPs

Diabetes Recognition Measure	Threshold (% of patients in sample)	Weight
HbA1c Control >9.0%	≤15%	15.0
HbA1c Control <7.0%	40%	10.0
Blood Pressure Control ≥140/90 mmHg	≤35%	15.0
Blood Pressure Control <130/80 mmHg	25%	10.0
LDL Control ≥130 mg/dL	≤37%	10.0
LDL Control <100 mg/dL	36%	10.0
Eye Examination	60%	10.0
Foot Examination	80%	5.0
Nephropathy Assessment	80%	5.0
Smoking Status and Cessation Advice or Treatment	80%	10.0
Total Points		**100.0**
Points Needed to Achieve Recognition		**75.0**

Virtuoso Teams

Publications on performance improvement have given much attention to teamwork. A recent book by Boynton and Fischer (2005) presents cases studying "virtuoso teams" that take a different approach to team membership and processes. The authors studied cases in businesses like Ford Motor Company, Cray Computers, IBM, and Microsoft (Boynton and Fischer 2005). Members of **virtuoso teams** were hand picked for their exceptional expertise in a particular field and given ambitious goals. Rather than selecting team members according to their availability and experience as is done with traditional teams, virtuoso teams "comprise the elite experts in their particular fields and are specially convened for ambitious projects" (Fischer and Boynton, 2005). The authors believe this group of hand-picked, elite experts "work best when members are forced together in cramped spaces under strict time constraints" (Boynton and Fischer 2005). "When virtuoso teams begin their work, individuals are in and group consensus is out" (Boynton and Fischer 2005). Leaders of these teams encourage collaboration and creative confrontation. Instead of relying on e-mail, phone calls, and occasional meetings, virtuoso teams engage in intense, face-to-face conversations. Where politeness and repression of individual egos is the norm in traditional teams, members of virtuoso teams celebrate individual egos, compete, and create opportunities for solo performances (Boynton and Fischer 2005). Virtuoso teams operate on the assumption that members have a stake in their reputation and are therefore energized to create notable results. This book was recommended to healthcare executives shortly after its publication, suggesting that healthcare executives will consider forming virtuoso teams for certain projects in the future. Leaders and participants in virtuoso teams will be expected to employ different skills and methods of interaction than they have experienced in previous team participation.

ISO 9000 Certification

If healthcare organizations expand into global entities, they will be required to deal with the same issues that other industries face when doing business outside the United States. **ISO 9000 certification** is part of a PI system that is required to conduct business in certain foreign countries. The International Organization for Standardization in Geneva, Switzerland, first published ISO 9000 standards in 1987. Into the 1990s, it was much more prevalent in European countries than in the United States. ISO 9000 sets specification standards for quality management with regard to process management and product control. In the healthcare setting, product control is quality control of patient care activities. Companies that document and demonstrate compliance with ISO 9000 standards can receive certification by independent ISO auditors.

In 1998, a few hospitals in the United States moved to adopt ISO 9002 standards, an enhancement of the original ISO 9000 standards. The American Legion Hospital in Crowley, Louisiana, dropped JCAHO accreditation and adopted ISO 9002. The Pulaski

Community Hospital in Virginia's New River Valley continued with the Joint Commission accreditation but also adopted ISO 9002 standards (Babwin 1998).

Whether other hospitals will follow the lead of these two remains to be seen. Although the American Legion Hospital in Louisiana must undergo a state audit to continue receiving Medicare payments, adopting ISO 9002 certification and dropping Joint Commission accreditation reportedly reduced its costs by $100,000 a year. These standards are very similar to those of The Joint Commission and incorporate the CMS requirements outlined in its Conditions of Participation. The actual survey process is also similar, and the NIAHCO uses the tracer methodology now familiar to all healthcare professionals who have participated in a Joint Commission survey (DNVHC 2012). In 2000, ISO made a significant revision to its 9000-level standards, discontinuing its 9002 and 9003 standard sets and refocusing its attention on the 9001 set. This is the current set that could be used for performance improvement purposes in healthcare organizations. The actual requirements for certification begin in the fourth chapter of the standards (with the first three chapters covering a variety of introductory and legalistic subjects):

- Chapter 4.1 Systemic Requirements sets forth standards for developing, implementing, and improving the quality management system; 4.2 sets forth standards for developing and maintaining quality system documents, manuals, and records.

- Chapter 5.1 sets forth standards for promoting and improving the quality management system; 5.2 sets standards for identifying, meeting, and enhancing customer expectations; 5.3 establishes the organization's quality policy and commitment to continual improvement; 5.4 requires a quality management system plan and objectives; 5.5 and 5.6 control and evaluate the quality management system.

- Chapter 6.1 through 6.4 provides for resources, personnel, infrastructure, and environment to support the quality management system.

- Chapter 7 is about making the quality management system a reality in terms of product/process development, purchasing, and operational activities.

- Chapter 8 is about monitoring and measuring product/process quality and identifying and making necessary quality improvements.

Real-World Case

Donna began her position as Director of Health Information Services at a large, metropolitan teaching hospital only one week ago. Arriving at work one morning during her second week, she found in her departmental mailbox a handwritten form with the title "Occurrence Report" in bold written across the top. Indeed, when she examined the contents of the recording, she realized that it was a report of occurrence regarding something that had happened with respect to HIS.

This particular hospital operated on the premises, in addition to its inpatient service, fifteen primary care and specialty clinics, for which HIS staff pulled 1,000 to 1,200 records per clinic day. The first order of business every morning was the delivery of the records to each clinic, some of which had to be transported via ancient, badly paved tunnels connecting the main hospital to clinics in peripheral buildings. Usually, the female clerks delivered to the main hospital and the male clerks delivered via the tunnels, but if staff were on vacation or out sick, it occasionally was necessary for the female clerks to use the tunnels. After delivery to a clinic, it was the responsibility of the clinic clerical staff to distribute the records to the appropriate provider or care area within the clinic.

The occurrence report received had been written by one of the supervisors of the General Medicine Clinic, one of the largest clinics on campus. It recounted, emphasizing that this was not the first time that this had happened, that the equipment used for transport of the records to the clinic the previous morning was in disrepair when used and had toppled over and injured one of the clinic staff. Donna contacted the supervisor of the file section of HIS and ordered that the offending piece of equipment be taken out of service and either repaired or discarded. Over the course of the following few weeks, the same scenario was repeated two times. Once again from the General Medicine Clinic (probably because its volume of records was so high), then from the OB-Gyn Clinic. Then, an HIS clerk returning in the evening from the clinic via the tunnels with a heavy load of returning records was injured when the equipment toppled over in the tunnel injuring his foot. It now became obvious to Donna that some comprehensive review of the equipment used was necessary.

Over many years, HIS at this institution had used carts designed for use in libraries to transport records to clinics. All of this type of equipment had open shelving top and front and sides, minimally soldered to uprights. Most were no taller than 4 feet. On all of them the wheels were removable. However, removable wheels meant that given an uneven surface they could fall out. Minimal soldering meant that under the pressure of hundreds of records the solder joints would break and the shelving would come loose from the uprights.

Donna decided to begin her investigation with the clinic supervisor. The story was pretty much as had been detailed in the occurrence reports. However, the same scenario had occurred multiple times over the last five years, but no one ever seemed to listen. The supervisor obviously harbored a lot of anger and hostility toward HIS for subjecting her staff to the inferior equipment. Next, Donna contacted the Director of Materials Management to see if she had resources other than the standard catalogues that had been used up until then to replace broken equipment. She did not, but she added that she had requested multiple times of the previous HIS Director not to continue to throw money away on the library type of equipment, again a request that went unheeded. She did give Donna the contact information for a materials consultant that the institution often used to find materiel that was difficult to identify through the usual channels. She also recommended that Donna discuss the situation with members of the occupational health team, one of whom was well-versed in ergonomic principles. Those folks also discussed the issue with the institution's worker's compensation insurer to see if they might be willing to fund a project to lessen the risk associated with the equipment now being used.

As the story played out, Donna had effectively put together an informal "virtuoso team." The materials management consultant knew of a sister institution nearby that had recently replaced transport equipment. She identified the company that had designed and built that equipment, and brought the owner/engineer of that company to review the situation. After interviewing HIS and clinic staff and the occupational health ergonomics expert, he designed and built several alternative prototypes, which he brought to the institution for review. The occupational health representative was successful in getting the worker's compensation insurer to fund the design and replacement of the transport equipment. After the prototypes had been delivered, Donna asked the occupational health expert to review the designs, demonstrate the equipment, and gain feedback from HIS and clinic staff on which design worked best in the multiple situations in which it had to be used. The occupational health expert would also be making ultimate recommendations regarding the ergonomic issues based on her own views about what was best for the individuals who actually had to use the equipment. Finally, the Director of Materials Management worked diligently to get the chosen prototype ordered, delivered, and paid for by the worker's comp insurer in a timely fashion.

The new clinic transport equipment—or carts, as some prefer to call them—worked out wonderfully. Built of heavy steel, they are enclosed on back, sides, top and bottom (also nice for HIPAA compliance). They are welded, not soldered, together in a manner that still allows some give to the structure when it is moving across uneven surfaces so that the welds do not fracture. Perhaps most important, the wheels, now heavy-duty casters, are solidly attached to the bottom so that they cannot pop out. The final product was a little heavy, but it moves smoothly down the halls and tunnels rather than bowing and scraping over every little flaw in the floor or pavement. Everyone is happy.

Summary

The pursuit of improvement in the US healthcare system has a long history and is itself based in the history of medicine. Methodologies for improvement have been put forward since the advent of Medicare, but the greatest focus has been developed over the last 20 years. Benefiting from the theoretical writings of industrial engineers like W. Edwards Deming and John Crosby and from the applications of the theory by many private, governmental, and accreditation entities, healthcare organizations have by and large come to be more adept at pursuing what is now most frequently called *performance improvement*. Knowledge of it is an important component of the practice of every healthcare professional. All must be able to participate in the common performance improvement cycles. All professionals should be able to design indicators and measures of the important functions of their organizational units. They should also be able to apply common performance improvement tools such as bar graphs, run charts, and affinity diagramming to participate in and assist their PI teams in improving the quality of the care provided by each individual in the organization. Taking these philosophies, tools, and techniques to heart is the only real way that determined and lasting improvement can be effectively accomplished in a healthcare organization today.

References

Agency for Healthcare Research and Quality. 2005. Clinical practice guidelines. http://www.ahrq.gov/clinic/cpgarchv.htm

Babwin, D. 1998. Move over, JCAHO. *Hospitals and Health Networks* 72(10):57–58.

Barton, E.J. 1997. Claims and litigation. In *Risk Management Handbook for Health Care Organizations,* 2nd ed. Edited by R. Carroll. Chicago: American Hospital Publishing.

Batalden, P.B., and P.K. Stoltz. 1993. A framework for the continual improvement of health care: Building and applying professional and improvement knowledge to test changes in daily work. *Journal on Quality Improvement* 19(10):424–447.

Berwick, D.M. 1989. Continuous improvement as an ideal in health care. *New England Journal of Medicine* 320(1):53–56.

Boynton, A., and B. Fischer. 2005. *Virtuoso Teams: Lessons from Teams that Changed Their Worlds.* New York: FT Prentice Hall.

Center for Case Management. nd. Welcome: About the Center for Case Management. http://cfcm.com/home.asp

Centers for Medicare and Medicaid Services. 2005. CMS home page. http://www.cms.gov

Department of Health and Human Services. 2011. Affordable Care Act to Improve Quality of Care for People with Medicare. http://www.hhs.gov/news/press/2011pres/03/20110331a.html

DNVHC, Inc. 2012. Dnvusa.com/focus/hospital_accreditation

Donabedian, A. 1988. The quality of care: How can it be assessed? *Journal of the American Medical Association* 260(12):1743–1748.

Fischer, B., and A. Boynton. 2005. Harvard Business Review. Virtuosis Teams. http://hbr.org/2005/07/virtuoso-teams/ar/1

Houk, C. 2003. From dispute resolution to conflict management. Presentation at NADRAC 2004 Conference, Sydney, Australia.

Imai, M. 1986. *Kaizen: The Key to Japanese Competitive Success.* New York: Random House.

Joint Commission. 2005. News release: Joint Commission hails enactment of Patient Safety and Quality Improvement Act of 2005.

Joint Commission. 2009a. *Comprehensive Accreditation Manual for Hospitals.* Oakbrook Terrace, IL.

Joint Commission. 2009b. Facts about patient safety. http://www.jointcommission.org/PatientSafety

Joint Commission. 2010. Inspiring health care excellence. http://www.jointcommission.org/NR/rdonlyres/3602CE1F-E2BB-4FF0-985E-49560E50DE1F/0/InspiringHCexcellenceweb1113.pdf

Kelly, D.L. 2003. *Applying Quality Management in Healthcare: A Process for Improvement.* Chicago: Health Administration Press.

Larsen-Denning, L., et al. 1997. Clinical practice guidelines. In *Risk Management Handbook for Health Care Organizations*, 2nd ed. Edited by R. Carroll. Chicago: American Hospital Publishing.

Longo, D. 1990. Integrating quality assurance into a quality management plan. In *Quality Assurance in Hospitals: Strategies for Assessment and Implementation.* Edited by N. Graham. Rockville, MD: Aspen Publishers.

McLaughlin, C.P., and A.D. Kaluzny. 2006. *Continuous Quality Improvement in Health Care: Theory, Implementation, and Applications,* 3rd ed. Gaithersburg, MD: Aspen.

Meisenheimer, C.G. 1997. *Improving Quality: A Guide to Effective Programs,* 2nd ed. Sudbury, MA: Jones and Bartlett.

National Academy of Engineering/Institute of Medicine. 2005. *Building a Better Delivery System.* Washington, DC: The National Academies Press.

Office of Inspector General. 2005. Consecutive Medicare inpatient stays. http://www.oig.hhs.gov/oei/reports/oei-03-01-00430.pdf

Omachonu, V.K. 1999. *Healthcare Performance Improvement.* Norcross, GA: Engineering and Management Press.

Pugh, M.D. 2005. Dashboards and scorecards: Tools for creating alignment. In *The Healthcare Quality Book: Vision, Strategy, and Tools.* Edited by S.B. Ransom, M.S. Joshi, and D.B. Nash. Chicago: Health Administration Press.

Shaw, P., and C. Elliott. 2012. *Quality and Performance Improvement in Healthcare: A Tool for Programmed Learning,* 5th ed. Chicago: AHIMA.

Shortell, S.M., and J. Selberg. 2002. "Working differently: The IOM's call to action." *Healthcare Executive* 17(1):6–10.

Additional Resources

American Society for Healthcare Risk Management. 2005. http://www.ashrm.org

Atlantic Information Services. 1995. A Guide to Patient Satisfaction Survey Instruments, 2nd ed. Washington, DC: Atlantic Information Services, 5–6.

Centers for Medicare and Medicaid Services. 2009. http://www.cms.gov/HospitalQualityInits

Fried, B., and W. Carpenter. 2006. Understanding and improving team effectiveness in quality improvement. In *Continuous Quality Improvement in Health Care: Theory, Implementation, and Applications,* 3rd ed. Edited by C.P. McLaughlin and A.D. Kaluzny. Boston: Jones and Bartlett.

Institute of Medicine. http://www.iom.edu

Institute of Medicine. 2001. *Crossing the Quality Chasm: New Health System for the 21st Century.* Washington, DC: National Academies Press.

Katzenbach, J.R., and D.K. Smith. 1993. *The Wisdom of Teams: Creating the High-performance Organization.* Boston: Harvard Business School Press.

Kohn, L.T., J.M. Corrigan, and M.S. Donaldson, eds. 1999. *To Err Is Human: Building a Safer Health System.* Washington, DC: National Academies Press.

McClanahan, S., S.T. Goodwin, and F. Houser. 1999. A formula for errors: Good people + bad systems. In *Error Reduction in Health Care: A Systems Approach to Improving Patient Safety.* Edited by P.L. Spath. San Francisco: Jossey-Bass.

McWay, D. 1997. *Legal Aspects of Health Information Management.* Albany, NY: Delmar.

White, Susan, Crystal Kallem, Allison Viola, and June Bronnert. "An ACO Primer: Reviewing the Proposed Rule on Accountable Care Organizations." *Journal of AHIMA* 82, no.6 (June 2011): 48–50.

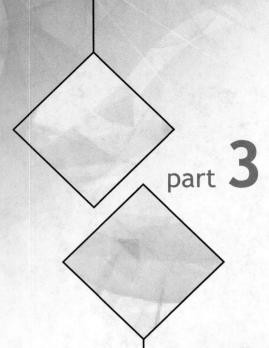

part **3**

Health Services Organization and Delivery

chapter 11

Healthcare Delivery Systems

Donald W. Kellogg, PhD, RHIA, CPEHR

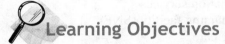

Learning Objectives

- Understand the history of the healthcare delivery system from ancient times until the present
- Understand the basic organization of the various types of hospitals and healthcare organizations
- Describe how internal and external forces have shaped the healthcare industry
- Differentiate the roles of various stakeholders throughout the healthcare delivery system
- Describe the influence of federal legislation on healthcare delivery
- Identify the various functional components of an integrated delivery system
- Describe the systems used for reimbursement of healthcare services
- Recognize the role of government in healthcare services

Key Terms

Accountable Care Organizations (ACOs)
Allied health professional
American Association of Medical Colleges (AAMC)

American College of Healthcare Executives (ACHE)
American Hospital Association (AHA)
American Medical Association (AMA)

American Nurses Association (ANA)

American Recovery and Reinvestment Act (ARRA)

Average length of stay (ALOS)

Case management

Chief executive officer (CEO)

Chief information officer (CIO)

Chief nursing officer (CNO)

Chief operating officer (COO)

Clinical privileges

Commission on Accreditation for Health Informatics and Information Management Education (CAHIIM)

Commission on Certification for Health Informatics and Information Management (CCHIIM)

Continuous quality improvement (CQI)

Continuum of care

Extended care facility

Health savings accounts

Health systems agency (HSA)

Hill-Burton Act

Home healthcare

Hospice care

Integrated delivery network (IDN)

Integrated delivery system (IDS)

Investor-owned hospital chain

Managed care organization (MCO)

Medical staff bylaws

Medical staff classifications

Mission

National Institutes of Health (NIH)

National Practitioner Data Bank (NPBD)

Peer review organization (PRO)

Public health services (PHS)

Quality improvement organization (QIO)

Reengineering

Rehabilitation services

Skilled nursing facility (SNF)

Subacute care

Utilization Review Act

Introduction

A broad array of healthcare services is available in the United States today, from simple preventive measures such as vaccinations to complex lifesaving procedures such as heart transplants. An individual's contact with the healthcare delivery system often begins before she or he is born, with family planning and prenatal care, and continues through the end of life, with long-term and hospice care.

Physicians, nurses, and other clinical providers who work in ambulatory care, acute care, rehabilitative and psychiatric care, and long-term care facilities provide healthcare services. Healthcare services also are provided in the homes of hospice and home care patients. In addition, assisted living centers, industrial medical clinics, and public health department clinics provide services to many Americans.

Integrated delivery systems (IDSs) offer a full range of healthcare services along a **continuum of care** to ensure that patients get the right care at the right time from the right provider. The continuum extends from primary care providers to specialist and ancillary providers. The goal of IDSs is to deliver high-quality, cost-effective care in the most appropriate setting (Sloane et al. 1999, 9).

Most hospitals are integrated into their communities through ties with area physicians and other healthcare providers, clinics and outpatient facilities, and other practitioners. Almost half the nation's hospitals also are tied to larger organizational entities such as multihospital and integrated healthcare systems (IHCSs), **integrated delivery networks** (IDNs), and alliances. An IDN comprises a group of hospitals, physicians, other providers, insurers, and/or community agencies that work together to deliver health services (AHA 2004).

In 2009, 1485 community hospitals (30 percent of the total) were in IDNs (AHA 2011). Multihospital systems include two or more hospitals owned, leased, sponsored, or contract managed by a central organization. In 1985, 27.5 percent of hospitals were system members, which rose to 58 percent by 2009 (AHA 2011). An alliance is defined as a formal organization, usually owned by shareholders/members, that works on behalf of its individual members in the provision of services and products and in the promotion of activities and ventures (AHA 2011).

This chapter traces the history of Western medicine to the present time. It discusses modern healthcare delivery in the United States, and how political, societal, and other factors have influenced its development. Well-known legislation affecting healthcare and healthcare information systems in the United States is examined. Different types of healthcare delivery facilities and the services they provide are explained.

Theory into Practice

In the 1990s, US hospitals faced growing pressure to contain costs, improve quality, and demonstrate their contributions to the health of the communities they serve. They adapted to these pressures in various ways. Some merged with or bought out other hospitals and healthcare organizations. Others created IDSs to provide a full range of healthcare services along the continuum of care, from ambulatory care to inpatient care to long-term care. Still others concentrated on improving the care they provided by focusing on patients as customers. Many hospitals responded to local competition by quickly entering into affiliations and other risk-sharing agreements with acute and nonacute care providers, physicians' groups, and **managed care organizations** (MCOs).

At the close of the first decade of 2000, healthcare organizations faced the challenges of a stressed economy. With higher unemployment rates and more uninsured individuals throughout the nation, hospital reimbursement payments continued to shrink and hospitals reached out for opportunities to control costs, streamline operations, implement efficient information technologies, engage in quality initiatives, and pursue joint ventures and consolidation. Healthcare costs in the United States are estimated to be about $2.2 trillion, representing 16 percent of the total economy. In response to increasing costs and shrinking access to care, the government initiated steps for reforming healthcare by instituting temporary measures to make healthcare coverage more affordable, providing incentives for computerizing health records, and investing in wellness and disease prevention.

In 2010, Congress passed healthcare insurance reform legislation with the goals of reducing healthcare costs, protecting and increasing consumers' choices, and guaranteeing access to quality, affordable healthcare for all Americans.

History of Western Medicine

Modern Western medicine is rooted in antiquity. The ancient Greeks developed surgical procedures, documented clinical cases, and created medical books. Before modern times, European, African, and Native American cultures all had traditions of folk medicine based on spiritual healing and herbal cures. The first hospitals were created by religious orders in medieval Europe to provide care and respite to religious pilgrims traveling back and forth from the Holy Land. However, it was not until the late 1800s that medicine became a scientific discipline. More progress and change occurred in the 20th century than during the preceding 2,000 years. The past few decades have seen dramatic developments in the way diseases are diagnosed and treated and in the way healthcare is delivered.

Before the advent of modern Western medicine, epidemics and plagues were common. Smallpox, measles, yellow fever, influenza, scarlet fever, and diphtheria killed millions of people. Bubonic plague spread periodically through Europe and killed millions more. Disease was carried by rodents and insects as well as by the travelers who moved along intercontinental trade routes.

The medical knowledge that had been gained by ancient Greek scholars such as Hippocrates was lost during the Middle Ages (400 to 1300 AD). Toward the end of the Middle Ages, medical schools were again being established with the first one in Salerno, Italy in 1085. The European Renaissance, a historical period beginning in the 14th century, revived interest in the classical arts, literature, and philosophy as well as the scientific study of nature. This period also was characterized by economic growth and concern for the welfare of workers at all levels of society. With this concept came a growing awareness that a healthy population promoted economic growth.

North America's First Hospitals

Early settlers in the British colonies of North America appointed commissions to care for the sick, provide for orphans, and bury the dead. During the mid-1700s, the citizens of Philadelphia recognized the need for a place to provide relief to the sick and injured. They also recognized the need to isolate newly arrived immigrants who had caught communicable diseases on the long voyage from Europe.

Benjamin Franklin and other colonists persuaded the legislature to develop a hospital for the community. The Pennsylvania Hospital was established in Philadelphia in 1752, the first hospital in the British colonies. (Almost 200 years earlier, Cortez established the first hospital in Mexico and it still serves patients today.)

In its first 150 years, the Pennsylvania Hospital was a model for the organization of hospitals in other communities. The New York Hospital opened in 1771 and started its first register of patients in 1791. Boston's Massachusetts General Hospital opened in 1821.

Standardization of Medical Practice

Human anatomy and physiology and the causes of disease were not well understood before the 20th century. At one time, it was believed that four basic fluids, called humors (yellow bile, black bile, phlegm, and blood), determined a person's temperament and health, and that imbalances in the proportion of humors in the body caused disease. The therapeutic bleeding of patients was practiced until the early 20th century. Early physicians also treated patients by administering a variety of substances with no scientific basis for their effectiveness.

An individual's early medical education consisted of serving as an apprentice to an established practitioner. Just about anyone could hang out a shingle and call himself a physician. The medical profession recognized that some of its members achieved better results than others, and leaders in the profession attempted to regulate the practice of medicine in the late 1700s. The first attempts at regulation took the form of licensure. The first licenses to practice medicine were issued in New York in 1760. By the mid-1800s, however, efforts to license physicians were denounced as being undemocratic and penalties for practicing medicine without a license were removed in most states.

As the US population grew and settlers moved westward, the demand for medical practitioners far exceeded the supply. To staff new hospitals and serve a growing population, private medical schools began to appear almost overnight. By 1869, there were 72 medical schools in the United States. However, these schools did not follow an established course of study and some graduated students with as little as six months of training. The result was an oversupply of poorly trained physicians.

The **American Medical Association** (AMA) was established in 1847 to represent the interests of physicians across the country. However, the AMA was dominated by members who had strong ties to the medical schools and the status quo. Its ability to lead a reform of the profession was limited until it broke its ties with the medical schools in 1874. At that time, the association encouraged the creation of independent state licensing boards.

In 1876, the **American Association of Medical Colleges** (AAMC) was established. The AAMC was dedicated to standardizing the curriculum for US medical schools and to developing the public's understanding of the need to license physicians.

Together, the AMA and the AAMC campaigned for medical licensing. By the 1890s, 35 states had established or reestablished a system of licensure for physicians. At that time, 14 states decided to grant licenses only to graduates of reputable medical schools. The state licensing boards discouraged the worst medical schools, but the criteria for licensing continued to vary from state to state and were not fully enforced.

By the early 20th century, it had become apparent that improving the quality of American medicine required regulation through curriculum reform as well as licensure. However, the members of the AMA were divided on this issue. Conservative members continued to believe that the association should stay out of the area of regulation, whereas progressive members supported continued development of state licensure systems and creation of a standardized model for medical education.

The situation attracted the attention of the Carnegie Foundation for the Advancement of Teaching. The president of the foundation offered to sponsor and fund an independent review of the medical colleges then operating in the United States. Abraham Flexner, an educator from Louisville, Kentucky, undertook the review in 1906.

Over the following four years, Flexner visited every medical college in the country and carefully documented his findings. In his 1910 report to the Carnegie Foundation, the

AMA, and the AAMC, he described the poor quality of the training being provided in the colleges. He noted that medical school applicants often lacked knowledge of the basic sciences. Flexner also reported how the absence of hospital-based training limited the clinical skills of medical school graduates. Perhaps most important, he reported that huge numbers of graduates were being produced every year and that most of them had unacceptable levels of medical skill. He recommended closing most of the existing medical schools to address the problem of oversupply.

Several reform initiatives grew out of Flexner's report and from recommendations made by the AMA's Committee on Medical Education. One of the reforms required medical school applicants to hold a college degree. Another required that medical training be founded in the basic sciences. Reforms also required that medical students receive practical, hospital-based training in addition to classroom work. These reforms were carried out in the decade following Flexner's report, but only about half the medical schools actually closed. By 1920, most of the medical colleges in the United States had met rigorous academic standards and were approved by the AAMC.

Today, medical school graduates must pass a test before they can obtain a license to practice medicine. The licensure tests are administered by state medical boards. Many states now use a standardized licensure test developed in 1968 by the Federation of State Medical Boards of the United States. However, passing scores for the test vary by state. Most physicians also complete several years of residency training in addition to medical school.

Specialty physicians also complete extensive postgraduate medical education. Board certification for the various specialties requires the completion of postgraduate training as well as a passing score on a standardized examination. The most common medical specialties include the following:

- Internal medicine
- Pediatrics
- Family practice
- Cardiology
- Psychiatry
- Neurology
- Oncology
- Radiology

The most common surgical specialties include:

- Anesthesiology
- Cardiovascular surgery
- Obstetrics/gynecology

- Orthopedics
- Urology
- Ophthalmology
- Otorhinolaryngology
- Plastic and reconstructive surgery
- Neurosurgery

Some medical and surgical specialists undergo further graduate training to qualify to practice subspecialties. For example, the subspecialties of internal medicine include endocrinology, pulmonary medicine, rheumatology, geriatrics, and hematology. Physicians also may limit their practices to the treatment of specific illnesses. For example, an endocrinologist may limit his or her practice to the treatment of diabetes. Surgeons can work as general surgeons or as specialists or subspecialists. For example, an orthopedic surgeon may limit his practice to surgery of the hand, surgery of the knee, surgery of the ankle, or surgery of the spine.

Some physicians and healthcare organizations employ physician assistants (PAs) and/ or surgeon assistants (SAs) to help them carry out their clinical responsibilities. Such assistants may perform routine clinical assessments, provide patient education and counseling, and perform simple therapeutic procedures. Most PAs work in primary care settings, and most SAs work in hospitals and ambulatory surgery clinics. PAs and SAs always work under the supervision of licensed physicians and surgeons.

Standardization of Nursing Practice

In the 19th century and the first part of the 20th century, religious organizations sponsored more than half the hospitals in the United States. Members of religious orders often provided nursing care in these organizations. As the US population grew and more towns and cities were established, new hospitals were built. Older cities also grew, and city hospitals became more and more crowded.

In the late 1800s, nurses received no formal education and little training. Nursing staff for the hospitals was often recruited from the surrounding community, and many poor women who had no other skills became nurses. The nature of nursing care at that time was unsophisticated. Indeed, the lack of basic hygiene often promoted disease. Many patients died from infections contracted while hospitalized for surgery, maternity care, and other illnesses.

In 1868, the AMA called the medical profession's attention to the need for trained nurses. During the years that followed, the public also began to call for better nursing care in hospitals.

The first general training school for nurses was opened at the New England Hospital for Women and Children in 1872. It became a model for other institutions throughout the country. As hospital after hospital struggled to find competent nursing staff, many institutions and their medical staffs developed their own nurse training programs.

The responsibilities of nurses in the late 19th and early 20th centuries included house-keeping duties. Nurses also cooked meals for patients in kitchens attached to each ward. Direct patient care duties included giving baths, changing dressings, monitoring vital signs, administering medications, and assisting physicians. During this time, nurses were not required to hold a license to practice.

In 1897, a group of nurses attending the annual meeting of the American Society of Superintendents of Training Schools for Nursing founded the Nurses Associated Alumnae of the United States and Canada. In 1911, the organization was renamed the **American Nurses Association** (ANA). During the early meetings of the association, members established a nursing code of ethics and discussed the need for nursing licensure and for publications devoted to the practice of nursing.

At the turn of the 20th century, nurses also began to organize state nursing associations to advocate for the registration of nurses. Their goal was to increase the level of competence among nurses nationwide. Despite opposition from many physicians who believed that nurses did not need formal education or licensure, North Carolina passed legislation requiring the registration of nurses in 1903. Today, all 50 states have laws that spell out the requirements for the registration and licensure of nursing professionals.

Modern registered nurses must have either a two-year associate's degree or a four-year bachelor's degree from a state-approved nursing school. Nurse practitioners, researchers, educators, and administrators generally have a four-year degree in nursing and additional postgraduate education in nursing. The postgraduate degree may be a master's of science or a doctorate in nursing. Nurses who graduate from nonacademic training programs are called licensed practical nurses (LPNs) or licensed vocational nurses (LVNs). Nondegreed nursing personnel work under the direct supervision of registered nurses. Nurses in all 50 states must pass an exam to obtain a license to practice.

Today's registered nurses are highly trained clinical professionals. Many specialize in specific areas of practice such as surgery, psychiatry, and intensive care. Nurse-midwives complete advanced training and are certified by the American College of Nurse-Midwives. Similarly, nurse-anesthetists are certified by the Council on Certification/Council on Recertification of Nurse Anesthetists. Nurse practitioners also receive advanced training at the master's level that qualifies them to provide primary care services to patients. They are certified by several organizations (for example, the National Board of Pediatric Nurse Practitioners) to practice in the area of their specialty.

The need for registered nurses is expected to rise over the next decade. Hospitals in the United States report continued vacancies for registered nurses. The Department of Health and Human Services estimates that over one million more nurses over the projected supply will be needed by 2020 (AHA 2011).

Standardization of Hospital Care

In 1910, Dr. Franklin H. Martin suggested that the surgical area of medical practice needed to become more concerned with patient outcomes. He had been introduced to this concept in discussions with Dr. Ernest Codman. Codman was a British physician who believed that hospital practitioners should track their patients for a significant amount of time after treatment to determine whether the end result had been positive or negative. Codman also supported the use of outcome information to identify the practices that led to the best results for patients.

At that time, Martin and other American physicians were concerned about the conditions in US hospitals. Many observers felt that part of the problem was related to the lack of organization in medical staffs and to lax professional standards. In the early 20th century, before the development of antibiotics and other pharmaceuticals, hospitals were used mainly by physicians who needed facilities in which to perform surgery. Most nonsurgical medical care was still provided in the home. It was natural, then, for the force behind improved hospital care to come from surgeons.

The push for hospital reforms eventually led to formation of the American College of Surgeons in 1913. The organization faced a difficult task. In 1917, the leaders of the college asked the Carnegie Foundation for funding to plan and develop a hospital standardization program. The college then formed a committee to develop a set of minimum standards for hospital care. It published the formal standards under the title of the Minimum Standards.

During 1918 and part of 1919, the college examined the hospitals in the United States and Canada just as Flexner had reviewed the medical colleges a decade earlier. The performance of 692 hospitals was compared to the college's Minimum Standards. Only 89 of the hospitals fully met the college's standards, and some of the best-known hospitals in the country failed to meet them.

Adoption of the Minimum Standards was the basis of the Hospital Standardization Program and marked the beginning of the modern accreditation process for healthcare organizations. Basically, accreditation standards are developed to reflect reasonable quality standards. The performance of each participating organization is evaluated against the standards. The accreditation process is voluntary; healthcare organizations choose to participate in order to improve the care they provide to their patients.

The American College of Surgeons continued to sponsor the hospital accreditation program until the early 1950s. At that time, four professional associations from the US and Canada joined forces with the college to create a new accreditation organization called the Joint Commission on Accreditation of Hospitals. The associations were the American College of Physicians, the AMA, the **American Hospital Association** (AHA), and the Canadian Medical Association. The new organization was formally incorporated in 1952 and began to perform accreditation surveys in 1953.

The Joint Commission continues to survey several different types of healthcare organizations today, including:

- Acute care hospitals
- Long-term care facilities
- Ambulatory care facilities
- Psychiatric facilities

- Home health agencies
- Rehabilitation Hospitals

Several other organizations also perform accreditation of healthcare organizations. These include the American Osteopathic Association (AOA), the Commission on Accreditation of Rehabilitation Facilities (CARF), and the Accreditation Association for Ambulatory Healthcare (AAAHC).

Professionalization of the Allied Health Professions

After the first World War, many roles previously played by nurses and nonclinical personnel began to change. With the advent of modern diagnostic and therapeutic technology in the mid-twentieth century, the complex skills needed by ancillary medical personnel fostered the growth of specialized training programs and professional accreditation and licensure.

According to the AMA, allied health incorporates the healthcare-related professions that function to assist, facilitate, and/or complement the work of physicians and other clinical specialists. The Health Professions Education Amendment of 1991 describes **allied health professionals** as health professionals (other than registered nurses, physicians, and physician assistants) who have received a certificate, an associate's degree, a bachelor's degree, a master's degree, a doctorate, or postdoctoral training in a healthcare-related science. Such individuals share responsibility for the delivery of healthcare services with clinicians (physicians, nurses, and physician assistants).

Allied health occupations are among the fastest growing in healthcare. The number of allied health professionals is difficult to estimate and depends on the definition of allied health. Unlike the case in medicine, women dominate most of the allied health professions, representing between 75 and 95 percent in most of the occupations. All 50 states require licensure for some allied health professions (physical therapy, for example). Practitioners in other allied health professions (occupational therapy, for example) may be licensed in some states but not in others. Significant shortages of personnel in many of the allied health disciplines are projected to reach 1.6 to 2.5 million by 2020 (US Census Bureau 2011).

The following list briefly describes some of the major occupations usually considered to be allied health professions (Jonas and Kovner 2005, 446–448):

- *Audiology:* Audiology is the branch of science that studies hearing, balance, and related disorders. Audiologists treat those with hearing loss and proactively prevent related damage. According to the American Speech-Language-Hearing Association, audiologists provide comprehensive diagnostic and treatment/rehabilitative services for auditory, vestibular, and related impairments. These services are provided to individuals across the entire age span from birth through adulthood; individuals from diverse language, ethnic, cultural, and socioeconomic backgrounds; and individuals who have multiple disabilities.

- *Clinical laboratory science:* Originally referred to as medical laboratory technology, this field is now more appropriately referred to as clinical laboratory science. Clinical laboratory technicians perform a wide array of tests on body fluids, tissues, and cells to assist in the detection, diagnosis, and treatment of diseases and illnesses.

- *Diagnostic medical sonography/imaging technology:* Originally referred to as x-ray technology and then radiologic technology, this field is now more appropriately referred to as diagnostic imaging. The field continues to expand to include nuclear medicine, radiation therapy, and echocardiography. These services are provided by physician specialists and technologists including radiation therapists, cardiosonographers (ultrasound technologists), and magnetic resonance technologists.

- *Dietetics and nutrition:* Dietitians (also clinical nutritionists) are trained in nutrition. They are responsible for providing nutritional care to individuals and for overseeing nutrition and food services in a variety of settings, ranging from hospitals to schools.

- *Emergency medical technology:* Emergency medical technicians (EMTs) and paramedics provide a wide range of services on an emergency basis for cases of traumatic injury and other emergency situations and in the transport of emergency patients to a medical facility.

- *Health information management:* Health information management (HIM) professionals (formerly called medical record administration) oversee health record systems and manage health-related information to ensure that it meets relevant medical, administrative, and legal requirements. Health records are the responsibility of registered health information administrators (RHIAs) and registered health information technicians (RHITs).

- *Occupational therapy:* Occupational therapists (OTs) evaluate and treat patients whose illnesses or injuries have resulted in significant psychological, physical, or work-related impairment.

- *Optometry:* Optometry is a health profession that is focused on the eyes and related structures, as well as vision, visual systems, and vision information processing in humans. Optometrists provide treatments such as contact lenses and corrective and low vision devices, and are authorized to use diagnostic and therapeutic pharmaceutical agents to treat anterior segment disease, glaucoma, and ocular hypertension. As primary eye care practitioners, optometrists often are the first ones to detect such potentially serious conditions as diabetes, hypertension, and arteriosclerosis.

- *Pharmacy:* The scope of pharmacy practice includes traditional roles such as compounding and dispensing medications, as well as modern services including reviewing medications for safety and efficacy, and providing drug information to physicians and patients. Pharmacists are the experts on drug therapy and are the primary health professionals who optimize medication use to provide patients with positive health outcomes.

- *Physical therapy:* Physical therapists (PTs) evaluate and treat patients to improve functional mobility, reduce pain, maintain cardiopulmonary function, and limit disability. PTs treat movement dysfunction resulting from accidents, trauma, stroke, fractures, multiple sclerosis, cerebral palsy, arthritis, and heart and respiratory illness. Physical therapy assistants (PTAs) work under the direction of PTs and help carry out the treatment plans developed by PTs.

- *Respiratory therapy:* Respiratory therapists (RTs) evaluate, treat, and care for patients with breathing disorders. They work under the direction of qualified physicians and provide services such as emergency care for stroke, heart failure, and shock, and treat patients with emphysema and asthma.

- *Speech-language pathology and audiology:* Speech-language pathologists and audiologists identify, assess, and provide treatment for individuals with speech, language, or hearing problems.

- *Surgical technologist:* Surgical technologists provide surgical care to patients in a variety of settings; the majority are hospital operating rooms. Surgical technologists work under medical supervision to facilitate the safe and effective conduct of invasive surgical procedures.

Check Your Understanding 11.1

1. What healthcare professional assists physicians in clinical assessments and patient education?

   A. Diagnostic Medical Sonographers
   B. Health information managers
   C. Clinical laboratory technicians
   D. Physician assistants

2. Licensure tests to practice medicine are administered by:

   A. Medical schools
   B. Federal licensure board
   C. Department of Health and Human Services
   D. State licensure boards

3. Which of the following statements is true about registered nurses?

   A. Nurses serve the same roles within an organization.
   B. Nurses are required to have a license in the state in which they practice.
   C. Nurses are graduates of nonacademic training programs.
   D. Nurses must have a bachelor's degree from an approved nursing school.

4. Which of the following professions is generally considered to be an allied health career?

   A. Clinical laboratory science

   B. Physician

   C. Nurse

   D. Medical student

5. To become board-certified in pediatrics, which of the following would an internal medicine physician need to do?

   A. Complete continuing education courses in pediatric medicine and pass a national examination

   B. Complete graduate training in pediatric medicine and pass a national examination

   C. Apply for a new credential from the state licensure board

   D. Attend continuing medical education programs

6. The adoption of the Minimum Standards marked the beginning of what modern practice for healthcare organizations?

   A. Accreditation

   B. Licensing

   C. Reform

   D. Educational

7. According to the AMA, which of the following incorporates the healthcare-related professions that function to assist, facilitate, and/or complement the work of physicians and other clinical specialists?

   A. Home health

   B. Nursing care

   C. Ambulatory care

   D. Allied health

Instructions: Indicate whether the statements below are true or false (T or F).

8. ____ Respiratory therapists treat patients with limited mobility.

9. ____ Physical therapy assistants develop treatment plans.

10. ____ A sonographer is a specialization of diagnostic imaging technologists.

Modern Healthcare Delivery in the United States

Until the second World War, most healthcare was provided in the home. Quality in healthcare services was considered a product of appropriate medical practice and oversight by physicians and surgeons. Even the Minimum Standards used to evaluate the performance of hospitals were based on factors directly related to the composition and skills of the hospital medical staff.

The 20th century was a period of tremendous change in American society. Advances in medical science promised better outcomes and increased the demand for healthcare services. But medical care has never been free. Even in the best economic times, many Americans have been unable to take full advantage of what medicine has to offer because they cannot afford it.

Concern over access to healthcare was especially evident during the Great Depression of the 1930s. During the Depression, America's leaders were forced to consider how the poor and disadvantaged could receive the care they needed. Before the Depression, medical care for the poor and elderly had been handled as a function of social welfare agencies. During the 1930s, however, few people were able to pay for medical care. The problem of how to pay for the healthcare needs of millions of Americans became a public and governmental concern. Working Americans turned to prepaid health plans to help them pay for healthcare, but the unemployed and the unemployable needed help from a different source.

Effects of the Great Depression

The concept of prepaid healthcare, or health insurance, began with the financial problems of one hospital, Baylor University Hospital in Dallas, Texas (AHA 1999, 14). In 1929, the administrator of the hospital arranged to provide hospital services to Dallas's schoolteachers for 50 cents per person per month. Before that time, a few large employers had set up company clinics and hired company physicians to care for their workers, but the idea of a prepaid health plan that could be purchased by individuals had never been tried before.

The idea caught on quickly, and new prepaid plans appeared across the country. Eventually, these plans became known as Blue Cross plans when the blue cross symbol used by some of the new plans was adopted officially as the trademark for all the plans in 1939.

Another type of prepaid plan, called the Blue Shield plan, was subsequently developed to cover the cost of physicians' services. The idea for the Blue Shield plans grew out of the medical service bureaus created by large lumber and mining companies in the Northwest. In 1939, the first formal Blue Shield plan was founded in California.

Growth in the number of Blue Cross/Blue Shield (BC/BS) plans continued through the Depression and boomed during the second World War. During the war-related labor shortages, employers began to pay for their employees' memberships in the Blues as a way to attract and keep scarce workers.

The idea of public funding for healthcare services also goes back to the Great Depression. The decline in family income during the 1930s curtailed the use of medical services by the poor. In ten working-class communities studied between 1929 and 1933, the proportion of families with incomes under $150 per capita had increased from 10 to 43 percent. A 1938 Gallup poll asked people whether they had put off seeing a physician because of the cost. The results showed that 68 percent of lower-income respondents had put off medical care, compared with 24 percent of respondents in upper-income brackets (Starr 1982, 271).

The decreased use of medical services and the inability of many patients to pay meant lower incomes for physicians. Hospitals were in similar trouble. Beds were empty, bills went unpaid, and contributions to hospital fundraising efforts tumbled. As a result, private physicians and charities could no longer meet the demand for free services. For the first time, physicians and hospitals asked state welfare departments to pay for the treatment of people on relief.

The Depression posed a severe test for the AMA. It was no easy matter to maintain a common front against government intervention when physicians themselves were facing economic difficulties. Because of the economic hardships, many physicians were willing to accept government-sponsored health insurance. In 1935, the California Medical Association endorsed the concept of compulsory health insurance because health insurance promised to stimulate the use of physicians' services and help patients pay their bills.

The AMA's response to the economic crisis emphasized restricting the supply of physicians, rather than increasing the demand for their services by instituting mandatory health insurance. The AMA reacted by pushing for the closure of medical schools and reductions in the number of new medical students.

By the mid-1930s, however, the AMA began to adjust its position on health insurance. Instead of opposing all insurance, voluntary or compulsory, it began to define the terms on which voluntary programs might be acceptable. Although accepting health insurance plans in principle, the AMA did nothing to support or encourage their development.

The push for government-sponsored health insurance continued in the late 1930s during the administration of President Franklin D. Roosevelt. However, compulsory health insurance stood on the margins of national politics throughout the New Deal era. It was not made part of the new Social Security program, and it was never fully supported by President Roosevelt.

Postwar Efforts toward Improving Healthcare Access

After the second World War, the issue of healthcare access finally moved to the center of national politics. In the late 1940s, President Harry S. Truman expressed unreserved support for a national health insurance program. However, the issue of compulsory health insurance became entangled with America's fear of communism. Opponents of Truman's healthcare program labeled it socialized medicine, and the program failed to win legislative support.

The idea of national health insurance did not resurface until the administration of Lyndon Johnson and the Great Society legislation of the 1960s. The Medicare and Medicaid programs were legislated in 1965 to pay the cost of providing healthcare services to the elderly and the poor. The issues of healthcare reform and national health insurance were again given priority during the first four years of President Bill Clinton's administration in the 1990s. However, the complexity of American healthcare issues at the end of the 20th century doomed reform efforts. In 2010, Congress passed health insurance reform legislation that was signed into law by President Barack Obama (Committee on Energy and Commerce 2010).

Influence of Federal Legislation

During the 20th century, Congress passed many pieces of legislation that had a significant impact on the delivery of healthcare services in the United States.

Biologics Control Act of 1902

Direct federal sponsorship of medical research began with early research on methods for controlling epidemics of infectious disease. The Marine Hospital Service performed the first research. In 1887, a young physician, Joseph Kinyoun, set up a bacteriological laboratory in the Marine Hospital at Staten Island, NY. Four years later, the Hygienic Laboratory was moved to Washington, DC. It was given authority to test and improve biological products in 1902 when Congress passed the Biologics Control Act. This act regulated the vaccines and sera sold via interstate commerce. That same year, the Hygienic Laboratory added divisions in chemistry, pharmacology, and zoology.

In 1912, the service, by then called the US Public Health Service, was authorized to study chronic as well as infectious diseases. In 1930, reorganized under the Randsdell Act, the Hygienic Laboratory became the **National Institutes of Health** (NIH). In 1938, the NIH moved to a large, privately-donated estate in Bethesda, Maryland (Starr 1982, 340).

Today, the mission of the NIH is to uncover new medical knowledge that can lead to health improvements for everyone. The NIH accomplishes its mission by conducting and supporting medical research, fostering communication of up-to-date medical information, and training research investigators. The organization has played a vital role in recent clinical research on the treatment of the following diseases:

- Heart disease and stroke
- Cancer
- Depression and schizophrenia
- Spinal cord injuries

Social Security Act of 1935

The Great Depression revived the dormant social reform movement in the United States as well as more radical currents in American politics. Unionization increased, and the American Federation of Labor (AFL) abandoned its long-standing opposition to social insurance programs. The Depression also brought to power a Democratic administration. The administration of Franklin D. Roosevelt was more willing than any previous administration to involve the federal government in the management of economic and social welfare.

Even before Roosevelt took office in 1933, a steady movement toward some sort of social insurance program had been growing. By 1931, nine states had passed legislation creating old-age pension programs. As governor of New York State, Roosevelt endorsed unemployment insurance in 1930. Wisconsin became the first state to adopt such a measure early in 1932.

Although old-age pension and unemployment insurance bills were introduced into Congress soon after his election, Roosevelt refused to give them his strong support. Instead, he created a program of his own. On June 8, 1934, he announced that he would appoint a committee on economic security to study the issue comprehensively and report to Congress in January 1935. The committee consisted of four members of the cabinet and the federal relief administrator. It was headed by the secretary of labor, Frances Perkins.

Although Roosevelt indicated in his June message that he was especially interested in old-age and unemployment programs, the committee included medical care and health insurance in its research. From the outset, the prevailing sentiment on the committee was that health insurance would have to wait. Abraham Epstein was the founder of the American Association for Social Security and a leading figure in the social insurance movement. In an article published in October 1934, he warned the administration that opposition to health insurance was strong. He advised the administration to be politically realistic and go slow on health insurance.

Sentiment in favor of health insurance was strong among members of the Committee on Economic Security. However, many members of the committee were convinced that adding a health insurance amendment would spell defeat for the entire Social Security legislation. Ultimately, the Social Security bill included only one reference to health insurance as a subject that the new Social Security Board might study. The Social Security Act was passed in 1935.

The omission of health insurance from the legislation was by no means the act's only conservative feature. It relied on a regressive tax and gave no coverage to some of the nation's poorest people, such as farmers and domestic workers. However, the act did extend the federal government's role in public health through several provisions unrelated to social insurance. It gave the states funds on a matching basis for maternal and infant care, rehabilitation of crippled children, general public health work, and aid for dependent children under the age of 16.

Hospital Survey and Construction Act of 1946

Passage of the **Hill-Burton Act** was another important development in American healthcare delivery. Enacted in 1946 as the Hospital Survey and Construction Act, this legislation authorized grants for states to construct new hospitals and, later, to modernize old ones. The fund expansion of the hospital system was to achieve a goal for 4.5 beds per 1,000 persons. The availability of federal financing created a boom in hospital construction during the 1950s. The hospital system grew from 6,000 hospitals in 1946 to a high of approximately 7,200 acute care hospitals.

Growth in Number of Hospitals

The number of hospitals in the United States increased from 178 in 1873 to 4,300 in 1909. In 1946, at the close of the second World War, there were 6,000 American hospitals, with 3.2 beds available for every 1,000 persons.

Of the $1.4 trillion spent on healthcare in 2001, hospital costs totaled $415 billion, or 32 percent. Most US hospitals are nonprofit or owned by local, state, or federal governments (Jonas and Kovner 2005, 224). In 2009, there were 5,795 hospitals in the United States, with a total of 944,277 beds (AHA 2011).

Decline in Number of Hospitals

During the 1980s, medical advances and cost-containment measures caused many procedures that once required inpatient hospitalization to be performed on an outpatient basis. Outpatient hospital visits increased by 40 percent with a resultant decrease in hospital admissions. Fewer patient admissions and shortened lengths of stay (LOS) resulted in a significant reduction in the number of hospitals and hospital beds. Healthcare reform efforts and the acceptance of managed care as the major medical practice style of US healthcare resulted in enough hospital closings and mergers to reduce the number of government and community-based hospitals in the United States to approximately 5,700 (Sultz and Young 2011, 71).

The advent of diagnosis-related groups (DRGs) in the mid-1980s resulted in the closure of many rural healthcare facilities. DRGs are discussed later in this chapter.

Public Law 89-97 of 1965

In 1965, passage of a number of amendments to the Social Security Act brought Medicare and Medicaid into existence. The two programs have greatly changed how healthcare organizations are reimbursed. Recent attempts to curtail Medicare/Medicaid spending continue to affect healthcare organizations.

Medicare (Title XVIII of the Social Security Act) is a federal program that provides healthcare benefits for people 65 years old and older who are covered by Social Security. The program was inaugurated on July 1, 1966. Over the years, amendments have extended coverage to individuals who are not covered by Social Security but are willing to pay a premium for coverage, to the disabled, and to those suffering from end-stage renal disease (ESRD).

The companion program, Medicaid, Title XIX of the Social Security Act, was established at the same time to support medical and hospital care for persons classified as medically indigent. Originally targeted recipients of public assistance (primarily single-parent families and the aged, blind, and disabled), Medicaid has expanded to additional groups so that it now targets poor children, the disabled, pregnant women, and very poor adults (including 65 and over). The only exception to these expansions was passage of the Personal Responsibility and Work Opportunity Reconciliation Act of 1996 (Public law 104-193), which changed eligibility for legal/illegal immigrants (Jonas and Kovner 2005, 56).

Today, Medicaid is a federally mandated program that provides healthcare benefits to low-income people and their children. Medicaid programs are administered and partially paid for by individual states. Medicaid is an umbrella for 50 different state programs designed specifically to serve the poor. Beginning in January 1967, Medicaid provided federal funds to states on a cost-sharing basis to ensure that welfare recipients would be guaranteed medical services. Coverage of four types of care was required: inpatient and outpatient services, other laboratory and x-ray services, physician services, and nursing facility care for persons over 21 years of age.

Many enhancements have been made in the years since Medicaid was enacted. Services now include family planning and 31 other optional services such as prescription drugs and dental services. With few exceptions, recipients of cash assistance are automatically eligible for Medicaid. Medicaid also pays the Medicare premium, deductible, and coinsurance costs for some low-income Medicare beneficiaries.

Four million individuals were enrolled in Medicaid in 1966, its first year of implementation. By 2011, 56 million people were enrolled in Medicaid programs. In 2007, the states and the federal government expended $319.6 billion on Medicaid. Elderly and disabled participants comprised about 65% of the expenditures while comprising only 14 percent of all enrollees (Kaiser Family Foundation 2011).

Public Law 92-603 of 1972

Utilization review (UR) was a mandatory component of the original Medicare legislation. Medicare required hospitals and **extended care facilities** to establish a plan for UR as well as a permanent utilization review committee. The goal of the UR process was to ensure that the services provided to Medicare beneficiaries were medically necessary.

In an effort to curtail Medicare and Medicaid spending, additional amendments to the Social Security Act were instituted in 1972. Public Law 92-603 required concurrent review for Medicare and Medicaid patients. It also established the professional standards review organization (PSRO) program to implement concurrent review. PSROs performed professional review and evaluated patient care services for necessity, quality, and cost-effectiveness.

Health Planning and Resources Development Act of 1974

The Health Planning and Resources Development Act of 1974 called for a new type of organization, the **health systems agency** (HSA), to have broad representation of healthcare providers and consumers on governing boards and committees. Although the governance structure required participation by consumers, interested parties from the provider groups dominated the discussions. HSAs were fundamentally unsuccessful in materially influencing decisions about service or technology expansion. Their decisions became undeniably political and attempts to achieve consensus based on real service needs were counterbalanced by community interests in economic and employment expansions.

Concurrent with attempts to slow cost increases through a planning approach, a number of other legislative initiatives took shape that were directly related to concerns over Medicare costs and service quality (Sultz and Young 2011, 41, 247). The legislation that created the HSAs or nationwide system of local health planning agencies was repealed in 1986.

Utilization Review Act of 1977

In 1977, the **Utilization Review Act** made it a requirement that hospitals conduct continued-stay reviews for Medicare and Medicaid patients. Continued-stay reviews determine whether it is medically necessary for a patient to remain hospitalized. This legislation also included fraud and abuse regulations.

Peer Review Improvement Act of 1982

In 1982, the Peer Review Improvement Act redesigned the PSRO program and renamed the agencies **peer review organizations** (PROs). At this time, hospitals began to review the medical necessity and appropriateness of certain admissions even before patients were admitted. PROs were given a new name in 2002 and now are called **quality improvement organizations** (QIOs). They currently emphasize quality improvement processes. Each state and territory, as well as the District of Columbia, now has its own QIO. The mission of the QIOs is to ensure the quality, efficiency, and cost-effectiveness of the healthcare services provided to Medicare beneficiaries in its locale.

Tax Equity and Fiscal Responsibility Act of 1982

In 1982, Congress passed the Tax Equity and Fiscal Responsibility Act (TEFRA). TEFRA required extensive changes in the Medicare program. Its purpose was to control the rising cost of providing healthcare services to Medicare beneficiaries. Before this legislation was passed, healthcare services provided to Medicare beneficiaries were reimbursed on a retrospective, or fee-based, payment system. TEFRA required the gradual implementation of a prospective payment system (PPS) for Medicare reimbursement.

In a retrospective payment system, a service is provided, a claim for payment for the service is made, and the healthcare provider is reimbursed for the cost of delivering the service. In a PPS, a predetermined level of reimbursement is established before the service is provided.

Prospective Payment Act (1982)/Public Law 98-21 of 1983

The PPS for acute hospital care (inpatient) services was implemented on October 1, 1983, according to Public Law 98-21. Under the inpatient PPS, reimbursement for hospital care provided to Medicare patients is based on diagnosis-related groups (DRGs). Each case is assigned to a DRG based on the patient's diagnosis at the time of discharge. For example, under inpatient PPS, all cases of viral pneumonia would be reimbursed at the same predetermined level of reimbursement no matter how long the patients stayed in the hospital or how many services they received.

PPSs for other healthcare services provided to Medicare beneficiaries have been gradually implemented in the years since 1983. Implementation of the ambulatory payment classification system for hospital outpatient services, for example, began in the year 2000.

Consolidated Omnibus Budget Reconciliation Act of 1985

The Consolidated Omnibus Budget Reconciliation Act made it possible for the Centers for Medicare and Medicaid Services (CMS) to deny reimbursement for substandard healthcare services provided to Medicare and Medicaid beneficiaries.

Omnibus Budget Reconciliation Act of 1986

The Omnibus Budget Reconciliation Act of 1986 requires PROs to report instances of substandard care to relevant licensing and certification agencies.

Healthcare Quality Improvement Act of 1986

The Healthcare Quality Improvement Act established the **National Practitioner Data Bank** (NPDB). The purpose of the NPDB is to provide a clearinghouse for information about medical practitioners who have a history of malpractice suits and other quality problems. Hospitals are required to consult the NPDB before granting medical staff privileges to healthcare practitioners. The legislation also established immunity from legal actions for practitioners involved in some peer review activities.

Omnibus Budget Reconciliation Act of 1989

The Omnibus Budget Reconciliation Act of 1989 instituted the Agency for Healthcare Policy and Research. The **mission** of this agency is to develop outcome measures to evaluate the quality of healthcare services.

Omnibus Budget Reconciliation Act of 1990

The Omnibus Budget Reconciliation Act of 1990 requires PROs to report actions taken against physicians to state medical boards and licensing agencies.

Mental Health Parity Act of 1996

The Mental Health Parity Act of 1996 (MHPA) is a federal law that may apply to large group self-funded group plans or large group fully insured group health plans. The purpose of the law is to provide equality (parity) for mental health benefits with medical/surgical benefits when applying aggregate lifetime and annual dollar limits under a group health plan. For example, if a health plan has a $500,000 lifetime limit on medical and surgical benefits, then it cannot apply a lower limit on mental health benefits. The law does not require group health plans to include mental health benefits in their plans and does not apply to employers who have less than 50 employees. Changes in the law occurred when the Mental Health Parity and Addiction Equity Act (MHPAEA) was signed into law in 2008.

Health Insurance Portability and Accountability Act of 1996

The Health Insurance Portability and Accountability Act of 1996 (HIPAA) addresses issues related to the portability of health insurance after leaving employment, establishment of national standards for electronic healthcare transactions, and national identifiers for providers, health plans, and employers. A portion of HIPAA addressed the security and privacy of health information by establishing privacy standards to protect health information and security standards for electronic healthcare information. HIPAA privacy and security standards are covered in chapters 14 and 17. Another provision of HIPAA was the creation of the Healthcare Integrity and Protection Data Bank (HIPDB) to combat fraud and abuse in health insurance and healthcare delivery. A purpose of the HIPDB is to inform federal and state agencies about potential quality problems with clinicians, suppliers, and providers of healthcare services. The American Recovery and Reinvestment Act (ARRA) discussed below includes important changes in HIPAA privacy and security standards that are discussed in chapters 13 and 17.

American Recovery and Reinvestment Act of 2009

In February 2009, President Barack Obama signed the **American Recovery and Reinvestment Act** (ARRA), one of the single largest health information technology laws in recent history. It provided stimulus funds to the US economy in the midst of a major economic downturn. A substantial portion of the bill, Title XIII of the Act entitled the Health Information Technology for Economic and Clinical Health (HITECH) Act, allocated funds for implementation of a nationwide health information exchange and implementation of electronic health records. The bill provides for investment of billions of dollars in health information technology and incentives to encourage doctors and hospitals to use information technology; $19.2 billion was dedicated to implementing and supporting health information technology. ARRA requires the government to take a leadership role in developing standards for exchange of health information nationwide, strengthens federal privacy and security standards, and establishes the Office of the National Coordinator for Health Information Technology (ONC) as a permanent office (Rode 2009). Four major components of the bill include: meaningful use (that providers are using certified EHRs to improve patient outcomes); EHR standards and certifications; Regional Extension Centers (used to assist providers with selection and implementation of EHRs); and breach notification guidance.

Patient Protection and Affordable Care Act, 2010

This federal statute was signed into law on March 23, 2010 and is the most significant healthcare reform legislation of the first decade of the 21st century. The Congressional Budget Office (CBO) projected savings of $143 billion over the first decade and a second decade deficit reduction of $1.2 trillion. Its major provisions include:

- Health insurance market reforms including:
  — Subsidized premiums for people with pre-existing conditions
  — Eliminating lifetime limits on benefits
  — The option of covering children on parents' insurance until the age of 26

- Development of state-based and state-administered health insurance exchanges

- Consumer Operated and Oriented Plan program

- Expansion of Medicaid to individuals under 65 with incomes up to 133 percent of federal poverty level

- Individual mandate to have minimum acceptable coverage or pay a tax penalty

- Employers with 50 or more employees must provide healthcare coverage

- Premium subsidies to individuals

- Small employer tax credits (AMA 2011)

A small part (7 pages) of this act will have a significant impact on physicians and hospitals: the establishment of **Accountable Care Organizations** (ACOs). ACOs are a healthcare model that develops a partnership between hospitals and physicians to coordinate and deliver quality care to Medicare patients. The Centers for Medicare and Medicaid Services (CMS) is to institute demonstration programs whereby participating ACOs would assume the accountability for improving quality care while reducing costs for a defined Medicare patient population. The beneficiaries will be assigned to the ACO based on utilization of primary care services provided by primary care physicians. CMS has outlined a series of 33 quality measures in four categories (patient/caregiver experience; care coordination/patient safety; preventative health; and at-risk population) to assess the quality of care furnished by the ACO (Slavkin et al. 2011). As of October 2011, approximately 6,000 groups have notified CMS of their intention to form an ACO or other shared savings program (Slavkin et al. 2011).

State of Healthcare Delivery

In 2006, the Commonwealth Fund Commission on a High Performance Health System developed a comprehensive method to measure and monitor various aspects of the healthcare system in the United States. The findings of the Commission's analysis are documented in an annual report called the National Scorecard on US Health System Performance.

The 2008 National Scorecard looked at five dimensions of health system performance including healthy lives, quality, access, efficiency, and equity. The average performance of US healthcare was evaluated against benchmarks from top-performing health providers in the United States and other top-performing countries. Findings from the Scorecard showed that out of a possible score of 100, the United States achieved an overall score of 65 and that performance had not improved from 2006 to 2008. Specifically, the Scorecard found that access to healthcare significantly declined and health system efficiency remained low. On a brighter side, quality metrics used in the Scorecard that had been the focus of national campaigns or public reporting efforts showed some significant gains (Commonwealth Fund Commission on a High Performance Health System 2008).

Poor healthcare system performance impacts individuals as well the nation as a whole. According to the 2011 Scorecard, expenditures on healthcare in the next decade are expected to increase to 18 percent of the Gross Domestic Product (GDP). It is also anticipated that there will be an increase in the population of uninsured individuals. If health system performance would improve, fewer people would die prematurely, more people would have access to primary care providers and receive preventative care, and cost savings could be realized in federal programs such as Medicare by reducing hospital readmissions and hospitalizations for preventable conditions.

Providing better primary care and care coordination by increasing patients' access to round-the-clock care, managing chronic conditions, and promoting efficient use of specialized and expensive resources are ways recommended to improve the healthcare system. There is hope for improvement as many of the performance targets listed in the 2008 Scorecard were included in the Patient Protection and Affordable Care Act of 2010 and the American Recovery and Reinvestment Act of 2009, including adoption of interoperable health information technology, and new payment reforms (Commonwealth Fund Commission on a High Performance Health System 2011).

Biomedical and Technological Advances in Medicine

Rapid progress in medical science and technology during the late 19th and 20th centuries revolutionized the way healthcare was provided (figure 11.1). The most important scientific advancement was the discovery of bacteria as the cause of infectious disease. The most important technological development was the use of anesthesia for surgical procedures. These 19th-century advances laid the basis for the development of antibiotics and other pharmaceuticals and the application of sophisticated surgical procedures in the 20th century.

To further medical advances in the 21st century, National Institutes of Health (NIH) sought the input of more than 300 recognized leaders in academia, industry, government, and the public to create a Roadmap program to accelerate biomedical advances, create effective prevention strategies and new treatments, and bridge knowledge gaps. The program, which involves a plethora of NIH institutes and centers, has three main strategic initiatives:

1. New Pathways to Discovery, which includes a comprehensive understanding of: building blocks of the body's cells and tissues; how complex biological systems operate; structural biology; molecular libraries and imaging; nanotechnology; bioinformatics; and computational biology
2. Research Teams of the Future, including interdisciplinary research and public–private partnerships
3. Re-engineering the Clinical Research Enterprise

Through these efforts, NIH will boost the resources and technologies needed for 21st-century biomedical science (NIH 2005).

Surgical procedures were performed before the development of anesthesia, so surgeons had to work quickly on conscious patients to minimize risk and pain. The availability of anesthesia made it possible for surgeons to develop more advanced surgical techniques. The use of ether as an anesthetic was first recorded in 1842. At about the same

Figure 11.1.   Key biological and technological advances in medicine

Time	Event
1842	First recorded use of ether as an anesthetic
1860s	Louis Pasteur laid the foundation for modern bacteriology
1865	Joseph Lister was the first to apply Pasteur's research to the treatment of infected wounds
1880s–1890s	Steam first used in physical sterilization
1895	Wilhelm Roentgen made observations that led to the development of x-ray technology
1898	Introduction of rubber surgical gloves, sterilization, and antisepsis
1940	Studies of prothrombin time first made available
1941–1946	Studies of electrolytes; development of major pharmaceuticals
1957	Studies of blood gas
1961	Studies of creatine phosphokinase
1970s	Surgical advances in cardiac bypass surgery, surgery for joint replacements, and organ transplantation
1971	Computed tomography first used in England
1974	Introduction of whole-body scanners
1980s	Introduction of magnetic resonance imaging
1990s	Further technological advances in pharmaceuticals and genetics; Human Genome Project
2000s	NIH creates roadmap to accelerate biomedical advances, create effective prevention strategies and new treatments, and bridge knowledge gaps in the 21st century

time, nitrous oxide was introduced for use during dental procedures, and chloroform was used to reduce the pain of labor. By the 1860s, the physicians who treated the casualties of the American Civil War on both sides had access to anesthetic and pain-killing drugs.

In the 1860s, Louis Pasteur began studying a condition in wine that made it sour and unpalatable. He discovered that the wine was being spoiled by bacterial growths. His research proved that tiny, living organisms (called bacteria) increase through reproduction and cause infectious disease. Pasteur also demonstrated that heat and certain chemicals such as alcohol could destroy bacteria. In doing so, he laid the foundation for modern bacteriology. After 20 years of research into the biology of microorganisms, Pasteur began studying human diseases. In 1885, he developed a vaccine that prevented rabies.

Although the importance of cleanliness had been known since early times, the role that microorganisms played in disease was not understood until Pasteur conducted his research. In 1865, Joseph Lister was the first to apply Pasteur's research to the treatment of infected wounds. Lister began by protecting open fractures from infection by treating the wounds with carbolic acid (a disinfectant). His discovery was called the antiseptic principle. Antisepsis reduced the mortality rate in Lister's hospital after 1865 from 45 to 12 percent. He published his results in 1868, and soon carbolic acid was being used to prevent bacterial contamination during surgery.

During the 1880s and 1890s, physical sterilization using steam was developed. This technological advance had a major impact on surgery and in other areas throughout the hospital. The sterile operative technique was further advanced through the introduction of rubber surgical gloves in 1898. Other advances included the use of sterile gowns, masks, antibiotics, and other drugs.

In 1895, the well-known physicist Wilhelm Roentgen made observations that led to the development of x-ray technology. He found that he could create images of the bones in his hand by passing x-rays through his hand and onto a photographic plate. Radiographic technology is used extensively to diagnose illnesses and injuries today.

Many advances in laboratory testing occurred during the 20th century. Equipment that allows the rapid laboratory processing of diagnostic and prognostic examinations was developed, and the number of diagnostic laboratory procedures increased dramatically. For example, studies of prothrombin time were first made available in 1940, electrolytes in the period 1941–1946, blood gas in 1957, creatine phosphokinase in 1961, serum hepatitis in 1970, and carcinoembryonic antigen (the first cancer-screening test) in 1974.

Diagnostic radiology and radiation therapy have undergone huge advances in the past 50 years. An enormous advance first used in 1971 in England is an imaging modality called computed tomography (CT). The first CT scanners were used to create images of the skull. Whole-body scanners were introduced in 1974. In the 1980s, another powerful diagnostic tool was added—magnetic resonance imaging (MRI). MRI is a noninvasive technique that uses magnetic and radio-frequency fields to record images of soft tissues.

Surgical advances have been remarkable as well. Cardiac bypass surgery was developed in the 1970s, as were the techniques for joint replacement. Organs are now successfully transplanted, and artificial organs are being tested. New surgical techniques have included the use of lasers in ophthalmology, gynecology, and urology. Microsurgery is now a common tool in the reconstruction of damaged nerves and blood vessels. The use of robotics in surgery holds great promise for the future (Sloane et al. 1999, 6–7).

Today, it is human genetics and progress toward sequencing the human genome that promise to change the healthcare paradigm. New research on cellular and molecular changes underlying disease processes will necessitate new approaches to diagnosis and treatment.

The current paradigm for treating disease is to meet with the patient, diagnose the patient's symptoms, and prescribe therapy to treat them. The hope is that genetic medicine will enable the provider to identify gene patterns that underlie the process of cellular dysfunction that leads to injury before even meeting with the patient. Thus, diseases will be diagnosed much earlier, enabling physicians to provide treatment to stop or slow the disease process.

The study of cell-based technologies is controversial. Cell-based technologies include:

- Tissue engineering, which involves the use of biomaterials to develop new tissue and even whole organs with or without transplanting cells

- Human embryonic stem cells and/or adult stem cells used for transplantation and in regenerative medicine

- Gene therapy/cell transplantation

Advances in cell-based technologies such as cell-signaling pathways, growth factors, and the human genome project are encouraging ongoing research in these areas (Elçin 2003).

The year 2003 saw completion of the Human Genome Project (HGP), a 13-year-long international effort with three principal goals: to determine the sequence of the three billion DNA subunits, to identify all human genes, and to enable genes to be used in further biological study. A process called parallel sequencing was used on selected model organisms to help develop the technology and interpret gene function. The US Human Genome Project was a joint venture of the Department of Energy's HGP and the NIH's National Human Genome Research Institute.

Check Your Understanding 11.2

1. Which of the following laws created the Health Insurance Portability and Accountability Act?

   A. Health Insurance Portability and Accountability Act
   B. American Recovery and Reinvestment Act
   C. Consolidated Omnibus Budget Reconciliation Act
   D. Healthcare Quality Improvement Act

2. What government agency supports medical research?

   A. Social Security Administration
   B. Centers for Medicare and Medicaid Services
   C. US Public Health Service
   D. National Institutes of Health

3. A HIT student has asked you why Medicare reimburses healthcare providers through prospective payment systems. Which of the following pieces of legislation would you use as your explanation?

   A. Peer Review Improvement Act of 1982
   B. Consolidated Budget Reconciliation Act of 1986
   C. Tax Equity and Fiscal Responsibility Act of 1982
   D. Omnibus Budget Reconciliation Act of 1986

4. A friend and I are debating cell-based technologies. Which of the following is a reason why I might argue for this technology?

   A. It uses magnetic and radio-frequency to record images of soft tissue.
   B. Diseases could be diagnosed earlier.
   C. It studies the blood to diagnose conditions.
   D. It looks for microorganisms.

5. Which of the following best describes Medicaid?

   A. Federal program targeted principally for those 65 years and older

   B. Federally mandated healthcare program for low-income people

   C. Healthcare program limited to those under 65 years of age

   D. Healthcare program for low-income persons regardless of age that is totally financially supported and operated by the states

Instructions: Match the descriptions with the appropriate legislation.

6. Healthcare Quality Improvement Act of 1986	a. Authorized grants for states to construct new hospitals
	b. Required concurrent review of Medicare and Medicaid patients
7. Omnibus Budget Reconciliation Act of 1990	c. Established the National Practitioner Data Bank
8. Public Law 92-603 of 1972	d. Required PROs to report actions taken against physicians to state medical boards and licensing agencies
9. Omnibus Budget Reconciliation Act of 1989	
10. Hill-Burton Act	e. Instituted and researched the Agency for Healthcare Policy

Professional and Trade Associations Related to Healthcare

A number of trade and professional associations currently influence the practice of medicine and the delivery of healthcare services in the United States. Descriptions of a few of these associations are provided below.

American Medical Association (AMA)

The AMA was founded in 1847 as a national voluntary service organization. Today, its membership totals approximately 215,000 physicians and medical students (approximately 23 percent of all physicians) from every area of medicine. The organization is headquartered in Chicago.

   Its mission is to promote the science and art of medicine and to improve public health. Its key objectives are:

- To become the world leader in obtaining, synthesizing, integrating, and disseminating information on health and medical practice

- To remain the acknowledged leader in promoting professionalism in medicine and setting standards for medical ethics, practice, and education

- To continue to be an authoritative voice and influential advocate for patients and physicians

- To continue to be a sound organization that provides value to its members, related organizations, and employees

In addition, the AMA acts as an accreditation body for medical schools and residency programs. It also maintains and publishes the *Current Procedural Terminology* (CPT) coding system. CPT codes are the basis of reimbursement systems for physician's services and other types of healthcare services provided on an ambulatory basis.

American Hospital Association (AHA)

The AHA was founded in 1899. At its first meeting, eight hospital superintendents gathered in Cleveland, OH, to exchange ideas, compare methods of hospital management, discuss economics, and explore common interests and new trends. Originally called the Association of Hospital Superintendents, its mission was "to facilitate the interchange of ideas, comparing and contrasting methods of management, the discussion of hospital economics, the inspection of hospitals, suggestions of better plans for operating them, and such other matters as may affect the general interest of the membership" (AHA 1999, 110).

The association adopted a new constitution in 1906 and a new name, the American Hospital Association. At that time, it had 234 members. Its major concerns were developing hospital standards and building the management skills of its members.

Today, the mission of the AHA is to advance the health of individuals and communities. The association's current membership includes approximately 5,000 hospitals and healthcare institutions, 600 associate member organizations, and 40,000 individual executives active in the healthcare field. Its headquarters are located in Chicago.

The AHA publishes *Coding Clinic,* which provides official ICD-9-CM coding advice.

The Joint Commission

Since 1952, the Joint Commission has continually evolved to meet the changing needs of healthcare organizations. The organization changed its name from the Joint Commission on Accreditation of Hospitals (JCAH) to the Joint Commission on Accreditation of Healthcare Organizations (JCAHO) in the late 1980s and more recently in 2009 to the Joint Commission. It is the nation's oldest and largest healthcare standards-setting body. It conducts accreditation surveys in more than 17,000 healthcare organizations and programs, including ambulatory care facilities, long-term care facilities, behavioral health facilities, healthcare networks, and MCOs in addition to acute care hospitals (Joint Commission 2009a). To earn and maintain accreditation by the Joint Commission Gold Seal of Approval, an organization must demonstrate compliance with its standards by successfully undergoing an on-site survey at least every three years and laboratories must be surveyed every two years.

The Joint Commission accredits the following types of healthcare organizations:

- General, psychiatric, children's, and rehabilitation hospitals
- Critical access hospitals
- Home care organizations, including medical equipment services, hospice services
- Nursing homes and other long-term care facilities
- Behavioral healthcare organizations, addiction services
- Ambulatory care providers, including group practices and office-based surgery practices
- Independent or freestanding clinical laboratories

A board of commissioners made up of clinicians, administrators, educators, and others governs the organization. The Joint Commission's corporate members are the American College of Physicians, the American College of Surgeons, the American Dental Association, the American Hospital Association, and the American Medical Association. The Joint Commission's central office is located in Oakbrook Terrace, IL (Joint Commission 2009a).

The Joint Commission sets standards to aid organizations in providing safe and high-quality healthcare. Standards are developed in consultation with a variety of healthcare experts and updated periodically. The standards set expectations for performance that affect the safety and quality of patient care. About 50 percent of standards relate to patient safety. In addition, the Joint Commission has instituted a number of patient safety programs including (Joint Commission 2009b):

- National Patient Safety Goals: Annually addresses specific patient safety concerns.

- Sentinel Event Policy: Designed to identify and prevent the occurrence of events that lead to unexpected deaths or events leading to or potentially leading to serious physical injuries. When a sentinel event occurs, a root cause analysis and identification of improvements to risks must be undertaken.

- Sentinel Event Alert: A newsletter that provides important information on specific types of sentinel events such as medication and blood transfusion errors and how to prevent their occurrences.

- Universal Protocol: Provides a protocol to prevent surgical mishaps such as procedures performed on the wrong person and wrong site.

In the late 1990s, the Joint Commission moved away from traditional quality assessment processes and began emphasizing performance and quality improvement. The ORYX initiative reflected the new approach. The goal of the ORYX initiative was to incorporate the ongoing collection of quality and performance data into the accreditation process. Outcome measures document the results of care for individual patients as well as for specific types of patients grouped by diagnostic category. For example, an acute care hospital's overall rate of postsurgical infection would be considered an outcome measure. Outcome measures must be reported to the Joint Commission via software from vendors that have been approved by the Joint Commission for this purpose.

Blue Cross and Blue Shield Association

The forerunner of the Blue Cross and Blue Shield Association was a commission instituted by the AHA in 1929. In 1960, the commission was replaced by the Blue Cross Association and ties to the AHA were broken. In 1982, the Blue Cross Association merged with the National Association of Blue Shield Plans to become the Blue Cross and Blue Shield Association, often referred to as the Blues. The Blue Cross and Blue Shield Association (BCBSA) is a national federation of 39 independent, community-based and locally operated Blue Cross and Blue Shield companies that collectively employ over 150,000 people nationwide.

As the nation's oldest and largest family of health benefits companies, the Blue Cross and Blue Shield Association prides itself on being the most recognized brand in the health insurance industry along with many other celebrated milestones. More than 96 percent of hospitals and 91 percent of physicians contract with BCBS companies in the United States, which is more than any other commercial insurer (BCBS 2012).

American College of Healthcare Executives

The **American College of Healthcare Executives** (ACHE) is an organization for healthcare administrators. Like most of the organizations already discussed, it is headquartered in Chicago. Its mission is to serve as "the professional membership society for healthcare executives; to meet members' professional, educational, and leadership needs; to promote high ethical standards and conduct; and to enhance healthcare leadership and management excellence" (ACHE nd).

ACHE has over 30,000 members and fellows internationally. It also publishes books and textbooks on healthcare services management.

American Nurses Association

The ANA was founded in 1897 and is headquartered in Washington, DC. It is a professional association as well as the strongest labor union active in the nursing profession, representing the interests of the nation's 3.1 million registered nurses. The ANA's mission is to work for the improvement of health standards and the availability of healthcare services, to foster high professional standards for nurses, to stimulate and promote the professional development of nurses, and to advance the economic and general welfare of its members.

American Health Information Management Association

The American Health Information Management Association (AHIMA) is the professional membership organization for managers of health record services and healthcare information. It was founded in 1928 under the name of the Association of Record Librarians of North America. In 1929, the association adopted a constitution and bylaws. The name of the association was changed to the American Medical Record Association in 1970 and then to the American Health Information Management Association in 1991.

Headquartered in Chicago, the association currently has more than 63,000 members. Its mission is "to lead the health informatics and information management community to advance professional practice and standards" (AHIMA 2011). The association's vision is "leading the advancement and ethical use of quality health information to promote health and wellness worldwide" (AHIMA 2011).

AHIMA is the founding corporate member for the **Commission on Accreditation for Health Informatics and Information Management Education** (CAHIIM). CAHIIM is an independent accrediting organization whose mission is to serve the public interest by establishing and enforcing quality accreditation *standards* for health informatics (HI) and health information management (HIM) educational programs. CAHIIM accredits associate, baccalaureate, and graduate programs in health information management and graduate-level educational programs in health informatics (CAHIIM 2011).

AHIMA also sponsors an approval process for certificate programs for coding specialists through a special program called the Coding Education Program Approval (CEPA).

The **Commission on Certification for Health Informatics and Information Management** (CCHIIM) is an AHIMA commission dedicated to assuring the competency of professionals practicing HIIM. CCHIIM serves the public by establishing, implementing, and enforcing standards and procedures for certification and recertification of HIIM professionals. Through certification, CCHIIM assures the competency of professionals practicing health informatics and information management worldwide. CCHIIM offers a variety of credentials in the areas of health information management, coding, health data analytics, and healthcare privacy and security (CCHIIM 2009).

Certification Commission for Health Information Technology (CCHIT)

Founded in 2004, the Certification Commission for Health Information Technology (CCHIT) is a nonprofit organization whose mission is to accelerate the adoption of health information technology. The Commission is recognized by the federal government as one of six organizations that can certify EHRs. The other five are: Surescripts; LLC, ICSA

Labs; SLI Global Solutions; InfoGard Laboratories, Inc.; and Drummond Group Inc. Currently 70 percent of attested EHRs are CCHIT Certified (CCHIT 2009).

The Commission offers a CCHIT Certified Comprehensive certification program that inspects health information technology products against criteria for functionality, interoperability, privacy, and security. Certification is offered for ambulatory, inpatient, emergency electronic health records, e-prescribing, health information exchange, long-term care, post-acute care, and behavioral health. More than 200 EHR products were certified by mid-2009, representing over 75 percent of the marketplace. In October 2009, CCHIT launched a second certification program called the Preliminary ARRA (2011) Certification. This program is a modular certification program for applications that address one or more of the meaningful use objectives of the American Recovery and Reinvestment Act (ARRA). CCHIT also offers the EACH (EHR Alternative Certification for Healthcare Providers) program that evaluates how a hospital's current EHR measures against HHS's meaningful use requirements and then allows the institution to pursue certification of an existing EHR that is not already certified through a previous vendor.

Other Healthcare-Related Associations

Many other healthcare-related associations serve their professional members by providing educational, certification, and accreditation services. The best known include:

- The American Osteopathic Association
- The American Dental Association
- The American College of Surgeons
- The American League for Nursing
- The American Society of Clinical Pathologists
- The American Dietetic Association
- The Commission on Accreditation of Rehabilitation Facilities
- The American Association of Nurse Anesthetists

Check Your Understanding 11.3

1. What organization has the mission of promoting the science and art of medicine and to improve public health?

   A. The Joint Commission
   B. American Medical Association
   C. American Hospital Association
   D. American College of Healthcare Executives

2. Which of the following organizations can certify the EHR?

   A. The Joint Commission
   B. Commission of Certification of Health Information Technology
   C. American Hospital Association
   D. American College of Healthcare Executives

3. A college wants to start a new HIT program. Who should the staff contact for program accreditation information?

   A. Commission on Certification for Health Informatics and Information Management
   B. Commission on Certification of Health Information Technology
   C. Commission on Accreditation for Health Informatics and Information Management Education
   D. The Joint Commission

4. At our hospital, a patient died in childbirth. As this is a sentinel event, what do we need to do?

   A. Check the National Patient Safety Goals
   B. Write an article in the next newsletter
   C. Check to see if there is a universal protocol to address this issue
   D. Perform a root cause analysis

5. I need to order the Coding Clinic for our coders. Who should I contact?

   A. The Joint Commission
   B. American Medical Association
   C. American Hospital Association
   D. American College of Healthcare Executives

Instructions: Match each organization with the description that best describes it.

6. The Joint Commission

7. Commission on Certification of Health Information Technology

8. American Nurses Association

9. American Medical Association

10. American Health Information Management Association

   a. This association was founded in 1928 under the name of the Association of Record Librarians of North America.

   b. Part of this organization's mission is to work for the improvement of health standards and the availability of healthcare services.

   c. This organization's mission is to certify electronic health records.

   d. This organization developed the National Patient Safety Guidelines.

   e. This organization shares information on health and medical practices.

Organization and Operation of Modern Hospitals

The term *hospital* can be applied to any healthcare facility that:

- Has an organized medical staff
- Provides permanent inpatient beds
- Offers around-the-clock nursing services
- Provides diagnostic and therapeutic services

Most hospitals provide acute care services to inpatients. Acute care is the short-term care provided to diagnose and/or treat an illness or injury. The individuals who receive acute care services in hospitals are considered inpatients. Inpatients receive room-and-board services in addition to continuous nursing services. Generally, patients who spend more than 24 hours in a hospital are considered inpatients.

The **average length of stay** (ALOS) in an acute care hospital is 30 days or less. (Hospitals that have ALOSs longer than 30 days are considered long-term care facilities. Long-term care is discussed in detail later in this chapter.) With recent advances in surgical technology, anesthesia, and pharmacology, the ALOS in an acute care hospital is much shorter today than it was only a few years ago. In addition, many diagnostic and therapeutic procedures that once required inpatient care now can be performed on an outpatient basis.

For example, before the development of laparoscopic surgical techniques, a patient might be hospitalized for 10 days after a routine appendectomy (surgical removal of the appendix). Today, a patient undergoing a laparoscopic appendectomy might spend only a few hours in the hospital's outpatient surgery department and go home the same day. The influence of managed care and the emphasis on cost control in the Medicare/Medicaid programs also have resulted in shorter hospital stays.

In large acute care hospitals, hundreds of clinicians, administrators, managers, and support staff must work closely together to provide effective and efficient diagnostic and therapeutic services. Most hospitals provide services to both inpatients and outpatients. A hospital outpatient is a patient who receives hospital services without being admitted for inpatient (overnight) clinical care. Outpatient care is considered a kind of ambulatory care. (Ambulatory care is discussed later in this chapter.)

Modern hospitals are extremely complex organizations. Much of the clinical training for physicians, nurses, and allied health professionals is conducted in hospitals. Medical research is another activity carried out in hospitals.

Rise and Fall in Numbers of Hospitals

During the 1980s, medical advances and cost-containment measures enabled many procedures that once required inpatient hospitalization to be performed on an outpatient basis. Outpatient hospital visits increased by 40 percent, resulting in a decrease in hospital admissions. Fewer admissions and shortened lengths of stay for patients resulted in a significant reduction in the number of hospitals and hospital beds. Healthcare reform efforts and the rise of managed care resulted in enough hospital closings and mergers to reduce the number of governmental and community-based hospitals in the United States to approximately 5,700 (Sultz and Young 2011, 71). In 2010 the number of hospitals in the United States reached 5,795. This figure includes, among others, community, federal, nonfederal psychiatric, and nonfederal long-term care hospitals (AHA 2011).

Types of Hospitals

Hospitals can be classified in many different ways, including by:

- Number of beds
- Types of services provided
- Types of patients served
- For-profit or not-for-profit status
- Type of ownership

Number of Beds

A hospital's number of beds refers to the number of beds that are equipped and staffed for patient care. The term *bed capacity* sometimes is used to reflect the maximum number of inpatients the hospital can care for. Hospitals with fewer than 100 beds are usually considered small. Most US hospitals fall into this category. Some large, urban hospitals may have more than 500 beds. The number of beds is usually broken down by adult beds and pediatric beds. The number of maternity beds and other special categories may be listed separately. Hospitals also can be categorized according to the number of outpatient visits per year.

Types of Services Provided

Some hospitals specialize in certain types of service and treat specific illnesses. For example:

- *Rehabilitation hospitals* generally provide long-term care services to patients recuperating from debilitating or chronic illnesses and injuries such as strokes, head and spine injuries, and gunshot wounds. Patients often stay in rehabilitation hospitals for several months.

- *Psychiatric hospitals* provide inpatient care for patients with mental and developmental disorders. In the past, the ALOS for psychiatric inpatients was longer than it is today. Rather than months or years, most patients now spend only a few days or weeks per stay. However, many patients require repeated hospitalization for chronic psychiatric illnesses. (Behavioral healthcare is discussed in more detail later in this chapter.)

- *General hospitals* provide a wide range of medical and surgical services to diagnose and treat most illnesses and injuries.

- *Specialty hospitals* provide diagnostic and therapeutic services for a limited range of conditions such as burns, cancer, tuberculosis, or obstetrics/gynecology.

Types of Patients Served

Some hospitals specialize in serving specific types of patients. For example, children's hospitals provide specialized pediatric services in a number of medical specialties and rehabilitation hospitals provide post-acute care for patients recovering from an injury, illness, or disease.

For-Profit or Not-for-Profit Status

Hospitals also can be classified based on their ownership and profitability status. Not-for-profit healthcare organizations use excess funds to improve their services and to finance educational programs and community services. For-profit healthcare organizations are privately owned. Excess funds are paid back to the managers, owners, and investors in the form of bonuses and dividends.

Type of Ownership

The most common ownership types for hospitals and other kinds of healthcare organizations in the United States include:

- *Government-owned hospitals* are operated by a specific branch of federal, state, or local government as not-for-profit organizations. (Government-owned hospitals sometimes are called public hospitals.) They are supported, at least in part, by tax dollars. Examples of federally owned and operated hospitals include those operated by the Department of Veterans Affairs to serve retired military personnel. The Department of Defense operates facilities for active military personnel and their dependents. Many states own and operate psychiatric hospitals. County and city governments often operate public hospitals to serve the healthcare needs of their communities, especially those residents who are unable to pay for their care.

- *Proprietary hospitals* may be owned by private foundations, partnerships, or investor-owned corporations. Large corporations may own a number of for-profit hospitals, and the stock of several large US hospital chains is publicly traded.

- *Voluntary hospitals* are not-for-profit hospitals owned by universities, churches, charities, religious orders, unions, and other not-for-profit entities. They often provide free care to patients who otherwise would not have access to healthcare services.

Organization of Hospital Services

The organizational structure of every hospital is designed to meet its specific needs. For example, most acute care hospitals are made up of a board of directors, a professional medical staff, an executive administrative staff, medical and surgical services, patient care (nursing) services, diagnostic and laboratory services, and support services (for example, nutritional services, environmental safety, and HIM services) (see figure 11.2).

Board of Directors

The board of directors has primary responsibility for setting the overall direction of the hospital. (In some hospitals, the board of directors is called the governing board or board of trustees.) The board works with the **chief executive officer** (CEO) and the leaders of the organization's medical staff to develop the hospital's strategic direction as well as its mission (statement of the organization's purpose and the customers it serves), vision (description of the organization's ideal future), and values (descriptive list of the organization's fundamental principles or beliefs).

Other specific responsibilities of the board of directors include:

- Establishing bylaws in accordance with the organization's legal and licensing requirements
- Selecting qualified administrators
- Approving the organization and makeup of the clinical staff
- Monitoring the quality of care

The board's members are elected or appointed for specific terms of service (for example, five years). Most boards also elect officers, commonly a chairman, vice-chairman, president, secretary, and treasurer. The size of the board varies considerably. Individual board members are called directors, board members, or trustees. Individuals serve on one or more standing committees such as the executive committee, joint conference committee, finance committee, strategic planning committee, and building committee.

The makeup of the board depends on the type of hospital and the form of ownership. For example, the board of a community hospital is likely to include local business leaders, representatives of community organizations, and other people interested in the welfare of the community. The board of a teaching hospital, on the other hand, is likely to include medical school alumni and university administrators, among others.

Increased competition among healthcare providers and limits on managed care and Medicare/Medicaid reimbursement have made the governing of hospitals especially difficult in the past two decades. In the future, boards of directors will continue to face strict accountability in terms of cost containment, performance management, and integration of services to maintain fiscal stability and to ensure the delivery of high-quality patient care.

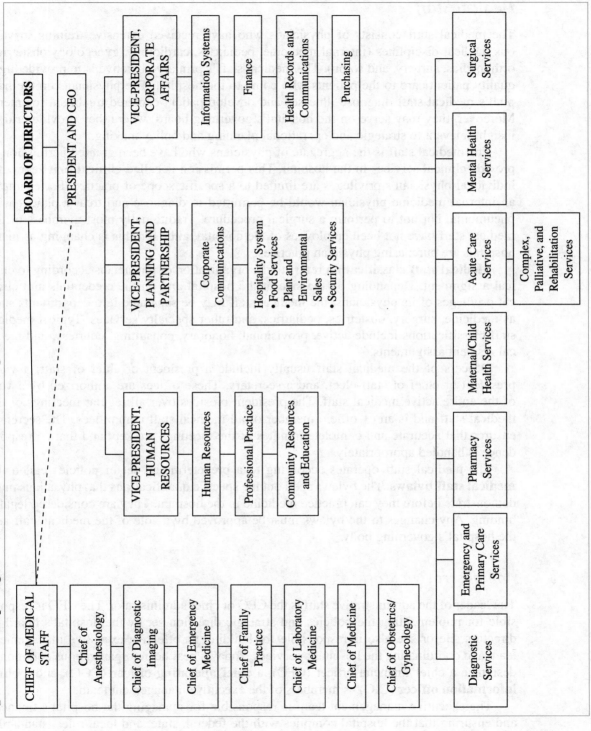

Figure 11.2.   Sample organizational chart for an acute care hospital with outpatient services

Medical Staff

The medical staff consists of physicians who have received extensive training in various medical disciplines (internal medicine, pediatrics, cardiology, gynecology/obstetrics, orthopedics, surgery, and so on). The medical staff's primary objective is to provide high-quality patient care to the patients who come to the hospital. The physicians on the hospital's medical staff diagnose illnesses and develop patient-centered treatment regimens. Moreover, they may serve on the hospital's governing board, where they provide critical insight relevant to strategic and operational planning and policy making.

The medical staff is the aggregate of physicians who have been granted permission to provide clinical services in the hospital. This permission is called **clinical privileges.** An individual physician's privileges are limited to a specific scope of practice. For example, an internal medicine physician would be permitted to diagnose and treat a patient with pneumonia, but not to perform a surgical procedure. Traditionally most members of the medical staff have not been employees of the hospital, although this is changing as many hospitals are purchasing physician practices.

Medical staff classification refers to the organization of physicians according to clinical assignment. Depending on the size of the hospital and on the credentials and clinical privileges of its physicians, the medical staff may be separated into departments such as medicine, surgery, obstetrics, pediatrics, and other specialty services. Typical medical staff classifications include active, provisional, honorary, consulting, courtesy, and medical resident assignments.

Officers of the medical staff usually include a president or chief of staff, a vice-president or chief of staff-elect, and a secretary. These offices are authorized by a vote of the entire active medical staff. The president presides over all regular meetings of the medical staff and is an ex officio member of all medical staff committees. The secretary ensures that accurate and complete minutes of the meetings are kept and that correspondence is handled appropriately.

The medical staff operates according to a predetermined set of policies called the **medical staff bylaws.** The bylaws spell out the specific qualifications that physicians must demonstrate before they can practice medicine in the hospital. They are considered legally binding. Any changes to the bylaws must be approved by a vote of the medical staff and the hospital's governing body.

Administrative Staff

The leader of the administrative staff is the CEO or chief administrator. The CEO is responsible for implementing the policies and strategic direction set by the hospital's board of directors. He or she also is responsible for building an effective executive management team and coordinating the hospital's services. Today's healthcare organizations commonly designate a chief financial officer (CFO), a **chief operating officer** (COO), and a **chief information officer** (CIO) as members of the executive management team.

The executive management team is responsible for managing the hospital's finances and ensuring that the hospital complies with the federal, state, and local rules, standards, and laws that govern the delivery of healthcare services. Depending on the size of the hospital, the CEO's staff may include healthcare administrators with job titles such as vice president, associate administrator, department director or manager, or administrative assistant. Department-level administrators manage and coordinate the activities of the highly specialized and multidisciplinary units that perform clinical, administrative, and support services in the hospital.

Healthcare administrators may hold advanced degrees in healthcare administration, nursing, public health, or business management. A growing number of hospitals are hiring physician executives to lead their executive management teams. Many healthcare administrators are fellows of ACHE.

Patient Care Services

Most direct patient care delivered in hospitals is provided by professional nurses. Modern nursing requires a diverse skill set, advanced clinical competencies, and postgraduate education. In almost every hospital, patient care services constitutes the largest clinical department in terms of staffing, budget, specialized services offered, and clinical expertise required.

Nurses are responsible for providing continuous, around-the-clock treatment and support for hospital inpatients. The quantity and quality of nursing care available to patients are influenced by a number of factors, including the nursing staff's educational preparation and specialization, experience, and skill level. The level of patient care staffing also is a critical component of quality.

Traditionally, physicians alone determined the type of treatment each patient would receive. However, today's nurses are playing a wider role in treatment planning and **case management.** They identify timely and effective interventions in response to a wide range of problems related to the patients' treatment, comfort, and safety. Their responsibilities include performing patient assessments, creating care plans, evaluating the appropriateness of treatment, and evaluating the effectiveness of care. At the same time that they provide technical care, effective nursing professionals also offer personal care that recognizes the concerns and emotional needs of patients and their families.

A registered nurse qualified by advanced education and clinical and management experience usually administers patient care services. Although the title may vary, this role is usually referred to as the **chief nursing officer** (CNO) or vice president of nursing or patient care. The CNO is a member of the hospital's executive management team and usually reports directly to the CEO.

In any nursing organizational structure, several types of relationships can be identified, including:

- *Line relationships* identify the positions of superiors and subordinates and indicate the levels of authority and responsibility vested with each position. For example, a supervisor in a postop surgical unit would have authority to direct the work of several nurses.

- *Lateral relationships* define the connections among various positions in which a hierarchy of authority is not involved. For example, the supervisors of preop and postop surgical units would have parallel positions in the structure and would need to coordinate the work they perform.

- *Functional relationships* refer to duties that are divided according to function. In such arrangements, individuals exercise authority in one particular area by virtue of their special knowledge and expertise.

Diagnostic and Therapeutic Services

The services provided to patients in hospitals go beyond the clinical services provided directly by the medical and nursing staff. Many diagnostic and therapeutic services involve the work of allied health professionals. Allied health professionals receive specialized education and training, and their qualifications are registered or certified by a number of specialty organizations.

Diagnostic and therapeutic services are critical to the success of every patient care delivery system. Diagnostic services include clinical laboratory, radiology, and nuclear medicine. Therapeutic services include radiation therapy, occupational therapy, and physical therapy.

Clinical Laboratory Services

The clinical laboratory is divided into two sections: anatomic pathology and clinical pathology. Anatomic pathology deals with human tissues and provides surgical pathology, autopsy, and cytology services. Clinical pathology deals mainly with the analysis of body fluids—principally blood, but also urine, gastric contents, and cerebrospinal fluid.

Physicians who specialize in performing and interpreting the results of pathology tests are called pathologists. Laboratory technicians are allied health professionals trained to operate laboratory equipment and perform laboratory tests under the supervision of a pathologist.

Radiology

Radiology involves the use of radioactive isotopes, fluoroscopic and radiographic equipment, and CT and MRI equipment to diagnose disease. Physicians who specialize in radiology are called radiologists. They are experts in the medical use of radiant energy, radioactive isotopes, radium, cesium, and cobalt as well as x-rays, radium, and radioactive materials. They also are experts in interpreting x-ray, MRI, and CT diagnostic images.

Radiology technicians are allied health professionals trained to operate radiological equipment and perform radiological tests under the supervision of a radiologist.

Nuclear Medicine and Radiation Therapy

Radiologists also may specialize in nuclear medicine and radiation therapy. Nuclear medicine involves the use of ionizing radiation and small amounts of short-lived radioactive tracers to treat disease, specifically neoplastic disease (that is, nonmalignant tumors and malignant cancers). Based on the mathematics and physics of tracer methodology, nuclear medicine is widely applied in clinical medicine. However, most authorities agree that medical science has only scratched the surface in terms of nuclear medicine's potential capabilities.

Radiation therapy uses high-energy x-rays, cobalt, electrons, and other sources of radiation to treat human disease. In current practice, radiation therapy is used alone or in combination with surgery or chemotherapy (drugs) to treat many types of cancer. In addition to external beam therapy, radioactive implants (as well as therapy performed with heat—hyperthermia) are available.

Occupational Therapy

Occupational therapy is the medically directed use of work and play activities to improve patients' independent functioning, enhance their development, and prevent or decrease their level of disability. The individuals who perform occupational therapy are credentialed allied health professionals called occupational therapists. They work under the direction of physicians. Occupational therapy is made available in acute care hospitals, clinics, and rehabilitation centers.

Providing occupational therapy services begins with an evaluation of the patient and the selection of therapeutic goals. Occupational therapy activities may involve the adaptation of tasks or the environment to achieve maximum independence and to enhance the patient's quality of life. An occupational therapist may treat developmental deficits, birth defects, learning disabilities, traumatic injuries, burns, neurological conditions, orthopedic conditions, mental deficiencies, and psychiatric disorders. Within the healthcare system, occupational therapy plays various roles. These roles include promoting health, preventing disability, developing or restoring functional capacity, guiding adaptation within physical and mental parameters, and teaching creative problem solving to increase independent function.

Physical Therapy and Rehabilitation

Physical therapy and rehabilitation have expanded into many medical specialties. Physical therapy can be applied in most disciplines of medicine, especially in neurology, neurosurgery, orthopedics, geriatrics, rheumatology, internal medicine, cardiovascular medicine, cardiopulmonary medicine, psychiatry, sports medicine, burn and wound care, and chronic pain management. It also plays a role in community health education. Credentialed allied health professionals administer physical therapy under the direction of physicians.

Medical **rehabilitation services** involve the entire healthcare team: physicians, nurses, social workers, occupational therapists, physical therapists, and other healthcare personnel. The objective is to either eliminate the patients' disability or alleviate it as fully as possible. Physical therapy can be used to improve the cognitive, social, and physical abilities of patients impaired by chronic disease or injury.

The primary purpose of physical therapy in rehabilitation is to promote optimal health and function by applying scientific principles. Treatment modalities include therapeutic exercise, therapeutic massage, biofeedback, and applications of heat, low-energy lasers, cold, water, electricity, and ultrasound.

Respiratory Therapy

Respiratory therapy involves the diagnosis and treatment of patients who have acute and/or chronic lung disorders. Under the direction of qualified physicians and surgeons, respiratory therapists provide services such as emergency care for stroke, heart failure, and shock patients. They also treat patients with chronic respiratory diseases such as emphysema and asthma.

Respiratory treatments include the administration of oxygen and inhalants such as bronchodilators. The therapists set up and monitor ventilator equipment and provide physiotherapy to improve breathing.

Ancillary Support Services

The ancillary units of the hospital provide vital clinical and administrative support services to patients, medical staff, visitors, and employees.

Clinical Support Services

The clinical support units provide the following services:

- Pharmaceutical services (provided by registered pharmacists and pharmacy technologists)
- Food and nutrition services (managed by registered dietitians who develop general and special-diet menus and nutritional plans for individual patients)
- HIM (health record) services (managed by RHIAs and RHITs)
- Social work and social services (provided by licensed social workers and licensed clinical social workers)
- Patient advocacy services (provided by several types of healthcare professionals, most commonly registered nurses and licensed social workers)
- Environmental (housekeeping) services
- Purchasing, central supply, and materials management services
- Engineering and plant operations

Administrative Support Services

In addition to clinical support services, hospitals need administrative support services to operate effectively. Administrative support services provide business management and clerical services in several key areas, including:

- Admissions and central registration
- Claims and billing (business office)
- Accounting

- Information services
- Human resources
- Public relations
- Fund development
- Marketing

Check Your Understanding 11.4

1. Which of the following is an example of a voluntary hospital?

   A. A hospital owned by a for-profit organization
   B. VA hospital
   C. Military hospitals
   D. A not-for-profit hospital owned by a church

2. I have been asked who has the primary responsibility to guide the direction of the hospital. My response should be:

   A. Board of directors
   B. Chief executive officer
   C. Medical staff
   D. Chief operating officer

3. The HIM Department is considered to be what type of department?

   A. Patient care services
   B. Diagnostic and therapeutic services
   C. Administrative support services
   D. Clinical support services

4. What service uses work and play to help the patient improve independent functioning?

   A. Occupational therapy
   B. Physical therapy
   C. Respiratory therapy
   D. Clinical laboratory services

5. Dr. Smith has been granted permission by Community hospital to perform cardiac catheterizations. This permission is called:

   A. Clinical privileges
   B. Clinical assignment
   C. Clinical classification
   D. Case management

Instructions: Indicate whether the statements below are true or false (T or F).

6. ____ General hospitals provide short-term care to diagnose and/or treat an illness.

7. ____ A registered nurse qualified by advanced education and clinical and management experience usually administers patient care services.

8. ____ Healthcare reform results in closing of some hospitals.

9. ____ The average length of stay for an acute care hospital is 21 days or less.

10. ____ Rehabilitation services include only physical therapy and occupational therapy.

Forces Affecting Healthcare Delivery

A number of recent developments in healthcare delivery have had far-reaching effects on the operation of hospitals and other healthcare delivery facilities and services in the United States. Many of these developments are discussed below.

Growth of Subacute Care

Subacute care represents a new movement in healthcare. In the past, the term was used in reference to the services provided to hospitalized patients who did not meet the medical criteria for needing acute care. Today, it refers to the level of skilled care needed by patients with complex medical conditions, typically Medicare patients with multiple medical problems.

Traditionally, nursing homes, home care providers, and rehabilitation facilities have provided subacute care. Now some hospitals are developing subacute units in response to changing demographics that make it a cost-effective alternative to inpatient acute care.

Development of Peer Review and Quality Improvement Programs

The goal of high-quality patient care is to promote, preserve, and restore health. High-quality care is delivered in an appropriate setting in a manner that is satisfying to patients. It is achieved when the patient's health status is improved as much as possible. Quality has several components, including:

- Appropriateness (the right care is provided at the right time)
- Technical excellence (the right care is provided in the right manner)
- Accessibility (the right care can be obtained when it is needed)
- Acceptability (patients are satisfied)

Peer Review

In peer review, a member of a profession assesses the work of colleagues within that same profession. Peer review traditionally has been at the center of quality assessment and assurance efforts. The medical profession's peer review efforts have emphasized the scientific aspects of quality. Appropriate use of pharmaceuticals, postoperative infection rates, and accuracy of diagnosis are among the measures of quality that have been used. Peer review is a requirement of both CMS and the Joint Commission.

Quality Improvement

Quality improvement (QI) programs have been in place in hospitals for years and have been required by the Medicare/Medicaid programs and accreditation standards. QI programs have covered medical staff as well as nursing and other departments or processes.

Efforts to encourage the delivery of high-quality care take place at the local and national levels. Such efforts are geared toward assessing the efforts of both individuals and institutions. Currently, professional associations, healthcare organizations, government agencies, private external quality review associations, consumer groups, MCOs, and group purchasers of care all play a role in trying to promote high-quality care. Discussion of quality improvement processes is provided in chapter 10.

Growth of Managed Care

Managed care is a generic term for a healthcare reimbursement system that manages cost, quality, and access to services. Most managed care plans do not provide healthcare directly. Instead, they enter into service contracts with the physicians, hospitals, and other healthcare providers who provide medical services to enrollees in the plans.

Managed care systems control costs primarily by presetting payment amounts and restricting patient access to healthcare services through precertification and utilization review processes. (Managed care is discussed in more detail in chapter 6.) Managed care delivery systems also attempt to manage cost and quality by:

- Implementing various forms of financial incentives for providers
- Promoting healthy lifestyles
- Identifying risk factors and illnesses early in the disease process
- Providing patient education

Although the most recent studies suggest that managed care results in lower costs with equal or better quality, most are limited because they have focused on short-term health outcomes (Weinerman et al. 1996). Very little is known about the long-term effects of specific reimbursement or organizational arrangements on quality of care. Further, recent evidence indicates that the quality of care provided under managed care systems may differ across population groups.

Efforts at Healthcare Reengineering

During the 1980s, healthcare organizations adopted **continuous quality improvement** (CQI) processes. Lessons learned from other areas of business were applied to healthcare settings. **Reengineering** came in many varieties, such as focused process improvement, major business process improvement and business process innovation, total quality management, and CQI. Regardless of approach, every healthcare organization attempted to look inside and to practice process as opposed to traditional department thinking. Healthcare organizations formed cross-functional teams that collaborated to solve organizational problems. At the same time, the Joint Commission reengineered the accreditation process to increase its focus on process and systems analysis. Gone were the days of thinking in a silo. All the silos were turned over, and healthcare teams learned from each other. The drivers of reengineering included cost reduction, staff shortages, and implementation of technology.

Emphasis on Patient-Focused Care

Patient-focused care is a concept developed to contain hospital inpatient costs and improve quality by restructuring services so that more of them take place in the nursing units (patient floors) and not in specialized units in dispersed hospital locations. The emphasis is on cross-training staff in the nursing units to perform a variety of functions for a small group of patients rather than one set of functions for a large number of patients. Some organizations have achieved patient-focused care by assigning multiskilled workers to serve food, clean patients' rooms, and assist in nursing care. However, some organizations have experienced low patient satisfaction with this type of worker because the patients are confused and do not know who to ask to do what.

Hospital staff spend most of their time performing activities in the following nine categories:

- Medical, technical, and clinical procedures
- Patient services
- Medical documentation
- Institutional documentation
- Scheduling and coordination
- Patient transportation
- Staff transportation
- Management and supervision
- Ready-for-action activities

A study at Lakeland Regional Medical Center, a 750-bed hospital in central Florida, found that medical, technical, and clinical activity consumed one-sixth of the center's personnel-related costs. The study also showed that almost twice that amount of time was spent writing things down. Scheduling and coordination took as much time as medical activity, and ready-for-action activities consumed even more.

The study suggested that restructuring services at Lakeland would reduce the number of staff required for patient care activities from 2,200 to 1,200 and improve care. The amount of physical space allotted to each unit would be sufficient to contain a minilab, diagnostic radiology rooms, linen and general supply, stockrooms, and so on. If such changes were carried out, medical documentation could be reduced by almost two-thirds, scheduling and coordination service by more than two-thirds, and ready-for-action time by two-thirds.

Hospitals have had difficulty in fully and rapidly implementing patient-focused care for the following reasons: the high cost of conversion; the extensive physical renovations required; resistance from functional departments; and other priorities for management, such as mergers and considering potential mergers.

Evidence-Based Best Practices and Outcomes

Evidence-based medicine is the conscientious, explicit, and judicious use of current best evidence in making decisions about the care of individual patients. The practice of evidence-based medicine means integrating individual clinical expertise with the best available external clinical evidence from systematic research (Sackett et al. 1996). Practicing evidenced-based medicine means that healthcare providers combine their individual experience and knowledge with clinically based research to make diagnoses and decisions about an individual's patient care.

Integrating individual expertise with clinically based research for making healthcare decisions is not a new concept. However, formalizing the use of clinically based research in day-to-day practice has received more attention during the past decade. For example, the Agency for Healthcare Research and Quality (AHRQ) in 1997 launched an initiative to promote evidence-based practice in everyday care. The goal of this initiative is to improve the quality of healthcare by facilitating the use of evidence-based research findings in everyday healthcare practice.

The AHRQ established 12 evidence-based practice centers (EPCs). Each of the EPCs develops evidence reports related to healthcare delivery issues that are common, expensive, and/or significant for the Medicare and Medicaid populations. These reports are used by federal and state agencies, private sector professional societies, health delivery systems, providers, payers, and others to develop evidenced base guidelines (Agency for Healthcare Research and Quality 2009).

Evidence-based guidelines suggest diagnostic or therapeutic interventions that a healthcare practitioner may use. For example, improvement of the palliative care of pain is a guideline that suggests clinicians monitor pain regularly and use therapies of proven effectiveness to manage pain (Oaseem et al. 2008). The purpose of such guidelines is to improve the quality of healthcare and patient's chances of getting as well as possible. Using evidence-based guidelines provide the following benefits when used for (National Institutes for Health and Clinical Excellence 2009):

- Recommendations for the treatment and care of people by health professionals
- Developing standards to assess the clinical practice of individual health professionals
- Education and training of health professionals
- Helping patients to make informed decisions
- Improving communication between patient and health professional

Development of Integrated Healthcare Delivery Systems

An integrated delivery system (IDS), also referred to as an Integrated Delivery Network or IDN, is a healthcare provider made up of a number of associated medical facilities that furnish coordinated healthcare services. Most IDSs include a number of facilities that provide services along the continuum of care (ambulatory surgery centers, physician office practices, outpatient clinics, acute care hospitals, **skilled nursing facilities** [SNFs], MCOs, and so on).

The purpose of an IDS is to organize the continuum of care, maximize effectiveness, and reduce costs. The continuum of care includes services for patients at different levels of the healthcare system. In an IDS arrangement, the focus is on holistic care rather than on fragmented care among specialists. Examples of different levels of care across the continuum are:

- Health promotion and disease prevention
- Primary care
- Acute care
- Tertiary care
- Long-term care
- **Hospice care**

Integrated healthcare information systems are needed to manage the continuum of care. The electronic health record (EHR) is essential for meeting IDS goals of effectively managing and delivering high-quality care. Timely, accurate, and accessible information is needed to manage care across all the different continuum of care levels. (Chapters 4 and 16 discuss many communication and interoperability issues associated with EHRs.)

Licensure, Certification, and Accreditation of Healthcare Facilities

Licensure, certification, and accreditation have had an enormous impact on the standardization and quality of healthcare services in the United States. Such programs require that high-performance standards be met in the provision of medical care and in the construction, maintenance, and management of the healthcare facility.

State Licensure

Licensure is a "process by which a governmental authority grants permission to an individual practitioner or healthcare organization to operate or to engage in an occupation or profession" (Quality Assurance Project 2005). State legislatures usually grant authority to a state agency to license healthcare facilities. For example, hospitals, nursing homes, home health agencies, ambulatory surgical facilities, and adult day-care/health facilities are usually licensed by state agencies.

Licensing agencies set standards that healthcare facilities must meet before being granted a license to operate. The standards are designed to promote the health, welfare, and safety of patients. Such standards may address staff levels, coordination of services, patient rights, quality assurance, safety of the environment, and adequacy of the physical plant. The licensing agency monitors compliance with the standards, usually through surveys and on-site inspections. The types of facilities licensed and the standards for licensure vary from state to state.

Although licensure requirements vary, healthcare facilities must meet certain basic criteria determined by state regulatory agencies. These standards address concerns such as adequacy of staffing, physical aspects of the facility (equipment and buildings), and services provided, including the maintenance of health records. Most licensing agencies perform reviews annually.

Certification for Medicare Participation

Certification is the procedure conducted by an authorized body in evaluating and recognizing whether an individual or institution meets predetermined requirements. To receive Medicare and Medicaid reimbursement, providers must prove that they follow the rules and regulations for participating in the Medicare program. Called the Medicare Conditions of Participation, these rules are set forth by CMS. Facilities that must meet the standards in the Conditions of Participation include hospitals, home health agencies, ambulatory surgical centers, and hospices.

Certification for Medicare reimbursement is the responsibility of the states. However, the Medicare act specifies that those facilities accredited by the Joint Commission and the AOA are deemed to be in compliance with the Conditions of Participation and do not have to undergo a separate certification process. Most recently in late 2009, DNV

Healthcare, Inc. was granted deeming authority by CMS in addition to the Joint Commission and the AOA.

Voluntary Accreditation

Accreditation is a voluntary system of institutional or organizational review performed by an independent body that has developed standards to measure and ensure the quality of healthcare services. Examples of accrediting organizations are The Joint Commission and the American Osteopathic Association (AOA).

The Joint Commission is a private, nonprofit organization that establishes guidelines and standards for the operation and management of healthcare facilities to ensure the quality and safety of care. It operates voluntary accreditation programs for hospitals, non-hospital-based psychiatric and substance abuse organizations, long-term care organizations, home care organizations, ambulatory care organizations, and organization-based pathology and clinical laboratory services.

Most state governments recognize the Joint Commission accreditation as a condition of licensure and receiving Medicaid reimbursement. Typically, organizations are inspected every three years with accreditation and survey findings made available to the public. When an organization is found to be in substantial compliance with the Joint Commission standards, accreditation may be awarded for up to three years.

The AOA sponsors a voluntary accreditation program for osteopathic healthcare facilities and medical schools. Its purpose is to advance the philosophy and practice of osteopathy. The AOA has developed accreditation requirements for osteopathic hospitals, ambulatory care/surgery, mental health, substance abuse, and physical rehabilitation medicine facilities. Like Joint Commission–accredited facilities, AOA- and now DNV Healthcare, Inc.–accredited facilities are considered to have deemed status and qualify to receive Medicare reimbursement.

Check Your Understanding 11.5

1. I have been asked to describe quality of healthcare. Which of the following would I include in my definition?

   A. Care that is provided at the lowest cost
   B. The right care is provided at the right time
   C. Care that is paid for by an insurance company
   D. Care that is administered only in an accredited healthcare facility

2. I work for an organization that owns a hospital, a skilled nursing facility, and physician practices. I work for what type of organization?

   A. A managed care organization
   B. A state department of public health
   C. An accreditation organization
   D. An integrated delivery system

3. Which of the following is true regarding Medicare certification of hospitals?

   A. Must be Joint Commission accredited
   B. Must be Joint Commission or AOA accredited
   C. Must be in compliance with the Conditions of Participation
   D. Must be accredited by the Joint Commission and the AOA

4. I have been asked what is the purpose of evidence-based guidelines. How would I respond?

   A. They organize the continuum of care.
   B. They help to improve the quality of patient care.
   C. They provide flexibility to the care provider.
   D. They are mandated by Medicare and Medicaid as well as many states.

5. At our facility, our staff on the nursing units are cross-trained to perform many tasks for a small group of patients. This concept is called:

   A. Continuous quality improvement
   B. Integrated delivery network
   C. Reengineering
   D. Patient-focused care

6. Quality has several components, including appropriateness, technical excellence, acceptability, and:

   A. Accuracy of diagnosis
   B. Continuous improvement
   C. Connectivity
   D. Accessibility

7. What type of program has been in place in hospitals for years and is required by the Medicare and Medicaid programs as well as accreditation standards?

   A. Quality improvement
   B. Patient-focused care
   C. Managed care
   D. Integrated delivery system

8. Which of the following is a true statement about peer review?

   A. Usually does not improve patient care
   B. Is not required by the Joint Commission or CMS
   C. Involves assessment of the work of colleagues by those in the same profession
   D. Involves assessment of the work of physicians by those outside of the medical profession

9. What program attempts to contain hospital inpatient costs and improve quality by restructuring services so that more is done in the nursing unit?

   A. Continuous quality improvement
   B. Patient-focused care
   C. Managed care
   D. Acute care

Other Types of Healthcare Services

Healthcare delivery is more than hospital-related care. It can be viewed as a continuum of services that cuts across care settings, including ambulatory, acute, subacute, long-term, and residential care, among others. Continuum of care has also been defined as "the totality of healthcare services provided to a patient and his or her family in all settings from the least extensive to the most extensive" (Shaw et al. 2009). Figure 11.3 shows various types of treatment settings available along the continuum of care.

Integrated Delivery Network/System

In an IDN/IDS, providers strive to meet every healthcare consumer's needs. This can be described as a full-service model of meeting patient needs from the cradle to the grave. IDNs develop a full continuum of care model, including acute care inpatient and outpatient services, a home health agency, a long-term care facility, and hospital-based durable medical equipment (DME) services. The continuum of care model can also be described as vertical integration whereas horizontal integration is when a company expands into similar businesses, such as a hospital network purchasing additional hospitals.

Ambulatory Care

Ambulatory care may be defined as the preventive and/or corrective healthcare provided in a practitioner's office, a clinic, or a hospital on a nonresident (outpatient) basis. The term

Figure 11.3.   The continuum of care

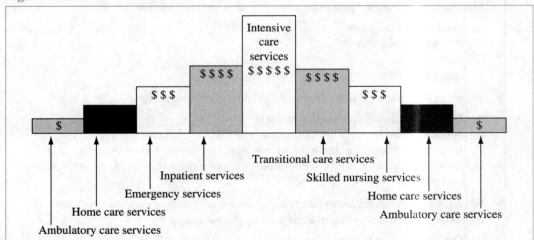

Source: Shaw et al. 2009, 107.

usually implies that patients go to locations outside their homes to obtain healthcare services and return the same day (HealthCare.com 2009).

It encompasses all the health services provided to individual patients who are not residents in a healthcare facility. Such services include the educational services provided by community health clinics and public health departments. Primary care, emergency care, and ambulatory specialty care (which includes ambulatory surgery) all may be considered ambulatory care. Ambulatory care services are provided in a variety of settings, including urgent care centers, school-based clinics, public health clinics, and neighborhood and community health centers.

Current medical practice emphasizes performing healthcare services in the least costly setting possible. This change in thinking has led to decreased utilization of emergency services, increased utilization of nonemergency ambulatory facilities, decreased hospital admissions, and shorter hospital stays. The need to reduce the cost of healthcare also has led primary care physicians to treat conditions they once would have referred to specialists.

Physicians who provide ambulatory care services fall into two major categories: physicians working in private practice and physicians working for ambulatory care organizations. Physicians in private practice are self-employed. They work in solo, partnership, and group practices set up as for-profit organizations.

Alternatively, physicians who work for ambulatory care organizations are employees of those organizations. Ambulatory care organizations include health maintenance organizations (HMOs), hospital-based ambulatory clinics, walk-in and emergency clinics, hospital-owned group practices and health promotion centers, freestanding surgery centers, freestanding urgent care centers, freestanding emergency care centers, health department clinics, neighborhood clinics, home care agencies, community mental health centers, school and workplace health services, and prison health services.

Ambulatory care organizations also employ other healthcare providers, including nurses, laboratory technicians, podiatrists, chiropractors, physical therapists, radiology technicians, psychologists, and social workers.

Private Medical Practice

Private medical practices are physician-owned entities that provide primary care or medical/surgical specialty care services in a freestanding office setting. The physicians have medical privileges at local hospitals and surgical centers but are not employees of the other healthcare entities.

Hospital-Based Ambulatory Care Services

In addition to providing inpatient services, many acute care hospitals provide various ambulatory care services.

Emergency Services and Trauma Care

More than 90 percent of community hospitals in the United States provide emergency services. Hospital-based emergency departments provide specialized care for victims of traumatic accidents and life-threatening illnesses. In urban areas, many also provide walk-in services for patients with minor illnesses and injuries who do not have access to regular primary care physicians.

Many physicians on the hospital staff also use the emergency care department as a setting to assess patients with problems that may either lead to an inpatient admission or require equipment or diagnostic imaging facilities not available in a private office or nursing home. Emergency services function as a major source of unscheduled admissions to the hospital.

Outpatient Surgical Services

Generally, the term *ambulatory surgery* refers to any surgical procedure that does not require an overnight stay in a hospital. It can be performed in the outpatient surgery department of a hospital and in a freestanding ambulatory surgery center. During the 1980s and 1990s, the percentage of surgeries done on an outpatient basis rose dramatically and this trend continues today. The increased number of procedures performed in an ambulatory setting can be attributed to improvements in surgical technology and anesthesia and the utilization management demands of third-party payers.

Outpatient Diagnostic and Therapeutic Services

Outpatient diagnostic and therapeutic services are provided in a hospital or one of its satellite facilities. Diagnostic services are those services performed by a physician to identify the disease or condition from which the patient is suffering. Therapeutic services are those services performed by a physician to treat the disease or condition that has been identified.

Hospital outpatients fall into different classifications according to the type of service they receive and the location of the service. For example, emergency outpatients are treated in the hospital's emergency or trauma care department for conditions that require immediate care. Clinic outpatients are treated in one of the hospital's clinical departments on an ambulatory basis. Referral outpatients receive special diagnostic or therapeutic services in the hospital on an ambulatory basis, but responsibility for their care remains with the referring physician.

Community-Based Ambulatory Care Services

Community-based ambulatory care services are those services provided in freestanding facilities that are not owned by or affiliated with a hospital. Such facilities can range in size from a small medical practice with a single physician to a large clinic with an organized medical staff.

Among the organizations that provide ambulatory care services are specialized treatment facilities. Examples of these facilities include birthing centers, cancer treatment centers, renal dialysis centers, and rehabilitation centers.

Freestanding Ambulatory Care Centers

Freestanding ambulatory care centers provide emergency services and urgent care for walk-in patients. Urgent care centers (sometimes called emergicenters) provide diagnostic and therapeutic care for patients with minor illnesses and injuries. They do not serve seriously ill patients, and most do not accept ambulance cases.

Two groups of patients find these centers attractive. The first group consists of patients seeking the convenience and access of emergency services without the delays and high costs associated with using hospital services for nonurgent problems. The second group consists of patients whose insurance treats urgent care centers preferentially compared with physicians' offices.

As they have increased in number and become familiar to more patients, many freestanding ambulatory care centers now offer a combination of walk-in and appointment services.

Freestanding Ambulatory Surgery Centers

Freestanding ambulatory surgery centers generally provide surgical procedures that take anywhere from 5 to 90 minutes to perform and require less than a 4-hour recovery period. Patients must schedule their surgeries in advance and be prepared to return home on the same day. Patients who experience surgical complications are sent to an inpatient facility for care.

Most ambulatory surgery centers are for-profit entities. Individual physicians, MCOs, or entrepreneurs may own them. Generally, ambulatory care centers can provide surgical services at lower cost than hospitals can because their overhead expenses are lower.

Public Health Services

The states have constitutional authority to implement public health measures, and many of them are assisted by a wide variety of federal programs and laws. The Department of Health and Human Services (HHS) is the principal federal agency that ensures health and provides essential human services. All HHS agencies have some responsibility for prevention. Through its 10 regional offices, HHS coordinates closely with state and local government agencies and many HHS-funded services are provided by these agencies as well as by private-sector and nonprofit organizations.

Two units in the Office of the Secretary of HHS are important to public health: the Office of the Surgeon General of the United States and the Office of Disease Prevention and Health Promotion (ODPHP). ODPHP has an analysis and leadership role for health promotion and disease prevention.

The surgeon general is appointed by the president of the United States and provides leadership and authoritative, science-based recommendations about the public's health. He or she has responsibility for the **public health service** (PHS) workforce (Jonas and Kovner 2005).

Home Care Services

Home healthcare is the fastest-growing sector to offer services for Medicare recipients. The primary reason for this is increased economic pressure from third-party payers. In other words, third-party payers want patients released from the hospital more quickly than they were in the past. Moreover, patients generally prefer to be cared for in their own homes. In fact, most patients prefer home care, no matter how complex their medical problems. Research indicates that the medical outcomes of home care patients are similar to those of patients treated in SNFs for similar conditions.

In 1989, Medicare rules for home care services were clarified to make it easier for Medicare beneficiaries to receive them. Patients are eligible to receive home health services from a qualified Medicare provider when they are homebound, when they are under the care of a specified physician who will establish a home health plan, and when they need physical or occupational therapy, speech therapy, or intermittent skilled nursing care.

Skilled nursing care is defined as both technical procedures, such as tube feedings and catheter care, and skilled nursing observations. *Intermittent* is defined as up to 28 hours per week for nursing care and 35 hours per week for home health aide care. Many hospitals have formed their own home healthcare agencies to increase revenues and at the same time to enable them to discharge patients from the hospital earlier.

Voluntary Agencies

Voluntary agencies provide healthcare and healthcare planning services, usually at the local level and to low-income patients. Their services range from giving free immunizations to offering family planning counseling. Funds to operate such agencies come from a variety of sources, including local or state health departments, private grants, and funds from different federal bureaus.

One common example of a voluntary agency is the community health center. Sometimes called neighborhood health centers, community health centers offer comprehensive, primary healthcare services to patients who otherwise would not have access to them. Often patients pay for these services on a sliding scale based on income or according to a flat rate, discounted fee schedule supplemented by public funding.

Some voluntary agencies offer specialized services such as counseling for battered and abused women. Typically, these are set up within local communities. An example of a voluntary agency that offers services on a much larger scale is the Red Cross.

Subacute Care

Patients needing ongoing rehabilitative care and/or treatments using advanced technology sometimes are eligible to receive subacute care. Subacute care offers patients access to constant nursing care while recovering at home. In the past, patients could receive comprehensive rehabilitative care only while in the hospital. Today, however, the availability of subacute care services allows patients to optimize their functional gain in a familiar and more comfortable environment. In essence, subacute care in most IDNs emphasizes patient independence. The patient is given an individualized care plan developed by a highly trained team of healthcare professionals. Patients considered appropriate for subacute care are those recovering from stroke, cardiac surgery, serious injury, amputation, joint replacement, or chronic wounds.

Long-Term Care

Generally speaking, long-term care is the healthcare rendered in a nonacute care facility to patients who require inpatient nursing and related services for more than 30 consecutive days. SNFs, nursing homes, and rehabilitation hospitals are the principal facilities that provide long-term care. Rehabilitation hospitals provide recuperative services for patients who have suffered strokes and traumatic injuries as well as other serious illnesses. Specialized long-term care facilities serve patients with chronic respiratory disease, permanent cognitive impairment, and other incapacitating conditions.

Long-term care encompasses a range of health, personal care, social, and housing services provided to people of all ages with health conditions that limit their ability to carry out normal daily activities without assistance. People who need long-term care have many different types of physical and mental disabilities. Moreover, their need for the mix and intensity of long-term care services can change over time.

Long-term care is mainly rehabilitative and supportive rather than curative. Moreover, healthcare workers other than physicians can provide long-term care in the home or in residential or institutional settings. For the most part, long-term care requires little or no technology.

Long-Term Care in the Continuum of Care

The availability of long-term care is one of the most important health issues in the United States today. There are two principal reasons for this. First, thanks to advances in medicine and healthcare practices, people are living longer today than they did in the past. The number of people who survive previously fatal conditions has been growing, and more and more people with chronic medical problems are able to live reasonably normal lives. Second, there was an explosion in birth rate after the second World War. Children born during that period (1946 to 1964), the so-called baby-boomer generation, are today in or entering their 50s and 60s. These factors combined mean that the need for long-term care will only increase in the years to come.

As discussed earlier, healthcare is now viewed as a continuum of care. That is, patients are provided care by different caregivers at several different levels of the healthcare system. In the case of long-term care, the patient's continuum of care may have begun with a primary provider in a hospital and then continued with home care and eventually care in an SNF. The patient's care is coordinated from one care setting to the next.

Moreover, the roles of the different care providers along the patient's continuum of care are continuing to evolve. Health information managers play a key part in providing consultation services to long-term care facilities with regard to developing systems to manage information from a diverse number of healthcare providers.

Delivery of Long-Term Care Services

Long-term care services are delivered in a variety of settings, including skilled nursing facilities/nursing homes, residential care facilities, hospice programs, and adult day-care programs.

Skilled Nursing Facilities and Nursing Homes

The most important providers of formal, long-term care services are nursing homes, which, provide medical, nursing, and/or rehabilitative care, in some cases, around the clock. Most SNF residents are over age 65 and often are classified as the frail elderly.

Many nursing homes are owned by for-profit organizations. However, SNFs also may be owned by not-for-profit groups as well as local, state, and federal governments. In recent years, there has been a decline in the total number of nursing homes in the United States, but an increase in the number of nursing home beds.

Nursing homes are no longer the only option for patients needing long-term care. Various factors play a role in determining which type of long-term care facility is best for a particular patient, including cost, access to services, and individual needs.

Residential Care Facilities

New living environments that are more homelike and less institutional are the focus of much attention in the current long-term care market. Residential care facilities now play a growing role in the continuum of long-term care services. Having affordable and appropriate housing available for elderly and disabled people can reduce the level of need for institutional long-term care services in the community. Institutionalization can be postponed or prevented when the elderly and disabled live in safe, accessible settings where assistance with daily activities is available.

Hospice Programs

Hospice care is provided mainly in the home to patients who are diagnosed with a terminal illness with a limited life expectancy of six months or less and to their families. Hospice is based on a philosophy of palliative care imported from England and Canada that holds that during the course of terminal illness, the patient should be able to live life as fully and as comfortably as possible, but without artificial or mechanical efforts to prolong life.

In the hospice approach, the family is the unit of treatment. An interdisciplinary team provides medical, nursing, psychological, therapeutic, pharmacological, and spiritual support during the final stages of illness, at the time of death, and during bereavement. The main goals are to control pain, maintain independence, and minimize the stress and trauma of death.

Hospice services have gained acceptance as an alternative to hospital care for the terminally ill. The number of hospices is likely to continue to grow because this philosophy of care for people at the end of life has become a model for the nation.

Adult Day-Care Programs

Adult day-care programs offer a wide range of health and social services to elderly persons during the daytime hours. Adult day-care services are usually targeted to elderly members of families in which the regular caregivers work during the day. Many elderly people who live alone also benefit from leaving their homes every day to participate in programs designed to keep them active. The goals of adult day-care programs are to delay the need for institutionalization and to provide respite for caregivers.

Data on adult day-care programs are still limited, but there were about 4,600 programs in 2010 providing services to 260,000 participants in a variety of programs (NADSA 2011). Most adult day-care programs offer social services, crafts, current events discussions, family counseling, reminiscence therapy, nursing assessment, physical exercise, activities of daily living, rehabilitation, psychiatric assessment, and medical care.

Behavioral Health Services

From the mid-19th century to the mid-20th century, psychiatric services in the United States were based primarily in long-stay institutions supported by state governments and patterns of practice were relatively stable. During the past 45 years, however, remarkable changes have occurred. These changes include a reversal of the balance between institutional and community care, inpatient and outpatient services, and individual and group practice.

Today, the number of long-stay residents in state mental hospitals is estimated to be well below 80,000. In 1955, it was more than 500,000. The shift to community-based settings began in the public sector and community settings remain dominant. The private sector's bed capacity increased in the 1970s and 1980s, including psychiatric units in nonfederal general hospitals, private psychiatric hospitals, and residential treatment centers for children. Substance abuse centers and child and adolescent inpatient psychiatric units grew particularly quickly in the 1980s, as investors recognized their profitability. In the 1990s, the growth of inpatient private mental health facilities leveled off and the number of outpatient and partial treatment settings increased sharply.

Some patients with treatment-resistant schizophrenia, severe mood disorders, or chronic cognitive impairment may be dangerous to themselves or others. State and county hospitals may be returning to their traditional role by providing asylum to disabled patients who are unable to function in their communities.

Residential treatment centers for emotionally or behaviorally disturbed children provide inpatient services to children under 18 years of age. The programs and physical facilities of residential treatment centers are designed to meet patients' daily living, schooling, recreational, socialization, and routine medical care needs.

Day-hospital or day-treatment programs occupy one niche in the spectrum of behavioral healthcare settings. Although some provide services seven days a week, many programs provide services only during business hours, Monday through Friday. Day-treatment patients spend most of the day at the treatment facility in a program of structured therapeutic activities and then return to their homes until the next day. Day-treatment services include psychotherapy, pharmacology, occupational therapy, and other types of rehabilitation services. These programs provide alternatives to inpatient care or serve as transitions from inpatient to outpatient care or discharge. They also may provide respite for family caregivers and a place for rehabilitating or maintaining chronically ill patients. The number of day-treatment programs has increased in response to pressures to decrease the length of hospital stays.

Insurance coverage for behavioral healthcare has always lagged behind coverage for other medical care. Although treatments and treatment settings have changed, rising healthcare costs, the absence of strong consumer demand for behavioral health coverage, and insurers' continuing fear of the potential cost of this coverage have maintained the differences between medical and behavioral healthcare benefits.

Although most individuals covered by health insurance have some outpatient psychiatric coverage, the coverage is often quite restricted. Typical restrictions include limits on the number of outpatient visits, higher copayment charges, and higher deductibles.

Behavioral healthcare has grown and diversified, particularly during the past 40 years, as psychopharmacologic treatment has made possible the shift away from long-term custodial treatment. Psychosocial treatments continue the process of care and rehabilitation in community settings. Large state hospitals have been supplemented—and in many cases replaced—by psychiatric units in general hospitals, new outpatient clinics, community mental health centers, day-treatment centers, and halfway houses. Treatment has become more effective and specific, based on our growing understanding of the brain and behavior.

Check Your Understanding 11.6

1. I am a patient. I went to see the doctor who owns her own office practice. This type of care is called which of the following?

   A. Hospital-based ambulatory care services
   B. Community-based ambulatory care services
   C. Private medical practice
   D. Freestanding ambulatory care center

2. My daughter fell and cut herself tonight. I believe that she needs stitches. It is not an emergency but I believe that she really needs to see someone tonight for treatment. What type of setting would I most likely access?

   A. Hospital-based ambulatory care services
   B. Community-based ambulatory care services
   C. Private medical practice
   D. Freestanding ambulatory care center

3. I work for a healthcare provider that provides ambulatory care to low-income patients. We receive funding from many sources. What type of setting do I work for?

   A. Voluntary agency
   B. Subacute care service
   C. Private medical practice
   D. Skilled nursing facility

4. A physician needs to find palliative care services for a terminally ill parent. What type of long-term care setting is the most appropriate?

   A. Residential care facilities
   B. Hospice
   C. Skilled nursing facilities
   D. Nursing home

5. Which of the following statements is true about behavioral health?

   A. It provides only day-hospital and day-treatment programs.
   B. The quality of the treatment provided has not changed in the past 20 years.
   C. Psychiatric care is restricted to ambulatory care settings.
   D. Insurance coverage generally places restrictions on the psychiatric care such as a limit on the number of outpatient visits.

Instructions: Match the descriptions provided with the terms to which they apply.

6. Day-treatment program

7. Skilled nursing facility

8. Residential care facility

9. Public health services

10. Continuum of care

a. Are designed to meet patient's daily living, schooling, recreational, socialization, and routine medical care needs

b. Has an analysis and leadership role for health promotion and disease prevention

c. Provides alternatives to inpatient care or serves as a transition from inpatient to outpatient care or discharge

d. Care provided by different caregivers at several different levels of the healthcare system

e. Healthcare rendered in a non-acute care facility to patients who require inpatient nursing and related services for more than 30 consecutive days

Reimbursement of Healthcare Expenditures

Reimbursement of healthcare expenditures has a long history in the United States. Traditionally healthcare services were paid for on a fee-for-service basis. However the entrance of third-party payer systems over 60 years ago has dramatically changed how expenditures of healthcare are reimbursed. (Reimbursement methodologies are thoroughly covered in chapter 6.)

Evolution of Third-Party Reimbursement

The evolution of third-party reimbursement systems for healthcare services began more than 60 years ago. It created a need for systematic and accurate communications between healthcare providers and third-party payers such as commercial health insurance companies (for example, Aetna) and medical plans similar to Blue Cross/Blue Shield (also called the Blues).

Most commercial health insurance is provided in the form of group policies offered by employers as part of their fringe benefit packages for employees. Unions also negotiate health insurance coverage during contract negotiations. In most cases, employees pay a share of the cost and employers pay a share.

Individual health insurance plans can be purchased but usually are expensive or have limited coverage and high deductibles. Individuals with preexisting medical conditions often find it almost impossible to get individual coverage.

Commercial insurers also sell major medical and cash payment policies. Major medical plans are directed primarily at catastrophic illness and cover all or part of treatment costs beyond those covered by basic plans. Major medical plans are sold as both group and individual policies. Cash payment plans provide monetary benefits and are not based on actual charges from healthcare providers. For example, a cash payment plan might pay the beneficiary $150 for every day he or she is hospitalized or $500 for every ambulatory surgical procedure. Cash payment plans are often offered as a benefit of membership in large associations such as the American Association of Retired Persons (AARP).

Like the Blues, commercial insurance companies are subject to supervision by state insurance commissioners. However, such supervision does not include rate regulation. One general requirement is that commercial plans establish premium rates high enough to cover all potential claims made under the insurance they provide.

Government-Sponsored Reimbursement Systems

Until 1965, most of the poor and many of the elderly in the United States could not afford private healthcare services. As a result of public pressure calling for attention to this growing problem, Congress passed Public Law 89-97 as an Amendment to the Social Security Act. The amendments created Medicare (Title XVIII) and Medicaid (Title XIX).

Medicare

Federal health insurance for the aged, called Medicare, was first offered to retired Americans in July 1966. Today, retired and disabled Americans who are eligible for Social Security benefits automatically qualify for Medicare coverage without regard to income. Coverage is offered under two coordinated programs: hospital insurance (Medicare Part A) and medical insurance (Medicare Part B).

Medicare Part A is financed through payroll taxes. Initially, coverage applied only to hospitalization and home healthcare. Subsequently, coverage for extended care in nursing homes was added. Coverage for individuals eligible for Social Security disability payments for over two years and those who need kidney transplantation or dialysis for end-stage renal disease also were added.

Medical insurance under Medicare Part B is optional. It is financed through monthly premiums paid by eligible beneficiaries to supplement federal funding. Part B helps pay for physician's services, outpatient hospital care, medical services and supplies, and certain other medical costs not covered by Part A. At the present time, Medicare Part B does not provide coverage of prescription drugs. The Balanced Budget Act of 1997 gave Medicare beneficiaries the option to receive their Medicare benefits through private health insurance plans, instead of through the original Medicare plan (Parts A and B). These programs were known as Medicare+Choice or Part C plans. The Medicare Prescription Drug, Improvement, and Modernization Act of 2003 made Medicare+Choice plans more appealing to Medicare beneficiaries because prescription drug coverage was made available. The prescription drug coverage was referred to as Medicare Advantage (MA). Effective January 1, 2006, any Medicare Advantage Plan that also included Part D prescription drug benefits is known as a Medicare Advantage Prescription Drug plan or a MA-PD. These plans are approved and regulated by the Medicare program, but are actually designed and administered by private health insurance companies. Unlike Medicare Parts A and B, Part D coverage is not standardized. Plans choose which drugs (or even classes of drugs) they wish to cover, at what level (or tier) they wish to cover them, and are free to choose not to cover some drugs at all. (Medicare Parts A, B, C, and D are discussed in greater detail in chapter 6.)

Medicaid

Medicaid is a medical assistance program for low-income Americans. The program is funded partially by the federal government and partially by state and local governments. The federal government requires that certain services be provided and sets specific eligibility requirements.

Medicaid covers the following benefits:

- Inpatient hospital care
- . Outpatient hospital care
- Laboratory and x-ray services

- SNF and home health services for persons over 21 years old
- Physician services
- Family planning services
- Rural health clinic services
- Early and periodic screening, diagnosis, and treatment services

Individual states sometimes cover services in addition to those required by the federal government.

Services Provided by Government Agencies

Federal health insurance programs cover health services for several additional specified populations.

TRICARE, originally referred to as the Civilian Health and Medical Program for the Uniformed Services (CHAMPUS), pays for care delivered by civilian health providers to retired members of the military and the dependents of active and retired members of the seven uniformed services. The Department of Defense administers the TRICARE program. It also provides medical services to active members of the military.

The Department of Veterans Affairs (VA) provides healthcare services to eligible veterans of military service. The VA hospital system was established in 1930 to provide hospital, nursing home, residential, and outpatient medical and dental care to veterans of the first World War. Today, the VA operates more than 950 medical centers throughout the country. The medical centers are currently being organized into 22 Veterans Integrated Service Networks (VISNs) to increase the efficiency of their services.

Through the Indian Health Service, HHS also finances the healthcare services provided to approximately 2 million American Indians and Alaskan Natives (AI/AN) living on and off reservations in the United States.

State governments often operate healthcare facilities to serve citizens with special needs, such as the developmentally disabled and mentally ill. Some states also offer health insurance programs to those who cannot qualify for private healthcare insurance. Many county and local governments also operate public hospitals to fulfill the medical needs of their communities. Public hospitals provide services without regard to the patient's ability to pay.

Workers' Compensation

Workers' compensation is an insurance system operated by the individual states. Each state has its own law and program. In 1910, New York enacted the first workers' compensation law. Workers' compensation programs cover healthcare costs and lost income associated with work-related injuries and illnesses. Federal government employees are covered by the Federal Employees' Compensation Act (FECA). Individual states pass legislation that addresses workers' compensation coverage for nonfederal government employees. Some states exclude certain workers (for example, business owners, independent contractors, farm workers, and so on). Texas employers are not required to provide workers' compensation coverage. (FECA is discussed in more detail in chapter 6.)

Managed Care

Managed care is a broad term used to describe several types of prepaid healthcare plans. Common types of managed care plans include health maintenance organizations (HMOs), preferred provider organizations (PPOs), and point-of-service (POS) plans. MCOs work to control the cost of, and access to, healthcare services while striving to meet high-quality standards. They manage healthcare costs by negotiating discounted providers' fees and controlling patients' access to expensive healthcare services.

The development of managed care was an indirect result of the federal government's enactment of the Medicare and Medicaid laws in 1965. Medicare and Medicaid legislation prompted the development of **investor-owned hospital chains** and stimulated the growth of university medical centers. Both furthered the corporate practice of medicine by increasing the number of management personnel and physicians employed by hospitals and medical schools (Kongstevdt 1993, 3–5).

Reimbursement by MCOs varies depending on the type of organization and the contract negotiated. For example, members of HMOs pay a set premium and are entitled to receive a specific range of healthcare services. In most cases, employers and employees share the cost of the plan. HMOs control costs by requiring members of the plan to seek services only from a preapproved list of providers, who are reimbursed at discounted rates. The plans also control access to medical specialists, expensive diagnostic and treatment procedures, and high-cost pharmaceuticals. They generally require preapproval for specialty consultations, inpatient care, and surgical procedures. Many other examples of reimbursement in managed care arrangements are presented in detail in chapter 6.

Further federal support for the corporate practice of medicine resulted from passage of the HMO Act of 1973. Amendments to the act enabled managed care plans to increase in numbers and to expand enrollments through healthcare programs financed by grants, contracts, and loans.

After years of unchecked healthcare inflation, the government authorized corporate cost controls on hospitals, physicians, and patients for reimbursement of government-sponsored healthcare such as Medicare. The use Prospective Payment Systems (PPS), Diagnostic-Related Groups (DRG) (a PPS used primarily in hospitals), and the resource-based relative value scale (RBRVS) are examples of these controls.

The growth of managed care seemed to reduce inflation of healthcare costs during the early and mid-1990s. However, healthcare costs are again rapidly rising. Higher costs are making employers ask workers to pay a larger share for healthcare services. MCOs face major challenges in remaining fiscally strong in the coming years.

Consumer-Driven Healthcare

Consumer-driven healthcare is a new strategy in the private insurance market. This method allows employees more choice in their healthcare decision making. Consumer-driven plans vary, but basically employers provide employees with a personal care account. This account is a fixed amount and offered in the form of a voucher, refundable tax credit, higher wages, or some other transfer of funds (Jonas and Kovner 2005).

Health Savings Accounts (HSA)

Health savings accounts, or HSAs (also called medical savings accounts or MSAs), offer their members the opportunity to control how their healthcare dollars are spent with a tax-advantaged savings account and comprehensive medical insurance coverage.

HSAs combine high-deductible health insurance with a tax-advantaged savings account. The money that a member saves in his or her account assists in paying the deductible. Most accounts limit the member to contributing the amount of the deductible into the tax-deferred account. This money is kept for medical expenses that qualify under the insurance plan.

The benefit of an HSA is that the member pays for this deductible with pretax dollars. This means that the member saves the money that ordinarily would have gone to pay taxes, which, in effect, decreases the cost of the deductible.

When the member has paid off the deductible, the insurance provider begins to pay. The money in the savings account earns interest and is owned by the member who holds the account. Approximately 17 percent of all employees are in HSAs, which allow their members to save approximately 70 percent or more on the cost of their health insurance (http://www.health-insurance-carriers.com/hsa.html).

Healthcare Reform Initiatives

The continuing high cost of healthcare has prompted calls for healthcare reform over the past several decades. The costs of healthcare have several impacts. Many families and individuals are unable to obtain healthcare insurance and forgo healthcare because of its high costs. The uninsured rate grew from 49 million in 2009 to 49.9 million in 2010 (US Census Bureau 2011). Illness and medical bills contribute to a large and increasing share of US bankruptcies with one study citing that 62.1 percent of all bankruptcies in 2007 were medically related (Himmelstein et al. 2009). In addition the United States spends over $2.2 trillion on healthcare each year. That number represents approximately 16 percent of the total economy and is growing rapidly (Office of Management and Budget 2009).

The following are among the steps taken in 2009 by the federal government to reform healthcare with the goals of alleviating escalating costs, improving access, and increasing quality:

- Instituting provisions to provide individuals who have lost or recently lost their jobs with a tax credit to keep their health insurance through COBRA

- Increasing healthcare coverage for children through the reauthorization of the Children's Health Insurance Program (CHIP) that provides support, options, and incentives for states to provide coverage for an additional four million children in CHIP and Medicaid who are uninsured

- Computerizing America's health records in five years
- Developing and disseminating information on effective medical interventions
- Investing in prevention and wellness

Congress also began to debate various pieces of healthcare reform legislation in 2009. The goals of reform included reducing healthcare costs, protecting and increasing consumers' choices, and guaranteeing access to quality, affordable healthcare for all Americans. President Barack Obama signed into law the Patient Protection and Affordable Care Act on March 23, 2010, and the Health Care and Education Reconciliation Act on March 30, 2010. Together, these acts include a number of healthcare provisions that are to be implemented within four years.

Check Your Understanding 11.7

1. A disadvantage of individual health plans is:

    A. They do not cover inpatient hospitalizations.
    B. They are part of fringe benefits.
    C. They have low deductibles.
    D. They cost more than group policies.

2. I am retired from the military. I am seeing a civilian healthcare provider for my care. What insurance do I most likely have?

    A. Medicaid
    B. Medicare
    C. TRICARE
    D. VA

3. An HMO is a model of a prepaid healthcare plan that falls under what type of reimbursement philosophy?

    A. Health savings account
    B. Managed care
    C. Commercial insurance
    D. Consumer-driven healthcare

4. Which of the following best describes workers' compensation insurance?

    A. Insurance plan administered by the federal government
    B. Insurance system covering healthcare costs associated with work-related injuries
    C. Insurance coverage restricted to Medicaid and Medicare recipients
    D. Insurance plan usually including all federal workers

5. Which of the following allows the patient to pay for the deductible with pretax dollars?

    A. TRICARE
    B. HMOs
    C. Medicare
    D. Health savings accounts

Instructions: Indicate whether the statements below are true or false (T or F).

6. ____ The development of managed care was a direct result of the federal government's enactment of the Medicare and Medicaid laws in 1965.

7. ____ Medicare Part B is optional.

8. ____ Workers' compensation plans are operated by the state governments.

9. ____ One of the disadvantages of the health savings accounts is that the deductible is paid with pretax dollars.

10. ____ Medicaid is co-funded by federal and state governments.

Real-World Case

This case study is extracted from a presentation at the 2004 IFHRO Congress and AHIMA Convention titled "e-HIM Framework and Case Study" (Cassidy 2004).

Evolution from e-Health Task Force to e-HIM Task Force

During the past decade, the Internet and its derived technologies have revolutionized the way business is conducted. In healthcare, the following examples illustrate this transformation:

- Increasing numbers of consumers access the Internet for information about healthcare providers, treatment options, and their own personal health information.
- Health websites provide consumers with tools to develop and maintain their own online health records through the use of patient portals, which allow the patient to interact with their medical information via the Internet.
- Consumers and health providers correspond via e-mail.
- Businesses and consumers purchase supplies and equipment over the Internet.
- Health information management (HIM) business processes, such as transcription and coding, use the Internet for off-site transaction processing.

The Internet and its derived technologies create a plethora of opportunities for HIM professionals. HIM professionals who understand and embrace this technology will harness and direct it to improve health information and the efficacy of healthcare for consumers, providers, vendors, payers, and all those in the healthcare supply chain. Those who fail to understand and embrace this technology will be left behind, and their opportunities will be forfeited to faster-moving, better-focused professionals.

The work of the AHIMA e-Health Task Force (2003) resulted in the following vision statement.

Vision for e-Health Information Management

E-health presents a new frontier for managing health information. HIM professionals will reinvent traditional HIM functions for a health record model in which the patient is part of the documentation team. In this model, the health record will be designed and/or maintained by a trusted third-party organization or by the patient. Individually identifiable data will be transmitted and accessed via the Internet.

HIM professionals will clearly define the mission-critical role of a cyber health record practitioner. They will develop standards of practice that support the implementation of AHIMA's tenets that its e-Health Task Force developed in 2000 and address the security, privacy, and quality standards for personal health information on the Internet.

In early 2003, AHIMA appointed a task force of experts to develop a vision of the e-HIM future.

The task force developed the following vision of the future of health information: "The future state of health information is electronic, patient-centered, comprehensive, longitudinal, accessible, and credible."

The task force's vision is not only theoretical, but it also offers practical guidance for anyone traveling the road toward e-HIM. Advancing the recommendations of the e-HIM Task Force, AHIMA created workgroups to develop practice standards that focus on areas that play an integral role in the transition from paper to electronic health records.

The following issues were selected for the initial standards development for the complete medical record in a hybrid electronic health record environment:

- Implementing electronic signatures

- E-mail as a provider–patient electronic communication medium and its impact on the electronic health record

- Electronic document management as a component of the electronic health record

- Core data sets for the physician-practice electronic health record

- Speech recognition in the electronic health record

Note: The outcomes are presented in a series of documents that can be found on the AHIMA website. To view more information about the e-HIM initiatives, go to http://www.ahima.org, select the Body of Knowledge at the top of the page and then search on the word "e-HIM."

From HIM to e-HIM

The knowledge and expertise for managing handwritten medical records containing source patient data have evolved through these steps:

- Independent management of paper medical records in settings across the continuum of care

- Scanning paper documents for multiple user access

- Entering data into automated systems that generate electronic patient data
- Integrated delivery systems that electronically manage the patient across the continuum of care
- Network integration and e-health information management

HIM professionals remain actively involved in developing effective processes to preserve patient privacy, confidentiality, and security. This is because the introduction of the Internet for accessing, transferring, and transmitting health information expanded the uses of source patient data (that is, the medical record as HIM professionals traditionally know it) as Internet-based business-to-business companies and business-to-consumer companies flourished.

Career Opportunities for e-HIM professionals

The application of HIM skills, expertise, and experience described in the previous section meet the job requirements of several roles in e-health businesses. This section discusses mission-critical functions and processes in e-health companies that HIM professionals can develop, manage, or perform. Some skills transfer easily into the e-health environment while some require translation due to the differences in the work setting or to accommodate differences in the capabilities of advanced technologies.

Many of these e-HIM processes are interrelated or complementary. Processes and/or functions may be decentralized in some e-health organizations and centralized in others in much the same way that HIM processes have always been a part of an HIM department in traditional healthcare provider organizations. In e-health companies as well as traditional settings, many HIM functions exist outside the HIM department. With e-health companies and providers varying in purpose and scope (from traditional healthcare provider organizations delivering services electronically, to clinical systems vendors, to application service providers, to consumer healthcare Internet websites), the concept of a professionally led HIM function or department will vary depending on the organization's structure, resources, and needs.

In the traditional and e-healthcare organizations, HIM professionals are responsible for managing two basic healthcare business objectives:

- Enabling the collection and storage of complete, accurate, and legal health information
- Facilitating the use of health information for patient care, quality evaluation, reimbursement, compliance, utilization management, education, research, funding, and in legal proceedings

The first objective is accomplished in the traditional setting through functions generally consolidated and managed under the auspices of the HIM director. It includes such functions as record assembly, analysis, coding and abstracting, correspondence, special registries, and medical transcription.

The second objective includes use of the information through functions such as creating and maintaining efficient filing and retrieval systems, master patient indices, chart and information retrieval and filing, release of information, and data retrieval for quality assurance, registries (for example, tumor or trauma registries), and other evaluative purposes.

These objectives are met within a highly regulated environment and managed with limited resources. This necessitates professional guidance by those with health information management skills, which includes knowledge in the administration of highly regulated activities.

Clearly, e-health companies, having many of the same business objectives and challenges as traditional healthcare organizations, need HIM knowledge and skills in developing processes that will meet their business objectives with a high level of quality and cost benefit.

Roles, Resources, and Competencies in e-HIM

Revolution is an overused word, but when applied to the effect of all that is digital, automated, or electronic in the healthcare industry, it is entirely accurate. Over the last decade, established relationships, value chains, and strategies have been radically altered or swept away.

As the revolution continues, the challenge to HIM professionals is clear. They can allow the technologies to roll uncontrolled through and around their organizations, in effect, handing over their rich knowledge base and expert skills to faster-moving, better-focused professionals in professions that don't even exist yet. Or they can understand the potential of the Internet and control and direct its power to the benefit of their customers, health plan members, and patients.

Future of e-HIM and Where You Might Work

Domain manager: Owns responsibility for a defined body of knowledge such as HIM, coding, laboratory, pharmacy, and so forth. Knowledge and authority may cross organizational lines as they maintain the integrity of the technical implementation of that body of knowledge. May work closely with product managers, operations staff, quality control, and so forth.

    Project manager: Manages the implementation of systems necessary to support personal health records, website content, and other projects.

    Medical language and classification expert: Employs skills in the design and use of medical vocabularies and classification; defines data and retrieves information from e-health systems.

    Compliance officer: Designs, implements, and maintains a compliance program that assures conformity to all types of regulatory and voluntary accreditation requirements governing the provision of healthcare products or services via the Internet.

    Information security expert: Designs, implements, or maintains an information security program that balances requirements of privacy, integrity, and availability of data. Understands the legal and social issues related to information security.

Patient information coordinator: Provides services to patients wanting to understand how to optimize their experience on the e-health website and create and maintain accuracy of their personal health records. Educates patients on protecting the privacy of their personal health information.

Reimbursement manager: Designs systems and procedures that assure generation of accurate clinical documentation needed to substantiate billing. Also involved in designing systems to efficiently classify information for billing. Develops and implements systems to assure the secure transfer of required data to billing centers, clearinghouses, or third-party payers.

Data quality manager: Ensures the quality of health information by performing quality reliability and validity checks. Develops reports and advises clinicians on identifying critical indicators.

Privacy officer: Oversees all ongoing activities related to the development, implementation, maintenance of, and adherence to the organization's policies and procedures covering the privacy of, and access to, patient health information in compliance with federal and state laws and the healthcare organization's information privacy practices.

Product manager: Responsible for overall implementation of a specific product or product line. This may include coordinating and managing the use, case design, development, quality control, version control, modifications and updates, and so forth.

The e-HIM Task Force (AHIMA) report outlines new roles and competency areas to help you envision ways to expand your scope of knowledge.

Business process engineer, information system designer, and consumer advocate are just a few new paths open to HIM professionals. Decision support is another important area where HIM professionals will be building, querying, and analyzing databases to give clinicians the information they need to decide how to treat current patients or analyze patterns in past patient care.

Coders will have several migration paths once code assignment becomes automated. Coders will play key roles as data quality and integrity monitors and data analysts. Others will become clinical vocabulary managers, helping to make the national information infrastructure a reality by ensuring consistency and linkages between different codes. Check out the AHIMA website to explore more information on these exciting emerging roles for HIM professionals.

Summary

Throughout history, humans have attempted to diagnose and treat illness and disease. As populations settled into towns and cities, early folk medicine traditions eventually led to the establishment of formalized entities specifically designed to care for the sick.

In the American colonies, enlightened thinkers such as Benjamin Franklin soon saw the need to establish hospitals and to regulate the practice of medicine. The 19th century saw the growth of organizations dedicated to standardizing medical practice and ensuring consistency in the quality of healthcare delivery. Organizations such as the American Medical Association and the American Nurses Association were created to represent the interests of their members and to further ensure the quality of their services.

The 20th century ushered in a completely new concept in the provision of healthcare: prepaid health plans. For the first time, Americans could buy health insurance. However, during the Great Depression of the 1930s and the second World War, it became obvious that millions of Americans could not afford to pay for healthcare. After the war, the federal government began to study the problem of healthcare access for all Americans. Finally, during the Johnson administration in the 1960s, Congress passed amendments to the Social Security Act of 1935 that created the Medicare and Medicaid programs. These programs were designed to pay for the cost of healthcare services for the elderly and the poor.

As the healthcare industry has grown, so have efforts to regulate it. Some regulation has come from professional and trade associations associated with the industry. However, much regulation has come from the federal government, particularly with regard to the Medicaid and Medicare programs. Moreover, the types and variety of healthcare services available today have increased dramatically. Every new type of service, and every new way to provide it, brings complex issues that must be addressed in order to ensure that Americans receive the highest-quality healthcare possible at the most affordable price.

Passage of the Medicare and Medicaid programs and establishment of the managed care industry have had a tremendous impact on the way that healthcare in the United States is delivered and paid for. Healthcare costs have continued to grow and outpace the growth rate in gross domestic product (GDP), inflation, and population for many years. Concern has risen about this situation as experts suggest that the continued rapid growth in spending may have many adverse impacts. Therefore, initiatives were intensified to pass healthcare reform legislation that would control costs and provide better access. One thing that is certain is that the American healthcare system continues to be a work in progress.

References

Agency for Healthcare Research and Quality. 2009. Evidence-based Practice Centers. http://www.ahrq.gov/clinic/epc/

AHIMA e-HIM Taskforce (2003). A Vision of the e-HIM Future. http://library.ahima.org/xpedio/groups/public/documents/ahima/bok1_020477.pdf

American College of Healthcare Executives. nd. Mission. http://www.ache.org/abt_ache/GovTaskForce/strat-op_overview.cfm

American Health Information Management Association. 2011. The mission of the American Health Information Management Association. http://www.ahima.org/about/mission.aspx

American Hospital Association. 1999. *100 Faces of Healthcare.* Chicago: Health Forum.

American Hospital Association. 2004. Fast facts on US hospitals from AHA hospital statistics. http://aha.org/aha/resource_center/fastfacts/fast_facts_US_hospitals.html

American Hospital Association. 2011. Fast facts on US hospitals from AHA hospital statistics. http://www.aha.org/aha/resource-center/Statistics-and-Studies/fast-facts.html

American Medical Association 2011. The Patient Protection and Affordable Care Act: Overview of major provisions relating to coverage. http://www.ama-org/ama1/pub/upload/mm/399/hsr-health-Insurance-coverage-reforms.pdf

The Blue Cross and Blue Shield Association. 2012. About the Blue Cross and Blue Shield Association. http://www.bcbs.com/about-the-association/

Cassidy, B.S. 2004. e-HIM framework and case study. 2004 IFHRO Congress & AHIMA Convention Proceedings.

Cassidy, B.S. 2011. "Healthcare Delivery Systems." Chapter 12 in *Health Information Management Technology: An Applied Approach*, 3rd ed. Edited by Johns, M. Chicago: AHIMA.

Certification Commission for Health Information Technology. 2009. http://www.cchit.org/about

Commission on Accreditation of Health Informatics and Information Management. 2011. http://www.CAHIIM.org

Commission on Certification of Health Informatics and Information Management. 2009. http://www.ahima.org/certification/about-cchiim.aspx

Committee on Energy and Commerce. 2010. http://docs.house.gov/energycommerce/SUMMARY.pdf

Commonwealth Fund Commission on a High Performance Health System. 2008. Why not the best? Results from the national scorecard on US health system performance. New York: The Commonwealth Fund.

Commonwealth Fund Commission on a High Performance Health System. 2011. Why not the best? Results from the national scorecard on US health system performance. New York: The Commonwealth Fund. http://www.commonwealthfund.org/Publications/Fund-Reports/2011/Oct/Why-Not-the-Best-2011.aspx?page=all

Elçin, Y.M., ed. 2003. *Tissue Engineering, Stem Cells and Gene Therapies: Advances in Experimental Medicine and Biology.* New York: Springer-Verlag.

HealthCare.com. 2009. What is ambulatory care? http://www.healthinsurancefinders.com/advice/ambulatory-care/

Health Insurance Carriers. 2007. Health Savings Accounts. http://www.health-insurance-carriers.com/hsa.html

Himmelstein, D., D. Thorne, E. Warren, and S. Woolhandler. 2009. Medical bankruptcy in the United States, 2007: Results of a national study. *The American Journal of Medicine* 122(8):741–746.

Joint Commission. 2009a. Facts About The Joint Commission. http://www.jointcommission.org/AboutUs/Fact_Sheets/joint_commission_facts.htm

Joint Commission. 2009b. Facts About Patient Safety. http://www.jointcommission.org/PatientSafety/

Jonas, S., and A.R. Kovner. 2005. *Healthcare Delivery in the United States,* 8th ed. New York: Springer-Verlag.

Kaiser Family Foundation statehealthfacts.org. 2011. http://www.statehealthfacts.org/index.jsp

Kongstevdt, P. 1993. *The Managed Care Handbook.* Gaithersburg, MD: Aspen.

National Adult Day Services Association. 2011. http://www.nadsa.org

National Institutes for Health and Clinical Excellence. 2009. http://www.nice.org.uk/aboutnice/whatwedo/aboutclinicalguidelines/about_clinical_guidelines.jsp

National Institutes of Health. 2005. http://www.nih.gov

Oaseem, A., V. Snow, P. Shekelle, D.E. Casey, T.J. Cross, and D.K. Owens. 2008. Evidence-based interventions to improve the palliative care of pain, dyspnea, and depression at the end of life: A clinical practice guideline from the American College of Physicians. *Annuals of Internal Medicine* 148(2):141–146.

Office of Management and Budget. 2009. http://www.whitehouse.gov/omb/fy2010_key_healthcare/

Quality Assurance Project. 2005. *Methods and Tools: A Glossary of Useful Terms.* Quality Research Project, University Research Company, LLC. http://www.qaproject.org/methods/resglossary.html

Rode, D. 2009. Recovery and privacy: Why a law about the economy is the biggest thing since HIPAA. *Journal of AHIMA* 80(5):42–44.

Sackett, D.L., W.M. Rosenberg, J.A. Gray, R.B. Haynes, and W.S. Richardson. 1996. Evidence based medicine: What it is and what it isn't. *British Medical Journal* 312(7023):71–72.

Shaw, P., C. Elliott, P. Isaacson, and E. Murphy. 2009. *Quality and Performance Improvement in Healthcare A Tool for Programmed Learning,* 3rd ed. Chicago: AHIMA.

Slavkin, R., E.F. Hodge, S.G. Prom, and J.W.N Rugg. 2011. The Affordable Care Act and Accountable Care Organization Final Regulations Released. http://www.jdsupra.com/post/documentViewer.aspx?fid=48f2bc80-1e49-4411-a23d-80f6ff52e313

Sloane, R.M., B.L. Sloane, and R. Harder. 1999. *Introduction to Healthcare Delivery Organization: Functions and Management,* 4th ed. Chicago: Health Administration Press.

Starr, P. 1982. *The Social Transformation of American Medicine.* New York: Basic Books.

Sultz, H.A., and K.M. Young. 2011. *Healthcare USA—Understanding Its Organization and Delivery,* 4th ed. Sudbury, MA: Jones and Bartlett.

US Census Bureau. 2011. Income, Poverty and Health Insurance Coverage in the United States: 2010http://www.census.gov/newsroom/releases/archives/income_wealth/cb11-157.htmlUS Department of Labor. 2010. Occupational Outlook Handbook 2010-11 edition. http://www.bls.gov/ooh/

Weinerman, E.R., R.S. Ratner, A. Robbins, and M.A. Lavenbar. 1996. Yale studies in ambulatory medical care: Five determinants of use of hospital emergency services. *American Journal of Public Health* 56:1037.

Additional Resources

Centers for Disease Control. 2004. Health care in America: Trends in utilization. http://www.cdc.gov/nchs/data/misc/healthcare.pdf

Centers for Medicare and Medicaid Services. 2010. The Mental Health Parity and Addiction Equity Act. http://www.cms.hhs.gov/HealthInsReformforConsume/04_TheMentalHealthParityAct.asp

Certification Commission for Health Information Technology. 2012. More Than 70 Percent of Attested EHRs are Dually Certified by CCHIT. http://www.cchit.org/press-releases/-/asset_publisher/l7V2/content/2012-02-13-more-than-70-percent-of-attested-ehrs-are-dually-certified-by-cchit?redirect=https%3a%2f%2fcchitstage.cchit.org%2fpress-releases%3fp_p_id%3d101_INSTANCE_l7V2%26p_p_lifecycle%3d0%26p_p_state%3dnormal%26p_p_mode%3dview%26p_p_col_id%3dcolumn-2%26p_p_col_pos%3d1%26p_p_col_count%3d2

Cofer, J., ed. 1994. *Health Information Management,* 10th ed. Berwyn, IL: Physicians' Record Company.

HBS Consulting. 2003. *Telehealth: A Keystone for Future Healthcare Delivery.* San Diego, CA: HBS Consulting.

Human Genome Project. 2005. Frequently asked questions. http://www.ornl.gov/sci/techresources/Human_Genome/faq/faqs1.shtml

Joint Commission. 2000. *2001 Comprehensive Accreditation Manual for Hospitals.* Oakbrook Terrace, IL: Joint Commission.

Leavitt, J.W., and R.L. Numbers, eds. 1997. *Sickness and Health in America: Readings in the History of Medicine and Public Health,* 3rd ed. Madison, WI: University of Wisconsin Press.

Plunkett Research. 2003. *Plunkett's Healthcare Industry Almanac,* 2004 ed. Houston, TX: Plunkett Research.

President's Advisory Commission on Protection and Quality in the Health Care Industry. 1998. Improving health care quality in an industry in transition. Chapter 2 in *Quality First: Better Health Care for All Americans.* http://www.hcqualitycommission.gov/final/chap02.html

Shryock, R.H. 1947. The beginnings: From colonial days to the foundation of the American Psychiatric Association. In *One Hundred Years of American Psychiatry,* edited by J.K. Hall, G. Zilboorg, and H.A. Bunker. New York: Columbia University Press.

Stevens, R. 1999. *In Sickness and in Wealth.* Baltimore, MD: Johns Hopkins University Press.

chapter 12

Ethical Issues in Health Information Management

Laurinda B. Harman, PhD, RHIA, FAHIMA

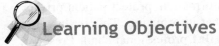

Learning Objectives

- Recognize and respond to health information ethical problems, including those related to privacy and confidentiality; compliance, fraud, and abuse; clinical code selection and use; quality review; research and decision support; public health; managed care; clinical care; electronic health information systems; the management of sensitive information; the roles of manager, entrepreneur, and advocate; and business relationships with vendors

- Recognize the historical problems of research and ethics and the importance of diligence for future research endeavors

- Recognize the problems associated with the emerging ethical problem of medical identity theft

- Identify ethical principles and professional values that can guide health information management (HIM) professionals who must confront and respond to ethical problems

- Apply the AHIMA Code of Ethics to guide behaviors such as protecting privacy, advancing HIM knowledge and practice, advocating for others, and refusing to participate in or conceal unethical behaviors

- Follow the steps in an ethical decision-making process that can be used to resolve complex ethical problems

Key Terms

Autonomy	Justice
Beneficence	Medical identity theft
Bioethics	Moral values
Blanket authorization	Need-to-know principle
Confidentiality	Nonmaleficence
Ethical agent	Privacy
Ethical decision making	Secondary release of information
Ethicist	Security
Ethics	

◆ Introduction

The responsibilities of the health information management (HIM) professional include a wide range of functions and activities. Regardless of the employer—such as healthcare facility, vendor, pharmaceutical company, or research firm—the HIM professional's core ethical obligations are to preserve the personal health information, protect patient privacy and confidential information and to assure security of that information. This is shown in the 2011 Code of Ethics as it specifically states that a HIM professional shall: Preserve, protect and secure personal health information (AHIMA 2011a).

The documentation in the paper and electronic health record (EHR) systems includes many sacred stories that must be protected on behalf of the individual patient and the aggregate community of patients and consumers served by the healthcare system. The obligation to protect this information is at the center of the decisions made on behalf of patients, the healthcare team, peers, colleagues, the public, or the many other stakeholders who seek access to patient and consumer information (AHIMA 2011a).

Moral intelligence is important for our understanding of the complexity of the issues that we face and how we can apply our values, goals and actions in ethical decision making (Lennick and Kiel 2008). There is also an increased understanding that technological systems require moral guidance in design and application. The focus on technology and human relationships increases ethical imperatives because what is done, how it is done, and what the intended (and sometimes unintended) outcomes are must be carefully examined (Van den Hoven and Weckert 2008).

The terms in this chapter describe ethical principles that most people already know, although the terms themselves may not be familiar. For example, recognizing the importance of individuals being able to decide what happens to them is autonomy, doing good is included in the ethical principle of beneficence, not harming others is nonmaleficence, and treating people fairly is justice (Beauchamp and Childress 2001). For example, with regard to one of the HIM professional's primary functions, how might ethical principles apply in the case of deciding whether to release patient information?

- **Autonomy** would require the HIM professional to ensure that the patient, and not a spouse or third party, makes the decisions regarding access to his or her health information.

- **Beneficence** would require the HIM professional to ensure that the information is released only to individuals who need it to do something that will benefit the patient (for example, to an insurance company for payment of a claim).

- **Nonmaleficence** would require the HIM professional to ensure that the information is not released to someone who does not have authorization to access it and who might harm the patient if access were permitted (for example, a newspaper seeking information about a famous person).

- **Justice** would require the HIM professional to apply the rules fairly and consistently for all and not to make special exceptions based on personal or organizational perspectives (for example, releasing information more quickly to a favorite physician's office).

This chapter provides the language and framework for understanding more about ethics within the context of dealing with complex health information issues. It also offers a step-by-step process that HIM professionals can use to make appropriate ethical choices and to analyze what is and is not justified from an ethical perspective.

Theory into Practice

The following discussion is extracted from "What the Seven Signs of Ethical Collapse Can Teach Us about Quality in Healthcare" (Tomzik 2008):

> Healthcare has much in common with the traditional business marketplace. What began as a means to meet the healthcare needs of the individual and promote health within the community has mushroomed into a steadily increasing $2.3 trillion dollar business enterprise. The temptations and ethical afflictions of traditional business activities are occurring within healthcare, setting a course for equally disastrous results. One strong indicator of impending demise is eroding quality. Healthcare can learn from its traditional counterparts who slowly drifted away from ethical values and failed to recognize or heed the ethical warning signs that eventually set the stage for their own demise. Restoring patient confidence and trust in quality of healthcare delivery requires more than adequate benefit coverage. Restoring patient confidence and trust in the quality of the healthcare delivery system requires a return to core values and a willingness to heed the ethical warning signs present in our midst to change course and position itself for return to solvency and success.

Moral Values and Ethical Competencies

Although most people probably have never undertaken a formal study of ethics, everyone is exposed to ethical principles, moral perspectives, and values throughout a lifetime. Individuals learn about basic **moral values** from families, religious leaders, teachers, the government, community organizations, and other groups that influence experiences and perspectives. Moral values are taught as "this is right and that is wrong." For example, some might consider it right to be nice to a neighbor and wrong to destroy the neighbor's property. However, these are not universal values. Others might consider it acceptable to be rude or mean to a neighbor they do not like and to destroy the neighbor's property. Applying this language to health information management, it is right—and a moral obligation—to protect the neighbor's privacy when you learn about diseases and conditions while working and it is wrong to share the neighbor's medical information with other neighbors, family, and friends.

HIM professionals should not make ethical decisions on behalf of others based solely on personal moral values or perspectives because not everyone shares the same moral perspectives or values. Professional responsibilities often require an individual to move beyond personal values. For example, an individual might demonstrate behaviors that are based on the values of honesty, providing service to others, or demonstrating loyalty. In addition to these, professional values might require promoting confidentiality, facilitating interdisciplinary collaboration, and refusing to participate or conceal unethical practices. Professional values could require a more comprehensive set of values than what an individual needs as an **ethical agent** in his or her personal life. For example, an HIM professional who hears information about a friend at a party has a range of options. He or she can share the information, share only part of it, change it, or not confirm or share it with anyone. However, that same individual in his or her role as an HIM professional cannot share overheard information under any circumstances. Optimally, the HIM professional will apply the same high standards in both personal and professional situations.

Ethics provides a language and a framework for formally discussing ethical issues, taking into account the values and obligations of others. Ethical discussion offers an opportunity to resolve conflicts when competing values are at stake. **Ethical decision making** requires people to explore choices beyond the perspective of simple right or wrong (moral) options. According to Glover, "ethics refers to the formal process of intentionally and critically analyzing the basis for our moral judgments for clarity and consistency" (Glover 2006, 34). When making health information decisions, HIM professionals must go beyond the personal right or wrong moral perspective and evaluate the many values and perspectives of others who are engaged in the decision to be made.

Ethical discussions outside the healthcare environment can be theoretical in nature, and the analysis of a problem does not necessarily result in an action. For example, **ethicists** could discuss whether to require all citizens living in a certain community to donate 10 hours a week to people in need as part of their civic duty. One ethicist might argue for a decision based on the ethical principle of beneficence, which would guide action to do good things for others. Another ethicist might argue for the same decision based on the principle of justice in which every citizen should contribute his or her fair share for the good of the community. These discussions and decisions would not necessarily require an action, but would help frame the ethical justification for a certain action.

In contrast, **bioethics** involves problems or issues regarding clinical care or the health information system that are never strictly theoretical in nature and must always result in a decision and an action. HIM professionals cannot merely deliberate whether to release patient information, assign the correct code, or purchase a new software system. Rather, they must apply ethical principles and then do something. In short, ethics applied in the work environment cannot remain theoretical and must result in an action.

Ethical Foundations in Health Information Management

Ethical principles and values have been important to the HIM profession since its beginning in 1928. The first ethical pledge was presented in 1934, by Grace Whiting Myers, a visionary leader who recognized the importance of protecting information in medical records. The HIM profession was launched with recognition of the importance of privacy and the requirement of an authorization for the release of health information (Huffman 1972, 135):

> I pledge myself to give out no information from any clinical record placed in my charge, or from any other source to any person whatsoever, except upon order from the chief executive officer of the institution which I may be serving.

Today, it is the patient who authorizes the release of information and not the chief executive officer (CEO) of the healthcare organization, as was stated in the original pledge. The most important values embedded in this pledge are to protect patient privacy and confidential information and to recognize the importance of the HIM professional as a moral agent in protecting patient information (Rinehart-Thompson and Harman 2006). The HIM professional has a clear ethical and professional obligation not to give any information to anyone unless the release has been authorized.

Protection of Privacy, Maintenance of Confidentiality, and Assurance of Data Security

The terms privacy, confidentiality, and security are often used interchangeably. However, there are some important distinctions, including:

- **Privacy** is "the right of an individual to be let alone. It includes freedom from observation or intrusion into one's private affairs and the right to maintain control over certain personal and health information" (Harman 2006, 634).

- **Confidentiality** carries "the responsibility for limiting disclosure of private matters. It includes the responsibility to use, disclose, or release such information only with the knowledge and consent of the individual" (Harman 2006, 627–628). Confidential information may be written or verbal.

- **Security** includes "physical and electronic protection of the integrity, availability, and confidentiality of computer-based information and the resources used to enter, store, process, and communicate it; and the means to control access and protect information from accidental or intentional disclosure" (Harman 2006, 635).

The HIM professional's responsibilities include ensuring that patient privacy and confidential information are protected and that data security measures are used to prevent unauthorized access to information. This responsibility includes ensuring that the release policies and procedures are accurate and up-to-date, that they are followed, and that all violations are reported to the proper authorities.

The Health Insurance Portability and Accountability Act (HIPAA) of 1996 established national standards for the protection of privacy and the assurance of the security of health information. This law deals with privacy, information standards, data integrity, confidentiality, and data security (Rinehart-Thompson and Harman 2006). Although HIPAA was passed in 1996, it took five years before the Privacy Rule became effective in April 2001, with an April 2003 compliance date. Congress passed the statute and the US Department of Health and Human Services (HHS) developed the regulations contained within the Privacy Rule (HHS 2003). The final HIPAA Security Rule regulations were published in the *Federal Register* in February 2003, and became effective in April 2005.

This legislation, which includes administrative simplification standards and security and privacy standards, has had a major impact on the collection and dissemination of information, and will continue to have this impact for years to come. This legislation has an enforcement program, and HIM professionals serve an important role that assures compliance, as indicated in the regulations. Preemptive federal legislation was needed so that all patient information would be protected regardless of where a patient lived or received healthcare. Moreover, this legislation protects individuals from losing their health insurance when leaving or changing jobs by providing insurance continuity (portability) and increases the federal government's authority over fraud and abuse in the healthcare arena (accountability) (Harman 2005). In addition to federal legislation, each state can pass its own legislation regarding access to patient information.

The American Recovery and Reinvestment Act of 2009 contains multiple provisions that affect the rights and obligations of certain parties under the privacy and security provisions of HIPAA. These changes relate to the application of the security and privacy provisions to business associates; the notification requirements in the event of a breach; the educational requirements regarding health information privacy; the restrictions on the disclosure and sale of health information; the accounting requirements of certain protected health information disclosures; auditing standards; and other related issues. The Department of Health and Human Services promulgated regulations to implement the provisions of this legislation over a multiyear period. It will be important to monitor these developments as they relate to the obligations of all parties affected by HIPAA. (HIPAA privacy and security standards are discussed more fully in chapters 13 and 17.)

Part of the impetus for HIPAA was the development of the electronic health record (EHR) (Amatayakul 2009; Dick et al. 1997; Hanken and Murphy 2006; Jones 2006; Murphy et al. 1999). As patient information was moved to the electronic medium, integrated systems across the continuum of care were developed and information was released and redisclosed to many people and agencies needing access to it. Thus, standardized federal legislation became an imperative. HIPAA was designed to guarantee that information transferred from one facility to the next would be protected. The National Committee on Vital and Health Statistics (NCVHS) supports a national health information infrastructure (NHII) so that patient care information can be transferred and protected in our integrated healthcare systems. As a result, patients benefit from the continuity of care and can control their personal health information (NCVHS 2001; Gellman 2004). In an electronic environment, protecting privacy has become extremely difficult and patients are becoming increasingly concerned about the loss of privacy and their inability to control the dissemination of information about them. As patients become more aware of the misuses of information, they may become reluctant to share information with their healthcare team. This may, in turn, result in problems with the healthcare provided and the information given to researchers, insurers, the government, and the many other stakeholders who legitimately need to access the information. Increasingly, patients are seeking anonymity and are responding to issues related to the use and disclosure of health information for directory purposes; to family and close personal friends; for notification purposes such as disasters; and for other disclosures required by law such as public health, employer medical surveillance, and funeral directors (Hughes 2002a; Hughes 2002b; Rhodes 2001; AHIMA 2002). Perhaps more importantly, the American Recovery and Reinvestment Act (ARRA), which was signed February 14, 2009 by President Barack Obama, includes legislative language that makes it clear that one of the key purposes of the act is that it "advances the delivery of patient-centered care." Part of laying that foundation includes some in-depth analysis about what it means to get consumers engaged in managing their health. It is imperative that principles such as patient-centered care get translated into policies that actually help to deliver it (Seidman 2009, 34). Accountable Care Organizations (ACOs) are intended to pay providers in a way that encourages collaboration, discourages supplier induced demand, and rewards high-quality care (AHIMA nd).

Professional Code of Ethics

HIM professionals used the pledge as the basis for guiding ethical decision making until 1957, at which time the American Association of Medical Record Librarians' (AAMRL 1957) House of Delegates passed the first Code of Ethics for the Practice of Medical Record Science (see figure 12.1). The first code of ethics combined ethical principles with a set of professional values to help support the decisions that HIM professionals had to make at work. The original code of ethics has been revised several times since 1957. Codes passed in 1977, 1988, 1998, and 2011 are included as good representations of how the codes changed to reflect the changes in the work responsibilities for the HIM professional. (See figures 12.2, 12.3, 12.4, and 12.5.) Other codes were passed during the timeframe but are not included in this chapter.

Upon being awarded the HIM credential of Registered Health Information Technician (RHIT) or Registered Health Information Administrator (RHIA); the coding credentials of Certified Coding Assistant (CCA); Certified Coding Specialist (CCS); Certified Coding Specialist-P (CCS-P); the health data analytics credential Certified Health Data Analyst (CHDA); the privacy and security credentials Certificate in Healthcare Privacy and Security (CHPS) or for clinical documentation improvement Certified in Healthcare Documentation Improvement (CDIP) by the American Health Information Management Association (AHIMA), the HIM professional agrees to follow the principles and values

Figure 12.1.   1957 Code of Ethics for the Practice of Medical Record Science

[Note: Gender-neutral language was not used in the 1950s, so the male pronoun should be read as "he or she."]

As a member of one of the paramedical professions he shall:

1. Place service before material gain, the honor of the profession before personal advantage, the health and welfare of patients above all personal and financial interests, and conduct himself in the practice of this profession so as to bring honor to himself, his associates, and to the medical record profession.

2. Preserve and protect the medical records in his custody and hold inviolate the privileged contents of the records and any other information of a confidential nature obtained in his official capacity, taking due account of the applicable statutes and of regulations and policies of his employer.

3. Serve his employer loyally, honorably discharging the duties and responsibilities entrusted to him, and give due consideration to the nature of these responsibilities in giving his employer notice of intent to resign his position.

4. Refuse to participate in or conceal unethical practices or procedures.

5. Report to the proper authorities, but disclose to no one else, any evidence of conduct or practice revealed in the medical records in his custody that indicates possible violation of established rules and regulations of the employer or of professional practice.

6. Preserve the confidential nature of professional determinations made by the staff committee which he serves.

7. Accept only those fees that are customary and lawful in the area for services rendered in his official capacity.

8. Avoid encroachment on the professional responsibilities of the medical and other paramedical professions, and under no circumstances assume or give the appearance of assuming the right to make determinations in professional areas outside the scope of his assigned responsibilities.

9. Strive to advance the knowledge and practice of medical record science, including continued self-improvement, in order to contribute to the best possible medical care.

10. Participate appropriately in developing and strengthening professional manpower and in representing the profession to the public.

11. Discharge honorably the responsibilities of any Association post to which appointed or elected, and preserve the confidentiality of any privileged information made known to him in his official capacity.

12. State truthfully and accurately his credentials, professional education, and experiences in any official transaction with the American Association of Medical Record Librarians and with any employer or prospective employer.

Copyright © 1957 by the American Association of Medical Libraries.

Figure 12.2.   1977 AMRA Bylaws and Code of Ethics

The medical record practitioner is concerned with the development, use, and maintenance of medical and health records for medical care, preventive medicine, quality assurance, professional education, administrative practices and study purposes with due consideration of patients' right to privacy. The American Medical Record Association believes that it is in the best interests of the medical record profession and the public which it serves that the principles of personal and professional accountability be reexamined and redefined to provide members of the Association, as well as medical record practitioners who are credentialed by the Association, with definitive and binding guidelines of conduct. To achieve this goal, the American Medical Record Association has adopted the following restated Code of Ethics:

1. Conduct yourself in the practice of this profession so as to bring honor and dignity to yourself, the medical record profession and the Association.

2. Place service before material gain and strive at all times to provide services consistent with the need for quality health care and treatment of all who are ill and injured.

3. Preserve and secure the medical and health records, the information contained therein, and the appropriate secondary records in your custody in accordance with professional management practices, employer's policies and existing legal provisions.

4. Uphold the doctrine of confidentiality and the individual's right to privacy in the disclosure of personally identifiable medical and social information.

5. Recognize the source of the authority and powers delegated to you and conscientiously discharge the duties and responsibilities thus entrusted.

6. Refuse to participate in or conceal unethical practices or procedures in your relationship with other individuals or organizations.

7. Disclose to no one but proper authorities any evidence of conduct or practice revealed in medical reports or observed that indicates possible violation of established rules and regulations of the employer or professional practice.

8. Safeguard the public and the profession by reporting to the Ethics Committee any breach of this Code of Ethics by fellow members of the profession.

9. Preserve the confidential nature of professional determinations made by official committees of health and health-service organizations.

10. Accept compensation only in accordance with services actually performed or negotiated with the health institution.

11. Cooperate with other health professions and organizations to promote the quality of health programs and advancement of medical care, ensuring respect and consideration for the responsibility and the dignity of medical and other health professions.

12. Strive to increase the profession's body of systematic knowledge and individual competency through continued self-improvement and application of current advancements in the conduct of medical record practices.

13. Participate in developing and strengthening professional manpower and appropriately represent the profession in public.

14. Discharge honorably the responsibilities of any Association position to which appointed or elected.

15. Represent truthfully and accurately professional credentials, education, and experience in any official transaction or notice, including other positions and duality of interests.

Figure 12.3.   1988 AMRA Code of Ethics and Bylaws

The medical record professional abides by a set of ethical principles developed to safeguard the public and to contribute within the scope of the profession to quality and efficiency in health care. This code of ethics, adopted by the members of the American Medical Record Association, defines the standards of behavior which promote ethical conduct.

1. The Medical Record Professional demonstrates behavior that reflects integrity, supports objectivity, and fosters trust in professional activities.

2. The Medical Record Professional respects the dignity of each human being.

3. The Medical Record Professional strives to improve personal competence and quality of services.

4. The Medical Record Professional represents truthfully and accurately professional credentials, education, and experience.

5. The Medical Record Professional refuses to participate in illegal or unethical acts and also refuses to conceal the illegal, incompetent, or unethical acts of others.

6. The Medical Record Professional protects the confidentiality of primary and secondary health records as mandated by law, professional standards, and the employer's policies.

7. The Medical Record Professional promotes to others the tenets of confidentiality.

8. The Medical Record Professional adheres to pertinent laws and regulations while advocating changes which serve the best interest of the public.

9. The Medical Record Professional encourages appropriate use of health record information and advocates policies and systems that advance the management of health records and health information.

10. The Medical Record Professional recognizes and supports the association's mission.

Copyright © 1988 by the American Medical Record Association.

discussed in this chapter and to base all professional actions and decisions on those principles and values. Even if federal or state laws did not require the protection of patient privacy, the HIM professional would be responsible for protecting it according to AHIMA's Code of Ethics (figure 12.5). Please see chapter 1 for a discussion of the credentials above.

Professional Values and Obligations

The ethical obligations of the HIM professional include the protection of patient privacy and confidential information. Important health information issues include what information should be collected, how the information should be handled, who should have access to the information, and under what conditions the information should be disclosed.

Ethical obligations are central to the professional's responsibility, regardless of the employment site or the method of collection, storage, and security of health information. Health information ethical and professional values are based on obligations to the patient, the healthcare team, the employer, the interests of the public, and oneself, one's peers, and one's professional associations (Harman 1999).

Based on an analysis of the AHIMA Code of Ethics for 1957, 1977, 1988, 1998, and 2004, the following themes and values were identified (Harman and Mullen 2006).

Figure 12.4.   **1998 AHIMA Code of Ethics and Bylaws**

AHIMA's Mission

The American Health Information Management Association is committed to the quality of health information for the benefit of patients, providers and other users of clinical data. Our professional organization:

- Provides leadership in HIM education and professional development
- Sets and promotes professional practice standards
- Advocates patient privacy rights and confidentiality of health information
- Influences public and private policies including educating the public regarding health information
- Advances health information technologies

Guiding Principles

We are committed to the:

- Creation and utilization of systems and standards to ensure quality health information
- Achievement of member excellence
- Development of a supportive environment and provision of the resources to advance the profession
- Provision of the highest-quality service to members and health care information users
- Investigation and application of new technology to advance the management of health information

We value:

- The balance of patients' privacy rights and confidentiality of health information with legitimate uses of data
- The quality of health information as evidenced by its integrity, accuracy, consistency, reliability, and validity
- The quality of health information as evidenced by its impact on the quality of health care delivery

This Code of Ethics sets forth ethical principles for the HIM profession. Members of this profession are responsible for maintaining and promoting ethical practices. This Code of Ethics, adopted by the American Health Information Management Association, shall be binding on health information management professionals who are members of the Association and all individuals who hold an AHIMA credential.

    I. Health information management professionals respect the rights and dignity of all individuals.

   II. Health information management professionals comply with all laws, regulations, and standards governing the practice of health information management.

  III. Health information management professionals strive for professional excellence through self-assessment and continuing education.

  IV. Health information management professionals truthfully and accurately represent their professional credentials, education, and experience.

   V. Health information management professionals adhere to the vision, mission, and values of the Association.

  VI. Health information management professionals promote and protect the confidentiality and security of health records and health information.

 VII. Health information management professionals strive to provide accurate and timely information.

VIII. Health information management professionals promote high standards for health information management practice, education, and research.

  IX. Health information management professionals act with integrity and avoid conflicts of interest in the performance of their professional and AHIMA responsibilities.

Source: AHIMA 1998.

Figure 12.5.   2011 American Health Information Management Association Code of Ethics

Preamble

The ethical obligations of the health information management (HIM) professional include the safeguarding of privacy and security of health information; disclosure of health information; development, use, and maintenance of health information systems and health information; and ensuring the accessibility and integrity of health information.

Healthcare consumers are increasingly concerned about security and the potential loss of privacy and the inability to control how their personal health information is used and disclosed. Core health information issues include what information should be collected; how the information should be handled, who should have access to the information, under what conditions the information should be disclosed, how the information is retained and when it is no longer needed, and how is it disposed of in a confidential manner. All of the core health information issues are performed in compliance with state and federal regulations, and employer policies and procedures.

Ethical obligations are central to the professional's responsibility, regardless of the employment site or the method of collection, storage, and security of health information. In addition, sensitive information (i.e., genetic, adoption, drug, alcohol, sexual, health, and behavioral information) requires special attention to prevent misuse. In the world of business and interactions with consumers, expertise in the protection of the information is required.

Purpose of the American Health Information Management Association Code of Ethics

The HIM professional has an obligation to demonstrate actions that reflect values, ethical principles, and ethical guidelines. The American Health Information Management Association (AHIMA) Code of Ethics sets forth these values and principles to guide conduct. (See also AHIMA Vision, Mission, Values.) The code is relevant to all AHIMA members and CCHIIM credentialed HIM professionals [hereafter referred to as certificants], regardless of their professional functions, the settings in which they work, or the populations they serve. These purposes strengthen the HIM professional's efforts to improve overall quality of healthcare.

The AHIMA Code of Ethics serves seven purposes:

- Promotes high standards of HIM practice
- Identifies core values on which the HIM mission is based
- Summarizes broad ethical principles that reflect the profession's core values
- Establishes a set of ethical principles to be used to guide decision-making and actions
- Establishes a framework for professional behavior and responsibilities when professional obligations conflict or ethical uncertainties arise
- Provides ethical principles by which the general public can hold the HIM professional accountable
- Mentors practitioners new to the field to HIM's mission, values, and ethical principles

The code includes principles and guidelines that are both enforceable and aspirational. The extent to which each principle is enforceable is a matter of professional judgment to be exercised by those responsible for reviewing alleged violations of ethical principles.

The Code of Ethics and How to Interpret the Code of Ethics

Principles and Guidelines

The following ethical principles are based on the core values of the American Health Information Management Association and apply to all AHIMA members and certificants. Guidelines included for each ethical principle are a non-inclusive list of behaviors and situations that can help to clarify the principle. They are not meant to be a comprehensive list of all situations that can occur.

    I.   *Advocate, uphold, and defend the individual's right to privacy and the doctrine of confidentiality in the use and disclosure of information.*

Figure 12.5. 2011 American Health Information Management Association Code of Ethics *(continued)*

A health information management professional **shall:**

1.1. Safeguard all confidential patient information to include, but not limited to, personal, health, financial, genetic, and outcome information.

1.2. Engage in social and political action that supports the protection of privacy and confidentiality, and be aware of the impact of the political arena on the health information issues for the healthcare industry.

1.3. Advocate for changes in policy and legislation to ensure protection of privacy and confidentiality, compliance, and other issues that surface as advocacy issues and facilitate informed participation by the public on these issues.

1.4. Protect the confidentiality of all information obtained in the course of professional service. Disclose only information that is directly relevant or necessary to achieve the purpose of disclosure. Release information only with valid authorization from a patient or a person legally authorized to consent on behalf of a patient or as authorized by federal or state regulations. The minimum necessary standard is essential when releasing health information for disclosure activities.

1.5. Promote the obligation to respect privacy by respecting confidential information shared among colleagues, while responding to requests from the legal profession, the media, or other non-healthcare related individuals, during presentations or teaching and in situations that could cause harm to persons.

1.6. Respond promptly and appropriately to patient requests to exercise their privacy rights (e.g., access, amendments, restriction, confidential communication, etc.). Answer truthfully all patients' questions concerning their rights to review and annotate their personal biomedical data and seek to facilitate patients' legitimate right to exercise those rights.

II. *Put service and the health and welfare of persons before self-interest and conduct oneself in the practice of the profession so as to bring honor to oneself, peers, and to the health information management profession.*

A health information management professional **shall:**

2.1. Act with integrity, behave in a trustworthy manner, elevate service to others above self-interest, and promote high standards of practice in every setting.

2.2. Be aware of the profession's mission, values, and ethical principles, and practice in a manner consistent with them by acting honestly and responsibly.

2.3. Anticipate, clarify, and avoid any conflict of interest, to all parties concerned, when dealing with consumers, consulting with competitors, in providing services requiring potentially conflicting roles (for example, finding out information about one facility that would help a competitor), or serving the Association in a volunteer capacity. The conflicting roles or responsibilities must be clarified and appropriate action taken to minimize any conflict of interest.

2.4. Ensure that the working environment is consistent and encourages compliance with the AHIMA Code of Ethics, taking reasonable steps to eliminate any conditions in their organizations that violate, interfere with, or discourage compliance with the code.

2.5. Take responsibility and credit, including authorship credit, only for work they actually perform or to which they contribute. Honestly acknowledge the work of and the contributions made by others verbally or written, such as in publication.

A health information management professional **shall not:**

2.6. Permit one's private conduct to interfere with the ability to fulfill one's professional responsibilities.

2.7. Take unfair advantage of any professional relationship or exploit others to further one's own personal, religious, political, or business interests.

(continued on next page)

Figure 12.5. **2011 American Health Information Management Association Code of Ethics** *(continued)*

III. *Preserve, protect, and secure personal health information in any form or medium and hold in the highest regards health information and other information of a confidential nature obtained in an official capacity, taking into account the applicable statutes and regulations.*

A health information management professional **shall:**

3.1.   Safeguard the privacy and security of written and electronic health information and other sensitive information. Take reasonable steps to ensure that health information is stored securely and that patients' data is not available to others who are not authorized to have access. Prevent inappropriate disclosure of individually identifiable information.

3.2.   Take precautions to ensure and maintain the confidentiality of information transmitted, transferred, or disposed of in the event of termination, incapacitation, or death of a healthcare provider to other parties through the use of any media.

3.3.   Inform recipients of the limitations and risks associated with providing services via electronic or social media (e.g., computer, telephone, fax, radio, and television).

IV. *Refuse to participate in or conceal unethical practices or procedures and report such practices.*

A health information management professional **shall:**

4.1.   Act in a professional and ethical manner at all times.

4.2.   Take adequate measures to discourage, prevent, expose, and correct the unethical conduct of colleagues. If needed, utilize the Professional Ethics Committee Policies and Procedures for potential ethics complaints.

4.3.   Be knowledgeable about established policies and procedures for handling concerns about colleagues' unethical behavior. These include policies and procedures created by AHIMA, licensing and regulatory bodies, employers, supervisors, agencies, and other professional organizations.

4.4.   Seek resolution if there is a belief that a colleague has acted unethically or if there is a belief of incompetence or impairment by discussing one's concerns with the colleague when feasible and when such discussion is likely to be productive.

4.5.   Consult with a colleague when feasible and assist the colleague in taking remedial action when there is direct knowledge of a health information management colleague's incompetence or impairment.

4.6.   Take action through appropriate formal channels, such as contacting an accreditation or regulatory body and/or the AHIMA Professional Ethics Committee if needed.

4.7.   Cooperate with lawful authorities as appropriate.

A health information management professional **shall not:**

4.8.   Participate in, condone, or be associated with dishonesty, fraud and abuse, or deception. A non-inclusive list of examples includes:

- Allowing patterns of optimizing or minimizing documentation and/or coding to impact payment
- Assigning codes without physician documentation
- Coding when documentation does not justify the diagnoses or procedures that have been billed
- Coding an inappropriate level of service
- Miscoding to avoid conflict with others
- Engaging in negligent coding practices
- Hiding or ignoring review outcomes, such as performance data
- Failing to report licensure status for a physician through the appropriate channels
- Recording inaccurate data for accreditation purposes

Figure 12.5.   2011 American Health Information Management Association Code of Ethics *(continued)*

- Allowing inappropriate access to genetic, adoption, health, or behavioral health information
- Misusing sensitive information about a competitor
- Violating the privacy of individuals

Refer to the AHIMA Standards for Ethical Coding for additional guidance.

4.9.   Engage in any relationships with a patient where there is a risk of exploitation or potential harm to the patient.

V.   *Advance health information management knowledge and practice through continuing education, research, publications, and presentations.*

A health information management professional **shall:**

5.1.   Develop and enhance continually professional expertise, knowledge, and skills (including appropriate education, research, training, consultation, and supervision). Contribute to the knowledge base of health information management and share one's knowledge related to practice, research, and ethics.

5.2.   Base practice decisions on recognized knowledge, including empirically based knowledge relevant to health information management and health information management ethics.

5.3.   Contribute time and professional expertise to activities that promote respect for the value, integrity, and competence of the health information management profession. These activities may include teaching, research, consultation, service, legislative testimony, advocacy, presentations in the community, and participation in professional organizations.

5.4.   Engage in evaluation and research that ensures the confidentiality of participants and of the data obtained from them by following guidelines developed for the participants in consultation with appropriate institutional review boards.

5.5.   Report evaluation and research findings accurately and take steps to correct any errors later found in published data using standard publication methods.

5.6.   Design or conduct evaluation or research that is in conformance with applicable federal or state laws.

5.7.   Take reasonable steps to provide or arrange for continuing education and staff development, addressing current knowledge and emerging developments related to health information management practice and ethics.

VI.   *Recruit and mentor students, staff, peers, and colleagues to develop and strengthen professional workforce.*

A health information management professional **shall:**

6.1.   Provide directed practice opportunities for students.

6.2.   Be a mentor for students, peers, and new health information management professionals to develop and strengthen skills.

6.3.   Be responsible for setting clear, appropriate, and culturally sensitive boundaries for students, staff, peers, colleagues, and members within professional organizations.

6.4.   Evaluate students' performance in a manner that is fair and respectful when functioning as educators or clinical internship supervisors.

6.5.   Report evaluation and research findings accurately and take steps to correct any errors later found in published data using standard publication methods.

6.6.   Serve an active role in developing HIM faculty or actively recruiting HIM professionals.

A health information management professional **shall not:**

6.7.   Engage in any relationships with a person (e.g., students, staff, peers, or colleagues) where there is a risk of exploitation or potential harm to that other person.

(continued on next page)

Figure 12.5.   2011 American Health Information Management Association Code of Ethics *(continued)*

VII.   *Represent the profession to the public in a positive manner.*

A health information management professional **shall:**

7.1.   Be an advocate for the profession in all settings and participate in activities that promote and explain the mission, values, and principles of the profession to the public.

VIII.   *Perform honorably health information management association responsibilities, either appointed or elected, and preserve the confidentiality of any privileged information made known in any official capacity.*

A health information management professional **shall:**

8.1.   Perform responsibly all duties as assigned by the professional association operating within the bylaws and policies and procedures of the association and any pertinent laws.

8.2.   Uphold the decisions made by the Association.

8.3.   Speak on behalf of the health information management profession and association, only while serving in the role, accurately representing the official and authorized positions of the association.

8.4.   Disclose any real or perceived conflicts of interest.

8.5.   Relinquish association information upon ending appointed or elected responsibilities.

8.6.   Resign from an association position if unable to perform the assigned responsibilities with competence.

8.7.   Avoid lending the prestige of the association to advance or appear to advance the private interests of others by endorsing any product or service in return for remuneration. Avoid endorsing products or services of a third party, for-profit entity that competes with AHIMA products and services. Care should also be exercised in endorsing any other products and services.

IX.   *State truthfully and accurately one's credentials, professional education, and experiences.*

A health information management professional **shall:**

9.1.   Make clear distinctions between statements made and actions engaged in as a private individual and as a representative of the health information management profession, a professional health information association, or one's employer.

9.2.   Claim and ensure that representation to patients, agencies, and the public of professional qualifications, credentials, education, competence, affiliations, services provided, training, certification, consultation received, supervised experience, and other relevant professional experience are accurate.

9.3.   Claim only those relevant professional credentials actually possessed and correct any inaccuracies occurring regarding credentials.

9.4.   Report only those continuing education units actually earned for the recertification cycle and correct any inaccuracies occurring regarding CEUs.

X.   *Facilitate interdisciplinary collaboration in situations supporting health information practice.*

A health information management professional **shall:**

10.1.   Participate in and contribute to decisions that affect the well-being of patients by drawing on the perspectives, values, and experiences of those involved in decisions related to patients.

10.2.   Facilitate interdisciplinary collaboration in situations supporting health information practice.

10.3.   Establish clearly professional and ethical obligations of the interdisciplinary team as a whole and of its individual members.

10.4.   Foster trust among group members and adjust behavior in order to establish relationships with teams.

Figure 12.5.   2011 American Health Information Management Association Code of Ethics *(continued)*

XI.   *Respect the inherent dignity and worth of every person.*

A health information management professional **shall:**

11.1.   Treat each person in a respectful fashion, being mindful of individual differences and cultural and ethnic diversity.

11.2.   Promote the value of self-determination for each individual.

11.3.   Value all kinds and classes of people equitably, deal effectively with all races, cultures, disabilities, ages and genders.

11.4.   Ensure all voices are listened to and respected.

The Use of the Code

Violation of principles in this code does not automatically imply legal liability or violation of the law. Such determination can only be made in the context of legal and judicial proceedings. Alleged violations of the code would be subject to a peer review process. Such processes are generally separate from legal or administrative procedures and insulated from legal review or proceedings to allow the profession to counsel and discipline its own members although in some situations, violations of the code would constitute unlawful conduct subject to legal process.

Guidelines for ethical and unethical behavior are provided in this code. The terms "shall and shall not" are used as a basis for setting high standards for behavior. This does not imply that everyone "shall or shall not" do everything that is listed. This concept is true for the entire code. If someone does the stated activities, ethical behavior is the standard. The guidelines are not a comprehensive list. For example, the statement "safeguard all confidential patient information to include, but not limited to, personal, health, financial, genetic and outcome information" can also be interpreted as "shall not fail to safeguard all confidential patient information to include personal, health, financial, genetic, and outcome information."

A code of ethics cannot guarantee ethical behavior. Moreover, a code of ethics cannot resolve all ethical issues or disputes or capture the richness and complexity involved in striving to make responsible choices within a moral community. Rather, a code of ethics sets forth values and ethical principles, and offers ethical guidelines to which a HIM professional can aspire and by which actions can be judged. Ethical behaviors result from a personal commitment to engage in ethical practice.

Professional responsibilities often require an individual to move beyond personal values. For example, an individual might demonstrate behaviors that are based on the values of honesty, providing service to others, or demonstrating loyalty. In addition to these, professional values might require promoting confidentiality, facilitating interdisciplinary collaboration, and refusing to participate or conceal unethical practices. Professional values could require a more comprehensive set of values than what an individual needs to be an ethical agent in one's own personal life.

The AHIMA Code of Ethics is to be used by AHIMA members and certificants, consumers, agencies, organizations, and bodies (such as licensing and regulatory boards, insurance providers, courts of law, government agencies, and other professional groups) that choose to adopt it or use it as a frame of reference. The AHIMA Code of Ethics reflects the commitment of all to uphold the profession's values and to act ethically. Individuals of good character who discern moral questions and, in good faith, seek to make reliable ethical judgments, must apply ethical principles.

The code does not provide a set of rules that prescribe how to act in all situations. Specific applications of the code must take into account the context in which it is being considered and the possibility of conflicts among the code's values, principles, and guidelines. Ethical responsibilities flow from all human relationships, from the personal and familial to the social and professional. Further, the AHIMA Code of Ethics does not specify which values, principles, and guidelines are the most important and ought to outweigh others in instances when they conflict.

Code of Ethics 2011 Ethical Principles

Ethical Principles: The following ethical principles are based on the core values of the American Health Information Management Association and apply to all AHIMA members and certificants.

A health information management professional **shall:**

1. Advocate, uphold, and defend the individual's right to privacy and the doctrine of confidentiality in the use and disclosure of information.

(continued on next page)

Figure 12.5.   2011 American Health Information Management Association Code of Ethics *(continued)*

2. Put service and the health and welfare of persons before self-interest and conduct oneself in the practice of the profession so as to bring honor to oneself, their peers, and to the health information management profession.

3. Preserve, protect, and secure personal health information in any form or medium and hold in the highest regards health information and other information of a confidential nature obtained in an official capacity, taking into account the applicable statutes and regulations.

4. Refuse to participate in or conceal unethical practices or procedures and report such practices.

5. Advance health information management knowledge and practice through continuing education, research, publications, and presentations.

6. Recruit and mentor students, peers and colleagues to develop and strengthen professional workforce.

7. Represent the profession to the public in a positive manner.

8. Perform honorably health information management association responsibilities, either appointed or elected, and preserve the confidentiality of any privileged information made known in any official capacity.

9. State truthfully and accurately one's credentials, professional education, and experiences.

10. Facilitate interdisciplinary collaboration in situations supporting health information practice.

11. Respect the inherent dignity and worth of every person.

Acknowledgement

Adapted with permission from the Code of Ethics of the National Association of Social Workers.

Resources

AHIMA Code of Ethics, 1957, 1977, 1988, 1998, and 2004.

Harman, L.B., ed. 2006. *Ethical Challenges in the Management of Health Information*, 2nd ed. Sudbury, MA: Jones and Bartlett.

McWay, D.C. 2010. *Legal and Ethical Aspects of Health Information Management*, 3rd ed. Clifton Park, NY: Cengage Learning.

National Association of Social Workers. "Code of Ethics." 1999. Available online on the NASW website.

Revised & adopted by AHIMA House of Delegates—October 2, 2011

Source: Copyright © 2011 by the American Health Information Management Association.

Obligations to the Patient and the Healthcare Team

With regard to the patient and the healthcare team, the HIM professional is obligated to:

- *Protect health, medical, genetic, social, personal, and adoption information:* Clinical information (for example, diagnoses, procedures, pharmaceutical dosages, or genetic risk factors) must be protected as well as behavioral information (for example, use of drugs or alcohol, high-risk hobbies, sexual habits). It is increasingly important to protect genetic and social information so that patients will not be vulnerable to the risks of discrimination.

- *Protect confidential information:* This involves ensuring that the information collected and documented in the patient information system is protected by all members of the healthcare team and by anyone with access to the information. This responsibility also includes protection of verbal communications on behalf of a patient and can involve communication with those in the legal profession, the media, or others who seek patient information.

- *Provide service to those who seek access to patient information:* Individuals who may request access to patient information include healthcare providers; insurance, research, or pharmaceutical companies; government agencies; and employers. Disclosure and redisclosure policies and procedures must be developed and followed. The HIM professional must ensure the honor of the profession before personal advantage and the health and welfare of patients before all other interests. He or she also must balance the many competing interests of all the stakeholders who want patient information, avoiding conflicts of interest.

- *Preserve and secure health information:* This includes obligations to maintain and protect the medium that stores the information, such as paper documentation and information stored in EHRs, including the protection of all databases and detailed secondary records and registries.

- *Promote the quality and advancement of healthcare:* As an important member of the healthcare team, the HIM professional provides valuable expertise in the collection of health information that will help providers improve the quality of care they deliver. The HIM professional might need to develop expertise in clinical medicine, pharmacology, biostatistics, and quality improvement methodologies so as to interpret clinical information and support research, based on work responsibilities.

- *Function within the scope of responsibility and restrain from passing clinical judgment:* Sometimes healthcare data may indicate a problem with a provider of care, the treatment of a diagnosis, or some other problem. The HIM professional's obligation is to provide the data; however, the obligation of evaluating the significance of the data rests with those held accountable for the review of the data. The HIM professional should repeatedly, consistently, and accurately report the results of studies, regardless of the volatility of the research outcomes.

Obligations to the Employer

With regard to the employer, the HIM professional is obligated to:

- *Demonstrate loyalty to the employer.* The HIM professional can do this by respecting and following the policies, rules, and regulations of employment unless they are illegal or unethical.

- *Protect committee and task force deliberations.* The HIM professional should be as committed to protecting committee conversations and decisions as he or she is to protecting patient information. These can include medical staff and employer committees.

- *Comply with all laws, regulations, and policies that govern the health information system.* The HIM professional should keep up-to-date with state and federal laws, accrediting and licensing standards, employer policies and procedures, and any other standards that affect the health information system.

- *Recognize both the authority and the power associated with the job responsibility.* The HIM professional is the expert on privacy and confidentiality and must be present at strategic meetings with clinical providers, administrative staff, and financial and operations management personnel to be sure that HIM expertise is presented and understood. Unethical behaviors would include avoidance of strategic meetings, waiting for the outcomes and decisions made by others, and then complaining about the decisions that were made. The HIM professional cannot remain quiet and let others have the power to decide what information is released, what software is installed, or other important HIM decisions. HIM professionals do have both the power and the authority to say, "This is inappropriate action and it is unethical."

- *Accept compensation only in relationship to work responsibilities.* Increasingly, there are groups or individuals who could benefit by having access to patient information and are willing to pay for such information. Access to databases with patient information on certain diagnoses such as AIDS or cancer could be sought by employers, commercial vendors, or others. The HIM professional must avoid the temptation to accept money for disclosing patient information or proprietary vendor secrets. This is especially important in the context of medical identity theft, which is discussed later in this chapter.

Obligations to the Public

With regard to the public interest, the HIM professional is obligated to:

- *Advocate change when patterns or system problems are not in the best interests of the patients.* The HIM professional should be a change agent and lead initiatives to change laws, rules, and regulations that do not ensure the integrity of patient information, including the protection of privacy and confidentiality. Moreover, the HIM professional should be proactive about protecting patients, the healthcare team, the organization, the professional association, peers, and himself or herself. State and national policy and legislative advocacy activities support this ethical obligation.

- *Report violations of practice standards to the proper authorities.* The HIM professional should not share information learned at work with family or friends or discuss such information in public places. The HIM professional should report the results of audits to the proper authorities only and bring potential or actual problems to the attention of those individuals responsible for the delivery and assessment of care and services.

- *Promote interdisciplinary cooperation and collaboration.* As an important member of the healthcare team, the HIM professional should work with others to analyze and address health information issues, facilitate conflict resolution, and recognize the expertise and dignity of his or her fellow team members.

Obligations to Self, Peers, and Professional Associations

With regard to self, peers, and professional associations, the HIM professional is obligated to:

- *Be honest about degrees, credentials, and work experiences.* The HIM professional should only report an acquired degree (such as a BS or MS) or successfully earned credentials (such as an RHIT, RHIA, or CCS). Work experiences must be reported accurately and honestly.

- *Bring honor to oneself, one's peers, and one's profession.* This obligation refers to personal competency and professional behavior. The HIM professional should ensure that peers and colleagues are proud to have him or her on the health information team.

- *Commit to continuing education and lifelong learning.* The HIM professional's education should not stop when he or she has earned a degree or a credential. Rather, the HIM professional should continue to attend educational sessions to keep abreast of changing laws, rules, and regulations that affect the health information system. The HIM professional should be a lifelong learner and contribute to improving the quality of healthcare service delivery. HIM professionals can keep their credentials by meeting the ongoing certification requirements of AHIMA. Maintaining competency through self-improvement is an important directive that ensures the continuance of the profession.

- *Strengthen health information professional membership.* This obligation includes belonging to professional associations, actively participating on committees, making presentations, writing for publications, and encouraging others to seek health information management as a career.

- *Represent the health information profession to the public.* The HIM professional has a responsibility to advocate for the public interest in areas related to the principles and values of HIM practice. For example, HIM professionals serve an important role when advocating for needed legislation to protect privacy and confidentiality, educational manpower funding, or appropriate EHR applications.

- *Promote and participate in health information research.* For example, when problems are discovered with the health information system, the HIM professional should conduct research to clarify the sources and potential solutions.

Ethical Responsibilities of the HIM Professional

In general, the HIM professional's primary responsibilities include those related to designing and implementing a system to ensure the completeness, accuracy, integrity, and timeliness of health information. In support of these responsibilities, the HIM professional is accountable for complying with laws, rules, regulations, standards, and policies from many sources, including the government, accreditation and licensure organizations, and the healthcare facility. Some of the HIM professional's core ethical responsibilities include the following:

- Protecting patient privacy and confidential information (Rinehart-Thompson and Harman 2006)

- Making appropriate decisions regarding the selection and use of clinical diagnostic and procedural codes (Schraffenberger and Scichilone 2006)

- Developing policies and procedures that ensure coding accuracy that supports clinical care and research and meets the requirements for reimbursement, while avoiding fraud and abuse violations (Rinehart-Thompson 2006)

- Reporting quality review outcomes honestly and accurately, even when the results might create conflict for an individual or an institution (Spath 2006)

- Ensuring that research and decision support systems are reliable (Johns and Hardin 2006)

- Releasing accurate information for public health purposes for patients with communicable diseases, such as AIDS or venereal disease, and assisting with the complexities of information management in the context of bioterrorism and the threat or reality of global diseases, such as smallpox or avian flu (Neuberger 2006)

- Supporting managed care systems by providing accurate, reliable information about patients and consumers, clinicians, healthcare organizations, and patterns of care, with special care devoted to issues related to access to information (Schick 2006)

- Facilitating the exchange of information for patients, families, and providers of care, especially for those affected by chronic and terminal illness, that ensures patient autonomy and beneficence (Tischler 2006)

- Ensuring that the EHR meets the standards of privacy and security according to HIPAA and other federal and state laws (Hanken and Murphy 2006), the standards of information security (Czirr et al. 2006), and software development (Fenton 2006)

- Ensuring that clinical data repositories, data marts, data warehouses, and EHRs meet the standards of the best practices of health information and database management (Lee et al. 2006)

- Participating in the development of integrated delivery systems so that patients can move across the continuum of care and the right information can be provided to the right people at the right time (Olson and Grant 2006)

- Working in the context of e-health technologies that allow consumers, patients, and caregivers to search for health information and advice, create and maintain personal health records, and conduct virtual consultations with their care providers (Baur and Deering 2006)

- Ensuring that health information technology systems, including EHRs, electronic prescribing, bedside barcoding, computerized provider order entry (CPOE), and clinical decision support systems reduce errors and improve quality (Bloomrosen 2006)

- Managing the protection of sensitive information, including genetic information (Fuller and Hudson 2006); drug, alcohol, sexual, and behavioral information (Randolph and Rinehart-Thompson 2006); and adoption information (Jones 2006)

- Developing moral awareness and nurturing an ethical environment in the context of managing a health information system (Flite and Laquer 2006)

- Serving as entrepreneur and advocate for patients, the healthcare team, and others who have interests in the health information system (Gardenier 2006; Helbig 2006)

- Working with vendors in the development of business relationships that ensure ethical processes when selecting and communicating with vendors, managing vendor relationships, and dealing with the contract negotiation process (Olenik 2006)

These continue to be important ethical issues. In response to the 2011 Code, important resources were created to further clarify the values, obligations and issues that are faced by HIM professionals. For a list of specific articles, please see References at the end of the chapter.

Ethical Issues Related to Medical Identity Theft

According to the Federal Trade Commission (FTC), medical identity theft is one of the fast growing ethical issues and is an information crime. Identity theft is on the rise, affecting almost 10 million victims in 2008 (a 22percent increase from 2007). It is relatively easy to do, the stakes are high, the financial temptations are huge, it is difficult to detect, and there are virtually no protections for the patient or providers who are victimized. The HIM professional must be familiar with what it is, who commits the crime, what protections can be put into place, and what HIM advocacy roles are needed (AHIMA e-HIM Workgroup on Medical Identity Theft 2008; Nichols et al. 2008).

The World Privacy Forum tracks medical identity cases and prepares important resources for consumers. Recent resources deal with HIPAA, genetic discrimination, facial recognition technology, Facebook protection, digital tracking systems, browser privacy settings, and cloud computing. The world Privacy Forum collects and reports on cases and trends with medical identity theft. A map gives the ability to look interactively at approximately one year of medical identity theft activity in the US, based on Federal Trade Commission complaints. The map reveals a strong geographic clustering of medical identity theft in Florida, California (especially southern California), New York, Arizona, and Texas (World Privacy Forum ndb), retrieved 2/24/12). There are thousands of patients who have been victimized by this crime. One received an alarming phone call from the local hospital one day claiming that her newborn baby had just tested positive for illegal drugs, even though she had not had any children in several years. Protective services threatened to take away her four children accusing her of being an unfit mother. It turned out that a 28 year-old alleged drug abuser had stolen the woman's driver's license, walked into a hospital, had the baby and left the hospital leaving a bill for $10,000. The victim has had to fight to clear her name (CBS 2009).

Medical identity theft occurs when someone uses a person's name and sometimes other parts of their identity—such as insurance information or Social Security number—without the victim's knowledge or consent to obtain medical services or goods, or when someone uses the person's identity to obtain money by falsifying claims for medical services and falsifying Medicare records to support those claims (World Privacy Forum 2006b, 16).

Medical identity theft can be committed by family, friends, and acquaintances. It can also be committed by strangers who steal someone's identity in order to obtain medical care, services, or equipment, either because they do not have medical care or their insurance does not cover the needed services. Medical identity theft creates an ethical dilemma for the healthcare system because those involved can be working within the healthcare delivery system, including doctors, nurses, administrative staff, and health information and billing employees. The World Privacy Forum (2006b, 14) notes that:

> All levels of the medical system may be involved in medical identity theft. Doctors, clinics, billing specialists, nurses and other members of the medical profession have taken part in this crime, as have criminals who work in administrative positions inside the healthcare system to collect information and to carry out their crimes.

There was one case in California in which it was determined that medical record and billing employees had copied the identity information for as little as $100 (Weaver 2000). Those who commit the crime can earn money by using the patient information fraudulently. Medical information systems have multiple access points across the continuum of the healthcare system, making it almost impossible to detect and correct fraud. Medical identify theft deserves the attention of the HIM professional because the central problem is falsification of medical documentation that could adversely affect patient safety. Inaccurate information, such as an incorrect blood type or inaccurate documentation of prescriptions can kill patients (World Privacy Forum 2006b; Weaver, 2000; Office of Inspector General 2005; *United States v. Sample* 2000). Also, the real patients can be denied needed equipment (wheelchairs or walkers, and the like) because their records show that they have already received the equipment, when, in fact, the fraudulent user of their health information received the equipment. Increasingly, physicians are becoming victims of this crime, with their name and license numbers stolen; and their signatures forged for writing prescriptions and documentation that will help criminals bill for services never rendered to patients.

The nationwide health information network (NHIN) and EHRs could exacerbate the ease of committing this crime. Electronic systems with multiple centralized and decentralized databases could facilitate both the commission and hiding of this crime. The government has passed red flag rules that require certain healthcare organizations to shelter patients from identity theft. Healthcare facilities will need to identify patterns, practices, and activities that could indicate identity theft, such as suspicious documents (altered or potential forgery), photographs or identification data that do not match, returned mail complaints, or other similar occurrence (Federal Trade Commission 2009).

HIPAA provides some modicum of protection, but cannot begin to truly protect patient information or patients from being harmed. The problem becomes almost unsolvable in the context of secondary releases of false information for insurance, the increasing number of integrated systems and the development of medical clearinghouses. HIM professionals are in a strong position to be advocates on behalf of patients who are victimized by this crime. In addition, it places an obligation on the profession to be diligent in hiring practices, especially with the employees that report directly to HIM professionals. Once hired, the employees must have ongoing educational sessions on the importance of ethical behavior.

The Patient's Perspective

Many patients have been victimized by medical identity theft and the overwhelming reality is that there are few who can assist them in resolving the problem, as opposed to those who are victimized by financial identity theft. There are inadequate resources and knowledge in the private sector (police departments, insurance companies, bankers, and the like) as well as the lack of laws specific to medical identity theft.

The HIM Professional's Perspective

Because of the unique aspects of this crime, HIM professionals must be vigilant in the case of medical identity theft and work with the real patient to confirm and correct inaccurate information. If there is no previous medical record, there must be a way to identify the record as being fraudulent and refuse further release of the false information. The HIM professional must be an advocate for the patient and find the time, resources, and expertise to substantiate valid identification. The HIM professional must seek assistance in this process, if necessary, rather than just sending the patient away. HIM professionals can exacerbate the problem by refusing to work with the real patient. Legal counsel should be sought if the HIM professional is unsure about what to do.

Once information is in a patient's medical record, it is difficult to amend or remove that information. HIM professionals cannot ignore the false documentation in the paper medical records and electronic information systems. Duplicating these false entries in multiple databases as a result of secondary data uses will increase the problem. The Code of Ethics requires attestation as to the accuracy and validity of the data.

Patients need to be able to access and amend their medical records if fraud has occurred. As patients maintain their own personal health record (PHR), they will become more aware of the fraud. They are in the best position to know that the documentation belongs to someone else, based on a review of medical or financial reports (AHIMA nd; World Privacy Forum 2006a).

The patient does have the right to request an amendment. The healthcare provider must respond but does not have to agree with the request. The patient then has the right to submit a statement of disagreement that must be added to the health record.

Covered entities are not required to account for disclosures related to treatment, payment, or healthcare. AHIMA (2006), as part of the 2006 State of HIPAA Compliance Survey noted:

> As in previous years, the accounting for disclosures requirement is reported to be a difficult one and is most often mentioned as needed modification. AHIMA and other groups have sought a recommendation for such an amendment from the National Committee on Vital and Health Statistics and the Office for Civil Rights, but at this time no amendment is expected in the near future. HITECH published NPRM titled, "HIPAA privacy rule accounting of disclosures under the HITECH Act" in 2011. As of early 2012, the final rule is still pending.
>
> This proposed rule includes two parts; the right to an accounting of disclosures and the right to a report on access. CEs would need to account for disclosures if such disclosures are made through an EHR. (AHIMA 2011b)

Given this, HIM professionals should work toward the solution that all HIM systems should track all disclosures, even if not required by HIPAA and there should be guaranteed protection of all information. Audit trails that identify both internal and external disclosures to prevent fraud, rather than allow the EHRs to exacerbate the problem (Sparrow 2000).

The health information system is extremely complex. Data can be entered manually, electronically, through PDAs, through wireless systems, or from laptops. Information systems cross geographical boundaries and utilize many different software and hardware applications for patient care and research. The AHIMA Code of Ethics requires the protection of information across this continuum. The adage a few years ago was follow the money. Today, the mantra must be follow the information (AHIMA e-Learning 2012).

What can HIM professionals do as part of advocacy roles? They can:

- Facilitate the patient's ability to review and correct errors in their medical records (not just the entries with which they disagree but those that are due to fraud and do not belong to their medical or treatment history). This information might also be in the pharmaceutical information system or within the insurance agency database.

- Prevent discrimination. Not only can medical errors affecting patient safety occur with medical identity theft, but there can also be discrimination in the life and health insurance systems. Do not obstruct patients' ability to review their records.

Pay attention to their pleas if they think that they are victims of medical identity theft, and make sure that patients have the right to amend their documentation and to assure systems that will facilitate this process.

- Reconsider the importance of analysis. The entire medical record used to be analyzed for accuracy and the medical record analyst could learn to identify falsification of information. Now, analysis often is limited to discharge summaries, operative reports, and other critical documents. Does the organization have systems in place, within the context of the EHRs, that will prevent medical identity theft?

- Consider advocacy to amend the HIPAA rules and regulations related to the accounting of disclosures to include problems related to internal participants.

- Participate in HIM research studies that will help identify occurrences and sources of medical identity theft. Build interdisciplinary collaborative teams to conduct this research, including healthcare providers; HIM professionals; privacy and security experts; legal representatives (both prosecution and defense); ethicists; HIPAA, identify theft, and fraud experts; and patients who have been victimized.

- Conduct needed risk assessments as the NHIN becomes more of a reality—the electronic health record (EHR), can make this crime easier. Document and quantify this problem. Improper access to information and disclosures of false information could increase in the future as a result of the EHR.

- Design systems that can assess employees' integrity and accountability. Make sure the healthcare team and employees that work on behalf of patients respect the importance and sacredness of the information in a patient's medical record. Give them an understanding of the importance of ethics so that they will avoid the temptation of taking money for the information in the system. Ensure that there are no pressures on employees that will tempt them to participate in the fraud.

- Design educational programs to ensure that colleagues understand and value the HIM Code of Ethics, which sets forth values and ethical principles and offers ethical guidelines to which professionals aspire and by which their actions can be judged. A code is important in helping guide the decision-making process and can be referenced by individuals, agencies, organizations, and bodies (such as licensing and regulatory boards, insurance providers, courts of law, agency boards of directors, government agencies, and other professional groups), among others (AHIMA Code of Ethics 2011a).

- Consider establishing policies so that patients who are victims of medical identity fraud do not have to pay for the costs of duplicating their files. A 2006 AHIMA survey found that 63 percent of providers charge patients for copies and these costs can be up to $5 per page (although $1 is more common) (AHIMA 2006). Increasingly, healthcare facilities have abandoned the practice of charging patients for copies of their medical information, based on a rationale that the information belongs to them and providing copies is an important customer service.

When HIM professionals think about identity, they typically think about the person and the story in an individual medical record. Emerging technologies are changing perceptions of a person's identity—the sum of our genetic and health information. HIM professionals are being challenged to understand and deal with issues that they have never faced before; and they must stay abreast of new and evolving issues that deal with identity. HIM professionals have ethical obligations to prevent problems with medical identity theft and to report those who participate in this crime. See chapter 13 for more detail on identity theft.

Ethical Issues Related to Documentation and Privacy

Just a few decades ago, only a few people created documentation in patient health records and still fewer wanted access to patient information after the episode of care was completed. In today's healthcare system, many providers document their decision-making process and patient outcomes in the health information system and many more people want access to that information. The HIM professional plays a critical role in developing policies and procedures to ensure the integrity of patient information, including appropriate and authorized access.

In addition to writing policies and procedures to ensure compliance with federal and state laws, accrediting and licensing agencies, and the bylaws of the healthcare facility, the HIM professional can serve many functions that support the integrity of data and the protection of privacy. The HIM professional can design and deliver educational sessions to the healthcare team to make them aware of the documentation and access rules and regulations. Sometimes educational sessions address the issue of avoiding participation in fraudulent or retrospective documentation practices. Retrospective documentation practices are those where healthcare providers add documentation after care has been given for the purpose of increasing reimbursement or avoiding a medical legal action.

Unacceptable documentation practices include backdating progress notes or other documentation in the patient's record and changing the documentation to reflect the known outcomes of care (versus what was done at the time of the actual care). It is the HIM professional's responsibility to work with others to ensure that patient documentation is accurate, timely, and created by authorized parties. The professional Code of Ethics requires the HIM professional to assure accurate and timely documentation.

Clinical documentation is essential to the expertise of HIM professionals. Increasingly, there are ethical issues which surface as a result of documentation, such as issues related to coding, reporting of data and inappropriate documentation and billing practices. AHIMA passed the Ethical Standards for Clinical Documentation Improvement (CDI) Professionals (2010). This ethical code is based on the principles and framework of the AHIMA Code of Ethics (2011a). See chapter's Appendix A for the complete set of CDI ethical standards.

Ethical Issues Related to Release of Information

Three primary ethical problems are pertinent to the release of information (ROI):

- Violations of the need-to-know principle
- Misuse of blanket authorizations
- Violations of privacy that occur as a result of secondary release of information procedures

In the past, the standard for ROI was the need to know. If an insurance company had a patient request to pay for surgery, the request was sent to the healthcare facility and the HIM professional carefully examined it for legitimacy. He or she would:

- Compare the patient's signature to the one collected upon admission to the facility
- Check the date to ensure that the request was dated after the occurrence so that the patient was aware of what was being authorized and released
- Verify the insurance company as the one belonging to the patient
- Review the request for what was wanted and whether the requestor was entitled to the information

The HIM professional then reviewed the documentation and provided the information requested. For example, the admission and discharge dates, the diagnoses of cholecystitis and cholelithiasis, and the surgical procedure of cholecystectomy were provided to the insurance company so that the bill could be paid.

Today, the process of abstracting needed information is virtually nonexistent, except for disability cases, and documentation is copied above and beyond the criterion of the **need-to-know principle.** For example, in response to the request to verify an admission for a cholecystectomy, the history and physical, the operative report, the discharge summary, and the laboratory report could be copied. That documentation could reveal social habits, genetic risks, and family history of disease that have nothing to do with the surgery. Patient privacy could be violated as a result of the release of the information through subsequent discrimination.

Another common ethical problem is misuse of **blanket authorizations.** Patients often sign a blanket authorization, which authorizes the release of information from that point forward, without understanding the implications. The requestor of the information then could use the authorization to receive health information for many years. The problem with the use of blanket authorizations is that there is no way for the patient to know that the information is being accessed. Patients cannot authorize the release of information in 2003 for diagnoses or care that has not yet been provided. For example, by 2011, the patient might have AIDS or cancer and might not want this information released.

A third problem is **secondary release of information** to others by the authorized recipient to an unauthorized party. This problem has increased in frequency in the context of EHRs since the computerization of health information. A legitimate request might be processed to pay for an insurance claim, but adequate safety and protections may not be in place for the information after it has been released. The initial requestor could then forward the information to others without patient authorization. The HIM professional cannot merely think about ROI within the context of the single request. The responsibility to follow the information beyond the walls of the healthcare facility is much more serious today than it was a few years ago. Does the HIM professional know who gains access to the information after it is released to an authorized requestor? If not, he or she may be contributing to the violations of patient privacy and discrimination by employers or insurance companies based on the information that was released.

Patients have increasingly expressed concerns about the use of blanket authorizations and secondary ROI by the initial requestor or receiving party. They fear that more information is being given out than is necessary and that they do not know about the many people and agencies that are gaining access to this information.

HIPAA has been designed to address several issues related to patient privacy, including a return to the need-to-know principle. The HIM professional needs to participate in the development of electronic systems that can replicate the original human decisions regarding ROI to release what is needed but not more. Although it is easier to just photocopy the information, the HIM professional needs to carefully consider the implications of doing this within the context of patient privacy. This situation has created an opportunity for HIM professionals to participate with other HIM professionals in efforts to correct these problems.

Because the HIM professional works in many employment sites throughout the healthcare delivery system, the ethical obligations extend into a variety of areas, as noted above. In fulfilling the responsibilities of the position, the HIM professional must apply ethical values when making decisions wherever he or she is positioned within the organization.

Check Your Understanding 12.1

1. The term that means the HIM professional applies rules consistently is:

    A. Nonmaleficence
    B. Beneficence
    C. Justice
    D. Moral values

2. An HIM professional's ethical obligations:

    A. Apply regardless of employment site
    B. Are limited to the employer
    C. Apply to only the patient
    D. Are limited to the employer and patient

3. Which of the following is the concept of the right of an individual to be left alone?

    A. Privacy

    B. Bioethics

    C. Security

    D. Confidentiality

4. An individual stole and used another person's insurance information to obtain medical care. This action would be considered:

    A. Violation of bioethics

    B. Fraud and abuse

    C. Medical identify theft

    D. Abuse

5. Which of the following threatens the need-to-know principle?

    A. Backdating progress notes

    B. Blanket authorization

    C. HIPAA regulations

    D. Surgical consent

Instructions: Match the HIM professional's obligations to the following groups with the professional values expressed in AHIMA's Code of Ethics.

6. Accept compensation only in relationship to responsibilities

7. Advocate change

8. Preserve and secure health information

9. Commit to continuing education and lifelong learning

    a. Patient and the healthcare team

    b. Employer

    c. Public interest

    d. Oneself and one's peers and professional associations

Ethical Decision-Making Matrix

HIM professionals must factor several criteria into their decision making, as illustrated in figure 12.6. These include, but are not limited to:

- *Cost:* Can the facility and the health information system afford the improvement in the system?

- *Technological feasibility:* Will the technological application provide accurate and reliable information for the decision-making process?

- *Federal and state laws:* Are there federal or state laws that must be considered before a change is made in the system?

- *Medical staff bylaws:* Are there rules or regulations unique to the facility that require or prohibit an action?

- *Accreditation and licensing standards:* Which agencies have standards that are important to the decision being made? Do the standards allow or prohibit a certain action?

- *Employer policies, rules, or regulations:* Does the facility have policies, rules, or regulations that require or prohibit a decision?

Although these criteria must be assessed in the decision-making process, they cannot be used alone. Virtually every decision the HIM professional makes also must be based on ethical principles and professional values.

Ethicists provide assistance in this process. Glover (2006, 35, 38, 50) has proposed a seven-step process to guide ethical decision making. When faced with an ethical issue,

Figure 12.6.   Ethical decision-making matrix

ETHICAL PROBLEM		
Steps	**Information**	
1. What is the question?		
2. What are the facts?	**KNOWN**	**TO BE GATHERED**
3. What are the values? Examine the shared and competing values, obligations, and interests in order to fully understand the complexity of the ethical problem(s).	**Patient:** **HIM Professional:** **Healthcare professionals:** **Administrators:** **Society:** **Other, as appropriate:**	
4. What are my options?		
5. What should I do?		
6. What justifies my choice?	*JUSTIFIED*	*NOT JUSTIFIED*
7. What can I do to prevent this ethical problem?		

Source: Glover 2006, p. 50.

the HIM professional should ask and answer all of the following questions. The questions represent the steps in the ethical decision-making process:

1. What is the ethical question?
2. What facts do you know and what do you need to find out?
3. Who are the different stakeholders, what values are at stake, and what are the shared and different obligations and interests of each of the stakeholders?
4. What options for action do you have?
5. What decision should you make and what core HIM values are at stake?
6. What justifies the choice and what are the value-based reasons to support the decision? What choice or choices cannot be justified?
7. What prevention options can be put into place so that this issue will not come up again?

When a decision must be made about an issue and only one choice is identified, the decision most likely will be based on an individual's narrow moral perspective of right or wrong. If it is an ethical problem, the decision makers must take into account the perspectives of competing stakeholders and their values. Decisions made without this model will not benefit from an ethical decision-making process that considers multiple options.

Check Your Understanding 12.2

1. Using A, B, C, and so on, rearrange the steps of the ethical decision-making process in the correct order.

____ What decisions should you make and what core HIM values are at stake?

____ What facts do you know and what do you need to find out?

____ What options for action do you have?

____ What is the ethical question?

____ What justifies the choice and what are the reasons to support the decision, based on values? What choice(s) cannot be justified?

____ What prevention options can be put into place so that this issue will not happen again?

____ Who are the different stakeholders, what values are at stake, and what are the different obligations and interests of each of the stakeholders?

Important Health Information Ethical Problems

Several problems face HIM professionals in today's complex world of work, including issues related to the use of information; electronic health information systems; the management of sensitive health information; process and strategies for decision making; and the HIM roles as manager, entrepreneur, and advocate. The business relationships with vendors can also create ethical tensions. There are issues raised because of the uses of information, including clinical code selection and use, quality review, research and decision support, public health, managed care, and clinical care (Harman 2006).

Ethical Issues Related to Coding

In the past, coding was done almost exclusively for clinical studies and quality assurance review processes. Although codes were provided for reimbursement purposes, the healthcare facility was reimbursed on the basis of usual, customary, and reasonable costs. The codes that were assigned became the basis of retrieval for clinical studies, quality reviews, and the reimbursement system. After the codes became the basis for reimbursement, there were inherent incentives to code so that the greatest amount of reimbursement could be acquired. This placed the importance of accurate coding at the forefront of the ethical issues facing HIM professionals.

Ethical problems have risen in the past few years as a result of the direct linkage between coding and payments for care. Increased pressure has been put on HIM professionals who are coding to transmit inaccurate information, creating problems that are legal and ethical in nature. Problems include pressure to code inappropriate levels of service, discovering misrepresentation in physician documentation, miscoding to avoid conflicts, discovering miscoding by other staff, lacking the tools and educational background to code accurately, and being required by employers to engage in negligent coding practices (Schraffenberger and Scichilone 2006). In response to these issues, AHIMA passed standards that specifically address coding issues (figure 12.7).

Failure to heed the complex rules of coding for reimbursement can lead to problems with compliance and with fraud and abuse for the HIM professional. If the HIM professional fails to establish adequate monitoring systems for accurate code assignment or submits a false claim, the consequences could include penalties such as fees and prison. The HIM professional must know the laws and the penalties for failure to follow the laws and have the expertise to develop preventive programs to ensure that submission of the false claim does not happen. Fraud and abuse problems include documentation that does not justify the billed procedure, acceptance of money for information, fraudulent retrospective documentation on the part of the provider to avoid suspension, and code assignment without physician documentation. An important role for the HIM professional is that of compliance officer (Rinehart-Thompson 2006).

Figure 12.7. AHIMA Standards of Ethical Coding

Coding professionals should:

1. Apply accurate, complete, and consistent coding practices for the production of high-quality healthcare data.

2. Report all healthcare data elements (e.g. diagnosis and procedure codes, present on admission indicator, discharge status) required for external reporting purposes (e.g. reimbursement and other administrative uses, population health, quality and patient safety measurement, and research) completely and accurately, in accordance with regulatory and documentation standards and requirements and applicable official coding conventions, rules, and guidelines.

3. Assign and report only the codes and data that are clearly and consistently supported by health record documentation in accordance with applicable code set and abstraction conventions, rules, and guidelines.

4. Query provider (physician or other qualified healthcare practitioner) for clarification and additional documentation prior to code assignment when there is conflicting, incomplete, or ambiguous information in the health record regarding a significant reportable condition or procedure or other reportable data element dependent on health record documentation (e.g. present on admission indicator).

5. Refuse to change reported codes or the narratives of codes so that meanings are misrepresented.

6. Refuse to participate in or support coding or documentation practices intended to inappropriately increase payment, qualify for insurance policy coverage, or skew data by means that do not comply with federal and state statutes, regulations and official rules and guidelines.

7. Facilitate interdisciplinary collaboration in situations supporting proper coding practices.

8. Advance coding knowledge and practice through continuing education.

9. Refuse to participate in or conceal unethical coding or abstraction practices or procedures.

10. Protect the confidentiality of the health record at all times and refuse to access protected health information not required for coding-related activities (examples of coding-related activities include completion of code assignment, other health record data abstraction, coding audits, and educational purposes).

11. Demonstrate behavior that reflects integrity, shows a commitment to ethical and legal coding practices, and fosters trust in professional activities.

Revised and approved by the House of Delegates 09/08.

Ethical Issues Related to Quality Management, Decision Support, Public Health, Managed Care, and Clinical Care

The pressures to conceal information, discovered as an outcome of quality reporting systems, that could be potentially harmful to an employer, and problems with patient safety require constant diligence and the courage to repeatedly report the truth. Many factors contribute to the ethical problems faced by quality management professionals, including the rising cost of healthcare, limited resources, and concerns with patient safety. Some of the common quality outcome problems include (Spath 2006):

- Inaccurate performance data that are inappropriately shared with the public

- Negative care outcomes, such as infections, that occur in the course of providing home healthcare

- Failure to check a physician's licensure status

- Incomplete health records hidden in preparation for accreditation or licensure surveys

- Patterns of inappropriate healthcare

Research and decision-support responsibilities include ensuring data integrity and confidentiality, assuring compliance with human subject research protocols, and maintaining and enhancing professional competence (Johns and Hardin 2006). Career opportunities for the HIM professional are growing in public health systems. Careers in this area require an understanding of the government's role in the collection and use of health information. The government's responsibility to protect the health of the public sometimes competes with the need to protect patient privacy, such as in the case of reporting HIV status. State and local mandatory reporting requirements exist for certain conditions, including infectious and communicable diseases. The government needs this information to monitor, investigate, and implement interventions, when necessary. Sometimes problems arise when the public's right to know or duty to one's employer conflicts with patient privacy (Neuberger 2006). The HIM professional can provide invaluable assistance with public health initiatives that will contribute to environmental and personal health. This role requires constant advocacy so that the interests of both the public and the individual patient can be served. New threats of bioterrorism and global infections (such as anthrax, SARS, H1N1, or avian flu) pose new ethical dilemmas in the management of health information. There will need to be a balance between protecting privacy of those injured and providing information to the government and healthcare professionals so that the medical crisis can be resolved.

There are many important ethical issues faced by the HIM professional working on behalf of managed care organizations. Problems arise if high-quality information is not provided to patients, clinicians, and communities. Access to information is key to the problems faced by the HIM professional as he or she helps with the organization's strategies regarding pricing, access to providers, and quality of care. Job responsibilities in this work context include providing information about provider practices, providing patient clinical and demographic information, and establishing policies and procedures that provide for patient privacy (Schick 2006).

There are an increasing number of patients who will require information in order to make difficult end-of-life decisions. Problems dealing with aging, frailty, autonomy of those near death, physician bias and equity, treatment choices, treatment goals and beneficence, advance care planning, palliative care, and managing pain are a few of the difficult decisions that must be made, and the availability of accurate information requires ethical decision making (Tischler 2006).

Ethical Issues Related to Sensitive Health Information

All health information must be protected, but additional ethical issues have emerged around the release of sensitive information such as genetic, drug and alcohol, and psychiatric; communicable disease; and adoption information. At least two levels of genetic information can be reported in an information system: presence of a disease, such as cystic fibrosis, and presence of a risk of disease, such as a genetic risk for breast cancer. Various state laws govern the use and release of genetic information and the HIM professional must be aware of them. In recent years, there have been growing concerns about discrimination in employment and insurance based on the misuse of genetic information (Fuller and Hudson 2006).

According to Fuller and Hudson (2006, 434), the HIM professional must be aware of the following issues related to genetic information:

1. Genetic research and testing can give researchers, clinicians, and patients a means to prevent, treat, or screen for a disease. Often, however, individuals are reluctant to participate in genetic research and testing because they believe they cannot be sure of the privacy of the genetic information that will be obtained from them and placed in their medical records or in research records.

2. Insurers and employers may seek genetic information to identify at-risk individuals and deny them employment or insurance coverage, fire them, or raise their insurance premiums. Genetic information may also be sought in custody battles or in cases of third-party liability. Even when this information is not used to discriminate, individuals may be concerned about its disclosure because of its possibility of causing psychosocial harm, such as harm to family relationships.

3. It is difficult to provide special protections for genetic information as a category because it cannot be clearly separated from other medical information. Therefore, the best way to protect genetic information is to strengthen privacy and confidentiality protections for medical information in general and to enact antidiscrimination legislation.

4. The HIPAA Privacy Rule provides a basic level of privacy and confidentiality protection for protected health information. The Privacy Rule does not preempt state laws (including genetic antidiscrimination laws) that offer a higher level of privacy protection.

5. The generation of experimental data by a research protocol is not specifically addressed by most state laws.

6. HIM professionals have the responsibility to ensure that their practices are guided by state and federal laws and regulations to protect genetic information and by the ethical imperative to protect the privacy and confidentiality of patients.

The Genetic Information Nondiscrimination Act was passed in 2008 (HHS 2008). This took many years to approve, and AHIMA worked extensively to facilitate passage of this important legislation. Other federal and state laws will need to be passed in order for patients to be fully protected in the context of genetic information and this is an important first step.

Federal and state laws also govern the use of behavioral health information and special concerns with its use. The HIM professional must respond to the government, the police, and other agencies that seek drug, alcohol, sexual, or other behavioral information (Randolph and Rinehart-Thompson 2006). The inappropriate release of information can have serious discriminatory consequences, such as:

- The police officer presents an arrest warrant to a behavioral health facility. Do you confirm that the patient has been treated? What are the implications for patient privacy if you do?

- A patient with schizophrenia and assaultive behavior is about to be released from a healthcare facility. Do you have a responsibility to inform the girlfriend who has been assaulted in the past? What are your obligations to protect the privacy of the patient being released?

The ROI dealing with substance abuse, sexually transmitted diseases, and mental health require extra caution on the part of the HIM professional when developing release policies and procedures. There are often competing interests between public safety and patient privacy. How does one deal with law enforcement officials within this context? Federal and state legislation can provide some guidance, but often additional legal counsel must be sought.

The release of adoption information is another example of an issue in which laws are necessary, but insufficient, for solving the problems. Decisions cannot be made merely by following the legal rules. More and more often, access to adoption information is being requested by adopted children seeking their biological parents, and vice versa. Biological parents often look for children who could be organ donors or for other assistance. This issue reflects the complexities of releasing genetic and behavioral information because, increasingly, self is defined within genetic parameters and biological heritage. Access to adoption information raises the larger issue of familial access to information, regardless of adoptive status. If biological children can gain access to health information for their biological parent(s), why can't all children gain access to familial information (Jones 2006)? HIM professionals must be alert to these special needs and refrain from processing requests for adoption information without carefully considering the risks for violations of patient privacy, discrimination, or inappropriate access.

Ethical Issues Related to Research

There are many past and present problems with research and ethics. Human subjects have been mistreated, misinformed, and harmed in recent years, even though there are ethical codes, national and international agreements, and agencies that review research proposals with a focus of protecting research participants. These include the Nuremberg Code, the Helsinki Agreement (also known as the Declaration of Helsinki), the National Research Act of 1974 (Public Law 93-348), the Belmont Report, bioethics commissions, HIPAA, and IRB processes (Harman and Nielsen 2008, 341).

The primary ethical principles that are engaged in research include respect for autonomy (self-determination); beneficence (promoting good); nonmaleficence (do no harm);

and justice (fairness) (Beauchamp and Childress 2001). The respect for autonomy requires an ability of the participant to understand and authorize the research through informed consent; beneficence means that benefit is possible; nonmaleficence means that patients will not be intentionally harmed; and justice requires fairness in the enrollment of participants (Harman and Nielsen 2008, 337).

Table 12.1 highlights some of the research projects and the ethical issues (Harman and Nielsen 2008).

As noted in table 12.1, mistreatment of vulnerable populations has happened too often. These populations include children, and persons who are cognitively impaired, comatose, drug addicts, economically disadvantaged, elderly, institutionalized, non-English speaking employees, low literacy persons, minorities, or involved in illegal activities. Other groups include pregnant women, fetuses, neonates, and in-vitro; prisoners; and students (over the age of 18) (Harman and Nielsen 2008). In 2010, the US government formally apologized for medical research on syphilis that was conducted in the 1940s because doctors had infected soldiers, prostitutes, prisoners, and mental patients with syphilis, without informed consent (McGreal 2010).

HIM professionals must be cautious when reviewing research protocols and take patient safety and protection seriously, so that unethical problems do not occur.

Ethical Issues Related to Electronic Health Record Systems

With a paper-based health record, access issues were relatively simple. Only one person at a time could access the information, and it was extremely difficult to collect and use data of an aggregate nature. With electronic systems, many requestors are allowed multiple, simultaneous access, it is relatively easy to share information across a continuum of care, and electronic systems may be well outside the boundaries of any individual care site. The advent of the electronic information system has presented complex challenges with regard to record integrity and information security, integrated linkage of information systems across a continuum of care, software development and implementation, and the protection of information in e-health systems. It is imperative for HIM professionals to be a part of the implementation team in order to advise their facilities on state and federal regulations regarding privacy/security so that these core principles are built into the system itself. At a very minimum, the HIM professional should ensure that the issues have been addressed by the team implementing the EHRs.

e-HIM affords information exchange that necessitates active participation on the part of HIM professionals, in both the public and private sectors. There are many ethical challenges, including developing and maintaining information and systems security, exchanging information within and across jurisdictions, executing technical and clinical services contracts, handling release of information, implementing and managing telehealth applications, maintaining and documenting compliance with HIPAA and state privacy rules, and maintaining the legal electronic medical record (Bloomrosen 2006).

As EHRs were developed and healthcare facilities began to link various health information systems, the temptation increased to sacrifice privacy and data integrity for the sake

Table 12.1.   **Vulnerable populations**

Vulnerable Populations	Issues to Consider Regarding Consent and How Attributes of the Vulnerable Population Manifest Themselves in the Consent Process
Children	Protected class of persons who cannot voluntarily consent without parental consent. Children may sign assent form depending on age; See Subpart D of Title 45, Part 46 of the Code of Federal Regulations.
Cognitively Impaired Persons	Cognitive skills may vary on a day-to-day basis and therefore the ability to understand consent and ongoing participation may change from week to week; ability to understand consent may be permanently impaired; judgment and reasoning affected. Assessment must occur so that the investigator knows the condition of each participant. Sometimes assessment must occur each time subject is seen as part of the study. Sometimes a legally authorized surrogate is utilized when research studies include persons with cognitive impairment.
Comatose Persons	Cannot give consent; need appropriate and legally authorized surrogate. Some research with comatose persons could be considered emergency research. See the OHRP guidance from 1996 on this topic.
Economically Disadvantaged Persons	May agree to be involved in a study only for free medical care or for payment made for participation when it may not be in the best interests of the individual.
Elderly Persons	Cognition levels may vary during the course of the study. Is informed consent still valid throughout the research study?
Employees	May feel coerced by employer to participate. Sometimes lab staff are asked to be normal subjects. There must not be any requirements of employment that coerce employees to participate if they don't want to.
Hearing-Impaired Persons	If a deaf person wishes to enroll in a study, how will the investigator make sure the consent process has been complete? It is not enough to have the consent form for the subject to read. How will questions be handled? How will future visits be handled? Does someone on the study staff know sign language? Note: The Deaf Pride movement may clash with the IRBs definitions of the hearing impaired and their ability to participate in research studies.
Institutionalized Persons	May not understand consent form, may be cognitively impaired, may not have autonomy, and may not be able to exercise free will (voluntariness).
Low Literacy Persons	May not understand the consent form.
Minorities	Not all minorities are considered vulnerable populations. The context of the study, why minorities are included, whether they are the targeted focus of the study are factors that must be considered and may impact informed consent.
Non-English Speaking Persons	Even though consent forms must be translated into the native language, without research staff that are fluent in the language, there is difficulty ascertaining whether non-English speaking participants truly understand their study involvement. How are participants informed, if they are illiterate in their native language?
Persons Involved in Illegal Activities	Could include: computer hackers, drug addicts, prostitutes, illegal immigrants, and other types of illegal activities. Collecting data from persons who are involved in illegal activities can be challenging. A foremost consideration must be that by signing a consent form, the subject is, in effect, agreeing to participate in a study about their illegal activities. Therefore the act of protecting subjects, making sure they understand their rights and explaining the study, and executing legally authorized consent may lead to disclosure and place the subject in more harm than non-participation would. Investigators need to carefully weigh what problems may be encountered if subjects are required to sign consent forms. It may be appropriate to ask for a waiver of written consent and employ the use of an information sheet for this type of research. A Certificate of Confidentiality may also be appropriate. "Certificates of Confidentiality are issued by the National Institutes of Health (NIH) to protect identifiable research information from forced disclosure. They allow the investigator and others who have access to research records to refuse to disclose identifying information on research participants in any civil, criminal, administrative, legislative, or other proceeding, whether at the federal, state, or local level." (DHHS, 2011)

Table 12.1. **Vulnerable populations** *(continued)*

Vulnerable Populations	Issues to Consider Regarding Consent and How Attributes of the Vulnerable Population Manifest Themselves in the Consent Process
Pregnant Women, Fetuses, Neonates, In-Vitro	In some instances, pregnant women must be included as would any other population; in other instances special protections for pregnant woman must be in place. Investigators who plan to use pregnant women, human fetuses, and neonates in research should be familiar with the government regulations described in 45 CFR 46, Subpart B.
	There are specific requirements for the wording in the consent form when using pregnant women in research. Problems with ethical research involving this population occur in third world research—promises of pregnancy care, if they participate in research.
Prisoners	Do not have free will as they are incarcerated. Prisoners may feel coerced into participating because they think the authorities may grant them special privileges. May agree to participate because they think it will reduce their sentence, earn favors with guards; See Subpart C of Title 45, Part 46 of the Code of Federal Regulations containing the federal policy on research that involves prisoners.
Students (over the age of 18)	May feel coerced because they think their grade may be affected if they don't agree to participate. The professor is always in power position over the student. Usually have another option for participation. Grade cannot be affected by non-participation.

Note: Vulnerable populations cannot be studied under an exemption certification. Additional current ethical violations are online from AHRP (2007).

Souce: Harman and Nielsen 2008.

of business efficiency and timely access to information. There is an exponential increase in the risk to privacy and the protection of confidential information (Hanken and Murphy 2006). The HIM professional must do a thorough systems analysis of the independent systems and ensure that the merged systems meet the criteria of data integrity, information security, and the ethical use of the information.

Information security carries additional burdens of ethical decision making. Many requestors such as insurance companies, government agencies, managed care organizations, and employers need health information to do their jobs. Unauthorized access to patient information becomes a constant challenge, given the need to balance the responsibility to protect information while giving others access to information within the context of job responsibilities. Internal requestors include, but are not limited to, patients, providers of care, financial agencies, and administrative and clinical personnel such as quality or risk management professionals. External stakeholders include other healthcare facilities, research institutes, accrediting and licensing agencies, and fiscal intermediaries (Czirr et al. 2006). The HIM professional must develop a comprehensive information security policy, including detailed audit trails of access and actions. Moreover, the policy must be monitored with consequences for violations. Increasingly, HIM professionals are being designated as the information security officers within a healthcare facility or healthcare system.

Development and implementation of software systems are inherently interdisciplinary in nature, and the process requires collaboration and conflict resolution. The physicians, the HIM professional, the information technology experts, and administrative personnel often have competing interests. The HIM professional is often in the position of carefully delineating the details of competing interests so that appropriate decisions can be made.

This role of being able to see the systems' implications within the context of protecting privacy is invaluable (Fenton 2006). The HIM professional's role as interdisciplinary facilitator is crucial, which is why educational sessions on organizational development, team building, and conflict resolution are often key components of the HIM professional's continuing education program.

The expertise of the HIM professional includes data resource management because EHRs generate data repositories and huge amounts of health information of interest to many people. A primary focus of the HIPAA legislation is to ensure that systems are developed that protect privacy, threats of violations of information integrity, and unauthorized access. Data resource managers must have both HIM technical expertise and information technology expertise so that they can design and monitor systems that ensure data security and patient privacy. These functions are accomplished through the use of many decision-making tools, including databases, clinical data repositories, and data-mining tools, among others. The primary ethical dilemma involves balancing the competing interests of access and appropriate use of information (Lee et al. 2006).

EHRs facilitated the capacity for developing integrated delivery systems across a continuum of care. HIM systems that relied on paper-based systems could only transmit information from one site of care to another was through copying procedures or faxing. Now, information can follow the patient and be instantly and simultaneously shared and made available as needed. The integrated computerized systems require HIM professional diligence to ensure protection of information and access to only those who have a need to know. Information management policies, rules, and procedures for individual healthcare entities must be compatible with those of other facilities, and often the issues of competing interests can create major ethical conflicts as to the appropriate action.

The master patient index presents a major problem because there is often no consistency among facilities in terms of how and what information is collected. If the information is to follow the patient, the individual systems must be accurate and compatible. AHIMA has developed the *HIM Principles in Health Information Exchanges: Data Quality Attributes Grid which identifies the following data quality attributes:* accuracy, accessibility, comprehensiveness, currency, consistency, definition, granularity, precision, relevancy, and timeliness (AHIMA Workgroup on Health Information Management in Health Information Exchange 2007).

Negotiation and problem-solving skills are an inherent requirement for the HIM professional working in an integrated delivery system (Olson and Grant 2006). The HIM professional must lead the organization in addressing data quality issues associated with implementing integrated information systems.

Last, but not least, the HIM professional's ethical expertise is needed in the burgeoning e-health systems. Some of the ethical issues the HIM professional faces in the work environment include the quality of online information, privacy protections, and equity and privacy. The issue of equity is important to e-health systems because not everyone has access to the information on the electronic systems. There cannot be equity when some patients can easily gain access to invaluable and voluminous information about symptoms, diseases, pharmaceutical interventions, and treatment options and others cannot. Privacy can be an issue when patients reveal sensitive information to a website and have no idea what will happen to the information or who will have access to it. The opportunities for the HIM professional are unlimited given the problems of consumer access to information, quality of information provided, and access to information. This nontraditional advocacy role for HIM professionals is important in this emerging technological advancement (Baur and Deering 2006).

Roles of Manager, Entrepreneur, and Advocate

The HIM professional deals with daily complexities that require the need for understanding ethics. Problems such as late and absent employees, temptations at conventions and meetings, employees who should be terminated, and poor work performance are a few of the many dilemmas facing the busy HIM manager (Flite and Laquer 2006). As an entrepreneur, the HIM professional must understand the complexities of business practices intersecting with professional values and ethical principles. Common ethical dilemmas occur when establishing contracts, clarifying the roles of intrapreneur and entrepreneur, or acting as an independent contractor. Difficulties may arise when consulting for competitors (having access to sensitive information that might be of value to the competition), dealing with advertising, confronting unrealistic client expectations, or confusing profit versus not-for-profit motivations for decisions (Gardenier 2006).

HIM professionals have always been advocates for patients and providers, and the advocacy role is important in today's healthcare delivery system. For the HIM professional, advocacy "is ethics in action: choosing to take a stand for and speak out for the rights or needs of a person, group, organization, or community" (Helbig 2006, 595). For example, HIM problems that require advocacy include:

- Protecting the privacy of prominent citizens because it is more tempting to want access to the information of prominent citizens, such as elected officials, famous actors, or sports heroes
- Demonstrating compassion for drug-dependent peers
- Protecting the work environment for HIM employees
- Ensuring that consent forms are properly designed so that patients understand what they are signing and so that patient information is protected from unauthorized secondary disclosure

The advocacy role requires HIM expertise, ethical expertise, and an understanding of the patient's bill of rights (Helbig 2006).

Business relationships with vendors also pose ethical dilemmas. What issues are raised when vendors are also friends? What is the appropriate use of gifts? Should some vendors be preferred when dealing with requests for proposals? How can you assure ethical dealings when negotiating contracts (Olenik 2006)?

Check Your Understanding 12.3

1. Which of the following is an example of ethical issues related to coding?

   A. Inaccurate performance data
   B. Fraud and abuse
   C. Release of sensitive data
   D. Mistreatment of vulnerability population

2. What has brought about changes based on access, security, linking data, and more?

   A. Electronic health record
   B. Research
   C. Law related to sensitive information
   D. Quality management

Instructions: Indicate whether the statements below are true or false (T or F).

3. _____ Protecting the work environment for HIM staff is part of advocacy.

4. _____ The advocacy role requires an HIM professional to understand HIM practices, ethics, and patient bill of rights.

Instructions: Match the ethical principle with its definition.

5. Beneficence   a. Fairness in applying rule
                                b. Right to be left alone
6. Nonmaleficence   c. Promote good
                                d. First do no harm
7. Justice

8. Privacy

Real-World Case

Carol Wright is an outstanding manager. She has worked for C&S Pharmaceuticals for 15 years. She has received five promotions and is currently responsible for abstracting and quality operations. Carol has been quick to identify personnel problems and provides educational and instructional support to her staff.

Carol supervises Joan, who is often absent or late for work. When she does come to work she makes many mistakes, but she always seems to meet work standards prior to her performance reviews. Various forms of motivation, education, and administrative support have been offered to Joan in the past. This week, Joan failed to show up for three days without notifying the office. The company policy states that if an employee does not show up for work for three consecutive days without notifying the office by the end of the third business day (5 p.m.), the employee's employment shall be terminated.

On the third day, some managers may be anxiously waiting for the employee to call and explain the absence, but this was not the case with Carol. Carol had recognized that this employee was nonproductive, noncompliant, and met the criteria for job abandonment. Carol was prepared to terminate Joan, because she repeatedly demonstrated a clear disregard for the policy related to reporting to work. Carol no longer had any patience for Joan's behaviors. Carol was confident that the employee was not going to comply with the policy and that this would be an easy termination. She completed the termination paperwork based on job abandonment at 3 p.m. and left it on her desk for the 5 p.m. submission to the human resources department. At 4:30 p.m., Carol's secretary told her that Joan was on the telephone, but Carol did not accept the call. The paperwork was sent to the human resources department at 5 p.m. and Joan's employment was terminated the next day due to her unethical behavior (Flite and Laquer, 2006, 510).

Summary

Ethical decision making is one of the health information professional's most challenging and rewarding job responsibilities. It requires courage because there will always be people who choose not tell the truth or do the right thing. HIM professionals must discuss these issues with their peer professionals and seek the advice of the professional association when necessary.

The HIM professional's job responsibilities inherently require an understanding of ethical principles, professional values and obligations, and the importance of using an ethical decision-making matrix when confronting difficult challenges at work. With this knowledge, the informed HIM professional can move from understanding problems based on a moral perspective to understanding the importance of applying an ethical decision-making process. Ethical decision making takes practice and discussions with peers will help the HIM professional to build competency in this important area.

When making ethical decisions, the HIM professional should use the complete ethical decision-making matrix to consider all the stakeholders and their obligations and the important HIM professional values. More than one response can be given for any ethical issue as long as the complete matrix is applied. Just as there can be more than one right answer to a problem, there can be wrong answers, especially when an answer is based only on a moral value or the perspective of one individual or when the action violates ethical principles.

There will always be ongoing ethical problems, such as the protection of human subjects in research, and emerging or new ethical problems, such as medical identity theft, which require the constant diligence of the HIM professional. HIM professionalism and the Code of Ethics will help with emerging issues, now and in the future.

Bioethical decisions involving the use of health information require action and such actions always require courage. The healthcare team, the patients, and the others who are served need to know that the HIM professional has the expertise and the courage to make appropriate ethical decisions.

References

American Health Information Management Association. nd Personal health record (PHR). http://www.myphr.com

American Health Information Management Association. 1998. Code of ethics and bylaws. Chicago: AHIMA.

American Health Information Management Association. 2002. Practice brief: Consent for uses and disclosures of information. Chicago: AHIMA.

American Health Information Management Association. 2004. Code of ethics. http://www.ahima.org/about/ethics.asp

American Health Information Management Association. 2006. HIPAA privacy and security compliance: A report by the American Health Information Management Association. Chicago: AHIMA.

American Health Information Management Association. 2011a. American Health Information Management Association Code of Ethics. http://library.ahima.org/xpedio/groups/public/documents/ahima/bok1_024277.hcsp?dDocName=bok1_024277#principle

American Health Information Management Association. 2011b. OCR Releases Proposed Rule on Accounting of Disclosure. http://journal.ahima.org/2011/05/27/ocr-releases-proposed-rule-on-accounting-of-disclosure/

AHIMA e-HIM Workgroup on Health Information Management in Health Information Exchange. 2007. Appendix to HIM Principles in Health Information Exchange (AHIMA Practice Brief), *Journal of AHIMA* 78(8):69–74.

AHIMA e-HIM Workgroup on Medical Identity Theft. 2008. Practice brief: Mitigating medical identity theft. *Journal of AHIMA* 79(7):63–69.

AHIMA e-Learning. 2012. Medical identity theft: Prevention in the EHR environment. http://www.ahima.org/advocacy

Amatayakul, M.K. 2009. *Electronic Health Records: A Practical Guide for Professionals and Organizations,* 4th ed. Chicago: AHIMA.

American Association of Medical Record Librarians. 1957. Code of ethics for the practice of medical record science.

American Medical Record Association. 1977. Bylaws and code of ethics.

American Medical Record Association. 1988. Code of ethics and bylaws.

Baur, C., and M.J. Deering. 2006. e-Health for consumers, patients and caregivers. Chapter 16 in *Ethical Challenges in the Management of Health Information,* 2nd ed. Edited by L.B. Harman. Sudbury, MA: Jones and Bartlett.

Beauchamp, T., and J. Childress. 2001. *Principles of Biomedical Ethics.* New York: Oxford University Press.

Bloomrosen, M. 2006. e-HIM: Information technology and information exchange. Chapter 17 in *Ethical Challenges in the Management of Health Information,* 2nd ed. Edited by L.B. Harman. Sudbury, MA: Jones and Bartlett.

CBS. 2009. Protect Against Medical ID Theft. http://www.cbsnews.com/stories/2006/10/09/earlyshow/living/ConsumerWatch/main2073225.shtml

Czirr, K., K. Rosendale, and E. West. 2006. Information security. Chapter 12 in *Ethical Challenges in the Management of Health Information,* 2nd ed. Edited by L.B. Harman. Sudbury, MA: Jones and Bartlett.

Department of Health and Human Services. 2003. Summary of the HIPAA Privacy Rule. *OCR Privacy Brief.* http://www.hhs.gov/ocr/privacy/hipaa/understanding/summary/privacysummary.pdf

Department of Health and Human Services. 2008. Genetic Information Nondiscrimination Act of 2008. http://frwebgate.access.gpo.gov/cgi-bin/getdoc.cgi?dbname=110_cong_bills&docid=f:h493enr.txt.pdf

Department of Health and Human Services. 2011 Certificates of Confidentiality Kiosk. http://grants.nih.gov/grants/policy/coc/

Dick, R.S., E.B. Steen, and D.E. Detmer, eds. 1997. *The Computer-Based Patient Record: An Essential Technology for Health Care.* Rev. ed. Washington, DC: The National Academies Press.

Federal Trade Commission. 2009. Fighting Fraud with the Red Flags Rule: A How-To Guide for Business. http://hawaii.bbb.org/Storage/55/Documents/business/Fighting%20Fraud%20with%20the%20Red%20Flags%20Rule%20-%20A%20How-To%20Guide%20for%20Business.pdf

Fenton, S.H. 2006. Software development and implementation. Chapter 13 in *Ethical Challenges in the Management of Health Information,* 2nd ed. Edited by L.B. Harman. Sudbury, MA: Jones and Bartlett.

Flite, C., and S. Laquer. 2006. Management. Chapter 21 in *Ethical Challenges in the Management of Health Information,* 2nd ed. Edited by L.B. Harman. Sudbury, MA: Jones and Bartlett.

Fuller, B.P., and K.L. Hudson. 2006. Genetic information. Chapter 18 in *Ethical Challenges in the Management of Health Information,* 2nd ed. Edited by L.B. Harman. Sudbury, MA: Jones and Bartlett.

Gardenier, M. 2006. Entrepreneurship. Chapter 22 in *Ethical Challenges in the Management of Health Information,* 2nd ed. Edited by L.B. Harman. Sudbury, MA: Jones and Bartlett.

Gellman, R. 2004. When HIPAA meets NHII: A new dimension for privacy. Presentation to US Department of Health and Human Services Data Council Privacy Committee, Washington, DC.

Glover, J.J. 2006. Ethical decision-making guidelines and tools. Chapter 2 in *Ethical Challenges in the Management of Health Information,* 2nd ed. Edited by L.B. Harman. Sudbury, MA: Jones and Bartlett.

Hanken, M.A., and G. Murphy. 2006. Electronic patient record. Chapter 11 in *Ethical Challenges in the Management of Health Information,* 2nd ed. Edited by L.B. Harman. Sudbury, MA: Jones and Bartlett.

Harman, L.B. 1999. HIM and ethics: Confronting ethical dilemmas on the job, an HIM professional's guide. *Journal of AHIMA* 71(5):45–49.

Harman, L.B. 2005. HIPAA: A few years later. Online *Journal of Issues in Nursing* 10(2). http://www.nursingworld.org/ojin/topic27/tpc27_2.htm

Harman, L.B., ed. 2006. *Ethical Challenges in the Management of Health Information,* 2nd ed. Sudbury, MA: Jones and Bartlett.

Harman, L.B., and V.L. Mullen. 2006. Professional values and the code of ethics. Chapter 1 in *Ethical Challenges in the Management of Health Information,* 2nd ed. Edited by L.B. Harman. Sudbury, MA: Jones and Bartlett.

Harman, L.B., and C.S. Nielsen. 2008. Research and ethics. In *Health Informatics Research Methods: Principles and Practice.* Edited by E.J. Layman and V.J. Watzlaf. Chicago: AHIMA.

Helbig, S. 2006. Advocate. Chapter 24 in *Ethical Challenges in the Management of Health Information,* 2nd ed. Edited by L.B. Harman. Sudbury, MA: Jones and Bartlett.

Huffman, E.K. 1972. *Manual for Medical Record Librarians,* 6th ed. Chicago: Physician's Record Company.

Hughes, G. 2002a. Practice brief: Laws and regulations governing the disclosure of health information. Chicago: AHIMA.

Hughes, G. 2002b. Practice brief: Required content for authorizations to disclose. Chicago: AHIMA.

Johns, M.L., and J.M. Hardin. 2006. Research and decision support. Chapter 7 in *Ethical Challenges in the Management of Health Information,* 2nd ed. Edited by L.B. Harman. Sudbury, MA: Jones and Bartlett.

Jones, M.L. 2006. Adoption Information. Chapter 19 in *Ethical Challenges in the Management of Health Information,* 2nd ed. Edited by L.B. Harman. Sudbury, MA: Jones and Bartlett.

Lee, F.W., A.W. White, and K.A. Wager. 2006. Data resource management. Chapter 14 in *Ethical Challenges in the Management of Health Information,* 2nd ed. Edited by L.B. Harman. Sudbury, MA: Jones and Bartlett.

Lennick, D., and F. Kiel. 2008. Moral intelligence: Enhancing busines performance and leadership success. New York: Wharton School Publishing.

McGreal, C. 2010 (October). US says sorry for "outrageous and abhorrent" Guatemalan syphilis tests. *The Guardian.* http://www.guardian.co.uk/world/2010/oct/01/us-apology-guatemala-syphilis-tests

Murphy, G., M.A. Hanken, and K.A. Waters. 1999. *Electronic Health Records: Changing the Vision.* Philadelphia: W.B. Saunders.

National Committee on Vital and Health Statistics. 2001. Information for health: A strategy for building the national health information infrastructure. http://www.aspe.hhs.gov/sp/nhii/Documents/ NHIIReport2001/report11.htm

Neuberger, B.J. 2006. Public health. Chapter 8 in *Ethical Challenges in the Management of Health Information,* 2nd ed. Edited by L.B. Harman. Sudbury, MA: Jones and Bartlett.

Nichols, C., N. Davis, C. Lemery, and C. Smith. 2008. *Medical Identity Theft.* Chicago: AHIMA.

Office of Inspector General, Department of Health and Human Services, Criminal Actions. 2005. http://oig.hhs.gov/fraud/enforcement/criminal/05/0905.html

Olenik, K. 2006. Vendor relationships. Chapter 23 in *Ethical Challenges in the Management of Health Information,* 2nd ed. Edited by L.B. Harman. Sudbury, MA: Jones and Bartlett.

Olson, B., and K.G. Grant. 2006. Integrated delivery systems. Chapter 15 in *Ethical Challenges in the Management of Health Information,* 2nd ed. Edited by L.B. Harman. Sudbury, MA: Jones and Bartlett.

Randolph, S.J., and L.A. Rinehart-Thompson. 2006. Drug, alcohol, sexual, and behavioral health information. Chapter 20 in *Ethical Challenges in the Management of Health Information,* 2nd ed. Edited by L.B. Harman. Sudbury, MA: Jones and Bartlett.

Rhodes, H. 2001. Practice Brief: Patient anonymity. Chicago: AHIMA.

Rinehart-Thompson, L.A. 2006. Compliance, fraud, and abuse. Chapter 4 in *Ethical Challenges in the Management of Health Information,* 2nd ed. Edited by L.B. Harman. Sudbury, MA: Jones and Bartlett.

Rinehart-Thompson, L.A., and L.B. Harman. 2006. Privacy and confidentiality. Chapter 3 in *Ethical Challenges in the Management of Health Information,* 2nd ed. Edited by L. B. Harman. Sudbury, MA: Jones and Bartlett.

Schick, I.C. 2006. Managed care: Lessons in integration. Chapter 9 in *Ethical Challenges in the Management of Health Information,* 2nd ed. Edited by L.B. Harman. Sudbury, MA: Jones and Bartlett.

Schraffenberger, L.A., and R.A. Scichilone. 2006. Clinical code selection and use. Chapter 5 in *Ethical Challenges in the Management of Health Information,* 2nd ed. Edited by L.B. Harman. Sudbury, MA: Jones and Bartlett.

Seidman, J.J. 2009. Big gamble: Will stimulus dollars pay off in health information consumers can use? *Journal of AHIMA* 80(6):34–36.

Sparrow, M.K. 2000. *License to Steal: How Fraud Bleeds America's Health Care System.* Boulder, CO: Westview Press.

Spath, P.L. 2006. Quality review. Chapter 6 in *Ethical Challenges in the Management of Health Information,* 2nd ed. Edited by L.B. Harman. Sudbury, MA: Jones and Bartlett.

Tischler, J.F. 2006. Clinical care: End of life. Chapter 10 in *Ethical Challenges in the Management of Health Information,* 2nd ed. Edited by L.B. Harman. Sudbury, MA: Jones and Bartlett.

Tomzik, K.M. 2008. What the seven signs of ethical collapse can teach us about quality in healthcare. 2008 AHIMA Convention Proceedings.

United States v. Sample, 213 F. 3d 1029 (2000).

Van den Hoven, J., and J. Weckert. 2008. Information technology and moral philosophy. New York: Cambridge University Press.

Weaver, L. 2000. Federal Trade Commission. Identity theft victim assistance workshop. http://www.ftc.gove/bcp/workshops/idtheft/comments/weaverlind.htm

World Privacy Forum. nda. What's New. http://www.worldprivacyforum.org/whatsnew.html.

World Privacy Forum. ndb. Medical Identity Theft, Mapped by city. http://www.worldprivacyforum.org/medicalidentitytheft-map.html

World Privacy Forum. 2006a. Access, amendment, and accounting of disclosures: FAQs for medical ID theft victims. http://www.worldprivacyforum.org/FAQ_medicalrecordprivacy.html

World Privacy Forum. 2006b. Medical identity theft: What to do if you are a victim (or are concerned about it). http://www.worldprivacyforum.org/medidtheft_consumertips.html

Additional Resources

American Health Information Management Association. nd. Advocacy and Public Policy. http://www.ahima.org/advocacy

American Health Information Management Association. 1998. Practice brief: Data quality management model. Chicago: AHIMA.

American Health Information Management Association. 2006. The state of HIPAA privacy and security compliance. http://www.ahima.org/emerging_issues/2006StateofHIPAACompliance.pdf

AHIMA House of Delegates. 2008. Standards of ethical coding. Chicago: AHIMA.

Dixon, P. 2006 (May 3). Medical identity theft: The information crime that can kill you. The World Privacy Forum.

Federal Trade Commission. 2003 (Sept.). Identity theft survey report. http://www.consumer.gov/idetheft/pdf/synovaterreport.pdf

Harman, L.B., and V.L. Mullen. 2007. Emerging HIM identity ethical issues. AHIMA's 79th National Convention and Exhibit Proceedings, October 2007.

Hornblum, A.M. 1999. *Acres of Skin: Human Experiments at Holmesburg Prison*. New York: Routledge.

Hornblum, A.M. 2007. *Sentenced to Science: One Black Man's Story of Imprisonment in America*. University Park, PA: Pennsylvania State University Press.

Appendix A: Ethical Standards for Clinical Documentation Improvement (CDI) Professionals

Introduction

The Ethical Standards for Clinical Documentation Improvement (CDI) Professionals are based on the American Health Information Management Association's (AHIMA's) Code of Ethics and the Standards for Ethical Coding. A Code of Ethics sets forth professional values and ethical principles and offers ethical guidelines to which professionals aspire and by which their actions can be judged. A Code of Ethics is important in helping to guide the decision-making process and can be referenced by individuals, agencies, organizations, and bodies (such as licensing and regulatory boards, insurance providers, courts of law, government agencies, and other professional groups).

The AHIMA Code of Ethics is relevant to all AHIMA members and credentialed HIM professionals and students, regardless of their professional functions, the settings in which they work, or the populations they serve. The AHIMA Ethical Standards for Clinical Documentation Improvement Professionals are intended to assist in decision-making processes and actions, outline expectations for making ethical decisions in the workplace, and demonstrate the professionals' commitment to integrity. They are relevant to all clinical documentation improvement professionals and those who manage the clinical documentation improvement (CDI) function, regardless of the healthcare setting in which they work, or whether they are AHIMA members or nonmembers.

Ethical Standards

1. Facilitate accurate, complete, and consistent clinical documentation within the health record to support coding and reporting of high-quality healthcare data.
2. Support the reporting of all healthcare data elements (e.g., diagnosis and procedure codes, and present on admission indicator) required for external reporting purposes (e.g., reimbursement and other administrative uses, population health, quality and patient safety measurement, and research) completely and accurately, in accordance with regulatory and documentation standards and requirements and applicable official coding conventions, rules, and guidelines.
3. Query provider (physician or other qualified healthcare practitioner), whether verbal or written, for clarification and additional documentation when there is conflicting, incomplete, or ambiguous information in the health record regarding a significant reportable condition or procedure or other reportable data element dependent on health record documentation (e.g., present on admission indicator).

4. Refuse to participate in or support documentation practices intended to inappropriately increase payment, qualify for insurance policy coverage, or distort data by means that do not comply with federal and state statutes, regulations and official rules and guidelines.

5. Facilitate interdisciplinary collaboration in situations supporting proper reporting practices.

6. Advance professional knowledge and practice through continuing education.

7. Refuse to participate in or conceal unethical reporting practices.

8. Protect the confidentiality of the health record at all times and refuse to access protected health information not required for job-related activities.

9. Demonstrate behavior that reflects integrity, shows a commitment to ethical and legal reporting practices, and fosters trust in professional activities.

How to Interpret the Ethical Standards

The following ethical principles are based on the core values of the American Health Information Management Association and the AHIMA Code of Ethics and apply to all clinical documentation improvement (CDI) professionals. Guidelines for each ethical principle include examples of behaviors and situations that can help to clarify the principle. They are not meant as a comprehensive list of all situations that can occur.

*1. **Facilitate accurate, complete, and consistent clinical documentation within the health record to support coding and reporting of high-quality healthcare data.***

Clinical documentation improvement professionals shall:

1.1. Facilitate documentation for the reporting of appropriate diagnoses, and procedures, as well as other types of health service related information (e.g., present on admission indicator).

1.2. Develop and comply with comprehensive internal reporting policies and procedures that are consistent with official coding rules and guidelines, reimbursement regulations and policies, and prohibit documentation practices that misrepresent the patient's medical conditions and treatment provided.

1.3. Foster an environment that supports honest and ethical reporting practices resulting in accurate and reliable data.

Clinical documentation specialists shall not:

1.4. Participate in improper preparation, alteration, or suppression of health record information.

2. *Support the reporting of all healthcare data elements (e.g., diagnosis and procedure codes, present on admission indicator) required for external reporting purposes (e.g., reimbursement and other administrative uses, population health, quality and patient safety measurement, and research) completely and accurately, in accordance with regulatory and documentation standards and requirements and applicable official coding conventions, rules, and guidelines.*

Clinical documentation improvement professionals shall:

2.1. Adhere to the official coding guidelines approved by the Cooperating Parties, the CPT rules established by the American Medical Association, and any other official coding rules and guidelines established for use with mandated standard code sets.

Example: Appropriate tools that assist clinical documentation improvement professionals with proper sequencing and reporting to stay in compliance with existing reporting requirements are available and used.

2.2. Comply with AHIMA's standards governing data reporting practices, including health record documentation and clinician query standards.

3. *Query provider (physician or other qualified healthcare practitioner) for clarification and additional documentation when there is conflicting, incomplete, or ambiguous information in the health record regarding a significant reportable condition or procedure or other reportable data element dependent on health record documentation (e.g., present on admission indicator).*

Clinical documentation specialists shall:

3.1. Participate in the development of query policies that support documentation improvement, AHIMA Practice Brief, (http://library.ahima.org/xpedio/groups/public/documents/web_assets/bok_home.hcsp), and meet regulatory, legal, and ethical standards for coding and reporting.

3.2. Query the provider for clarification when documentation in the health record impacts an externally reportable data element is illegible, incomplete, unclear, inconsistent, or imprecise.

3.3. Use queries as a communication tool to improve the quality of health record documentation, not to inappropriately increase reimbursement or misrepresent quality of care.

Example: Policies regarding the circumstances when clinicians should be queried are designed to promote complete documentation, regardless of whether reimbursement will be affected.

Clinical documentation improvement professionals **shall not**:

3.4. Query the provider when there is no clinical information in the health record prompting the need for a query.

Example: Query the provider regarding the presence of gram-negative pneumonia on every pneumonia case, regardless of whether there are any clinical indicators (including treatment) of gram-negative pneumonia documented in the record.

Query the provider for sepsis when the clinical indicators are only suggestive of urinary tract infection, such as low grade fever, increased WBCs, no blood cultures obtained, and physician documentation stated urosepsis.

4. *Refuse to participate in or support documentation practices intended to inappropriately increase payment, qualify for insurance policy coverage, or skew data by means that do not comply with federal and state statutes, regulations and official rules and guidelines.*

Clinical documentation improvement professionals shall:

4.1. Facilitate documentation that supports reporting of diagnoses and procedures such that the organization receives the optimal payment to which the facility is legally entitled, remembering that it is unethical and illegal to increase payment by means that contradict regulatory guidelines.

Clinical documentation improvement professionals shall not:

4.2. Misrepresent the patient's clinical picture through intentional incorrect documentation or omission of diagnoses or procedures, or the addition of unsupported diagnoses or procedures to inappropriately increase reimbursement, justify medical necessity, improve publicly reported data, or qualify for insurance policy coverage benefits.

5. *Facilitate interdisciplinary collaboration in situations supporting proper documentation and reporting practices.*

Clinical documentation improvement professionals shall:

5.1. Assist and educate physicians and other clinicians by advocating proper documentation practices, further specificity, and re-sequence or include diagnoses or procedures when needed to more accurately reflect the acuity, severity, and the occurrence of events.

Example: Failure to advocate for ethical practices that seek to represent the truth in events as expressed by the associated code sets when needed is considered an intentional disregard of these standards.

6. ***Advance professional knowledge and practice through continuing education.***

Clinical documentation improvement professionals shall:

6.1. Maintain and continually enhance professional competency and maintain professional certifications and licensure (e.g., through participation in educational programs, reviewing official coding publications such as the Coding Clinic for ICD-9-CM) in order to stay abreast of changes in coding guidelines, and regulatory and other requirements.

7. ***Refuse to participate in or conceal unethical reporting practices.***

Clinical documentation improvement professionals shall:

7.1. Act in a professional and ethical manner at all times.

7.2. Take adequate measures to discourage, prevent, expose, and correct the unethical conduct of colleagues.

7.3. Be knowledgeable about established policies and procedures for handling concerns about colleagues' unethical behavior. These include policies and procedures created by AHIMA, licensing and regulatory bodies, employers, supervisors, agencies, and other professional organizations.

7.4. Seek resolution if there is a belief that a colleague has acted unethically or if there is a belief of incompetence or impairment by discussing their concerns with the colleague when feasible and when such discussion is likely to be productive. Take action through appropriate formal channels, such as contacting an accreditation or regulatory body and/or the AHIMA Professional Ethics Committee.

7.5. Consult with a colleague when feasible and assist the colleague in taking remedial action appropriate to the organization and credentialing licensing body when there is direct knowledge of a professional colleague's incompetence or impairment.

Clinical documentation improvement professionals shall not:

7.6. Participate in, condone, or be associated with dishonesty, fraud and abuse, or deception. A non-exhaustive list of examples includes:

- Allowing inappropriate patterns of retrospective documentation to increase reimbursement

- Encouraging documentation that does not justify the diagnoses and/or procedures that have been provided

- Encouraging documentation for an inappropriate level of service

- Adding, deleting, and altering health record documentation

- Copying and pasting another clinician's documentation without identification of the original author and date
- Knowingly supporting documentation practices that result in reporting incorrect present on admission indicator

8. ***Protect the confidentiality of the health record at all times and refuse to access protected health information not required for job-related activities.***

Clinical documentation improvement professionals shall:

8.1. Protect all confidential information obtained in the course of professional service, including personal, health, financial, genetic, and outcome information.

8.2. Access only that information necessary to perform their duties.

9. ***Demonstrate behavior that reflects integrity, shows a commitment to ethical and legal reporting practices, and fosters trust in professional activities.***

Clinical documentation improvement professionals shall:

9.1. Act in an honest manner and bring honor to self, peers, and the profession.

9.2. Truthfully and accurately represent their credentials, professional education, and experience.

9.3. Demonstrate ethical principles and professional values in their actions to patients, employers, other members of the healthcare team, consumers, and other stakeholders served by the healthcare data they collect and report.

Resources

ACDIS Code of Ethics. http://www.hcpro.com/acdis/code_of_ethics.cfm

AHIMA Code of Ethics. http://www.ahima.org/about/ethicscode.aspx

AHIMA Standards of Ethical Coding. http://library.ahima.org/xpedio/groups/public/documents/ahima/bok1_040394.hcsp

AHIMA's position statement on Data Stewardship. http://www.ahima.org/dc/positions

AHIMA's position statement on Quality Health Data and Information. http://www.ahima.org/dc/positions

AHIMA Practice Brief: Managing an Effective Query Process. http://library.ahima.org/xpedio/groups/public/documents/ahima/bok1_040394.hcsp

ICD-9-CM Official Guidelines for Coding and Reporting. http://www.cdc.gov/nchs/datawh/ftpserv/ftpicd9/ftpicd9.htm#guidelines

chapter 13

Legal Issues in Health Information

Laurie A. Rinehart-Thompson, JD, RHIA, CHP

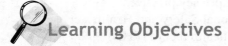

Learning Objectives

- Identify legal issues related to ownership, control, and confidentiality of health information

- Become familiar with the types of laws that govern the healthcare industry

- Understand the significance of statutes, administrative laws, and regulatory agencies with regard to the maintenance, use, and disclosure of health information

- Understand policies and procedures with regard to health information use and disclosure

- Discuss the HIPAA Privacy Rule with regard to health information use and disclosure, including requirements implemented by the American Recovery and Reinvestment Act such as breach notification

- Describe types of medical identity theft and understand actions required by the Red Flags Rule

- Identify legal issues relating to the workforce, including employees and the medical staff

Key Terms

Access report
Administrative law
Administrative simplification
Age Discrimination in Employment Act

American Recovery and Reinvestment Act (ARRA)
Americans with Disabilities Act of 1990 (ADA)

Appeal
Appellate court
Arbitration
Authenticate
Authorization
Bench trial
Breach
Breach notification
Business associate (BA)
Business associate agreement
Causation
Cause of action
Clinical privileges
Collective bargaining
Complaint
Consent
Constitutional law
Counterclaim
Court order
Courts of appeal
Covered entity
Credentialing
Cross-claim
Defendant
Deidentified information
Department of Health and Human
   Services (HHS)
Deposition
Designated record set (DRS)
Discovery
District court
Diversity jurisdiction
Duty
Equal Employment Opportunity Act
Equal Pay Act
Express contract
Fair and Accurate Credit Transactions Act
   (FACTA)
Fair Labor Standards Act
False Claims Act
Federal Trade Commission (FTC)
Health Information Technology for
   Economic and Clinical Health Act
   (HITECH)
Implied contract
Individual

Individually identifiable health information
Injury (harm)
Intentional tort
Joinder
Judicial law
Jurisdiction
Legal health record
Litigation
Malfeasance
Mediation
Medical identity theft
Medical malpractice
Minimum necessary standard
Misfeasance
National Labor Relations Act (NLRA)
Negligence
Nonfeasance
Notice of privacy practices
Occupational Safety and Health Act
Personal health record (PHR)
Personal representative
Petition for writ of certiorari
Plaintiff
Preemption
Privacy officer
Private law
Protected health information
Public law
Red Flags Rule
Rehabilitation Act
Right-to-work laws
Rules and regulations
Standard of care
Statutory law
Subject matter jurisdiction
Subpoena ad testificandum
Subpoena duces tecum
Summons
Supreme Court
Tort
Treatment, payment, and operations (TPO)
Trial court
Use, disclosures, and requests
Voir dire
Workforce members

Introduction

The health information technician (HIT) must be familiar with the legal requirements for compiling and maintaining patient health records. In addition, as a health record custodian, the HIT must be concerned with how health information is used and when it can be disclosed.

The main purpose of collecting and storing health information is to provide direct, high-quality patient care and serve the interests of the patient. The healthcare organization must ensure information in the patient health record is complete, accurate, and timely. Use of patient information is not confined exclusively to the delivery of direct patient care, however. A healthcare organization may use such information internally to assess quality of care and operations (for example, infection control), to process billing information, to support institutional research, and to compile reports for government agencies and accrediting organizations.

Moreover, the use of patient information is not limited to organizations that provide direct patient care. Insurance companies, medical claims processing bureaus, third-party payers, employers, and pharmaceutical companies all may have access to patient health information. Further, because health information provides critical evidence in the legal process, the HIT must be familiar with the use of the health record and health information in judicial or quasi-judicial proceedings. In light of the many uses and disclosures of health information, the threat of medical identity theft and appropriate protective measures must also be considered.

It is important for the HIT to be familiar with pertinent federal regulations and statutes, including the federal Privacy Rule of the Health Insurance Portability and Accountability Act (HIPAA) and the American Recovery and Reinvestment Act (ARRA), which provides changes to the original HIPAA provisions.

State laws are critical, too, because healthcare organizations that do not abide by state regulations and statutes could have their licenses suspended or revoked. In addition to federal and state laws, healthcare organizations may be subject to the standards of accrediting bodies such as the Joint Commission or the American Osteopathic Association (AOA).

This chapter discusses the legal aspects surrounding the maintenance, use, disclosure, and protection of health information. It identifies the HIT's role in these functions and emphasizes the importance of developing and following policies and procedures that guide the the handling of health information to prevent inappropriate use and improper disclosure.

Theory into Practice

The privacy of patient information first gained widespread attention with the implementation of federal regulations resulting from passage of the Health Insurance Portability and Accountability Act of 1996 (HIPAA). With passage of the American Recovery and Reinvestment Act (2009), significant revisions to the HIPAA privacy regulations were introduced. Further, to combat the rising incidence of medical identity theft and to protect patient identity, many healthcare providers have had to comply with the **Red Flags Rule** of the Fair and Accurate Credit Transaction Act (FACTA). An important part of all of these legal updates is the electronic health record challenge. How does the health information management (HIM) professional begin to track statutory and regulatory changes, and then translate them into actual practice?

First, the HIM professional needs to be very familiar with existing HIPAA privacy and security requirements, as well as other applicable state and federal statutes and regulations. Second, the individual must stay abreast of changes by making diligent use of available professional resources. Such references include AHIMA publications, electronic networking tools on the AHIMA website, the Body of Knowledge, other resources located on the AHIMA website such as the Advocacy and Public Policy section, and the actual text of statutory and regulatory changes. The US Department of Health and Human Services (HHS) also maintains a wealth of information on its website. The HIM professional must have excellent oral and written communication skills, experience dealing with the public, and a good understanding of information technology and its relationship to compliance with legal requirements. Each of these skills is necessary to effectively implement changes required by law.

Turning theory into practice requires an understanding that the rules governing the protection of patient information are dynamic and require a commitment to lifelong learning.

Overview of Legal Issues in Health Information Management

For the HIM professional, legal aspects of health records and health information present three primary concerns:

- Compilation and maintenance of health records
- Ownership and control of health records, including use and disclosure
- Use of health records and health information in judicial proceedings

Compilation and Maintenance of Health Records

Requirements for compiling and maintaining health records are usually found in state rules and regulations. They are typically developed by state administrative agencies responsible for licensing healthcare organizations and usually specify only that health records be complete and accurate. However, they may specify categories of information to be kept or outline the detailed contents of the health record.

In some circumstances, the federal government stipulates specific requirements for maintaining health records. For example, the Medicare Conditions of Participation contain specific requirements that must be satisfied by healthcare organizations that treat Medicare or Medicaid patients.

In addition to state and federal requirements, accrediting bodies have established standards for maintaining health records. Specifically, the Joint Commission's standards relate to information management through its Information Management (IM) and Record of Care (RC) chapters. Acute, long-term care, home health, and behavioral health providers, among others, must follow these standards if they are to be accredited by the Joint Commission. In addition to regulatory and accrediting bodies, professional organizations such as the American Health Information Management Association (AHIMA) publish best practice information.

Besides defining the content of health records, states usually have laws that address how long records must be kept. Some state laws designate how long health records must be retained in their original form and specify whether they can be stored on other media, such as digitally or on microfilm.

HITs are responsible for knowing and applying pertinent state and federal laws and accreditation standards that apply to their specific practice settings. Because each practice setting (acute, long-term care, home health, and behavioral health) has different requirements, HITs must update their knowledge regularly through education and reading.

HITs must also be aware of state and local laws that require information be maintained for reporting to public authorities (for example, vital statistics and public health data). Reporting, a type of disclosure, is detailed in the next section.

Complete, accurate, and timely health record documentation is extremely important. It contributes to high-quality patient care and can protect a healthcare organization in civil malpractice litigation. Because health records are frequently admitted into evidence in medical malpractice suits, the absence of complete, accurate, and timely documentation can result in a verdict against the healthcare organization.

Ownership and Control of Health Records, Including Use and Disclosure

HITs also must understand rules, regulations, and statutes affecting the use and disclosure of health information. Use and disclosure are usually associated with the concepts of ownership and control. *Use* is how health information is used internally; *disclosure* is how health information is disseminated externally. Medical records, x-rays, laboratory reports, consultation reports, and other physical documents relating to the delivery of patient care are owned by the healthcare organization. However, ownership and physical control do not mean that the patient and other legitimately interested third parties do not have an ownership interest in the content and, therefore, a legal right to access these documents (Showalter 2008).

State Laws Involving Use and Disclosure

Most states have laws that protect patient confidentiality (Brodnik et al. 2012.) Known as privileged communication statutes, they generally prohibit medical practitioners from disclosing information arising from the parties' professional relationship and relating to the patient's care and treatment (Showalter 2008). If patients waive their privilege, the medical provider is not prohibited from making disclosures.

State law may specifically provide a patient with the right to access his or her health information. Even without state law, however, the HIPAA Privacy Rule grants an individual the right to access his or her health information for as long as it is maintained, with limited situations where access may be denied. It also establishes standards by which others may access an individual's health information. The Privacy Rule is a federal regulation that covers all types of healthcare providers. It is central to the health information profession and is discussed in detail later in this chapter.

Disclosure of health information without patient authorization may be required under specific state statutes. As described in the section on record maintenance, examples include reporting vital statistics (births, deaths, and autopsies) and other public health, safety, or welfare situations. For example, healthcare providers may be required to provide information to the appropriate state agency about patients who suffer from venereal and other communicable diseases, have been injured by knives or firearms, or have wounds that suggest some type of violent criminal activity. The treatment of suspected victims of child abuse or neglect also must be reported. Because requirements vary by state, the HIT must know the reporting requirements for the state in which he or she practices. Health information has a variety of purposes, from the provision of direct patient care to use by outside entities such as insurance and pharmaceutical companies, and those uses and disclosures must be appropriate. The HIT must ensure compliance with legal requirements for appropriate use and disclosure, and adherence to the profession's ethical principles of practice.

Use of Health Records and Health Information in Judicial Proceedings

The health record of an individual who is a party to a legal proceeding is usually admissible in **litigation** or judicial proceedings provided they are material or relevant to the issue (Showalter 2008). Either a **court order** or **subpoena duces tecum** is used to obtain medical information for a court that has **jurisdiction** (legal authority to make decisions) over the pending litigation. A court order and a subpoena are not the same and must be handled differently. A court order is issued by a judge and must be complied with or the records custodian faces contempt-of-court sanctions, possibly including jail time. Conversely, a subpoena is issued on behalf of one of the parties in the case. In most instances, a subpoena for the disclosure of an individual's health information must be accompanied by an **authorization** from that individual. Although court orders and subpoenas are official documents issued through the court, the HIT must carefully review any document when it is received to determine which type it is.

Responses to court orders and subpoenas depend on state regulations. In some instances, states allow copies of health records to be certified and mailed to the clerk of the court or other designated individuals. In other instances, however, original records must be produced in person and the records custodian is required to **authenticate** the records through testimony.

Check Your Understanding 13.1

Instructions: Select the phrase that best completes the following statements.

1. HIT professionals must have knowledge of:

    A. privacy issues with regard to the management of health information
    B. laws affecting the use and disclosure of health information
    C. AHIMA's professional ethical principles of practice regarding the use and disclosure of health information
    D. all of the above

2. A medical record is owned by

    A. the patient who is the subject of the record
    B. the healthcare organization that created it
    C. the staff members who document in it
    D. all of the above parties equally own it

3. The HIPAA Privacy Rule:

    A. applies only to certain states
    B. applies only to healthcare providers operated by the federal government
    C. applies nationally to healthcare providers
    D. serves to limit access to an individual's own health information

4. A subpoena requesting patient records:

    A. is issued by a judge
    B. is also referred to as a court order
    C. has less legal weight than a court order
    D. must usually be accompanied by patient authorization

5. The principal purpose of collecting and storing health information is to:

    A. serve as evidence in litigation
    B. support statistical analysis and research
    C. provide direct patient care and serve the patient's interests
    D. provide a record for reimbursement purposes

Introduction to the US Legal System

With direct responsibility for the maintenance and use of business records (namely, health records), HITs are likely to be involved in situations involving state and federal regulations and statutes. Therefore, they need to have a basic understanding of the US legal system.

The Source and Making of Laws

Law can be classified as public or private. **Public law** involves the government and its relationship with individuals and business organizations. Its purpose is to define, regulate, and enforce rights where any part of a government agency is a party (Showalter 2008). The most familiar type of public law is criminal law, where the government is a party against an accused who has been charged with violating a criminal statute. In healthcare, Medicare is a public law. Public law includes both criminal and civil actions.

Private law is concerned with rights and duties among people and among private businesses. For example, private law applies when a contract for the purchase of a house is written between two parties. Normally, private law encompasses issues related to contracts, property, and **torts** (injuries). In the medical arena, it often applies when there is a **breach** of contract or when a tort occurs through malpractice. Private law includes civil actions.

There are four sources of public and private law: constitutions, statutes, **administrative law,** and judicial decisions.

Constitutions

Constitutional law deals with the amount and types of power and authority that governments are given.

The US Constitution defines and lays out the powers of the three branches of the federal government. The legislative branch (the House of Representatives and the Senate) creates **statutory laws** (statutes). Examples include Medicare and HIPAA. The executive branch (the president and staff, namely cabinet-level agencies) enforces the law. For example, the Centers for Medicare and Medicaid Services (CMS) is contained within the **Department of Health and Human Services** (HHS), a cabinet-level agency that reports to the president. CMS enforces the Medicare laws. The judicial branch (composed of federal and state courts) interprets laws passed by the Congress and signed by the president (federal courts) and those passed by state legislatures and signed by governors (state courts).

In addition to defining the three branches of government, the Constitution includes twenty-seven amendments. These include the Bill of Rights (the first ten amendments) and seventeen additional amendments.

Each state also has a constitution. The state constitution is the supreme law of each state but is subordinate to the US Constitution, the supreme law of the nation.

Statutes

Statutes (statutory laws) are enacted by a legislative body. Congress and state legislatures are legislative bodies. Local bodies, such as municipalities, also can enact statutes, sometimes referred to as ordinances.

Administrative Law

Administrative law falls under the umbrella of public law. As already noted, the executive branch of government is responsible for enforcing laws enacted by the legislative branch. Administrative agencies (part of the executive branch) often develop **rules and regulations** that carry out the intent of statutes. For example, Congress directed the secretary of HHS to develop rules and regulations to carry out the intent of the HIPAA statute. These rules and regulations are administrative law. The federal Food and Drug Administration (FDA), another agency within HHS, has the power to develop rules that control the manufacture of drugs. Thus, the legislative branch of the federal government has given a number of administrative agencies the power to establish regulations.

Judicial Decisions

The fourth major source of law is **judicial law,** which is law created from court (judicial) decisions. Courts interpret statutes, regulations and constitutions, and resolve individual conflicts. Judicial decisions are the primary source of private law (Showalter 2008).

The Handling of Legal Disputes

The traditional method of resolving legal disputes is through court systems. In the United States, one court system exists at the federal level. As described below, certain requirements must be met for a case to be filed in the federal court system. The 50 states, the US territories, and the District of Columbia have their own court systems as well. Although the court system is the most familiar method for resolving legal disputes, there is growing reliance on alternative dispute resolution to lighten court dockets and provide less costly alternatives for parties to settle their differences. Alternative dispute resolution methods are described below.

Court System

The US court system consists of state and federal courts. The federal court system has a three-tier structure:

- **District courts** are the lowest tier in the federal court system. They have jurisdiction to hear cases involving felonies and misdemeanors under federal statutes **(subject matter jurisdiction)** or suits where a citizen of one state sues a citizen of another state and the amount in dispute exceeds $75,000 **(diversity jurisdiction).** District courts are established geographically throughout the United States.

- **Courts of appeal** have the power to hear **appeals** on final judgments of the district courts.

- The **Supreme Court** is the highest court in the system. It hears appeals from the US courts of appeal and from the highest state courts in cases generally involving federal statutes, treaties, or the US Constitution.

Thousands of cases are submitted to the Supreme Court annually by parties who have lost at the lower court level and are requesting review. Such requests are **petitions for writ of certiorari.** The Supreme Court may deny the petition and refuse to review the case (informally referred to as *cert denied*) or grant the petition and agree to review the case (informally referred to as *cert granted*). The Supreme Court has broad discretion to decide which cases to review and which to deny.

State court systems usually use the same three-tier system as the US court system:

- **Trial courts** are at the lowest tier of state courts. In many states, trial courts are divided into two courts. Courts of limited jurisdiction hear cases that pertain to a particular subject matter (for example, landlord/tenant or juvenile) or involve crimes of lesser severity or civil matters of lower dollar amounts. Courts of general jurisdiction hear more serious criminal cases or civil cases that involve large amounts of money.

- Many states have appellate courts similar to the federal courts of appeal. **Appellate courts** hear appeals on final judgments of the state trial courts.

- The state supreme court is the highest tier. It hears appeals from the appellate courts or from trial courts when the state does not have appellate courts.

Cases presented to federal and state appellate courts are not trial reenactments. Legal documents are prepared by each party's attorney(s), who argue the merits of the case before a panel of appellate judges. Appeals are designed nearly exclusively to address legal errors or problems alleged to have occurred at the lower court.

Dispute Resolution

Disputes are resolved in the court system through trial or through settlement. However, the legal system provides for disputes to be resolved outside the court system, through **arbitration** or **mediation.**

In *arbitration,* a dispute is submitted to a third party or a panel of experts who are not judges. The process only works when the parties to the dispute agree to have their differences heard and settled by an arbitrator or arbitration panel and agree that the settlement will be binding.

In *mediation,* a dispute is also submitted to a third party. However, the outcome of mediation occurs by agreement of the parties, not by a decision of the mediator. The role of the mediator is to facilitate agreement between the disputing parties.

Arbitration and mediation offer several advantages over the court system, including time and cost savings, and additional privacy. Smaller tort claims are often handled through arbitration and criminal misdemeanors may be handled through mediation.

Legal Proceedings

HITs may prepare health records for judicial proceedings, either civil or criminal. Proceedings may involve malpractice, accidents, workers' compensation, criminal activity, or other litigation. Consequently, HITs should be familiar with various legal procedures, particularly deposition and other methods of **discovery.**

The Lawsuit

The **plaintiff** initiates a lawsuit against the **defendant** by filing a **complaint** in court. After being filed, a copy of the complaint is served on the defendant along with a **summons.** Through this process, the defendant is given notice of the lawsuit and what it pertains to, and is informed that the complaint must be answered or some other action taken. If the defendant fails to answer the complaint or take other action, the court grants the plaintiff a judgment by default.

Usually, the defendant answers the complaint in one of four ways: by denying, admitting, or pleading ignorance to the allegations or by bringing a countersuit (**counterclaim**) against the plaintiff by filing a complaint. A defendant may file a complaint against a third party (**joinder**) or against another defendant (**cross-claim**). The defendant can ask the court to dismiss the plaintiff's complaint, but not without substantial reason.

The Discovery Period

The next stage of litigation is discovery, where parties use various strategies to discover information about a case prior to trial and determine the strength of an opposing party's case. It is during this period that health records are usually subpoenaed. There are several different types of discovery methods, but most common to the HIT are the deposition and an associated discovery tool, the subpoena duces tecum.

In a **deposition,** a subpoena is issued for an individual to appear at an appointed time and place and testify under oath before a reporter who transcribes the testimony. Usually, the attorneys for both plaintiff and defendant are present. Sometimes HITs are subpoenaed to testify as to the authenticity of the health records by confirming that they were compiled in the normal course of business and have not been altered in any way. A subpoena that seeks testimony is a **subpoena ad testificandum.**

More frequently, as records custodian, HITs are served a subpoena duces tecum. *Duces tecum* means to bring documents and other records with oneself. These subpoenas may direct the HIT to bring originals or copies of health records, laboratory reports, x-rays, or other records to a deposition or to court. Each state has different rules governing the production of health records in litigation. Many component state HIM associations of AHIMA have legal handbooks that outline various situations and how HITs should respond to a subpoena.

The Trial

The next stage is the trial. A jury is selected through a process called **voir dire** or, if a jury is waived, a judge hears the case **(bench trial).** Evidence is then presented. The plaintiff's attorney is the first to call witnesses and present evidence. In turn, the defendant's attorney calls witnesses and presents evidence. Typically, the HIT is called as a witness by one party or the other to testify as to the authenticity of the health record being sought as evidence. Testifying as to a record's authenticity means the HIT is verifying that the record contains information about the individual in question, was compiled in the usual course of business, and is reliable and truthful as evidence. Because individuals who document in a health record do not typically falsify their entries, the truthfulness of a health record is generally not questioned. Parties to litigation often agree (stipulate) as to a record's authenticity and allow it to be entered into evidence without requiring the HIT to appear in court and testify. The parties may also agree to allow a photocopy of the record, or a printed version of an electronic health record, to be introduced into evidence rather than the original. This generally requires the HIT to certify in writing that the copy is an exact duplicate of the original. Note that state laws vary on the admissibility of electronic health record printouts.

Many times, a case is settled before it reaches trial. This saves time, money, and emotional hardship on the parties. A settlement may be reached between or among parties and their attorneys with or without intervention from a third party.

The Appeal and Collection of the Judgment

After the court (either a jury or the judge) has rendered a verdict, the next stage in litigation is the appeal. A case may or may not be appealed to the next court for review. The final stage of litigation is the collection of the judgment, which may be in equity (that is, the defendant is required to do or refrain from doing something) or monetary. Examples of collection of monetary judgments include single payments, garnishment of wages (by court order), seizure of property, or a lien on property.

Professional Liability and the Physician-Patient Relationship

Medical malpractice is the professional liability of healthcare providers—physicians, nurses, therapists, or others involved in the delivery of patient care. Breach of contract, **intentional tort,** and **negligence** are all **causes of action**, or theories under which lawsuits are brought that are related to professional liability. To understand how these causes of action apply, let's first examine the elements of the physician-patient relationship.

A physician-patient relationship is established by either an **implied contract** or an **express contract**. Implied contracts are created by the parties' behaviors. Express contracts are articulated, either in writing or verbally. A contract is usually created by the mutual agreement of the parties involved—in this case, the patient and the physician or other healthcare provider.

An example of an *implied contract* is where an individual with symptoms of a cold comes to the doctor's office for treatment. If the doctor examines the patient and provides treatment, an implied contract exists between the two parties. An example of an express contract is where an individual comes to the doctor's office with specific symptoms and agrees beforehand about the terms of payment for treatment. When either type of contract is established, an expectation of the scope of duty arises. Termination of the contract usually occurs when the patient either gets well or dies, the patient and the physician mutually agree to terminate, the patient dismisses the physician, or the physician withdraws from providing care for the patient.

No medical liability for breach of contract can exist without a physician-patient relationship. However, when this relationship does exist, the physician's failure to diagnose and treat the patient with reasonable skill and care may cause the patient to sue the physician for breach of contract.

Healthcare providers also can be held responsible for professional liability when they harm another person. This is a tort. A tort is a wrongful act that results in injury to another. An intentional tort is where a healthcare provider purposely commits a wrongful act that results in injury. Usually, however, professional liability actions are brought against a healthcare provider because of the tort of negligence.

Negligence occurs when a healthcare provider does not do what a prudent person would normally do in similar circumstances. There are three types of negligence: failure to act **(nonfeasance),** a wrong or improper act **(malfeasance),** or improper performance during an otherwise correct act **(misfeasance).** An example of nonfeasance is failure to order a standard diagnostic test. An example of malfeasance is removal of the wrong body part. An example of misfeasance is nicking the bladder during a surgery in which the gallbladder was appropriately removed.

For a negligence lawsuit to be successful, the plaintiff must prove four elements:

1. The existence of a **duty** to meet a **standard of care** (degree of caution expected of an ordinary and reasonable person under given circumstances)
2. Breach or deviation from that duty
3. **Causation,** which is a relationship between the defendant's conduct and the harm that was suffered
4. **Injury (harm),** which may be economic (medical expenses and loss of wages) and/or noneconomic (pain and suffering)

The causes of actions mentioned above are not the only ones that can be brought against a healthcare provider. Others include assault and battery, defamation, invasion of privacy, wrongful disclosure of confidential information, and abandonment. Invasion of privacy and wrongful disclosure of confidential information are specific issues of concern for HITs and are discussed in greater detail in this chapter.

Check Your Understanding 13.2

Instructions: Select the phrase that best completes each of the following sentences.

1. Law can be classified as:

   A. public or private
   B. public or criminal
   C. criminal or medical malpractice
   D. trial or appeal

2. The purpose of private law is to:

   A. define, regulate, and enforce rights where any government agency is a party
   B. define rights and duties among private parties
   C. create statutes
   D. convict individuals charged with crimes

3. The sources of law are:

   A. constitutions
   B. statutes and administrative law
   C. judicial decisions
   D. all of the above

4. Statutes are laws:

   A. created by an administrative body
   B. between private parties
   C. created by trial and appellate courts
   D. created by legislative bodies

5. Administrative law falls under the umbrella of:

   A. criminal law
   B. private law
   C. public law
   D. statutory law

6. Arbitration is the submission of a dispute to a:

   A. mediator
   B. third party or a panel of experts
   C. judge, without a jury
   D. judge, with a jury

7. Medical malpractice:

   A. refers to the professional liability of healthcare providers
   B. includes breach of contract
   C. includes intentional torts and negligence
   D. all of the above

8. In a deposition:

   A. a subpoena is issued
   B. an individual appears at an appointed time and place to testify under oath
   C. a reporter transcribes the testimony
   D. all of the above

9. Mrs. Elfman has filed a medical malpractice lawsuit against Dr. Quinn. She accomplishes this through a mechanism called a:

   A. counterclaim
   B. voir dire
   C. cross-claim
   D. complaint

10. A tort is:

   A. a wrongful act that results in injury to another
   B. a purposeful wrongful act against another
   C. mutual consent between two parties
   D. the professional liability of healthcare providers

Form and Content of the Health Record

The form and content of the health record are determined in a number of ways. State and federal statutes, regulations (for example, the Medicare Conditions of Participation), accreditation bodies such as the Joint Commission, and third-party payers all play a significant role in establishing requirements. Failure to comply with the requirements of any of these groups will likely result in some type of penalty such as loss of licensure or accreditation, non-payment of claims, or fines. Thus, health information must be compiled and maintained appropriately and in compliance with legal and ethical standards. Healthcare organizations establish their own requirements to ensure the uniformity of health record format and content. They do this in the form of organizational policies and procedures. Each of the influential factors listed above should be incorporated into policies and procedures, as well as professional practice standards such as those established by AHIMA. HITs must be familiar with their organizational requirements.

The primary purpose of the health record is to document the care provided to a patient. It also serves several other purposes, including (Odom-Wesley and Brown 2009):

- Ensuring the continuity of patient care among providers and along the continuum of care

- Providing a means for evaluating outcomes, quality, and peer review

- Providing documentation to substantiate reimbursement claims and medical necessity of care

- Protecting the legal interests of customers, caregivers, and healthcare organizations
- Providing clinical data for biomedical research
- Supporting professional education and training for physicians, nurses, and allied health professionals
- Supporting operational management of healthcare organizations
- Providing health-services data for public health planning and governmental policy making

Following are general guidelines for determining acute care health record form and content:

- The health record should be organized systematically to facilitate the retrieval and compilation of data.
- Only persons authorized by the hospital's policies to document in the health record should do so. Such authority should be recorded in the medical staff rules and regulations and/or the hospital's administrative policies.
- Hospital policy and/or medical staff rules and regulations should specify who may receive and transcribe a physician's verbal orders.
- Health record entries should be documented at the time the treatment they describe is rendered.
- The authors of all entries should be clearly identifiable.
- Abbreviations and symbols should be used in the health record only when approved according to hospital and medical staff bylaws, rules, and regulations. The Joint Commission's list of prohibited abbreviations must be taken into consideration when the facility's approved list is created and updated.
- All entries in the health record should be permanent.
- To correct errors or make changes in the paper health record, a single line should be drawn in ink through the incorrect entry. The word error should be printed at the top of the entry along with a legal signature or initials; the date, time, title, and reason for the change; and the discipline of the person making the change. The existing entry should be left intact and corrections should be entered in chronological order. Late entries should be labeled as such. Error correction in electronic health records (EHRs) is particularly important because courts have historically viewed their integrity as suspect. Thus, procedures must be developed to control, check, and track changes made to data housed in the electronic record.

- In the event the patient wishes to change information in his or her record, the change should not be made to the original entry but, rather, should be made as an addendum. The information should be clearly identified as an additional document appended to the original health record at the direction of the patient, who will thereafter bear responsibility for explaining the change.

- The HIM department should develop, implement, and evaluate policies and procedures related to the quantitative and qualitative analysis of health records.

- Any requirements outlined in state law, regulation, or healthcare facility licensure standard should be reviewed as they relate to documentation requirements. Where the state requires verbal orders to be authenticated within a specified time frame, accrediting and licensing agencies will survey for compliance with that requirement.

Legal Health Record

The **legal health record** is the official business record created by or for a healthcare organization (Odom-Wesley and Brown 2009). It is the record that will be disclosed upon request by third parties. It includes documentation about health services provided and can be stored on any media (for example, paper, microfilm, electronic). The legal health record is organization-specific; therefore, its content is defined by the organization rather than by law. Organizations should develop and maintain an inventory of documents and data that comprise the legal health record and consider whether other types of information that are not document-based are part of the legal health record (for example, e-mail, electronic fetal monitoring strips, diagnostic images, digital photography, and video) (Dougherty and Washington 2008).

The legal health record distinction is important because it can be differentiated from other types of records that are integral to health information such as:

- Designated record set: The designated record set, described later under the HIPAA discussion, also includes billing records, which are not ordinarily considered to be part of the legal health record.

- Electronic health records: Electronic health records contain components, such as metadata (which can reveal changes and access patterns to health information) that are not ordinarily considered to be part of the legal health record.

- **Personal health records** (PHR): Personal health records are owned and managed by the individual who is the subject of the record—they are not created by or for the healthcare organization. Therefore, they are not legal health records.

Figure 13.1.   Comparison of designated record set and legal health record

Designated Record Set versus the Legal Health Record		
This side-by-side comparison of the designated record set and the legal health record demonstrates the differences between the two sets of information, as well as their purposes.		
	Designated Record Set	**Legal Health Record**
Definition	A group of records maintained by or for a covered entity that is the medical and billing records about individuals; enrollment, payment, claims adjudication, and case or medical management record systems maintained by or for a health plan; information used in whole or in part by or for the HIPAA covered entity to make decisions about individuals.	The business record generated at or for a healthcare organization. It is the record that would be released upon receipt of a request. The legal health record is the officially declared record of healthcare services provided to an individual delivered by a provider.
Purpose	Used to clarify the access and amendment standards in the HIPAA Privacy Rule, which provide that individuals generally have the right to inspect and obtain a copy of protected health information in the designated record set.	The official business record of healthcare services delivered by the entity for regulatory and disclosure purposes.
Content	Defined in organizational policy and required by the HIPAA Privacy Rule. The content of the designated record set includes medical and billing records of covered providers; enrollment, payment, claims, and case information of a health plan; and information used in whole or in part by or for the covered entity to make decisions about individuals.	Defined in organizational policy and can include individually identifiable data in any medium collected and directly used in documenting healthcare services or health status. It excludes administrative, derived, and aggregate data.
Uses	Supports individual HIPAA right of access and amendment.	Provides a record of health status as well as documentation of care for reimbursement, quality management, research, and public health purposes; facilitates business decision-making and education of healthcare practitioners as well as the legal needs of the healthcare organization.

Source: Dougherty and Washington 2008.

Figure 13.1 provides a comparison between the designated record set and the legal health record content and purposes. Additional information about the legal health record in the context of an EHR is discussed in chapter 16.

Retention of the Health Record

Health record retention policies depend on a number of factors. They must comply with federal and state statutes and regulations. Retention requirements vary by state and possibly by organization type.

Health records should be retained for at least the period specified by the state's statute of limitations for malpractice, and other claims must be taken into consideration when determining how long to retain records as evidence (for example, under the **False Claims Act** [31 USC 3729], claims of fraud may be brought for up to 10 years after the incident).

Payer requirements must also be considered (for example, the Medicare Conditions of Participation require five-year retention for hospital records). In particular, the health information of a minor should be retained until the patient reaches the age of majority (as defined by state law) plus the period of statute of limitations, unless otherwise provided by state law. A longer retention period is prudent because the statute may not begin to run until a potential plaintiff learns of the causal relationship between an injury and the care received. HITs must know the laws of the state in which they practice and be familiar with the retention standards of groups such as The Joint Commission and the AOA.

Health record retention also depends on how the healthcare organization uses the information. For example, an acute care facility may have very different retention policies than a long-term care facility that provides geriatric nursing care. Further, an organization that provides care exclusively to children may have different retention policies than a home health agency. Healthcare organizations with significant educational and research operations may need to retain health records for longer periods than other healthcare organizations.

Governing boards and medical staffs of every healthcare organization must analyze the organization's medical and administrative needs to ensure that health records are available for peer review, quality assessment, and other activities. These needs must be considered in conjunction with legal and accreditation requirements. In many instances, healthcare organizations retain health records longer than the law requires.

AHIMA Retention Recommendations

AHIMA publishes recommendations for the retention of health records (AHIMA 2011a). HITs can use these to determine how their organizations compare with industry-wide best practices. AHIMA recommends, at a minimum, record retention schedules:

- Ensure patient health information is available to meet the needs of continued patient care, legal requirements, research, education, and other legitimate uses of the organization

- Include guidelines that specify what information is kept, the time period for which it is kept, and the storage medium on which it will be maintained (i.e., paper, microfilm, optical disk, magnetic tape)

- Include clear destruction policies and procedures that include appropriate methods of destruction for each medium on which information is maintained

Further, Table 13.1 shows AHIMA's retention recommendations for various types of health information.

Table 13.1. AHIMA retention standards

Health Information	Recommended Retention Period
Diagnostic images (such as x-ray film)	5 years
Disease index	10 years
Fetal heart monitor records	10 years after the infant reaches the age of majority
Master patient/person index	Permanently
Operative index	10 years
Patient health/medical records (adults)	10 years after the most recent encounter
Patient health/medical records (minors)	Age of majority plus statute of limitations
Physician index	10 years
Register of births	Permanently
Register of deaths	Permanently
Register of surgical procedures	Permanently

Source: AHIMA 2011b.

Check Your Understanding 13.3

Instructions: Select the one best answer to each of the following questions.

1. Which of the following determines the content of the health record?

   A. State law
   B. Federal regulations
   C. Accrediting body regulations
   D. All of the above

2. AHIMA recommends that the operative index be retained

   A. 5 years
   B. 7 years
   C. 10 years
   D. permanently

3. Erin is a health information professional. She is teaching a class to clinicians about proper documentation in the health record. Which of the following would she *not* instruct them to do?

   A. Obliterate errors.
   B. Leave existing entries intact.
   C. Label late entries as being late.
   D. Ensure the legal signature of an individual making a correction accompanies the correction.

4. The legal health record
   A. must be electronic
   B. includes the designated record set
   C. is the record disclosed upon request
   D. includes a patient's personal health record

5. Which of the following is *not* true about health information retention?
   A. Retention depends on state, federal, and accreditation requirements.
   B. Retention is the same for all types of healthcare facilities.
   C. Retention depends on the needs of the healthcare facility.
   D. Retention periods are frequently longer for health information about minors.

The HIPAA Privacy Rule

The HIPAA Privacy Rule is a key law that governs the confidentiality of **protected health information** (PHI). This chapter provides an overview of HIPAA legislation (namely, the Privacy Rule).

HIPAA Overview

The Privacy Rule is only part of HIPAA legislation passed by Congress in 1996.

As shown in table 13.2, HIPAA contains five titles. Title II is the most relevant title to the HIT. It contains provisions relating to the prevention of healthcare fraud and abuse and medical liability (medical malpractice) reform, as well as **administrative simplification.** The HIPAA Privacy Rule resides in the Administrative Simplification provision of Title II along with the HIPAA security standards, national provider identifiers, and transaction and code set standardization requirements. *Administrative simplification* is HIPAA's attempt to streamline and standardize the healthcare industry's nonuniform business practices, such as billing, including the electronic transmission of data.

Historical Context of the HIPAA Privacy Rule

Federal Legislation

Before HIPAA was enacted, no federal statutes or regulations generally protected the confidentiality of health information. Specific laws applied only in particular circumstances, such as to providers of Medicare services or to those receiving federal funds to provide substance abuse treatment.

Table 13.2. HIPAA structure

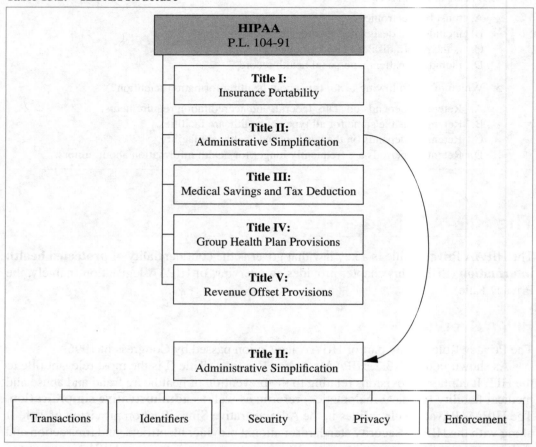

State Legislation

Patient privacy protection laws governing access, use, and disclosure had largely resided with the individual states. They varied considerably, creating a patchwork of laws across the United States. Many states had passed laws to protect highly sensitive health records such as mental health and HIV/AIDS, but no laws existed in many states to protect health information generally. With the Privacy Rule, protection was achieved uniformly across all the states through a consistent set of standards affecting providers, healthcare clearing-houses, and health plans.

The legal doctrine of **preemption** means that federal law (for example, the HIPAA Privacy Rule) may supersede state law. However, the Privacy Rule is only a federal floor, or minimum, of privacy requirements so it does not preempt, or supersede, stricter state statutes (or other federal statutes). The term *stricter* refers to state or federal statutes that provide individuals with greater privacy protections or give individuals greater rights with respect to their PHI. Thus, HITs must still review state and federal legal requirements, as well as consult with their legal counsel, to determine which law prevails.

American Recovery and Reinvestment Act of 2009

On February 17, 2009, President Obama signed the **American Recovery and Reinvestment Act** (ARRA) into law. With significant funding for health information technology and other stimulus funding, it provided important changes to the HIPAA Privacy and Security Rules. These changes are located in the **Health Information Technology for Economic and Clinical Health Act** (HITECH), which is a part of ARRA. The compliance date for ARRA provisions affecting HIPAA was set at February 17, 2010, one year after the law was signed. However, varying timelines for rule drafting and review have resulted in staggered compliance deadlines. Rules are still pending in some areas. Additional information can be obtained at http://www.hhs.gov/ocr/privacy.

Major revisions, to be addressed by section in this chapter, include provisions relating to deceased individuals' health information; business associate requirements; the minimum necessary requirement for individual rights (namely access, accounting of disclosures, and the right to request restrictions); the Notice of Privacy Practices; student immunization records; research authorizations; breach notification; personal health record vendors; marketing; fundraising, and the sale of information; and increased enforcement and penalties for noncompliance.

Office of the National Coordinator for Health Information Technology (ONC)

Previously established by an executive order, the Office of the National Coordinator for Health Information Technology (ONC) was codified by ARRA and now recognized by statute. The ONC has an expanded role in supporting the implementation of health information technology (HHS 2009). A HIT Policy Committee addresses technologies to promote EHR privacy and security, and a HIT Standards Committee consists of members with expertise in healthcare privacy and security. Provisions also include the appointment of a Chief Privacy Officer of the ONC to advise on electronic health information privacy, security, and data stewardship (AHIMA 2009).

Applicability of the Privacy Rule

This section discusses those entities (covered entities, business associates, and workforce) that are subject to the Privacy Rule and the types of information the Privacy Rule protects (PHI).

Covered Entities

The Privacy Rule applies to any **covered entity** involved, either directly or indirectly, with transmitting or performing any electronic transactions specified in the act. Transactions include those related to:

- Health claims and encounter information
- Health plan enrollment and disenrollment
- Eligibility for a health plan
- Healthcare payment and remittance advice
- Health plan premium payments
- Health claim status
- Referral certification
- Coordination of benefits

Covered entities include healthcare providers (such as hospitals, long-term care facilities, physicians, pharmacies, insurance carriers, and so forth), health plans, and healthcare clearinghouses. Thus, HITs will likely be working for organizations that are covered by the Privacy Rule.

Business Associates

The Privacy Rule also applies to entities that are business associates of HIPAA covered entities. A **business associate** (BA) is a person or organization, other than a member of a covered entity's workforce, that performs functions or activities on behalf of or for a covered entity that involve the use or disclosure of PHI. Common BAs include consultants, billing companies, transcription companies, accounting firms, and law firms. Per ARRA, the BA definition also includes patient safety organizations (PSOs), which receive and analyze patient safety issues; health information organizations (HIOs), e-prescribing gateways and persons who facilitate data transmissions; as well as personal health record (PHR) vendors that, by contract, enable covered entities to offer PHRs to their patient as part of the covered entity's EHR (HHS 2010, 40872). Per ARRA, a BA's subcontractors are BAs under HIPAA if they require access to an individual's protected health information, regardless of whether an agreement has actually been signed (HHS 2010, 40873). ARRA requires BAs and their subcontractors to comply with certain HIPAA provisions and subjects them to the same civil and criminal penalties that covered entities face for violating the law. The administrative, physical, and technical safeguards; and policies, procedures, and documentation requirements of the HIPAA security regulations apply to BAs. So too do privacy requirements such as breach notification, which is described later in this chapter (AHIMA 2009). Under HITECH, a BA's workforce includes paid and unpaid individuals working under the BA's direct control (HHS 2010, 40874).

The Privacy Rule does not allow covered entities to disclose PHI to BAs unless the two enter into a written contract (**business associate agreement**) that meets HIPAA and ARRA requirements. The BA may use or disclose PHI once it agrees to the covered entity's requirements to protect the information's security and confidentiality. Covered entities must respond to BA noncompliance, and ARRA requires BAs to respond to covered entity noncompliance. They do this by corrective action or severing the relationship with the covered entity. Per HITECH, entities that meet the definition of a BA are obligated as BAs by definition, even if they have not entered into an agreement with a covered entity as ARRA requires.

Business associate agreements must be updated to comply with ARRA. At a minimum, the agreement between the covered entity and business associate should:

- Prohibit the business associate from using or disclosing the PHI for any purpose other than that stated in the contract, and pursuant to the Privacy Rule and minimum necessary standard

- Prohibit the business associate from using or disclosing the PHI in a manner that would violate the requirements of the HIPAA Privacy Rule

- Require the business associate to maintain safeguards, as necessary, to ensure that the PHI is not used or disclosed except as provided by the contract

- Require the business associate to report to the covered entity any use or disclosure of the PHI that is not provided for in the contract

- Clarify that the business associate is responsible to report breaches of unsecured PHI

- Clarify that the business associate must adhere to policy and procedure, and documentation requirements imposed by the HIPAA Security Rule

- Establish how the covered entity would provide access to PHI to the individual whom the information is about when the business associate has made any material alterations to the information

- Require the business associate to make available its internal practices, books, and records relating to the use and disclosure of PHI received from the covered entity to HHS or its agents

- Establish how the entity would provide access to PHI to the individual whom the information is about in circumstances where the business associate holds the information and the covered entity does not

- Require the business associate to incorporate any amendments or corrections to the PHI when notified by the covered entity that the information is inaccurate or incomplete

- At termination of the contract, require the business associate to return or destroy all PHI received from the covered entity that it still maintains and prohibit the associate from retaining it

- State that individuals who are the subject of disclosed PHI are intended third-party beneficiaries of the contract

- Authorize the covered entity to terminate the contract when it determines that the business associate has repeatedly violated a term required in the contract

- State the business associate is subject to the HIPAA Security Rule, including implementation of administrative, technical, and procedural safeguards, and procedural and documentation requirements

- State that the business associate will receive satisfactory assurances from its subcontractors that the subcontractors will appropriately safeguard protected health information

- State that subcontractors of the business associate are responsible for complying with HIPAA, and are directly liable for HIPAA violations, as is the business associate, even if the business associate has not entered into a contractual agreement with the subcontractor

- Clarify that the business associate is responsible to take action, possibly including termination, against a subcontractor if it violates HIPAA or provisions of the BAA

- Clarify that the business associate is subject to civil monetary penalties for violation of the Privacy Rule or the Security Rule

(Adapted from Cassidy 2000; updated 2010 per ARRA/HITECH requirements (NPRM 40872-40874.)

Workforce Members

A covered entity is responsible under the Privacy Rule for its **workforce members.** A covered entity's workforce consists not only of employees, but also volunteers, student interns, trainees, and even employees of outsourced vendors who routinely work on-site in the covered entity's facility.

To illustrate this, examine the following scenario. Ted is employed as a custodial worker by Tidy Team, a company that contracts with Mercy Hospital to provide janitorial services. Ted has been assigned to Mercy Hospital. As part of his duties, he routinely cleans the floors and empties the trash in the HIM department. What is Tidy Team's relationship with Mercy Hospital? What is Ted's relationship with Mercy Hospital? Does a business associate relationship exist here?

In this example, Tidy Team was contracted to clean the hospital, not to use or disclose individually identifiable health information. The fact that Ted is in close proximity to such information on a regular basis does not make him (or Tidy Team) a business associate. More appropriately, because he routinely works in Mercy Hospital's HIM department, he would be treated as a workforce member and should be trained as such.

Protected Health Information

The Privacy Rule defines *protected health information (PHI)* as **individually identifiable health information** transmitted by electronic media, maintained in any electronic medium, or maintained in any other form or medium (section 160.103). This includes paper and oral forms. To be individually identifiable, the information must either identify the person or provide a reasonable basis to believe the person could be identified from the information. It must also relate to one's past, present, or future physical or mental health condition; the provision of healthcare; or payment for the provision of healthcare. To meet the definition of PHI, the information must be held or transmitted by a covered entity or a BA in any of the forms listed above. Per a 2010 proposed rule (HHS 2010), not originally part of ARRA, individually identifiable health information of deceased persons would no longer be protected by HIPAA after the individual has been deceased more than fifty years.

Deidentified Information

Not all patient information is PHI. PHI either *identifies an individual or provides a reasonable basis to believe the person could be identified from the information given.* This definition does not include **deidentified information,** which the Privacy Rule does not protect.

Deidentified information does not identify an individual because personal characteristics have been stripped from it. Deidentified information cannot be later constituted or combined to reidentify an individual. It is commonly used in research.

Information technology is powerful in assisting with the collection and analysis of data, so it is possible to identify individuals by combining specific data. Therefore, the HIPAA Privacy Rule requires the covered entity to do one of the following things to ensure deidentification:

- The covered entity can strip off certain elements to ensure that the patient's information is truly deidentified. These elements are listed in figure 13.2 (Brodnik et al 2012, 223).

- The covered entity can have an expert apply generally accepted statistical and scientific principles and methods to minimize the risk that the information might be used to identify an individual.

Other Basic Concepts

In addition to understanding the individuals and organizations that are subject to the Privacy Rule and the types of information the Privacy Rule protects, it is important to understand other basic HIPAA concepts.

Individual

The Privacy Rule defines an **individual** as the person who is the subject of the PHI (section 160.103).

Figure 13.2.   Data elements to be removed for deidentification of information

Eighteen identifiers must be removed for deidentification. They pertain to the individual, relatives, employers, and household members:

- Names

- Geographic identifiers including subdivisions smaller than a state, street addresses, city, county, precinct and zip code if the geographic unit contains fewer than 20,000 people (the initial three digits of the zip code must be changed to 000 or zip codes with the same three initial digits may be combined to form a unit of more than 20,000 people).

- All elements of dates, except the year, directly related to an individual including birth, admission, discharge, and death dates. In addition, all ages over 89 and all elements of dates (including the year) that would identify such age cannot be used. However, individuals over 89 can be aggregated into a single category of 90 and over.

- Telephone numbers

- Fax numbers

- E-mail addresses

- Social Security numbers

- Medical record numbers

- Health plan beneficiary numbers

- Account numbers

- Certificate/license numbers

- Vehicle identifiers and serial numbers, including license plates

- Device identifiers and serial numbers

- Web universal resource locators (URLs)

- Internet protocol (IP) address numbers

- Biometric identifiers, including fingerprints and voiceprints

- Full-face photographic images and any comparable images

- Any other unique identifying number, characteristic, or code except for permissible reidentification to match information back to the person (code must not be derived from or related to information about the individual, cannot be translated to her or her identity, may not be used for any other purpose, and may not disclose the reidentification mechanism)

Personal Representative

A **personal representative** is a person who has legal authority to act on another's behalf. Per the Privacy Rule, a personal representative must be treated the same as an individual regarding use and disclosure of the individual's PHI.

Designated Record Set

A **designated record set (DRS)** includes the health records, billing records, and various claims records that are used to make decisions about an individual (section 164.501).

Use, Disclosures, and Requests

The Privacy Rule affects three situations in which PHI is handled: **use, disclosures, and requests.** *Use* is internal to a covered entity or its business associate. *Disclosure* is the dissemination of PHI from a covered entity or its business associate to an outside person or organization. The Privacy Rule applies to PHI requests made by covered entities and their business associates. The Privacy Rule emphasizes use and disclosure.

Minimum Necessary

Per the **minimum necessary standard,** healthcare providers and other covered entities must limit uses, disclosures, and requests to only the amount needed to accomplish an intended purpose. For example, for payment purposes, only the minimum amount of information necessary to substantiate a claim for payment should be disclosed.

Use applies to individuals who work for an organization. For example, policies and procedures should identify those persons or classes of persons who work for the covered entity who need to access PHI to perform their duties. Also, the categories of PHI that each person or class of persons can access and use should be identified. For example, employees working in the housekeeping department would not have the same level of access to PHI as a nurse working in critical care.

Because "minimum necessary" has been somewhat unclear, ARRA seeks to further clarify its definition. Until a final determination is made, covered entities are to use the limited data set (PHI with certain specified direct identifiers removed) for using or disclosing only minimum necessary information, while reverting back to the "amount needed to accomplish the intended purpose" definition when the limited data set definition is inadequate (AHIMA 2009).

Treatment, Payment, and Operations

Treatment, payment, and operations (TPO) is an important concept because the Privacy Rule provides a number of exceptions for PHI that is being used or disclosed for TPO purposes. *Treatment* means providing, coordinating, or managing healthcare or healthcare-related services by one or more healthcare providers. For example, treatment includes caring for patients admitted to the hospital or coming for an appointment with a physician. Treatment also includes healthcare provider consultations and referrals of patient from one provider to another.

Payment includes activities by a health plan to obtain premiums, billing by healthcare providers or health plans to obtain reimbursement, claims management, claims collection, review of the medical necessity of care, and utilization review.

The Privacy Rule provides a broad list of activities that are healthcare *operations.* They include quality assessment and improvement, case management, review of healthcare professionals' qualifications, insurance contracting, legal and auditing functions, and general business management functions such as providing customer service and conducting due diligence.

Individual Rights

There are two key goals to the Privacy Rule: to provide an individual with greater rights with respect to his or her health information; and to provide greater privacy protections for one's health information (this also serves to limit access by others). HIPAA's individual rights further these goals. Those rights include right of access, right to request amendment of PHI, right to accounting of disclosures, right to request restrictions of PHI, right to request confidential communications, and right to complain of Privacy Rule violations. These rights are described below. Further, table 13.3 details all individual rights except the right to complain of Privacy Rule violations.

Right of Access

The Privacy Rule allows an individual to inspect and obtain a copy of his or her own PHI contained within a designated record set, such as a health record (section 164.524). The individual's right extends as long as the PHI is maintained. There are exceptions. For example, psychotherapy notes; information compiled in reasonable anticipation of a civil, criminal, or administrative action or proceeding; or PHI subject to the Clinical Laboratory Improvements Act (CLIA) are all exceptions. ARRA requires covered entities with EHRs to make PHI available electronically or, if the individual requests, to send PHI to a designated person or entity electronically (Nunn 2009).

Grounds for Denial of Access

Per the Privacy Rule, there are times when a covered entity can deny an individual access to PHI. These are described below and are generally categorized as "no opportunity to review" or "opportunity to review."

No Opportunity to Review

There are times when a covered entity can deny an individual access to PHI without providing him or her an opportunity to review or appeal the denial. These include:

- access to PHI in psychotherapy notes

- where covered entities that are correctional institutions or providers who have acted under the direction of a correctional institution (for example, an inmate's request to obtain a copy of his or her own PHI may be denied under certain circumstances without an appeal)

- where PHI is created or obtained by a covered healthcare provider in the course of research that includes treatment (if an individual receiving treatment as part of a research study agrees to suspend his or her right to access PHI temporarily, to protect the integrity of the research study, the covered entity may deny access to PHI as long as the research is in progress)

- when the PHI was obtained from someone other than a healthcare provider under a promise of confidentiality and the access requested would be reasonably likely to reveal the source of the information

- when the PHI is contained in records that are subject to the federal Privacy Act (5 U.S.C. 552a) if the denial of access under the Privacy Act would meet the requirements of that law

Opportunity to Review

In two instances, the Privacy Rule requires a covered entity to give an individual the right to review a denial of access. These are situations where a licensed healthcare professional determines that access to PHI as requested by the individual or his or her personal representative (1) would likely endanger the life or physical safety of the individual or another person or (2) would reasonably endanger the life or physical safety of another person mentioned in the PHI.

When a denial is made, the covered entity must write the denial in plain language and include a reason. Second, it must explain that the individual has the right to request a review of the denial. Third, it must describe how the individual can complain to the covered entity and must include the name or title and phone number of the person or office to contact. Finally, it must explain how the individual can lodge a complaint with the secretary of HHS.

The individual has the right to have the denial reviewed by a licensed healthcare professional who did not participate in the original denial and is designated by the covered entity to act as the reviewing official. The covered entity must grant or deny access in accordance with the reviewing official's decision.

Requesting Access to One's Own PHI

HIPAA gives individuals the right to request access to their PHI, but the covered entity may require that requests be in writing. An individual's request for review of PHI must be acted on no later than 30 days after the request is made (or 60 days if the PHI is not onsite). This may be extended once by a maximum of 30 additional days if the individual is given a written statement (within the 30 days) explaining the reasons for the delay and the date by which the covered entity will respond. A covered entity must arrange a convenient time and place for an individual to inspect his or her PHI; otherwise, a copy of the PHI must be mailed if requested. HIPAA allows a reasonable cost-based fee when the individual requests a copy of PHI or agrees to accept summary or explanatory information. The fee may include the cost of:

- Copying, including supplies and labor of copying

- Postage, when the individual has requested that the copy or summary or explanation be mailed

- Preparing an explanation or summary, if agreed to by the individual

Table 13.3.   Individual rights under the HIPAA Privacy Rule

Patient Rights at a Glance

Right	Request	Acceptance	Termination	Timeliness	Fee	Denial	Review
Right to request restriction of uses and disclosures	Provider must permit request, but does not have to be in writing.	Provider generally not required to agree, but if accepted, must not violate restriction except for emergency care. However, requests must be complied with (unless otherwise required by law) if disclosure would be to a health plan for payment or operations purposes and the individual has paid for the service or item completely out of pocket.	Provider may terminate if individual agrees or requests in writing, oral agreement is documented, or written notice for information created after it has informed the individual.	There is no provision for addressing timeliness.	There is no provision for a fee.	There are no requirements associated with denying restriction.	Not applicable
Right to receive confidential communications	Provider may require written request for receiving communications by alternative means or locations.	Provider must accommodate reasonable requests and may condition how payment will be handled but may not require explanation.	There is no provision for termination.	There is no provision for addressing timeliness.	There is no provision for a fee.	Not applicable	Not applicable
Right of access to information	Provider must permit request for copying and inspection and may, upon notice, require requests in writing. Provider may supply a summary or explanation of information, instead, if individual agrees in advance.	Provider may deny access without opportunity for review if information is: psychotherapy notes, compiled for legal proceeding, subject to CLIA, about inmate and could cause harm, subject of research to which denial of access has been agreed, subject to Privacy Act, or obtained from someone else in confidence. Provider may deny access with opportunity to review if licensed professional determines access may endanger life or safety, there is reference to another person and access could cause harm, or request made by personal representative who may cause harm. Covered entities with EHRs must make information available electronically or must send it electronically upon the individual's request.	Individuals have right of access for as long as information is maintained in designated record set.	Provider must act upon a request within 30 days. If information is not maintained on site, provider may extend by no more than 30 days if individual is notified of reasons for delay and given date for access.	Provider may impose reasonable, cost-based fee for copying, postage, and preparing an explanation or summary.	If access is denied, provider must provide timely written explanation in plain language, containing basis for denial, review rights if applicable, description of how to file a complaint, and source of information not maintained by provider if known. Provider must also give individual access to any part of information not covered under grounds for denial.	An individual may request a review of a denial by a different healthcare professional.

Right to amend information	Provider must permit requests to amend a designated record set and may, upon notice, require request in writing and a reason.	If amendment is accepted, provider must append or link to record set and obtain and document identification and agreement to have provider notify relevant persons with which amendment needs to be shared. Provider may deny amendment if information was not created by the provider unless individual provides reasonable basis that originator is no longer available to act on request, is not part of designated record set, would not be available for access, or is accurate and complete.	Amendment applies for as long as information is maintained in designated record set.	There is no provision for a fee.	Provider must act upon a request within 60 days of receipt. If unable to act on request within 60 days, provider may extend time by no more than 30 days provided individual is notified of reasons for delay and given date to amend.	If amendment is denied, provider must provide timely written explanation in plain language, containing basis for denial, right to submit written statement of disagreement, right to request provider include request and denial with any future disclosures of information that is subject of amendment, and description of how to file a complaint.	Provider must accept written statement of disagreement (of limited length). Provider may prepare written rebuttal and must copy individual. Provider must append or link request, denial, disagreement, and rebuttal to record and include such or accurate summary with any subsequent disclosure. If no written disagreement, provider must include request and denial, or summary, in subsequent disclosures only if individual has requested such action.
Right to accounting of disclosures	Provider must provide individual with written accounting including date of disclosure, name and address of recipient, description of information disclosed, purpose of disclosure or copy of individual's written authorization or other request for disclosure.	Provider must provide individual and retain documentation of written accounting of disclosures of PHI made in three years prior to date of request, except for disclosures (1) to carry out treatment, payment, and healthcare operations (this exception will not apply to covered entities with EHRs); (2) to the individuals themselves; (3) incident to a use or disclosure otherwise permitted or required; (4) pursuant to an authorization; (5) for the facility's director or to persons involved in the individual's care or other notification purposes; (6) for national security or intelligence purposes; (7) to correctional institutions or law enforcement as permitted; (8) as part of a limited data set; or (9) that occurred prior to the compliance date for the covered entity.	Not applicable	First accounting in any 12-month period must be provided without charge. A reasonable, cost-based fee may be charged for subsequent accountings in 12-month period if individual is notified in advance.	Provider must act upon request within 60 days of receipt. If unable to provide accounting, provider may extend time by no more than 30 days provided individual is notified of reasons for delay.	Provider must temporarily suspend right to receive an accounting of disclosures to health oversight agency or law enforcement official if agency or official provides written statement that accounting would impede their activities.	There is no provision for review of temporary suspension.

Adapted from Amatayakul 2001 and AHIMA 2009.

HIPAA does not permit retrieval fees to be charged to patients. However, they are permitted for nonpatient requests.

A covered entity must provide access to the PHI in the format requested if it is readily producible in such form or format. If not, it must be produced in a readable hard-copy form or other format agreed to by the covered entity and the individual.

Right to Request Amendment of PHI

The Privacy Rule allows an individual to request that a covered entity amend PHI or a record about the individual in a designated record set (section 164.526). The covered entity may deny the request when it determines that the PHI or the record:

- Was not created by the covered entity

- Is not part of the designated record set

- Is not available for inspection as noted in the regulation of access (for example, psychotherapy notes, inmate of a correctional institution, and so on)

- Is accurate or complete as is

A covered entity may require the amendment request to be in writing and to include a rationale if the requirement was communicated in advance (usually in the Notice of Privacy Practices, discussed later in the chapter).

An individual's amendment request must be acted on no later than 60 days after receipt by allowing it or denying it in writing. The covered entity may extend its response once, by 30 days, if it explains the reasons for the delay in a written statement and gives a date by which it will act. If an amendment is granted, the Privacy Rule requires a covered entity to:

- Identify the records in the designated record set that are affected by the amendment and append the information through a link to the amendment's location. For example, if the diagnosis were incorrect, the amendment would have to appear and/or be linked to each record/report in the designated record set.

- Inform the individual that the amendment was accepted and have him or her identify the persons with whom the amendment needs to be shared and then obtain his or her agreement to notify those persons. The covered entity must make reasonable efforts to provide the amendment within a reasonable amount of time to anyone who has received the PHI.

Denials must be made within 60 days of the request, be written in plain language and contain (section 164.526):

- The basis for the denial

- The individual's right to submit a written statement disagreeing with the denial

- The process by which the individual can submit his or her disagreement

- A statement explaining how, when the individual does not submit a disagreement, he or she may request that both the original amendment request and the covered entity's denial accompany any future disclosures of the PHI that is the subject of the amendment

- A description of how the individual may complain to the covered entity, including the name or title and telephone number of the contact person or office

The covered entity can prepare a written rebuttal to the individual's disagreement statement but must provide the individual with a copy.

All requests for amendments, denials, the individual's statement of disagreement, and the covered entity's rebuttal (if one was created) must be appended or linked to the record or PHI that is the subject of the amendment request. Future disclosures of the subject information must include this material or a summary. If a request for amendment was denied and the individual did not write a statement of disagreement, the request for amendment and denial must only accompany future disclosures if the individual requests such action. In cases where the disclosure is made using a HIPAA standard electronic transaction, the covered entity may transmit the material that pertains to the standard transaction separately.

Right to Request Accounting of Disclosures

Maintaining some type of accounting procedure for monitoring and tracking PHI disclosures has been a common practice in HIM departments. However, the Privacy Rule has a specific standard with respect to such recordkeeping. An individual has the right to receive an accounting of certain disclosures made by a covered entity (section 164.528). HIPAA originally required an accounting of all disclosures within the six years prior to the date on which the accounting was requested, but ARRA proposes to decrease it to three years (AHIMA 2009). A covered entity may either account for the disclosures of its BAs or require the BA to make its own accounting. Per ARRA, BAs must respond to accounting requests that are made directly to them (AHIMA 2009).

The types of disclosures that must be accounted for are limited but include those made erroneously (that is, breaches, which will be discussed later in the chapter); for public interest and benefit activities (discussed later in this chapter) where patient authorization is not obtained; and pursuant to a court order. Disclosures for which an accounting is *not* required (that is, exceptions) are disclosures:

- needed to carry out treatment, payment, and healthcare operations (although a proposed access report, discussed below, would essentially negate this exception for covered entities with EHRs)

- to individuals to whom the information pertains, or the individual's personal representative

- incidental to an otherwise permitted or required use or disclosure

- pursuant to an authorization

- for use in the facility's directory, to persons involved in the individual's care, or for other notification purposes

- to meet national security or intelligence requirements

- to correctional institutions or law enforcement officials

- as part of a limited data set

- that occurred before the compliance date for the covered entity (section 164.528)

Per ARRA as originally written, covered entities using or maintaining an electronic health record would be required to include (in an accounting of disclosures) any disclosures made for TPO. Compliance dates depended on when covered entities acquired an electronic health record (AHIMA 2009). A subsequent rule issued in 2011, however, proposes to exclude use, as well as TPO, from an accounting for both paper and electronic records. Instead, individuals (upon request) would be able to receive a separate **access report** from covered entities with EHRs. This report would allow an individual to see a record of every person who viewed the individual's DRS during the previous three years. TPO disclosures would therefore be displayed in the access report rather than in the accounting of disclosures, as earlier suggested. This proposal is pending (HHS 2011a).

The definition of healthcare operations is broad, but HIPAA has carved out exceptions to this definition. For example, mandatory public health reporting is not part of a covered entity's operations (this includes state requirements to report births [birth certificates]; communicable diseases; and incidents of abuse or suspected abuse of children, mentally disabled individuals, and the elderly). As a result, these disclosures must be included in an accounting of disclosures. Also, if a physician's office reports a case of tuberculosis to a public health authority, that disclosure must be included if the patient requests an accounting. If a covered entity provides PHI to a third-party public health authority to review, but the third party does not actually review it, the third-party's access must be included in an accounting of disclosures.

Disclosure pursuant to a court order (if without a patient's written authorization) is also subject to an accounting. However, disclosure pursuant to a subpoena that is accompanied by a patient's written authorization is not subject to an accounting because the authorization exempts the disclosure from the accounting requirement. The accounting requirement includes disclosures made in writing, by telephone, or orally. In some situations, an individual's right to an accounting of PHI disclosure may be suspended at the written request of a health oversight agency or law enforcement official indicating that an accounting would impede its activities and specify how long such a suspension is required. HIPAA has provided a list of exceptions to the accounting requirement, but has not included a list of which disclosures must be accounted for. ARRA proposes to explicitly list that which is to be included.

What elements must be included in the accounting? HIPAA specifies the date of disclosure, the name and address (when known) of the entity or person who received the information, and a brief statement of the purpose of the disclosure or a copy of the individual's written authorization or request be included. ARRA proposes to relax this specificity to some extent.

A covered entity must act on a request for an accounting of disclosures no later than 60 days after receipt (extended by no more than 30 days if the covered entity notifies the individual in writing of the reasons for the delay and the date by which the accounting will be made available). HITECH proposes to limit the response period to 30 days, with one 30-day extension.

The first accounting within any 12-month period must be provided without charge. Additional requests within a 12-month period may be assessed a reasonable, cost-based fee if the individual is informed in advance and given an opportunity to withdraw or modify the request or avoid or reduce the fee.

The Privacy Rule requires documentation to be maintained on all accounting requests, including information included in the accounting, the written accounting that was provided to the individual, and the titles of persons or offices responsible for receiving and processing requests for an accounting. Policies and procedures must be developed to ensure that PHI disclosed from all areas of an organization, which very likely may include departments outside HIM, can be tracked and compiled when an accounting request is received.

Right to Request Restrictions of PHI

An individual can request that a covered entity restrict the uses and disclosures of PHI to carry out treatment, payment, or healthcare operations (section 164.522(a)). ARRA requires that requested restrictions be complied with (unless otherwise required by law) if the disclosure would be made to a health plan for payment or operations purposes and the individual had paid for the healthcare service or item completely out of pocket (AHIMA 2009).

When a covered entity agrees to a restriction, whether voluntarily or as required by ARRA, it must live up to the agreement. The restriction can be terminated by either the individual or the covered entity. When the covered entity initiates termination of the agreement, it must inform the individual that it is doing so. However, the termination is only effective with respect to the PHI created or received after the individual has been informed (section 164.522(a)).

To illustrate this, examine the following scenario. A patient, Mr. Smith, agrees to allow a hospital to tell callers that he has been admitted to the hospital and therefore is in the patient directory. Such notification is a hospital operation. However, he requests that this information be restricted/withheld only from his Aunt Mary and Uncle Jack, if they should call. What would you do if you were responsible for making the decision about a restriction such as this?

In this scenario, the hospital is not required to agree to this request for a restriction. In fact, the hospital probably should not agree to this request because of the administrative difficulty of informing certain individuals, but not others, as well as the risk of accidentally violating the request. It would be difficult for every receptionist to recall this small restriction, particularly if other patients had similar restrictions on their information. The risk of violation simply becomes too great.

Right to Request Confidential Communications

Healthcare providers and health plans must give individuals the opportunity to request that communications of PHI be routed to an alternative location or by an alternative method (section 164.522(b)). Healthcare providers must honor such a request without requiring a reason if it is reasonable. Health plans must honor such a request if it is reasonable and if the requesting individual states that disclosure could pose a safety risk. However, providers and health plans may refuse to accommodate requests if the individual does not provide information as to how payment will be handled or an alternative address or method by which he or she can be contacted.

An example of a request for confidential communications would be a woman who requests that billing information from her psychiatrist, from whom she is seeking treatment because of a domestic violence situation, be sent to her work address instead of to her home.

Right to Complain of Privacy Rule Violations

A covered entity must provide a process for an individual to lodge a complaint about the entity's policies and procedures, its noncompliance with them, or its noncompliance with the Privacy Rule (section 164.530(d)). The covered entity's **notice of privacy practices,** described later in this chapter, must contain contact information at the covered entity level and inform individuals of the ability to submit complaints to HHS. All complaints must be documented along with their disposition.

HIPAA Privacy Rule Documents

The Privacy Rule contains parameters for three key documents that serve to inform patients and give them a degree of control over their PHI. Two of these documents, the notice of privacy practices and the authorization, are required. The consent document is optional.

Notice of Privacy Practices

Except for certain variations or exceptions for health plans and correctional facilities, an individual has the right to a notice explaining how his or her PHI will be used and disclosed (section 164.520). This is the notice of privacy practices. It also must explain the patient's rights and the covered entity's legal duties with respect to PHI. Healthcare providers with a direct treatment relationship with an individual must provide the notice of privacy practices by the first service delivery date (for example, first visit to a physician's office, first admission to a hospital, or first encounter at a clinic), including service delivered electronically. Notices must be available at the site where the individual is treated and must be posted in a prominent place where patients can reasonably be expected to read them. If the facility has a website with information on the covered entity's services or benefits, the notice of privacy practices must be prominently posted to it. Per ARRA, the notice of privacy practices must be updated. It must state that uses and disclosures not described in the notice will require an authorization. It must also address the ARRA marketing update and the right to opt out of fundraising communications (both of which will be explained later in this chapter). A covered entity's obligation to comply with a restriction request if the item or service is paid in full must also be included in the notice:

1. AHIMA outlines the requirements for the content of the notice of privacy practices (AHIMA 2011c). In general, the notice is to include the following: A header such as "THIS NOTICE DESCRIBES HOW INFORMATION ABOUT YOU MAY BE USED AND DISCLOSED AND HOW YOU CAN GET ACCESS TO THIS INFORMATION. PLEASE REVIEW IT CAREFULLY."

2. A description, including at least one example of the types of uses and disclosures that the covered entity is permitted to make for treatment, payment, and healthcare operations

3. A description of each of the other purposes for which the covered entity is permitted or required to use or disclose PHI without the individual's written consent or authorization

4. A statement that other uses and disclosures will be made only with the individual's written authorization and that the individual may revoke such authorization

5. When applicable, separate statements that the covered entity may contact the individual to provide appointment reminders or information about treatment alternatives and other health-related benefits and services that may be of interest to the individual; or to raise funds for the covered entity, the group health plan or health insurance issuer or health maintenance organization may disclose PHI to the sponsor of the plan

6. A statement of the individual's rights with respect to PHI and a brief description of how the individual may exercise these rights including:

   - The right to request restrictions on certain uses and disclosures as provided by 45 CFR 164.522(a), including a statement that the covered entity is not required to agree to a requested restriction and (b) those services for which the individual has paid him- or herself

   - The right to receive confidential communications of PHI as provided by 164.522(b), as applicable

   - The right to inspect and copy PHI as provided by 164.524

   - The right to amend PHI as provided in 164.526

- The right to receive an accounting of disclosures as provided in 164.528

- The right to obtain a paper copy of the notice upon request as provided in 164.520

7. A statement that the covered entity is required by law to maintain the privacy of PHI and to provide individuals with a notice of its legal duties and privacy practices with respect to PHI

8. A statement that the covered entity is required to abide by the terms of the notice currently in effect

9. A statement that the covered entity reserves the right to change the terms of its notice and to make the new notice provisions effective for all PHI that it maintains

10. A statement describing how the covered entity will provide individuals with a revised notice

11. A statement that individuals may complain to the covered entity and to the Secretary of Health and Human Services if they believe their privacy rights have been violated; a brief description of how one files a complaint with the covered entity; and a statement that the individual will not be retaliated against for filing a complaint

12. The name or title and the telephone number of a person or office to contact for further information

13. An effective date, which may not be earlier than the date on which the notice is printed or otherwise published

A sample notice of privacy practices (which may also be referred to as a notice of health information practices) is available in appendix B.

Consent to Use or Disclose PHI

Under the Privacy Rule healthcare providers are not required to obtain patient **consent,** which is the patient's agreement to use or disclose personally identifiable information for treatment, payment, and healthcare operations (section 164.506(b)). However, some providers obtain consents as a matter of policy. Except for special circumstances such as emergencies (discussed in this section), patient consent is usually obtained at the time care is provided and has no expiration date (figure 13.3). However, it can be revoked by the individual as long as the revocation is in writing. Consents should be written in plain language. The covered entity must document and retain signed consents and revocations. A sample consent is provided in figure 13.3.

Figure 13.3.   Sample consent for the use or disclosure of individually identifiable health information

Consent to the Use and Disclosure of Health Information
for Treatment, Payment, or Healthcare Operations

I understand that as part of my healthcare, this organization originates and maintains health records describing my health history, symptoms, examination and test results, diagnoses, treatment, and any plans for future care or treatment. I understand that this information serves as:

- A basis for planning my care and treatment
- A means of communication among the many health professionals who contribute to my care
- A source of information for applying my diagnosis and surgical information to my bill
- A means by which a third-party payer can verify that services billed were actually provided
- A tool for routine healthcare operations such as assessing quality and reviewing the competence of healthcare professionals

I understand and have been provided with a Notice of Information Practices that provides a more complete description of information uses and disclosures. I understand that I have the right to review the notice prior to signing this consent. I understand that the organization reserves the right to change its notice and practices and prior to implementation will mail a copy of any revised notice to the address I've provided. I understand that I have the right to object to the use of my health information for directory purposes. I understand that I have the right to request restrictions as to how my health information may be used or disclosed to carry out treatment, payment, or healthcare operations and that the organization is not required to agree to the restrictions requested. I understand that I may revoke this consent in writing, except to the extent that the organization has already taken action in reliance thereon. Therefore, I consent to the use and disclosure of my healthcare information.

☐ I request the following restrictions to the use or disclosure of my health information.

Signature of Patient or Legal Representative

_____

Witness _____

Date Notice Effective _____

Date or Version _____

☐ Accepted   ☐ Denied

Signature _____

Title _____

Date _____

Source: HHS 2000, 82818.

Authorization

The Privacy Rule generally requires that an authorization for uses and disclosures be obtained from an individual (section 164.508). However, there are a number of exceptions, which are outlined later in this chapter.

Under the Privacy Rule, an authorization must be written in plain language. A valid authorization is one that contains at least the following elements (section 164.508(c)):

- A description of the information to be used or disclosed that identifies the information in a specific and meaningful fashion

- The name or other specific identification of the person(s), or class of persons, authorized to make the requested use or disclosure

- The name or other specific identification of the person(s), or class of persons, to whom the covered entity may make the requested use or disclosure

- An expiration date or event that relates to the individual or the purpose of the use or disclosure

- A statement of the individual's right to revoke the authorization in writing and the exceptions to the right to revoke, together with a description of how the individual may revoke

- A statement that information used or disclosed pursuant to the authorization may be subject to redisclosure by the recipient and no longer protected by this rule

- Signature of the individual and date

- When the authorization is signed by a personal representative of the individual, a description of the representative's authority to act for the individual

An authorization is considered invalid (defective) when any one of the following defects exists (section 164.508(b)):

- The expiration date has passed or the expiration event is known by the covered entity to have occurred.

- The authorization has not been filled out completely.

- The authorization is known by the covered entity to have been revoked.

- The authorization lacks a required element (for example, appropriate signature).

- The authorization violates the compound authorization requirements, if applicable.

- Any material information in the authorization is known by the covered entity to be false.

Authorizations are always required for the use or disclosure of psychotherapy notes except to carry out treatment, payment, or healthcare operations for (section 164.508(a)):

- Use by the originator of the psychotherapy notes for treatment

- Use or disclosure by the covered entity in training programs for students, trainees, or practitioners in mental health

- Use or disclosure by the covered entity to defend a legal action or other proceeding brought by the individual

- Use or disclosure that is required or permitted with respect to the oversight of the originator of the psychotherapy notes

An individual may revoke an authorization at any time if it is in writing. However, revocation does not apply to prior disclosures.

The Privacy Rule requires that authorizations be obtained for uses and disclosures of PHI in research unless the covered entity obtains documentation that an Institutional Review Board (IRB) or privacy board has approved an alteration or waiver. Where authorizations are required, the Privacy Rule requires that they contain the required core elements.

The Privacy Rule also provides other specifications for authorization, including those requested by a covered entity for its own uses and disclosures and those requested for disclosures by others. This section of the Privacy Rule also generally prohibits requiring an authorization as a condition of treatment and allows authorizations to be combined only in certain situations (section 164.508). Covered entities must document and retain signed authorizations and permit individuals to review what was disclosed.

Differences among Notice of Privacy Practices, Consent, and Authorization

Table 13.4 outlines differences among these three key documents.

Uses and Disclosures of Health Information

As table 13.5 shows, PHI may not be used or disclosed by a covered entity unless the individual who is the subject of the information authorizes the use or disclosure in writing or the Privacy Rule *requires or permits* such use or disclosure without the individual's authorization. The Privacy Rule *requires* such use or disclosure in only two situations: when the individual or individual's personal representative requests access to or an accounting of disclosures of the PHI (with the exceptions detailed earlier in this chapter), and when HHS is conducting an investigation, review, or enforcement action.

Uses and Disclosures for Which Authorization Is Not Required

In addition to the two situations where use or disclosure is *required* without the individual's authorization (section A in table 13.5), there are many situations where the Privacy

Table 13.4. Differences among notice of privacy practices, consent, and authorization

	Notice of Privacy Practices	Consent	Authorization
Required?	Required by HIPAA	Optional	Required by HIPAA
Requirements regarding TPO	Must explain TPO uses and disclosures, along with other types of uses and disclosures	Only obtains patient permission to use or disclose PHI for TPO purposes	Is used to obtain for a number of types of uses and disclosures, although it not required for TPO uses and disclosures
PHI that this document addresses	Provides prospective and general information about how PHI might be used or disclosed in the future (and includes information that may not have been created yet)	Provides prospective and general information about how PHI might be used or disclosed in the future for TPO purposes (and includes information that may not have been created yet)	Obtains patient permission to use or disclose specific information that generally has already been created and for which there is a specific need
Required for treatment?	May not refuse to treat an individual because he or she declines to sign this form	May condition treatment on individual signing this form	May not refuse to treat an individual because he or she declines to sign this form
Time limit on document validity	No time limit on validity of the document	No time limit on validity of the document	Time limit on validity of document (specified by an expiration date or event)

Adapted from Brodnik et al. 2012, 228.

Rule *permits* a covered entity to use or disclose PHI without an individual's written authorization (HHS 2003). These exceptions to the patient authorization requirement are summarized in section B of table 13.5.

Permitted Uses and Disclosures without Written Patient Authorization

- Patient has opportunity to agree or object (informal agreement) in the following situations:

  — Patient directory

  — Notification of relatives and friends

- Patient does not have opportunity to agree or object in the following situations:

  — Public interest and benefit (12 situations)

  — Treatment, payment, and operations

  — To the individual

  — Incidental disclosures

  — Limited data set

Table 13.5. **Authorization requirements for use and disclosure of PHI**

I. Patient Authorization Required:
All situations except those listed in Part II

II. Patient Authorization Not Required:

    A. When use or disclosure is *required*, even without patient authorization
- When the individual/patient or individual's/patient's personal representative requests access or accounting of disclosures (with exceptions)
- Dept. of HHS investigation, review, or enforcement action

    B. When use or disclosure is *permitted*, even without patient authorization
- Patient has opportunity to informally agree or object
  - patient directory
  - notification of relatives and friends
- Patient does not have opportunity to agree or object
  - Public interest and benefit
    1. As required by law
    2. For public health activities
    3. To disclose PHI regarding victims of abuse, neglect, domestic violence
    4. For health oversight activities
    5. For judicial and administrative proceedings
    6. For law enforcement purposes (six specific situations)
    7. Regarding decedents
    8. For cadaveric organ, eye, or tissue donation
    9. For research, with limitations
    10. To prevent or lessen serious threat to health or safety
    11. For essential government functions
    12. For workmen's compensation
    13. TPO
    14. To the individual/patient
    15. Incidental disclosures
    16. Limited data set

Patient Has Opportunity to Agree or Object

The Privacy Rule lists two circumstances where PHI can be used or disclosed without the individual's authorization (although the individual must be informed in advance and given an opportunity to agree or object (section 164.510). The covered entity may inform the individual verbally and obtain his or her verbal agreement or objection.

The first circumstance is when the healthcare facility wants to keep a directory of patients for clergy or other persons who ask for the individual by name. The information may include the patient's name, location in the facility, condition described in general terms, and religious affiliation. Disclosure of an individual's religious affiliation is limited to members of the clergy.

The covered entity must inform the patient of the information to be included in the directory and people to whom information may be disclosed. The patient must be given the opportunity to restrict or prohibit some or all of the uses or disclosures.

When it is not possible to get the patient's agreement (for example, in emergencies), the organization can use and disclose PHI in the directory if the disclosure is consistent with the prior expressed preference of the patient or the organization has determined that it is in the patient's best interest. When it becomes possible after the emergency situation, the healthcare organization must inform the patient and give him or her the opportunity to object to such use and disclosure.

The second circumstance is disclosing to a family member or a close friend PHI that is directly relevant to his or her involvement with the patient's care or payment. Likewise, a covered entity may disclose PHI, including the patient's location, general condition, or death, to notify or assist in the notification of a family member, personal representative, or some other person responsible for the patient's care (section 164.510(b)).

If the patient is present and able to make healthcare decisions, the covered entity may use or disclose the PHI in the above situations only if it has done one of the following:

- Obtained the patient's agreement

- Provided the patient with the opportunity to object to the disclosure and the patient has not objected

- Reasonably inferred from the circumstances that the patient does not object to the disclosure

The covered entity also may use or disclose PHI to a public or private entity authorized by law or by its charter to assist in disaster relief efforts.

Patient Does Not Have Opportunity to Agree or Object

There are 16 circumstances where PHI can be used or disclosed without the individual's authorization and the individual does *not* have the opportunity to agree or object. The first 12 circumstances are sometimes referred to as public interest and benefit circumstances because they are of benefit to society (section 164.512). Although the Privacy Rule permits the 12 public interest and benefit uses or disclosures without an individual's authorization, if it would violate a state law that otherwise protects the patient's information, the information cannot be legally used or disclosed.

A use or disclosure may meet more than one of the 12 public interest and benefit situations. They are:

1. As required by law: Disclosures are permitted when required by laws that meet the public-interest requirements of disclosures relating to victims of abuse, neglect, or domestic violence; judicial and administrative proceedings; and law enforcement purposes (section 164.512(a)). These three areas are detailed more fully below.

2. Public health activities: This includes preventing or controlling diseases, injuries, and disabilities, and reporting disease, injury, and vital events such as births and deaths. Examples include the reporting of adverse events or product defects to comply with FDA regulations and, when authorized by law, reporting a person who may have been exposed to a communicable disease and may be at risk for

contracting or spreading it (section 164.512(b)). Per a 2010 proposed rule (HHS 2010), not originally part of ARRA, disclosure of students' immunization records would be considered a public health disclosure. This would eliminate the requirement that an authorization be obtained prior to this information being disclosed to the student's school, although an oral agreement would still be required.

3. Victims of abuse, neglect, or domestic violence: An example is the reporting to authorities authorized by law to receive information about child or other abuse or neglect. In non-child abuse situations, the Privacy Rule requires the covered entity to promptly inform the individual that such a report has been or will be made unless it believes that doing so would place the individual at risk of serious harm or not be in his or her best interest. An example might be when the covered entity would be informing the personal representative it reasonably believes is responsible for the abuse, neglect, or other injury (section 164.512(c)).

4. Healthcare oversight activities: An authorized health oversight agency may receive PHI for activities authorized by law such as audits, civil or criminal investigations, licensure, and other inspections (section 164.512(d)).

5. Judicial and administrative proceedings: Disclosures of specified PHI are permitted in response to an order of a court or an administrative tribunal. For subpoenas and discovery requests, the party seeking the PHI must assure the covered entity that it has made reasonable efforts to make the request known to the subject individual. The covered entity also must be assured that the time for the individual to raise objections to the court or administrative tribunal has elapsed and that either no objections have been filed, all objections have been resolved, or a qualified protective order has been secured (section 164.512(e)).

6. Law enforcement purposes: The Privacy Rule specifies six instances when disclosures to law enforcement do not require patient authorization or the patient has no opportunity to agree or object:

   • Pursuant to legal process or otherwise required by law: Examples of legal process include a court order, a court-ordered warrant, or a subpoena or a summons issued by a judicial officer. For otherwise required by law, for example, a law may exist that requires the reporting of certain types of wounds or other physical injuries to law enforcement.

   • In response to a law enforcement official's request for the purpose of identifying or locating a suspect, fugitive, material witness, or missing person. Only the following information may be disclosed:

     — Name and address

     — Date and place of birth

     — Social Security number

     — ABO blood type and Rh factor

     — Type of injury

— Date and time of treatment

— Date and time of death, if applicable

— Description of distinguishing physical characteristics, including height, weight, gender, race, hair and eye color, and presence or absence of facial scars or tattoos

- In response to a law enforcement official's request about an individual who is, or suspected to be, a victim of a crime (when the individual agrees to the disclosure or when the covered entity is unable to obtain the individual's agreement because of incapacity or other emergency circumstance). The law enforcement official must show such information is needed to determine whether a violation of law has occurred, that immediate law enforcement activity depends on the disclosure, and that disclosure is in the best interest of the individual as determined by the covered entity.

- About a deceased individual when the covered entity suspects that the death may have resulted from criminal conduct.

- To a law enforcement official when the covered entity believes in good faith that the information constitutes evidence of criminal conduct that occurred on the covered entity's premises.

- To a law enforcement official in response to a medical emergency when the covered entity believes that disclosure is necessary to alert law enforcement to the commission and nature of a crime, the location or victims of such crime, and the identity, description, and location of the perpetrator of such crime. Further, it is permitted when the covered entity believes the medical emergency was the result of abuse, neglect, or domestic violence. (Section 164.512(f))

7. Decedents: Disclosures to a coroner or medical examiner are permitted to identify a deceased person, determine a cause of death, or accomplish other purposes as required by law. In accordance with applicable law, disclosures to funeral directors are permitted, as necessary, to allow them to carry out their duties with respect to the decedent. This type of information also may be disclosed in reasonable anticipation of an individual's death (section 164.512(g)).

8. Cadaveric organ, eye, or tissue donation: PHI may be disclosed to organ procurement agencies or other entities to facilitate the procurement, banking, or transplantation of cadaveric organs, eyes, or tissue (section 164.512(h)).

9. Research: Authorizations for the use of PHI in research are required except where the covered entity obtains documentation that an IRB or privacy board has altered or waived (in whole or in part) authorization. Many documentation requirements must be met for either board to decide about waiving authorization (see section 164.512(i)). Table 13.6 provides a detailed analysis of the responsibilities of both the IRB and the researcher under the Privacy Rule requirements. Per a 2010 proposed rule (HHS 2010), not originally part of ARRA, a covered

entity would be permitted to combine conditioned authorizations (that is, those that condition research-related treatment upon research participation) and unconditioned authorizations (that is, those that do not condition research-related treatment upon research participation) as long as the conditioned and unconditioned components were clearly distinguished and the individual was able to opt in to the unconditioned research activities.

10. Threat to health and safety: Use or disclosure is allowed if thought necessary to prevent or lessen a serious and imminent threat to the health or safety of an individual or the public. Disclosure must be made to a person who can reasonably prevent or lessen the threat. Disclosures also are permissible when law enforcement officials must apprehend an individual who may have caused harm to the victim being treated or when the individual appears to have escaped from a correctional institution or lawful custody.

    For correctional institutions or to a law enforcement official who has lawful custody of an inmate, the Privacy Rule allows disclosures if the institution states that the information is necessary to provide continuing healthcare; to secure the health and safety of the individual or other inmates, officers, employees, transportation personnel, or law enforcement on the premises; or to ensure the administration and maintenance of the institution's safety, security, and good order (section 164.512(j))

11. Specialized government functions: These include information regarding armed forces personnel for military and veterans activities, for purposes of national security and intelligence activities, for protective services for the president of the United States and others, and for public benefits and medical suitability determinations (section 164.512(k)).

12. Workers' compensation: The Privacy Rule permits the disclosure of PHI relating to work-related illness or injury or a workplace-related medical surveillance if the disclosure complies with workers' compensation laws (section 164.512(l)).

The remaining four types of uses and disclosures that do not require patient authorization or an opportunity for the patient to agree or object are TPO; disclosure to the subject individual; incidental disclosures; and limited data set. The first two have been discussed at length in this chapter; the latter two are examined here.

- *Incidental uses or disclosures* occur as part of a permitted use or disclosure (164.502(a)(1)(iii)). For example, calling out patients' names in a physician office is an incidental disclosure because it occurs as part of office operations. It is permitted as long as the information disclosed is the minimum necessary (for example, the patient's name with no diagnostic information).

- A *limited data set* is PHI that excludes direct identifiers of the individual, the individual's relatives, employers, or household members without deidentifying it (164.514(e)(2)). Such PHI may be used or disclosed, provided it is used or disclosed only for research, public health, or healthcare operations.

Table 13.6.   Actions required for use of PHI in research

Type of Information	IRB	Researcher	Research Subject (patient or decedent)
PHI preparatory to research	None*	Representation that use is solely and necessary for research and will not be removed from covered entity	None
Deidentified health information	None*	Removal of safe-harbor data or statistical assurance of deidentification	None
Limited data set	None*	Removal of direct identifiers and data use agreement	None
Individually identifiable on health information on decedents	None*	Representation that use is solely and necessary for research on decedents and documentation of death upon request of covered entity	None
PHI of human subjects (whether research is interventional or record review)	Waive authorization requirement if determined that risk to privacy is minimal	Representation that: 1. Privacy risk is minimal based on: • plan to protect identifiers • plan to destroy identifiers unless there is a health or research reason to retain • written assurance that PHI will not be reused or redisclosed 2. Research requires use of specifically described PHI 3. Justify the waiver 4. Obtain IRB approval under normal or expedited review procedures	None
	Approve alteration of authorization (e.g., to restrict patient's access during study) if determined that risk to privacy is minimal	Same as above	Sign altered authorization form
	Approve research protocol ensuring that there is an authorization for use either combined with consent for and disclosure of PHI research or separate		Sign authorization combined with consent for research or sign standard authorization for use and disclosure of PHI for research as described in authorization

Source: Amatayakul 2003.
* There may be requirements imposed by the IRB, but there are none imposed by HIPAA.

ARRA prohibits both covered entities and BAs from selling PHI without patient authorization. In the authorization, the patient must declare whether the recipient of the PHI can exchange the PHI further for payment. Exceptions to this prohibition include public health and research data; treatment and healthcare operations; to a BA pursuant to a business associate agreement; to an individual who is receiving a copy of his or her own PHI; and for other exchanges deemed by the Secretary of HHS to be permissible (AHIMA 2009).

Check Your Understanding 13.4

Instructions: Select the best response to the following questions.

1. An accounting of disclosures must include disclosures:

   A. made for public health reporting purposes
   B. for use in the facility's patient directory
   C. to the individual about whom the information pertains
   D. none of the above

2. The Privacy Rule establishes that a patient has the right of access to inspect and obtain a copy of his or her PHI:

   A. For as long as it is maintained
   B. For six years
   C. Forever
   D. For 12 months

3. HIPAA regulations:

   A. Never preempt state statutes
   B. Always preempt state statutes
   C. Preempt less strict state statutes where they exist
   D. Preempt stricter state statutes where they exist

4. The Privacy Rule applies to:

   A. All covered entities involved with transmitting or performing any electronic transactions specified in the act
   B. Healthcare providers only
   C. Only healthcare providers that receive Medicare reimbursement
   D. Only entities funded by the federal government

5. The Privacy Rule extends to protected health information:

   A. In any form or medium, except paper and oral forms
   B. In any form or medium, including paper and oral forms
   C. That pertains to mental health treatment only
   D. That exists in electronic form only

6. Mrs. Guindon is requesting every piece of health information that exists about her from Garrett Hospital. The Garrett Hospital privacy officer must explain to her that, under HIPAA privacy regulations, she does not have the right to access her:

   A. History and physical report
   B. Operative report
   C. Discharge summary
   D. Psychotherapy notes

7. A provider may deny a patient's request to review and copy his or her health information if:

   A. The patient agreed to temporarily suspend access during a research study.
   B. The patient requests his psychotherapy notes.
   C. A licensed healthcare professional determines that access to PHI would endanger the life or physical safety of the patient or another person.
   D. All of the above

8. When an individual requests a copy of the PHI or agrees to accept summary or explanatory information, the covered entity may:

   A. Impose a reasonable cost-based fee
   B. Not charge the individual
   C. Impose any fee authorized by state statute
   D. Charge only for the cost of the paper on which the information is printed

9. Mr. Martin has asked his physician's office to review a copy of his PHI. His request must be responded to no later than _____ after the request is made.

   A. 90 days
   B. 60 days
   C. 30 days
   D. 6 weeks

10. The term *minimum necessary* means that healthcare providers and other covered entities must limit use, access, and disclosure to the minimum necessary to:

    A. Satisfy one's curiosity
    B. Accomplish the intended purpose
    C. Treat an individual
    D. Perform research

11. Notices of privacy practices must be available at the site where the individual is treated and:

    A. Must be posted next to the entrance
    B. Must be posted in a prominent place where it is reasonable to expect that patients will read them
    C. May be posted anywhere at the site
    D. Do not have to be posted at the site

12. Calling out patient names in a physician's office is:

   A. An incidental disclosure
   B. Not subject to the "minimum necessary" requirement
   C. A disclosure for payment purposes
   D. All of the above

13. A notice of privacy practices:

   A. Is to be given to patients upon their first contact with the covered entity
   B. Does not have to be given to inmates who are patients
   C. Explains an individual's rights under the HIPAA Privacy Rule
   D. All of the above

14. Janice is a well-informed patient. She knows that the Privacy Rule requires that individuals be able to:

   A. Request restrictions on certain uses and disclosures of PHI
   B. Request amendment of their PHI
   C. Receive a copy of the notice of privacy practices
   D. All of the above

15. A valid authorization must contain:

   A. A description of the information to be used or disclosed
   B. An expiration date or event
   C. A statement that the information being used or disclosed may be subject to redisclosure by the recipient
   D. All of the above

16. Consents:

   A. Are the same as authorizations
   B. Expire 60 days after they are executed
   C. Are required under the HIPAA Privacy Rule
   D. Are generally not required to permit use and disclosure of PHI for treatment, payment, or operations

17. When a covered entity has given a patient a notice of privacy practices:

   A. A consent to use or disclose information for purposes of treatment, payment, or operations is not required
   B. A consent to use or disclose information for purposes of treatment, payment, or operations is also required
   C. An authorization to use or disclose information for the purpose of treatment, payment, or operations is also required
   D. No authorizations are required for any subsequent use or disclosure of PHI

18. Disclosure in a facility's patient directory:

   A. Can occur only with the patient's written authorization
   B. Is automatic upon a patient's admission to a healthcare provider
   C. Is subject to the patient having had the opportunity to informally agree or object
   D. Can include all PHI in the patient's designated record set

19. An individual may:

   A. Revoke an authorization in writing
   B. Never revoke a valid authorization
   C. Not specify an expiration date on an authorization
   D. None of the above

20. When an individual requests that PHI be routed to an alternative location:

   A. A health plan must honor reasonable requests necessary to minimize a safety risk
   B. Both health plans and healthcare providers may deny a request if information regarding payment is not provided.
   C. Both health plans and healthcare providers may deny a request if no alternative contact information is provided.
   D. All of the above.

21. The Privacy Rule public interest and benefit purposes include:

   A. Facilitating organ donations
   B. Information about decedents
   C. Information provided to law enforcement
   D. All of the above

22. Jennifer's widowed mother is elderly and often confused. She has asked Jennifer to accompany her to physician office visits because she often forgets to tell the physicians vital information. Under the Privacy Rule, the release of her mother's PHI to Jennifer is:

   A. Never allowed
   B. Allowed when the information is directly relevant to Jennifer's involvement in her mother's care or treatment
   C. Allowed only if Jennifer's mother is declared incompetent by a court of law
   D. None of the above

23. Which of the following may be part of Hillside Hospital's workforce?

   A. Nursing employees
   B. Volunteers
   C. Employees who work on-site for a contractor of the hospital
   D. All of the above

24. Deidentified information:

   A. Does not identify an individual
   B. Is information from which personal characteristics have been stripped
   C. Cannot be later constituted or combined to reidentify an individual
   D. All of the above

25. Under the Privacy Rule, a code to reidentify deidentified information:

   A. Is never allowed
   B. Is allowed if it cannot be translated to the individual's identity
   C. May disclose the mechanism for reidentification
   D. None of the above

26. Business associate agreements are developed to cover the use of PHI by:

    A. The covered entity's employees
    B. Organizations outside the covered entity's workforce that use PHI to perform functions on behalf of the covered entity
    C. The covered entity's entire workforce
    D. The covered entity's janitorial staff

27. Release of birth and death information to public health authorities:

    A. Is prohibited without patient consent
    B. Is prohibited without patient authorization
    C. Is a public interest and benefit disclosure that does not require patient authorization
    D. Requires both patient consent and authorization

28. Patient authorization is required to release:

    A. An individual's name and address to a law enforcement official who needs it to identify or locate a suspect
    B. PHI to the patient's family physician for follow-up treatment
    C. PHI that is relevant to national security
    D. PHI to the patient's attorney

29. The Privacy Rule permits use or disclosure without written patient authorization:

    A. For specific law enforcement purposes specified by the Privacy Rule
    B. For incidental disclosures
    C. To prevent or lessen serious threats to health or safety
    D. All of the above

30. Protected health information (PHI):

    A. Relates to one's past, present, or future mental health condition
    B. Relates to one's past, present, or future physical condition
    C. Relates to payment for the provision of healthcare
    D. All of the above

31. Under the Privacy Rule, a healthcare provider who chooses to obtain a patient's consent does so in order to use or disclose PHI for:

    A. Fundraising activities
    B. Marketing activities
    C. Treatment, payment, or healthcare operations
    D. None of the above

32. An individual's request that a covered entity attach an amendment to his or her health record:

    A. Must always be honored
    B. Can always be denied
    C. Can be denied if the PHI in question was not created by the covered entity
    D. Must be acted on no later than six months after the request was made

33. The Privacy Rule states that an individual has the right to receive an accounting of certain disclosures made by a covered entity:

   A. Within the 12 months prior to the date on which the accounting is requested
   B. Since the covered entity came into existence
   C. Within the three years prior to the date on which the accounting is requested
   D. None of the above

Breach Notification

ARRA added **breach notification** requirements for entities with custody of PHI. HIPAA-covered entities and BAs are subject to HHS-issued regulations, and noncovered entities and non-BAs (including PHR vendors) are subject to **Federal Trade Commission** (FTC)–issued regulations.

Definition of Breach under ARRA

A breach is an impermissible use or disclosure that compromises the privacy or security or PHI and poses a significant risk of harm to the individual, including financial harm or harm to one's reputation. This is known as the risk of harm threshold. It excludes disclosures to unauthorized persons if they would not reasonably be able to retain the information (Subtitle D, 13400, 13402). It also excludes "unintentional acquisition, access or use by a workforce member acting under the authority of a covered entity or business associate." Finally, it excludes disclosures by a person authorized to access PHI to another authorized person at the covered entity or business associate. In the second and third exceptions, the information cannot be further used or disclosed in a way that the Privacy Rule does not allow (HHS 2011b).

Breach notification only applies to unsecured PHI, which technology has not made unusable, unreadable, or indecipherable to unauthorized persons. Covered entities should have mechanisms in place to identify incidents that meet the breach definition, determine whether any exceptions apply, and assess whether the risk of harm threshold has been met. Further, per their agreements business associates must notify covered entities of breaches. Finally, all workforce members must be educated to notify the appropriate contact person within the covered entity when they learn of a breach so appropriate notifications can be made.

Notification Requirements

Breaches by covered entities and BAs (both are governed by HHS breach notification regulations) are deemed discovered when the breach is first known or reasonably should have been known. All individuals whose information has been breached must be notified without unreasonable delay, and not more than 60 days, by first-class mail or a faster method (such as telephone) if there is the potential for imminent misuse. If 500 or more individuals are affected they must be individually notified immediately and media outlets must be used as a notification mechanism as well. The Secretary of HHS must specifically be notified of the breach (AHIMA 2009). All breaches affecting fewer than 500 people must be logged by the covered entity in an online reporting system and submitted annually as a report not later than 60 days after the end of the calendar year (AHIMA 2009).

Individuals who are notified that their PHI has been breached must be given a description of what occurred (including date of breach and date that breach was discovered); the types of unsecured PHI that were involved (such as name, Social Security number, date of birth, home address, account number); steps that the individual may take to protect himself or herself; what the entity is doing to investigate, mitigate, and prevent future occurrences; and contact information for the individual to ask questions and receive updates.

Companion breach notification regulations by the Federal Trade Commission (FTC) are applicable to noncovered entities and non-BAs that are PHR vendors, third-party service providers of PHR vendors, or other non-HIPAA covered entities or BAs that are affiliated with PHR vendors (AHIMA 2009). In addition to notifying the individuals affected by the breach, the FTC must also be notified. Third-party PHR service providers shall notify the PHR vendor or entity of the breach. Other notification requirements, such as the content and nature of breach notices, parallel HHS requirements (AHIMA 2009).

HIPAA Requirements Related to Marketing and Fundraising

The Privacy Rule defines marketing as communication about a product or service that encourages the recipient to purchase or use that product or service (section 164.501). PHI use or disclosure for marketing requires an authorization from the individual except in certain cases. Marketing activities that do not require authorization are those that:

- Occur face to face between the covered entity and the individual, or
- Concern a promotional gift of nominal value provided by the covered entity

Some activities look like marketing but do not meet the Privacy Rule's definition of marketing. As a result, no authorization is required for:

- Communications to describe health-related products and services provided by, or included in the plan of benefits of, the covered entity itself or a third party
- Communication for treatment of the individual
- Case management or care coordination for the individual, or to direct or recommend alternative treatments, therapies, healthcare providers, or care settings (Section 164.501)

Per ARRA unless a communication fits in one of the categories above, it is not a healthcare operation. Additionally, even these categories are not healthcare operations if the covered entity was paid for making the communication. There are exceptions, however. If a communication describes a currently prescribed drug; if the payment was reasonable (and the covered entity made the communication and received an authorization from the recipient); or the communication was made by a BA on behalf of a covered entity and is consistent with a business associate agreement, then the communication will be considered a healthcare operation despite payment (AHIMA 2009). If the covered entity has received—or will receive—direct or indirect payment in exchange for making a communication to an outside entity, this must be prominently stated.

In addition to the above, when the communication is directed toward a specific target audience (for example, not a broad spectrum or cross-section of patients), it must instruct individuals how to opt out of future communications.

If a covered entity uses PHI to target an individual or group based on health status or condition, it must determine that the product or service being marketed may be beneficial to the health of the type of individual being targeted before it makes the communication. Then, the communication must explain why the individual has been targeted and how the product or service relates to his or her health. Related to the concept of marketing is the sale of information. This is addressed specifically by ARRA, which prohibits a covered entity or BA from receiving direct or indirect compensation in exchange for an individual's PHI without that individual's authorization. The authorization must also state whether the receiving entity can further exchange the PHI for compensation.

For fundraising activities that benefit the covered entity, the covered entity may use or disclose to a business associate or an institutionally related foundation, without authorization, demographic information and dates of healthcare provided to an individual. However, the covered entity must inform individuals in its notice of privacy practices that PHI may be used for this purpose. It must also include in its fundraising materials instructions on how to opt out of receiving materials in the future. If a fundraising activity targets individuals based on diagnosis (for example, patients with kidney disease for a new kidney dialysis center), prior authorization is required. Per ARRA, fundraising communications that meet the definition of healthcare operations must clearly and conspicuously provide the opportunity to opt out of future communications. This opt-out is a revocation of authorization (AHIMA 2009).

HIPAA Privacy Rule Administrative Requirements

HIPAA provides several standards regarding administrative requirements that are important to the HIT, including:

- Designation of a **privacy officer** and a contact person for receiving complaints
- Requirements for privacy training
- Requirements for establishing privacy safeguards for handling complaints
- Standards for policies and procedures and changes to policies and procedures

Like most of the requirements, HIT professionals may find the scope of their responsibilities encompasses functions that relate to the Privacy Rule.

Designation of Privacy Officer and Contact Person

The Privacy Rule requires covered entities to designate an individual as a chief privacy officer. This position is ideally suited to the background, knowledge, and skills of the HIM professional because the role includes developing and implementing privacy policies and procedures; facilitating organizational privacy awareness; performing privacy risk assessments; maintaining appropriate forms; overseeing privacy training (discussed below); participating in compliance monitoring of business associates; ensuring that patient rights are protected; maintaining knowledge of applicable laws and accreditation standards; and communicating with the OCR and other entities in compliance reviews and investigations of alleged privacy violations (AHIMA 2001).

Additionally, the covered entity must designate a person or office as the responsible party for receiving initial complaints about alleged privacy violations. This individual must be able to provide further information about matters covered by the entity's notice of privacy practices.

Privacy Training

Every member of the covered entity's workforce must be trained in PHI policies and procedures to include maintaining the privacy of patient information, upholding individual rights guaranteed by the Privacy Rule, and reporting alleged breaches and other Privacy Rule violations. Each new employee must be trained within a reasonable period of time after joining the workforce. When material changes are made to policies or procedures regarding privacy, employees must receive additional training. It is also recommended that refresher training be provided to all workforce members at least annually.

Further, the covered entity must maintain documentation showing that privacy training has occurred. Although not required, a signed acknowledgement of training by each workforce member is helpful to show compliance. It is also recommended that training be conducted for new employees, but as a refresher for all workforce members at least annually.

Privacy Safeguards

A covered entity must have safeguards and mechanisms to protect the privacy of PHI. This includes appropriate administrative, technical, and physical safeguards. These safeguards should work hand in hand with those specified in the HIPAA Privacy Rule. (Chapter 17 contains additional information on HIPAA security regulations.)

Standards for Policies and Procedures

The covered entity must implement policies and procedures to ensure compliance with the Privacy Rule. This process includes an ongoing review of privacy policies and procedures and ensuring that all policy changes are consistent with changes in the privacy and security regulations. Any regulatory changes that materially affect the covered entity's notice of privacy practices must be reflected in the notice; thus the notice may have to be updated. All revisions must be noted on the policies, procedures, or notice of privacy practices. HIM professionals are ideally qualified for developing and overseeing policies and procedures.

Enforcement of Federal Privacy Legislation and Rules

Per ARRA, legal responsibility for HIPAA violations is not limited to covered entities. Employees or other individuals can be individually prosecuted. Civil and criminal penalties also apply to both business associates and covered entities.

Tiered Penalties

ARRA establishes tiered penalties, with a range of $100–$25,000/violation for unknowing violations; $1,000–$100,000/violation if due to reasonable cause; $10,000–$250,000 for willful neglect that was corrected; and $50,000–$1,500,000 for willful neglect that was uncorrected. The nature and extent of both the violation and the harm determine the amount assessed within each statutory range. A method for compensating individuals harmed by HIPAA and ARRA provisions is to be recommended.

Legal Action by State Attorneys General

ARRA also grants state attorneys general the ability to bring a civil action in federal district court on behalf of residents believed to have been negatively affected by a HIPAA violation. The OCR offered training to all state attorneys general in the spring of 2011. Topics included an introduction to the Privacy and Security Rules; investigative techniques to identify and prosecute alleged violations; a review of the relationship between HIPAA and state law; OCR's enforcement role; the roles and responsibilities of state attorneys general under both HIPAA and ARRA/HITECH; and available resources (HHS 2011c). To date there have been few actions brought under this new provision.

Audits

Enforcement is no longer solely a complaint-based system (AHIMA 2009). Unannounced audits to detect Privacy and Security Rule violations have been mandated for covered entities and BAs under ARRA, although the focus will be on covered entities. HHS awarded a contract to KPMG, an audit, tax, and advisory firm, to conduct up to 150 audits by the end of calendar year 2012. Each audit, which will consist of both a site visit and audit report, will determine whether comprehensive policies and procedures are in place and whether they have been implemented to comply with the Privacy and Security Rules. At this point, the OCR has indicated the purpose of the audits is more focused on prevention and education, but serious noncompliance issues will be referred to OCR for investigation and enforcement (Greene 2011).

Medical Identity Theft

Another challenge for the HIM professional is a sinister one: **medical identity theft.** Medical identity theft is a crime that presents significant patient care, legal, and financial challenges for the healthcare industry and for the health information profession in particular. It is a type of healthcare fraud with many types of perpetrators and victims.

Definition of Medical Identity Theft

Medical identity theft includes both financial fraud and identity theft. It involves the inappropriate or unauthorized misrepresentation of one's identity. Its victims include patients, providers, and insurers.

The World Privacy Forum has identified two primary types of medical identity theft. First is the use of a person's name and, at times, other identifiers such as Social Security number, without the knowledge or consent of the victim, to obtain medical services or goods. Second is the use of a person's identity to obtain money by falsifying claims for medical services. In a subset of the first type, a person's name or other identifier is used with that individual's consent but without the individual's full understanding of the ramifications (for example, allowing an uninsured family member to use one's insurance card so that medical services will be covered).

Medical identity theft does not include situations where patient information is inappropriately changed without the assumption or abuse of the patient's identity. Likewise, the use of a patient's financial information to purchase goods or services that are not medical in nature is not medical identity theft because of the financial, but not medical, consequences.

Medical identity theft can be internal or external. Internal medical identity theft is committed by insiders in an organization, such as clinical or administrative staff with access to patient information. Sophisticated crime rings may infiltrate an organization to commit internal medical identity theft. External medical identity theft is committed by individuals outside an organization.

The extent to which uninsured Americans are committing external medical identity theft out of a sense of need (that is, to obtain covered medical services) may be increasing. Nonetheless, the World Privacy Forum suggests that internal crimes occur more frequently than external ones (Dixon 2006). Further, there is concern that the evolution of the electronic health record may assist perpetrators by granting them broad access to patient information.

It is important to perform adequate pre-employment and ongoing background checks to minimize access to medical and financial information by those who will misuse it.

Implications of Medical Identity Theft

Medical identity theft is distinguished from other types of identity theft because of negative consequences to both the victim's financial status and medical information. A victim may face financial consequences such as debt collection, monetary losses, damaged credit, and insurance denials (possibly due to lifetime caps being reached). A victim could also receive improper medical treatment if incorrect medical information (that of the perpetrator) has been inserted in the victim's health record. For example, if the medical identity theft victim is given a blood transfusion based on the different, and incompatible, blood type of a perpetrator whose medical information has wrongfully been entered into the victim's health record, the result could be life-threatening.

Many states have data breach notification laws, but very few address medical information. Also, although financial industry regulations protect consumers against lost or stolen credit cards, no corollary exists for medical identity theft victims. HIPAA, when applied to medical identity theft, has also been inadequate. First, the right to request an accounting of disclosures has not been used extensively. Second, medical identity theft may involve the insertion of the perpetrator's medical information into the victim's health record rather than a disclosure, rendering an accounting irrelevant. Under ARRA, covered entities with electronic health records must include payment disclosures in an accounting of disclosures, which will detect disclosures to payers for services the victim did not receive. However, the victim must request an accounting and study the disclosures to find these.

As consumers seek more control over their healthcare and look for convenient storage and portability of their health information, many are creating vendor-sponsored web-based personal health records (PHRs). Although many of these PHRs have not been subject to HIPAA regulations in the past, ARRA's breach notification requirements apply to PHR vendors and third-party service providers (AHIMA 2009).

Fair and Accurate Credit Transactions Act (FACTA)

Under the federal **Fair and Accurate Credit Transactions Act** (FACTA), financial institutions and creditors must develop and implement written identity theft programs that identify, detect, and respond to red flags that may signal the presence of identity theft. Although this law does not specifically address medical identity theft, many healthcare organizations meet the definition of creditor, which is anyone who meets one of the three following criteria:

- Obtains or uses consumer reports in connection with a credit transaction
- Furnishes information to consumer reporting agencies in connection with a credit transaction
- Advances funds to—or on behalf of—someone, except for funds for expenses incidental to a service provided by the creditor to that person

The law consists of five categories of red flags (16 CFR Part 681), which include:

- Alerts, notifications, or warnings from a consumer reporting agency
- Suspicious documents
- Suspicious personally identifying information such as a suspicious address

- Unusual use of, or suspicious activity relating to, a covered account

- Notices from customers, victims of identity theft, law enforcement authorities, or other businesses about possible identity theft in connection with an account

Meeting the Red Flags Rule

In addition to mandated red flags, healthcare providers must act to prevent, detect, and mitigate activities that address both external and internal incidents. Employee awareness and training, and implementation of organization-wide policies and procedures, are important.

Certain types of external medical identity theft can be detected when a perpetrator presents for service or seeks to obtain benefits such as medical equipment. Providers often require a driver's license to verify a patient's identity and registration personnel may take photographs of patients for inclusion in their health records for future reference. More sophisticated, and costly, options include biometric identifiers such as fingerprint, handprint, or retinal scans. Patient signatures from previous encounters may also be compared with the signature of the patient presenting for the current episode of care. All of these measures, however, are dependent on valid baseline information. If the information relied upon by the provider is the perpetrator's signature, photograph, or biometric identifier, all future encounters will be based on fraudulent information, decreasing the chances of detecting the fraud. This may also wrongfully identify the true patient as the perpetrator when and if he comes to that provider for treatment.

Measures that verify patient identity are ineffective for internal medical identity theft. Ongoing review and revision of policies related to system security and access are important. The AHIMA e-HIM Work Group on Medical Identity Theft (2008) has identified best practices to minimize internal medical identity theft. These include performing background checks for employees and business associates; minimizing the temporary hiring of individuals who are not licensed, credentialed, or bound by professional codes of ethics; minimizing the use of Social Security numbers as patient identifiers; and avoiding Social Security numbers on any data collection field. Other practices applicable to the protection of electronic patient data include strict application of access levels based on role or other need factors, and automatic log-out procedures and screen savers. The AHIMA Work Group also recommends that the three areas of the HIPAA Security Rule, administrative, technical, and physical safeguards, be included in a risk analysis, which identifies system vulnerabilities to medical identity theft. Other areas that it recommends in a risk analysis include:

- Limit access to the minimum necessary

- Require user identification and passwords

- Implement encryption devices for transmitted data

- Install protective hardware and software devices, including firewalls

- Eliminate open network jacks in unsecured areas

- Routinely audit access to patient information through audit trails

When medical identity theft occurs, a response plan is necessary. In addition to breach notification requirements, mitigation (including the separation of the intermingled health information of the victim and the perpetrator) is necessary to lessen the intensity or minimize the damage. As medical identity theft continues to challenge the healthcare industry and is centered in the health record itself, the health information professional will often be involved in developing solutions through effective prevention, detection, and mitigation protocols (Rinehart-Thompson and Harman 2009).

Medical Staff Appointments and Privileges

Another area with significant legal implications that the HIT may become involved in is medical staff appointments, also referred to as **credentialing.** A basic understanding of the legal issues and some of the functions in the credentialing process is important.

As a legal entity, the healthcare facility is ultimately responsible for the quality of care it provides. This includes the quality of the medical staff, which is the aggregate of physicians who have been given permission to provide a healthcare facility's clinical services. A healthcare facility's governing board is accountable to establish policies and procedures that ensure reasonable care in the appointment of medical practitioners to the facility's medical staff and the granting of clinical privileges. **Clinical privileges** are the defined set of services a physician is permitted to perform in that facility such as admitting patients, performing surgeries, or delivering infants.

Credentialing includes both the initial appointment and reappointment of individuals to the medical staff and determination of the extent of their privileges. The customary process by which an application for medical staff appointment and privileges is reviewed involves several levels. These include the appropriate clinical departments, the credentials committee, the medical staff executive committee, and the board of directors. Although the board of directors relies on the advice and recommendations of the medical staff, ultimate responsibility for making appointments and reappointments and for ensuring the medical staff members are qualified to perform the functions for which they have been granted privileges rests with the board (Pozgar 2007).

As described in chapter 7, an important part of the credentialing process is the National Practitioner Data Bank (NPDB) established by the federal Health Care Quality Improvement Act of 1986. One goal of the NPDB is to limit the movement of physicians throughout the United States where their negative histories such as medical malpractice lawsuits and loss of privileges at other healthcare facilities may go undetected. NPDB regulations include requirements for reporting information to the NPDB and querying information from the NPDB prior to granting medical staff privileges (Pozgar 2007). Penalties and liability can result from failure to use the NPDB.

The HIT may serve as the medical staff coordinator, involving the collection, organization, verification, and storage of all information associated with credentialing. This includes information about the individual staff member's professional background, credentials, previous professional experience, and quality profiles. All this information, including that obtained from the NPDB, is confidential. Therefore, policies and procedures must be in place to specify who may have access to what information and under what circumstances.

Labor Laws and Unionized Personnel

In addition to the appointment of individuals to a health organization's medical staff, the HIT may be responsible for supervising his or her own staff. There are additional requirements when an organization's employees belong to unions or professional associations that represent their members through the **collective bargaining** process.

The most pervasive federal labor law is the **National Labor Relations Act** (NLRA) and its amendments. The act provides procedures for union representation and prohibits unfair labor practices by unions such as coercing nonstriking employees, and by employers, such as interfering with the union selection process and discriminating against employees who support a union. However, employers may restrict union activity to prevent disruption of the organization's operations. Further, the NLRA allows employers to prohibit supervisors, as stewards of the employer, to be involved in union activity. Supervisors are thus differentiated from the NLRA definition of employee (Pozgar 2007).

Other federal labor laws that are significant to the HIT who supervises employees who are union members include (Pozgar 2007):

- The **Americans with Disabilities Act** (1990), which is described fully in the following section. The **Fair Labor Standards Act** (1938) defines the minimum wage and maximum hours of employment.

- The **Equal Pay Act** (1963) prohibits discrimination in payment of wages based on gender.

- The **Equal Employment Opportunity Act** (1972) is the amendment to the Civil Rights Act of 1964 (Title VII) that prohibits discrimination on the basis of age, race, color, religion, sex, or national origin.

- The **Age Discrimination in Employment Act** (1967) prohibits employment discrimination against workers at least 40 years of age.

- The **Occupational Safety and Health Act** (1970) develops and enforces safe and healthy workplace environments.

- The **Rehabilitation Act** (1973) protects handicapped employees against discrimination.

Managers also need to be familiar with state labor laws. Because the NLRA does not apply to public organizations at the state or local level, individual state labor relations laws may fill that void. Other labor laws that are handled by individual states include workers' compensation, child labor laws, and minimum wage laws where states have established a rate higher than the federal rate. States may also prohibit labor contracts that require union membership for employment. Such laws are called **right-to-work laws** (Pozgar 2007).

Americans with Disabilities Act

The **Americans with Disabilities Act of 1990** (ADA) applies to both private and public employers by prohibiting discrimination against qualified individuals who have disabilities with respect to hiring, promotion, and other employment actions. When reviewing the job application of an individual with a disability, the employer must focus on the individual's ability to perform the required job duties rather than on his or her disability. For example, it is an ADA violation to ask whether an individual has a disability. However, it is appropriate to determine whether that person is able to perform the functions required by a particular job (Pozgar 2007).

An employer must, if possible, make reasonable accommodations or alterations that allow an individual with a disability to perform the necessary job functions. An example of a reasonable accommodation may be a larger computer monitor for a visually impaired employee. Accommodations may not be reasonable if an employer is able to show that they are cost prohibitive or negatively affect the completion of one's job duties. If an accommodation is not possible or reasonable, an employer has a valid defense against a claim that the ADA was violated. However, what is considered reasonable differs from one court to another.

Check Your Understanding 13.5

Instructions: Select the answer that best completes the following statements.

1. The use or disclosure of PHI for marketing:

   A. Always requires written authorization from the patient
   B. Does not require written authorization for face-to-face communications with the individual
   C. Requires written authorization from the patient when products or services of nominal value are introduced
   D. None of the above

2. With regard to training in PHI policies and procedures:

   A. Every member of the covered entity's workforce must be trained.
   B. Only individuals employed by the covered entity must be trained.
   C. Training only needs to occur when there are material changes to the policies and procedures.
   D. Documentation of training is not required.

3. The privacy officer is responsible for:

   A. Handling complaints about the covered entity's violations of the Privacy Rule
   B. Developing and implementing privacy policies and procedures
   C. Providing information about the covered entity's privacy practices
   D. All of the above

4. Credentialing applies to:

   A. Medical staff appointments
   B. Medical staff reappointments
   C. The granting of specific clinical privileges
   D. All of the above

5. Per the HITECH breach notification requirements, what is the threshold for the immediate notification of each individual?

   A. 1000 individuals affected
   B. 500 individuals affected
   C. 250 individuals affected
   D. Any number of individuals affected requires individual notification

6. The maximum penalty per violation for HIPAA violations due to willful neglect with correction is

   A. $1000
   B. $250,000
   C. $1,500,000
   D. there is no maximum penalty

7. Medical identity theft includes all of the following *except* use of another person's

   A. name to obtain durable medical equipment
   B. insurance policy number to undergo reconstructive surgery
   C. financial information to purchase expensive handbags
   D. identity to falsify claims for medical services

8. Per the Fair and Accurate Credit Transactions Act (FACTA), which of the following is a red flag category?

   A. suspicious documents
   B. warnings from a consumer reporting agency
   C. unusual activity relating to a covered account
   D. all of the above are red flag categories

9. Medical staff credentialing refers to

   A. awarding physicians who have treated the most patients
   B. appointing and granting clinical privileges to physicians
   C. renewing physicians' medical licenses
   D. establishing physicians' medical malpractice premiums

10. Per the Americans with Disabilities Act (ADA), a person with a documented disability

   A. may not be denied a job
   B. may not be denied a job if a reasonable accommodation is possible
   C. receives no special legal protections
   D. none of the above

Real-World Case

LaVonne Wieland, health information privacy director at HealthEast Care System in St. Paul, MN, has spent considerable time addressing the significant privacy provisions of the American Recovery and Reinvestment Act (ARRA), which makes changes to HIPAA (Wieland 2009). Her systematic approach includes reading the applicable provisions, determining how each is going to affect the organization, and identifying steps for preparation.

HealthEast Care System includes three acute care hospitals, a long-term acute care hospital, multiple physician clinics, medical transportation, home care, and other services. It has more than 7,000 employees. Its HIPAA compliance task force has seen increased activity with the ARRA privacy provisions. The approach to ARRA has been twofold: identifying the big topics and determining the timelines for action.

Three changes were effective immediately and could only be responded to by making sure that staff was aware of:

- Enhanced enforcements via tiered penalties

- The ability of state attorneys general to bring civil lawsuits on behalf of residents in their respective states

- Periodic audits by the Department of Health and Human Services (HHS) to assess privacy and security compliance

Thereafter, the top priority became addressing the security breach notification changes. With the rules not finalized, the organization still had to act, including:

- Determining which actions fit the ARRA definition of a security breach

- Training staff on what is or is not a security breach

- Establishing a process for staff to report breaches so they could be tracked and reported to the federal government and to the individuals whose information was breached

Examples of clear security breaches included misdirected external faxes, misdirected copies of health records, and unauthorized and inappropriate employee access of a patient health record. Other situations, such as the ARRA exception of inadvertent disclosures to unauthorized persons who would not reasonably be able to retain the disclosed information, were more difficult to ascertain. It is difficult to determine whether an individual retained information or unwittingly passed it along to someone else. In light of these murky situations, HealthEast nonetheless continued to categorize potential privacy or security breaches by type. These included inappropriate disclosure, inappropriate access, or theft.

Also, notification of individuals following a breach of their information had to be implemented. Processes were put in place to make sure that individuals would be notified within 60 days after discovery of the breach. The privacy office was involved to determine annual reporting and immediate reporting to HHS or the local media. The privacy office was also responsible for initiating patient notification letters.

Wieland lists other topics that need to be handled to ensure ARRA compliance, but will need to be addressed as guidelines are issued. These topics are:

- Business associate agreements
- Request for restrictions
- Disclosures limited to the limited data set or minimum necessary
- Accounting of disclosures
- Access to PHI electronically

Summary

The health information technician is on the front line as a champion for health information privacy. Requirements for the maintenance of medical records and health information are only one important matter with which HITs must be concerned. How health information is used and under what circumstances it can be disclosed are equally important. The HIPAA Privacy Rule and changes provided by ARRA underscore the importance of health information privacy and have increased the responsibilities of HIM professionals. So, too, have ongoing challenges such as medical identity theft.

Thus, HITs must thoroughly understand the legal issues involved in maintaining, using, disclosing, and protecting health information. Knowing the contents of this chapter is only the beginning. Because practices and regulations are constantly evolving, the HIT must engage in constant learning. Keeping up-to-date in practice in this essential and important area is among the HIT's key responsibilities.

References

5 USC 552a: Privacy Act (1974).

31 USC 3729: False Claims Act (1986).

AHIMA e-HIM Work Group on Medical Identity Theft. 2008. Mitigating medical identity theft. *Journal of AHIMA* 79(7):63–69.

American Health Information Management Association. 2001. Sample (chief) privacy officer job description. *Journal of AHIMA* 72(6):39.

American Health Information Management Association. 2009. Analysis of health care confidentiality, privacy, and security provisions of the American Recovery and Reinvestment Act of 2009, Public Law 111-5. http://library.ahima.org/xpedio/groups/public/documents/ahima/bok1_044016.pdf

American Health Information Management Association. 2011a. Retention and Destruction of Health Information (updated August 2011). http://www.ahima.org

American Health Information Management Association. 2011b. Retention and Destruction of Health Information. Appendix D: AHIMA's Recommended Retention Standards (updated August 2011). http://www.ahima.org

American Health Information Management Association. 2011c. Notice of Privacy Practices (updated February 2011). http://www.ahima.org

Amatayakul, M. 2001. HIPAA on the job: Managing individual rights requirements under HIPAA privacy. *Journal of AHIMA* 72(6):16A–16D.

Amatayakul, M. 2003. HIPAA on the job: Another layer of regulations: Research under HIPAA. *Journal of AHIMA* 74(1):16A–16D.

Brodnik, M., L. Rinehart-Thompson, and R. Reynolds. 2012. *Fundamentals of Law for Health Informatics and Information Management*. Chicago: AHIMA.

Cassidy, B. 2000. HIPAA on the job: Update on business partner/associate agreements. *Journal of AHIMA* 71(10):16A–16D.

Department of Health and Human Services. 2000. *Federal Register* 65(250):82818.

Department of Health and Human Services. 2003. OCR privacy brief: Summary of the HIPAA Privacy Rule. 2003. http://www.hhs.gov/ocr/privacy/hipaa/understanding/summary/privacysummary.pdf

Department of Health and Human Services. 2009. The Office of the National Coordinator for Health Information Technology: Background. http://healthit.hhs.gov/

Department of Health and Human Services. 2010 (July). Modifications to the HIPAA Privacy, Security, and Enforcement Rules Under the Health Information Technology for Economic and Clinical Health Act; Proposed Rule. 45 CFR Parts 160 and 164. *Federal Register* 75(134): 40868–40924.

Department of Health and Human Services. 2011a (May). HIPAA Privacy Rule Accounting of Disclosures Under the Health Information Technology for Economic and Clinical Health Act. 45 CFR Part 164. *Federal Register* 76(104):31426–31449.

Department of Health and Human Services. 2011b. Health Information Privacy. http://www.hhs.gov/ocr/privacy/hipaa/administrative/breachnotificationrule/index.html

Department of Health and Human Services. 2011c. HIPAA Enforcement Training for State Attorneys General. http://www.hhs.gov/ocr/privacy/hipaa/enforcement/sag/sagmoreinfo.html

Dixon, P. 2006 (May 3). Medical identity theft: The information crime that can kill you. *World Privacy Forum*. http://www.worldprivacyforum.org/medicalidentitytheft.html

Dougherty, M., and L. Washington. 2008. Defining and disclosing the designated record set and the legal health record. *Journal of AHIMA* 79(4):65–68.

Greene, Adam H. 2011 (October). HHS steps up HIPAA audits: Now is the time to review security policies and procedures. *Journal of AHIMA* 82(10):58–59.

Nunn, S. 2009. Integrating ARRA: Leveraging current compliance efforts to meet the new privacy provisions. *Journal of AHIMA* 80(10):50–51.

Odom-Wesley, B., and D. Brown. 2009. *Documentation for Medical Records*. Chicago: AHIMA.

Office of Civil Rights, Department of Health and Human Services. http://www.hhs.gov/ocr/privacy/

Pozgar, G.D. 2007. *Legal Aspects of Health Care Administration,* 10th ed. Sudbury, MA: Jones and Bartlett.

Rinehart-Thompson, L., and L. Harman. 2009. Medical identity theft: The latest information crime. Prepared with funding from 3M per contract with AHIMA.

Showalter, J.S. 2008. *The Law of Healthcare Administration,* 5th ed. Chicago: Health Administration Press.

Standards for Privacy of Individually Identifiable Health Information. 2003. 45 CFR Parts 160 and 164.

Wieland, L.R. 2009. Tackling ARRA's privacy provisions: How one organization is addressing the new requirements. *Journal of AHIMA* 80(10):52–53, 58.

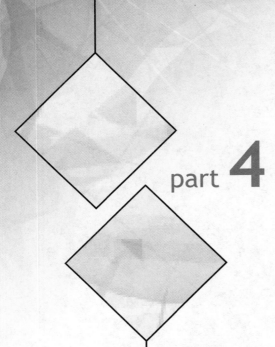

part **4**

Information Technology and Systems

chapter 14

Fundamentals of Electronic Information Systems

Martin J. Smith, MEd, RHIT, CCA

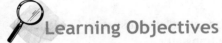

Learning Objectives

- Discuss the major components of an information system
- Identify principal activities of information systems
- Describe the major types of information systems and give an example of each
- Distinguish between the purposes and functions of MIS, DSS, ES, and KMS
- Differentiate between the various types of computers
- Describe the steps in the systems development life cycle
- Explain the vendor selection process
- Identify the three main types of system software and provide an example of each
- Discuss the purpose of an electronic database
- Describe the purpose of a database management system (DBMS)
- Explain the use and components of a data dictionary (DD)
- Summarize the purpose and benefits of a data warehouse
- Understand the functions of a communications system's components
- Compare and contrast clients and servers
- Describe the general practices used to ensure data and computer security

- Compare and contrast local-area networks, wide-area networks, intranets, extranets, and the Internet
- Become acquainted with the policies that must be incorporated into the use of an information system
- Describe functions associated with the management of computer systems
- Identify new and emerging personal productivity software

Key Terms

Application service provider (ASP)
Application software
Artificial intelligence
Assembler
Assembly language
Barcode
Bus topology
Business process
Business-to-business (B2B)
Business-to-customer (B2C)
Chief information officer (CIO)
Client
Cloud computing
Column/field
Communications technology
Dashboard
Data dictionary
Data mining
Data type
Data warehouse
Database
Database management system (DBMS)
Decision support system (DSS)
Direct cutover conversion
E-health
Encoder
Enterprise-wide system
Executive information system (EIS)
Expert system (ES)
Extranet
Foreign key
Graphical user interface (GUI)
Hardware

Health information exchange (HIE)
Information system (IS)
Information technology (IT)
Inputs
Integrity constraints
Internet
Intranet
Key field
Knowledge management system (KMS)
Language translator
Local-area network (LAN)
Machine language
Mainframe
Management information systems (MIS)
Management support information system
Mesh topology
Minicomputer
Natural language
Network
Network protocol
Object
Object-oriented database
Object-relational database
Operating system
Operation support systems
Outputs
Parallel conversion
Peripheral
Phased conversion
Physical topology
Primary key
Productivity software
Programming language

Relational database
Ring topology
Row/record
Screen prototype
Secondary storage
Sequence diagram
Server
Software
Specialty software
Star topology
Strategic information systems planning
Structured query language (SQL)

Supercomputer
System software
Telecommunications
Transaction-processing system (TPS)
Turnkey systems
Unified modeling language (UML)
Use case diagram
Utility program
Wide-area network (WAN)
Wireless network
Workstation

Introduction

The computer is now an essential component for the collection and management of health information. While the planning for the widespread use of electronic health records has covered several decades, recent federal initiatives and legislation has ensured that the use of computers in healthcare delivery is now a requirement for healthcare providers.

Computers comprise a major portion of an organization's **information system** (IS). The IS helps healthcare organizations meet the growing demands of patients, providers, and payers for electronic information. Efficient management and distribution of information are indispensable to a healthcare organization's operation. Because of the principal role that computers play in an organization's healthcare information system, it is vital that HIT professionals understand what makes up a well-constructed computer IS.

It is also essential that health information technicians (HITs) understand their evolving roles and responsibilities in working in this new **e-health** environment. To be effective workers, in addition to knowing the basic structure of an electronic information system and how it is applied to the healthcare environment, HITs must also understand the language of IS. This chapter introduces the primary components of an IS and discusses its essential elements, including data, people, processes, and computer systems. The chapter serves as a foundation for chapters 15 and 16 of this text.

Theory into Practice

Every healthcare provider must adopt an electronic health record no matter what setting they practice medicine in. Although the following example refers to the physician office setting, the challenges faced apply to all settings. This case study from the August 2009 edition of the *Journal of AHIMA* discusses a systematic planning process for successful EHR implementation in physician practices (Gaudreau and Palermo 2009, 80).

One consistent theme emerges from EHR implementations in physician practices: almost everyone underestimates the complexity, time, and effort required.

Implementing ambulatory EHRs includes all the challenges of acute EHR implementations with the potential for many more issues. Delivering an EHR program to scores of ambulatory practices requires enterprise-grade IT scaled down to the practice level at a reasonable cost. The sweep of EHRs includes many aspects of the way healthcare is delivered, affecting processes developed informally over decades. To translate so many manual processes into a tightly defined EHR is a major undertaking.

To deal with the complexity, time, and costs of EHR implementation within a short time period, a solid planning method must be in place. A rapid implementation planning process, called EHR RIP, can focus organizations and guide them in developing a plan that will help bring success.

RIP is a systematic approach that helps organizations establish their EHR objectives, translate them to functional and technical requirements, and identify all resources needed to implement an EHR. RIP also helps to establish realistic budgets, define roles and responsibilities, identify additional resources that need to be hired or contracted, and schedule every element in a detailed timeline.

RIP is a workshop-based process that unfolds in four to six weeks. The working sessions focus on gaining agreement on the strategy, defining functional requirements, and setting the scope of the program. As the plan takes shape, the process delves into the stated and implied assumptions, bringing them to the surface to ensure they will be addressed during the detailed planning.

The process begins with stakeholder executives and the implementation team at a kickoff meeting that establishes overall program objectives at the 40,000-foot level. The first working session descends to 10,000 feet to translate strategic objectives into strategic requirements that will fulfill each high-level goal grouped into program phases. The focus then descends to treetop level in subsequent workshops to map strategic requirements to specific functional requirements for data, access, and security. The rollout's scope is defined in terms of the number of practices, providers, and users; their locations; and the interfaces they will use. The process drills down to illuminate all required resources and identify their likely costs.

RIP contains several important steps. These include: planning, design, building, and implementation. Each of these steps is successively broken down into activities. The following are examples of activities within each step:

- Planning:

  — Validation of existing EHR planning against best practices

  — Establish project governance

  — Develop high-level budget

  — Establish project management

- Design:

  — High-level technology and requirements design

  — Clinical standards design

- — Budget refinement
- — Implementation plan finalization
- ● Building:
  - — Clinical buildout
  - — Integration and testing
  - — Implementation budget finalization
- ● Implementation:
  - — Pilot rollout
  - — Pilot assessment
  - — Refinement
  - — Implementation and design changes
  - — Budget review
  - — Implementation

Basic Concepts of an Information System

An IS is the integration of several elements of a **business process** to achieve a specific outcome. The system receives and processes **input** and provides **output.** For instance, a physician ordering a lab test is a business process. The input is the order for the lab test. The output is a report from the laboratory. An IS is essential in integrating all the elements of the process so that the laboratory test is performed. For the system to work, the physician must provide the laboratory with specific information about what test is to be performed, when it needs to be performed, and on whom it is to be performed. The laboratory must schedule the requested test, collect the sample, analyze the sample (usually with the aid of a computer system), and finally report the test results to the physician. As you can see, the IS integrates all of the steps of the test-ordering process.

A well-designed and well-managed IS is critical for supporting the purposes of the health record. Accurate data can provide physicians, nurses, and administrators with information to make sound decisions. Bad data, on the other hand, can create bad decisions that can affect the health of patients. In *Computers, Communications & Information*, Hutchinson and Sawyer (2000, 9.2) define an information system "as a collection of related components that interact to perform a task in order to accomplish a goal." All organizations generate information that must be managed and used in ways that allow them to accomplish their goals. "In addition to coordination among elements, systems must also be adaptive. That is, they must be able to respond to environmental changes by self-correcting the relationships among their internal elements" (Johns 1999, 368). Computers often are used to assist organizations with this challenging task.

Information System Components

An IS consists of data, people, and work processes and a combination of **hardware** (machines and media), **software** (computer programs), and **communications technology** (computer networks) known as **information technology** (IT).

Data, or raw facts, are provided to the IS by end users. These raw facts (also called inputs) have no meaning of their own. The IS refines them into meaningful information. For example, an end user may input the number 103 into the IS. The raw fact of 103 does not have any specific meaning of its own. However, when the IS system associates the fact as a patient's temperature and compares the fact to the normal temperature range of 98.6 degrees Fahrenheit, the raw fact is transformed into meaningful information, in this case, indicating that the patient's temperature is above normal.

In addition to data, an IS also consists of people. Users work with the IS to accomplish a variety of tasks. In healthcare, users include providers such as doctors and nurses, health data managers, technicians, therapists, oncology registrars, unit secretaries, case managers, chief information officers, and others who add data to the patient's health record. Because the IS must satisfy their needs and solve their problems, users should be a part of the team that designs the IS. Their tasks and goals should be included in the system's initial concept, and the users should be able to suggest changes as the system is being developed.

The last component of an IS is work business processes. Processes are the policies and procedures that users must follow to do their work. An IS automates many processes that are performed by end users. For example, procedures that are followed to assign an ICD code to a diagnosis would be considered a process. A coding **encoder** automates many of the procedures used to assign an ICD code number.

Information System Activities

An IS performs five specific activities: input, processing, output, storage, and controlling. Typically, the first activity an IS performs is accepting input (for example, a patient's identification, temperature, blood pressure, and heart rate).

The second activity is processing the input. Processing can include performing calculations, making comparisons, or selecting alternative actions. For instance, the patient's temperature and blood pressure readings may be compared against the normal values to determine if his or her vital signs are within normal range.

The third activity is producing meaningful output (such as providing a report of a patient's vital signs). The output of an IS is usually considered information to be used in making decisions.

In addition to accepting input and processing it into meaningful output, an IS performs storage and control activities. In an EHR, the computer would store a patient's physical exam on specific storage media such as a hard disk so that many users can retrieve it or so that it can be accessed at a later time.

The final activity of an IS is to control its own performance. For example, a hospital administrator might discover that the daily census output does not add up to the correct monthly census. This may indicate that data-entry or data-processing procedures need to be corrected.

Check Your Understanding 14.1

Instructions: Choose the correct answer for the following questions.

1. What is an information system?

   A. A collection of related components that interact to perform a task in order to accomplish a goal
   B. The integration of several elements in a business process to effect a specific outcome
   C. A process that refines raw facts into meaningful information
   D. All of the above

2. What are the components of an information system?

   A. Computer servers, networks, and wiring along with personal computers
   B. A combination of hardware, software, and communications technology
   C. Data, people, and processes and a combination of hardware, software, and communications technology
   D. Collecting, maintaining, analyzing, and disseminating information

3. What is the difference between data and information?

   A. Data are composed of numbers, and information is composed of words.
   B. Data represent raw facts and figures, and information represents the meaningful interpretation of data.
   C. There is no difference between data and information.
   D. All of the above.

4. Which of the following is an information system activity?

   A. privacy
   B. security
   C. quality
   D. input

5. A physician ordering a lab test is an example of:

   A. business process
   B. input
   C. output
   D. storage

Types of Information Systems

In healthcare organizations, computer-based information systems have historically been used to help managers at different levels to do their work. Physicians used specialized computer systems called decision support systems (DDSs) to help them make important decisions about the care of patients. The managers of the nursing, physical therapy, and health information management (HIM) departments often used computer systems called management information systems (MISs) to manage budgets, create work schedules, perform employee evaluations, and so on.

Coders, on the other hand, still use transaction systems. Every record is coded and entered into the database as part of an ongoing, daily activity. Eventually, the billing department uses the codes to submit bills to insurance companies and patients. The computer system stores this vast amount of data and makes them available for reuse for a variety of purposes.

Information systems usually fall into one of several categories. These include operation support systems, enterprise-wide systems, management support information systems, expert systems, and knowledge management systems. With the advance of sophisticated information technologies some of these boundaries are becoming blurred. However, the categorization is still useful in identifying the primary functions of specific systems. The following sections examine the different types of information systems in detail.

Operation Support Systems

When ISs are used to process data created and used by business operations, they are referred to as **operation support systems.** The role of an operations support system is to efficiently process business transactions, support communication and collaboration among business units, and update business databases (O'Brien 2002, 26). A registration, admission, discharge, and transfer (R-ADT) system is an example of an operation support system. It is used to process data created and used for the registration, admission, discharge, and transfer of patients. Outputs of an R-ADT system would include the daily admission, census, and discharge reports.

Transaction-Processing System

A **transaction-processing system** (TPS) is an example of an operations support system. A TPS manages the different kinds of transactions that occur in a healthcare facility. Patient admissions, employee time cards, and supply purchases are examples of transactions that take place in a healthcare facility.

The characteristics of a TPS include the following:

- Inputs and outputs: Examples include patient admissions, discharges, and transfers.

- Users: The users of a TPS are mainly lower-level managers who make daily operational decisions.

- Products: These are detailed reports on transactions. A dictation-monitoring system reports the number of dictated events by type and by physician. A transcription supervisor can see how much work is left to do, what each transcriptionist has done, and other important data that can be used to determine how many transcriptionists are needed, how much overtime is required to handle the workload, and so on.

- Support MISs and DSSs (discussed later): For example, the database for the R-ADT transaction system in a hospital supports higher-level decision-making support systems. The R-ADT system can send its data through an interface to an

MIS software application. The MIS software turns the data into information such as average daily census, average length of stay, percentage of occupancy, and bed turnover rates and provides this information to management decision makers.

Enterprise Collaboration Systems

Enterprise collaboration systems are another type of operations support system. These systems typically enhance teamwork and are sometimes called office automation systems. Examples include electronic mail and appointment scheduling, project management software to coordinate tasks and schedules, and videoconferencing systems to hold electronic meetings.

Enterprise-wide System

An **enterprise-wide system,** sometimes referred to as an enterprise resource planning (ERP) system, is a large IS that manages data for an entire healthcare business. It helps automate information at the point of service and analyzes business and clinical practices for outcome and cost improvements. It is intended to solve enterprise-wide, rather than department, problems. Enterprise-wide systems are products that allow an organization to perform activities such as:

- Human resource management
- Financial management
- Customer relationship management (CRM)
- Supply chain planning
- Sales and logistics

These systems enable a hospital to gather and manage data from across a health system providing administrators with consolidated data to evaluate operations by a variety of measures such as patient volumes, procedures, care sites, and other factors. This type of information helps administrators make decisions about standardization, productivity improvement, and cost reductions.

It is interesting to note that the electronic health record is a network connected enterprise-wide information system. It is the traditional record transformed into digital format and can be shared across different healthcare settings, because it is embedded in this type of system. Records may include a whole range of data including demographics, medical history, medication and allergies, laboratory test results, radiology images, and all the billing information for any particular patient.

Management Support Information Systems

Information systems that provide information primarily to support manager decision making are called **management support information systems.** The three major information systems fall into these categories: **management information systems** (MIS), **decision support systems** (DSS), and **executive information systems** (EIS).

Management Information System

An MIS is supported by a Transaction Processing System (TPS) which collects, stores, modifies, and retrieves the transactions of an organization to help middle managers make decisions about their departments' objectives. MISs are usually specialized and designed to support a particular area of the business. For example, there are accounting management information systems, financial management information systems, marketing management information systems, and so on. The features of an MIS include the following:

- Transaction data input

- The users of an MIS include middle managers, such as directors of HIM departments.

- The products of the system include summary, exception, periodic, and on-demand reports. An exception report might be a monthly report that lists the percentage of incomplete records by clinical department specialty.

In an HIM MIS, for example, input data might include admission, discharge, and transfer data; and data on the number of dictated reports, coded records, filed records, and incomplete records. Examples of the outputs would include structured reports, production schedules, and productivity analysis so that the HIM director can make management decisions.

Decision Support System

A DSS provides information to help users make accurate decisions. To the healthcare provider, this means using a product that goes beyond supplying facts about a patient's medical condition. One example of a clinical DSS (CDSS) is a special type of DSS that helps a provider make decisions about patient care. It may alert the physician when a lab result is outside the normal range, for instance.

Moreover, reminders help physicians comply with clinical practice guidelines in the management of certain disease processes, such as diabetes mellitus. In addition, DSSs are used to link physicians via the World Wide Web to clinical knowledge databases. One such database is the National Library of Medicine, which enables physicians to search the literature to learn about the latest research. Top management also uses DSSs in planning for the future.

The general characteristics of a DSS include the following:

- The inputs and outputs of a DSS include summarized reports, transaction data, and perhaps external data such as the ORYX performance measurement data developed by The Joint Commission (TJC).

- The users of a DSS include top and middle managers and clinicians. Information from the system can help users make decisions about unexpected, and sometimes isolated, problems.

- The products of a DSS include analytic models. Analytic models are mathematical interpretations of real systems such as pharmacy drug inventory systems. They help users manage inventory, predict customer needs, and make informed business decisions.

Executive Information System

An executive information system (EIS) is a type of management information system intended to facilitate and support the information and decision-making needs of senior executives by providing easy access to both internal and external information relevant to meeting the strategic goals of an organization. For example, an EIS can assist marketing executives in making effective marketing decisions as it provides an approach to sales forecasting, which can allow the market executive to compare a sales forecast with past sales.

The user interface is usually a series of interactive, interconnected, and cascading **dashboards** providing information that is relevant to specific executives and managers. For top executives the dashboard allows access to high-level information in addition to the ability to drill down to departmental-level data. See chapter 10 for additional information on dashboards.

Expert System

An **expert system** (ES) is a knowledge system built from a set of rules applied to specific problems. It can take the place of a human expert when it comes to problem solving. The system simulates the reasoning process of human experts in certain well-defined areas. "Knowledge engineers interview the expert or experts and determine the rules and knowledge that must go into the system. Programs incorporate not only surface knowledge ('textbook knowledge') but also deep knowledge ('tricks of the trade')" (Hutchinson and Sawyer 2000, 11.19).

Dr. Larry Weed's knowledge coupler system (Weed 1991) is an example of an expert system applied to the practice of internal medicine. Much of the knowledge built into the system comes from his experience as a practicing physician as well as from common medical theory. Expert systems are also discussed in chapter 15.

Knowledge Management System

A **knowledge management system** (KMS) is a more recent type of information system that has the potential to increase work effectiveness. This type of system supports the creation, organization, and dissemination of business or clinical knowledge and expertise to providers, employees, and managers throughout the healthcare enterprise.

A KMS is usually composed of an electronic library or central repository of best practices that offers enhanced search capabilities. Information is organized by specific business domain in the electronic library. Most IT-based KMS in healthcare are web-based technologies. Employees can access the electronic library through the **Internet** or an **extranet** to search for information. KMSs also use special software that enables employees to collaborate in teams to use or add to the knowledge in the electronic library.

An example of a KMS is one developed at Partners Healthcare in Boston. This system integrates the clinical database and patient electronic records and embeds drug information into the physician order-entry process. Using this type of system, the physician is alerted to potential drug interactions before an order is processed. This system has reportedly reduced medication errors by 55 percent (Davenport and Glaser 2002).

Instructions: Match the type of information system with the scenario in which it would be used.

1. Dr. J is treating a patient with a rare disease. He enters the patient's signs and symptoms into a computer program that indicates the probability of the correct diagnosis with its treatment regime. The doctor then uses this information to determine the best treatment protocol for the patient.

2. Every week, an HIM department director receives statistical information on the number of incomplete medical records for discharged patients. Summary reports show totals and trends by the physician responsible for completing each patient record.

3. Dr. J orders a series of lab tests on his patient with a rare disease. The computer-generated results signal several abnormal values. This prompts the physician to add three new medications to the patient's treatment protocol. The computer then reminds Dr. J that serious drug interactions could occur when the new medications are combined with the original drug protocol. In response to this reminder, he stops the order for the new medications.

4. The HIM department director receives daily reports on the number of new admissions to and discharges from the hospital.

A. Transaction-processing system
B. Management information system
C. Executive information system
D. Expert system
E. Decision support system

Development of Information Systems

Information systems must be created in a logical manner. The system development life cycle (SDLC) is the traditional way to plan and implement an IS in an organization. The major phases of the cycle are planning, analysis, design, implementation, and maintenance. Figure 14.1 shows the five phases of the system development life cycle. The case presented in Theory into Practice at the beginning of this chapter is a modification of the traditional system development life cycle.

Planning Phase

Given the size and complexity of healthcare organizations and the number of emerging technologies, **strategic information systems planning** is an essential first step in adopting new IS technology. Strategic information systems planning is the process of identifying and assigning priorities to the various upgrades and changes that might be made in an organization's ISs. Its goal is to ensure that all changes contribute to the achievement of the organization's strategic goals and objectives by developing a strategic information systems plan.

The financial and human resources of most healthcare organizations are limited. Different functional areas may want or need to upgrade or replace current ISs with new ones. All the competing requests may be valid and appropriate. For example, the pharmacy director may want to replace an outdated pharmacy IS with state-of-the-art handheld devices designed to allow electronic prescribing. At the same time, the laboratory director may request funds to upgrade the laboratory IS to the latest version. The health information manager may wish to implement a document-imaging system to address space constraints within the health information services department. The vice president for finance may want to install a decision support system on the desktop of every administrator. The whole organization might also need to install a facility-wide electronic healthcare system. How can the organization decide which of these requests is the most important to implement?

The IS strategic plan can be thought of as something like a blueprint for remodeling a house. A blueprint that incorporated all the wishes and needs of the family members— enlarged kitchen for mom, new garage for dad, additional bedrooms for the kids, new roof, third bathroom—probably would be too expensive to build and the resulting house might not function well. Family members would need to consider their long-term priorities before deciding how best to invest their limited resources. Similarly, an IS strategic plan should be based on the needs of the organization as a whole and its long-term priorities.

Figure 14.1. Phases in the system development life cycle

1. Planning	4. Implementation
2. Analysis	5. Maintenance and evaluation
3. Design	

In the earlier example, implementing all the requests for a pharmacy IS, an administrative decision support system and so on probably would be too expensive and might not support the organization's long-term goals. If the hospital's long-range strategy were to implement a nonproprietary EHR system within two years, each director's request should be considered within the context of how each application would contribute to that goal. Priority would be given to those projects that support the future implementation of an enterprise-wide EHR system.

Adopting new information technology represents an enormous investment in terms of staff time, hardware and software costs, and consulting fees. Establishing enterprise-wide priorities for IS development is not an easy task. As stated earlier, every area of the organization may be able to make a compelling case for why a new IS or new technology is needed and how a new system would help the area contribute to the organization's strategic goals. Many factors come into play. And priorities do change in response to political pressure, patient safety issues, new federal regulations, and other factors.

One approach is to compile a comprehensive list of all of the proposed changes to the organization's ISs. The list would include a description of every proposed change along with information on the new technology's availability and ease of implementation, expected benefits and cost savings, and estimated acquisition and maintenance costs. The list then could be distributed to a broad sample of clinicians, managers, and end users. They would be asked to rank the different systems. The steering committee might oversee such a process under the leadership of the **chief information officer** (CIO) or some other top-level clinician or administrator. For clinical systems, it is critical that the initiative be clinician driven, not IS driven.

The strategic IS plan should serve as a guide to making difficult decisions about where, when, and how an institution should allocate resources for the management of information. The interdisciplinary IS steering committee and its role in setting priorities and managing projects are discussed in more detail later in this chapter.

Analysis Phase

Analysis phase of the SDLC is usually initiated by the submission of a project requisition or request from a department for the development, modification or purchase of an information system. The request typically includes an overview of the system purpose, desired functions, anticipated benefits, and costs. The request is generally reviewed by an organization-wide information systems planning or steering committee that determines how the proposed system supports the organization's information systems strategic plan. Before approval additional information may also be obtained, including detailed cost estimates, resource requirements, and timeline.

Once the request is approved a systems analysis is performed. It is very likely that the HIM professional will be involved in the analysis phase of systems development. HITs may participate in this phase as end users who identify necessary functions of a new or existing IS for a particular HIM function. If the system is part of the HIM department, the

HIT may be a member of the HIM team that determines the costs and benefits of the new system and prepares a report that justifies proceeding with analysis and design of the new system. Therefore, it is important that the HIT be familiar with the various steps in the systems analysis process.

The systems analysis defines the whats of the proposed IS project. The whats are based on asking some of the following questions:

- What are the current healthcare business practices the IS will support?
- What areas of the healthcare organization will be using the IS?
- What are the IS project's schedule and budgetary constraints?
- What training methods are used currently in the healthcare organization?
- What are the users' needs for this system?
- What system interfaces will be needed for this IS (for example, user interfaces, system-to-system interfaces, and so on)?
- What legal issues are involved with this IS project (for example, patient confidentiality, physicians' signatures, and so on)?

How do systems analysts collect information about the requirements for an IS project? Several methods are available to them. One very useful method for collecting data is to review existing documentation, forms, and databases. In the healthcare industry, paper forms are vital tools in understanding healthcare processes.

Another useful method is to do research and make site visits. Systems analysts must observe the work environment and learn how existing computer screens, data, and forms are used in the organization. The users of an IS can be invaluable to analysts. Users know their jobs well and can help analysts determine the system's requirements. Users can show analysts how they do the jobs in question. This enables the analysts to understand the processes firsthand.

Conducting a joint application development (JAD) session is a valuable technique used to identify the goals, objectives, and required functions of a proposed IS. A JAD session is made up of a group of end users, system analysts, and technical development professionals who are brought together to analyze the strengths and weaknesses of the current IS and to propose functionalities for the new system. It is very likely that an HIT will participate as an end user in a JAD session.

A trained facilitator conducts the JAD session, which usually spans a period of several days. The session is held away from the organizational campus in a specially prepared meeting room so that participants will not be distracted or interrupted. At the conclusion of the JAD session, the essential functions are identified. The strength of the JAD method is that end users, analysts, and developers are brought together to collaborate in analysis of the IS. This allows for the free exchange and input of information among all concerned groups. The premise underlying JAD is that a group of individuals working together at the same time can perform an analysis faster and better than individuals working independently.

Prototyping is another analysis technique. A prototype is a model or example of what a completed IS may look like. Prototyping a system allows for maximum end-user input while speeding up the analysis and development process by simulating potential end versions of the system. End users and analysts work together to develop the external features of the IS, such as input screens and reports. These external features provide the look and feel of the proposed system but do not include actual program application codes that would make the IS work. The strength of the prototyping method is that it allows the end user to critique the functionalities of the system before time and expense are put into programming efforts. When the basic functionality of the system is prototyped, developers and computer programmers can develop application program codes and databases to support the new system.

As the systems analyst collects data for the IS project, he or she needs a way to document the system's requirements in an easy-to-use graphical manner. Many graphical techniques are available to assist systems analysts. One technique is the **unified modeling language** (UML). The UML is an object-oriented modeling language that assists in the documentation of a software project by specifying, visualizing, modifying, constructing, and documenting the artifacts of a system under development.

An important part of the documentation process is the **use case diagram.** A use case documents the functions of a system from the user's point of view. The use case is similar to a scenario or story that describes the functions of the system and is often used with a **sequence diagram** and sequence table. Figure 14.2 shows a complete use case. In this example the use case shows the interaction between a physician end user and the IS function of searching for a patient. The sequence table in the use case shows how the interaction between the physician and system unfolds (that is, similar to a story). Other documentation may include process flowcharts which are charts that are graphical in nature and provide a symbolic representation of the processing activities performed on the work piece; data flow diagrams (DFD) that are a graphical representation of the flow of data through an information system, modeling its process aspects; and conceptual data models that are maps of concepts and their relationships.

The output of the analysis phase usually results in identification of what the system is to accomplish; its functions; models describing process flow, data flow, and entity-relationship diagrams (ERD), a database modeling method used to produce a type of conceptual schema or semantic data model of a system; and its requirements in a top-down fashion that identifies data items to be included in the IS.

Design Phase

When the analysis phase has been completed and IS functions identified, the system must be designed. The systems design phase specifies the functions of the system and provides

Figure 14.2.   **Example of a complete use case with sequence diagram and sequence table**

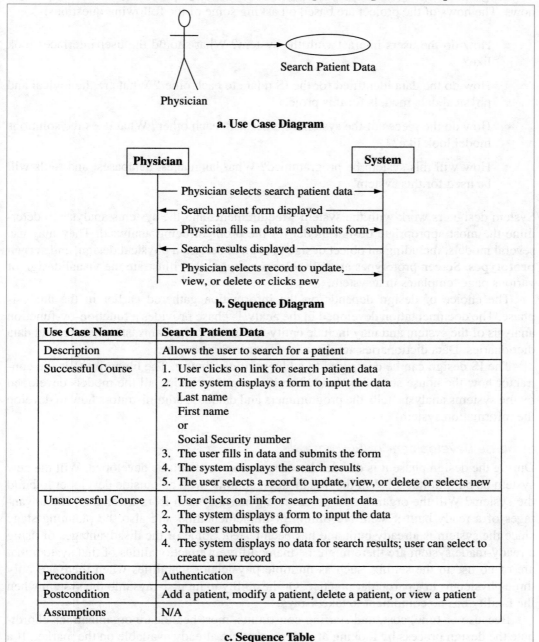

a. Use Case Diagram

b. Sequence Diagram

Use Case Name	Search Patient Data
Description	Allows the user to search for a patient
Successful Course	1. User clicks on link for search patient data 2. The system displays a form to input the data Last name First name or Social Security number 3. The user fills in data and submits the form 4. The system displays the search results 5. The user selects a record to update, view, or delete or selects new
Unsuccessful Course	1. User clicks on link for search patient data 2. The system displays a form to input the data 3. The user submits the form 4. The system displays no data for search results; user can select to create a new record
Precondition	Authentication
Postcondition	Add a patient, modify a patient, delete a patient, or view a patient
Assumptions	N/A

c. Sequence Table

the design or blueprint of the proposed system. The design phase describes the system's hows. The hows of the project are based on asking some of the following questions:

- How do the users interact with the system? What should the user interfaces look like?

- How do the data identified for the IS relate to each other? What are the logical and physical data models for this project?

- How do the pieces of the system interact with each other? What does the solutions model look like?

- How will this system be programmed? What languages, databases, and tools will be used for this system?

System designers work with the system's requirements and the systems analysts to determine the most appropriate design model for the problem being analyzed. They may use several models, including an object design or logical design, a physical design, and **screen prototypes.** Screen prototypes are full-color prototypes that illustrate the visual design of various page templates in a system.

The choice of design depends on the information gathered earlier in the analysis phase. The documentation developed in the analysis phase provides a function-by-function analysis of the system and may include entity-relationship diagrams, storyboards, and data dictionaries. Data dictionaries are discussed later in this chapter.

The IS design can be compared to a blueprint of a house. The blueprint tells the contractor how the house should be built. The IS design, including all the models developed by the systems analysts, tells the programmers and database administrators how to develop the information system.

In-House Development or Purchase

During the design phase it is decided how the new system will be developed. Will the new system be built in-house? Will the organization contract with an outside developer to build the system? Will the organization purchase a generic system from a vendor? The advantages of a ready-built system are timing of implementation and also the planning stage since the system is already built and has been tested. Some of the disadvantages of using a ready-made system are there might be many different functionalities of that system that are of no use in the setting, such as multiple physician capabilities when there are only three physicians in a particular practice. Or the ability to input x-rays into the system when the facility has no equipment to take x-rays.

Because of time, cost, and staffing constraints, most healthcare organizations coordinate the design process by looking at systems that are already available on the market. If a decision is made to purchase an already developed system, then the organization must go through a vendor analysis and selection process. Figure 14.3 describes the vendor analysis and selection process.

Cloud Computing

The expense barrier in the 1960s and 1970s led to the emergence of so-called shared systems. Shared systems were developed by data-processing companies to provide computing power simultaneously to several healthcare organizations within a local or regional area. Healthcare organizations were charged for using the shared-system company's data-processing centers and, usually, their applications. Like the mainframe systems used by hospitals that could afford them, most shared-system products began as administrative and financial systems. During the 1970s, the systems gradually migrated toward department-level clinical systems such as laboratory, radiology, and pharmacy systems. Shared systems came to be known as **application service providers** (ASPs). Today this is known as **cloud computing.** Cloud computing "denotes the use of cloud- or Internet-based computers for a variety of services" (Shimrat 2009, 27). The Internet is used to access systems such as EHR, financial information systems, CPOEs, and other healthcare information systems software that are located at a remote site.

Turnkey Systems

Turnkey systems also began to emerge in the 1970s. Turnkey systems were actually developed by IS vendors and installed on the hospitals' computers. Essentially the healthcare institution purchased a complete system of hardware and software that was installed by the vendor and ready to implement. Typically, the hospital's data-processing staff maintained the systems (Johns 1997; Wager et al. 2005). However, most turnkey systems could not be modified.

Implementation Phase

The implementation phase is a complex undertaking and includes the development of the computer programs, testing of the system, and development of system documentation, user training, and system conversion. Typically, the organization designates an interdisciplinary implementation team led by a project manager to develop a plan for implementing the new system. Selecting an effective project manager is critical to successful system implementation. Ideally, the project manager should be a knowledgeable individual with past experience in similar implementation projects. The project manager should be someone who is highly respected by others in the organization. Some of the typical functions of an implementation project manager include overseeing the entire project from conception to completion, controlling the budget, resources, timelines, and coordinating project status meetings. Finally, he or she should have strong organizational and communication skills and the political influence and authority necessary to get the project done.

A well-executed implementation does not guarantee that users will accept a new system. Problems during implementation can lead to user frustration, dissatisfaction, and disillusionment. Indeed, some organizations never recover fully from disastrous system implementations. Some of the potential problems facing the implementation are

Figure 14.3.   **Vendor selection process**

Identify Vendors

The selection process begins with the organization identifying a number of vendors that can meet the requirements of a new system. Information about IS vendors is available from a number of sources such as exhibits at professional association conferences, publications, consulting firms, and professional colleagues. Often the organization sends a request for information (RFI) to a list of vendors known to offer products or systems that may meet its needs. The RFI asks for general product information and is a good tool for prescreening vendors. Responses to the RFI can be used to narrow the list of potential vendors who will receive a request for proposal (RFP).

Request for Proposal

Next the organization issues a request for proposal (RFP) to the narrowed down list of vendors. The RFP is a written document that generally includes a detailed description of the requirements for the system and gives guidelines for vendors to follow in bidding for the contract. For example, the RFP might request the vendor provide the following (Wager, Lee, and Glaser 2005, 156):

- Vendor qualifications: general background of vendor, experience, number of installations, financial stability, list of current clients, standard content, and implementation plan.
- Proposed solutions: how vendor believes its product meets the goals and needs of the healthcare organization. Vendor may include case studies, results from system analysis projects, and other evidence of the benefits of its proposed solution.
- General contractual requirements: such as warranties, payment schedule, penalties for failure to meet schedules specified in contract, vendor responsibilities, and so forth.
- Pricing and support: quote on cost of system, using standardized terms and forms.

Vendors are usually given a specified time in which to respond to the RFP.

Evaluation Vendors

After the RFP has been distributed to the vendors, the organization may hold a bidders' conference to answer vendors' questions about the RFP. This gives all the vendors the opportunity to receive the same information.

The organization should assess the reliability, cost, and projected benefits of each product. However, evaluation of the vendor and its products may not depend solely on the vendor's response to the RFP. Other formal and informal mechanisms may be used to assess the vendor's fit with the organization and the product's capabilities. For example, it is a good idea to hold vendor presentations, attend user group meetings, and make site visits to other facilities that use the product. The purpose of these activities is to gain as much relevant information as possible. Clinicians and other end users should participate throughout the vendor selection process.

Contract Negotiations

After the top two or three vendors have been identified, the contract negotiation process can begin. The contract generally addresses numerous technical issues, everything from when the system is to be delivered and installed to who is responsible for ensuring that the product works with the organization's other ISs. Internal legal counsel should review the contract carefully before it is signed and binding agreements are made.

Implementation

Once contract negotiations are completed, system implementation follows specified steps and a timeline, stipulated in the contract. Typically, the organization designates an interdisciplinary implementation team led by a project manager to develop a plan for implementing the new system. Implementation of a vendor system should include the usual implementation steps including coding, loading of data, testing, and user training.

overspending of the budget, delays affecting the installation of equipment, and clients requesting last minute changes. Of course, the larger the healthcare entity, the higher the stakes for a successful implementation.

The project manager and the implementation team should begin the implementation process by making a list of the tasks to be completed. The scope and complexity of the process depend on the type of system, the number of users, and the complexity of the conversion process. Typical milestones in the implementation process for healthcare information systems include:

- Preparation of the site (for example, remodeling work spaces and installing telephone lines, computer cables, and electrical power lines)
- Installation of hardware and software
- Preparation of data tables
- Construction of system interfaces
- Development of a network infrastructure to support the system
- Training for managers, technical staff, and other end users who will test the new system
- Testing of the new system to identify and correct problems
- Preparation of support documentation (for example, procedure manuals)
- Development of backup and disaster recovery procedures
- Training for other end users
- Data conversion
- Conversion to the new system

Many implementation activities take place simultaneously. Others need to be completed before other activities can begin. It is generally a good idea for the project manager to use a Gantt chart or another project management tool to schedule and track the milestones in the implementation process. The tool should list the activities to be completed along with the estimated start and completion dates for each, the names of the individuals responsible for each activity, and the resources needed to complete each task. Project management software (for example, Microsoft Project) is useful for creating Gantt charts and tracking project resources (for example, staff, equipment) and expenditures.

All the implementation tasks are important. However, three are especially critical to the success of the project: testing the new system, training the end users, and converting to the new system.

Testing of the New System

Thorough testing of new systems (hardware and/or software) before the actual conversion date is critical. Systems testers test the cases developed in the design phase against the system's requirements. These testers should be users of the system. If a requirement fails, the tester reports the problem to the technical staff. The technical staff then fixes the problem and completes their report. Based on this report, the testers retest the requirement until it passes.

Testing should be conducted using actual patient data, not sample data the vendor has provided or the organization has created for training purposes. Correcting a problem in the test mode is often easier than correcting it after the system is fully operational. Even though it is nearly impossible to identify and correct every potential problem before a new system goes live, it is essential to identify and correct as many of them as possible. It is very unlikely that any errors will be found once the system has been through the testing phase. Problems that are not identified and resolved prior to implementation could end up with the system causing major problems and even could result in having to take the system down if the problems are significant.

It is very likely that an HIT professional will participate in systems testing, particularly when the IS is part of the HIM department or electronic health record. For example, the HIT professional may be asked to put test data into the new IS, such as an electronic master patient index, and determine whether the system provides the expected output.

Training for End Users

It is critical to provide adequate training for the end users of the new system. For any new system to be successful, it must be accepted and used by the staff. This includes physicians and other caregivers in the healthcare setting. When staff is not thoroughly trained, the result may be low morale and dissatisfaction with the system. Some of the resources required for training will be system manuals, training software (potentially online through the vendor), and customer service support. It is important to have policies and procedures and other documentation available during training so that staff can be trained on the entire process—not just the computer system.

One common approach to staff training is a train-the-trainer program. In this approach, key people in the various functional areas (for example, nursing, laboratory, and billing) are identified and trained first. They then train the other users in their area. This approach is effective because the trainers are still available to help the staff after the system has been installed and the vendor is no longer on-site to answer questions.

It is equally critical to allow adequate time for training. Staff should not have to squeeze in training during their lunch breaks. They will need time to practice using the new system. Just as it is important to use actual data to test the system, it is also important for staff to practice using the new system with actual data on real patients. One other method to ensure staff receive the necessary training is to negotiate a training package with the vendor who is supplying the hardware and/or software.

Conversion to the New System

Conversion to a new IS often requires significant changes in workflow and organizational structure. The process also demands a lot of staff time and disrupts productivity and business processes if not properly executed and resourced. Adequate technical support staff must be available to assist managers and end users as needed.

Several different approaches may be used to make the conversion from an old IS to a new one. In deciding which approach to use, it is important to consider the nature of the application, the risks and costs associated with each alternative, and the resources available. The most common approaches are parallel, phased, and direct cutover conversions (Wold and Shriver 1994).

The **parallel** approach involves running both the old and the new systems until the managers and staff are confident that the new system works. This approach is costly and can be confusing to staff, but it ensures that a backup system would be available if needed, which makes it the safest implementation approach.

One type of **phased** approach involves implementing portions of the new system over time instead of installing the entire system all at once. Another type of phased approach involves implementing systems in selected locations instead of at all locations at the same time. For example, a document-imaging system might be implemented in one clinic as a pilot site, with future plans to deploy the system to other clinics within the facility. Converting in phased stages helps the staff gain confidence in the new system, helps the implementation team learn from the experience at the pilot site, and ensures that sufficient time is allowed to make the transition smoothly.

Finally, with the **direct cutover** approach, the organization stops using the old system and starts the new one on a specified date. This approach is risky, but can work effectively when sufficient testing was done and adequate backup procedures are in place. In fact, it may make more sense to convert via the direct cutover method when the old system is quite different from the new one.

Maintenance and Evaluation Phase

The last phase of the systems development life cycle is system maintenance and evaluation. Maintenance and evaluation activities ensure both the short- and long-term success of the information system. Problems inevitably show up after a new IS is put into operation. Adequate IS support staff must be available to identify potential problems and take steps to correct them.

Technical support for critical systems should be available 24 hours a day, 7 days a week. The patient care IS is probably the most vital system in a healthcare organization. Sufficient technical staff also should be available to oversee the following activities:

- System backups
- Software upgrades

- Equipment maintenance and replacement
- Ongoing user training and assistance
- Disaster recovery

Some IS experts estimate that at least 25 percent of the technical staff's time should be devoted to maintenance activities (Austin and Boxerman 2003). System maintenance can be either performed by full-time employees or contracted out to the system vendor.

Every organization that maintains electronic health information is required by federal law to develop emergency backup procedures and a disaster recovery plan. (See the discussion of the Health Insurance Portability and Accountability Act in chapters 13 and 17.) Staff training in emergency procedures also is required. Written backup and emergency procedures should be made readily available to staff.

Maintaining and supporting new systems is not enough, however. The effectiveness of every IS should be evaluated on a continuous basis. Continuous evaluation activities ensure that the organization's ISs support its overall mission and goals and meet users' needs.

Healthcare administrators today demand information on the organization's return on investment (ROI) when new technological systems are implemented. The ability to measure ROI is increasingly important as healthcare institutions struggle to manage limited resources more effectively. Consequently, as a part of the system evaluation process, organizations are looking at the organizational, technological, and economic impact of ISs on the enterprise as a whole (Friedman and Wyatt 1997; Anderson and Aydin 2005).

Evaluation measures how well the original ambitions of the new system (i.e. the logical design laid down during the analysis phase) have been achieved. Evaluation doesn't really serve to improve the system that is being evaluated; it serves to improve the *next* system that will be worked on. Different systems will have different criteria that demonstrate their effectiveness or efficiency. For example, if you buy a cow, you don't evaluate its speed, and if you buy a greyhound, you don't evaluate its milk output.

Once you know what criteria you need to evaluate, you need to devise a *way* to evaluate them. There are two main ways: *objective* and *subjective*. Objective evaluation involves collecting facts, figures, and measurements. Subjective evaluation involves finding out opinions. Where possible, objective measurements are preferred because they are more reliable.

So how long after implementation should you start the evaluation phase? If you wait too long, users remember less about the development process and how it might be improved, but if you start too soon, users have insufficient time to assess system strengths and weaknesses. A good rule of thumb is six months, but pressure to finish sooner often exists. A client should wait until the system is "bedded down" and users are familiar with it, then evaluate whether it has solved the original problem. Has it achieved the goal specified in the Problem Analysis? If not, it should be fixed as soon as possible. Don't sit around with a new system that is as bad, maybe worse, than the old system.

Ideally, the post-implementation evaluation should be performed by people who were not involved in the development process. External auditors often are involved, since they are impartial and don't have a stake in the success or failure of the system.

Check Your Understanding 14.3

Instructions: Choose the best answer to complete the following statements.

1. The systems development life cycle (SDLC):

   A. Is the traditional way to plan and implement an IS
   B. Takes at least three years to complete
   C. Is primarily transaction oriented
   D. Is a never-ending process

2. The first phase of the SDLC is the _____ phase.

   A. Design
   B. Planning
   C. Implementation
   D. Maintenance

3. End-user requirements are identified in the _____ phase of the SDLC.

   A. Design
   B. Analysis
   C. Implementation
   D. Maintenance

4. The method(s) used to identify requirements for a proposed IS is (are):

   A. Conducting site visits
   B. Conducting a JAD
   C. Developing a prototype
   D. All of the above

5. Testing the new IS system is part of the _____ phase.

   A. Design
   B. Planning and analysis
   C. Implementation
   D. Maintenance

6. Instructions: Following is a list of the different tasks or activities that might need to be done to implement an automated coding system. Number the tasks in the order in which they should be carried out. Assign the same number to any tasks that can be done simultaneously.

_____ a. Establish an implementation team and develop a project timeline

_____ b. Assess the coders' needs

_____ c. Determine whether the proposed coding program is in line with the organization's strategic plan and mission

_____ d. Hold bidders' conferences for potential vendors

_____ e. Prepare a list of users' specifications

_____ f. Negotiate a contract with the system vendor

_____ g. Prepare documentation and procedures to support the new system

_____ h. Determine the date of implementation

_____ i. Submit an RFI to potential vendors

_____ j. Train staff on how to use the new system

_____ k. Test the new system

_____ l. Submit an RFP to potential vendors

_____ m. Identify problems with current coding processes and opportunities for improvement

_____ n. Contact other sites that use the products or systems being considered

_____ o. Determine conversion plans

_____ p. Conduct cost-benefit analysis of the different products or systems being considered

Information Architecture

Information architecture (IA) is the art and science of organizing and labeling websites, intranets, online communities and software to support usability. As information proliferates exponentially, usability is becoming the critical success factor for websites and software applications. Good IA lays the necessary groundwork for an information system that makes sense to users. Information technology (IT) encompasses a wide range of topics. This section limits examination to the basic functions of the hardware and software used in information systems.

Categories of Computers

Even though they perform basically the same functions, computers come in various size categories. The different sizes of computers are discussed in the following subsections.

Supercomputers

Supercomputers are the fastest and highest-capacity machines built today. They can cost millions of dollars and are used in large-scale activities such as weather forecasting and mathematical research.

Mainframe Systems

Mainframes were the only computers available until the late 1960s. They can perform millions of instructions per second, are designed to connect input/output devices over long distances, and can handle hundreds or thousands of users at the same time. Mainframe systems vary in size from middle to large capacity, depending on the number of concurrent stations they serve. They are generally used in healthcare to handle input/output-intensive transactions.

Most hospitals use mainframes to store payroll, personnel, billing, and accounting data. The challenge for today's systems engineers is to interface newer technologies for clinical information systems with the older legacy systems stored within the mainframes.

Midrange Systems

There are two types of midrange systems: minicomputers and workstations. **Minicomputers** can support hundreds of connected users at the same time via terminals consisting of a keyboard and a video screen. They are cheaper than mainframes.

A more recent introduction in the 1980s was the workstation. A **workstation** is a very powerful desktop computer used mainly by power users such as graphics specialists for multimedia production. Workstations are comparable to midsize mainframes but sit on a desktop. They also may be used as servers to microcomputers connected through a network.

Microcomputers

Microcomputers, also called personal computers (PCs), were introduced in the early 1970s and are the fastest-growing type of computer today. They come in a variety of sizes, including desktop, laptop, palmtop, and pen-based. Microcomputers can be used in a stand-alone environment or connected to a network.

Handheld Devices

These devices are lightweight mobile devices that provide special functions such as taking notes, organizing telephone numbers and addresses, and calendaring. Other **application software** such as word processing and spreadsheets are now widely available. Today's devices, such as iPads and Kindles include thousands of applications that enable users to perform job functions, search the Internet, and can act as a truly portable computer. Importantly, these devices can exchange data with a desktop computer and can be used alone or in a networked environment.

The vast majority of these devices have web-based capabilities allowing them to send or receive e-mails and access the Internet. Similarly, some devices also provide video conferencing capabilities. Today's devices have a user-friendly interface that includes touch screen capabilities and a stylus input device. The stylus is used to navigate the PDA and write notes.

The use of these devices in healthcare is growing rapidly and computer vendors are now producing them specifically for the healthcare market. These devices may allow clinicians to:

- Track patients and write, upload, and retrieve clinical notes
- Enter laboratory orders and check results
- Access reference materials to perform medical calculations, such as determining drug dosages
- Write prescriptions
- Record and verify charge capture

Specific privacy and security policies and procedures should be in place for control of protected health information that may reside on a particular device.

Cellular Phones

A cellular phone can be a web-based telephone having features of analog and digital devices, also referred to as a smart phone. In addition to basic phone capabilities, a smart phone also provides the functions to receive and send e-mails and faxes and access the Internet. Cell phones allow patients to look up information on conditions, schedule appointments, communicate with healthcare providers, and more. Cell phones can also have special applications. Most recently MIT Media Lab's NextLab program is developing cell phone applications geared toward the developing world. The software would allow patients to transmit their health information, including pictures, to a doctor or nurse in a remote location in order to receive a preliminary diagnosis and to find out whether the condition warrants a trip to the clinic (Merrill 2009).

Types of Computers

Computers can also be divided into three categories depending upon their instruction and form of input data that they accept and process. These are analog computers, digital computers, and hybrid computers.

Analog Computers

The word *analog* means continuously varying in quantity. Analog computers accept input in continuous analog signal form, and output is obtained in the form of scaled graphs. Voltage, current, sound, speed, temperature, and pressure values are examples of analog data. These values continuously increase and decrease. The thermometer is an example of an analog device because it measures continuously the length of a mercury column. Another example is the analog clock because it measures the time by means of the distance continuously covered by the needle around a dial. Similarly speedometer and tire-pressure gauges are also examples of analog devices.

Analog computers have low memory size and have fewer functions. They are very fast in processing, but output return is not very accurate. They are used in industrial units to control various processes and also used in some fields of engineering.

Digital Computers

The word *digital* means discrete. It refers to the binary system, which consists of only two digits (that is, 0 and 1). Digital data consists of binary data represented by OFF (low) and ON (high) electrical pulses. These pulses are increased and decreased in discontinuous form rather than in continuous form.

In digital computers, quantities are counted rather than measured. A digital computer operates by counting numbers or digits and gives output in digital form. A digital computer represents the data in digital signals 0 and 1 and then processes it using arithmetic and logical operations. Examples of digital devices are calculators, personal computers, digital watches, digital thermometers, and so forth. Today, most of the computers used in offices and homes are digital computers.

The main features of these computers are that they give accurate results, they possess high-speed data processing, they can store large amounts of data, they are easy to program and use, and finally, they consume low energy.

Hybrid Computers

The hybrid computers have the best features of both analog and digital computers. These computers contain both the digital and analog components. In hybrid computers, the users can process both the continuous (analog) and discrete (digital) data. These are special purpose computers and are very fast and accurate. They are used in scientific fields and in hospitals, and are used to watch the patient's health condition in the ICU (intensive care unit). These are also used in telemetry, spaceships, missiles, and so forth.

Computer Peripherals

The different pieces of hardware that are connected to central processing units (CPUs) to make them more functional and user-friendly are called peripherals. **Peripherals** are usually described in terms of the five basic computer functions: input, processing and memory, output, storage, and communications.

Input Devices

Input devices include keyboards; microphones; scanners; pointing devices such as mice, trackballs, light pens, and intelligent tablets; sensors; and biometrics such as fingerprints, handprints, and iris scans. Sensors are important in healthcare because they can read a patient's physiological data and transmit them to a computer database. A common example is the use of monitoring systems in critical care units.

The selection of the appropriate type of input device for an IS depends on the user's workflow. If the user moves around a lot (as a nurse does, for example), an input device that allows data entry while moving from place to place is ideal. Headsets with speech input are often used in a mobile work environment.

Barcodes are being used more frequently in healthcare for data capture. **Barcodes** are machine-readable representations of data, typically dark ink on a light background. Barcodes are recognized by scanners as narrow and wide, or 0 or 1. Using appropriate barcode software, these data are then interpreted into meaningful information. In HIM department electronic document management systems, barcodes are used to eliminate the manual indexing of document type, patient name, provider name, medical record number, and other information, as well as medical record separator sheets during the digital scanning process (Kohn 2009).

Output Devices

An output device is any piece of computer hardware equipment used to communicate the results of data processing carried out by an information-processing system (such as a computer) to the outside world. The most common output device is the screen of the visual display unit. The processor is continually addressing the screen to send it signals whenever the results of an instruction have to be communicated to the user. Other output devices include printers, faxes, and speakers. The function of these devices is to translate the machine's response to a usable form for the user.

Data Storage Devices

Secondary storage devices include a flash drive, hard disk drive, magnetic tape, and an optical disk drive. The drives may be internal or external. Digital data can be stored permanently on any of these media, although the life span of each medium varies. This type of device has come into notoriety since they can be easily lost or misplaced.

Optical storage allows for extremely large quantities of data to be stored on one CD. This medium is very useful for storing image and sound data and has the longest life span of secondary storage media.

Processors

A processor is a microchip implanted in a CPU's hard drive that processes instructions sent to it by the computer and software programs. Processors come in a number of sizes. The greater the gigahertz capacity of the processor, the quicker the computer will be able to process instructions sent to it. Some corporations have developed a dual processor, which allows one processor to process multiple instructions at the same time without slowing down performance.

Communications Devices

Communications devices are used to assist communications among different computers. Modems translate digital data into analog data so that the data can be transmitted over telephone lines and received by a remote computer. At the receiving end, the modems reverse the process by turning the analog signal back to digital.

Transmission speeds are very important to the transmission of data. They are expressed in terms of bits per second (bps) or kilobits per second (kbps). Many phone lines max out at 28.8 kbps. Thus, even though the user may have a 56K modem, the rate of transmission will still be 28.8K. Newer technologies in communications include integrated services digital network (ISDN) lines that allow digital data to be transmitted through copper wire telephone lines. This is a dedicated line that can be very costly compared to normal telephone service, but it is five times faster than the fastest modem.

Another technology is the asymmetric digital subscriber line (ADSL). This is thought to be the successor to the ISDN and also functions on standard telephone lines. Cable modems are connected through TV cable lines. This technology is faster than ADSL. Cable modems can download data at a million bits per second (mbps).

Finally, satellite dishes, a wireless connection, offer the fastest transmission. Clients subscribe through a service provider. These are entities that provide web services but can also provide communications, storage, or processing services. One example is an Internet Service Provider or ISP.

The advances in the portfolio of communication technologies (that is, faster broadband wireless networks, smart phones, and data compression techniques) have made it possible to put together a suite of telemedicine applications. For example, communications technologies support emergency medical services (EMS) in a variety of ways including transmission of real-time physiologic data and real-time video from ambulance to emergency room. Communication technologies also support telemedicine services, connecting rural health clinics to clinical specialists and services at urban centers.

Computer Programming Languages and Software

To make all these devices work together, the equipment must use a set of instructions called software. The software programs (or directs) the hardware components to perform the tasks required of them. Software is an ordered sequence of instructions and is developed by using programming languages.

An overview of programming languages and software categories is provided in this section.

Programming Languages

Software programmers who write instructions to the computer use highly specialized languages. The relative ease with which people can interact with and instruct computers has progressed dramatically—from very difficult hardwiring instructions to the use of natural languages.

Since they were introduced in 1945, **programming languages** have gone through five generations of development, including:

1. **Machine languages:** The first generation of programming languages, machine language, consists of ones and zeros.

2. **Assembly languages:** The second generation, assembly language, uses a standard set of abbreviations to replace some of the ones and zeros of machine language. Assembly languages are usually defined by the hardware manufacturer and therefore are not portable to different computers.

3. **High-level languages:** High-level languages use words and arithmetic phrases to construct programs. Examples of third-generation languages include COBOL and BASIC.

4. **Very high-level languages:** The fourth generation of programming languages includes report generators, query languages, data management languages, and application generators. These languages were developed to reduce programming effort, time, and costs. They are easier to use and require fewer commands to execute programs. **Structured query language** (SQL), Report Builder, and SPPS are just a few examples of a fourth-generation language.

5. **Natural languages:** Natural programming languages allow users to speak in a more conversational way with the computer and are part of the expanding field of **artificial intelligence** (AI). "One of the most successful natural language systems is LUNAR, developed to help users analyze the rocks brought back from the moon" (Hutchinson and Sawyer 2000, 13.14). AI is used widely to develop expert systems that help physicians manage patient care, telemedicine, teleradiography, and other e-health and telemedicine activities.

Software

Software can be categorized into three major classes based on the software's function. These broad classes include: system software, computer programming software, and application software, although the boundaries between them at times are often fuzzy.

System Software

In an orchestra, the different musical instruments are played in complete synchronization. How does this happen? A composer writes a set of instructions for each instrument using the language of music. In a sense, a computer programmer is a composer except that the programmer writes a set of instructions for computer hardware. Like the conductor guiding the orchestra through a musical composition, the **system software** acts as the conductor for all the hardware components and the application software. It essentially tells the computer when to start, what to do, and when to stop. Without system software, nothing would happen.

System software has three basic pieces. These are discussed in the following subsections.

Operating System

The **operating system** "consists of the master programs, called the supervisor, that manage the basic operations of the computer. These programs reside in RAM [random access memory] while the computer is on and provide resource management services of many kinds; for example, they run and store other programs and store and process data. The operating system includes BIOS (the basic input/output system), which manages the essential peripherals such as the keyboard, screen disk drives, and parallel and serial ports" (Hutchinson and Sawyer 2000, 5.4–5.5).

Common microcomputer operating systems include DOS (disk operating system), Windows, and earlier versions—OS/2, Unix, and Macintosh.

User interfaces are an important software support for an operating system because they determine how the user communicates with the computer. The DOS system, for example, uses a command-driven interface that requires instructions to be typed in at a command prompt. A second type of interface is the menu-driven approach. This approach allows the user to select choices using a mouse or some other non-keyboard pointer. Presently, the **graphical user interface** (GUI) is the standard microcomputer interface. It operates on the basis of icons that represent different computer tasks and programs. The GUI allows for keyboard as well as point, click, and drag functions.

a. Utility Programs

Utility programs "are generally used to support, enhance, or expand existing programs in a computer system" (Hutchinson and Sawyer 2000, 5.8). Examples of utilities include:

- Backup processes that store data in more than one location

- Virus protection that protects computer programs and data

- Data recovery that prevents the loss of data in the event of physical or software accidents

b. Language Translator

The **language translator** "is software that translates a program written by a programmer in a language such as C++ into **machine language,** which the computer can understand. All system software and applications software must be turned into machine language for execution by the computer" (Hutchinson and Sawyer 2000, 5.12). According to Hutchinson and Sawyer (2000, 10.15–10.16), language translators include **assemblers**, compilers, and interpreters.

Application Software

Application software can be further categorized into four different types:

- **Productivity software** products are used in almost all businesses to assist with word processing, accounting, database management, graphics presentations, scheduling, e-mail, time management, and other functions performed in offices and homes.

- **Specialty software** includes programs designed for a specific industry. For example, in health information management, encoders are designed to accelerate the medical coding process. Other types of specialty software in other industries include multimedia authoring, desktop publishing, and CAD/CAM products.

- **Education and reference software** includes encyclopedias, anatomy atlases, and library searches. One very successful library search program is Medline, which is offered through the Internet site of the National Library of Medicine.

- **Entertainment software** includes games and audio/video entertainment.

Check Your Understanding 14.4

Instructions: Indicate whether the following statements are true or false (T or F).

1. _____ Computer peripherals such as mice, printers, and monitors control the computer's operating system.

2. _____ Common utility programs include virus checkers, backup, and recovery.

3. _____ DOS stands for disk operating standard.

4. _____ The user communicates with the computer through an interface (Windows, for example).

5. _____ Machine languages use a standard set of abbreviations to replace some of the ones and zeros used in assembly language.

6. _____ The increasing use of wireless technology is one of the hottest technology trends today.

7. _____ Artificial intelligence is one type of natural programming language.

8. _____ Education and reference software is one category of application software.

9. _____ The three basic pieces of system software are the operating system, the language translator, and the utility program.

Databases

The most critical resource in healthcare is patient data. An argument can be made that data is actually more valuable than money since you can only use money once before it is gone whereas data can be used over and over again. The most important functions of any healthcare information system involve being able to create, modify, delete, and view patient data. And the most important storage mechanism used to perform these functions is a database. As discussed in chapter 4, databases are essential in the development of EHR systems.

A **database** is an organized collection of data saved as a binary-type file on a computer. Users cannot read a binary-type file because it contains only ones and zeros. A database management system provides the ability to perform the functions mentioned earlier. Many different kinds of database management system vendors are available in the marketplace, including Oracle, SQL Server, Sybase, and Access.

Database Approach

There are three popular types of databases: relational databases, object-oriented databases, and object-relational databases.

A **relational database** stores data in predefined tables that contain rows and columns similar to a spreadsheet. The kinds of data that can be stored in a relational database are currency, real numbers, integers, and strings (characters of data). They are used for the storage of information in databases used for financial records, manufacturing and logistical information, personnel data, and much more. This type of database is a popular model used in healthcare applications.

An **object-oriented database** stores objects of data. An **object** is a discrete or abstract thing such as a car or a line at the grocery store. Data objects can model relational data or advanced **data types** such as graphics, movies, and audio. Objects are used in object-oriented languages such as Smalltalk, C++, Java, and others

Finally, the **object-relational database** combines the best of the relational and object-oriented databases. It uses both traditional data types (such as currency, integers, and strings) and advanced data types (such as graphics, movies, audio, and so on). They can be used to build database management system and can connect to a company's website and allow updates to items such as their inventory records.

Database Purpose and Activities

The purpose of a database is to store and retrieve data. A popular common language called structured query language (SQL) is used to store and retrieve data in relational databases. SQL gives the information system the ability to query and report on data and to insert, update, and delete data from the database.

A **database management system** (DBMS) is a collection of computer programs that controls the creation, maintenance, and use of a database. The DBMS allows different application programs to access the database. An important purpose of a DBMS is to maintain the data definitions (data dictionary) for all the data elements in the database. It also enforces data integrity and security constraints.

Relational Database

The relational database, as stated earlier, is one of the most popular database architectures used in healthcare. Relational databases perform the following activities:

- Store data in tables consisting of rows and columns. Figure 14.4 shows the hierarchy of data in a relational database. A column consists of a name and a data type (the kind of data being stored in the column). A row in a table consists of data values in the various columns. A row would be the values of these columns, such as "John" for the first name and "Smith" for the last name.

- Retrieve and store data in tables using SQL to insert, update, delete, and query data from tables.

- Provide a level of security, usually by user and by table and column that each user is allowed to access. In healthcare systems, access to health records must be limited to only certain users in order to protect patient privacy.

A table is a two-dimensional structure made up of rows and columns. Table 14.1 shows an example of a table that stores information about a patient.

A **column/field** is a basic fact such as LAST_NAME, FIRST_NAME, DOB, RACE. A **row/record** is a set of columns or a collection of related data items. An example of a row in the PATIENTS table is: Smith, Keith, 2/13/70, White.

Figure 14.4. **Storage hierarchy of a relational database**

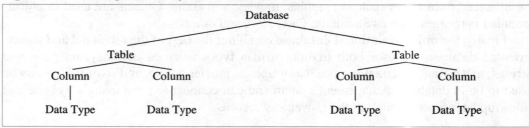

Table 14.1. **Example of a PATIENTS table**

PATIENT_ID	LAST_NAME	FIRST_NAME	DOB	RACE	DOCTOR_ID
1	Smith	Keith	2/13/70	White	1
2	Roberts	Debbie	7/30/70	Black	1
3	Morrison	Rebecca	2/4/99	White	1
4	James	Sally	7/29/50	Black	1

A **key field** uniquely identifies each row in a table. There are two types of keys:

- **Primary keys** ensure that each row in a table is unique. A primary key must not change in value. Typically, a primary key is a number that is a one-up counter or a randomly generated number in large databases. A number is used because a number processes faster than an alphanumeric character. In large tables, this makes a difference. In the PATIENTS table, the PATIENT_ID is the primary key. It is good programming practice to create a primary key that is independent of the data in a table.

- A **foreign key** is a column of one table that corresponds to a primary key in another table. Together, they allow two tables to join together. For example, say we have two tables, a CUSTOMER table that includes all customer data, and an ORDERS table that includes all customer orders. The intention here is that all orders must be associated with a customer that is already in the CUSTOMER table. To do this, we will place a foreign key in the ORDERS table and have it relate to the primary key of the CUSTOMER table.

The cancer registry is an example of a health record database that can be computerized. A manual registry is already organized logically by site of the neoplasm. Imagine that a two-drawer file cabinet is being used for the cancer registry. The entire file cabinet is considered the database. The first drawer contains a set of abstracts by site of the neoplasm. Within each file folder are the abstracts or records kept on each patient. Each record contains a collection of data fields or facts about the patient.

The second file drawer is organized by month. Each month is one file folder. Within each month's folder are the cases that need to be followed for that month. Each case is considered a record. Within each record are the necessary pieces of information, or data fields, required to contact the patient and update the medical data.

In a computerized IS, each case is stored in one table and each patient is stored in another table. Case and patient have to be related to each other so that the user can look up the case and also locate the patient information. For example, if the cases were stored in a CASES table (with a primary key of CASE_ID) and the patients were stored in a PATIENTS table (with a primary key of PATIENT_ID), a foreign key would be needed to relate the case to the patient. If the patient were to have many cases, a foreign key of PATIENT_ID would have to be located in the CASES table in order to create the one-to-many relationship. Thus, when a user queries a case, he or she can easily use the foreign key PATIENT_ID to find the patient information. (Relational databases are also covered in chapter 16.)

Data Models

Data models provide a contextual framework and graphical representation that aid in the definition of data elements. In a relational database, the data model lays the foundation for the database and identifies important entities, their attributes, and the relationships among entities (Johns 2002). An entity is anything about which data can be stored and can be a concept, person, place, thing, or event. In the cancer registry example above, "PATIENT" and "CASES" would both be entities. Data models are usually constructed by data administrators after a thorough analysis of the business processes has been performed. A sample data model for the entity "Person" is shown in figure 14.5.

Data Dictionary

Databases are only as good as the data they contain. Without a mutually agreed upon set of data elements with clearly defined names and definitions, the validity and reliability of the data contained in a system are suspect at best and must be discounted at worst. The **data dictionary** is a central building block that supports communication across business processes (AHIMA e-HIM Workgroup on EHR Data Content 2006). A data dictionary improves data validity and reliability within, across, and outside the enterprise because it ensures that each piece of data can only mean one thing. It also improves communication in clinical treatment, research, and business processes because terms are defined and used the same way by everyone in the organization. Standardization provides developers with a common road map to promote consistency across applications. For example, the data element "PATIENT" would have the same field length and definition across all applications in the organization.

Lack of a sound data dictionary can cause problems within and across organizations. For example, in an organization one department may use the term "PATIENT" while another department may use the term "CLIENT" and yet another department may use the term "CUSTOMER" to define the same entity. Clearly this situation makes it difficult for an organization to collect all of the information it needs, and it may make it impossible to combine or map data across systems because the definitions are not identical. A worse possibility is that an organization may combine data elements it believes to be equivalent and draw incorrect inferences from the invalid data. Multiple users entering data may have different definitions or perceptions of what goes into a data field, thereby confounding the data. For example, are "reason for visit" and "chief complaint" the same or different?

Table 14.2 provides an example of a data dictionary. Maintaining the data dictionary frequently is an HIM function. A data dictionary is essential in ensuring consistent definitions of what data names mean and making sure that data are accurate. A data dictionary is critical in the development of EHR systems.

The content structure of a data dictionary may vary among organizations. Data dictionary content depends on the use of the dictionary and the specific notation method used to develop the dictionary. A good dictionary defines each data field or column according to the following information:

- Name of field
- Type of data field
- Length of data field
- Edits placed on the data field

Figure 14.5. **Sample data model for the entity "person"**

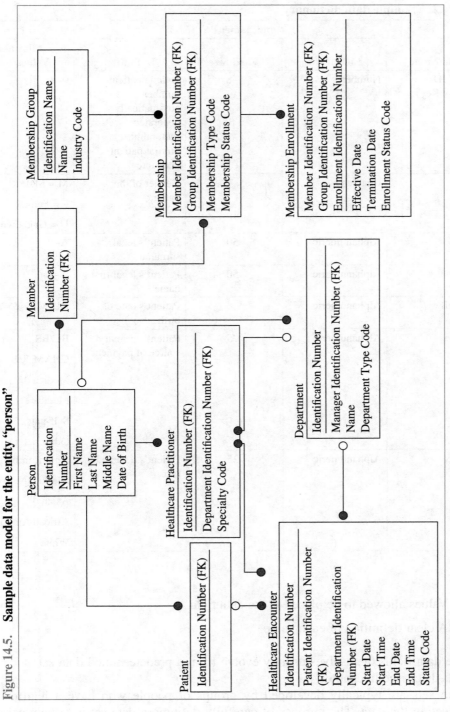

Source: Shakir 1999.

Table 14.2.   **Sample data dictionary**

Table Name: PATIENT				
Field Name	**Field Type**	**Field Size**	**Definition**	**Allowable Values/Edits**
Patient_ID (Primary Key)	Number	8	Unique patient number automatically generated (autonumber) on first patient encounter	0–9
Gender	Character	1	Gender of the patient	M = Male F = Female U = Unknown
PT_LN	Alphanumeric	50	Patient's legal surname	A–Z
PT_FN	Alphanumeric	50	Patient's legal first name	A–Z
PT_DOB	Alphanumeric	8	Patient's date of birth	DD-MM-YYYY
PayType	Alphanumeric	25	Patient's primary source of payment	BC/BS CHAMPUS Medicaid Medicare Self-pay Other
PT_Race	Alphanumeric	25	Patient's declared race	American Indian Alaskan Native Asian African American White

- Values allowed to be placed in the data field
- A clear definition of each value

The data fields themselves usually evolve from a predetermined data set, such as the data sets discussed in chapter 4.

Data sets are typically developed by groups of people who have a legitimate use for collecting the data. The purpose of carefully defining a data set is to help ensure the accuracy of the data collected and the usefulness of the statistics obtained from the collection of the data.

HIT professionals can play a vital role in the development of data sets and data dictionaries because they possess the knowledge and terminology that are recognized throughout their particular healthcare setting. Their involvement will help healthcare organizations to create clear and nonredundant electronic patient records in the future. Additional information on the data dictionary use in the EHR is provided in chapter 16.

Techniques for Database Integrity

Because databases are the backbone of an EHR, careful attention must be given to ensure that data stored in a database have the data quality characteristics described in chapter 2. These include accuracy, accessibility, comprehensiveness, consistency, currency, definition, granularity, precision, relevancy, and timeliness. The following discussion is a guide for achieving these characteristics in a database.

Good Database Design

Good database design is a process that involves a team of individuals who have good relational database knowledge and extensive technical database design expertise. In addition, the database development team needs to include end users who have knowledge of the real world or domain, which the database will describe. It is very rare to find one person with knowledge in both technical database design and the described domain.

Usually the end user describes the domain, its elements, and the data that needs to be stored to the database designer. This step is very important as it defines the goals and the requirements of the database. Because of their experience and knowledge with healthcare information, HIM professionals should take the lead in being the interface between the domain and technical experts in documenting the data dictionary.

Good database design relies heavily on development of accurate data models (figure 14.5). Data models, as stated earlier, are the blueprint of the database and describe database entities and their relationships. Data models are usually developed by individuals with expertise in data modeling who identify entities and their relationships with help of the individual who has the domain knowledge.

A good database design implements exactly the data requirements of the end users (the ones with the domain knowledge). A proper database design ensures that there are minimal redundant data in the database and that the data structure is flexible enough to easily handle change in the database requirements.

Integrity Constraints

Using **integrity constraints** is extremely important. Integrity constraints provide a way of ensuring that data that are entered or updated in a database by authorized users do not result in a loss of data quality. Integrity constraints could either be a specification of uniqueness for values of a column (for example, only allowing the input of "M" for male or "F" for female in a gender field) or validation for values of a column (for example, allowing only a specified range of values for a field that records a patient's temperature). Referential integrity is another strategy that is used to ensure data quality in relational databases. Referential integrity ensures that there is consistency between tables that are linked in the relational database. HIM professionals are frequently involved in helping to develop integrity constraints in a database.

Database Management Systems

Database management systems (DBMSs) fall into two categories: a personal DBMS, which runs on a client; and a server-based DBMS, which runs on a server.

Personal DBMS

A personal DBMS is used for small projects such as storing contact information (for example, in a personal address book). It should not be used for systems that require large amounts of storage and 24/7 access. Most healthcare systems would not use a personal DBMS. Personal DBMSs are tempting to use because (1) they are inexpensive and (2) most people already have access to one with an office software package such as Microsoft Office. Microsoft Access only supports a few gigabytes of storage. Today, databases span terabytes of storage. These types of databases require the use of a server-based DBMS.

Server-Based DBMS

A server-based database management system runs on a server computer. It also runs as a separate application from a personal system. This allows the DBMS to run faster and more efficiently than the personal DBMS. A question might take minutes to answer on a personal DBMS, but only seconds on a server-based DBMS. Examples of a server-based DBMS are Oracle, SQL Server, Sybase, and Informix. A server-based DBMS also allows data to be retrieved by multiple end users. Such a database system is essential in an EHR system.

Server-based database management systems provide support for 24/7 access with large amounts of storage in the terabyte range or higher. They are very expensive compared to personal database management systems.

Data Warehouses

Today, most organizations use multiple databases in their daily business operations. Many of these are separated from each other and the data are not available in a consolidated form to help managers and others make decisions. A **data warehouse** is a special type of database that alleviates this problem by consolidating and storing data from various databases throughout the enterprise. Data warehouses are designed to perform data analysis rather than to support routine operations (figure 14.6).

Figure 14.6.   **Example of a data warehouse**

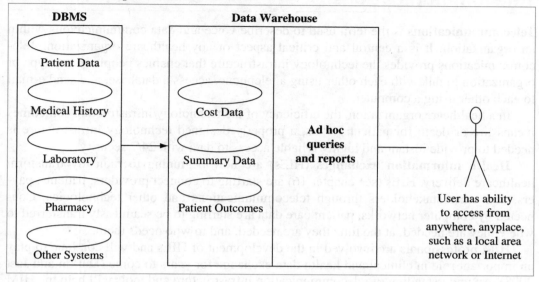

The principal purpose of the data warehouse is to provide data for improved decision support. A data warehouse usually contains historical data that are derived from operation (transaction) systems and is optimized for speed of retrieval of data. "A data warehouse enables users to tap into knowledge hidden in the massive amounts of data to understand business trends and make timely strategic decisions. The data warehouse allows decision makers to perform simple reporting, complicated analysis, multidimensional analysis, population analysis, physician analysis and benchmarking, clinical protocol development, reimbursement/cost analysis, and much more" (Farishta 2001, 28–32).

The benefits of a data warehouse include better customer service, lower production costs, increased profitability, and quicker turnaround times for making decisions. One of the most powerful applications of a data warehouse is to engage in data mining.

Data Mining

Data mining is associated with data warehouses. Data mining is a process that identifies patterns and relationships by searching through large amounts of data. Because data warehouses contain large amounts of data, data mining processes are frequently used to systematically analyze these data. In healthcare, data mining is used to identify methods for cutting healthcare costs, suggest more appropriate medical treatments, and predict medical outcomes. It has also been used by the federal government to help identify fraud and abuse practices and evaluate and reduce Medicare payment errors.

Typically, data mining is performed by individuals with a background in statistical analysis. An evolving role for the HIM professional is in data analytics. A certified health data analyst (CHDA) manages, analyzes, interprets, and transforms data into accurate, consistent, and timely information.

Telecommunications

Telecommunications is the term used to describe voice and data communications within an organization. It is a central and critical aspect of any healthcare organization. Telecommunications provides the technology infrastructure that enables people in any type of organization to talk with each other using a telephone, access a database, and send e-mail to each other using a computer.

In a healthcare organization, the efficiency of the technology infrastructure sometimes means life or death for patients. Thus, a properly designed technology infrastructure is needed to provide instant and highly reliable access to data with 24/7 security.

Health information exchanges (HIEs) are now beginning to radically transform healthcare delivery. HIEs (see chapter 16) are starting to connect providers, patients, payers, and other stakeholders through telecommunications and other technologies. Connected by computer networks, patient care data are starting to be seamlessly transferred to where they are needed, at the time they are needed, and to who needs them.

HIM professionals are involved in the development of HIEs and will continue to play an important role in clinical and health data exchange for years to come (Durkin and Just 2008). An understanding of telecommunication infrastructure and tools will help the HIM professional in this role.

Network Fundamentals

A computer network, often simply referred to as a network, is a collection of hardware components and computers interconnected by communication channels that allow sharing of resources and information. Where at least one process in one device is able to send and receive data to and from at least one process residing in a remote device, then the two devices are said to be in a network. They may be classified according to a wide variety of characteristics such as the medium used to transport the data, communications protocol used, scale, topology, and organizational scope.

To understand the nature of a computer network, it is important to first understand the nature of communications systems. As shown in figure 14.7, a communications system is made up of four components:

- The transmitter is the device that sends information.

- The receiver is the device that receives information.

- The medium is the mechanism that connects the transmitter to the receiver. It may be a cable (for example, the twisted-pair cable commonly used to connect workstations in an office building) or the air (in the case of cellular phone transmissions).

- Data create the message that is transferred from the transmitter to the receiver as electrical pulses.

One very common communications system is the telephone. The handset of a typical telephone acts as both transmitter and receiver. The cables and telephone wires that

Figure 14.7.   **Components of a communications system**

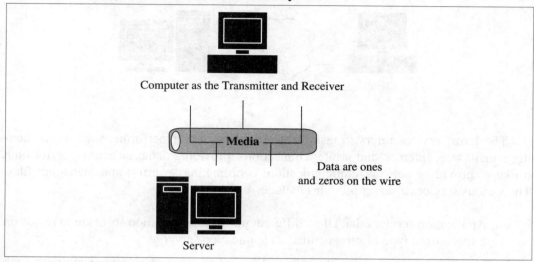

connect one telephone to another are the media. Voice signals, such as words and other sounds, are the data.

It is possible to create a communication system by connecting one computer to another to form a network. The users of computers in the network then can share information and resources. In a computer network, a computer functions as both transmitter and receiver.

The specific type of communication that takes place on a computer network is often called data communication. Data communication involves transferring information in binary form, which is the electronic equivalent of ones and zeros. In addition to computers, a network can incorporate a variety of computer devices (called nodes) such as printers, fax modems, scanners, CD-ROM drives, tape backup units, and plotters. The collection of computers and devices that make up a network are sometimes called the network's resources.

The purpose of a **network** is to allow users to share its resources easily and efficiently. For example, any network user can access the network printer, not just the user sitting behind the computer to which the printer is attached.

Clients, Peers, and Servers

Network computers play one of two roles: client or server. **Clients** are computers that access shared resources. **Servers** are computers that share resources such as printers or hard-disk space across the network. For example, a user interacts with the client computer to request something from the network (for example, e-mail messages). The server responds by supplying the e-mail messages the user requested. People often refer to this interaction as the client-server relationship (figure 14.8).

Figure 14.8. **Client-server network relationship**

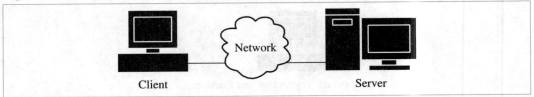

The term services refers to tasks that a network server performs, such as facilitating e-mail, web, Internet, and printer connections; providing database access; performing backups; providing network communication; coordinating security; and managing files. The various services a server provides include:

- Application services that allow different pieces of application software to reside on a specialized type of server called an application server

- Communication services that allow different systems to communicate with each other

- E-mail services that permit the exchange of correspondence electronically

- Internet services that let users transfer files and other information via the Internet

- Web services that allow users to use a browser and a server to access the World Wide Web (a system of Internet servers that support specially formatted documents called web pages, although some Internet servers are not part of the web)

- Printer services that enable users to access a printer from anywhere on the network

- Database services that store and retrieve information such as accounting and financial data

- Backup services that routinely create backup copies of information

- Network management services that make it possible to manage network resources from a central location

- Security services that prevent unauthorized users from accessing the network

- File services that allow anyone with access to a server to store and retrieve files

Because network computers can act in only one of two roles, the peer-to-peer relationship is an extension of the client/server model. In a peer-to-peer relationship, a networked computer acts as both client and server.

Network Architectures

The way a computer network is set up is its basic design or architecture. There are three main types of network architectures: local-area networks, wide-area networks, and wireless networks.

Local-Area Networks

The **local-area network** (LAN) connects computers in a relatively small area (for example, within one room or one building). It can take the form of a client/server network, a peer-to-peer network, or a hybrid network. A hybrid network is a mixture of client/server and peer-to-peer networks.

One special form of a LAN is an intranet. An **intranet** is a specialized client/server network that uses Internet technologies. An intranet provides information within the organization. This information can include policies and procedures, cafeteria menus, forms, training, and more.

Intranets let corporations supply Internet services over their LANs. Essentially, intranets are private Internets with the security required to protect a corporation's assets. An extranet, on the other hand, provides network connectivity between suppliers to allow direct connection to each other's network.

Wide-Area Networks

The **wide-area network** (WAN) connects devices across a large geographical area (for example, across a state or even the world). WANs can take several forms but often simply consist of two or more LANs connected by telephone lines.

The world's largest public WAN is the Internet. The Internet consists of hundreds of thousands, if not millions, of interconnected LANs around the world. By connecting private LANs to the Internet, individuals and corporations can create a relatively inexpensive WAN. However, the Internet is a very insecure environment. Thus, LANs connected via the Internet may be subject to intrusion from unauthorized users.

Wireless Networks

The **wireless network** refers to any type of computer network that is not connected by cables of any kind. It is a method by which homes, telecommunication networks and enterprise (business) installations avoid the costly process of introducing cables into a building, or as a connection between various equipment locations.

Network Topologies

Computer networks consist of a configuration of cables, computers, and other devices. How data flow through a network is referred to as **physical topology.** For example, in star topology, data transferred between one computer and another must first flow through a central connection point called a hub. There are four types of physical network topologies that are commonly used. Each of these, described below, has its strengths and weaknesses. Selection of a topology is based on the purpose of the network, size of the network, and cost, among other considerations. The main types of physical topologies are **star, ring, bus,** and **mesh.** Figure 14.9 shows three of these topologies.

Bus Topology

Bus technology is an older topology where each computer is connected to a common backbone or trunk through some kind of connector. A signal or message from the source computer travels along the backbone in both directions to all machines. If the machine address (that is, MAC or IP address) does not match the intended address for the data, the machine ignores the data. Where the machine address matches, the data are accepted. Bus topology is inexpensive to implement and works best with a limited number of devices. A disadvantage of this topology is that the central cable is a single point of failure. If this cable fails for any reason then the entire network goes down.

Figure 14.9.   Common network topologies

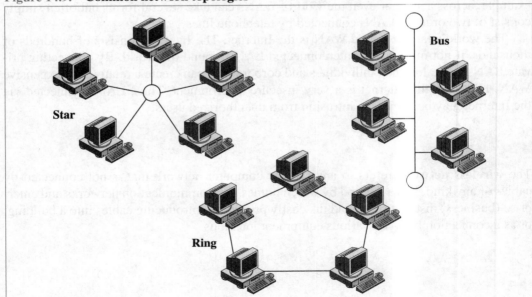

Source: Durkin and Just 2008.

Star Topology

In a star topology each machine is connected to a central hub. All of the data on the network have to pass through the hub, which forwards those data to the correct destination. The star topology is easy to design and install, and adding nodes (computers or other devices) to the network is less difficult than other topologies. Like the bus topology, the star topology has a single point of failure, which is the hub. If the hub fails, the entire network would go down.

Ring

In the ring topology each device is connected to the network in a closed loop or ring. Each machine is identified by a unique address. The signal passes through each machine or computer connected to the ring in one direction. Ring topology usually uses a token passing scheme. A token is essentially an empty container to transport data. To use the network a machine has to capture an empty token and insert its message. The token is then passed from machine to machine sequentially on the network until it reaches its correct destination. Only one machine can transmit on the network at a time. Ring topology is good for small networks and not costly to install, and it is easy to add new nodes to the ring. The primary disadvantage of ring topology is the failure of one machine will cause the entire network to fail.

Mesh

A mesh topology combines characteristics of bus, ring, and star topologies, but allows for redundant routes for data transfer. Essentially each node in a mesh topology is interconnected to all the other nodes. Even if one node fails on the network, the network will not go down because there is more than one path from one node to another. Mesh topologies allow for the expansion of an existing network, and enable companies to configure a network to meet their needs. The Internet is the most famous example of a mesh topology. The disadvantages include the overall length of each segment is limited by the type of cabling used; if the backbone line breaks, the entire segment goes down; and they are more difficult to configure and wire than other topologies.

Data Transfer

Network protocols enable computers on the network to communicate with each other. The computers have to use the same language, just as people have to speak the same language in order to understand each other. Network protocols provide computers with a common language.

The variety of network types, computers, operating systems, and browsers available today greatly complicates the exchange of information between computers. To facilitate this exchange, networks rely on some basic protocols, or rules, to govern the organization and transmission of data. Most protocols apply to three distinct phases of the data exchange process:

1. Connection setup phase: Just as a telephone uses ringing to request a connection to another telephone, a protocol must first initiate a connection between computers on the network.

2. Data transfer phase: After setting up the connection, the protocol allows the computers to transfer data. After the data are transmitted, the receiving computer decides whether to accept or reject them.

3. Connection release phase: After the data transfer is complete, the protocol allows the computers to terminate the connection.

The following are common network protocols:

- Transmission Control Protocol/Internet Protocol (TCP/IP) is the basic communication language or protocol of the Internet. It is also used as a protocol in a private network such as an intranet or extranet.

- File Transfer Protocol (FTP) is a protocol used to exchange and manipulate files over a TCP/IP network.

- Hypertext Transfer Protocol (HTTP) is a protocol used to transfer and display information in the form of web pages on browsers.

- Simple Mail Transfer Protocol (SMTP) is an Internet standard for electronic mail transmission across Internet Protocol (IP) networks.

HL7

Health Level Seven (HL7), founded in 1987, is a not-for-profit, ANSI-accredited standards developing organization that provides comprehensive standards for the exchange, integration, sharing, and retrieving of electronic health information that supports patient care. The HL7 standard allows exchange of data between common systems that make up the EHR such as radiology, laboratory, pharmacy, and other systems.

As described in chapter 16, Health Level Seven (HL7) is a family of standards that aid the exchange of data among hospital systems and, more recently, physician practices and other types of provider systems. HL7 is used by almost every EHR vendor in the United States and its version 3 is web-based and has been adopted in several other countries around the world.

Check Your Understanding 14.5

Instructions: Match the following terms with their definitions.

1. Intranet

2. World Wide Web

3. Extranet

4. LAN

5. WAN

6. Data warehouse

7. Clients

8. Telecommunications

9. Relational database

10. Data dictionary

a. Type of database that stores data in predefined tables made up of rows and columns

b. Storage device for multiple databases that can be accessed via a single question-and-report interface

c. Type of network that works as a private Internet

d. Computer network that connects devices in a small geographical area

e. System of Internet servers that supports specially formatted documents

f. Description of the structure of a specific database

g. Type of network that allows the networks of separate organizations to communicate with one another

h. Term used to describe a system of voice and data transmission

i. Computers that are used to access shared resources in a network

j. Computer network that connects devices across a large geographical area

Electronic Commerce in Healthcare

"E-commerce is a euphemism for conducting business via Internet tools, especially the World Wide Web, and to a lesser extent, e-mail" (McLendon 2000, 22). Electronic commerce (e-commerce) has revolutionized healthcare. E-commerce uses both the web and electronic data interchange (EDI) as the means for conducting business. Traditionally a web-based platform has been used for **business-to-customer** (B2C) transactions while EDI has been used for **business-to-business** (B2B) transactions. However, with advances in web and related technologies, a web-based platform is being used increasingly for both B2C and B2B transactions.

A special task force (AHIMA e-Health Task Force 2002) predicted that e-commerce would have a tremendous impact on healthcare delivery. Specifically the task force provided the following examples:

- Increased numbers of consumers will access the Internet for information about healthcare providers, treatment options, and their own personal health information.
- Health websites will provide consumers with tools to develop and maintain their own online health records.
- Consumers and health providers will correspond via e-mail.
- Businesses and consumers will purchase supplies and equipment over the Internet.
- Health information management (HIM) business processes will use the Internet for off-site transaction processing.

All of the above examples are common today. B2B e-commerce is routinely conducted between healthcare facilities, vendors, suppliers, insurance companies, and others. B2B e-commerce focuses on improving the efficiency of providing products, services, and information among businesses. Some examples include web-enabled online claims handling, online medical supply purchasing, web-enabled medical record systems for individual physicians, and remote HIM support services such as transcription, coding, release of information, and billing to healthcare providers or organizations. Streamlining the processes involved in the ordering, purchasing, and delivery of products and services through the use of e-commerce can save millions of dollars.

B2C e-commerce today includes a variety of applications to help improve the participation of the patient in the delivery of care. Among the many healthcare examples are websites that educate consumers on disease prevention and wellness promotion, portals for communities of interest, online provider directories, customer service portals (that is, making an appointment with a healthcare provider), and portals for managing individual health information (that is, personal health records).

While the media and means of maintaining and transporting health information and services may have changed, the challenges of delivering quality information and protecting the confidentiality and security of information have not changed. HIM professionals should be in the forefront of developing standards of practice that address the security, privacy, and quality standards of health information in an e-commerce environment.

Management of Information Technology

Information technology by itself cannot fulfill its potential unless it is appropriately organized and managed as a system to meet the goals of the organization. Formal organizational structures for the planning and management of information systems are required. Modern healthcare organizations recognize that information is a critical resource to be managed as carefully as human, financial, and capital resources. In large part, the organization's ability to provide high-quality and cost-effective healthcare services depends on the availability of accurate information.

The specific organizational structure for managing information resources varies among organizations. For example, a small community-based clinic would have a different organizational structure for information systems management than a large urban acute care facility. Regardless of size, there is a set of functions that be must organized and executed to ensure information resources management. Among these are:

- Information systems strategic planning and enterprise-wide oversight of the organization's information systems functions. In smaller organizations, this responsibility might be assumed by the top manager or director with assistance from a consultant. In larger organizations, this role might be filled by a chief information officer (CIO).

- Management of the technical infrastructure and staff to support an organization's information systems including such areas as data administration, network administration, database management, and end-user support. This responsibility usually is assumed by an information systems director or department. In smaller organizations a manager may oversee these responsibilities in conjunction with a consultant or outsourcing company.

- Management of security and privacy of healthcare and other information. In larger organizations, these responsibilities are usually assumed by individuals with titles of chief security officer (CSO) and a chief privacy officer (CPO). In smaller organizations, the functions may be assumed by management staff with the assistance of consultants or professional health information managers.

- Health record information management functions such as managing health record content, retention, retrieval, diagnostic and procedural coding, and compliance with accreditation and legal standards. Management of these functions should be performed by qualified health information professionals.

Additional information on the management and organization of information system resources is provided in chapter 17.

Personal Productivity Software

Personal productivity software is software applications designed for individual use on personal computers to improve the efficiency and productivity of work. The variety and sophistication of personal productivity software has grown over the past few years. Just a decade ago these systems principally consisted of word-processing, spreadsheet, and simple database and project management applications. Today, however, productivity software consists of powerful applications brought to a user's desktop that frequently come in a bundle, called an application suite.

Many of these applications are used to support health information management functions. Therefore the HIT professional should know the purpose of these software applications and have a working knowledge of when and how to use them. Some of the more popular of these are described below.

Database Systems

Database applications designed for personal computer systems have the same purpose as the large database systems described earlier in this chapter. The principal functions of a database system are to organize and store data so that they can be readily retrieved in a meaningful way by end users.

Personal databases usually are complete database management systems and provide functions for the creation, storage, and use of data. These systems are fairly sophisticated with user-friendly interfaces that allow for easy and quick defining and development of database structures such as tables and relationships. These systems also provide functions for the development of forms, reports, screens, and queries for the input and output of data, and can be used for the development of smaller, complete applications.

These database applications are appropriate for individual, small group, or team level work. The drawback of such systems is that they do not have the flexibility, security, or performance of larger and more sophisticated systems. HITs may use this type of database application for small departmental or research projects. One of the most popular examples of this type of system is Microsoft Access.

Spreadsheets

Spreadsheets are computer applications designed for use on personal computer systems and networks and are used for business analysis, planning, and modeling. A spreadsheet is an electronic worksheet of rows and columns that simulates a paper accounting worksheet. The user designs the format of the spreadsheet by identifying variables and entering associated data. Associations between cells are defined through formulas. For example, a column of numbers can be related by a formula to sum (add) all the numbers in that column.

Most spreadsheet applications include functions for statistical analyses and for developing displays of spreadsheet data such as charts and graphs. The strength of spreadsheet software is that numerical data can be modeled and analyzed. HITs may use spreadsheets to collect and analyze data for smaller research projects or to analyze business processes associated with HIM functions. Popular spreadsheets include Microsoft Excel, IBM Lotus 1-2-3, and Apple Numbers.

Presentation Software

Presentation software is used to support a public presentation by creating multiple computer screens that display text and graphical information. Presentation software usually has functions that allow a user to insert and format text, graphics, and sound or video clips. The software allows the user to navigate from one screen to the next, in effect creating a slide show to support a presentation. Using specialized projection equipment, the slide show can be projected on a screen to accommodate large audiences. Slide shows can be uploaded as web pages and be viewed on the web. Electronic presentations can be used to supplement or replace traditional presentation materials such as chalkboards, overhead transparencies, and flip charts. HITs are likely to use presentation software in conducting privacy and security or other HIM-related training or in providing information to health-care organization staff and management. Microsoft PowerPoint is one of the most popular presentation software packages.

Project Management Software

Project management software provides functions for the planning, organizing, and managing of resources to complete a project. Most project management software includes applications for planning, scheduling, and tracking tasks through the use of automated GANTT or PERT charts. More sophisticated packages add tools to simulate the project and can readjust schedules, budget, and personnel assignments as well as provide sophisticated tracking and analysis of project progress. HITs frequently work with project teams whose management is supported by project management software. Microsoft Project is one of the most popular products for small- to medium-sized projects.

Groupware

Groupware is another category of productivity software. It helps increase efficiency within work groups and teams by facilitating the exchange of information and supporting real-time collaboration. The software can support teams who are both located onsite and off-site. Groupware can include functions that allow users to share documents, post notes, receive notifications, plan meetings and events in a group calendar, access e-mail, track schedules, and store document versions. Many groupware applications include discussion boards and chat rooms. Lotus Notes is one of the more popular groupware packages.

Real-World Case

This case is based on article in AHIMA's *79th National Convention and Exhibit Proceedings* (Nugent et al. 2007).

Developing and Implementing Telehealth Program: The VA's Story

The VA's Office of Care Coordination's (OCC) Home Telehealth (HT) Program is currently putting medical devices in patient homes to improve the quality of care and standard of living for veterans throughout the United States. Veterans use these home devices to capture various measurements including blood glucose, blood pressure, pulse from the blood pressure device, temperature, weight, pain, and pulse from the pulse oximetry device. All these measurements are obtained from measurement devices (except pain, which is subjective) that are connected to the home device. The home device sends the measurements to a national vendor server located within the VA network, and it sends those measurements to VHA systems where their VA providers can view them.

Summary

Well-managed information systems are even more critical to the success of today's healthcare organizations than ever before. Information systems are the integration of people, data, processes, and technology to affect specific outcomes. These systems can be categorized as operation support, enterprise-wide, and management systems. The traditional way to manage information systems is through the systems development life cycle. The SDLC is a four-step process that takes the organization from system planning and design through implementation and maintenance. As the seismic shift for health information rapidly continues to change from paper to electronic, the health information management professional is at the forefront in the planning, design, development, and implementation of information systems. A variety of computer hardware and software components are available to ensure the effective storage, management, and transmission of healthcare data. Moreover, advances in programming languages are enabling users to communicate with and through computers with greater ease and efficiency.

The database is the primary foundation of the electronic health record. The most important functions of any healthcare information system involve being able to create, modify, delete, and view patient data. And the most important storage mechanism used to perform these functions is a database. The relational database is the most common type of database system. Most healthcare organizations maintain several different databases to serve different functions in their day-to-day operation. These databases are managed by a collection of computer programs called a database management system. The DBMS allows different application programs to access the database. An important purpose of a DBMS is to maintain the data definitions (data dictionary) for all the data elements in the database. It also enforces data integrity and security constraints. Increasingly, healthcare organizations are using data warehousing technology to access data from different databases for analyzing patient care delivery and business processes. The health information professional provides key support in the development and maintenance of databases and data warehouses.

Healthcare organizations must also have a technology infrastructure in place that provides the users of healthcare and business data with a communications system that enables them to share information. One example of such a system is a computer network in which computers are either clients or servers. The two main types of computer network setups are local-area networks (LANS) and wide-area networks (WANs).

Electronic commerce is revolutionizing healthcare in many ways through both business-to-customer and business-to-business transactions. The impact of e-commerce growth is reflected in increased numbers of consumers accessing the Internet for information, growth of health websites, increased use of portals by healthcare organizations providing a variety of healthcare services, and increased management of the supply chain through business-to-business applications. Health information management professionals play a principal role in planning, designing, and implementing e-health applications using electronic commerce technologies.

References

AHIMA e-Health Task Force. 2002. Report on the roles and functions of e-health information management. Chicago: AHIMA.

AHIMA e-HIM Work Group on EHR Data Content. 2006. Guidelines for developing a data dictionary. *Journal of AHIMA* 77(2):64A–64D.

Anderson, J.G., and C. Aydin. 2005. *Evaluating the Organizational Impact of Health Care Information Systems,* 2nd ed. New York: Springer.

Austin, C.J., and S.B. Boxerman. 2003. *Information Systems for Health Services Administration,* 6th ed. Chicago: Health Administration Press.

Davenport, T.H., and J. Glaser. 2002. Just-in-time delivery comes to knowledge management. *Harvard Business Review* 80(7).

Durkin, S., and B. Just. 2008. An IT primer for health information exchange. *Journal of AHIMA* 79(1):38–42.

Farishta, M. 2001. More than a database: Mining your data for decision-making success. *Journal of AHIMA* 72(10):28–32.

Friedman, C.P., and J.C. Wyatt. 1997. *Evaluation Methods in Medical Informatics.* New York: Springer.

Gaudreau, E., and D. Palermo. 2009. EHR fast track: Fundamentals of rapid implementation planning. *Journal of AHIMA* 80(8):40–43.

Hutchinson, S.E., and S.C. Sawyer. 2000. *Computers, Communications & Information.* Boston: Irwin McGraw-Hill.

Johns, M. 1999. The electronic health record process for health services delivery. In *Electronic Health Records: Changing the Vision,* edited by G.F. Murphy, M.A. Hanken, and K.L. Waters. Philadelphia: W.B. Saunders.

Johns, M.L. 1997. *Information Management for Health Professions.* Albany, NY: Delmar.

Johns, M.L. 2002. *Information Management for Health Professions,* 2nd ed. Albany, NY: Delmar Thomson Learning.

Kohn, D. 2009. How information technology supports virtual HIM departments. *Journal of AHIMA* 80(3):Web extra.

McLendon, K. 2000. E-commerce and HIM: Ready or not, here it comes. *Journal of AHIMA* 71(1):22–23.

Merrill, M. 2009. MIT ventures explore cell phone use in developing countries. *Healthcare IT News.* http://www.healthcareitnews.com/news/mit-ventures-explore-cell-phone-use-developing-countries

Nugent, L., M. Johnson, D. Maloney, and P. Goyal. 2007. Developing and implementing telehealth program: The VA's story. *AHIMA's 79th National Convention and Exhibit Proceedings.*

O'Brien, J.A. 2002. *Management Information Systems: Managing Information Technology in the E-Business Enterprise.* New York: McGraw-Hill.

Shakir, A.M. 1999. Tools for defining data. *Journal of AHIMA* 70(8):48–53.

Shimrat, O. 2009. Cloud computing and healthcare: Bad weather or sunny forecast. http://www.himss.org/content/files/Code%2093_Shimrat_CloudComputingandHealthcare_2009.pdf

Wager, K.A., F.W. Lee, and J.P. Glaser. 2005. *Managing Health Care Information Systems: A Practical Approach for Health Care Executives.* San Francisco: Jossey-Bass.

Weed, L. 1991. *Knowledge Coupling.* New York: Springer-Verlag.

Wold, G.H., and R.F. Shriver. 1994. *The Healthcare Systems Planning Manual: Evaluating, Selecting, and Implementing Information Systems throughout the Organization.* Chicago: Probus Publishing.

Additional Resources

Amatayakul, M. 1999. *The Role of Health Information Managers in CPR Projects.* Chicago: AHIMA.

Andrews, D., and S. Stalick. 2000. BPR project management: A radical approach to project team organization. *American Programmer* 8(6).

Briggs, B. 1999. *1999 Comprehensive Guide to Electronic Health Records.* Edited by B. Hoehn. New York: Faulkner and Gray.

Burke, L., and B. Weill. 2000. *Information Technology for the Health Professions.* New York: Prentice-Hall.

DeJesus, E. 2000. The wireless e-connection. *Healthcare Informatics* 2:67–70.

Duggan, C.M. 2004. The constancy of change. *Journal of AHIMA* 75(1):40.

Goodman, P.S. 2000. Hello, Internet? Talking Web sites next challenge. *Washington Post.*

Hoehn, B, ed. 1999. *1999 Comprehensive Guide to Electronic Health Records.* New York: Faulkner and Gray.

Loshin, D. 2004. Issues and opportunities in data quality management coordination. *DM Review Magazine.*

Morneau, K. 2000. *MCSD Guide to Solutions Architectures.* Boston: Thompson Course Technology.

Nakamoto, G. 2000. Building a legacy system. *Health Management Technology* 21(10):56.

Rollins, G. 2009. ARRA and the HIM workforce. *Journal of AHIMA* 80(10):26–30.

Welch, J.J. 1999. CPR systems: Which one is right for your organization? *Journal of AHIMA* 70(8):24–26.

chapter 15

Introduction to Electronic Health Information Systems

Nanette B. Sayles, EdD, RHIA, CCS, CHPS, CPHIMS, FAHIMA

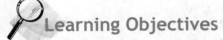

Learning Objectives

- Describe the evolution of information systems in healthcare
- Identify the three major types of information system applications and their general functions used in healthcare organizations
- Discuss the purpose, functions, and use of the major types of clinical information systems
- Describe the purpose and function of the major types of electronic systems that support administrative functions in a healthcare organization
- Describe information resource management
- Identify the key roles needed to manage information resources effectively
- Understand the organizational structure utilized in information resource management
- Identify the purpose, function, and trends of information systems in nonacute healthcare settings
- Recognize emerging trends affecting the development of healthcare information systems
- Understand the role of the health information technician in information systems planning and development

Key Terms

Administrative information systems

Admission-discharge-transfer (ADT)

Aggregate information

Ambulatory care information system

Barcode-enabled devices

Care pathways

Chief financial officer (CFO)

Chief information officer (CIO)

Chief information security officer (CISO)

Chief medical informatics officer (CMIO)

Chief privacy officer

Clinical decision support system (CDSS)

Clinical information systems (CIS)

Comparative information

Computerized provider order entry (CPOE)

Computers on wheels (COWs)

Data mart

Data mining

Data warehouse

Digital dictation

Electronic document management system (EDMS)

Electronic medication administration record (eMAR)

Enterprise content and record management (ECRM)

Executive information system (EIS)

Expert knowledge-based information

Financial information system

Home health information system

Information resource management (IRM)

Information services department

Interoperability

Laboratory information system (LIS)

Long-term care information system

Management information system (MIS)

Materials management system

Nursing information system (NIS)

Online analytical processing (OLAP)

Patient-specific information

Pharmacy information system

Picture archiving and communication systems (PACSs)

Point-of-care charting

Radiology information system (RIS)

Strategic decision support system

Structured data

Telematics

Telesurgery

Unstructured data

Introduction

Healthcare information systems (ISs) run the gamut from patient-specific clinical ISs to administrative or financial systems to fully integrated systems that combine clinical and administrative/financial information. Such systems can exist within a single institution or across organizations. The development and use of healthcare information systems is not new. ISs were first introduced in healthcare in the 1960s. Since then, advances in computer technology, coupled with the increasing demand for clinical and administrative information, have grown exponentially. Despite these advances, however, many healthcare organizations today continue to maintain paper-based health record systems.

The reasons for the predominance of paper-based health records are many. Healthcare organizations are enormously complex, both in their organizational structure and in terms of the information they manage. The complexity makes it difficult to implement healthcare information systems effectively. Healthcare ISs can be costly to implement and support, and many small providers may not have the resources or technical expertise to maintain and support them. Unprecedented attention at the national level has been directed toward the expanded use of information technology (IT) in healthcare and, most recently, the adoption of electronic health records (EHRs). This push toward the EHR is driving the implementation of supporting systems such as those described in this chapter. For information on EHR and related federal initiatives, please see chapter 16.

In addition to the national and regional efforts, a great deal of work must be done at the institutional level. Healthcare organizations must adopt appropriate planning strategies and methods and put the necessary resources in place to support any healthcare IS, large or small. Selecting the most up-to-date and appropriate IS is not always adequate to ensure successful implementation of a new system. Healthcare organizations must continually evaluate the extent to which their ISs are meeting the needs of users. Sufficient financial, personnel, and other resources must be available to support the system and its users.

Health information management (HIM) professionals play an important role in the selection, development, implementation, and support of healthcare ISs. Their roles depend on individual work responsibilities and on the size, scope, and complexity of the organization in which they work. In one setting, a health information technician (HIT) whose main responsibility is coding may be asked to participate in evaluating an automated coding system as a component of an integrated health record system. In another setting, an HIT in a supervisory position may offer input on user needs and expectations of an EHR system. Regardless of the setting, HIM professionals should understand the major types of healthcare ISs available, the process of selecting and implementing such systems, and the resources needed to support them.

Chapter 16 discusses the evolution, development, and implementation of the electronic health record. This chapter gives a general overview of the types of clinical systems that support the EHR, cites examples of other electronic systems that support the operations of a healthcare enterprise, and discusses the usual organizational structures that support the management of all of these systems. Specifically, the chapter reviews the history of healthcare ISs and describes the major IS applications used by healthcare organizations and HIM departments today. This discussion includes a description of the people, policies, and organizational structure needed to manage information resources in today's healthcare environment. Several examples that demonstrate the importance of appropriate planning and user buy-in also are offered.

Theory into Practice

John Smith, a Medicare patient, went to his physician office yesterday. The physician ordered some tests and was able to schedule the tests for today through the hospital's central registration. When John arrived at the hospital for the tests, he went to centralized registration and registered for the chest x-ray and a complete blood count. Even though John had never been to this facility, he only had to provide a minimum amount of information since his physician's ambulatory care information system had exchanged electronically his demographic and insurance information as well as the physician orders with the hospital.

John had the tests performed and went home. A radiology information system was used to manage the chest x-ray and a laboratory information system was used to manage the complete blood count. The x-ray taken was digital which allowed the radiologist to review it through a picture archival and communications system. The radiologist used a digital dictation system to dicate the x-ray report. Two days later, John received a phone call from the physician's office telling him the results of his tests. John was able to get the test results quickly because the physician office had been sent the test results electronically from the hospital laboratory. The physician had reviewed the test results and notified the nurse electronically to call the patient. The physician also prescribed a new medication, which was submitted electronically to the pharmacy and was waiting for pickup by John. The coder used the encoder and grouper to assign the code number and the Ambulatory Payment Classifications. The codes were submitted electronically by the financial information system. After Medicare paid the hospital for John's care, the financial information system submitted a bill to John for his share.

Evolution of Information Systems in Healthcare

Information systems (ISs) are not new to healthcare. Early automated systems were implemented almost 50 years ago. Despite this long history, the majority of health record systems in place today are still predominately paper-based (Hillestad et al. 2005). An overview of the evolution of healthcare ISs may explain why full implementation is taking so long (figure 15.1).

The first computer systems used in healthcare date to the early 1960s. A small number of hospitals began to develop in-house administrative and/or financial systems. The systems were used primarily to perform payroll and patient accounting functions (Glandon et al. 2008). The reason these early systems focused on financial applications was primarily

Figure 15.1.   Evolution of healthcare information systems

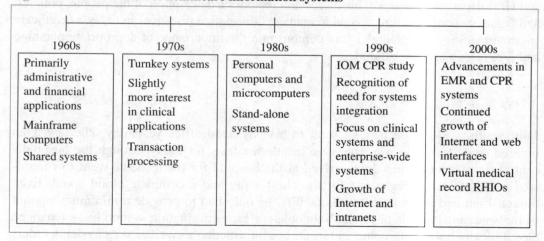

1960s	1970s	1980s	1990s	2000s
Primarily administrative and financial applications Mainframe computers Shared systems	Turnkey systems Slightly more interest in clinical applications Transaction processing	Personal computers and microcomputers Stand-alone systems	IOM CPR study Recognition of need for systems integration Focus on clinical systems and enterprise-wide systems Growth of Internet and intranets	Advancements in EMR and CPR systems Continued growth of Internet and web interfaces Virtual medical record RHIOs

because financial applications were being used in other industries and it made sense to transfer this technology to healthcare.

The nature and scope of computer technology at the time also supported data-processing systems rather than more sophisticated information systems (Johns 2002). Hospitals with sufficient resources maintained data-processing departments with in-house computer programmers. The data-processing unit typically reported to the finance department or the **chief financial officer** (CFO) because healthcare institutions relied on revenue generation and volume-of-service statistics. This reporting structure may have contributed to the slow growth of clinical information systems (Johns 2002). The administrative and financial systems used in hospitals during this era ran on large, centralized mainframe computers. The cost of the computers made it prohibitively expensive to develop multiple departmental systems (Kennedy et al. 1992).

Development of Clinical Systems

By the 1980s, healthcare institutions were beginning to change their focus from maximizing revenues to minimizing expenses. There was still a financial focus, but more progress was being made in the development of clinical systems. Hospitals were under pressure to decrease their average lengths of stay and to shift patient care from inpatient to outpatient settings. Clinical departments also were under pressure to increase productivity.

At the same time, advances were being made in computer technology. The development of personal computers, enabled healthcare institutions to purchase relatively inexpensive desktop computers. The new computers had computing power and storage capacity equivalent to that of the early mainframe computers.

Stand-alone systems supported functional tasks for specific departments and units. Departments controlled their own information because they collected and maintained it. However, the use of stand-alone systems led to duplication of effort and redundant files. There was little, if any, effort to integrate the data among systems. Even today, hospitals and other healthcare organizations struggle with integrating data from separate ISs within the same organization.

The early 1990s brought further changes in the healthcare industry with the advent of market-driven healthcare reform, the growth of managed care, and the development of integrated delivery systems. As a result, much more attention was given to the development of clinical systems and the integration of clinical and financial data for decision-making purposes. **Clinical information systems** (CISs) collect and store information related to patient care (Sayles and Trawick 2010). Little clinical information was collected and maintained, and few clinical information systems were available during this time. Clinical information systems will be discussed in more detail later in this chapter.

Electronic Health Record Systems

In 1991, the Institute of Medicine (IOM) published its landmark report outlining the need for computer-based patient record (CPR) systems (Glandon et al. 2008). The IOM report brought national attention to the problems with paper-based systems. It also challenged private and public sectors to work together to develop an electronic, longitudinal health record. The goal of developing longitudinal records was to capture information about the health of individuals throughout their lifetime.

By the late 1990s, the widespread use of home computers and the Internet began to change how healthcare institutions delivered services and managed health-related information. The growth of the World Wide Web (WWW) and other Internet technologies led to the development of easy-to-access healthcare ISs in many organizations. These systems range from web pages that provide consumers with information on health issues and the services provided by the sponsoring healthcare organization to sophisticated, interactive, web-based clinical ISs.

The electronic health record (EHR) is defined as "An electronic record of health-related information on an individual that conforms to nationally recognized interoperability standards and that can be created, managed, and consulted by authorized clinicians and staff across more than one healthcare organization" (AHIMA 2012, 119). With the EHR, clinicians and others no longer need to be physically present in the healthcare organization to view or even record patient data. Web interfaces have led to the development of virtual health records. In these systems, the web-based interface brings together information from different databases and data repositories, links the data by patient, and displays them on a single workstation. These different databases come from many of the systems described in this chapter.

Chapter 16 provides a detailed description of the evolution, development, and implementation of the EHR.

Electronic Healthcare Information Applications

Many IS applications are used in healthcare today and can be classified in many ways. For simplicity's sake, this chapter groups them into four broad categories:

- Clinical information systems
- Administrative information systems
- Management support systems
- Research and data analytics systems

Many of the functions identified for the following categories apply regardless of whether the system supports healthcare delivery in an inpatient or outpatient setting. Clinical ISs include systems that support patient care including the following functions:

- EMRs, EHRs, and CPRs
- Patient care management
- Computerized provider order entry (CPOE)

- Results reporting
- Nursing services
- Departmental clinical management
- Laboratory services
- Medication administration (using barcoding technology)
- Pharmacy services
- Radiology services
- Clinical decision support

Administrative information systems, which support the business functions of the organization, have the following functions:

- Patient registration
- Financial management
- Human resource management
- Materials management
- Facilities management

Management support systems, which assist in organizational planning, are applied in the following areas:

- Executive decision making
- Financial modeling
- Planning and marketing
- Resource allocation (labor, supplies, and facilities planning)
- Expert systems

Research and data analytics systems, which turn data into information, are used to:

- Study diseases
- Analyze data
- Perform research

To realize the full potential of each system, the system must be fully integrated. In other words, it must be possible to combine information from any system with information from any other system. For example, when healthcare practitioners are expected to control costs and provide high-quality care at the same time, they must have access to both clinical *and* financial information. Access to both types of data allows the facility to analyze their services to determine many things such as which services are profitable and which ones suffer losses. Similarly, when administrators are making difficult decisions about the future direction of their enterprises, they need access to decision support systems that provide timely, relevant, and meaningful clinical and administrative information.

The following section discusses the various types of ISs as well as some other IS applications that are commonly used in healthcare facilities. It should be kept in mind that the goal in today's healthcare environment is to create fully integrated ISs. Although these systems can be described as separate entities with specific functions, they should be viewed as part of the enterprise-wide IS.

Clinical Information Systems

One of the major categories of information systems used in healthcare is the clinical information system. Clinical ISs are designed primarily to support patient care by providing healthcare practitioners with access to timely, complete, and relevant clinical information. Healthcare practitioners use clinical information to diagnose, treat, and manage patient care.

In addition to patient care, clinical ISs also may be used for quality improvement, peer review, research, and other purposes. Clinical ISs include a broad range of applications such as patient records, patient care management, departmental clinical management (also known as ancillary systems), computerized provider order entry, medication administration, and clinical decision support. All of these systems and more feed the EHR (figure 15.2).

Patient Registration Systems

According to the Office of the National Coordinator,

> Going to the doctor or hospital often requires filling out multiple forms. These forms collect information such as name, address, insurance, medications, allergies, etc. Then, when an individual requires lab work or other testing, the same information has to be collected again. A single electronic health registration will make it easier for individuals to give their information and for clinicians to use it. Additionally, the consumer could update the information once and share it with all providers immediately as needed (ONC 2006).

Today, most hospitals and other healthcare facilities use computer systems for registering patients and tracking their encounters that require multiple points for data input. Within hospitals, these systems are commonly known as **admission-discharge-transfer** (ADT) systems or registration-admission-discharge-transfer (R-ADT) systems. Diagnostic

Figure 15.2. **Source systems feeding data to the inpatient EHR**

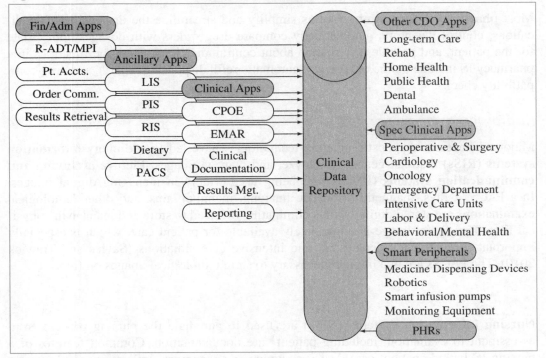

Copyright © 2012, Margret\A Consulting, LLC.

and length of stay (LOS) information also can be stored in ADT systems. In ambulatory care and outpatient settings, similar registration systems are used to collect relevant demographic and insurance information.

Patient registration systems must be linked with other ancillary departments in order to coordinate the patient's care. Similarly, they are often used to generate a set of documents that require the patient's signature. Examples of such documents are a consent to treatment, an authorization to release medical information for insurance purposes, and advance directives for care. Chapter 7 provides additional information about the operation of these systems and the role of the HIM professional in management of them.

Laboratory Information Systems

Laboratory information systems (LISs) are used for collecting, verifying, and reporting test results. Systems today use computer technology to process specimens and analyze data, monitor test quality, control inventory, monitor workflow, and assess laboratory productivity (Sayles and Trawick 2010).

Pharmacy Information Systems

Most **pharmacy information systems** simplify and streamline the dispensing of medications, control inventory, automatically compare drug orders with dosages appropriate for the patient, and provide information about contraindications. Common functions in a pharmacy IS include online order entry, automatic refill dispensing reports, and drug compatibility checks.

Radiology Information Systems

Major advances in diagnostic imaging technologies have led to **radiology information systems** (RISs) that can generate, analyze, and manage images. **Picture archiving and communication systems** (PACSs) are being used widely in managing digital images. In a PACS, x-rays, magnetic resonance imaging, mammograms, and other radiological examinations are stored digitally, thus eliminating the need to store and manage the physical film. The digital image is immediately available for patient care, which is especially important in emergency department and intensive care situations (Sayles and Trawick 2010). The PACSs are making it unnecessary to store radiological images on film.

Nursing Information Systems

Nursing information systems (NISs) are used to automate the nursing process from assessment to evaluation, including patient care documentation. Common features of a nursing IS include patient care decision support, management applications, and nursing education and research.

Emergency Medical Systems

Emergency medical systems provide the necessary information to healthcare providers in the emergency room. Not only would the emergency medical system include patient information, it would also include decision support alerts based on the patient's illness, charting functionality, and workflow support. The emergency medical systems would also provide the patient with discharge instructions and follow-up information (Hebda and Czar 2009).

Patient Monitoring Systems

Patient monitoring systems automatically collect and store patient data from various systems used in healthcare. These systems include:

- Fetal monitoring
- Vital signs
- Oxygen saturation rates

Patient monitoring systems are typically used in the intensive care units and other specialty areas such as operating and recovery rooms (Sayles and Trawick 2010).

Electronic Clinical Order Entry and Results Reporting

A **computerized provider order entry** (CPOE) system is a computer application that accepts physician orders electronically, replacing handwritten or verbal orders and prescriptions. Most CPOE systems provide physicians with decision-support capabilities during the ordering process and are used to facilitate patient care and decrease medical errors (Sayles and Trawick 2010). The CPOE utilizes alerts and reminders to assist the care provider in the decision-making process.

Alerts are a type of decision support that uses messages to notify the user of a problem. For example the problem may be that a contraindicated medication is being ordered or that the patient is allergic to the medication, or even that the physician needs to order lab tests to monitor the blood level of a particular medication. As more documentation is performed electronically (and because it has been demonstrated that alerts improve patient safety), the use of alerts is becoming increasingly important.

Reminders notify the care provider of care that should be provided. For example, if a patient is 50 or older, the system may remind the provider that the patient is due for a colonoscopy.

Electronic Documentation

Many clinical information systems support the electronic documentation of patient information. These systems are specially designed to meet the needs of the users such as nurses, physicians, respiratory therapy, and more. The documentation systems may use structured data entry, free text, or templates (which is a combination of both).

Structured data entry allows the user to pick and choose from predesigned selections, such as male and female for the gender field. Free text allows the user to type in any information necessary to describe the patient's care. Templates utilize both structured data entry and free text and are designed based on the needs of the user (Sayles and Trawick 2010).

To meet the needs of a user, for example, a template for documenting the history and physical might be developed. Each body system would be listed and common entries for each body system would be listed. The physician would point and click to document a cough, heart murmur, and more. **Point-of-care charting** (POC) is documentation performed at the bedside or wherever the patient is located. From the bedside, the care provider can order tests and medication, document care provided, and review documentation made by other members of the healthcare team. There may be separate systems for physicians, nurses, physical therapists, respiratory therapists, and others. These systems may use bedside terminals, personal digital assistants, and other wireless devices to allow for the care provider to document in the health record as the information is obtained from the patient. Handheld wireless devices are frequently utilized (LaTour and Eichenwald-Maki 2010). The quality of the documentation is improved as patient care is documented immediately rather than later when the details of the care may become forgotten. One form of POC is **computers on wheels** (COWs), which involves a computer on a moveable cart that can be moved from patient to patient. One of the advantages of POC charting is that it utilizes alerts and reminders to assist the care provider in providing the best care possible for patients by identifying problems before they can occur (Amatayakul 2009).

These systems generally allow entry of both structured and unstructured data. **Structured data** are generally found in checkboxes, drop-down boxes, and other data entry means whereby the user chooses from options already built into the system. **Unstructured data,** also called narrative data, can be entered in a free text format by the user usually by typing (Amatayakul 2009).

Unstructured Data Entry

Unstructured data is also called narrative or free text data. It is usually entered using a keyboard, but other methods such as dictation or voice recognition may also be used (Amatayakul 2009). Unstructured data allows the data entered to be more specific and detailed for each patient than structured data. In these fields, the provider could enter a patient's history of present illness, level of compliance with medical regimen, or anything else not captured in the structured data. The level of detail is much greater with unstructured data because the choices designed in the system are not limited. The user can use his/her own words. A disadvantage of unstructured data is that it is not beneficial for reporting purposes. Because unstructured data does not have a data model, it is difficult for the system to identify and gather desired information provided in a report.

Structured Data Entry

Drop-down lists, check boxes, radio buttons, and other forms of controlled data entry are used in structured data entry. The choices must be clearly defined, comprehensive, and applicable. Use of structured data entry allows quickness, but there is a learning curve in the beginning while users get familiar with the choices and the graphical user interface (GUI) (Amatayakul 2009). AHIMA defines a GUI as a "style of computer interface in which typed commands are replaced by images that represent tasks (for example, small pictures [icons] that represent the tasks, functions, and programs performed by a software program)" (2012, 149). For example, when entering a patient's gender, the options would be male and female or if the data being entered were the number of dilation centimeters for an obstetric patient, the choices would range from 0 to 10.

Structured data entry is frequently used for physician EHRs, with the menus developed specifically for the physicians' medical or surgical specialty. Because it is easy for the user to overlook entry, defaults should not populate an entry but rather should be left blank and force the user to address the field. The EHR should be able to convert structured data into a narrative format (Amatayakul 2009). An example would be structured data of "no tobacco use" and "no alcohol use" converts to "Patient denies the use of tobacco and alcohol". One of the advantages of structured data is that it can easily be used for reporting purposes. Data can also be graphed allowing for trending. An example of the use of graphing is the ability to trend blood sugar or blood pressure levels over time.

Template-Based Entry

Templates are a cross between free text and structured data entry. The user is able to pick and choose data that are entered frequently, thus requiring the entry of data that change from patient to patient (Amatayakul 2009). Templates can be customized to meet the needs of the organization as data needs change by physician specialty, patient type (surgical/medical/newborn), disease, and other classification of patients. Templates may be used to cut and paste words from one note and place them into another note, thus saving time. This option should be used judiciously because the wrong data could be copied and/or pasted into the wrong patient's record. All templates have predefined parameters that are checked as data are entered. They can check for logic but not accuracy (Amatayakul 2009). For example, it can prevent a data entry that shows a patient has a temperature of 200°F, but would not catch entering 100.4°F instead of 100.8°F. Also, too many checks can slow down the system, so templates should be used judiciously.

As the documentation is entered, the care provider is able to access clinical practice guidelines. Clinical practice guidelines are recommendations for the patient's care. They are embedded into documentation systems, which allows the care provider to consult them quickly and easily. There are challenges in embedding guidelines into documentation systems because there are differences in documentation and terminology and problems translating the detailed clinical guidelines into a format appropriate for the computer (LaTour and Eichenwald-Maki 2010). Physicians, nurses, and other healthcare professionals follow standards of care when they treat patients. **Care pathways** merge these standards of care together to integrate and improve the care provided to the patient. The pathway would indicate treatments to be performed, tests and medications to order, monitoring to be performed, and more by each member of the healthcare team.

Care pathways are different from clinical practice guidelines in two ways. First care pathways are used by multidisciplinary teams. The care pathways also consider the quality of care provided as well as coordination of the care provided to the patient (Open Clinical, nd).

Electronic Medication Administration Systems

Like CPOE systems, **electronic medication administration record** (eMAR) systems are barcode-enabled point-of-care software designed to improve patient safety. **Barcode-enabled devices** when utilized at the point of care, ensure that the right patient gets the right dose at the right time and through the right route. Medication administration systems that use barcode-enabled point-of-care technology can be highly effective in reducing all types of medication errors (Sayles and Trawick 2010). For example, if a nurse is about to administer an incorrect medication or an incorrect dosage of a medication, the system can notify the nurse of the error before the medication is administered.

Clinical Decision Support Systems

The more advanced clinical information systems generally include decision support capabilities. **Clinical decision support systems** (CDSS) assist healthcare providers in the actual diagnosis and treatment of patients. CDS systems integrate data from a number of systems to assist with charting, CPOE, and identifying drug contraindications. The CDSS uses alerts and reminders to assist heathcare providers in decision making (LaTour and Eichenwald-Maki 2010). As discussed above, a message can be triggered by an information system to notify the healthcare provider of information required to provide quality care (Amatayakul 2009). Reminders notify the healthcare provider of tests or other bits of information necessary for quality care. These alerts or reminders can perform a wide range of functions, from indicating potential drug interactions to recommending a plan of care based on the patient's health history and clinical assessment.

Studies have shown that CDS systems can save lives, reduce healthcare costs, improve communication, increase clinician and patient satisfaction, and enhance the overall process of care (Bates and Gawande 2003).

Electronic Document Management Systems

Electronic document management systems (EDMSs) scan documents into the computer and create a picture of the document. This image can be retrieved by any authorized user from essentially any location. Multiple users can also view the same image at the same time, enhancing communication between care providers. The scanned document cannot be searched, edited, or changed. Although an EDMS is not an EHR, it is a valuable tool for healthcare facilities that do not have the space needed to store paper records and that do not want to use microfilm. Many of the healthcare facilities that elect to implement an EDMS use it as an intermediate step toward the EHR (Sayles and Trawick 2010). EDMS is also used in the EHR to accommodate documents that come from outside the organization or that must be signed by the patient. A number of advantages exist, such as immediate access to patient information, space savings, and multiple users can access the same patient or even the same document at the same time. Chapter 7 provides a detailed discussion of these types of systems.

Digital Dictation

The **digital dictation** system is used by physicians and other healthcare providers to dictate various medical reports such as the operative report, history and physical, and the discharge summary. The dictation may be transcribed by a transcriptionist, but if the facility utilizes voice recognition, the voice is automatically converted into text, which must be reviewed by an editor to ensure that the voice was converted correctly (Sayles and Trawick 2010). Chapter 7 provides a detailed discussion about digital dictation.

Multimedia and Telematics Systems

In today's digital age, multimedia and telematic systems are an important part of healthcare. **Telematics** systems, which may also be called telehealth, can be defined as "the use of telecommunication technologies and computers to exchange healthcare information and to provide services to clients at another location" (Hebda and Czar 2009). These locations can be across town or across the world. Most specialists are located in urban areas, leaving patients in rural areas without easy access to them. Telehealth allows a physician to examine and treat a patient without either party traveling. Multimedia is often used in telehealth and can utilize video, telephone, images, audio, and more to be able to evaluate and diagnose a patient. A nurse may be required to interact directly with the patient in order to support the physician's evaluation and treatment.

Physicians find clinical telehealth a benefit in giving patients living in rural areas or those who are homebound medical consultations and monitoring. Telemonitoring is used at the patient's home to monitor cardiac rhythms, blood sugar, blood pressure, and other values to be submitted to the care provider. This type of monitoring can be performed through the use of the telephone or the computer. The data collected at the patient's home are digitally submitted into a CIS and thus made a part of the EHR.

Telehealth is a very sophisticated technology. Technology used includes virtual reality and robotics, which may be used to assist with the examination or treatment of a patient. Virtual reality is the use of technology to make the user feel a part of the situation. In this situation, the physician or other care provider would feel like he is in the same room with the patient. The use of robotics to perform surgery is called **telesurgery.** This allows surgery to be performed on a patient in a different location (Sayles and Trawick 2010).

One of the newest technologies is a shirt that monitors a patient's blood pressure, temperature, and other vital signs. This shirt can also determine the location and position (such as standing or sitting) of the patient. This shirt can also allow healthcare professionals to monitor the patient remotely (iHealthBeat 2011).

Telehealth provides many advantages such as improved access to care, treatment provided via communication tools, and home monitoring. The problem is that the infrastructure is expensive and because physicians are licensed to practice medicine by state, the geographic range in which the physician can consult is limited.

Toward an Electronic Health Record System

The transition from the paper-based health record to the EHR is a complex endeavor, usually taking years to achieve. As noted earlier a small percentage of hospitals in the United States have comprehensive EHRs. Many healthcare facilities are currently operating in a hybrid environment. In a hybrid environment, some of the health record is still paper-based while other components are electronic. Some of these electronic systems communicate with each other while others do not. For example, a transcribed report is frequently accessible through the EHR, but the inpatient EHR and outpatient EHR may not share information between the two. A healthcare organization will have multiple information systems that must be able to share information. Figure 15.3 shows the various formats used in the electronic health record during this time of hybrid records. Chapter 7 provides a detailed examination of hybrid systems and the role of the HIM professional in managing paper, hybrid, and electronic systems.

One of the popular concepts in the industry now is interoperability. The NCVHS defines **interoperability** as "the ability of one computer system to exchange data with another computer system" (2000, 8). This sharing of information along with standardization is necessary for all of the systems to work together, thus providing us with a seamless integration of data."

Figure 15.3.   **Formats used in the hybrid health record**

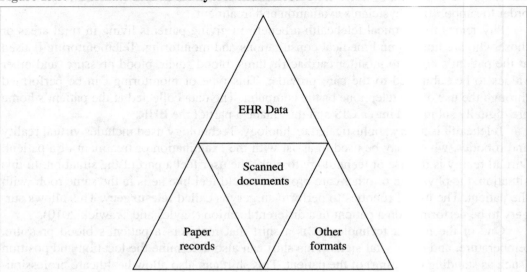

Check Your Understanding 15.1

1. Which clinical information system assists the physician in recording orders and in the decision-making process?

   A. Clinical provider order entry
   B. Order entry/results reporting
   C. Clinical decision support system
   D. Point-of-care charting

2. I need a system that allows me to treat patients located at a different site. I should use:

   A. Patient monitoring system
   B. Multi-professional care pathways
   C. Clinical decision support systems
   D. Telematics

3. A medication being ordered is contraindicated due to a patient allergy. The physician is notified. This is an example of a(n):

   A. Reminder
   B. Order entry/results reporting
   C. Alert
   D. Clinical decision support system

4. Dr. Rogers is sitting in his home office and reviewing digital images from a patient's MRI. He must be using a(n):
   A. Laboratory information system
   B. Radiology information system
   C. Picture archival communication system
   D. Electronic documentation

5. Which of the following systems would be an intermediate step toward the EHR?
   A. Digital dictation
   B. Multi-professional care pathways
   C. Electronic document management system
   D. Point-of-care documentation

Instructions: Indicate whether the following statements are true or false (T or F).

6. _____ I need to look up the results of an H1N1 blood test. I would look this up on an emergency medical system.

7. _____ A clinical decision support system will identify a medication contraindication.

8. _____ Electronic document management system is the same as the EHR.

9. _____ Telematics is an example of a clinical information system.

10. _____ Embedded guidelines are recommendations for patient care.

Administrative Information Systems

Administrative information systems comprise another major category of IS used in healthcare. Often called management information systems (MISs), these systems are used to manage the financial, personnel, materials, facilities, and other resources used in the delivery of healthcare services. In other words, administrative information systems support the daily management-related operations of the healthcare enterprise. Additional information about some of these systems such as MIS, EIS, and DSS is provided in chapter 14.

Financial Information Systems

As discussed earlier, administrative systems and financial information systems were the first computer systems used by healthcare organizations. **Financial information systems** typically include functions such as payroll preparation and accounting; accounts payable; patient accounting, including billing and accounts receivable processing; cost accounting;

general ledger accounting; budgeting; and financial statement preparation (Malec 1998). All these functions provide essential information to the healthcare managers who plan, monitor, and control the financial resources of the enterprise.

Human Resource Management Systems

Today, personnel expenses make up 60 to 70 percent of the operating budgets of healthcare institutions. Consequently, healthcare managers rely increasingly on ISs not only to maintain personnel records, but also to enable them to create management reports.

A wide range of human resource management applications are available. Reports can be created to track staff productivity, analyze labor expenses by cost center, monitor turnover and absenteeism, assess training and continuing education needs, and forecast staffing needs. Some healthcare organizations use human resource management programs to review applicants' qualifications and experience and match them with current job openings.

Materials Management Systems

Healthcare organizations also use computer systems to manage materials and supplies. **Materials management systems** may include electronic purchasing and inventory control software and barcoding and wireless devices for tracking supplies and materials. The benefits of using materials management systems include cost savings, reductions in inventory, greater efficiency, fewer lost charges, and lower labor costs (LaTour and Eichenwald-Maki 2010).

Facilities Management Systems

In today's competitive environment, well-maintained physical facilities are critical to providing high-quality patient care and a safe, comfortable environment for patients and their families. In fact, in recent years, many healthcare organizations have invested considerable resources in upgrading their physical facilities in an effort to make patients feel more at home. Automated facilities management systems can help organizations plan, manage, and maintain physical facilities. Common functions include preventative maintenance, energy management, and project management and scheduling (Malec 1998).

Management Information Systems

Management information systems (MISs) focus on providing reports and information to managers for day-to-day operations of the organization. The types of common reports produced by an MIS include:

- *Periodic scheduled reports:* Periodic scheduled reports are the most traditional type of reporting system. The content and the time schedule for production of the reports are prespecified. Examples of periodic scheduled reports are the daily hospital census and the financial monthly reports of the organization. The content and the format of these reports are specified in advance, as is the time period in which they will be produced.

- *Exception reports:* An MIS also may include reports that are produced only when exceptional or out-of-the-ordinary conditions are met or occur. An example of an exception report is an accounting report of past-due bills. In this case, the report is only generated for accounts that are past due. The out-of-the-ordinary occurrence and content and format of the report are predefined, and only cases or records meeting the predefined criteria are reported.

- *Demand reports:* As opposed to periodic and exception reports, demand reports, also known as ad hoc, are produced as needed, whenever a manager demands or asks for it. Usually, demand reports are produced through report generators or database query languages and are customized by the manager.

Strategic Decision Support System

Another category of management reports is the **strategic decision support system,** otherwise known as a decision support system (DSS). There are several differences between an MIS and a DSS. A DSS is geared toward supporting strategic decisions of managers, analysts, and executives, whereas the MIS produces reports for operational and tactical decision making. MIS reports are less dynamic than DSS reports. DSSs are interactive systems that allow managers and analysts to manipulate data using analytical models and statistical techniques. The benefit to the DSS is that it may be used to allocate resources or improve overall operations and efficiency within the healthcare enterprise. One way of improving operations and efficiency is to ask what-if questions. For example, if the manager of the emergency department wanted to determine the best staffing pattern to ensure that patients are seen as quickly as possible, he or she might enter the number of patient visits, the type of visit (emergency or urgent), and the top waiting period in minutes. Using a mathematical or statistical model, the DSS could calculate the optimal number and mix of employees (physicians, nurses, and technicians) needed to staff the emergency department.

Some common features of DSS systems include the ability to:

- Monitor and evaluate key performance indicators and trends

- Perform simulations of revenue and expense patterns based on various assumptions

- Estimate potential demand for services within different market areas

Although these systems are not currently used as widely as clinical and administrative ISs, they are emerging as a vital resource that helps healthcare executives make sound strategic decisions.

Executive Information Systems

Executive Information Systems (EISs) are a type of decision support system used by high-level managers. Like other decision support systems, an EIS draws data from the organization's other databases. An executive information system combines many of the features of the management information and decision support systems. It can produce standard, scheduled, and periodic reports but is not limited to producing them. Executive information systems are easier to use than decision support systems. For example, they allow executives to choose from among numerous tabular or graphical formats. The EIS is programmed to reorganize and distill large quantities of data into a form that meets the executive's information needs. Another important feature of an EIS is a capability called *drill down*. Drill down enables the user to find even more detailed information. For example, a CEO reading a computer management report showing a decline in average daily census over the past month might decide to investigate why the decline has occurred. With drill-down capabilities, the CEO would immediately be able to look at more specific details to determine whether all or only certain hospitals are contributing to the decline. The ability to look at key information in a concise format is why these types of ISs are often referred to as dashboard reports or balanced scorecard reports.

Research and Data Analytics Systems

With the EHR, other clinical information systems, and administrative systems, there is an enormous amount of data available. These data have to be turned into information so that they can be used to make decisions on patient care, services provided at the healthcare facility, and more. These data can be used to study diseases, treatments, quality of care, and many other issues related to healthcare. There are a number of tools that assist in data analysis. Two of these are data warehouses and data mining. These are valuable tools used to analyze data for decision-making purposes. The information is important for medical research and public health purposes. Public health systems may utilize geographic information systems (GISs). GISs can be used to monitor patterns of disease to track epidemics or to look for anomalies in cancer incidence or other trends.

Data Warehouses

AHIMA defines a **data warehouse** as a "database that makes it possible to access data from multiple databases and combine the results into a single query and reporting interface" (2012, 98). In a data warehouse, selected data are extracted from multiple sources in the organization's IS. A data warehouse, therefore, is a consolidated database maintained separately from the organization's operational systems. The data contained in the data warehouse depends on how the data warehouse will be used and may include both clinical and administrative data. The organization will need to determine how the system will be used and then choose the various information systems that will be loaded into the data warehouse. The source data may come from the EHR, financial information system, human resources, CPOE, and others. Data in such a warehouse are updated periodically and are essentially a snapshot in time of the organization's data. Such warehouses are used primarily for managerial decision support purposes.

Data warehousing is gaining in popularity. This is particularly true in healthcare, where decision makers rely on accurate and timely information, both financial and clinical. Pharmaceutical manufacturers are using data warehousing for marketing and research. Insurance companies are using it to form clinical repositories, merging their members' claims and clinical data. Such information can provide a better understanding of cost-effectiveness and quality of care. Futures studies performed by AHIMA indicate that HIM professionals will have jobs that encompass roles in developing data warehouses (Sayles and Trawick 2010).

Data Mart

A **data mart** is a subset of the data warehouse designed for a single purpose or specialized use. The data mart performs the same type of analyses as a data warehouse; however, the target area is narrower. There are a number of reasons why a data mart is desired; for example, the costs of managing the data mart are lower than those associated with the data warehouse, and the data in the system can be scaled down to only those data required for the project. The facility may choose to develop the data warehouse before the data mart, or the data mart can be developed first—or both can be developed at the same time. The order of development depends on the needs of the organization. Examples of how a data mart may be used include patient satisfaction and research. Patient satisfaction would not require the patient-specific information that would be stored in the data warehouse, but it would include the types of services, nursing unit, and other basic information in addition to the patient survey or other patient satisfaction information collected. The data mart can be used in research because it can be used to provide deidentified information and the limited information required to conduct the research, and protect the confidentiality of the patient by providing only the minimum information necessary (Sayles and Trawick 2010).

Data Mining

Data mining is the process of extracting and analyzing large volumes of data from a database for the purpose of identifying hidden and sometimes subtle relationships or patterns and using those relationships to predict behaviors (AHIMA 2012, 95–96). Data mining may also be called database exploration or information discovery. Data mining is used to analyze data to identify patterns that would be unnoticed without analysis. Data mining requires sophisticated software such as decision trees, genetic algorithms, neural networks, predictive models, rule induction, and fuzzy logic. These techniques are described as follows:

- A decision tree is visually diagrammed as a tree-shaped configuration. This configuration allows rules to be defined that are used to make a decision.

- Genetic algorithms determine the best model to be used because they are able to enhance other algorithms.

- Neural networks are used to predict actions and classify data. They are nonlinear predictive models that improve with practice.

- Predictive models identify patterns. Once a pattern is identified, the model is able to calculate the odds that a specific action will occur.

- Rule induction identifies patterns from if/then statements. Statistical significance tests are used on the data.

- Fuzzy logic is the method of data mining used when concepts are imprecise.

Once the data pattern has been identified, the facility must decide how to use the information (Sayles and Trawick 2010).

Online Analytical Processing

LaTour and Eichenwald-Maki define **online analytical processing** (OLAP) as "a database architecture that allows the user to retrieve specific information from a large volume of data" (2010, 984). The use of OLAP turns the data warehouse into a decision support tool because it can analyze large amounts of data quickly by drilling down into the data. It can help the facility use operational data that it already has to make strategic decisions.

Check Your Understanding 15.2

1. Which of the following systems would be used to manage productivity?

   A. Financial information system
   B. Human resource system
   C. Embedded guidelines
   D. Facility management

2. What is the difference between the executive information system and decision support system?

   A. There is no real difference since both are decision support systems.
   B. The decision support system is designed to be used by high-level management.
   C. The executive information system is designed to be used by high-level management.
   D. The executive information system is a strategic decision support system, and the decision support system is a clinical decision support system.

3. I will be conducting some analysis of data, but I only need a limited amount of data that are contained in the data warehouse. What system should I utilize?

   A. Data mart
   B. Data mining
   C. Online analytical process
   D. Management information system

4. We receive a report each morning listing all of the admissions from the day before. This is an example of what type of report?

   A. Ad hoc
   B. Demand
   C. Exception
   D. Periodic scheduled

5. Which of the following is an example of when an executive decision support system should be used?

   A. To develop the nursing schedule
   B. To order food and other supplies for the cafeteria
   C. To identify a new service for the hospital to implement
   D. To prepare for hospital accreditation

Instructions: Match the descriptions with the appropriate terms.

6. Uses models and statistical analysis to help decision makers solve problems

7. Displays concise information and may be called a dashboard report

8. Tracks productivity and turnover

9. Is updated periodically and used for strategic decision support

10. Creates reports needed to manage the day-to-day activities of the organization

a. Human resource management system
b. Decision support system
c. Data warehouse
d. Executive information system
e. Management information system

Overview of Electronic Clinical Information Applications in Nonacute Care Settings

Clinical information applications are not limited to the inpatient environment, but are used in other healthcare settings. These settings include, but are not limited to, ambulatory care and long-term care. Although nonacute care settings may use many of the same type of systems as acute care, the systems need to support the specific functions of these facilities and must be specially customized for their use. For example, an appointment scheduling system in a clinic would be different from a registration system in an acute care facility.

Ambulatory Care

Ambulatory care settings have functional needs that are different from other settings. **Ambulatory care information systems** are information systems utilized in the ambulatory setting. This type of system frequently contains administrative and clinical functions. Many of the functions in these systems are the same as inpatient settings, such as documentation, billing, decision support, and security. However, outpatient systems must be tailored to the needs of the ambulatory care environment. For example, an ambulatory EHR frequently contains a practice management function that combines the clinical and administrative requirements where an inpatient system would not.

Functionalities

Depending on the type of outpatient service (physician office, clinic, dental office, and so on), the type of functionality in the ISs will vary. In general, however, outpatient IS will include the following functionalities:

- Appointment scheduling
- Patient billing
- Electronic claims submission for health plans
- Automatic charge and payment posting
- Patient collection and mail-merge systems
- Health record data capture and retrieval
- Prescription writing
- Report generation
- Interface with hospital
- Ability to link to a health information exchange
- Clinical decision support
- Health maintenance programs

Trends

Ambulatory settings are more likely to have practice management systems than an EHR. This may be changing with the incentives offered by Medicare to encourage adoption of the EHR in physician practices. Younger physicians are adopting the use of technology in their practices more than older physicians (Congress of the United States Congressional Budget Office 2008). Incentives provided by the American Recovery and Reinvestment Act (ARRA) to physicians to implement EHRs in their practices are anticipated to dramatically increase the use of ambulatory care information systems.

Challenges

Some of the challenges that face ambulatory systems face any implementation of information systems. These include concerns about data quality, privacy and security, workflow, and the inability to capture the expected financial returns. Also, many physicians are waiting until their peers adopt technology before they decide to adopt. One of the biggest challenges to ambulatory information systems is the cost. Physician offices generally do not have the support and infrastructure to support systems. The costs of the hardware, software, implementation, and other costs prevent many physicians from implementing the system. One cost that is frequently overlooked is the reduction in productivity that occurs initially during the learning process (Congress of the United States Congressional Budget Office 2008).

Long-Term Care

Long-term care (LTC) facilities are behind other healthcare providers in the adoption of information systems. The LTC facilities could benefit from the implementation of information systems because of the improved communications that will result in improved efficiency and improved compliance with federal guidelines and more. Some other benefits of IS in long-term care is improved quality, reduced care disparities, and the use of HIEs to facilitate communication among providers.

Functionalities

Much of the focus of **long-term care information systems** includes census management, patient assessments, documentation, orders, nutritional assessments, and pharmacy. Other functions include the communication between the admitting physician and the facility, including remote access to patient information (Glandon et al. 2008). LTC systems have many of the same functions as other healthcare facilities, such as order entry, documentation, developing care plans, and more. There are functions unique to LTC systems, such as collecting MDS data and calculating RUGS (HealthMEDX nd).

Trends

LTC organizations are becoming part of the integrated delivery system. Being a part of the integrated delivery system demands the connectivity between the hospitals, physician offices, and other components to facilitate the sharing of information (Glandon et al. 2008). Many of the information systems designed for the LTC facilities are adapted from systems designed for inpatient or other healthcare settings, so the systems do not meet the needs of the organization (AHRQ 2009). A number of drivers are compelling LTC facilities and communities to adopt EHRs, including:

- Changing consumer expectations
- Quality of care and patient safety

- Administrative efficiency and effectiveness
- New business models (AHIMA 2011)

Challenges

LTC facilities face the same challenges as other healthcare facilities regarding money, lack of standards, and more. There are other challenges specific to LTC. Frequently they do not have their own information system department to support the implementation and maintenance of the EHR or other systems. Also, many of the systems available on the market are not designed with the LTC environment in mind and so do not meet their needs, and physicians are frequently not at the LTC facility when making decisions about patient care (AHRQ 2009). Since the EHRs available to the LTC facility are adapted from systems designed for other healthcare settings, the EHRs are not designed to accommodate the unique processes of the LTC industry, such as collecting and managing the LTC data sets process, thus making it difficult to locate a system to meet the needs of the LTC organization.

Home Health

Home health organizations have very specific demands in an information system since the care is provided in the patient's home, which may or may not have computers and/or Internet access. Many home health agencies utilize laptops or other mobile devices to access patient information and to document the care provided. These mobile devices may use cellular or other wireless connectivity, or the data may be downloaded into the home health agency's system at the end of the day.

Functionalities

In addition to the ability to document and manage patient care, **home health information systems** should be able to transmit monitoring results. The patient or his or her representative may submit data for review by the nurses or other healthcare professionals (Glandon et al. 2008). An example of monitoring results would be cardiac monitoring. An example of the data that may be submitted by the patient is blood sugar. Other functions are patient education materials, teaching guidelines, and outcome pathways (McKesson 2010).

Trends

More and more, care is being performed in the patient's home, so the home health systems must be able to accommodate the documentation of this care. This care includes telehealth, so the systems must be able to accommodate the recording of data, video, audio, and other tools utilized in telehealth.

Healthcare Information Resources Management

All the healthcare information systems discussed cannot be operated efficiently or effectively on their own. These systems must be coordinated and managed through policies and procedures and an appropriate organizational structure that assigns responsibility and accountability for systems planning, management, and operation. Effectively managing its information resources is just as important to the healthcare organization as keeping its information systems up-to-date. Modern healthcare organizations recognize that information is a critical resource to be managed as carefully as human resources, financial resources, and capital equipment. In large part, the organization's ability to provide high-quality, cost-effective healthcare services depends on the availability of accurate and accessible information.

One of the most important concepts about managing information systems is **information resource management** (IRM). IRM assumes that information is a valuable resource that must be managed no matter what form it takes or what medium it is stored in.

However, healthcare organizations have not always valued information as an essential resource. The modern notion of managing information resources emerged during the late 1980s. At that time, healthcare organizations were being forced to become more competitive in order to survive in the marketplace. They came to recognize the value of an enterprise-wide perspective on information as well as the need to integrate clinical and administrative information (Johns 2002). Before that time, most clinical information was managed at the departmental level or stored in paper-based patient records housed in the health record department. The IS departments of this era were chiefly concerned with processing data and played only a minor role in deciding how to use information within the organization.

IRM is a broad concept that encompasses the creation, use, storage, and eventual disposal of all information, whether it is captured and maintained in a paper-based system or a computer-based system. This broad view is congruent with the philosophy of information management adopted by The Joint Commission. The Joint Commission encourages healthcare organizations to develop ISs that support their needs and those of the patients they serve.

IRM has as its foundation the development of an information systems strategic plan. The strategic plan, discussed later in this chapter, assesses the organization's information needs, establishes IS priorities, and oversees IS implementation projects. The goal of IRM is to coordinate all information processes, both automated and manual, and integrate all information technologies. The key question that IRM answers is "How can we coordinate and control all information activities throughout the enterprise" (Johns 2002). Typically, IRM includes responsibility for ensuring an appropriate information system infrastructure; administering information technology principles for data structures such as databases; developing policies, procedures, and standards that support information systems operations; protecting and maintaining the quality of data; and fostering technological ideas and solutions that benefit the entire organization. An important element of IRM is the establishment of a management structure headed by a chief information officer. This position is discussed in more detail below.

One of the most important aspects of IRM is ensuring data quality. In healthcare organizations, the healthcare professionals who provide services to patients in a number of different care settings need information. They also need information to meet the reporting requirements of external accreditation and regulatory agencies and to carry out performance improvement activities. Several categories of information can be captured and used to satisfy these needs, including:

- *Patient-specific information* consists of data that are linked to individual patients. For example, a blood glucose level for Mr. Smith would be considered patient-specific information.

- *Aggregate information* consists of detailed data sets that are combined to provide a summarization. For instance, adding the numbers of all the female and male patients for a specific month to arrive at a total number of patients is an example of aggregate information.

- *Expert knowledge-based information* is a database of specialized facts about a specific subject area. In healthcare, this information can be used by expert decision support systems to assist physicians in the diagnosis and treatment of patients. The information would include recent research findings and other information to assist the physician in making decisions about the patient's care.

- *Comparative information* consists of data sets that have the same attributes but are from different sources and are evaluated or compared against each other. For example, one hospital might want to compare its average length of stay for patients who experienced myocardial infarctions with the average stays of patients in other, similar hospitals.

Each category of information must be managed at multiple points. IRM assumes an important role in ensuring optimal information management at each point. First, the appropriate sources of data must be identified, and the data must be captured and stored. Data can be defined as uninterpreted facts, images, and sounds that must be analyzed, interpreted, and transformed into information. This information then must be transmitted to the appropriate users for functions such as clinical decision making, administrative decision making, research, performance improvement, and patient education (Clark and Cofer 2000). Thus, information is interpreted data or sets of data whose content is useful to some specific task.

Organizational Structures

Managing information at the enterprise level is not an easy task. Healthcare organizations need an organizational structure that facilitates effective information resource management. Figure 15.4 provides an example of an organizational model that supports enterprise-wide IRM.

Figure 15.4.   **Sample organizational model for managing information resources**

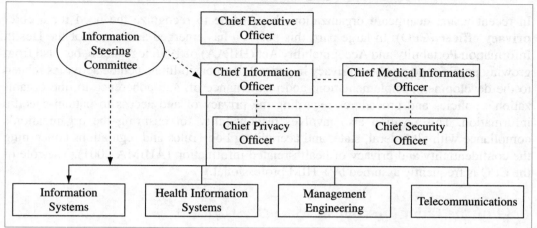

Role of the Chief Information Officer

The **chief information officer** (CIO) is a senior-level executive. He or she is responsible for leading the strategic IS planning process, for assisting the leadership team in using ISs in support of strategic planning and management, and for overseeing the organization's IRM functions. These functions are performed by the IS department as well as by the telecommunications, management engineering, and HIM departments.

The CIO typically reports directly to the organization's chief executive officer (CEO). Through the CIO's efforts as a senior manager, IS activities can be aligned with the organization's mission and strategic priorities. Frequently the HIM department reports directly to the CIO position.

Role of the Information Systems Steering Committee

The CIO does not determine the strategic vision for information systems or information management alone. Most healthcare organizations establish an IS steering committee to take on this responsibility. The committee includes clinicians and administrators from key areas throughout the enterprise as well as IS professionals and the CIO. Working as a team, the IS steering committee assesses the organization's information needs, establishes IS priorities, and oversees IS implementation projects. As stated earlier, the information systems strategic plan is essential to the IRM philosophy. To be successful, the committee needs senior-level support from the medical staff, nursing, and other clinical areas. All plans for new IS or technology projects should be channeled through the IS steering committee to ensure that they are in line with the organization's strategic vision.

Role of the Chief Privacy Officer

In recent years, healthcare organizations have come to recognize the need for a **chief privacy officer** (CPO). In large part, this position has emerged as a result of the Health Information Portability and Accountability Act (HIPAA) of 1996 legislation, but also from growing public concern about privacy in general. Responsibilities include activities related to the development, implementation, and maintenance of, and adherence to, the organization's policies and procedures regarding the privacy of and access to patient-specific information. This position also involves responsibility for ensuring the organization's compliance with all federal, state, and accrediting body rules and regulations concerning the confidentiality and privacy of health-related information (AHIMA 2001). The role of the CPO is frequently assumed by a HIM professional.

Role of the Chief Information Security Officer

As information management has become more complex and information technology has taken on more strategic importance, a new information management position has emerged: the **chief information security officer** (CISO). The CISO may report directly to the CIO or the CEO. The typical CISO is responsible for overseeing the development, implementation, and enforcement of the organization's security policies. He or she manages the security of all patient-identifiable information, whether it is stored in paper-based or computer-based systems.

Recently, the CISO role has become better recognized within healthcare organizations in the context of the new security and confidentiality regulations. Federal agencies developed these regulations in response to passage of the HIPAA. HIPAA security regulations apply to all patient-identifiable healthcare information created, maintained, or stored in an electronic format. They require administrative, physical, and technical services and mechanisms to safeguard the confidentiality, availability, and integrity of health information. ARRA also addresses security. (Information security and privacy issues within the healthcare organization are discussed in detail in chapters 14 and 17.)

Like the CIO, the CISO does not develop policies or make decisions alone. Most healthcare institutions already have or plan to establish information security committees or patient information confidentiality councils. These groups oversee the development and implementation of policies related to the security and confidentiality of patient information. In addition to policy development and enforcement, the committee or council may develop and implement employee education and training programs. The goal of the training programs is to ensure that anyone who creates or uses information understands the importance of protecting it from unauthorized access or disclosure.

Role of the Chief Medical Informatics Officer

The **chief medical informatics officer** (CMIO) is another relatively new position within the information services organizational structure. This position emerged as healthcare organizations recognized the need to have physician leadership in the adoption of clinical ISs. A physician will staff the CMIO position. In some cases, the CMIO is a member of the healthcare organization's medical staff who fulfills this role on a part-time basis. Wager, Lee, and Glaser cite several examples of responsibilities that might be assumed by the CMIO (2005, 288), including:

- Leading the implementation of an EMR system

- Engaging physicians and other healthcare professionals in the development and use of the EMR system

- Leading the clinical informatics steering committee or other designated group that serves as the central governance forum for establishing the organization's clinical IS priorities

- Keeping pulse on the national efforts to develop EHR systems, assuming a leadership role in areas where the national effort and the organization's agenda are aligned

- Being highly responsible to user needs, such as training, to ensure widespread use and acceptance of clinical ISs

Other IS Leadership Roles

Other leadership roles that have emerged recently within healthcare IS organizational structures are chief technology officer and chief nursing informatics officer. The number and type of formal leadership positions will depend on the type and size of the healthcare organization. The chief technology officer is generally an IT or network specialist whose focus is on the technical infrastructure of the IS system. The chief nursing informatics officer would fill a similar role as the CMIO, but with a focus on nursing ISs. The chief records officer manages records across the entire organization, which can assist with retention, legal compliance, and other broad record-management issues (AHIMA 2008a, 98).

Role of the Information Services Department

The **information services department** is generally responsible for ensuring that the organization has the technical infrastructure and staff required to support its healthcare information systems. Common functions of the department include data administration, network administration, network security, database management, systems integration, programming, end-user support, and IS development.

Traditionally, the staff working in the information services department had technical backgrounds in computer science, programming, network administration, and database management. However, managers of information services departments today recognize that technical expertise alone may not be sufficient to support the needs of end users.

Consequently, information services managers are hiring healthcare professionals (physicians, nurses, and laboratory technicians) who understand clinical data and patient care processes and also have a background in IS technology (database management, systems analysis and design, or network management). These healthcare professionals often have job titles such as clinical systems analyst.

Role of the Health Information Management Department

The HIM department plays an integral role in the management of information and, in particular, the management of patient records. Common functions of the HIM department include management of record retention and retrieval in all formats, diagnostic and procedural coding, medical transcription, release of information, and data management. Increasingly, many of the traditional functions of HIM are performed outside the boundaries of a single department. As the fully developed EHR is implemented, the functions performed by HIM professionals often cross departmental boundaries and frequently are performed remotely. This is frequently referred to as virtual HIM. This situation provides even greater prospects for HIM professionals to assume leadership roles in IRM activities in the organization.

HITs have the opportunity to provide leadership in the planning, selection, implementation, and evaluation of enterprise-wide healthcare ISs. HIM professionals bring to the table expertise in classification systems, patient confidentiality, documentation, accreditation standards, and regulations. Chapter 8 provides a detailed discussion of HIM functions.

Enterprise Content and Records Management Department

Enterprise content and records management (ECRM) is the "strategy, technology, and processes for managing information assets facilitated by information technology" (Strong 2008, 39). It also facilitates achieving the goals of IRM. This combines two areas: electronic record management and content management. Electronic record management utilizes accepted practices of record management to retain, use, and dispose of records. Content management is more focused on the tools and methods used to capture, manage, store, preserve, and deliver content across an enterprise rather than the practice of records management (AHIMA 2008a).

A healthcare organization has many information assets, such as health records, business documents, e-mail, and more. This information includes both paper and electronic information. All of these information resources must be managed. This is the role of the ECRM department. This management includes retaining the data, providing access, managing multiple versions of information, reducing risks resulting from poorly managed information, and more. ECRM works with information across the organization—not just the HIM or other departments. Examples of processes conducted by the ECRM include policies and procedures, inventories, training, and standardization (Strong 2008).

Check Your Understanding 15.3

1. What individual or group is responsible for developing the strategic vision for the organization's information?

    A. Steering committee
    B. Chief information security officer
    C. Chief medical information system officer
    D. Chief information officer

2. Information resource management addresses information in what form?

    A. Information stored electronically
    B. Information stored on paper
    C. Information stored in both electronic and paper formats
    D. Information stored in any format

3. Which role works with physicians to assist in the implementation of the EHR?

    A. Chief information officer
    B. Chief information security officer
    C. Chief medical information system officer
    D. Chief privacy officer

4. What individual or group is knowledgeable on accreditation and classification systems?

    A. Chief information officer
    B. Health information management department
    C. Chief medical information system officer
    D. Information systems department

5. Fifty percent of patients treated at our facilities have Medicare as their primary payer. This is an example of what type of information?

    A. Patient-specific
    B. Expert knowledge
    C. Comparative
    D. Aggregate

Roles of HIM Professionals in Electronic Health Information Systems

According to Watzlaf et al. (2009), the changes in technology and the increase in the amount of information collected will only create new roles for HIM professionals who can adapt to the changes facing the profession. In a recent marketing campaign, AHIMA reported 125 different job titles in 40 different work settings. These figures indicate the wide range of opportunities for HIM professionals. Many of these roles are related to information systems in some way. The roles selected here are only a small sample of the available roles for the HIM professional.

Data Management

Data management is a very broad term. It includes functions such as data retention, data storage, data quality, data analysis, and data collection. These are functions that the HIM professional has been performing for decades. The advent of information systems has provided the HIM professional with much more data to manage. These digital data allow the data to be managed in a way that paper records never could. Examples include audit trails to monitor access, retrieval of information in seconds, and the ability of access to the same information by multiple people at the same time.

Data Quality

Physicians and other healthcare providers rely heavily on quality data in order to make the right decisions on patient care. Administration relies on quality data in order to make decisions on the future of the healthcare facility. The HIM professional has the skills necessary to ensure the quality of the data used in these decision-making processes. Data quality begins with data collection and continues through the processing of the data, interfaces transmission of data from one point to another, data storage, and retrieval. The HIM professional utilizes data standards, messaging standards, data dictionaries, data quality checks, and more to assist in ensuring data quality (AHIMA 2007). The HIM professional can also work with patients to prepare them to be more participative in their care (Rulon 2009a).

Data Collection and Analysis

The knowledge that the HIM professional has on the content of the health record, data quality, data sets, and more allows him or her to play a key role in data collection and analysis. This role is not new. HIM professionals have abstracted data manually. Now, the role focuses more on mining data to be used in the reporting and analysis of data (AHIMA 2007).

Data Privacy

HIM has always led the way in protecting the privacy of patient information. With the knowledge of state and federal laws and regulation related to HIM and the content of the health record, no one is better prepared to control access to health information. The HIM professional in this role may monitor compliance with HIPAA, ARRA, and other laws. They may work with others in the organization to assess risks to the health information. They also develop the policies and procedures required to minimize the risks to health information. Another task for the HIM professional in a data privacy role is to develop and monitor the training programs to ensure that they are effective in educating the staff on the privacy requirements. Privacy issues would include protecting portable devices, watching for identity theft, controlling access to the EHR and other information systems, and much more (AHIMA 2008b). HIM professionals should also strive to identify risks to patient information as well as educate healthcare professionals and the public on privacy (Rulon 2009b).

Data Security

The HIM professional has the necessary skills to manage the access controls to the EHR and other information systems. Other tasks include managing the disaster recovery and incident response plans for the organization (AHIMA 2008b). The HIM professional must identify and address risks for medical identity theft as more and more patient information is exchanged electronically (Rulon 2009b).

Electronic System Design and Development

HIM professionals do not usually perform the actual programming required to develop an electronic system. The HIM professional is more likely involved in determining what functions are needed within the system, screen design, data capture, the reports needed, and more. They would also be involved in the development of security and other administrative features. The HIM professional is ideal for this role because of his or her knowledge of data, legal issues, data quality, and data collection. HIM professionals who work in this role generally work for an information system vendor.

Other HIM Roles

Many other roles exist for the HIM professional within the e-HIM area. These roles include an emphasis in consumer health informatics, data integrity, and data mining, among others.

One of the newest roles for HIM professionals is to work in regional extension centers. The HIM professionals can perform a number of tasks including implementation of the EHR, data management, privacy and security, community education, data quality, information exchange, and more (AHIMA 2009).

The HIM profession will also be a valuable player in consumer health informatics. Consumer health informatics is defined as "a subspecialty of medical informatics which studies from a patient/consumer perspective the use of electronic information and communication to improve medical outcomes and the healthcare decision-making process" (AMIA nd). This opens up roles such as PHR liaison, which would assist patients in gathering and organizing their PHR, and the patient information coordinator, which would assist patients and families in obtaining the health information about the healthcare provided (Dolan et al. 2009).

Data integrity is another area in which the HIM professional can excel. No one knows the data like the HIM professional, so it is logical for the HIM professional to be in a role that ensures the accuracy of the data contained in the EHR. In this role, the HIM professional would look for discrepancies in data. For example, they would identify overlays in the master patient index or illogical diagnoses, such as a newborn having coronary artery disease (Dimick 2007).

Data mining is another opportunity for the HIM professional. In this role, the HIM professional would use data mining tools such as online analytical processing in order to manipulate and then analyze the data to look for trends that can assist management and care providers in decision making (Sayles and Trawick 2010).

Check Your Understanding 15.4

1. What HIM role determines what functions should be added to an information system?
   A. Data quality
   B. Data collection and analysis
   C. Electronic system design and development
   D. Data management

2. What HIM role is involved with the personal health record?
   A. Data quality
   B. Data collection and analysis
   C. Consumer health informatics
   D. Data management

3. Critique the following statement: Ambulatory information systems are the same as inpatient information systems.
   A. This is a false statement. They have many functions in common, but they each have unique functions as well.
   B. This is a true statement.
   C. This is a false statement. Ambulatory systems do not have a need for administrative systems like inpatient systems do.
   D. This is a false statement. Ambulatory systems do not allow for electronic documentation like inpatient systems do.

4. In what type of setting(s) are mobile devices critical to the efficient use of information systems?
   A. Home health
   B. Long-term care
   C. Ambulatory care
   D. Both home health and long-term care

5. As data quality coordinator for our facility, when does my responsibility/concern for data quality begin?
   A. At the time of patient discharge
   B. After the data are entered
   C. At the time of data usage
   D. At the time that the data are collected

Real-World Case

The following is adapted from the presentation "In Search of eHIM: A Case Study of Transformation to a Centralized HIM Record Archival and EDMS Processing Center in a Multihospital Network" at AHIMA's 79th National Convention (Grzybowski 2007).

Mercy Health Partners in southwest Ohio decided to implement an electronic document management system on their migration to the electronic health record. They wanted a system that would fit into their long-term information system strategic plan. They also wanted the support from physicians and other staff. The first phase focused on the storage of the paper record as well as other administration records. A consulting firm was hired to assist in the system selection process, and the decision was made to centralize the document management system for three of the hospitals in their system. A number of challenges were identified, including:

- Increased volume of paper
- Storage of paper records in about 40 different locations
- Increased patient load
- Inability to locate records more than 40 percent of the time

The system selected was expected to improve efficiency, reduce costs, and protect the records. These benefits were realized upon implementation with an annual cost savings of $200,000, improved record retrieval, and better record management. They were also able to open up space at the facilities for use by patient care areas. Much of the success of the project is attributed to their planning for not only the electronic document management system but the long-term storage as well.

Summary

Early computer systems were introduced to healthcare in the 1960s. These systems were predominately mainframe systems used to support financial and/or administrative functions. The 1970s saw the introduction of turnkey systems. These systems also ran on large mainframe systems that often were not flexible enough to address the information needs of individual departments. By the 1980s, personal computers were being used in healthcare, and smaller-scale, stand-alone systems for department applications had been introduced. This put information in the hands of the users but led to the development of many separate systems throughout the organization that could not talk to each other. In the 1990s, integrated healthcare information systems that supported clinical, administrative, and decision support functions evolved. These systems use advanced network technologies such as the Internet to ensure seamless operations across the healthcare enterprise.

Healthcare information system (IS) applications can be categorized as clinical, administrative, and management support. To be used to their full potential, these systems should be integrated into an enterprise-wide IS that supports the organization's mission.

Healthcare organizations today recognize that information is an essential resource that must be managed just as other valuable resources are. This recognition has led to new organizational structures that support information resource management. Some of the key positions in these new structures include the chief information officer (CIO), the IS steering committee, the chief security officer (CSO), and the chief privacy officer (CPO). In many organizations, the health information management and IS departments report directly to the CIO.

Other information technologies also can support managerial and clinical decision making. Decision making, however, is not limited to managers and clinicians. Increasingly, patients are becoming more involved in making decisions about their own healthcare. Many technologies can help patients access healthcare information and increase timely and efficient communication with healthcare providers.

The growth of decision support systems and consumer health informatics has opened up a number of career opportunities for health information management professionals. Moreover, these opportunities are likely to expand as technology evolves to make information available to healthcare decision makers in new and more effective ways.

References

Agency for Healthcare Research and Quality. 2009. Implementation of health information technology in long-term care settings: Findings from the AHRQ health IT portfolio. http://healthit.ahrq.gov/portal/server.pt/gateway/PTARGS_0_907434_0_0_18/08-0087-EF.pdf

Amatayakul, M.K. 2009. *Electronic Health Records: A Practical Guide for Professionals and Organizations*. Chicago: AHIMA.

American Health Information Management Association. 2001. Sample chief privacy officer job description. http://ahima.org/downloads/pdfs/resources/POjobdesc.pdf

American Health Information Management Association. 2007. Beyond the buzz: data quality dissected. *AHIMA Advantage* 11:3.

American Health Information Management Association. 2008a. Enterprise content and record management for healthcare. *Journal of AHIMA* 79(10):91–98.

American Health Information Management Association. 2008b. HIM and health IT: Discovering common ground in an electronic healthcare environment. Appendix A roles and job elements that support EHR management. *Journal of AHIMA* 79(11):69A–69C.

American Health Information Management Association. 2009. The HIM role in assisting regional extension centers. http://www.ahima.org/arra/documents/TheHIMRoleinAssistingRegional ExtensionCentersJuly09.pdf#pagepercent3D1

American Health Information Management Association. 2011. EHR Adoption in LTC and the HIM Value. *Journal of AHIMA* 82(1):46–51 (expanded online edition).

American Health Information Management Association. 2012. *Pocket Glossary for Health Information Management and Technology.* Chicago: AHIMA.

American Medical Informatics Associations. nd. Consumer health informatics. https://www.amia.org/working-group/consumer-health-informatics

Bates, D.W., and A. Gawande. 2003. Improving safety with information technology. *New England Journal of Medicine* 348(2):526–534.

Clark, J.S., and J. Cofer. 2000. *Information Management: The Compliance Guide to the JCAHO Standards,* 3rd ed. Marblehead, MA: Opus Communications.

Congress of the United States Congressional Budget Office. 2008. Evidence on the costs and benefits of health information technology. http://www.cbo.gov/ftpdocs/91xx/doc9168/05-20-HealthIT.pdf

Dimick, C. 2007. Documentation detectives: Data integrity specialists track down data gone bad. *Journal of AHIMA* 78(8):48–52.

Dolan, M., J. Wolter, C. Nielsen, and J. Burrington-Brown. 2009. Consumer health informatics: Is there a role for HIM professionals? http://perspectives.ahima.org/index.php?option=com_content&view=article&id=155:consumer-health-informatics-is-there-a-role-for-him-professionals&catid=49:workforce&Itemid=94

Glandon, G.L., D.H. Smaltz, and D.J. Slovensky. 2008. *Austin and Boxerman's Information Systems for Healthcare Management.* Chicago, IL: Hospital Administration Press.

Grzybowski, D. 2007. In search of eHIM: A case study of transformation to a centralized HIM record archival and EDMS processing center in a multihospital network. *AHIMA's 79th National Convention and Exhibit Proceedings.*

HealthMEDX. nd. http://www.healthmedx.com/solutions/LongTermCare.aspx

Hebda, T., and P. Czar. 2009. *Handbook of Informatics for Nurses & Healthcare Professionals.* Upper Saddle River, NJ: Pearson Prentice Hall.

Hillestad, R., J. Bigelow, A. Bower, F. Girosi, R. Meili, R. Scoville, and R. Taylor. 2005. Can electronic medical record systems transform health care? Potential health benefits, savings, and costs. *Health Affairs* 24(5):1103–1117.

iHealthBeat. 2011. New "Smart" T-Shirt Could Monitor Patients' Vital Signs Remotely. http://www.ihealthbeat.org/articles/2011/9/27/new-smart-tshirt-could-monitor-patients-vital-signs-remotely.aspx

Johns, M.L. 2002. *Information Management for Health Professions*, 2nd ed. Albany, NY: Thompson-Delmar.

Kennedy, O.G., G.M. Davis, and S. Heda. 1992. Clinical information systems: 25-year history and the future. *Journal of the Society for Health Systems* 3(4):49–60.

LaTour, K.M., and S. Eichenwald-Maki. 2010. *Health Information Management: Concepts, Principles, and Practice*. Chicago: AHIMA.

Malec, B.T. 1998. Administrative applications. In *Information Systems for Health Services Administration*. Edited by C.J. Austin and S.B. Boxerman. Chicago: Health Administration Press.

McKesson. 2010. Horizon Homecare. http://www.mckesson.com/en_us/McKesson.com/ For+Healthcare+Providers/Home+Care/Agency+Management/Horizon+Homecare.html

National Committee on Vital and Health Statistics. 2000. Report to the Secretary of the U.S. Department of Health and Human Services on Uniform Data Standards for Patient Medical Record Information as Required by the Administrative Simplification Provisions of the Health Insurance Portability and Accountability Act of 1996. http://www.ncvhs.hhs.gov/hipaa000706.pdf

Office of the National Coordinator. 2006. Harmonized use case for consumer empowerment (registration and medication history). http://healthit.hhs.gov/portal/server.pt/gateway/ PTARGS_0_10731_848102_0_0_18/ConsumerEmpowerment.pdf

Open Clinical. nd. Clinical pathways. http://www.openclinical.org/clinicalpathways.html

Rulon, V. 2009a. HIM's role in ensuring patient safety: Reducing medical errors requires a cultural and technological shift in healthcare. *Journal of AHIMA* 80(10).

Rulon, V. 2009b. HIM's role in maintaining privacy and security. *Journal of AHIMA* 80(8).

Sayles, N.B., and K.C. Trawick. 2010. *Computers in Healthcare*. Chicago: AHIMA.

Strong, K.V. 2008. Enterprise content and records management. *Journal of AHIMA* 79(2):38–42.

Wager, K.A., F.W. Lee, and J.P. Glaser. 2005. *Managing Health Care Information Systems: A Practical Approach for Health Care Executives*. San Francisco: Jossey-Bass.

Watzlaf, V.J.M., W.J. Rudman, S. Hart-Hester, and P. Ren. 2009. The progression of the roles and functions of HIM professionals: A look into the past, present and future. *Perspectives in Health Information Management* (6): Summer.

Additional Resources

American Health Information Management Association. 2007. Practice brief: HIM principles in health information exchange. *Journal of AHIMA* 78(8).

Austin, C.J., and S.B. Boxerman. 2003. *Information Systems for Health Services Administration*, 6th ed. Chicago: Health Administration Press.

Barlas, S. 2002 (September). Report from the FDA's bar coding initiative. *Healthcare Informatics*, pp. 17–18.

Bates, D.W. 2005. Physicians and ambulatory electronic health records. *Health Affairs* 24(5):1,180–189.

Foundation of Research and Education of AHIMA. 2008. The state-level health information exchange consensus project: HIE policies and practices: developing options and implementation guidance to foster consistency interim report. http://library.ahima.org/xpedio/groups/public/documents/ahima/bok1_043512.pdf

Fox, S., and L. Rainie. 2000. *The Online Health Care Revolution: How the Web Helps Americans Take Better Care of Themselves.* Washington, DC: Pew Charitable Trusts.

Garets, D., and M. Davis. 2005. EMRs and EHRs: Concepts as different as apples and oranges at least deserve separate names. *Healthcare Informatics* 22(10):53–54.

Gilbert, F.E. 2000. Demystifying HIPAA. Presentation to Association of Pathology Chairs West and Midwest Regional Meeting.

HIMSS. nd. http://www.himss.org/ASP/topics_eprescribing.asp

Hunter, R.L. 1999. The past and future of laboratory information systems. *Annals of Clinical and Laboratory Science* 29(3):176–184.

Institute of Medicine, Committee on Data Standards for Patient Safety. 2003. *Key Capabilities of an Electronic Health Record System.* Washington, DC: National Academies Press.

Kelly, P., and G. Legrow. 2000. *Medicaid Health Plans: Are Application Service Providers Right for You? A Market Segment Report.* Oakland, CA: California Healthcare Foundation.

Teich, J.M., and M.M. Wrinn. 2000. Clinical decision support systems come of age. *MD Computing* 17(1):43–46.

Wager, K.A., F.W. Lee, A.W. White, D.M. Ward, and S.M. Ornstein. 2000. Impact of an electronic medical record system on community-based primary care practices. *Journal of the American Board of Family Practice* 13(5):338–348.

Wager, K.A., F.W. Lee, and A.W. White. 2001. Life after a disastrous electronic medical record implementation: One clinic's experience. *Annals of Cases on Information Technology* 3:153–368.

Whitten, J.L., L.D. Bentley, and K.C. Dittman. 2005. *Systems Analysis and Design Methods,* 6th ed. New York: McGraw-Hill.

Electronic Health Records

Margret K. Amatayakul, MBA, RHIA, CHPS, CPHIT, CPEHR, FHIMSS

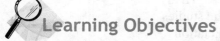

Learning Objectives

- Introduce the definition of the electronic health record (EHR) and describe its various components

- Describe challenges to developing EHRs and how they have evolved to their current state of implementation in hospitals, ambulatory care, and other settings

- Identify various initiatives to promote adoption of EHR and health information technology (HIT)

- Describe the technologies that support the EHR and their impact on HIM functions

- Develop an appreciation for the planning, selection, implementation, and ongoing management aspects of EHRs

- Discuss the roles of health information management professionals with respect to privacy, security, legal aspects, and data quality in an electronic environment

Key Terms

Access control
Accountable care organization (ACO)
Accredited Standards Committee X12 (ASC X12)
Affordable Care Act (ACA)

Alert fatigue
American National Standards Institute (ANSI)
American Recovery and Reinvestment Act (ARRA)

Ancillary systems
Architecture
ASTM International
Audit log
Authentication
Automated drug dispensing machines
Barcode medication administration record
  (BC-MAR)
Billing system
Business intelligence (BI)
Certification
Change control
Charge capture
Chart conversion
Chart deficiency system
Chief medical informatics officer (CMIO)
Claim
Claims attachment
Claims data
Claims status inquiry and response
Client/server architecture
Clinical data repository (CDR)
Clinical data warehouse (CDW)
Clinical decision support (CDS)
Clinical decision support system (CDSS)
Clinical Document Architecture (CDA)
Clinical documentation system
Clinical information system (CIS)
Clinical messaging
Clinical transformation
Clinician
Closed-loop medication management
Cloud computing
Coding and abstracting systems
Complete EHR
Computer output to laser disk (COLD)/
  enterprise report management (ERM)
Computerized provider order entry
  (CPOE)
Configuration management
Consent directive
Consistent federated model (of HIE)

Contextual
Continuity of care document (CCD)
Continuity of care record (CCR)
Contraindication
Controlled vocabulary
Core measures
Data availability
Data center
Data comparability
Data conversion
Data dictionary
Data exchange standards
Data Use and Reciprocal Support
  Agreement (DURSA)
Database
Database management system (DBMS)
Department of Health and Human
  Services (HHS)
Diagnostic studies
Digital dictation
Digital images
Digital Imaging and Communications in
  Medicine (DICOM)
Discrete reportable transcription (DRT)
Disease management (DM)
Document imaging management system
  (DIMS)
Drug knowledge database
Electronic date interchange (EDI)
Electronic document/content management
  (ED/CM)
Electronic document management system
  (EDMS)
Electronic funds transfer (EFT)
Electronic health record (EHR)
Electronic medical record (EMR)
Electronic medication administration
  record (E-MAR)
Electronic (or enterprise) report
  management (ERM)
Electronic signature authentication (ESA)
Eligibility verification

Encoded
Encoder
Encryption
e-Prescribing (e-Rx)
Evidence-based medicine
e-visits
Federated model (of HIE)
Flat file
Health information exchange (HIE)
Health information exchange organization (HIEO)
Health information technology (HIT)
Health Information Technology for Economic and Clinical Health (HITECH)
Health Insurance Portability and Accountability Act of 1996 (HIPAA)
Health Level Seven (HL7)
Hierarchical database
Hospital information system (HIS)
Hospitalist
Human–computer interface
Hybrid record
Identity management
Identity matching algorithm
Institute of Medicine (IOM)
Interface
International Classification of Diseases, Ninth Revision, Clinical Modification (ICD-9-CM)
International Classification of Diseases, Tenth Revision, Clinical Modification (ICD-10-CM)
International Health Terminology Standards Development Organization
Interoperability
Issues management
Kiosk
Laboratory information system (LIS)
Logical Observations, Identifiers, Names and Codes (LOINC)
Meaningful use

Medical devices
Medication Five Rights
Medication reconciliation
Message format standards
Metadata
Migration path
Modular EHR
Multi-dimensional database
National Alliance for Health Information Technology (NAHIT)
National Committee for Quality Assurance (NCQA)
National Council for Prescription Drug Programs (NCPDP)
National Drug Codes (NDC)
National health information infrastructure (NHII)
Nationwide health information network (NHIN)
National Library of Medicine (NLM)
Natural language processing (NLP)
Nursing information system
Office of the National Coordinator (ONC) for Health Information Technology
ONC authorized testing and certifying body (ONC-ATCB)
Online analytical processing (OLAP)
Online transaction processing (OLTP)
Operating rules
Opt-in/opt-out
Order communication
Patient acuity staffing
Patient-Centered Medical Home (PCMH)
Patient financial system (PFS)
Patient portal
Patient safety
Personal health record (PHR)
Pharmacy benefits manager (PBM)
Pharmacy information system
Physician champion
Physician Quality Reporting System (PQRS)

Picture archiving and communications
     system (PACS)
Point of care (POC)
Point-of-care charting
Portals
Practice guidelines
Practice management system (PMS)
Primary care physician (PCP)
Print file
Prior authorization
Process improvement
Proprietary vocabulary
Protocol
Provider
Radio-frequency identification (RFID)
Radiology information system (RIS)
Record locator service (RLS)
Redundant arrays of independent (or
     inexpensive) disks (RAID)
Registration-Admission, Discharge,
     Transfer (R-ADT)
Registry
Relational database
Release of information system
Remittance advice
Remote patient monitoring device
Report cards
Results management
Results retrieval
Retention schedule
Revenue cycle management (RCM)
RxNorm

Server failover
Server redundancy
Source systems
Speech dictation
Speech recognition
Standard vocabulary
Storage area network (SAN)
Storage management
Storage management software
Structured data
System
Systematized Nomenclature of Medicine-
     Clinical Terms (SNOMED-CT)
Telehealth
Template
Textual
Thick client
Thin client
Transaction
Transactional database
Unintended consequence
Uninterruptable power supply (UPS)
Unstructured data
Value
Vocabulary standards
Voluntary Universal Health Identifier
     (VUHID)
Web services architecture (WSA)
Wireless on wheels (WOWs)
Workflow
Workflow and process management

Introduction

The **Health Information Technology for Economic and Clinical Health** (HITECH)
component of the **American Recovery and Reinvestment Act** (ARRA) of 2009 states
that a qualified **electronic health record** (EHR):

> includes patient demographic and clinical health information, such as medical history and
> problem lists; and has the capacity to provide clinical decision support, support physician
> order entry, capture and query information relevant to healthcare quality, and exchange
> electronic health information with and integrate such information from other sources.

There have been a number of different terms and descriptions used over the years to describe what is currently called EHR. The HITECH description reflects a growing interest in a broader purpose for the EHR than in past uses of paper records or even early electronic record systems. The goal now is for the health record to not only be a place where health information about a person is documented, stored, and referenced for later episodes of care, but to be a tool that provides support for changing how medicine is practiced. The intent is to improve the value of healthcare delivered in the United States. **Value** is the combination of quality and cost. EHRs help achieve better healthcare value through support for clinical decision making, alerts to avoid errors, reminders about preventive services needed, improved coordination of care, opportunities for greater productivity, and better data with which to conduct quality measurement, clinical research, and business intelligence.

This chapter describes the components of EHRs in depth. The EHR is not a single computer application, but a complex system of hardware technology and multiple software applications, supported by people, policies, and processes. Also discussed is the role health information management professionals play in acquiring, implementing, gaining adoption, and optimizing use of EHR.

Theory into Practice

Consider the scenario where a diabetic patient, John, moves to a new city and logs on to the Internet to select a local **primary care physician** (PCP) to manage his overall care, making referrals to specialists as needed. He is able to select one who appears to have strong outcomes in diabetes and positive patient satisfaction scores on **report cards** that describe the quality of care they provide for several types of chronic conditions. John schedules an appointment via the physician's website and is set up with a user ID and password to link the PCP with his **personal health record** (PHR), which he maintains on his own by uploading copies of records from various **provider**s he has seen over the years. This enables the PCP to view and retrieve pertinent information from other providers as well as information John has recorded about his diet, over-the-counter medications being taken, and other information relating to compliance with his diabetic treatment regimen.

John also asks his former hometown physician to send information to this new PCP. This physician does this using the standard **continuity of care document** (CCD) content and format specifications for exchanging referral information between providers. With the information supplied by the PHR and the CCD, the new PCP's EHR is prepopulated with a current problem list, recent laboratory results, and other data. Additionally, John's medication history can be directly supplied to his new PCP's EHR by the PCP linking to information available from the **pharmacy benefits manager** (PBM) that John's health plan uses to evaluate which drugs the health plan will pay for and what co-pay may be required from the patient.

When John visits the new PCP, data from these various sources will be validated and updated. The new PCP is able to document all components of John's visit at the **point of care** (POC), including demonstrating medical necessity for lab work by applying ICD diagnosis codes and generating appropriate evaluation and management (E/M) codes for the level of service provided. The PCP decides to put John on a strict smoking-cessation program and exercise routine, with plans to adjust medications according to John's vital signs and HgA1c (blood sugar) levels, which will be monitored remotely through a **remote patient monitoring device.**

All is going well until John has an accident at work that requires a visit to the emergency service, subsequent admission to the hospital, and outpatient physical therapy. All his providers, however, are members of a **health information exchange organization** (HIEO); thus, each provider has immediate access to the specific information needed to treat John throughout his care and for which John has provided a **consent directive** to opt-in to the sharing of such information with all participants in the HIO.

At the hospital, a **hospitalist** (a physician dedicated to hospital-based care services) is able to reconcile all of John's medications in accordance with the Joint Commission requirements and to select medications that have been screened against John's known allergies. The hospital is also part of an **accountable care organization** (ACO), which is a health reform mechanism that ties reimbursement to quality metrics and reduced costs in an assigned population of patients. As a result, the hospital has access to John's previous lab and x-ray results, so repeating these **diagnostic studies** is not necessary, saving John time and potential health risks and reducing overall costs. In selecting the physical therapy referral, the hospitalist has access to John's health plan benefits information, so no time is wasted in arranging for the physical therapy to begin.

Because John's PCP meets the requirements of NCQA as a **Patient-Centered Medical Home** (PCMH) Recognized Practice by the **National Committee for Quality Assurance** (NCQA nd), the PCP is continuously monitoring the impact of the accident on John's diabetes during his hospitalization and makes appropriate adjustments. After John is discharged and in physical therapy, the health plan conducts **disease management** (DM), which observes whether he is following the prescribed exercise routine and can notify the PCP to follow up if necessary. John can access tailored discharge instructions that superimpose his picture on the exercise instructions so that it is clear how to avoid further injury. In addition, each provider John encountered throughout this episode of care follows up with him on the smoking-cessation program he started with his PCP, motivating him to keep from smoking.

The EHR System

The term **system** refers to a set of components that work together to accomplish a goal. An EHR system may be considered, in a narrow sense, as the major clinical applications that are often acquired towards the end of an automation journey in a healthcare organization. However, in the broadest sense, an EHR system includes these major clinical applications plus connection points to many other applications in a healthcare organization and with other healthcare and related organizations. In addition, an EHR system includes not only software applications and computer hardware, but operational elements associated with people, policies, and processes such that the system is adequately staffed and there is leadership commitment to the project, appropriate guidance for use is supplied, and attention to **workflow and process management** ensures that the components work together to achieve their intended purpose.

EHR Definition

The definition of EHR has been evolving over time and is becoming increasingly complex. One of the earliest terms used to describe EHR is *computer-based patient record* (CPR), used in the 1980s by the **Institute of Medicine** (IOM). This is a nonprofit organization that is part of the National Academies that provides advice to lawmakers and the public. Even though the capabilities of systems at the time were not as robust as today, the IOM provided a very sophisticated vision that reflects the HITECH description of EHR today.

The IOM described "a system specifically designed to support users through availability of complete and accurate data, practitioner reminders and alerts, clinical decision support, links to bodies of medical knowledge, and other aids" (1997, 1991). The IOM further noted that "this definition encompasses a broader view of the patient record than is current today, moving from the notion of a location or device for keeping track of patient care events to a resource with much enhanced utility in patient care (including the ability to provide an accurate longitudinal account of care), in management of the healthcare system, and in extension of knowledge" (1997, 1991).

These observations made by the IOM have been reaffirmed in all of their subsequent work, including their letter report *Key Capabilities of an Electronic Health Record System* (2003) that laid the groundwork for today's EHR product certification and more recent works such as edited by Stead and Lin (2009) recommending immediate steps and strategic directions for better use of *Computational Technology for Effective Health Care*. This work also contributed to the development of an EHR-System Functional Model by **Health Level Seven** (HL7) (2007) standards development organization.

The term **electronic medical record** (EMR) is another early term, often used to describe systems that integrated dictation, transcription, scanned documents, and **print files** (which is an image of information created when commanding a computer to print). Some hospitals use the term today to distinguish between such a system and an EHR that is a system used by clinicians at the POC and across care settings to aid in clinical decision support. Many physician offices, outpatient departments, clinics, and other ambulatory care facilities (collectively referred to as physician practices) as well as vendors, however, continue to use the term EMR by habit. Such systems range from "lite" products that may only be a word-processing file to the most sophisticated vision of EHR as originally described by the IOM and now by the federal government.

One final distinction between EMR and EHR was made by the **National Alliance for Health Information Technology** (NAHIT 2008) for the **Office of the National Coordinator (ONC) for Health Information Technology.** Within the **Department of Health and Human Services** (HHS), ONC provides leadership for the development and implementation of an interoperable health information technology infrastructure nationwide to improve healthcare quality and delivery. NAHIT recommended the following distinction (with differences relating to how well the systems are able to exchange data across health-care organizations highlighted in italics):

- Electronic *medical* record: "An electronic record of health-related information on an individual that can be created, gathered, managed, and consulted by authorized clinicians and staff *within one healthcare organization*"

- Electronic *health* record: "An electronic record of health-related information on an individual that *conforms to nationally recognized* **interoperability** *standards* and that can be created, managed, and consulted by authorized clinicians and staff *across more than one healthcare organization*"

HIT Definition

Health information technology (HIT) is another commonly used term. HIT encompasses not only the EHR components but other, broader uses of information technology (IT) in healthcare. For example, many hospitals have a set of applications that support collection of patient demographics and insurance information, billing, and processing of diagnostic studies, and drug ordering, collectively referred to as a **hospital information system** (HIS). Likewise in a physician practice, a **practice management system** (PMS) would support collection of patient demographic and insurance information, scheduling visits, and billing. Other HIT might include PHRs; **telehealth** that delivers healthcare services remotely; **health information exchange** (HIE) services that support sharing health information across different healthcare organizations; **medical devices** that are instruments that collect or supply health information as they monitor patients' vital signs, aid in analyzing lab specimens, and perform other diagnostic and therapeutic support; and others.

This chapter references HIT to describe the broadest scope of information technology used in healthcare. It adopts the term EHR consistent with the federal government's definition and use in the incentive program for making meaningful use of a certified EHR. The incentives were initiated in 2011 under regulations issued by the Centers for Medicare and Medicaid Services (CMS 2012). The program, commonly referred to as **meaningful use** (MU), is set to roll into sanctions on Medicare reimbursement in 2015. The ultimate goal is to provide seamless exchange of information among providers (including hospitals, physicians, and other healthcare professionals who bill or get paid directly for their services) at all levels of the healthcare continuum and provide support for fully integrated evidence-based medicine. **Evidence-based medicine** (EBM) is the practice of medicine utilizing guidance gleaned from research studies. In the absence of such research, **practice guidelines** may be used. These draw from experts in the field who reach consensus on best practices. This means that **clinicians** (healthcare professionals who provide direct patient care support, whether they bill directly for their services or are employed by a provider organization, including physicians, nurses, pharmacists, allied health professionals, and others) must interact directly with the EHR as they care for patients at the POC. Information is accessed as needed and documentation is made directly into the system, either as **unstructured data** (dictated, keyed as text, or scanned) or **structured data** (discrete facts, figures, observations, or findings entered via **templates** [that direct what data should be entered] that are able to be processed by the computer). The EHR combines structured data from many sources, such as that entered at the POC along with drug information from **drug knowledge databases** (that provides references to information about drugs, their active ingredients, side effects, and other information), lab results from a laboratory system, and vital signs from a medical device for patient monitoring. These data are then able to be processed into alerts, such as potential drug **contraindications** or reminders about lab tests that need to be performed.

EHR System Applications

The development of an EHR system most often begins in a healthcare organization with acquisition of source systems, including administrative and financial systems and ancillary or departmental systems. From there and depending on the size and type of healthcare organization, other systems are acquired, including the core EHR applications, specialty systems, medical devices, and connectivity systems. Throughout this process, supporting infrastructure (computers, network devices, cables, and many other technical tools) must also be acquired. Figure 16.1 summarizes these applications and how they relate to one another.

Source Systems

Source systems are so named because they supply the EHR and other applications with data. Source systems may include administrative and financial systems as well as ancillary, or departmental, systems.

Administrative and Financial Systems

Administrative and financial systems typically have been among the first systems implemented by healthcare organizations. While each of the systems within this category is usually managed by a specific department, such as admitting, patient financial services, and health information management, they are not considered departmental systems because they manage patient-specific data needed for all other applications, and do not process data that aid in management of the departments as do ancillary, or departmental, systems. Administrative and financial systems include:

- **Registration, admission, discharge and transfer** (R-ADT) systems in hospitals, which register patients for admission or outpatient services, capturing demographic and insurance data and supplying this data to all other applications as needed. An R-ADT system tracks when patients are admitted and opens an account for them. It also tracks all transfers within the hospital, such as to and from an intensive care unit. Finally, the R-ADT system closes the account when a patient is discharged. Other related systems keep track of the organization's census, track who is in what bed, compile length of stay information, and maintain a master person index. In

Figure 16.1. **EHR system application**

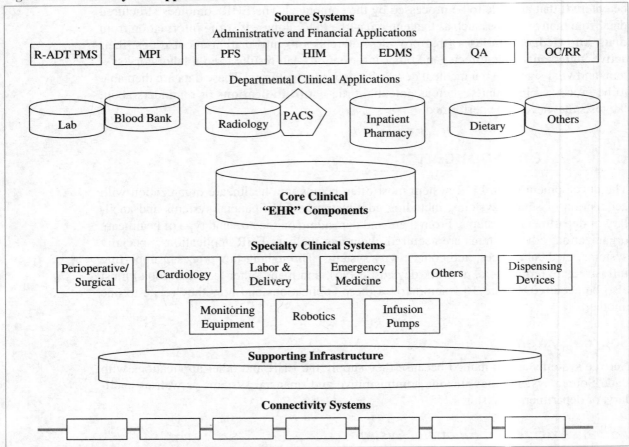

a physician practice, an equivalent system would be a PMS, or just a scheduling system.

- **Patient financial systems** (PFSs), frequently called **billing systems** in a physician practice, aid **revenue cycle management** (RCM). RCM refers to the entire process of creating, submitting, analyzing, and obtaining payment for healthcare services (TripleTree 2006). RCM includes **charge capture** to collect information about services performed from **ancillary systems** and the EHR; **claim** generation for reimbursement by a health plan (and patient); **claims status inquiry and response,** posting **remittance advice** reflecting actual fees reimbursed to the organization, receiving **electronic funds transfers** (EFTs); and other related processes.

Other related systems also aid RCM, such as **encoders** to support accurate coding of diagnoses and procedures, **eligibility verification** systems to determine if a patient's health plan will provide reimbursement for services to be performed, **prior-authorization** management systems where a health plan requires review and approval of a procedure prior to its performance, **claims attachment** systems where additional information required by the health plan to pay the claim can be sent electronically, collections services, and others. Many of these functions have mandated standards for use under the **Health Insurance Portability and Accountability Act** of 1996 (HIPAA). These standards have been or are being updated or added to under the **Affordable Care Act** (ACA) of 2010. ACA requires standard **operating rules** that further explain the standards so their use is consistent across health plans. ACA also imposes penalties for health plan noncompliance with the standards.

As a result of increasing standardization of **claims data** (information required to be reported on a healthcare claim for service reimbursement), there is increasing convergence of claims data with health data (see figure 16.2 that illustrates the HIPAA **transactions** and their relationship to clinical data). As claims data and clinical data are used together, healthcare quality and cost improvements can be made. This integration of financial and clinical data provides **business intelligence** (BI) that helps support business decisions by both the administrative and clinical leadership of healthcare organizations. For example, with more complete clinical information available at the time of admission, a hospital is better able to verify a patient's eligibility for health plan benefits so that it is not faced with a denied claim later. Information that shows the hospital how many and what type of patients are readmitted within 30 days of discharge for the same condition is another example of BI that will enable a hospital to take proactive measures to monitor these patients more closely after discharge.

- Form creation systems are those that automate some of the authorization, consent (McKenzie and Karnstedt 2010), advance directive, and other administrative forms used to manage healthcare administrative processes. These systems provide information to the patient, capture an electronic signature from the patient, and supply the patient with a copy of the signed form if requested.

Ancillary or Departmental Systems

Ancillary systems, also called clinical departmental systems, serve primarily to manage the department in which they exist, while at the same time providing key clinical data for the EHR. There are three main departmental systems that are necessary for an EHR to function in a hospital. These include:

- **Laboratory information system** (LIS) will receive an order for a lab test; generate a work list for specimen collection, labeling, and accessioning; retrieve results from an auto-analyzer (device that analyses the specimen); perform quality control; maintain an inventory of equipment and supplies needed to perform lab tests;

Figure 16.2.   HIPAA transactions and clinical data

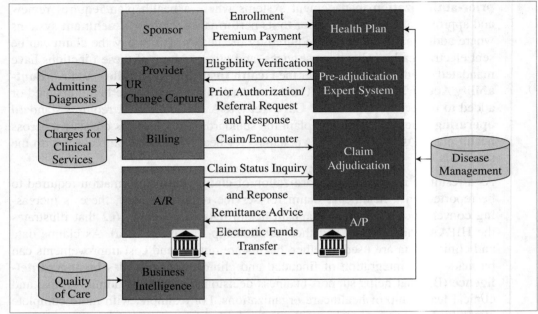

Copyright © 2012 Margret\A Consulting, LLC. Reprinted with permission.

and manage information on departmental staffing and costs. Of course, the LIS supplies the lab results to the user, either as a printout or print file and/or as structured data to an EHR. Note that blood-banking and clinical pathology are often separate systems in addition to the LIS.

- **Radiology information systems** (RISs) perform similar functions, receiving an order for a procedure; scheduling it; notifying hospital personnel or the patient, if performed as an outpatient, how to prepare for the procedure; tracking the performance of the procedure and its output (that is, images in analog or digital form); tracking preparation of the report; performing quality control; maintaining an inventory of equipment and supplies; and managing departmental staffing and budget.

- **Pharmacy information system,** which receives an order for a drug; aids the pharmacist in checking for contraindications; directs staff in compounding any drugs requiring special preparation; aids in dispensing the drug in the appropriate dose and for the appropriate route of administration; maintains inventory; supports staffing and budgeting; and performs other departmental operations.

Other clinical departments in a hospital, such as dietary/food and nutrition, have similar information systems that both receive orders and supply results (or services) to users, as well as manage the respective department.

Small physician practices are unlikely to have any clinical departmental systems, although larger practices may have LIS, RIS, and potentially others depending on their specialty.

Health information management (HIM) departments typically do not have a specific departmental information system, although sometimes the different applications managed in HIM departments may be referred to as HIM applications. Instead of a single HIM information system, HIM departments manage some of the administrative and financial systems, support applications that complement the EHR, and retain responsibility for the content and quality of the EHR. HIM applications vary by how far along the organization is in implementing its EHR applications. For example, if the organization continues to retain some paper charts, the HIM department may have a chart tracking system to manage location of paper records. Many organizations do not yet have all the EHR components to be completely paperless, so they need to complement the EHR components with systems to support dictation, transcription, and electronic document and content management. There are also HIM functions that may not yet be able to be fully addressed by the EHR. As a result, **chart deficiency systems, release of information systems, coding and abstracting systems,** and others are not likely to go away very soon, although there may be a transition in how they are managed. These are discussed in a later section in this chapter.

Core EHR Applications

There are generally five main components necessary to consider when an organization has an EHR. These include: (1) **results management;** (2) clinical documentation; (3) closed-loop medication management; (4) **clinical decision support** (CDS); and (5) analytics and reporting. These are illustrated in figure 16.3.

These applications include the functionality required for earning federal meaningful use (MU) incentives—and more. The MU incentive program does not require all EHR functionality that is available, or even that is common in hospitals and physician practices today. For example, MU includes **computerized provider order entry** (CPOE) but does not at this time include **electronic medication administration record** (E-MAR) or **barcode medication administration record** (BC-MAR). Similarly, MU does not include support for E&M coding despite that most physician practices find this an essential part of their EHR.

It is also important to note that there are some variations in the core EHR applications as they are used in a hospital or physician practice. One main difference is that in a hospital, the EHR applications are often implemented separately; whereas in a physician practice EHR the applications tend to be more integrated. Other differences are noted below as each of these core applications is described more fully.

Finally, the core EHR applications are listed in the sequence in which they are typically acquired by a hospital or used in a physician practice—although this varies considerably as well.

Figure 16.3.   **Core clinical EHR systems**

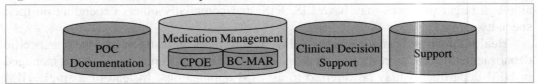

Results Management

Results management is an application that enables diagnostic study results (primarily lab results) to be both reviewed in a report format and the data within the reports to be processed. In fact, results retrieval systems came before results management systems. **Results retrieval** systems only allowed reports of results to be viewed and/or printed. Normal ranges were printed alongside of the patient's results and often a flag was used to show out-of-range results. Results management systems enable lab results to be used in interactive ways. For example, a physician could automatically send a page or text message when specified results are abnormally high. Users can compare, trend, and graph the results. Depending on their level of sophistication, results management systems may also be able to compare lab results with other clinical data. For example, a graphic display could depict lab results as a function of medications administered, or be compared with a patient's vital signs. Lab results can also be used directly without requiring abstraction in quality measurement studies, clinical research, and business intelligence systems—such as to evaluate the cost-effectiveness of one type of test in comparison to another. In order for a healthcare organization to have results management, all data to be processed must be in structured format and ideally stored together in one data repository.

The importance of results management cannot be emphasized enough. It has been observed that 70 percent of the ability to reach a diagnosis for a patient depends on lab results (Wians 2009). Similarly, as medications are increasingly powerful in their impact on the human body, monitoring vital signs and lab results in association with medication administration is critical to appropriate medication management. In fact, in one, widely-publicized hospital incident, not taking appropriate action when a baby's blood test showed an extraordinarily high level of sodium chloride from a drug being administered caused the baby to die (Graham and Dizikes 2011).

Clinical Documentation

Another EHR component is clinical documentation. These systems are also called **point-of-care charting** systems because the intent of these applications is to direct what documentation needs to be recorded for the patient, and is the means to supply CDS at the time when the clinician is able to be most responsive to alerts and reminders. **Clinical documentation systems** are those that supply templates to the user to be completed primarily via point-and-click, drop-down, type-ahead, and other data-entry tools. Usually the EHR has a library of templates. The user may choose the appropriate template, or may have displayed the appropriate template based on the user's profile as indicated via the login as well as the patient's admitting diagnosis or chief complaint at the time of a physician office visit. Some templates are very sophisticated and as the user enters data will adjust the data fields displayed accordingly. As a simple example, a template for conducting a history and physical exam for a male patient would not display data fields applicable to females. If the system detects that the patient's condition involves heart disease, additional data fields may be displayed for associated signs, symptoms, and potential complications. The result is structured data that the computer is essentially processing into clinical documentation.

Clinical documentation systems in a hospital may initially include only those for nursing staff, such as for nurse admission assessments, nursing problem lists, nurses' notes, vital signs (which may also be captured directly from patient monitoring systems), intake/output records, and other nursing documentation. Medication administration is also a nursing documentation requirement, but such systems are typically grouped under medication management systems, as described next.

However, a **nursing information system** is generally considered a departmental system, not a clinical documentation system. Similar to LIS, RIS, and pharmacy information systems, a nursing information system manages the nursing department, including staffing, credentialing, training, budgeting, and other managerial functions. Clinical data may be combined with department operations data in a nursing information system to provide **patient acuity staffing** levels, where the number of staff needed for any shift or day is determined by how acutely ill the current patients are.

In a hospital, physicians are increasingly expected to document orders in a computerized provider order entry (CPOE) system, although this is also more specifically considered a part of a medication management system described below. Physician documentation of the history and physical exam, consults, operative reports, and discharge summary in a hospital are still largely dictated and electronically fed as an image into the EHR. Progress notes may be handwritten and scanned into the EHR. The problem list may be handwritten, although increasingly managed through a combination of sources including the admission order for the admitting diagnosis and directly from a drop-down menu for discharge diagnoses and procedures. Such structured data links to ICD-9-CM and/or **SNOMED-CT** codes.

In physician practices, however, clinical documentation is much more often entered directly as structured data into the EHR by both physicians and nurses. In part this is due to the fact that physician coding for services performed in the practice can be drawn directly from the EHR. It is also due to the fact that visit notes, orders, prescriptions, and CDS are more integrated in ambulatory EHRs.

Closed-loop Medication Management

Closed-loop medication management refers to the use of certain systems that help assure **patient safety** from the point a drug is ordered to the point it is administered. These systems include CPOE, **e-prescribing** (e-Rx) as a special type of CPOE, electronic medication administration record (E-MAR) or barcode medication administration record (BC-MAR), **medication reconciliation** systems, and automated drug dispensing machines as well as the policies, procedures, and **workflows** associated with ensuring proper drug ordering, dispensing, administering, and monitoring of reactions. Although there is no recommended sequence for implementing these systems, many hospitals in the past implemented CPOE last because it is difficult to get physicians to use such systems in the hospital. This is changing as MU incentives require use of a CPOE system (and, as noted above, not E-MAR or BC-MAR systems). In the ambulatory setting, e-Rx has sometimes been implemented as a standalone system before an EHR (and its CPOE functionality) because some insurers and Medicare were providing incentives for its use.

CPOE systems can be used for entering all orders, such as patient admission, laboratory tests, x-rays and other diagnostic studies, dietary/food and nutrition, therapies, nursing services, consults, discharge of patient, referrals, and even building personal task lists, as well as entering orders for medications. In the past, physicians typically handwrote these orders and they were either internally faxed to various departments as applicable or were transcribed by nursing personnel (such as ward secretaries or unit clerks) into an order communication system. The **order communication** system, however, only enabled transmission of the order to various departments' information systems. There was no CDS in the order communication system. In fact, one of the issues physicians have with CPOE today is that they view themselves as now having to perform clerical tasks. As a result, some hospitals have eased in implementation of CPOE, requiring its use—at least initially—only for medication ordering. The CPOE functionality in an ambulatory EHR is much more likely to be used by physicians, because the scope of the types of orders placed is more limited.

In addition to concerns by physicians that CPOE systems require them to perform clerical tasks, there have been other concerns. Rudimentary CDS is built into these systems so that drug-allergy and drug-drug contraindication checking against a drug knowledge database is provided. Alerts and reminders about medication issues can be very useful, if set up properly. If not, however, the alerts and reminders can be annoying and often ignored. For example, an alert that reminds a physician that aspirin should not be given to patients with gastrointestinal bleeding or uncontrolled hypertension—unless the specific patient has one of these conditions—is an alert that many physicians believe is unnecessary and becomes annoying. In fact, this has become such a problem in some CPOE systems that the term **alert fatigue** is used to describe this issue. Another concern with CPOE systems is that they are often based on standard order sets. These order sets reflect the current thinking about patient care from research and other forms of evidence-based medicine (EBM). Despite that EBM may reflect the best scientific evidence on how to treat a patient with a specific condition, there is rarely one size fits all for human beings. A patient with a specific condition frequently has other conditions, which may not have been taken into account when the research study was performed. As a result, most standard orders need to be modified for each patient. In haste a physician may accept the standard orders or may make an error in modifying them—which may result in **unintended consequences.** An unintended consequence is an unanticipated and undesired effect of implementing and using an EHR (Rollins 2012). These are often attributed to the EHR software even though they reflect that a user may not have applied professional judgment or due diligence in using the system.

CPOE systems also generate the patient's medication list. Caution must also be applied here, as the medication list will only be as accurate and complete as all systems contributing information to it. For instance, if a medication is ordered prior to surgery, suspended during surgery, reinstated after surgery but then changed before administration, not only must the CPOE and E-MAR/BC-MAR contribute correct medication information, but the surgery information system may also need to be linked to the medication management systems, which is not always the case.

E-Rx is a special type of CPOE used exclusively to make a prescription and transmit it electronically to retail pharmacies. As such, they are used in ambulatory settings, including not only the physician practice but when a patient is discharged from the hospital or emergency service with a prescription and in hospital outpatient departments or clinics. The e-Rx system includes medication alerts and reminders just as the hospital-based CPOE system, but also includes formulary information that identifies whether the patient's health plan covers the cost of a drug and what co-pay may be required. Physicians can then work with their patients to find the most cost-effective as well as clinically-suitable drug. Because e-Rx systems are able to transmit prescriptions directly to retail pharmacies, physicians find benefit from fewer calls from pharmacies not able to read their handwriting or needing to advise the physician that a drug ordered is off formulary for a patient. Physicians are also able to receive electronic communications from retail pharmacies, such as for renewal approvals that can significantly save time in a practice. Recently, the Drug Enforcement Administration (DEA), which previously banned use of e-Rx for controlled substances (such as narcotics), set special requirements, including use of a product that provides identity proofing and two-factor authentication to enable such use.

Medication administration recording is a function performed by nurses in a hospital. The frequency and care which must be taken to assure that a nurse administers the right drug, in the right dose, through the right route, at the right time, and to the right patient (the **Medication Five Rights**) is critical to avoid medication errors. As a result, computerized systems have been created. Early E-MAR systems were simply electronically generated paper lists of medications from the pharmacy information system after it processed physician orders. Later, the lists were retained on the computer and nurses were expected to post the date and time of medication administration to the computer. Any exceptions or issues with medication administration, however, were still included in handwritten nurses' notes. Most importantly, these systems, while providing a legible list of medications did not fully address the Medication Five Rights.

Today, many hospitals are moving to BC-MAR systems. These require the hospital to have each patient identified with a barcode (usually on a wrist band) and to package (or buy pre-packaged) drugs in unit dose form, each with a barcode or **radio-frequency identification** (RFID) tag that identifies the drug, dose, and intended route of administration. At the time the drug is to be administered to a patient, the nurse logs onto the BC-MAR system and scans the patient's wrist band and unit dose package. The system automatically dates and time-stamps the entry made through this process. As a result, the Medication Five Rights have been followed. Most BC-MAR systems also enable notes to describe exceptions, such as the fact that the patient was in surgery at the time the next dose was to be administered. BC-MAR systems provide some CDS as do CPOE systems, often including links to additional information about drugs. BC-MAR systems also generate reports on timely administration of drugs.

There are some issues with using BC-MAR systems. One is that the bags that contain specially compounded drugs administered intravenously require special labels, which not all hospital pharmacy information systems can accommodate. In this case, special care must be taken to manually check and enter the medications being administered. The other important issue associated with using BC-MAR systems is that of bringing the computer, barcode wand, and medication to the patient bedside. Some hospitals use wireless **workstations on wheels** (WOWs), although these can be heavy to push once fully loaded with these devices as well as a long-life battery. An alternative is to carry, sometimes by wearing a sling, a tablet computer that may be outfitted with a wanding device and the medication. Walking around all day with such equipment on one's person, however, is also not comfortable. Finally, it is very important for the hospital to fully define what constitutes a medication administration error, a wrong time, for instance, may or may not be due to an error but rather the availability of the patient.

The medication reconciliation process also can be automated, although not as easily as the other elements of medication management. Each time a patient is transferred across levels of care, such as when admitted, transferred into an intensive care unit, sent to surgery, and so on, the medications the patient should be taking needs to be reviewed. This is because very often certain medications must be discontinued or a dose changed as a result of the change in level of care. In addition, the clinicians working with the patient are different at different levels of care. Connecting all the systems at the different levels of care has been a challenge that only a few hospitals have been able to fully achieve as yet.

Finally with respect to medication management, **automated drug dispensing machines** are available that both secure and make drugs more readily available to nursing staff. These machines are typically filled by pharmacy department staff based on the physician orders.

Clinical Decision Support

CDS is a key component of the EHR, and sets it apart from simply automating paper documents. CDS functionality in the EHR helps physicians, nurses, and other clinical professionals, collectively referred to as clinicians, as well as patients themselves make decisions about patient care. Some examples of CDS as previously discussed include alerts about potential drug contraindications and out-of-range lab results as well as standard order sets in CPOE. In addition, CDS templates can help determine what documentation of clinical findings is necessary; provide suggestions for prescribing less expensive, but equally effective, drugs; supply protocols for certain health maintenance procedures; and alert that a duplicate lab test is being ordered. There are countless other decision-making aids for all stakeholders in the care process.

CDS may be built into each of the core applications of EHR. However, CDS is also acquired as separate systems that work in conjunction with the EHR applications. In general, the CDS found in the core EHR applications is fairly rudimentary because they typically are able to only process data within the given application. More sophisticated CDS requires the convergence of different types of data from the various EHR components. As a result, separate applications are typically used to help integrate and analyze these data.

Separate CDS applications may be fully integrated with the core EHR applications, or be used in a standalone fashion. An example of a separate CDS application is one that provides drug-lab checking, such as whether a drug is contraindicated for a patient with poor liver function. This is not a routine function of CPOE or LIS, but requires the combination of data from both sources and the ability to deliver the alert back to the appropriate system or systems. This is then commonly referred to as a separate **clinical decision support system** (CDSS), even though it may be fully integrated into the core EHR applications through supporting infrastructure. Other examples of separate CDSS that are integrated into the EHR include the templates used in clinical documentation, the standard order sets used in CPOE, and the clinical pathways that guide nursing services. While some EHR products build a basic set of templates directly into their clinical documentation systems, others require a separate CDSS to generate the templates, or provide more sophisticated and customizable templates than exist in the basic clinical documentation applications.

CDSS that are used in a standalone fashion are often those specific to a unique function. For example, a CDSS that is used in a standalone fashion in a hospital includes a system to alert infection control nurses of a potential hospital-acquired infection. It provides advice on which medication may be most effective in combating the infection given the causative agent. Such a system compiles data from clinical documentation (such as documentation of a high temperature), lab results (such as the strain of bacteria that is causing the infection), x-ray results (such as a finding of pneumonia), and other sources processed against automated clinical reference information to produce the specific findings.

An example of a CDSS that is used in a standalone fashion by physicians is a differential diagnosis system. Some of these compare diagnostic images against a library of images and their known conditions, especially useful for radiologists, dermatologists, pathologists, and others. Other differential diagnosis CDS systems compare data from clinical documentation, especially the history of present illness and review of systems, with a library of known symptoms and signs for specific diagnoses. Some of these are used only when the differential diagnosis is obscure. Others may be a routine part of a **protocol**, such as for assessing a patient presenting to the emergency service with chest pain. Still another CDS system can aid in identifying whether a patient's symptoms are due to a new condition or are the result of an adverse reaction to a medication. Figure 16.4 summarizes the different forms of CDS.

It should be noted that despite the advantages CDSS can offer, many clinicians are still resistant to entering data into the computer system at the point of care, especially when the system requires a lot of structured data. This is both a workflow issue for which many clinicians have not been trained to overcome as well as a system design issue. As a result, in a number of both hospitals and physician practices, clinical information is still dictated and turned into typed reports or handwritten and scanned into an electronic document management system. However to take advantage of CDS, the data required for the system to work must be captured in or converted at some point to a structured data format.

Figure 16.4. **Types of clinical decision support**

Data Display
- Data always available
- Flow sheets (e.g., problem list, medication list)
  - —Maintain longitudinally
  - —Across continuum
- Dynamic displays
  - —Flow sheet/graphic/table/narrative—helps review data
  - —Clinical imaging integration
  - —Search tools
  - —Query support
- Summaries/abstracts
  - —Quickens access, supports continuity of care
  - —Flags problems

Workflow
- In-basket
  - —Reminders in support of timeliness, compliance
- Schedule/patient list
  - —Patient status continuously
- Workgroup tools
  - —Easy handoffs
- Refills choice lists
- Integrated clinical/financial
  - —Medical necessity checking
  - —Overcomes inability to pay for treatment
- Telephony, e-mail/visits, instant messaging
  - —Quick response

Data Retrieval
- Single sign-on (for multiple applications)
  - —Overcomes interface vs. integration (through one system or repository) issues
- Ease of navigation aids adoption
- Density of screen
  - —"Flip-ability"
  - —Avoids getting lost in "drill downs"
- Specialized formats focus information
- Customized screens
  - —Standards vs.
  - —Personal preference (convenience? adoption?)

Data Entry
- Context-sensitive templates/order sets guide documentation
- Provides immediate access to active decision support
  - —Alerts and reminders
  - —Clinical calculations
  - —Therapy critiquing and planning
- Patient self-assessment/PHR
- Medication list maintenance (by patient or claims consolidator)
- Structured data/registry support
  - —Contributes to downstream knowledge
  - —Wellness or disease management reminders/interventions due/recalls
- Access to reference information
  - —Context-insensitive/portal
  - —Context-sensitive/direct links

Structured data are discrete data points that are **encoded** by and can be processed in the computer. A number of examples have been provided. Another example is social history of smoking, where use of a template to indicate whether a patient smokes and perhaps the number of cigarettes smoked per day are discrete data points. These can then generate an alert that smoking cessation counseling should be given, which is one of the clinical quality measures for earning MU incentives. Another example might be the ability of the system to calculate the patient's body mass index (BMI) and recommend weight counseling. Many ambulatory EHR systems include reminders for preventive or chronic care services, such as dates when a vaccine, cancer screening, diabetes care, and other services are due.

Analytics and Reporting

Analytics and reporting are a final core EHR application. Analytics refers to statistical processing of data to reveal new information. This goes beyond the simple use of descriptive statistics, such as how many patients were seen for a specific condition; to questions such as which form of treatment for the specific condition had the best outcomes. The ability to produce such reports is increasingly important as there is ever more pressure to improve quality and reduce the cost of healthcare. Analytics, however, entails sophisticated processes to be performed on data, such as data mining, forecasting, neural networks (mathematical modeling that makes connections between data to discover relationships), and others.

In healthcare, analytics has been primarily performed in academic and research institutions, by health plans, at pharmaceutical manufacturers, and for public health departments. Analytics has brought the healthcare industry many clinical benefits, such as in genomic research and personalized medicine (SAS nd). It is also used to create business intelligence, such as in predicting prescribing patterns of physicians, or the impact of a disaster on local emergency services (Strome 2011).

Although most information systems are able to generate some data for analysis and reporting, there has been strong interest for the EHR to provide more robust analysis of data. Unfortunately, the nature of the **database** required for POC charting and CDS, that are key elements of an EHR, does not support analytics and reporting as well. Very often it is necessary to move data from the EHR system to a separate database that has been optimized to perform analytics and reporting. In addition, healthcare organizations that want to perform sophisticated analytics will need staff highly skilled in such statistical techniques. It may be that a given hospital or physician practice cannot perform the analytics and reporting itself, but sends data to a vendor who performs the analytics. An increasing number of EHR vendors are supplying such services, often aggregating data from many of its customers so the data have greater reliability and validity.

An appreciation for analytics and reporting and the need for good data are important to hospitals and physician practices even if they do not perform analytics themselves. It is very important to consider the types of information ultimately needed for analytics so that the data can be captured in the EHR. The quality of the data being captured must also be assured.

Health plans have analyzed data from healthcare claims for a long time; now they are getting additional data in the form of feeds from commercial labs, claims attachments, and other sources to perform even more sophisticated analytics. Such information may impact whether the hospital or physician practice gets a favorable discount rate on its fees for services. Quality benchmarking depends on analytics. Consumers are beginning to look at which hospital excels in cardiac care or has a center of excellence for orthopedics. Having aggregated data to understanding why one healthcare organization is ahead in its quality metrics over another can help poorer performers improve. But the data must also be recorded accurately and precisely. For example, a physician practice may routinely report CPT codes describing where their diabetic patients are on their HbA1c results. There are three codes for reporting HbA1c results: one code reflects results of less than 7.0, a second code reflects results between 7.0 and 9.0, and a third code reflects results greater than 9.0. However, if clinical research causes a change in the metrics, such as identifying that a successful outcome of diabetic care requires the HbA1c to only be less than 7.5, or to increase the target to 6.5, the ability to trend improvement over time using only the three CPT codes will not be feasible (Frei et al. 2010).

Analytics and reporting is not only used for retrospective quality or research studies. An important set of reports include rule-based lists for patient follow-up. Patient follow-up lists have not been very easy to generate. In the past much of the data had to be manually abstracted from paper records, transcription, and/or scanned images of documents. However, the ability to identify all patients requiring follow-up after discharge, for chronic disease care, to notify them of a drug or device recall, to send preventive care reminders, or any of many other similar types of reports or lists is integral to quality patient care.

Most analytics implementations are still retrospective. However, it can be anticipated that the use of data mining at the POC will be able directly improve clinical decision making, such as in selecting affordable therapies (Chaiken 2011) and earlier diagnosis of complex conditions such as rheumatoid arthritis and multiple sclerosis (Kalatzis, et al. 2009).

Today, the federal government is putting increased emphasis on using EHR for quality improvement. For a number of years hospitals have been required to report quality measures to the Joint Commission to retain accreditation; and to the Centers for Medicare and Medicaid Services (CMS) in order to earn full reimbursement for their services under Medicare. These measures were consolidated as **core measures** for both programs, and are reported to the public by CMS on its HospitalCompare website. Physician quality reporting to earn incentives under the federal government's **Physician Quality Reporting System** (PQRS) was started more recently. Reporting clinical quality measures is also a requirement for earning MU incentives. However, going forward, it is anticipated that not only must quality measures be *reported*, but there must be the ability to demonstrate *improvement* in the measures over time. As health reform legislation encourages new and risk-based forms of reimbursement structures, such as ACOs, bundled payments, and PCMH, the ability to predict patient volumes, outcomes, and improve quality will directly impact a healthcare organization's bottom line.

Specialty Systems and Automated Medical Devices

Specialty systems are those which support documentation of patient care in specialty areas, such as intensive care units, emergency services, respiratory and other therapy services, rehabilitative care, behavioral healthcare, hospice, and many others. These systems might be like a "mini-EHR" for the specialty area, although ideally should not replicate information collection and services provided by other source systems in the organization. This is not always feasible, as many vendors that supply the mainstream source systems and core EHR applications do not also supply specialty systems. In other cases, the specialty systems require such different types of data and processes that it is difficult to fully integrate them into the core EHR applications. Finally, specialty applications are often found in specialty locations not integrated with general medical services. For example, most dentists practice in offices or clinics separate from their medical colleagues. It is only in the small percentage of federal qualified health centers, for example, where dental services are integrated with medical services.

Picture archiving and communications systems (PACSs) are yet another form of specialty information system. They capture **digital images** from various modalities, such as x-ray, ultrasound, and others and provide special viewing capabilities of these images via a computer. Some of these also have the ability to connect directly with a radiology information system.

Automated medical devices, until recently, have generally not been considered information systems, even though they have generated information—sometimes only in the form of a blood pressure on a display screen and other times in the form of a continuous feed of data such as a fetal monitoring strip. Other examples of such medical devices include vital signs monitors, cardiac output monitors, defibrillators, electrocardiographs, infusion pumps, physiologic monitors, ventilators, and others (HIMSS Analytics 2010). Today, however, many healthcare organizations would like to connect these devices to their EHR, but the technology to do so, called medical device integration, requires special technical infrastructure. Hospitals and other healthcare provider settings are just beginning to prioritize integration of these medical devices into their EHR infrastructures (ECRI Institute 2012).

Supporting Infrastructure

Supporting infrastructure refers to the technology that allows the various applications to work. This includes both hardware and additional software, both of which are described more fully in a later section of this chapter. Infrastructure also must consider the policies for using the applications, address workflow changes, and provide training and support to users. For example, the medical device integration described above requires not only special hardware and software, but inventory controls on the devices, identification of associated IP addresses, policies on how long the data may be retained, and changes to processes people use to review the results. Suffice it to say, a supporting infrastructure is vital to manage the different applications necessary for today's health information needs. Large hospitals may have close to a thousand applications, with hundreds of applications being common in medium-sized hospitals. Physician practices may have only one combined PMS-EHR system, but frequently have some ancillary and specialty systems—potentially accumulating 10 to 20 or more systems.

Connectivity Systems

Connectivity systems enable the exchange of data across separate information systems both within a healthcare organization and across organizations.

Essentially computer systems contain data in incompatible formats unless all the systems are acquired from the same vendor who took the time to enable connectivity across its different applications. Connectivity systems support the ability, for example, for the R-ADT system from vendor A or PMS from vendor B to share patient demographic data with the CPOE system from vendor C, or to share a single patient's data in a provider setting with a health plan for reimbursement, with a separate provider for continuity of care, and with the patient or patient's designated representative. Connectivity systems are also required to contribute data about many patients to a **registry** or data collection vendor to conduct quality measurement and reporting, for research, and/or to public health for biosurveillance and other public health functions. Connectivity systems range from legacy structures, such as **interfaces** using **message format standards,** to new web-based services and XML. They also include PHRs and other means to supply health information to patients and others who are authorized to have such information. Systems integrators, registries, and health information exchange organizations provide connectivity services.

Check Your Understanding 16.1

1. Which of the following is a source system:

   A. Laboratory information system
   B. Results management system
   C. Clinical decision support system
   D. Input devices

2. Which of the following is *not* considered a core EHR component:

   A. Computerized provider order entry
   B. Pharmacy information system
   C. Electronic medication administration record
   D. Point-of-care charting

3. Dr. Smith always orders the same 10 things when a new patient is admitted to the hospital in addition to some patient-specific orders. What would assist in assuring that the specific patient is not allergic to a drug being ordered?

   A. Drug knowledge database
   B. Standard order set
   C. Pharmacy information system
   D. Electronic medication administration record system

4. What provides alerts and reminders to clinicians?

   A. Clinical decision support system
   B. Electronic data interchange
   C. Point-of-care charting system
   D. Workflow system

5. Point-of-care charting systems in hospitals today are primarily used by:

   A. Physicians
   B. Pharmacists
   C. Nurses
   D. All of the above

Instructions: Indicate whether the following statements are true or false (T or F).

6. _____ E-MARs that utilize barcodes or RFID technology support Medication Five Rights.

7. _____ Medication reconciliation is the most difficult function of closed-loop medication management systems to implement.

8. _____ The meaningful use incentive program requires all medication management components to be present and used in a hospital.

9. _____ Templates utilize free text but not data-entry tools like drop-down boxes.

10. _____ The EHR itself does not have to perform analytics for complex analysis of data to be available to the healthcare organization.

Evolution of the Electronic Health Record

Achieving comprehensive EHR systems has been very much a journey. There has been increased emphasis on EHRs since 2004 when President Bush included their promotion in an executive order to create the Office of the National Coordinator (ONC) for Health Information Technology; however, the concept of an EHR is not new.

The earliest efforts to address **clinical information systems** (CISs) occurred in the mid-1960s. Clinical data are **textual** and contextual, making it difficult to develop systems that can collect and process these data effectively and efficiently. Clinical data are largely **textual** because clinicians often (and prefer to) describe patient conditions in narrative form. Narrative data also depend on context or situation to make the data meaningful. For example, when a patient is described as "having a red face," but the situation is not explained, we do not know whether the patient is embarrassed, angry, hot, burned, or has a rash.

As a result of the difficulty in developing complex information systems that could handle textual and **contextual** data, the automation process of healthcare data started with simpler financial and administrative systems, such as patient registration, census, and billing. The healthcare delivery system is fragmented by departments within an organization and across the continuum of care. As a result, information systems initially focused on solving departmental and institutional business-related functions like those in other industries, such as materials and inventory management. Consequently, information systems to manage pharmacy inventory or lab specimen collection mimicked similar systems in other industries.

By the mid-1980s, the Institute of Medicine (IOM 1991) indicated that new technologies should be considered for improving the state of medical records. A committee formed to make recommendations and produced a report in 1991 entitled "The Computer-based Patient Record: An Essential Technology for Health Care." The concept of what the IOM called a CPR, described at the start of this chapter, was an important result of the report, changing the thinking about the purpose, characteristics, and features of an automated medical record.

Subsequent IOM reports focusing on quality of care and patient safety have emphasized that EHR systems can make a difference. In their first report in 1999 on "To Err is Human: Building a Safer Health System," the IOM exposed the fact that between 44,000 and 98,000 hospitalized Americans die every year from medical mistakes. They cited a number of factors that needed improvement in the US healthcare system, including adoption of information technology.

The IOM subsequently published a series of "quality chasm" reports addressing medication errors, poor workflow, and other gaps that require addressing to ensure good quality healthcare. To this day, the IOM has been a staunch supporter of using information technology.

In 2003, the IOM report entitled "Patient Safety: Achieving a New Standard for Care" addressed many of the standardization issues that were needed to improve patient safety through the use of the EHR and, in a report appended to the work, defined the key capabilities of an EHR system (figure 16.5).

In their 2009 study "Computational Technology for Effective Health Care: Immediate Steps and Strategic Directions," members of IOM/National Research Council observed that there have been a number of success stories in implementing HIT, but these still fall significantly short of what is needed (Stead and Lin 2009). The IOM described a "healthcare IT chasm" much like the quality chasm.

The evolution of EHR has not been smooth, has varied by type of organization, and is continuing to evolve.

Evolution of EHRs in Hospitals

Many hospitals began their journey to EHR long before EHR was even considered an important goal. Hospitals generally acquired administrative and financial systems first in order to track patient admissions and discharges and manage the filing of claims for reimbursement of their services. Once these were in place, departmental systems were adopted, generally first with an LIS, next RIS, and then a pharmacy information system. These are considered the big three ancillary systems necessary to support the majority of clinical processes other than physician and nurse documentation.

However, once the basic applications were in place, many physicians wanted electronic access from their offices to the hospital's lab and x-ray results (through PACS).

Figure 16.5.   **IOM key capabilities of an EHR system**

1. Health information and data	5. Electronic communication and connectivity
2. Results management	6. Patient support
3. Order entry/management	7. Administrative processes
4. Decision support	8. Reporting and population health management

Source: Adapted from Kohn 2000.

Hospitals generally provided these through a physician portal that enables the physician or office staff to login to the hospital and view and/or download results. In some cases, the **portals** also enabled physician practices to enter data about their patients they were admitting, sign transcribed documents, and perform other chart completion activities.

As more data became available electronically, hospitals grew frustrated with part of their data on paper and part electronic (a situation described as a **hybrid record**). They wanted to be able to make everything electronic, but knew it would take some time to acquire, implement, and convince clinicians to adopt the core EHR applications. As a result, most hospitals adopted some form of document imaging. Some of these are very basic and others more complex. They are summarized in figure 16.6. Early in the evolution, **document imaging management systems** (DIMSs) and **computer output to laser disk** (COLD) systems were adopted. These would allow clinicians to continue documenting on paper, but would also make the paper documents more accessible. DIMS involve scanning documents created on paper and making their images available on a computer monitor. COLD systems capture print images of lab results and other documents that are in standalone electronic systems and make them available for viewing on a computer monitor. Because of the use of newer, magnetic storage media, COLD systems are more commonly referred to as **electronic (or enterprise) report management** (ERM) systems.

DIMS have become more sophisticated and today are called **electronic document management systems** (EDMSs). They can manage many types of digital documents, including e-mails and e-faxes. When EDMSs are well indexed, certain content within the documents can be uniquely retrieved. **Electronic document/content management** (ED/CM) systems, for example, may include barcoding on the forms to identify specific content, such as the name of the form (for example, nurse assessment, emergency services report) or part of a form, such as the section of a history and physical exam containing

Figure 16.6.   Forms of document imaging systems

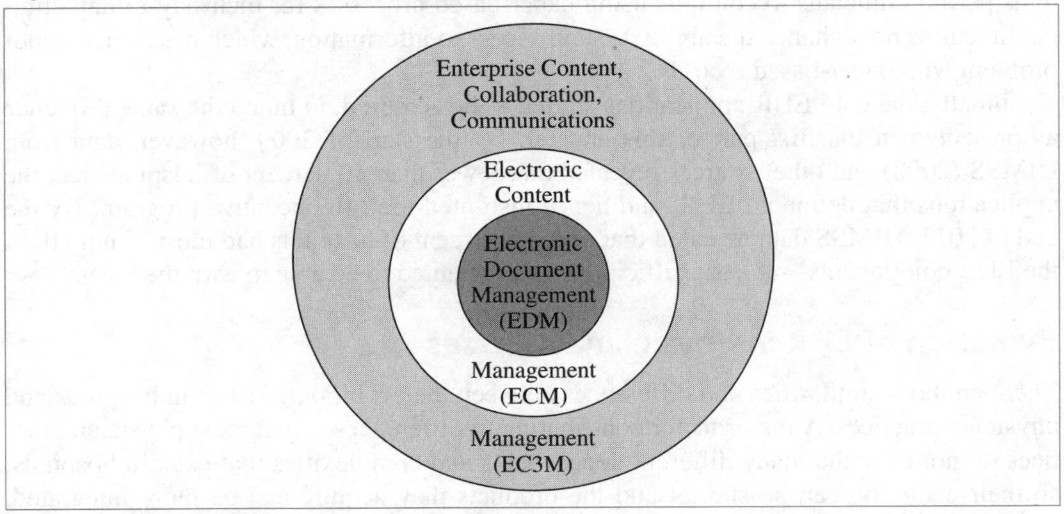

Enterprise Content, Collaboration, Communications

Electronic Content

Electronic Document Management (EDM)

Management (ECM)

Management (EC3M)

allergy information. When information on a patient's allergies is needed, it can be selected for viewing.

Workflow support also has been added to EDMSs. This means that the EDMS facilitates various functions that must be performed, often simultaneously or in a specific sequence. For example, upon patient discharge, a notification is sent to an analyst that the record is ready for analysis and coding. The analyst can retrieve the electronic images and analyze and code the patient stay. When the coding is completed, a notification is sent to financial services for the next function to be performed. Because the images are in electronic form, patient care areas for follow-up by quality departments or any other locations that require access can also access them.

Simultaneously, the chart deficiency system can identify what documents require signature by which physicians and make them available at any computer workstation for electronic signature. **Electronic signature authentication** (ESA) systems require the author to sign onto the system using a user ID and password, review the document to be signed, and indicate approval. The system annotates that the review and approval took place by the specified individual at the date and time performed.

Digital dictation systems also became popular, where the dictation files could be accessed for listening by clinicians prior to being transcribed. Today, many hospitals (and physician practices) use **speech recognition** systems where dictation automatically converts to text. Dictators themselves can make any necessary corrections as they are dictating or transcriptionists can make corrections for them. Even newer technology, **discrete reportable transcription** (DRT) combines speech recognition with basic **natural language processing** (NLP) techniques to create structured data from the dictation. NLP is the ability for a computer to evaluate narrative information and structure it given sophisticated rules for addressing context. Although highly sophisticated NLP is still in its infancy, DRT systems require the dictation to follow a specific template. The result is a narrative note plus structured data that follows the requirements of the specific template. Such systems permit clinicians to continue using paper-based processes for their day-to-day clinical functions but enhance the ability to gain access to information, which has been a major problem with paper-based records.

Finally, the core EHR applications started to be acquired, in much the same sequence as presented in the first part of this chapter. By the start of 2009, however, data from HIMSS (2008) and other sources revealed that fewer than 10 percent of hospitals had the applications that define an EHR, and hence instituted the MU incentive program. By the end of 2011, HIMSS data revealed that over 25 percent of hospitals had most, if not all, of the EHR components—at least sufficiently implemented to be able to earn the incentives.

Evolution of EHR in Physician Practices

There are both similarities and differences between the evolution of EHR in hospitals and physician practices. A major factor contributing to differences is that most physician practices do not have the many different departments and complexities that exist in hospitals, so their evolution can be shorter and the products they acquire can be more integrated. Although HIMSS does not track physician adoption of EHR, a comprehensive study was conducted between late 2007 and early 2008 by researchers in Boston (DesRoches et al. 2008) revealed that only 4 percent of physicians reported having an extensive, fully functional EHR, and 13 percent reported having a basic system. These numbers were very similar to hospitals and also contributed to the creation of the MU incentive program. At the end of 2011, a study conducted for the Centers for Disease Control and Prevention (CDC) by Hsiao et al. found that EHR usage in physician practices had jumped to 57 percent. While other reports concur that there has been an increase in physician adoption of EHR due to the MU incentive program, other studies show a somewhat lower rate of implementation, typically in the 33 percent range.

The fact that it is difficult to assess the rate of adoption of EHR by physicians reveals that, despite specific functionality required of certified EHR products for use in the MU incentive program, the actual products being acquired and used have vastly different levels of sophistication. Certified products may only have the minimum necessary functionality for the MU incentives, or may have much more functionality. It is also noted that physicians do not have to use the EHR for 100 percent of their patients or functions performed in order to earn the incentives.

Despite the difficulty in describing physician adoption of EHR and the fact that EHR product offerings can be highly integrated, it is also known that many physicians have eased into EHR. They often have started with using the physician portal offered by their hospital. They may have exchanged data with their hospital and other providers through a **clinical messaging** system. This would be a secure means to exchange e-mail, either through a portal or simply using e-fax or encrypted e-mail. They then may have acquired a smart phone with access to drug knowledge information; later, moving to a standalone e-Rx system either on their smart phones or on a workstation in the office. Some physicians, especially in smaller practices, moved to a "lite" EHR. Such a system was largely comprised of **speech dictation,** word processing, document scanning, and/or optical character recognition (OCR). For example, some lite EHRs utilized encounter forms where structured data could be entered through OCR, viewed, and then printed out again to provide another set of encounter forms for the next time the patient visited. A surprising number of physicians attempted to create their own EHR using a Microsoft Access database. Along the path toward EHR many physician practices acquired a PMS. Larger physician practices tended to acquire more sophisticated EHRs when they made the leap to automation.

Evolution of EHR in Other Care Settings

EHR adoption in other care settings has not been tracked as closely as in hospitals or physician practices, but many long-term and post-acute care (LTPAC) facilities, behavioral healthcare providers, dentists, and others have had an interest in and have begun moving toward EHR. Specialty EHR systems are available for these providers. Much like hospitals, LTPAC begin their migration to EHR with administrative and financial systems. LTPAC have had mandatory data reporting for some time, and this has often been facilitated by some rudimentary information systems capabilities. Behavioral health providers, dentists, and other highly specialized professionals have had more limited product offerings available to them, but they are recognizing the importance of tracking patient care needs with their systems. Many other types of care settings, from ambulance services to retail clinics have begun to enter the automation age with products that tend to be "lite" in comparison to hospital products, but are beginning to grow in their sophistication—especially with increased interest in connecting systems and sharing data across the continuum of care.

Implementation versus Adoption versus Optimization

A description of the evolution toward EHR would not be complete without observing that there is a significant difference between a system that has been implemented, one that has been adopted, and one that is optimally used.

Implementation refers to a system having been installed and configured to meet a specific organization's needs. Users have begun to be trained and are beginning to use the system. However, during implementation an organization may not have rolled out use of the system to all potential users. It may be used on only one or a few nursing units, or on all nursing units but only for certain functions (such as only medication ordering in CPOE). In a teaching hospital, house staff (physicians in training) may fully use the system but the attending physicians may not use it at all, or only to view reports. In physician practices, the EHR may be used at one site, or only by primary care physicians, or only by certain physicians who have personally decided to use the system. New workflows and process changes may have been introduced, but users are still experimenting with them. Implementation, then, is a period of time in which the organization is still working on some aspects of deployment before every user has become fully acclimated to the system and the changes in workflows and processes that accompany use of the EHR. Many healthcare organizations have implemented systems but do not have full adoption. Full implementation can take several months and often several years. It is estimated that by the end of 2011, only about 25 percent of hospitals had fully implemented EHR systems. Adoption refers to the state of EHR where every intended user is using the basic functionality of the system. Frequently adoption requires a period of acclimation where users need time to work through how they are going to use the system and what further personal configuration may be desired. This can be aided with the help of workflow and process analysts, but often requires individual acceptance of these changes that just takes time. Adoption may also require retraining, reinforcement (of change), further re-design of workflows and processes, and even a system of rewards. Rewards should not be monetary, but ones that acknowledge the work effort required to make changes in ingrained habits, praise positive outcomes that result from use of the system, and contribute to a health competitive spirit so that everyone keeps pushing forward. Adoption may overlap with implementation, as those who are trained and brought live on the system first are often technology leaders who will also be early adopters. Unfortunately, some users may never reach full adoption, in which case counseling, workarounds, sanctions, termination, or other strategies may be necessary to achieve the results needed by all.

Optimization includes activities that extend use of EHRs beyond the basic functionality. Optimization of technology use frequently includes changes in the clinical practice of medicine. Sometimes a profound change in how medicine is practiced due to significant changes in technology is referred to as **clinical transformation.** For example, if a physician has always prescribed a certain medication for a given condition, the physician who has optimized use of the EHR will follow evidence-based medicine guidelines in selecting the appropriate medication. This may sometimes be the same medication as always and other times may be a medication that is more targeted, more aggressive, less expensive, or more expensive due to having better information available about the patient, condition, drug, and health plan formulary requirements. A clinical transformation often leads to acquisition of additional technology, such as more sophisticated CDS, different input devices, medical device integration, data analytics, or additional applications as they become available on the market. It could be said that optimization is an ongoing state.

Challenges to Implementation and Adoption

Despite federal incentives, health reform, and even peer pressure that are causing significant improvement in implementation and adoption of EHR, there remain challenges. These include their cost, questions about their true benefits, workflow changes, impact on productivity, and unintended consequences of their use.

Cost of EHR

Cost is definitely an impediment to acquiring EHR, even with the federal incentives, which are temporary. Costs vary tremendously. For very small hospitals (such as critical access hospitals with fewer than 25 beds) EHRs could cost between $350,000 and $2 million. At the higher end, large hospitals and integrated delivery systems could spend between $10 million to $70 million or more (Congdon 2009). For physician practices, the average cost of software is between $8,000 and $12,000 per physician; although systems can be acquired for free if the physicians are willing to receive advertising and have their patients' data deidentified and sold. EHRs could also cost physicians as much as $25,000 to $40,000 or more per physician (Hoyt 2011). For both hospitals and physician practices there is also ongoing maintenance at about 20 percent of the base cost plus the cost of staffing and user time.

It should be evident that EHR systems are highly sophisticated. As a result, they generally have a high cost. Higher-priced systems will have greater technical capabilities that extend the system beyond the basic requirements. They will also enable a high degree of customization. It is possible to buy lower-cost products. In many cases, lower-cost products are less sophisticated, will have less ability to be customized to user preferences, may not easily scale up to new requirements for the next stage of incentives or other new uses, and generally include very little training and virtually no workflow and process redesign support. Cloud-based EHRs also can lower the cost. Traditional EHR vendors sell the organization a license to use the software. This may be loaded on the organization's computers or housed at the vendor's company and accessed remotely. **Cloud computing** refers to the delivery of computing resources over a network sold as a metered service, much like buying electricity. To keep costs low, the cloud computing vendor provides the same service to every client, so customization is not possible—at least for the low price charged. Customization could be possible, but then a much higher price is charged.

Benefits of EHR

Benefits from using an EHR have been questioned. Most hospitals consider an EHR a cost of doing business today and do not anticipate very much financial return on the investment. Due to the nature of the US reimbursement system and the high cost of the systems, a net monetary value is elusive and most cost savings associated with clinical changes often accrue more directly to health plans. For example, if a hospital is able to reduce repeat testing, use lower cost drugs, apply more cost-effective treatments, keep people out of acute care beds, and reduce readmissions, it is actually losing revenue unless there is form of incentive or sanction applied by health plans as a share of their savings. A number of commercial health plans will negotiate more favorable contracts with hospitals if they demonstrate such cost savings. Medicare is establishing a rule that will not reimburse hospitals for readmissions that are within 30 days of discharge for the same condition.

However, most hospitals do find some cost savings in administrative functions, and believe that it is virtually impossible anymore to do so without an EHR. For example, hospitals may realize savings from the impact of the EHR system on the clerical workforce, admissions personnel, billers, transcriptionists, couriers, and other support staff. While some of these staff members will be retained and often redeployed, others are lost through attrition. Storage of paper charts and therefore warehousing costs should be reduced (although as previously noted this depends on the hybrid record situation and may even increase). Although nurses are rarely, if ever, eliminated, overtime and temporary staffing costs may be reduced or eliminated. The impact on nursing is related much more to productivity and reduced need to perform fewer administrative functions.

Hospitals also generally find improvements in increased charge capture and can reduce the number of denied claims, bad debt, and collections services costs. The EHR helps provide better business intelligence to reduce losses.

Alternatively, many physician practices are finding direct cost savings, in addition to the indirect savings from being able to prove the quality of their care to health plans. A study conducted by the Medical Group Management Association (MGMA 2011) reported that in practices surveyed, 39.7 percent found a decrease in total practice operating costs. These often derive from reduced transcription and clerical expenses associated with paper record maintenance; increased revenue from more accurate coding, better patient follow-up, and being able to see more patients in a day; and improved revenue cycle management.

Still, proving that the overall quality of care has been impacted by EHR is somewhat elusive. To date, quality improvements in *process* measures are fairly common, whereas improvements in *outcomes* measures have been more difficult to identify. For example, a study conducted by the Robert Wood Johnson Foundation (2010) found that 51 percent of diabetes patients treated at practices with EHRs in Cleveland received all the care they needed, as opposed to only 7 percent in practices with paper records. While **process improvement** is important and ideally contributes to positive outcomes, there are very few studies on the impact of EHR on outcomes, and what studies exist show mixed results (for example, Johns and Sayles 2010).

It is also important to recognize that these studies were generally conducted in the mid-2000s but are only now being published (Romano and Stafford 2011). At that time, there were many hospitals and practices that were just getting started implementing their EHRs. The EHRs may have been less mature than those available today and time may not have been given to work through adoption and optimization stages. In fact, it has been suggested (Collier 2011) that there are two types of organizations that have implemented EHR. Those with very high scores on quality measures to begin with were among early adopters—but their incremental improvement is naturally going to be lower than those with lower quality measure scores. Unfortunately, the other category of EHR implementer is the more typical organization—wherein there have been a number of poorly managed projects and many projects that have not addressed workflow changes.

Workflow and Process Changes

Workflow and process changes come about when the tasks to be performed or their sequence is altered by the EHR or other HIT. Much as workflow technology associated with EDMS, workflow and process changes in an EHR help better direct work, but the changes in EHR more directly impact the users. For example, if a physician is notified that a transcribed discharge summary is available for signature from an EDMS, the physician is relieved of going to the HIM department and can sign the document at his or her convenience. But, if a CDS reminder about the need for seasonal flu vaccination appears at the time a physician opens a patient record, this may not be the desirable time for this reminder. It may interrupt the thought flow of the physician with respect to addressing the patient's chief complaint. Changes in workflow and processes are the primary reason for lack of better results with EHRs for both hospitals and physician practices. Virtually every article that describes EHR implementation identifies workflow improvement as a "golden rule" for EHR (McNickle 2011b) or states that assuming the EHR is a magic bullet and therefore not addressing workflow changes is a common practice (McNickle 2011a). An EHR is not an automated form of the paper health record. Instead, it is automation of health information, much of which resided in the paper record but some of which was not captured via the paper record or at least was not readily accessible or processable in paper. The result is that the EHR should now be used in new and improved ways—a fact that many organizations have not fully embraced. However, the technology should not drive workflow and process changes either. Such changes can result in quality improvement (such as to be reminded about the seasonal flu vaccination), but their timing should be able to be customized to the needs of the physician and patient.

There are many potential reasons for not addressing workflow changes (Amatayakul 2011). These include the fact that it takes a long time just to install and configure an EHR system, so many organizations shortchange themselves in training and workflow and process redesign. Most EHR vendors do not support workflow and process redesign as they barely have sufficient staff to get systems installed and configured. Vendors view workflow and process redesign as the responsibility of the organization. Workflow and process redesign is either new to healthcare organizations or they lack the expertise to redesign workflows in an EHR environment. Part of the problem is also that vendors have attempted to replicate the paper world with their EHRs thinking that would help organizations adopt them better—only to find that little gets changed and so little benefit results. Finally, while much is written about the need to address workflows and processes in an EHR environment, there is very little concrete advice and assistance available.

Productivity

In general, productivity refers to how effectively and efficiently people can perform their work. In hospitals, nurses very often find their productivity decreases as they are learning how to use the EHR. In some cases, the length of time it takes to document in the EHR will always be longer than on paper because more data are collected—although often more data result in better patient care. In general, however, nurse productivity either returns to normal or may result in downstream time savings.

Productivity loss with an EHR is the number one complaint in physician practices. Almost all physicians find initial reduction in productivity as measured by the number of patients they can see in a day, which in turn directly reduces their reimbursement. However, the MGMA study previously cited also reveals that after optimization, 41.1 percent of practices reported that productivity increased over baseline, 42.4 percent reported that productivity returned to normal, and only 16.5 percent indicated productivity was reduced. It was also found that practice ownership influenced EHR optimization, with independent practices more likely to have optimized their EHR use than those that are owned by hospital systems. This suggests that optimization is a factor of motivation, not lack of feasibility.

Unintended Consequences from EHR

Unintended consequences from EHR have occurred and have been widely published since the mid-2000s. As previously defined, an unintended consequence is an unanticipated and undesired effect of implementing and using an EHR. Unintended consequences may include not only generation of new kinds of errors that harm patients, but many other issues that result in poor use of the systems and contribute further to harmful errors. A panel of experts (Campbell et al. 2006) categorized the unintended consequences, as shown in figure 16.7. One commenter on unintended consequences (Sanders 2010) likens the EHR to early use of seatbelts that were only lap belts. While they did provide some of the safety improvements desired, they also caused new forms of injuries. As a result, shoulder straps were added. Others (Sittig and Classen 2010) have observed that the National Transportation Safety Board (NTSB) and the Federal Aviation Administration (FAA) investigate transportation accidents much more thoroughly than healthcare investigates its errors, and that an NTSB-like organization for EHRs would provide a reporting mechanism to track incidents and police vendors and providers who repeatedly ignore

Figure 16.7. **Categories of causes of unintended consequences of EHR**

• More or new work for clinicians	• Negative emotions
• Unfavorable workflow issues	• Generation of new kinds of errors
• Never ending system demands	• Unexpected changes in the power structure
• Problems related to paper persistence	• Overdependence on the technology
• Untoward changes in communication patterns and practices	

Source: Campbell et al. 2006.

dangers. To help reduce unintended consequences, the Agency for Healthcare Research and Quality (AHRQ 2011) developed a guide to help identify and remediate problems related to unintended consequences.

As a consequence of the concern over unintended consequences and the federal government's push to promote EHR, Tom Marino (R-PA) has introduced legislation (referred to as the Safeguarding Access for Every Medicare Patient Act [SAFE Medicare Patient Act]). This bill would offer legal protection to Medicare and Medicaid providers who participate in the MU incentive program to help ensure patient safety. Among other things, the proposed legislation would create a system for reporting errors and potential errors that occur when using EHR or HIE.

Check Your Understanding 16.2

1. A transition technology used by many hospitals to increase access to health record content during the evolution to EHR is:

   A. EMR
   B. EDMS
   C. HIE
   D. PACS

2. The EHR component that is often the most challenging for which to gain adoption in a hospital is:

   A. Computerized provider order entry
   B. Electronic medical records
   C. Electronic medication administration record
   D. Point-of-care charting for nurses

3. A system that is used by all intended users for at least basic functionality is:

   A. Complete
   B. Implemented
   C. Adopted
   D. Optimized

4. Unintended consequences from using EHR technology are primarily due to issues with:

   A. Technology
   B. Human users
   C. System design
   D. Lack of patient cooperation

5. The biggest complaint physicians have with using an EHR already installed relates to:

   A. Cost
   B. Productivity
   C. Lack of real benefits
   D. Workflow

Instructions: Indicate whether the following statements are true or false (T or F).

6. _____ Cloud computing can reduce cost of EHR if customization capability is not required.

7. _____ In 2011, about half of all hospitals had implemented an EHR.

8. _____ Many physicians eased into acquiring an EHR by starting with e-prescribing.

9. _____ The primary benefit of an EHR in a hospital is quality improvement.

10. _____ Notifying a coder that the physician has completed the discharge summary is an example of workflow in EDMS.

Initiatives and Framework for the Electronic Health Record

Despite challenges, the transition to EHR is moving forward. To aid in gaining full adoption, several initiatives are under way in order to reach the goal where health information is fully automated, can be exchanged safely and securely, and provides decision-making support in an intuitive and meaningful way.

Governmental Initiatives

The 1991 IOM study urged adoption of EHRs within a decade. As a nonprofit organization that provides unbiased and authoritative advice to Congress and the public, the IOM's work was instrumental in focusing the Administrative Simplification part of HIPAA on "encourage[ing] the development of a health information system through the establishment of standards and requirements for the electronic transmission of certain health information." While many consider HIPAA to be only about privacy and security, HIPAA is actually based on automating financial and administrative transactions (for example, claims, eligibility verification, and explanation of benefits) and is being updated under HITECH and ACA legislation. ACA is adding new standards and operating rules. HIPAA also called recommendations relating to uniform data standards for what it called patient medical record information (PMRI). These recommendations are embedded in the criteria for EHR product certification under the HITECH MU incentive program. The privacy and security requirements of HIPAA were added to ensure that such exchange of health information would be adequately protected, and these are being updated under HITECH to reflect enhanced health information exchange.

Office of the National Coordinator (ONC)

More than a decade after the first IOM study and HIPAA, in 2004, President George W. Bush laid out a 10-year EHR adoption plan. This included creating the Office of the National Coordinator (ONC). During the Bush administration, ONC largely promoted adoption of EHR through supporting regulatory exceptions to anti-kickback laws so that hospitals could make limited donations of EHRs and e-prescribing systems to physicians and by promoting a **certification** process in which vendor products were evaluated against a set of published criteria to ensure that such EHRs would be sufficiently robust as to provide value.

Health Information Exchange

George W. Bush's administration also launched the definition and testing of a strategic national agenda for HIE. Various models of HIE and the organizations that provide HIE services are currently being established. Figure 16.8 describes the three primary types of HIE models.

In the **federated model,** there is no central location of data. An HIO serves to manage patient identity, record location, and security—including **consent directives** where patients may **opt in or opt out** of having their data exchanged through the HIO. Health information is exchanged in a point-to-point manner. Most consider this a more private and secure model of HIE, even though it is often necessary to review actual patient records before identifying the correct patient and the overall security is only as strong as the weakest link across participating organizations. This model may also be less efficient, with the potential for not finding all desired information about a patient.

The consolidated model is one in which there is a central store of data in one large database. While the misperception is that these data are co-mingled, they are not. Rather, they are logically separated with **access controls** requiring specific authorization to gain access to any data. Because security controls are centralized, they can be made stronger by a single, rather than dispersed, investment. Still, the fear is that the consolidated model could be used to compile massive amounts of data about individuals to be used against them, or to be hacked and wrongfully accessed or disclosed.

Figure 16.8. HIE models

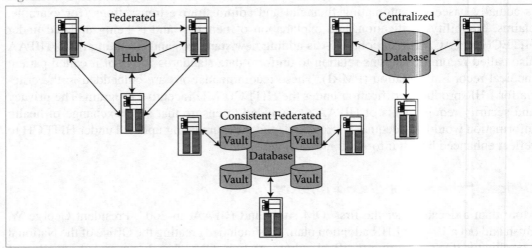

In reality, most HIOs have a hybrid structure. This structure may be some of both the federated and consolidated model, or it may be a **consistent federated model** wherein independent vaults or databases are managed by the HIO, so the data are centrally managed but both logically and physically separated. The hybrid structure or consistent federated model is often necessitated by how data are supplied and used. For example, lab results for all participating organizations in the HIO may be supplied to the HIO from a commercial lab, to be distributed by the HIO. This enables faster dissemination of results and easier updating of results. At the same time, information about patient hospitalizations and visits would be accessed in a point-to-point manner from the respective organizations.

In general, an HIO requires several important structures, shown in figure 16.9. First, there needs to be a specific form of governance, agreements, and policies and procedures for exchanging health information. Sometimes the governance structure is under the jurisdiction of the state government, although more often the HIO is a private entity. Whatever structure it takes, HITECH has deemed that it is a business associate under HIPAA. Usually the HIO requires all participants to sign a participation agreement that spells out the policies and procedures for exchanging information.

A second important element in forming an HIO is to determine what services it will supply. All HIOs will supply some basic services. These include patient identification, usually using an **identity matching algorithm** in which specified patient demographic information is compared to select the patient for whom information is to be exchanged. The algorithmic process is determined by the vendor supplying the service, but uses sophisticated probability equations to identify patients. There is increasing interest in using a unique patient identifier, despite the US Congress prohibition on spending any federal money to create such a national identifier. The **voluntary universal health identifier** (VUHID) is being promoted as a solution that combines an enumeration and a registration process.

Figure 16.9. **HIO services**

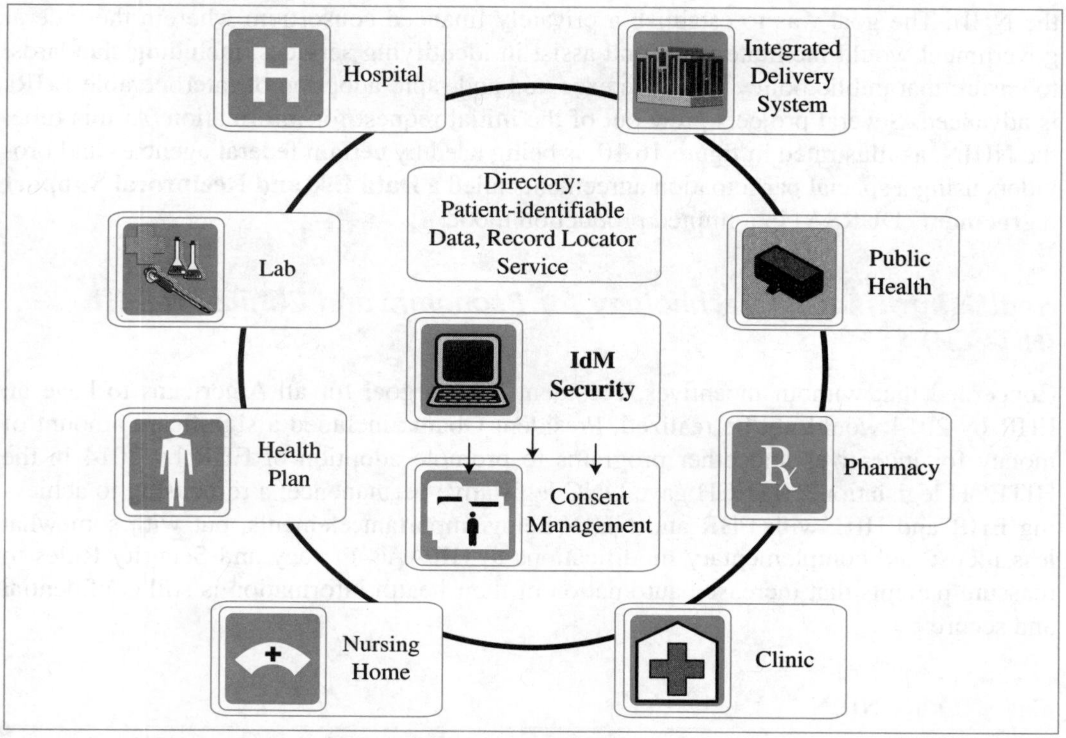

Copyright © 2012 Margret\A Consulting, LLC. Reprinted with permission.

Another important service an HIO provides is a **record locator service** (RLS). The RLS is a process that seeks information about where a patient, once identified, may have a health record available to the HIO.

Yet another critical service is identity management. Not to be confused with patient identification, **identity management** provides security functionality, including determining who (or what information system) is authorized to access information, **authentication** services, audit logging, **encryption,** and transmission controls.

Consent management is yet another HIO service. In consent management, patients may opt in or opt out of having their health information exchanged. As noted above, the patient will often provide a consent directive for this purpose.

ONC also expanded the vision for HIOs to a national focus. In 2001, the National Committee on Vital and Health Statistics (NCVHS) proposed a **national health information infrastructure** (NHII) that would be a set of technologies, standards, applications, systems, values, and laws that support all facets of provider healthcare, individual health, and public health. A comprehensive knowledge-based network of interoperable systems of clinical, personal, and public health information would improve decision making by making health information available when and where it is needed. In 2004, ONC released a request for information to seek ideas on how a NHII could be translated into a **nationwide**

health information network (NHIN). A NHIN would provide the technology to support the NHII. The goal was to establish a privately financed consortium wherein the federal government would facilitate work and assist in identifying services, including standards, to ensure that public policy goals are executed and rapid adoption of interoperable EHRs is advanced. Several projects grew out of the initial request for information. At this time, the NHIN, as illustrated in figure 16.10, is being used by certain federal agencies and providers using a special participation agreement called a **Data Use and Reciprocal Support Agreement** (DURSA) in a limited production mode.

Health Information Technology for Economic and Clinical Health (HITECH)

Concerned that without incentives, President Bush's goal for all Americans to have an EHR by 2014 would not be realized, President Obama included a significant amount of money for incentives and other programs to promote adoption of EHR by 2014 in the HITECH legislation. HITECH gave ONC legislative permanence; a refocusing to achieving EHR and HIE, with PHR and NHIN being important elements, but with somewhat less focus; and complementary modifications to HIPAA's Privacy and Security Rules to reassure patients that increased automation of their health information is still confidential and secure.

Figure 16.10.   NHIN

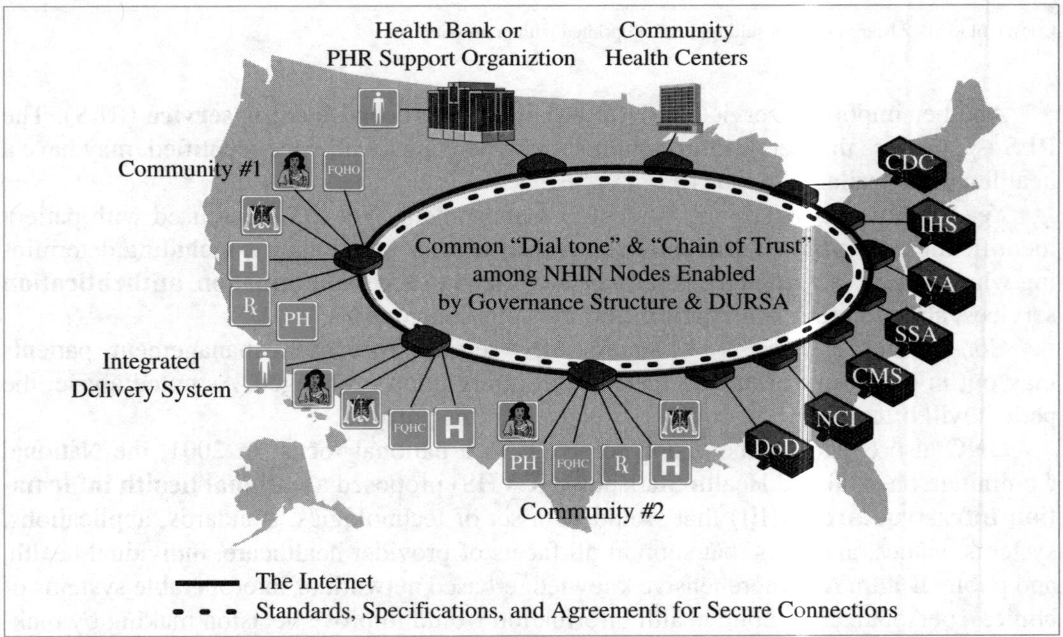

Source: http://healthit.hhs.gov/portal/server.pt/community/healthit_hhs_gov__nhin_exchange/1407.

Meaningful Use Incentives

To achieve the goal of EHRs for all, HITECH is providing incentives for "meaningful use of certified EHR technology," starting in 2011 and running through 2014, with sanctions thereafter for those who have not adopted an EHR. These sanctions are in the form of a downward adjustment to Medicare reimbursements.

This MU initiative has three components: standards for MU of EHR, certification that EHR technology meets the standards, and criteria for earning MU incentives.

Standards for MU of EHR are provided in regulation released by ONC and include those to support structures to ensure that health data can be exchanged between systems and their use integrated, vocabulary standards to ensure consistent meaning across applications, and specific functionality. Not all the standards are new. For example, without a common structure, it would be impossible for an R-ADT system to supply a lab system with patient demographics. That has been occurring for some time. However, for one provider's problem list for a patient to be compared with another provider's problem list for the patient, there needs to be not only common structures but common terminology used. The result is that the problem list required for MU must be encoded with ICD-9-CM or SNOMED-CT.

Certification of EHR technology also comes from regulation released by ONC. In 2006, prior to the MU incentive program, the federal government supported the development of a private sector initiative called the Certification Commission for Health Information Technology (CCHIT). It began certifying EHR products primarily to aid consumers make smart acquisition decisions. Under the MU incentive program, the certifying entity must be approved by the ONC as an **ONC authorized testing and certifying body** (ONC-ATCB). This certification has resulted in a streamlined certification process, several organizations providing certification, and many more vendor products being certified. It is important to note two things about the certification itself. First, products may be certified as complete or modular. A **complete EHR** product meets all the requirements; a **modular EHR** product meets only one or more but not all of the requirements. Providers must combine modular products such that they have a complete solution in order to earn the incentives. A second thing to observe about certification is that a product certified for the MU incentive program only needs to meet the specific MU requirements. The requirements do not include all functionality that is frequently considered to be core components of EHR or that may even be necessary to achieve other goals for EHR, such as return on investment. For example, hospital EHRs certified for MU are not required to have electronic or barcode medication administration record systems. Ambulatory EHRs are not required to have physician progress notes. The federal government recognizes that the MU requirements are limited, but wants to focus initially on just getting providers to adopt the systems and then expects to expand the requirements.

An interesting phenomenon and potential problem has occurred as a result of the changes in the certification requirements. This is the fact that there has been an explosion of EHR vendors. CCHIT estimated there were potentially 24 hospital EHR vendors, having certified about half of them; and about 250 ambulatory EHR vendors of which it had certified about 80. By early 2012, there were over 300 hospital EHR vendors certified for MU and over 700 certified ambulatory EHR vendors. In fact, this has led some industry observers (Tholemeier 2011) to note that market consolidation is inevitable—potentially impacting vendors' interest in survival over enhancing research and development to improve upon products. This state of affairs can also put providers at risk when many vendors can be expected to be acquired or go out of business.

Criteria for MU have been specified by CMS and identify the extent to which the functionality must be used. For example, the criteria for use of CPOE only requires that more than 30 percent of patients with an EHR have at least one medication order directly entered by any licensed healthcare professional into the CPOE application. As a result, physicians could use nurses to enter these orders for them, and orders for labs, x-rays, and other care services will not have the benefit that the CDS in the CPOE system could afford. It is anticipated that as the subsequent two stages of MU are rolled out, the criteria will become tighter.

The MU program is generally considered successful, as by the start of 2012 a significant amount of federal dollars had been supplied providers as incentives. However, it has been found that over half of providers earning the incentives already had an EHR and were essentially being reimbursed for their past efforts. While this is not necessarily bad, it may not have had the intended effect of stimulating the rest of the provider community to move forward with EHR. As a result, stage 2 of the incentive program, scheduled to begin in 2013, was delayed by a year. This gives both providers and vendors an opportunity to catch up and address the new stage 2 requirements.

Affordable Care Act (ACA)

The Affordable Care Act (ACA) actually does not address EHR technology, although it does include small, but important sections on enhancing the administrative simplification provisions of HIPAA. ACA completes the adoption of financial and administration transactions and code sets under HIPAA and adds to these an electronic funds transfer (EFT) standard and operating rules for the standard transactions. Important to EHR, however, is that ACA introduces new Medicare reimbursement structures that essentially depend on having automated health information. Where in the past financial and clinical data were separate with diagnostic and procedural codes determining reimbursement, under ACA, providers who are willing to take a risk for higher reimbursement will need to improve their overall quality in order to achieve these higher rates. Financial and clinical data will need to become much more integrated and analyzed when providers participate in ACOs, bundled payments, and/or PCMH structures.

Initiatives Directed toward Consumers

State and Private-Sector Initiatives

Although many states are taking an active role in promoting HIE and (partially) funding state HIOs, and one state (Minnesota) has mandated use of EHR by all providers, most efforts to promote EHR and other forms of HIT have either occurred through federal initiatives or at the local provider level. Many local providers have spearheaded HIO formation. A few states but even more so integrated delivery networks have initiated or begun to participate in voluntary quality reporting efforts either through recognition programs such as Thomson Reuters "100 Top Hospitals" or various healthcare report card programs, such as Minnesota HealthScores.

Consumerism

Until recently, patients have had little interaction with EHRs. Those who are computer savvy may recognize the benefits of EHRs but are often unaware whether EHRs are being used. In fact, many patients assume that because a computer is in the registration area, everything else is computerized. Alternatively, patients may be fearful of EHRs and not fully understand the privacy and security protections put into these systems. They may see news stories about patient data being inadvertently e-mailed to others or left on a laptop that is stolen out of someone's car and assume (sometimes correctly) that the systems are not as secure as they could be. To help overcome these myths and realities, care delivery organizations need to find better ways of engaging their patients in EHR and HIT.

One way is to provide more direct communication to patients about the EHR. Some organizations are distributing brochures about the EHR, including information about privacy and security. Another key element is making sure that clinicians who use the systems use them at the POC as intended. This often requires special training, and many vendors have started using role-playing to get clinicians to understand how to use the EHR in front of the patient, what to say to the patient, and in general to overcome the notion that the patient has no business knowing what is in the health record.

The idea of allowing patient-generated data into the EHR is also emerging. Some organizations support a **patient portal** that is special software that enables patients to log on to a website from home or a **kiosk** (special form of input device geared more to people less familiar with computers) in a provider's waiting room to schedule appointments, pay bills, obtain patient educational material, sign informed consents, request release of information, or enter their own health history using a context-specific template. Some providers are supporting **e-visits**, where existing patients can exchange e-mail in lieu of visiting the physician office for follow-up or recurring care needs. E-visits are now reimbursable by some insurance companies.

Personal Health Records

The personal health record (PHR) is a relatively new concept that encourages patients to take an active role in their health information. AHIMA defines the PHR as an electronic, universally available, lifelong resource of health information needed by individuals to make health decisions. Although use of an electronic system for PHRs is encouraged, many more patients use a paper-based file folder as their PHR rather than an electronic offering. Whether electronic or paper-based, patients are expected to own and manage the information in the PHR, which comes from both healthcare providers and the individual. The PHR is maintained in a secure and private environment, with the patient determining rights of access. It is separate from and does not replace the legal health record of any provider (AHIMA e-HIM Personal Health Record Workgroup 2005) or their EHR. AHIMA has taken a very active role in promotion of PHR. AHIMA maintains a PHR website (MyPHR), which provides the public with free educational resources about personal health information and PHRs. In 2005, AHIMA formulated the definition provided above and described minimum common data elements.

Just like EHRs, PHRs are also in transition. Although there is a fair amount of interest in PHRs by consumers, the vast majority still do not use PHRs. As a result, care delivery organizations may still find that patients are bringing paper copies of documents to them for incorporation into the health records. Few providers offer PHRs to their patients, often putting this application off until their EHRs are more complete and fully adopted.

There are generally considered to be two main types of electronic PHRs: integrated and standalone. Integrated, sometimes referred to as tethered, PHRs are essentially a spin-off of the EHR in the hospital or clinic system. However, there may also be such PHRs offered by insurance companies, in which case they are pre-populated for the patient with data from claims. The second form of PHR is completely standalone. In this case the patient adopts a commercial vendor's PHR, usually through a website, although it could be on a CD or paper. Sometimes providers or health plans may recommend that the patient retain a PHR and then refer the patient to a specific commercial vendor that the provider or plan may or may not populate the PHR for the patient.

PHRs have been most popular with patients who have chronic illnesses or with caretakers of elderly patients having to manage multiple providers, many drugs, and much other data.

PHRs get mixed reviews by providers. Some providers believe that they empower the patient to be a more informed consumer of healthcare and actually improve compliance with treatment regimens. Other providers, however, are skeptical and believe that PHRs will inundate providers with more information than they have time to address. This attitude is changing considerably as a better understanding develops of what constitutes a PHR, their role in a disaster situation, and how they can support health information exchange.

Standards have also been developed to provide a foundation for what a PHR should include. The standards development organization Health Level Seven (HL7) has developed a PHR-System Functional Model (HL7 2008). It describes the functionality one should expect to find in a PHR.

Continuity of Care Record/Continuity of Care Document

In effort to supply patients with more information about their healthcare and without directly promoting a PHR, the federal MU incentive program is requiring that providers supply patients, upon their request, electronic clinical summaries using the **Continuity of Care Record** (CCR) standard or Continuity of Care Document (CCD) standard.

The CCR was created by physicians from the Massachusetts Medical Society and other organizations working under the auspices of the **ASTM International** standards development organization. The initial purpose of the CCR was to eliminate data inconsistencies when patients were referred from one provider to another. In the past when a patient was to be referred to another provider, the originating provider would dictate a letter describing the patient's case. There was no consistency across physicians as to what might be included in this referral letter. To eliminate this problem, the CCR standard recommends specific categories of information to include in referral letters. The developers of the standard emphasize that the CCR is not an EHR. Rather, it is a subset of data from an EHR; or, if an organization does not yet have an EHR, it may be generated through dictation, scanned documents, and/or reports from various source systems. Many PHR vendors picked up on the CCR and have incorporated it into their commercial offerings, even though it is not considered a PHR standard.

As the federal government learned of this initiative, it encouraged ASTM International to work with HL7 to develop a transport mechanism for the CCR. HL7 had already developed a **Clinical Document Architecture** (CDA) standard. This is an XML-based markup standard that provides structure (including a description of document content for users and discrete data for computer processing), vocabulary standards (such as SNOMED-CT and **Logical Observations, Identifiers, Names and Codes** (LOINC)), and codes (to represent the vocabulary and other concepts, such as a code structure for representing dates and units of measure) for sharing clinical documents.

The result of using HL7's CDA with the CCR from ASTM International is called the Continuity of Care Document (CCD). The CCD may be transmitted electronically via HL7 standard messages, in attachments to e-mail, or via standard Internet file transfer protocols, such as File Transfer Protocol (FTP).

Check Your Understanding 16.3

1. Exchange of a standard set of health information content between providers and with patients is facilitated by:

    A. Continuity of care document
    B. Data set
    C. Electronic health record
    D. Personal health record

2. In what form of health information exchange are data centrally located but physically separated?

    A. Consolidated
    B. Centralized
    C. Consistent federated
    D. Federated

3. The function used to provide access controls, authentication, and audit logging in an HIE is:

   A. Patient Identification
   B. Record Locator Service
   C. Identity Management
   D. Consent Management

4. In order for hospitals or physicians to earn meaningful use, their EHR technology must be:

   A. Certified
   B. Interoperable
   C. Used in a meaningful way
   D. All of the above

5. In order to participate in the nationwide health information network, providers must:

   A. Have certified EHR technology
   B. Sign a special participation agreement
   C. Utilize the voluntary universal health identifier
   D. All of the above

Technologies That Support Electronic Health Records

Technologies that support EHRs include databases and data storage devices, data exchange and comparability standards, and hardware infrastructure.

Databases and Data Storage

Databases

A database is an organized collection of data. There are different types of databases. The form of database used may also depend on the purpose of the database. **Database management systems** (DBMSs) are software applications that organize, provide access to, and otherwise manage a database.

The earliest form of database was called a **flat file** because it stored data in a plain text file, where each line of text holds one record, with fields separated by delimiters, such as commas or tabs. While this structure is a simple way to store files, there are no folders or paths to organize the data. Despite that there are many newer, much more functional forms of databases, there are a surprisingly large number of flat file databases still used, especially by health plans, and in some healthcare provider organizations for patient accounting systems.

Most database systems in use today for EHRs and other HIT are relational databases. A **relational database** stores data in predefined tables that contain rows and columns similar to a spreadsheet. The kinds of data that can be stored in a relational database are currency, real numbers, integers, and strings (characters of data). Each table is a set of rows and columns that relate to one another. Rows represent a single record, such as for a given patient. Each column has a unique name and the content within it must be of the same type. For example, there may be columns for patient name, age, diagnosis, allergies, blood pressure, and so on. Because no single table can contain every piece of data collected about a patient, several tables are usually created and related to one another in a variety of ways. Many tables are relatively stable; that is, they contain information that does not change frequently, such as a table of all physicians on the medical staff and their credentials. Other tables are being populated (updated) constantly with new information, such as those that collect the lab results for a given patient over the course of a hospitalization.

Figure 16.11 illustrates some of these database concepts. In this very simple example, a patient demographic table is linked to the physician table and both are linked to a results table. In this case, Dr. Smith is John's PCP. If the physician table were used for messaging, Dr. Smith could be alerted that there is a new result and that the new result may be an image of a chest x-ray for John. Structured data elements also are recorded in the results table, including blood pressure and hemoglobin results taken at 9:00 a.m. Note that the hemoglobin results have been marked with a down arrow, indicating that this is a low result. This would have been processed by the results being compared with yet another table of normal values (not shown).

Other forms of databases include **hierarchical** and **multi-dimensional.** Where relational databases attempt to store each piece of data only one time, hierarchical and multi-dimensional data may purposefully duplicate data in the database.

Figure 16.11. Database concepts

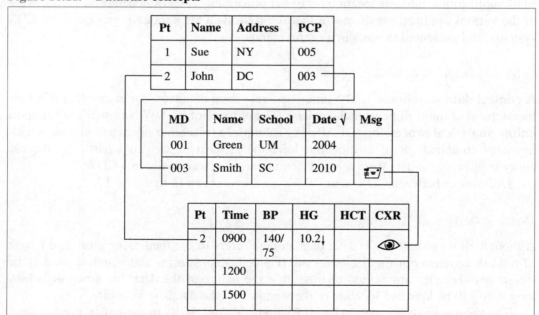

Clinical Data Repository (CDR)

Today, EHR systems are generally based on the use of a special kind of relational database referred to as a **clinical data repository** (CDR). This database helps manage data that come from many different sources, ancillary systems in the hospital, or other provider settings as well as from direct entry of structured data by the clinician. CDRs can make this data rapidly available and process this data in CDS. For example, if a physician wants to see both the patient's lab results and vital signs in a graph, the CDR more quickly and easily can pull the data together from the LIS and the nursing system to generate such a graph. Where the CPOE system may be able to compare a drug being ordered to the drugs to which the patient is allergic because both the order and the allergies are contained in the same CPOE database, a CDR type of database would make it easier to compare the drug being ordered to the patient's lab results that come from the separate LIS and provide a CDS alert or reminder.

CDRs are often referred to as **transactional databases** because they aid **online transaction processing** (OLTP). A transaction is nothing more than an entry, retrieval, or process on data. A physician entering a drug order for a patient, the nurse (or patient monitoring device) entering vital signs, the pharmacist retrieving data on patient allergies, the coder calling up the patient's problem list, or the R-ADT system calculating the patient's age from the birthdate and current date are all examples of transactions.

CDRs also can store and make accessible paper document images and clinical images such as those from PACS. However, merely having a CDR does not equate with having an EHR. A CDR helps combine data from multiple source systems, including the various EHR applications, into one location for easier processing. A CDR depends on the software in the various applications to ensure that the right data are captured, processed by CDS systems, and presented to users in a useful manner.

Clinical Data Warehouse (CDW)

A **clinical data warehouse** (CDW) may be a relational database, but more often will be a hierarchical or multi-dimensional database. The purpose of a CDW is primarily to support **online analytical processing** (OLAP). For example, a researcher interested in understanding what combinations of medications have the greatest impact on a particular disease entity could analyze data from many different patients more easily in a CDW.

Differences between CDRs and CDWs are summarized in figure 16.12.

Data Storage Technology

Although all databases retain data, data storage refers to the media, location, and length of time the contents of the databases are retained. Repositories and warehouses may be stored anywhere for any period of time. It is the nature of the data that determines how long they will be kept and location of the storage, not the database structure.

The volume of data captured by HIT in general, and EHRs in particular, is enormous. There is a growing expectation that data should be accessible in real time for very long periods of time. As clinicians become dependent on the computer for all their data needs,

Figure 16.12.   **CDR vs. CDW**

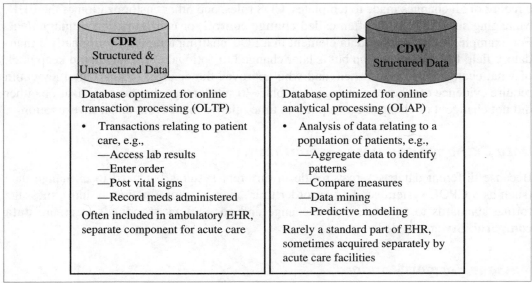

they will not tolerate downtime or delays for retrieving archived data. As a result, managing data storage is an increasingly important issue. Unlike in the past when data were retained online for only a few days after discharge and backups were stored on tape, an EHR virtually demands that data be retained online for a very long period of time and be instantaneously retrievable and backed up continuously.

A storage device is a machine that contains nothing but storage media. Tape drives are the oldest form of storage device and are rapidly becoming obsolete. Disk drives are the most common storage device today. Disk technology, however, has moved rapidly from magnetic disks to optical disks of many different forms. Many servers contain optical disk drives that can store very large volumes of data. Storing data on the same server used to process data slows response time. As a result, disks are being arrayed in **redundant arrays of independent (or inexpensive) disks** (RAID) so that a great volume of data can be stored. Storage devices also are being organized into their own **storage area networks** (SANs) so that they can be accessible from any server in the network. When such technology is deployed, however, **storage management software** must be available to manage the SAN, to keep track of where data are stored, and to move older data to less expensive, but still accessible, storage locations. Storage management is becoming an entire domain within information systems management.

Thus, although storage media are cheap and healthcare has had a tendency to store all electronic data, **storage management** is becoming a more expensive proposition. The introduction of an EHR should trigger a review of the organization's **retention schedule** with an eye toward enabling a realistic retention schedule for electronic data. Another element of the retention schedule should be the retention of **metadata,** including both **audit**

logs and the data about data that supports the **data dictionary.** It is also important to keep a record of all changes made to templates, CDS rules, and other customization of the EHR. Managing such changes is often called **change control,** or **configuration management.** For example, if a structured data element in a POC charting template is originally a mandatory field for documentation but is later changed to optional, it is essential to keep track of what change was made, when, and who approved the change. A smart attorney could require evidence of when the change took place to substantiate that the organization either did not change it or changed it at a point in time relative to an event under investigation.

Data Exchange and Data Comparability

Because different databases may reside in different systems but need to exchange data (such as a CPOE system sending an order to a laboratory information system), message format standards to facilitate data exchange and **vocabulary standards** to assure **data comparability** are needed.

Message Format Standards

There are two primary ways different systems can exchange data with one another. One way is by simply sending a copy of data needed from one system to the other system. This method requires that the two systems be structured in exactly the same way, or be integrated. This would be the ideal way to exchange data, but because it is very common to have systems that come from different vendors, or even from the same vendor but are not structured in the same way, it is necessary to exchange data through an interface. An interface is a special program where specific data are identified as needing to be exchanged and then rules about how those data must be structured to make the exchange happen.

In order for an interface to be written, however, the two systems that are intended to exchange data must both follow the same protocol (predefined way to do something) established by a message format standards organization. For example, if John's medical record number (012345) is to be exchanged with another system it must be interpreted as the medical record number and cannot be interpreted as John's date of birth. **Data exchange standards** provide a protocol for writing software applications. For EHRs, HL7 provides the standard protocols to which EHR vendors should write their applications so that, in fact, medical record number and date of birth are distinguishable.

It should be obvious from this example that a repository that can collect all data, once without repetition, would make it easier to use the data. Unless the repository is an integral part of the source systems, however, there needs to be an interface from each system that contributes data to the repository in order for the repository to receive the data.

The most common message format standards used in the US healthcare system are:

- Health Level Seven (HL7) is a family of standards that aid the exchange of data among hospital systems and, more recently, physician practices and other types of provider systems. Version 2.x is used by almost every EHR vendor in the United

States. Version 3 is web-based and has been adopted in several other countries around the world that do not have the investment in older systems that characterize the United States.

- **Digital Imaging and Communications in Medicine** (DICOM) helps exchange clinical images such as x-rays, CT scans, and so on.

- **National Council for Prescription Drug Programs** (NCPDP) enables the communication of retail pharmacy eligibility inquiries and claims (as mandated by HIPAA) and more recently provides a standard for the exchange of prescriptions from a physician practice electronic prescribing system directly to the retail pharmacy's information system (that has been proposed for use under the Medicare Part D drug program).

- **American National Standards Institute** (ANSI) **Accredited Standards Committee X12** (ASC X12) provides **electronic data interchange** (EDI) standards for hospital, professional, and dental claims, eligibility inquiries, electronic remittance advice, and other standards (as mandated by HIPAA).

The need for message format standards in healthcare is especially important because so many different systems are used. Unfortunately, not all vendors have been good about adopting message format standards. Some believe the only way to keep market share is to have a highly proprietary set of systems so that customers are dependent on buying additional systems from only that vendor. Furthermore, because message format standards are generally created in a group process often including competing vendors, the standards themselves may reflect only the minimal requirements everyone can agree on. The EHR initiatives discussed earlier in this chapter are urging vendors to adopt more open systems that comply more closely with standards and use web-based services.

Vocabulary Standards

Until recently, message format standards have been limited to exchanging whatever data were sent from one system to another. There was no reconciliation of vocabulary used in one system with another system. In other words, although the types and formats of the data elements were standardized, the data values themselves were not standardized. Ensuring that the meaning of a term is consistent across all users is especially important in healthcare and is referred to as data comparability. Data comparability is achieved through vocabulary standards, ideally embedded in the message being exchanged. *Semantics* is the term used to describe the fact that the value of the data in the message conforms to a standard vocabulary such that it has a standardized meaning. When a message format standard specifies the vocabulary with which the data are encoded, the functionality is called semantic interoperability.

The vocabulary used in an EHR system should, at a minimum, be a controlled vocabulary. A **controlled vocabulary** means that a specific set of terms for specified data is used and that any additions or changes to the terms and/or their meanings must be formally approved, for example, by the vendor that has developed the vocabulary (which is then referred to as a **proprietary vocabulary**) or by a standards organization (see also next paragraph on standard vocabulary). A controlled vocabulary is essential to ensure common meaning for all users. For example, if the term *fall* is currently used in a template for physical therapists to describe the reasons for a patient's injury, but a group of nurses want to add *slip* as a synonym, there should be consensus that these two terms mean the same thing. Otherwise, when any one group wants to perform analysis on the data and does not realize that *fall* and *slip* are used as synonyms, only part of the data may be retrieved for the analysis.

A **standard vocabulary** is developed through a process that confirms consensus on the meaning of the terms included in the vocabulary. Standard vocabularies are, by definition, controlled vocabularies, but are not owned and managed by only one vendor (which would be the proprietary vocabulary). Standard vocabularies help not only assure common meaning within a given organization or by clients of a particular vendor, but across all users of any EHR. They achieve data comparability. The MU incentive criteria require standard vocabulary usage, where the problem list is required to be recorded in either ICD-9-CM or SNOMED-CT, laboratory results must be expressed as LOINC codes, and medications must be documented using terms from **RxNorm.**

SNOMED-CT (formerly known as the Systematized Nomenclature of Medicine-Clinical Terms) was originally developed by the College of American Pathologists (CAP) in the 1960s and is now maintained by a separate company based in Denmark, the **International Health Terminology Standards Development Organization.** Initially it was a robust set of multi-axial codes that could identify the topography, morphology, etiology, and function associated with pathological specimens. SNOMED-CT has subsequently grown into the most comprehensive effort to standardize vocabulary for the representation of medical knowledge. It has been licensed by the **National Library of Medicine** (NLM) so that it is now freely available to US vendors as the basis for clinical data dictionaries in EHR systems. The NLM has also mapped SNOMED-CT to other vocabularies and classification systems, such as **ICD-9-CM** and **ICD-10-CM.** Such mapping may assist in data comparability and in transition to new versions.

Logical Observation, Identifiers, Names and Codes (LOINC), developed by the Regenstrief Institute, provides names and codes for laboratory test results and other observations. To earn meaningful use incentives, EHRs must be able to accept structured lab results encoded with LOINC.

RxNorm is a standardized nomenclature for clinical drugs and drug delivery devices (such as syringes). The codes are used in a variety of drug knowledge databases developed by different companies. RxNorm was developed jointly between the NLM and the Veterans Health Administration, and is available from the NLM.

There are many other healthcare vocabularies and classification systems that may or may not be standard vocabularies, but may be used in EHR systems or other health information technology. Some are widely used, such as the **National Drug Codes** (NDC) for maintaining inventories of drugs in pharmacies, or Current Procedural Terminology (CPT) used to code physician services for reimbursement. Others are less widely used or are used for specific purposes. For example, ABC Codes is a vocabulary and code system for integrative care that provides codes for billing and research from alternative and complementary medicine, such as acupuncture and aromatherapy. Medcin is a computer-based nomenclature developed and maintained by Medicomp Systems, Inc. It is widely used for the recording of history and physical exam findings, even though it is not a standard vocabulary.

Hardware Infrastructure

Hardware infrastructure includes computers to process data and computers to deliver data to or receive data from users, as well as networking and communications technology. The backbone of an EHR obviously is the hardware and software on which the system runs. The term *architecture* refers to the configuration, structure, and relationships of all components of a computer system. Two main types of architecture may be used in creating an EHR:

- **Client/server** (C/S) **architecture** uses a combination of computers to capture and process data. Server computers are powerful processors. They typically house all the application software and store all active data captured by all the client computers throughout the network. They then serve multiple client computers, which have less powerful processors.

- **Web services architecture** (WSA) is an emerging architecture that utilizes web-based tools to permit communication among different software applications. While client and server computers are still needed, there is not the one-to-one relationship of a client to a server.

Processing, Data Capture, and Retrieval Technology

Servers are typically kept in a **data center** with special temperature, humidity, and power controls and where they can be specially secured. Very often there is one server devoted to one application, although this is changing as servers can be logically divided into sections. This is called server virtualization.

As EHRs are being implemented without paper backup, contingency planning and disaster recovery is becoming increasingly important. Not only must a healthcare organization be able to replace data if a server or storage device is destroyed in some manner, but organizations need to be able to instantaneously failover to another server during a server crash. Back up of stored data has been routinely performed by most healthcare organizations. To reduce the risk of downtime, healthcare organizations now must also have **server redundancy** with **server failover.** This means that at least two if not more servers are performing the same processing on data simultaneously. If one server goes down, processing is still occurring at another server. Users are not interrupted, and in fact will not even be aware that there was a server crash. While servers can crash for any number of reasons, one is loss of power. In this case, many healthcare organizations are building backup power supply as well. All hospitals have diesel generators to run lifesaving equipment in case of a power outage. Many hospitals and larger clinics are also getting backup power systems. For smaller organizations, at least an **uninterruptable power supply** (UPS) device operating on a battery would be able to help power down computer equipment such that preparations can be made for alternative power sources or to close the facility.

The computers that users use to retrieve and enter data are called clients. The clients rely upon the servers to process data. The choice of **thick client** (with full processing capability) versus **thin client** (with minimal processing capability) is often dependent upon how the application software is designed. Client computers may be desktops, laptops, various forms of tablets, and in some cases smart phones, with the choice sometimes being left to the individual user or users collectively, often with the advice or assistance from the information technology (IT) department. Client computers also typically include various types of data capture aids such as keyboards, navigational devices, microphones, and speakers. Hardware infrastructure also includes other types of computing devices, such as storage devices, printers, scanners, cables, and network devices.

With the exception of the most current generation of users, many clinicians have never learned to type and consider typing or any other form of keyboard use to be a clerical function. Even clinicians who are willing and able to type still often find data entry on a computer more challenging and time-consuming than handwriting or dictating.

Unfortunately, no ideal solution has yet been found to support data capture effectively for all users in all environments. However, there are a few key considerations that must be met in order to more closely meet this goal. Most important, data entry must return value to the user. If the user can obtain decision support at the time of data entry that is valuable, he or she is more likely to perform data entry. Clinicians are more inclined to do data entry when they can see that the direct result of their data entry is a benefit to their subsequent work (for example, if the system automatically generates tailored instructions for the patient when discharge information is entered). If data entry is perceived to take longer than traditional recording, even when its purpose is laudable (such as to have more legible data to improve patient safety), it will be a hard sell.

Several technologies can help make data capture easier. Collectively, these are often called **human–computer interfaces.** They include:

- *Structured data entry through point-and-click fields, drop-down menus, structured templates, or macros:* These make data entry and processing easier. Devices supporting such data entry include the mouse, light pens, and touch screens.

- *Speech and handwriting recognition:* Speech recognition can be very effective in certain situations when data entry is fairly repetitive and the vocabulary used is fairly limited. As speech recognition improves, it is becoming a replacement for other forms of dictation. In some cases, the user reviews the speech as it is being converted to type and makes any needed corrections; in other cases, the speech is sent to a special device where it generates type for another individual to review and edit. Handwriting recognition is similar to speech recognition, where the system learns to recognize a user's handwriting. Some tablet computers have been able to convert handwriting to type fairly successfully, but because of the need for somewhat greater precision than normal handwriting, most tablet computers are used today to capture discrete data through point-and-click or simply retain the handwriting.

- *Handheld and wireless devices:* Handheld devices, such as tablet computers and PDAs, may use any of the other forms of data entry, from keying and selecting from a list to speech and handwriting recognition. Although their use is growing in popularity, they still are not necessarily the answer for everyone. Tablets are generally easy for mobile professionals to have readily available, although they are still fairly heavy. PDAs may be limited in the size of both the screen and the keypad. Unless tablets or PDAs are wireless, their ability to communicate or link to primary information systems is limited to when they are docked to a workstation. Handheld devices can run out of power, requiring extra batteries and charging. However, handheld devices are ideal for certain limited functions, such as for writing prescriptions or capturing a home health data set; and as they are becoming more sophisticated and wireless, they are becoming very popular. Still, many healthcare organizations find it just as effective to mount a notebook computer to a cart and move it with the user. These are affectionately called WOWs **(wireless, or workstations, on wheels).** For the less mobile healthcare professional, desktop computer workstations are still the mainstay, often enhanced with keyboards that can be rolled out of the way into a drawer and monitors on swing arms that can be rotated to engage the patient in the documentation process.

- *Direct data capture from a medical device attached to a patient:* This is yet another important means of capturing certain kinds of data, such as vital signs. Special medical devices (such as a pacemaker) can even be connected to a standard telephone for capturing data or checking on the device's status from a remote location.

- *Patient data entry:* Incorporating patient-generated data into the EHR discussed previously is just now starting to be used. In the past, providers have been somewhat reluctant to incorporate patient-generated information. There were misunderstandings that the patients could access and change the entire content of the provider's records. There also were misperceptions that the information may be too voluminous or erroneous. As patients continue to be seen by an ever-increasing number of providers, however, it is now recognized that the patients are the only source of at least where all their information is located, if not what the information is.

- *Natural language processing (NLP):* Considered a special form of data entry, NLP is the capability of a computer to apply very sophisticated mathematical and probabilistic formulas to narrative text and convert them to structured data. Although text processing is becoming more feasible, the technology still has a way to go before it can be used routinely for all data entry.

Networks and Communications Technology

Whatever architecture is deployed, it is necessary to share data among different users, whether they are internal to an organization, or across an HIO or even the NHIN. When one computer is linked to another computer, a network exists. Network devices link computers to one another and one network to another. For additional information, please see chapter 14.

Check Your Understanding 16.4

1. A clinical data warehouse is:

    A. Storage device
    B. Database for online analytical processing
    C. EHR
    D. Company that stores paper records

2. A computer that has minimal processing capability of its own is a:

    A. Human–computer interface
    B. Thin client
    C. Server
    D. Web service architecture

3. Which of the following technologies would reduce the risk that information is not accessible during a server crash:

    A. RAID
    B. Storage area network
    C. Server redundancy
    D. Tape or disk backup

4. A part of storage management that assures documentation is retained about changes is called:

    A. Auditing
    B. Database management
    C. Data dictionary
    D. Change control

5. What form of database does online analytical processing typically require:

    A. Relational database
    B. Hierarchical database
    C. Database management system
    D. Analytical database

Instructions: Match the message format standard or vocabulary standard to its purpose.

6. ASC X12

7. HL7

8. RxNorm

9. DICOM

10. NDC

a. Claims
b. Clinical drug names
c. Drug inventory
d. Data exchange
e. Clinical images

Acquisition of Electronic Health Record Systems

Acquiring an EHR system for a hospital or physician practice requires extensive planning and organizational commitment. Figure 16.13 illustrates the steps required to successfully determine organizational readiness for an EHR, develop strategic and tactical plans, select a vendor, implement and maintain the system, and ensure ongoing value.

Readiness Assessment

While virtually every healthcare organization recognizes that an EHR is likely to be in their future if not present already, determining readiness for EHR is an important first step in either adopting automation in general or adding the core clinical applications that comprise an EHR.

Readiness assessment helps an organization prepare users to better adopt an EHR. Many agree that readiness assessment starts at the top, with an assessment of the organization's leadership and culture. In fact, one physician (Adler 2007) observes that many healthcare organizations are dysfunctional, and that a dysfunctional organization will have a dysfunctional EHR. To improve upon executive leadership readiness for an EHR it may be necessary to use an outside facilitator to evaluate the organization's governance structure and walk leaders through a culture assessment, sometimes even including coaching leaders on newer approaches to management. Leadership must be supportive of and committed to assuring the resources necessary for EHR. Those who cut corners, want to apply blame for broken processes, or even those who totally abdicate responsibility for EHR will not have a successful implementation. Excellent communications, clear lines of authority, and an explicit decision-making process are essential.

Attitudes and beliefs about EHR among users also should be assessed and education supplied to help ready everyone for using an EHR. Many myths have materialized about EHRs, and even where some of the myths may be partially true, no organization wants to have a self-fulfilling prophecy. Determining how users feel about an EHR's security,

Figure 16.13.   EHR planning steps

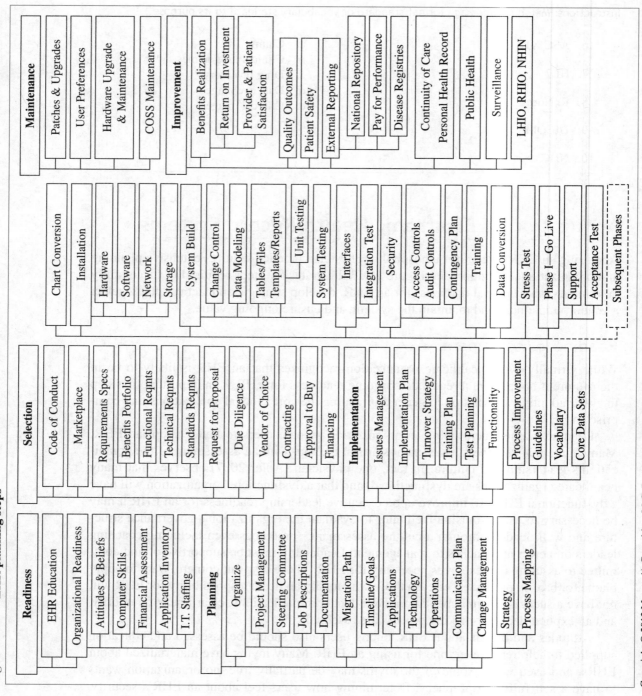

impact on productivity, use of evidence-based medicine, and many other factors can help pinpoint and then head off potential issues.

An EHR results in changes. Many clinicians are not very familiar with computers and may have never used a computer as part of their work. In addition, an EHR is not just about changing from paper to computer, but changing how medicine is practiced. Everyone in the organization needs to understand change and have support for making changes. Understanding the degree to which an organization as a whole is prepared to make a change can help set a timetable and **migration path** for making changes in stages. If there are lessons learned from past changes, these need to be recognized and addressed as part of the readiness for making such a huge change.

Obviously, EHR costs a lot of money, not only in actual expenditure for the software and hardware but also for new staff, training, and many other costs. An organization needs to assess its readiness for such a financial investment and plan accordingly. The MU incentive program is urging fairly rapid implementation of EHR. Unfortunately, some organizations may be moving too rapidly through an EHR implementation only because the financial resources to do it correctly are not present.

Workflow and process changes are very specific focuses that an organization should assess. Understanding current workflows and processes will highlight where there can be improvements. This can also direct a vendor selection process if an EHR has not already been acquired. If one has been acquired but is not being used very well, workflow and process assessment can help identify course corrections to be taken.

IT infrastructure should also be assessed prior to moving ahead with EHR. While the current data center may be adequate for the applications currently in place, it may need upgrading. Many more interfaces will be required. Full redundancy and other contingency planning must be done. An assessment of the hardware and staff skills that exist and what is needed for the future is critical.

Strategic and Tactical Plans

When a decision is made in a healthcare facility that it is ready to move forward with acquiring the components for an EHR, it is important to put resources into planning. Virtually everyone who has conducted an EHR project has wished they had spent more time on planning. Planning includes organizing the project and staffing, setting goals, developing a migration path, communicating to stakeholders, and developing plans for implementation and to manage change.

Organizing and Staffing the EHR Project

Most organizations create an EHR steering committee to engage all the various stakeholders. This ensures that the EHR planning is comprehensive and also starts the process of introducing change and gaining buy-in. In addition to the EHR steering committee, various domain teams, implementation teams, and other such groups are formed as the need for more specific focus arises.

The EHR project also needs support staff other than just IT staff. Certainly, the project needs a project manager. (A very large project might need a project management office.) Project managers ensure that the steps in the project are performed and coordinate the various committees and vendor staff. Project plans, budgets, staff resource utilization, issues logs, change control records, installation manuals, user manuals and training tools, and various forms of communications about the project are just one part of the overall documentation needed in developing an EHR project. Because the EHR is a clinical project, there should be clinical staff engaged in the project. Many hospitals and physician practices hire or appoint a **chief medical informatics officer** (CMIO) or medical director of information systems (MDIS). If such a position is not feasible in a small organization, at a minimum a **physician champion** should be identified. Nurse informatics and health informatics personnel are also important. Job descriptions also should be available for all persons filling new positions and may be helpful in describing the roles played on various committees.

Goal Setting

Setting specific, measurable, achievable, realistic, and time-based (SMART) goals helps the organization envision the future, establish target milestones, and benefit from the realization process. Goals should direct the results of using the EHR. Some organizations set goals that describe what the EHR should do, but not its outcomes. More meaningful are goals that describe the quality and cost improvements that should result from the EHR.

Migration Path

Developing a migration path to describe the strategic approach to EHR is an often-overlooked planning activity. A migration path is a strategic plan that outlines the major components to be implemented. It should describe the phases over which the organization intends to implement its EHR components. In addition, each phase should have specific goals.

A good way to construct an EHR migration path is to list all the current applications, technology, and operations the organization has in place or is starting to roll out. Each phase can be populated with plans for subsequent rollout of applications, technology, and operations to support them. Figure 16.14 illustrates a sample migration path. The plan for the hospital in this illustration extends over three phases. The hospital has separated technology into three categories: database, network, and interfaces. It should be noted that this is an example of a plan and is not necessarily the right plan for everyone. The nature of the current applications and technical infrastructure needs to be considered. For example, it may be determined that some of the source systems need to be upgraded because they are not compliant with message format standards, or use a proprietary and not standard vocabulary. Interfaces will be needed between applications and the CDR. Telecommunications capabilities may need to be upgraded. The readiness of the organization's clinicians to adopt various types of applications plays an important role in what the migration path will look like. Other operational elements should address all aspects of people, policy, and

Figure 16.14.   **Migration path**

Phases	Current	Phase 1	Phase 2	Phase 3
Applications	ADT	Outpt Registration	E-registration	
	MPI		E-MPI	
	Digital dictation	Speech dictation		
	Abstracting		Document Imaging	
	Encoder			
	Pt accts			
	Lab			
	Pharmacy	E-MAR		
	Radiology	PACS		Integrated RIS+PACS
	Materials mgt			
	Strategic planning			Exec Dec Support
	Order communication		CPOE	
		Nurse charting	Physician charting	CDSS
Database	Vendor proprietary	Drug Knowledgebase		
		CDR		CDW
Network	Wired		Wireless	
Interfaces	Primarily one vendor	Connect w/Ref Lab	Connect Pharmacy to CPOE	HIE standards
Operations	EHR Steering	Physician champion	Evidence-based guideline review	HIE Participation HIPAA security risk analysis
		MPI clean up		
	Manual pathways	Process mapping		

Copyright © 2012 Margret/A Consulting, LLC. Reprinted with permission.

process. But the key point of an EHR migration path is that it is an overarching plan that everyone can understand and follow.

Communicating to Stakeholders

There is often a lot of buzz surrounding early discussion of acquiring an EHR. Then as the real work starts to occur, everyone is very busy doing the work. As a result, the intended users who are waiting to be trained are not told about what is happening. They do not know if the project was abandoned or something really horrible is going to happen to them and no one wants to tell them. These are not healthy feelings. Communication about the status of the project and true engagement of as many stakeholders as possible is very important. This alleviates concerns, debunks myths, and prepares users to be ready for the changes about to happen.

Using a communication plan can be very effective. This should identify who will communicate about what activities, when, where, and how. The more who can formally communicate about the project the more widely the right messages will spread.

Plans for Implementation and Managing Change

While planning should begin early, planning for the specific implementation process and managing detailed changes should be a key part of the overall planning for EHR. Plans will include:

- Total cost of ownership and budgets. Total cost of ownership refers to the identification of all costs associated with the EHR implementation. Most organizations recognize they have to pay the EHR vendor and buy hardware. Many organizations, however, fail to anticipate the cost of extra staff, consultants, construction, furniture, and other costs associated with things like a parking lot for the WOWs while their batteries are being charged, lower desks or trays for keyboards, facilitators to analyze workflows, and many other costs. Once all costs are identified, budgets should be compiled and managed.

- Implementation plans direct the work of the implementation. Although much of this detailed planning will need to wait until a product has been selected, being prepared and anticipating the nature of the implementation can be very helpful. The EHR vendor will have an implementation plan; but the organization is advised to have its own plan as well. This will entail many of the items on the vendor's plan but other tasks as well, such as communications with board members, review of templates by physicians, establishing policies on definition of medication error, and many others. Implementation plans for EHRs often entail thousands of steps.

- **Chart conversion** plans are something many organizations think about very early in their planning and should plan for even before vendor selection, even though such plans would not be implemented until after the EHR has been installed. The nature of the conversion desired, however, may influence the choice of EHR. For hospitals, chart conversion generally refers to how to handle paper chart documentation not yet automated. Chart conversion, often in the form of document scanning and COLD feed will go on for many years after the start of the EHR implementation. For physician practices, chart conversion refers more to how to bring important information from old paper charts directly into the EHR. This often entails both scanning/COLD feed as well as abstracting critical data.

- **Data conversion** planning is necessary if data in an existing computer application must be moved to a new application. For example, frequently a physician practice will have a billing system, but then acquire a combined PMS and EHR. Deciding whether or not to move billing data from the old system to the new system should be planned for fairly early in the implementation, if not even prior to selection.

- Phasing implementation and go-live is another worrisome task, which can be planned far in advance of implementation, although it obviously depends on the installation of the product. Some organizations plan to phase-in their EHR by nursing unit or other location-based organizational structure. Other organizations decide to phase in their EHR by function, with all nursing first, then all physician orders, then physician documentation. Still others use a hybrid of these approaches.

- **Issues management** plan is another very specific task that can wait until implementation begins, although some suggest that keeping track of all internal and vendor selection issues can be insightful. Every EHR process will have issues. For example, specific hardware is delayed in delivery, the EHR vendor has forgotten to arrange for an interface, or several physicians were on vacation when training occurred. Issues should be documented so that their resolution can be tracked. Documenting issues also helps a project manager identify patterns. For example, Nurse A calls IT every day with a question that can be answered by hovering the mouse over a cell or selecting online help. Once this is observed, it may be prudent to provide Nurse A with remedial training on computers; or counseling for change management.

- Change management planning is another critical step in preparing for EHR. Change management is both formal and informal. Specific visioning exercises, education, engagement in implementation activities, and training are all formal aspects of change management. But a pat on the back, an acknowledgment that the change is large but support will be provided, and many other informal strategies are potentially even more important. How an organization helps people through the process of change is often a matter of culture. Despite the fact that healthcare organizations intend to be caring organizations, caring about making changes is often overlooked. Workflow and process change has been highlighted elsewhere in this chapter. Very few vendors address workflow and process changes, leaving these to the organization. Unfortunately, with all of the other tasks needing to be done as part of an EHR implementation, workflow and process improvements are the most overlooked aspects of change management. Time must be allotted for attention to how work changes for every user.

Information Management in an Electronic Environment

The electronic environment presents many new roles for HIM professionals. AHIMA has done a tremendous amount of work in identifying, describing, sponsoring training for, and introducing these new roles to HIM professionals and the facilities for whom HIM professionals work, as well as those organizations that accredit and license those facilities. AHIMA envisions HIM professionals as data analysts, information brokers, data set developers, data miners, workflow analysts, data security managers, database administrators, and in many other capacities that support EHRs. Not only do HIM professionals have the expertise to fill these roles, but they also have demonstrated an appreciation for data quality, confidentiality, and data security that is unparalleled in any other healthcare profession.

Data Quality

In 1998, AHIMA developed a data quality management model (figure 16.15). Appreciating the various characteristics of data quality is essential to making the EHR work. An EHR depends on data that are complete and accurate to function appropriately. In an electronic environment, there are both more potential areas for poor data quality but also more controls able to ensure data quality.

One area for poor data quality surrounds the need for making data entry easier. These include copy and paste, macros, standard orders, and other techniques that reuse data. These techniques can make data entry faster, but care must be taken to ensure appropriate modification to the specific patient. Copying the note about the four-year-old boy with an infection in the left ear for the three-year-old girl with an ear infection in the right ear is dangerous without appropriate controls being built into such copying. Even where a macro is used into which the user is expected to insert the appropriate variables can be risky if a variable is missed. Consider the following:

This is a <3> year old <female> child with <otitis media> in the < > ear.

Figure 16.15. **Data quality management model**

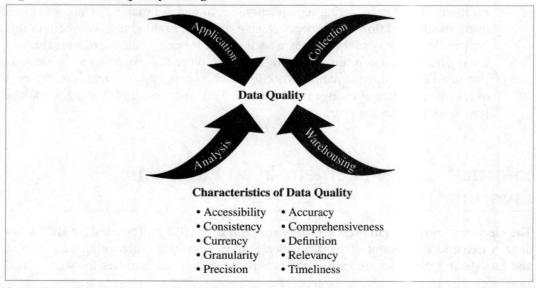

Source: Copyright © 2012 Margret/A Consulting, LLC. Reprinted with permission.

Some data quality controls can be implemented in the macro—where, perhaps, the user is not able to sign off on the note until all elements (such as which ear in the above example) are completed. Many clinicians do not like this, however, because they may feel compelled to complete a note prior to having full information. Something most EHRs cannot do, however, is to check the accuracy of all variable data. While the sex of the child could be prepopulated from other information in the chart and the age of the child computed from the birth date and entered automatically, the fact that the child actually had otitis externa and not otitis media would be difficult if not impossible for an EHR to validate. Some provider settings are starting to evaluate use of data quality monitoring programs, where a sample of records that have used such data-entry techniques are reviewed in depth.

Another data quality issue relates to use of comment fields and potential for discrepancies between what is entered as structured data and what is entered in comment fields. Comment fields can be very helpful for describing nuances not able to be captured through drop-down menus or check boxes. But, there are numerous potential issues. For example, they can be used as substitutes for discrete data entry because of lack of understanding that one term is synonymous with another. More seriously, they can potentially contradict what is entered as discrete data. The content of comment fields may not be visible to every user, and hence information recorded there essentially lost. And, data entered into comment fields are not discrete and cannot be processed in CDS or reports. Periodically, an attempt should be made to evaluate usage of comment fields and corrective action taken. It may be necessary to reword or add data elements to discrete data-entry fields. It may be necessary to educate users. It may even be necessary to limit the size of the comment field and require the vendor to display it on every applicable screen.

Another data-entry issue is determining whether entries are made by legitimate users. Unfortunately, there are some users who prefer not to use the EHR, or may occasionally give their password to someone else to enter data for them if they are in a hurry or for other reasons. This is harder to detect, but not impossible. If such a practice is suspected, it may be necessary to review audit logs for how frequently certain users are accessing the system. For example, if there are orders that appear to have been entered by a provider, but the provider had not been present in the hospital that day, it is possible someone else entered the order under the provider's access.

Handling amendments, corrections, and deletions is yet another data quality challenge. In the paper chart, a line can be drawn through an erroneous entry, initialed, and the correction made along the margin. But in EHRs, lines cannot be drawn and there are no margins. The result is often a cumbersome process at best for handling a correction, and in some cases almost impossible.

The fact that there was a correction to any entry must be visible to users, but not confusing to them. When an error is corrected, where the correction is placed also needs to be considered. If the correction is placed in the wrong sequence, this may adversely impact patient care. For example, in one EHR, making a correction to an erroneous vital sign put the correct data at the time the correction was made, not when the data were originally entered. The result was a distorted trend line of vital signs data. These issues should be identified during system build, but frequently are not or are not corrected at that time.

Future Directions in Information Technology

Every 18 months, some form of the technology becomes obsolete or at least is replaced with new technology. When one considers the fate of the floppy disk or magnetic tape as examples, it is clear that the future of HIM professionals is one of continuous need. Each change in technology presents new challenges that a background in health information management can support.

Exactly what the future holds is, of course, uncertain. General trends suggest that devices will get smaller and more user-friendly. Ways to process data will become more and more sophisticated. Today's speech and handwriting recognition are far better than they used to be and will likely get better. Natural language processing, where it is possible to extract discrete data from narrative data, also will continue to get better. In fact, all the effort put into screen design to capture discrete data will no longer be necessary if natural language processing really succeeds in the years to come.

Much of the new technology today is coming from Internet and web-based technologies. The tools available to present dynamic, context-driven information to users are only just beginning to be invented. If it is feasible today to conduct a search on the web for a specific topic that yields not only national, but also international, results in different languages, it is certainly conceivable that health information can be made available to any provider with a legitimate need to know and protected from individuals without a legitimate need for it.

Even as the promise of the future draws near, the challenges are ever present and must be addressed. Hackers with all sorts of new malware and spyware will continue to exploit systems, especially when humans make decisions not to protect them to their fullest extent or create workarounds to avoid hassles. In some cases, it seems as though systems are needed to protect humans from themselves. Still, the power of information technology will only continue to grow, especially in healthcare, which is one of the last frontiers for its adoption.

Check Your Understanding 16.5

1. Determining an organization's readiness for EHR is:
   A. Not needed if the organization already has some information technology
   B. May be optional if users are familiar with EHR and appear excited about using it
   C. Essential for every organization to ensure that everyone from top management down is prepared for the level of change
   D. Often performed by the vendor, who manages the workflow and process improvements that can occur with EHR

2. Which of the following is a plan to provide access to content of previous visit information in an EHR?

    A. Change management
    B. Chart conversion
    C. Data conversion
    D. Phasing

3. A strategic plan that identifies applications, technology, and operational elements needed for the overall information technology program in a healthcare organization is:

    A. Implementation plan
    B. Information Technology plan
    C. Migration Path
    D. Transition strategy

4. Which of the following make data entry easier but may harm data quality?

    A. Use of templates
    B. Copy and paste
    C. Drop-down boxes
    D. Structured data

5. A potential problem with reuse of data in an EHR is:

    A. Correcting entries
    B. Documentation compliance
    C. Privacy
    D. All of the above

Real-World Case

Community Hospital has a single-vendor hospital information system (HIS) that provides typical financial and administrative information systems services, including laboratory, radiology, and pharmacy information systems, and order-entry/results review. Other ancillary departments such as nutrition, physical therapy, and nursing are not online. The hospital, however, is considering acquiring a CPOE system to reduce medication errors and to earn the MU incentives. The hospital participates in a cardiac care registry but abstracts data from their paper charts to contribute to the registry. The health plans serving the community are starting to offer incentives for use of health information technology if positive patient outcomes can be identified.

Physicians who are affiliated with Community Hospital have expressed interest in acquiring EHR systems for their practices but are waiting for the hospital to make a vendor decision concerning CPOE. They believe that if they acquire an EHR from the same vendor as the hospital, they will be able to write orders from their practices for patients who are in the hospital, have better access to the information they need to monitor their patients, and be able to tap into other providers' EHR systems when they are covering in the emergency department.

The hospital and representative physicians are reviewing vendor products but are confused by what various vendors are telling them. One vendor has suggested that the hospital does not have the type of pharmacy information system that would support CPOE and thus would have to also buy a new pharmacy system. A vendor selling EDMS has suggested scanning and COLD feeding all the current chart forms from all provider settings into one repository so that they would be readily available when needed in an emergency. In the meantime, a couple of physicians purchased a standalone electronic prescribing device. They can send prescriptions to the major chain pharmacies in the community, but not to the community pharmacy, nor can they get an interface written between the device and the clinical pharmacy in the hospital that would be needed for CPOE.

Summary

Many hospitals and physician practices are in the throes of analyzing their current information systems environment and assessing how to move forward to achieve an electronic health record (EHR). An EHR is a major investment, a complex undertaking, and involves all the organization's stakeholders, especially clinicians. The EHR also is touching others in the healthcare community, including payers, employers, and, most important, patients who are learning that EHRs contribute to increased patient safety and quality healthcare. The federal government is now taking a significantly greater role in promoting adoption of EHR through incentive programs, training initiatives, and other funding opportunities—all tied to improving quality and patient safety.

Ensuring that data can be collected from all the various source systems and that there are applications to provide reminders and alerts when needed most by the clinician is a laudable goal and may seem easy. However, such an undertaking requires hardware and software that adhere to standards for interoperability and data comparability, as well as active engagement of all potential users, appropriate policies for adoption and use, and change management to use the computer to improve processes. Implementing an EHR is a clinical transformation; it truly changes how clinicians think and act—indeed, how they practice medicine.

Most hospitals cannot migrate to such systems overnight, which results in hybrid records that challenge the HIM professional's skills in managing the two worlds of paper and computer. Moreover, some are concerned that the electronic systems may not be receiving the data quality attention previously given paper records, which is even more acutely needed in the electronic environment. Many physician practice systems are highly sophisticated, but its users less informed about how to effectively use the systems. Such challenges point to the enhanced need for HIM professionals to understand and lead their organization's adoption of health information technology.

References

Adler, K.G. 2007. How to Successfully Navigate Your EHR Implementation. http://www.aafp.org/fpm/2007/0200/p33.pdf

Agency for Healthcare Research and Quality. 2011 (Aug.). Guide to Reducing Unintended Consequences of Electronic Health Records. http://psnet.ahrq.gov/resource.aspx?resourceID=23191

AHIMA e-HIM Personal Health Record Workgroup. 2005. Defining the Personal Health Record. http://library.ahima.org/xpedio/groups/public/documents/ahima/bok1_027351.hcsp?dDocName=bok1_027351

Amatayakul, M. 2011. *A Stepwise Approach to Workflow and Process Management for Health Information Technology and Electronic Health Records*, Boca Raton, FL: Productivity Press.

American Recovery and Reinvestment Act of 2009, Title XIII Health Information Technology.

Campbell, E.M., et al. 2006 (Sept.–Oct.). Types of unintended consequences related to computerized provider order entry. *Journal of the American Medical Informatics Association*. 13(5):547–556.

Center for Medicare and Medicaid Services. 2012. EHR Incentive Programs. https://www.cms.gov/Regulations-and-Guidance/Legislation/EHRIncentivePrograms/index.html?redirect=/EHRIncentivePrograms/

Chaiken, B. 2011. Web 3.0 Data-mining for comparative effectiveness and CDS. *Patient Safety & Healthcare Quality* 8(5):10–11.

Collier, R. 2011. Why quality did not improve with hospital EHR implementation. Kevinmd.com. http://www.kevinmd.com/blog/2011/05/quality-improve-hospital-ehr-implementation.html

Congdon, K. 2009 (Sept. 14). How much will an EHR cost you? Healthcare Technology Online. http://www.healthcaretechnologyonline.com/article.mvc/How-Much-Will-An-EHR-System-Cost-You-0001

DesRoches, C.M., et al. 2008. Electronic health records in ambulatory care: A national survey of physicians. *The New England Journal of Medicine* 359:50–60.

ECRI Institute. 2012. CERI Institute's Top 10 C-Suite Watch List: Hospital Technology Issues for 2012. Plymouth Meeting, PA: ECRI Institute. http://www.ecri.org

Frei, A., et al. 2010. The Chronic CARe for diAbeTes study (CARAT): a cluster randomized controlled trial. *Cardiovascular Diabetology* 9(23). http://www.cardiab.com/content/9/1/23

Graham, J., and C. Dizikes. 2011 (Jun. 27). Baby's death spotlights safety risks linked to computerized systems. *Chicago Tribune*. http://articles.chicagotribune.com/2011-06-27/news/ct-met-technology-errors-20110627_1_electronic-medical-records-physicians-systems

Health Level Seven. 2007. EHR-System Functional Model. http://www.hl7.org/ehr/downloads/index_2007.asp

Health Level Seven. 2008. PHR-System Functional Model. http://www.hl7.org/ehr/index.asp

HIMSS Analytics. 2008, 2011. US EMR Adoption Model. HIMSS Analytics Database. http://www.himssanalytics.org/

HIMSS Analytics. 2010 (Dec. 1). Medical Devices Landscape: Current and Future Adoption, Integration with EMRs, and Connectivity. A HIMSS Analytics White Paper. http://www.himssanalytics.org/docs/medicaldevices_landscape.pdf

Hoyt, B. 2011. Low cost electronic health records. Health informatics in developing countries. http://www.healthinformaticsforum.com/forum/topics/low-cost-electronic-health

Hsiao, C., et al. 2011 (Nov.). Electronic health record systems and intent to apply for meaningful incentives among office-based physician practices: United States. NCHS Data Brief. No. 70.

Institute of Medicine. 1991. *The Computer-Based Patient Record: An Essential Technology for Health Care.* Washington, DC: National Academies Press.

Institute of Medicine. 1997. *The Computer-Based Patient Record: An Essential Technology for Health Care.* Washington, DC: National Academies Press.

Institute of Medicine.1999. To Err is Human: Building a Safer Health System. http://www.iom.edu/Reports/1999/To-Err-is-Human-Building-A-Safer-Health-System.aspx

Institute of Medicine. 2003. *Key Capabilities of an Electronic Health Record System.* http://www.iom.edu/Reports/2003/Key-Capabilities-of-an-Electronic-Health-Record-System.aspx

Johns, Merida, and Nanette Sayles, eds. 2010. *Health Information Management Technology: An Applied Approach,* third edition. Chicago: AHIMA.

Kalatzis, F.G., et al. 2009. Developing a genomic-based point-of-care diagnostic system for rheumatoid arthritis and multiple sclerosis. *Conf Proc IEEE Eng Med Biol Soc.* 827–830.

McKenzie, K., and P. Karnstedt. 2010 (Sept.–Oct.). Automated informed consent: Patients and institutions benefit alike. *Patient Safety & Quality Healthcare* 7(4):38–45.

McNickle, M. 2011a. The 7 deadly sins of EMR implementation, *Healthcare IT News.* http://www.healthcareitnews.com/print/33547

McNickle, M. 2011b. 6 golden rules of EMR implementation. *Healthcare IT News.* http://www.healthcareitnews.com/print/37726

Medical Group Management Association. 2011. Electronic Health Records: Status, Needs and Lessons: 2011 Report Based on 2010 Data, Englewood, CO: MGMA.

National Alliance for Health Information Technology. 2008. Defining key health information technology terms. http://healthit.hhs.gov/portal/server.pt/gateway/PTARGS_0_10741_848133_0_0_18/10_2_hit_terms.pdf

National Committee for Quality Assurance. nd. Physician Practice Connections: Patient-Centered Medical Home. http://www.ncqa.org/tabid/631/Default.aspx

Robert Wood Johnson Foundation. 2010. Reform in action: Does use of EHRs help improve quality? http://www.rwjf.org/files/research/72480af4qehr201106.pdf

Rollins, G. 2012 (Jan.). Unintended consequences: Identifying and mitigating unanticipated issues in EHR use. *Journal of AHIMA* 83(1):28–32.

Romano, M.J., and R.S. Stafford. 2011 (Jan. 24). Electronic health records and clinical decision support systems: Impact on national ambulatory care quality. *Archives of Internal Medicine.* doi:10.1001/archinternmed.2010.527

Sanders, D. 2010 (Apr. 4). Patient safety and electronic health records: healthsystemcio.com. http://healthsystemcio.com/2010/04/20/patient-safety-and-electronic-health-records/

SAS. nd. Analytics In Healthcare. A SAS White Paper. http://jonhunt.org/resources/HealthcareAnalytics_eHR_EMR.pdf

Sittig, D.F., and D.C. Classen. 2010 (Feb.). Safe electronic health record use requires a comprehensive monitoring and evaluation framework. *Journal of the American Medical Association* 303(5):450–451.

Stead, W.W., and H.S. Lin, eds. 2009 (Jan. 9). Computational Technology for Effective Health Care: Immediate Steps and Strategic Directions. Washington, DC: The National Academies Press.

Strome, T. 2011 (Feb. 25). Moving to predictive analytics in healthcare. Healthcare Analytics.com. http://healthcareanalytics.info/2011/02/moving-to-predictive-analytics-in-healthcare/

Tholemeier, R. 2011. HIT Vendors Scramble for Positioning. http://www.healthdatamanagement.com/issues/19_6/health-information-technology-vendor-acquisitions-42542-1.html

TripleTree. 2006. Healthcare Revenue Cycle Management. Spotlight Report. http://www.connexions.com/files/TripleTreeRevenueCycle.pdf

Wians, F.H. 2009 (Feb.). Clinical laboratory tests: Which, why, and what do the results mean? *LAB Medicine* 40(2):105–106.

Additional Resources

Acker, B. 2009. Medical device deliberations: Data issues to consider when purchasing and implementing new devices. *Journal of AHIMA* 80(11):54–55.

AHIMA Data Quality Management Task Force. 1998. Practice brief: Data quality management model. *Journal of AHIMA* 69(6).

AHIMA e-HIM Personal Health Record Workgroup. 2005. The role of the personal health record in the EHR. *Journal of AHIMA* 76(7):64A–D.

AHIMA e-HIM Task Force. 2003. A Vision of the e-HIM Future. *Journal of AHIMA:* Supplement.

AHIMA e-HIM Workgroup: Best Practices for Electronic Signature and Attestation. 2009. Electronic signature, attestation, and authorship (Updated). *Journal of AHIMA* 80(11): expanded online edition.

Amatayakul, M.K. 2010. Electronic Health Records: Transforming Your Medical Practice, 2nd ed. Denver, CO: Medical Group Management Association.

Amatayakul, M.K. 2012. *Electronic Health Records: A Practical Guide for Professionals and Organizations,* 5th ed. Chicago: AHIMA.

American College of Physicians, Physician's Information and Education Resource. http://pier.acponline.org/index.html

American Health Information Management Association. 2008. Enterprise content and record management for healthcare. *Journal of AHIMA* 79(10):91–98.

Berner, E.S. 2009. Clinical decision support systems: State of the art. Agency for Healthcare Research and Quality. http://www.ahrq.gov/

Congressional Budget Office. 2008. Evidence on the costs and benefits of health information technology. http://www.cbo.gov/doc.cfm?index=9572&zzz=37777

Connecting for Health. 2004. Financial, legal, and organizational approaches to achieving electronic connectivity in healthcare. http://www.connectingforhealth.org/assets/reports/flo_sustain_healtcare_rpt.pdf

Connecting for Health. 2005. Linking health care information: Proposed methods for improving care and protecting privacy. http://www.connectingforhealth.org/assets/reports/linking_report_2_2005.pdf

Dimick, C. 2008. Documentation bad habits: Shortcuts in electronic records pose risk. *Journal of AHIMA* 79(6):40–43.

Dimick, C. 2008. Record limbo: Hybrid systems add burden and risk to data reporting. *Journal of AHIMA* 79(11):28–32.

Dimick, C. 2009. Fear factor: Ambiguities in state law leave some providers hesitant to adopt EHRs. *Journal of AHIMA* 80(11):50–51.

eHealth Initiative. 2009. Migrating toward meaningful use: The state of health information exchange. http://www.ehealthinitiative.org/HIESurvey/

Fahrenholz, C.G., and S.L. Buck. 2007. PHRs and physician practices. *Journal of AHIMA* 78(4): 71–75.

Goodson, J., and R.A. Steward. 2009. *The Data Access Handbook: Achieving Optimal Database Application Performance and Scalability.* Upper Saddle River, NJ: Prentice Hall.

Health and Human Services. 2005. Press release: HHS Awards Contracts to Advance Nationwide Interoperable Health Information Technology. http://www.hhs.gov/news/press/2005pres/20051006a.html

Health Level Seven. 2005. CDA Release 2. http://www.hl7.org/implement/standards/cda.cfm

Health Level Seven. 2007. EHR-System Functional Model. http://www.hl7.org/ehr/downloads/index_2007.asp

Institute of Medicine. 1999. *To Err Is Human: Building a Safer Health System.* Washington, DC: The National Academies Press.

Institute of Medicine. 2003. *Key Capabilities of an Electronic Health Record System, Letter Report. Patient Safety: Achieving a New Standard of Care.* Washington, DC: The National Academies Press.

Lormand, J. 2005. Bringing patient safety technology to the bedside. *Health Management Technology* 24–27. http://www.healthmgttech.com/

Miller, R.A., et al. 2005. Clinical decision support and electronic prescribing systems: A time for responsible thought and action. *Journal of the American Medical Informatics Association* 12(4):403–409.

National Committee on Vital and Health Statistics. 2001. Information for health: A strategy for building the national health information infrastructure. http://aspe.hhs.gov/sp/NHII/Documents/NHIIReport2001/default.htm

National Quality Forum. 2010. National Voluntary Consensus Standards for Ambulatory Care. http://www.qualityforum.org/Projects/Ambulatory_Care_2010.aspx

National Research Council. W.W. Stead and H.S. Lin, eds. 2009. *Computational Technology for Effective Health Care: Immediate Steps and Strategic Directions.* Washington, DC: The National Academies Press.

Nunn, S. 2008. Tools of the e-discovery trade. *Journal of AHIMA* 79(11):54–55, 62–63.

Parmigiani, J. 2009. Communicating security efforts: Informing consumers of data protection programs helps build trust. *Journal of AHIMA* 80(11):56–57.

Presidential Executive Order 13335: Incentives for the use of health information technology and establishing the position of the national health information technology coordinator. http://edocket.access.gpo.gov/2004/pdf/04-10024.pdf

Roszell, S., and C. Stewart. 2008. E-charting point-of-care data entry dilemma. *Journal of Nursing Administration* 38(10):417–418.

Strong, K. 2008. Enterprise content and records management. *Journal of AHIMA* 80(2):38–42.

Tang, P.C., and T.H. Lee. 2009. Your doctor's office or the Internet? Two paths to personal health records. *The New England Journal of Medicine* 360:1276–1278.

Thompson, T.G., and D.J. Brailer. 2004. The decade of health information technology: Delivering consumer-centric and information-rich health care, framework for strategic action. http://healthit.hhs.gov/portal/server.pt

Washington, L., E. Katsh, and N. Sondheimer. 2009. Dispute resolution: Planning for disputed information in EHRS and PHRS. *Journal of AHIMA* 80(11):25–30.

chapter 17

Information Security

Sheila Carlon, PhD, RHIA, FAHIMA, CHPS

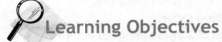

Learning Objectives

- Understand the differences among the terms *confidentiality, privacy,* and *security*
- Describe the elements of a data security program
- Identify the greatest threats to the security of health information
- Discuss methods for minimizing threats to data security
- Discuss monitoring methods for enforcement of security policies and procedures
- Participate in security audits and breach prevention strategies
- Describe the primary components of the security provisions of the Health Insurance Portability and Accountability Act and extensions by the HITECH Act and American Recovery and Reinvestment Act
- Understand the roles and responsibilities of health information technicians with regard to data and information security

Key Terms

Access control	Audit controls
Access safeguards	Audit trails
Administrative safeguards	Authentication
American Recovery and Reinvestment Act (ARRA)	Authorization
	Biometrics
Application controls	Breaches

Breach notification
Business associates
Business continuity plan
Contingency and disaster planning
Cryptography
Data availability
Data integrity
Data security
Department of Health and Human
   Services Office for Civil Rights (OCR)
Digital certificate
Digital signatures
Encryption
Firewall
Flexibility of approach
General Rules
Health Information Technology for
   Economic and Clinical Health
   (HITECH)
Health Insurance Portability and
   Accountability Act of 1996 (HIPAA)
Implementation specifications

Incident detection
Information Technology Asset Disposition
   (ITAD)
Integrity controls
Intrusion detection
Malware
Medical identity theft
Network controls
Password
Physical safeguards
Public Law 104-191
Risk analysis
Risk management
Security breach
Security program
Security threat
Single sign-on
Technical safeguard provisions
Transmission security
Unsecured electronic personal health
   information (e-PHI)

Introduction

In the past 30 years there has been significant growth in the collection and use of personal healthcare data. This data continues to be used in the delivery of patient care, but is growing because a significant number of companies and agencies such as third-party payers, employer healthcare benefit plans, government programs, research programs, and public health interests are using the data for reasons not directly related to patient care. And recently, with the development of Regional Health Information Organizations (RHIOs) and Health Information Exchanges, data sharing among providers is increasing. There are also increasing demands by government agencies and the public health sector for biosurveillance data in order to keep the public and medical communities informed of disease outbreaks and bioterrorist threats.

The sophistication of information technologies also has contributed to the growth in the collection and use of patient data. Because today's computers and networks are faster and can store and move greater amounts of data, it is much easier to collect, maintain, aggregate, and disseminate personal healthcare data today than it was even a decade ago.

The collection and storage of personal health data, however, has elevated the need for increased protection of this data while still allowing data and information sharing.

The Markle Foundation, in recent congressional testimony (Ten Years 2011), began their report on the current state of information sharing with this quote "it is clear that our failure to discover the September 11th plot was in many ways a failure of information sharing and a failure to empower our best and brightest." Their point, in this testimony, illustrates the risks inherent in data sharing. There are risks in sharing sensitive data, but also risks in not sharing data. The de-centralization and distribution of data is increasing and demands higher levels of sensitivity and security than previously existed.

Who is actually collecting and seeing all these data on patients? Providers of health-care services have always had access to patient data. These providers include physicians, consultants, nurses, ancillary providers, and those who need access to the data for administrative and operational functions. The **Health Insurance Portability and Accountability Act** (HIPAA) of 1996 restricted access to patient information on a "need to know" basis or more specifically, only those directly involved in the care of the patient were given legitimate access. Operational and administrative users were also restricted under this provision. However, many secondary users also collect information kept in the patient's health record. These users include researchers (those engaged in pure research and those doing research on clinical outcomes for evidence-based practice), pharmaceutical companies, health and life insurance companies, credit card agencies, financial institutions, and the civil and criminal justice systems (US Congress 1993, 2–3). Indeed, some secondary users and other private companies have "begun to act on the commercial incentive" to gather and sell aggregate healthcare data without the patient's knowledge. However language in the HIPAA Privacy Rule has restricted the access and use of such data and the Notices of Privacy Practices (NOPPs) previously mentioned in chapter 13 help patients understand how their information is being used.

In the past decade new entrants into the information-sharing market have emerged. These new users of health information typically are companies that have significant business interests in the collection of individually identifiable health information. In the main, they provide products and services to the healthcare industry. Examples of such companies are medical and surgical suppliers, pharmaceutical companies, reference laboratories, and businesses that offer information technology services.

Until 1996, with the passage of the Health Insurance Portability and Accountability Act (HIPAA), no uniform national standard was in place to protect the privacy and security of patient information. HIPAA contained provisions that would lead to the development of **data security** standards on a national level. The standards that grew out of this legislation were published on February 20, 2003, and were based on sound data security practices and required compliance by certain healthcare and healthcare-related entities regardless of size. The HIPAA privacy and security standards were further strengthened when the **Health Information Technology for Economic and Clinical Health** (HITECH) Act was enacted on February 17, 2009. The HITECH Act is part of the **American Recovery and Reinvestment Act** (ARRA) of 2009, which is addressed in chapter 13.

This chapter, then, examines the basic elements of data security and data security programs and explains why each element of those programs is important for ensuring the integrity and availability of patient data and protecting it from unauthorized access. The provisions of the Security Rule and strategies for risk management and breach preventions are discussed as well as examples of the disastrous consequences of not instituting effective data security practices.

Theory into Practice

The following real life case illustrates what can happen to data security when security and e-PHI policies are not followed leading to breaches of protected health information on a large scale. This case was reported to the Office of Civil Rights and also reported in *Health Data Management* (Goedert 2010).

A large health plan in Florida reported that two laptops were missing or stolen. One was subsequently recovered. While initial numbers of those potentially affected were not known, it was estimated at around 330,000. It was later reported that closer to 1.2 million subscribers were at risk from the loss of the data on the laptops, which contained names, addresses, Social Security numbers, and health details.

A lawsuit was filed on behalf of the claimants saying the insurer violated federal health privacy laws, industry standards, and its own company procedures by not securing information stored on the two laptops. The president and COO of the company reported they were "strengthening their data security capabilities and procedures to ensure this kind of incident did not recur."

Confidentiality, Privacy, and Security

Privacy

Confusion about the meanings of the terms *privacy, confidentiality,* and *security* frequently result in their misuse. As discussed in chapter 12, in the healthcare context, privacy is usually understood to mean the right of an individual to limit access to information about his or her person. The Privacy Act of 1974 was enacted to safeguard an individual's privacy from potential misuse of federal records and to give individuals access to records that are maintained by federal agencies about them. The act also established a Privacy Protection Safety Commission designed to address the right to privacy as a personal and fundamental right under the Constitution thereby protecting individuals identified in information systems maintained by federal agencies. It also provided safeguards for the individual against an invasion of personal privacy.

Confidentiality

Confidentiality, on the other hand, refers to the expectation that information shared by an individual with a healthcare provider during the course of care will be used only for its intended purpose. Physicians have always had a duty to keep a patient's information confidential. In essence, the physician's duty to maintain confidentiality means that a physician may not disclose any medical information revealed by a patient or discovered by the physician in connection with the treatment of a patient. In general, the AMA's *Code of Medical Ethics* states that the information disclosed to a physician during the course of the patient-physician relationship is confidential to the utmost degree (AMA-assn.org). Other providers and employees in healthcare settings, specifically those that have access to e-PHI in patient records or reports, are also required to ensure patient confidentiality with respect to the contents of those records. AHIMA's Code of Ethics (AHIMA.org) also contains a standard that relates to maintaining confidentiality and ensuring privacy of patient information. Thus, disclosure of information beyond its intended purpose without the patient's knowledge and consent is a violation of confidentiality.

Security

Security can be defined as the protection measures and tools for safeguarding information and information systems. Specifically, as defined by the US Code on Information Security (NIST 2008, A-6), information security means:

- Protecting information and information systems from unauthorized access, use disclosure, disruption, modification, or destruction and includes ensuring information non-repudiation and authenticity through the following:
  - Integrity, which means guarding against improper information modification or destruction, and includes ensuring information non-repudiation and authenticity
  - Confidentiality, which means preserving authorized restrictions on access and disclosure, including means for protecting personal privacy and proprietary information
  - Availability, which means ensuring timely and reliable access to and use of information

Information security includes a variety of protection measures that safeguard data and computer programs and resources from undesired access and exposure. These measures include:

- *Management practices,* such as prohibiting employees from sharing their passwords
- *Physical safeguards,* such as ensuring that doors to areas that house major computer systems are locked or otherwise secured to keep out unauthorized persons
- *Technical measures* (including computer software), such as ensuring that only certain passwords allow an individual access to patient data

Thus, a healthcare data security system is concerned with implementing security measures that safeguard both the data and the systems that collect, maintain, and store the data.

Elements of a Security Program

What elements of a **security program** could help prevent system or access errors from occurring? A good data security program embodies three basic concepts:

- Protecting the privacy of data
- Ensuring the integrity of data
- Ensuring the availability of data

Protecting the Privacy of Data

Within the context of data security, protecting data privacy basically means defending or safeguarding access to information. In other words, only those individuals who need to know information should be authorized to access it.

Also, protecting informational privacy usually refers primarily to patient-related data. However, the privacy of other information in the healthcare organization should be protected as well. For example, certain information about providers (physicians, nurses, therapists, and so on), employees, and the organization itself should be considered confidential. Information leaked to unauthorized individuals about providers, employees, or the organization can have as devastating an effect as information leaked about patients.

Ensuring the Integrity of Data

Data integrity means that data is complete, accurate, consistent, and up-to-date. The Security and Privacy Rule (45 C.F.R.) Part 164.304 defines data integrity as data that has not been altered or destroyed in an unauthorized manner. Ensuring the integrity of healthcare data is important because providers use them in making decisions about patient care. For example, an error made in recording a drug dosage that caused the wrong amount of medication to be given to a patient could result in significant injury or even loss of life. Thus, one important aspect of any security program is to put in place measures that protect the integrity of data.

The issue of data integrity and accuracy should not be taken lightly. Studies on data accuracy in healthcare indicate that it is a major issue of concern. In a recent Consensus Report and press release, the IOM stated that "health IT can help improve provider performance and communication between providers and patients and that health IT can also help reduce costs and enhance patient safety" (IOM 2011). The report goes on to say that the number of patients who receive the correct medication increases when hospitals use well-designed, robust computerized drug ordering systems and barcodes, but poorly designed systems can create hazards in an already "complex delivery system." Thus, a security program is as much about ensuring data quality and accuracy as it is about maintaining informational privacy.

Ensuring the Availability of Data

Ensuring **data availability** means making sure the organization can depend on the information system to perform exactly as expected, without error, and to provide information when and where it is needed. Some studies have indicated that information required for patient care is unavailable in up to 30 percent of patient visits (IOM 1991, 62).

Problems with the retrieval of information can happen in both paper and computer formats. For example, paper records may be misfiled or being used by another provider. Retrieval problems occur when the computer system is unreliable or unavailable. For example, sometimes the system experiences unscheduled downtime and is unable to process or provide access to information. A good security program will ensure that data are available seven days a week, 24 hours a day. To accomplish this effectively, organizations must have backup and downtime procedures in place. Data backup procedures may involve server redundancy or duplexing (duplicate information on one or more servers) and sending data to offsite contracted vendors or data warehouses for safe and secure storage and access. Backup policies and procedures for all systems (including non-networked computers such as laptops) should be in place. Backup procedures are necessary to ensure that the organization's business can continue in the event of a disruption. Backup procedures are also necessary to be in compliance with federal and state regulations.

Backup policies and procedures should specify what files and programs require backup, what type of backup should be performed, how frequently the backup should occur, and how the backup is to be conducted. For example, a backup policy may require that all data, operating systems, and utility files be adequately and systematically backed up including all patches, fixes, and updates. The policy may also indicate whether a full or incremental backup procedure be performed and the frequency of the backup (such as daily or weekly).

Records should be kept of what is backed up and where it is maintained. Copies of backup media and records of backups should be stored at a secure off-site location. This action is taken so that if a disaster occurs at the main site, backup copies will be unaffected. There are many companies that specialize in digital off-site storage.

Backed up media is only good if it can be used in the event of an emergency. Therefore, regular tests of restoring data and software from backed up copies should be performed to ensure that they work in an emergency.

Downtime procedures for both planned and unplanned system availability should be part of the regular IT infrastructure as well as incorporated into the security program.

To summarize, a data security program must:

- Protect informational privacy by ensuring that data cannot be accessed by unauthorized persons

- Build in safeguards to ensure that data are altered or disposed of by only authorized means

- Employ mechanisms to ensure that computer systems operate effectively and can provide information when and where it is needed

Every organization is subject to **security breaches** by people from both inside and outside the organization. It is essential to recognize the scope of data security needs and to develop a systematic and comprehensive program to deal with them. Security breaches also can occur through hardware or software failures and when an intruder hacks into the system. More often, however, they occur when an employee of the organization either accesses information without authorization or deliberately alters or destroys information. A 2007 report from the Federal Bureau of Investigation (FBI) shows that 70 percent of all security problems begin inside the organization (Patel 2009). In healthcare, hospital employees have been reported to comprise the largest known group of individuals involved in **medical identity theft** and fraud (Johnson 2009, 4).

Therefore, an organization's security program must have protections in place to keep its employees honest as well as to keep outsiders from harming or accessing information resources. Good data security does not just happen. It requires planning and the implementation of realistic policies and procedures that address both internal and external threats.

Check Your Understanding 17.1

Instructions: Select the best answer to each question.

1. Which term is defined as ensuring timely and reliable access to and use of information?

   A. Availability
   B. Confidentiality
   C. Integrity
   D. Security

2. Which of the following is an example of a technical measure?

   A. A policy that states that passwords cannot be shared
   B. A policy that states that only authorized people can access the data center
   C. Locking the door of the data center
   D. Assigning passwords that limit access to computer stored information

3. Which statement is true about data security?

   A. Data availability means that data should be complete, accurate, consistent, and up to date.
   B. Data availability means that an organization must be able to depend on the information system to function appropriately.
   C. Most data security problems are due to hackers and external threats.
   D. The privacy of data only concerns patient information.

Instructions: Indicate whether the following statements are true or false (T or F).

4. _____ One of the most important jobs of the health information technician is to ensure that health data are protected from unauthorized use.

5. _____ Confidentiality is the right of an individual to limit access to information about his or her person.

6. _____ Data security includes all the protection measures and tools for safeguarding information.

7. _____ Prohibiting an employee from sharing his or her computer password is an example of a physical safeguard.

8. _____ Protection of the privacy of information may be defined as the safeguard of information from unauthorized access.

Data Security Threats

Before implementing a security program, it is important to understand the potential threats to **data security.** Threats from a number of sources can cause the loss of informational privacy, compromise data integrity and/or the availability of data.

Basically, threats to data security from people can be classified into five categories (figure 17.1). These include:

- *Threats from insiders who make unintentional mistakes:* Such threats could be employees who accidentally make a typographical error, inadvertently delete files on a computer disk, or unknowingly give out confidential information. Unintentional error is one of the major causes of security breaches.

- *Threats from insiders who abuse their access privileges to information:* Such threats could be employees who knowingly disclose information about a patient to individuals who do not have proper authorization. They also could be employees with access to computer files who purposefully snoop for information they do not need to perform their jobs. However one of the biggest threats from employees who may abuse their access to information is storing it on a thumb or flash drive, removing it from the facility on a laptop or other storage device, and subsequently losing the device or having it stolen.

- *Threats from insiders who access information or computer systems for spite or profit:* Generally, such employees seek information for the purpose of committing fraud or theft. Identity theft, or stealing information from patients, their families, or other employees is on the rise and in some cases has resulted in prosecution of those employees who obtained that information unlawfully.

- *Threats from intruders who attempt to access information or steal physical resources:* Individuals may physically come onto the organization's property to access information or steal equipment such as laptop computers or printers. They also may loiter in the organization's buildings hoping to access information from unprotected computer terminals or to read or take paper documents, computer disks, or other information.

- *Threats from vengeful employees or outsiders who mount attacks on the organization's information systems:* Disgruntled employees might destroy computer hardware or software, delete or change data, or enter data incorrectly into the computer system. Outsiders might mount attacks that can harm the organization's information resources. For example, malicious hackers could plant viruses in the computer system or break into telecommunications systems to degrade or disrupt system availability.

Threats Caused by People

Three of the threats listed in figure 17.1 involve the organization's employees. Thus it is important for an organization to assure that their employees and others with routine access to patient data are vigilant in their use of this data.

Threats Caused by Environmental and Hardware or Software Factors

People are not the only threats to data security. Natural disasters such as earthquakes, tornadoes, floods, and hurricanes can demolish physical facilities and electrical utilities. According to the Federal Emergency Management Agency (FEMA), there has been a yearly average of 33 declared disasters in the United States during the past two decades. However, FEMA reported in 2010 75 declared emergencies in 2008, 59 in 2009, 81 in 2010 and 99 in 2011 for an average of 78 per year, an indication that disasters may be increasing. On August 29, 2005, a Category 5 Hurricane devastated coastal Louisiana, Mississippi, and neighboring states. New Orleans was hit hard and damage was significant particularly due to flood waters after the hurricane passed. Included in the loss of life and property was damage to medical practices and hospitals and their patient records. Many of the facilities and practices had paper records that were completely destroyed and those that did exist on computer hard drives were destroyed by winds, water, and other forces.

Figure 17.1.   **Categories of people-oriented security threats**

• Insiders who make innocent mistakes	• Physical intruders who steal or otherwise harm systems
• Insiders who abuse their privileges	• Vengeful employees or outsiders who mount attacks
• Insiders who access or alter data for spite or profit	

Patient care was severely compromised because of the lost records that contained information on patient's diagnoses, medications, lab tests, and such.

On May 22, 2011, an EF 5 tornado ripped through Joplin, Missouri, literally decimating St. John's Regional Medical Center with a direct hit. The winds were so powerful that items from the hospital, like medications, x-rays and medical records, were found in neighboring counties.

While this kind of devastation is not ordinary, facilities must begin to protect themselves against this kind of loss. Facilities in California and other earthquake prone areas send backup information to vaults offsite to assist in the recovery of data should an earthquake or other untoward event destroy onsite computer systems.

To recover from the devastation that natural disasters can cause, organizations must have good backup and recovery procedures in place both for paper and electronic medical records and other important facility data.

Other causes of security breaches are utility, software, and hardware failures. These include hardware breakdowns and software failures that cause information systems to shut down or malfunction unexpectedly. Examples would be a hard-disk crash that destroys or corrupts data, a program code that does not execute properly and alters or destroys information, a failed, weak, or poorly configured firewall and unsecured browsers.

Electrical outages and power surges also can cause problems. When an electrical outage occurs, for example, information is unavailable to the end user. In addition, data might be corrupted or even lost. Power surges also can destroy or corrupt information. Thus, organizations must have the appropriate equipment to protect information systems from power surges and backup equipment to keep them running during an outage.

Yet another type of threat is a hardware or software malfunction. Security breaches may be introduced when new software or hardware is added to the system or when it is not correctly tested. One well-publicized case occurred when a software upgrade in the computer system of a health insurance company was not properly tested. During the implementation, mailings of Explanation of Benefits (EOBs) were sent to the wrong addresses by mistake. The EOBs may have included e-PHI. The state insurance commissioner stated that the breach was the worst in 14 years and although it was unintentional it was a violation of both state and federal law. Basically, the security breach was caused by poor practice (Krigsman 2008). Thus, organizations must follow good configuration management procedures to ensure that software and hardware malfunctions do not seriously affect data security.

While malfunctions of various software applications can corrupt data, another type of threat is caused by intentional software intrusions known as malicious software or **malware.** These software applications can take over partial or full control of a computer and can compromise data security and corrupt both data and hard drives.

Some examples of malware include:

- Computer viruses: A computer virus is a program that reproduces itself and attaches itself to legitimate programs on a computer. A virus can be programmed to change or corrupt data. Frequently viruses can slow down the performance of a computer system.

- Computer worms: A computer worm is a program that copies itself and spreads throughout a network. Unlike a computer virus, a computer worm does not need to attach itself to a legitimate program. It can execute and run itself.

- Trojan horse: A Trojan horse is a program that gains unauthorized access to a computer and masquerades as a useful function. A Trojan horse virus is capable of compromising data by copying confidential files to unprotected areas of the computer system. Trojan horses may also copy and send themselves to e-mail addresses in a user's computer.

- Spyware: Spyware is a computer program that tracks an individual's activity on a computer system. Cookies are a type of spyware. These programs can store authentication information such as an individual's password.

- Backdoor programs: A backdoor is a computer program that bypasses normal authentication processes and allows access to computer resources, such as programs, computer networks, or entire computer systems.

- Rootkit: A rootkit is a computer program designed to gain unauthorized access to a computer and gain control over the operating system and modify the operating system.

Malware usually gains access to computers via the Internet as attachments in e-mails or through browsing a website that installs the software after the user clicks on a popup window. To prevent the intrusion of malware, organizations should establish antivirus policies and procedures. The policy should establish the use of antivirus software and specify: (1) what devices should be scanned, such as file servers, mail servers, desktop computers; (2) what programs, documents, and files should be scanned; (3) how often scans should be scheduled; (4) who is responsible for ensuring that scans are completed; and (5) what action should be taken when malware is detected. In addition, filters can be used to filter both incoming and outgoing e-mail so that malware is quarantined.

In addition to an antivirus policy, organizations should have in place security awareness policies and training that deal with prevention of and identification of malware.

Strategies for Minimizing Security Threats

The first and most fundamental strategy in minimizing security threats is to establish a secure organization that is responsible for managing all aspects of computer security. This usually involves appointing someone in the organization to coordinate the development of security policies and to ensure that they are followed. Generally, this individual is called the chief security officer (CSO).

In addition to appointing someone to the CSO position, the organization should appoint an advisory or policy-making group. This group is often called the Information Security Committee. This committee usually works with the CSO to evaluate the organization's security needs, to establish a security program, develop associated policies and procedures including monitoring and sanction policies, and ensure that the policies are followed. Sanction policies and procedures are important to develop and enforce so that employees understand the penalties for noncompliance with security and privacy rules.

The Security Rule does not specify the roles and composition of an Information Security Committee, but the responsibilities extend well beyond the protection of the data and involve Human Resources, which typically assists in workforce clearances, employee termination procedures, and applications of sanctions to employees who violate established policies (Miaoulis 2011). Other roles include executive-level managers who should have a high level understanding of the data security policies and procedures and approve security budgets. In addition, the Health Information Management Director or designee should sit on the Information Security Committee and assist in determining levels of access, authorization, and audit trail reviews. Other management positions involved in the Information Security Committee are the CIO, IT system directors, network engineers, and representatives from ancillary departments (lab, pharmacy, radiology) as appropriate.

What strategies should organizations use to protect their information systems? Figure 17.2 lists some of the most common approaches. Taken together, they form a data security program.

Components of a Security Program

A good security program should contain the following components:

- Employee awareness including ongoing education and training
- Risk management program
- Access safeguards
- Physical and administrative safeguards
- Software application safeguards
- Network safeguards
- Business continuity plan
- Data quality control processes

Figure 17.2.   Common approaches to protecting information systems

• Implementing an employee security awareness program	• Implementing software application controls
• Conducting regular risk analyses and assessments	• Developing a disaster recovery and business continuity plan
• Establishing access controls	• Implementing network controls
• Implementing physical and management controls	• Implementing policies on mobile devices
	• Implementing policies on social media use

Each component will be discussed as it relates to the establishment of an organization's security program. Some of these same elements will also be discussed in relation to the provisions of the Security Rule later in this chapter.

Employee Awareness

As discussed above, employees are often responsible for threats to data security. Consequently, employee awareness is a particularly important tool in reducing security breaches.

The organization should offer a formal program that educates every new employee on the confidential nature of patient and organization data. The program should inform employees about the organization's security policies and the consequences of failing to comply with them. The organization should give each employee a copy of its security policies as they relate to the employee's job function. It also should require every employee to sign a yearly confidentiality statement. Finally, because data security is such an important part of everyone's job, employees should receive periodic and ongoing security reminders.

Included in the employee awareness program should be policies and procedures regarding mobile devices and the use of e-mail and faxed information, and social media. According to a survey by Price Waterhouse Coopers (pw.com), less than 50 percent of organizations include approved uses of social media and mobile devices in privacy and security training.

Risk Management Program

Another strategy in protecting the organization's data is to establish a risk management program. **Risk management** encompasses the identification, management, and control of untoward events. Healthcare entities must take steps to prevent, detect, and mitigate both external and internal incidents. A well-conceived risk management program can aid prevention, intrusion detection, and mitigation of security breaches including identity theft.

Risk Analysis

The Security Rule requires an organization to implement security measures that are sufficient to reduce risk and vulnerabilities but may use a flexible and reasonable approach to do so [164.308(a)]. Given the applicability of the rule to various sizes of healthcare organizations from small physician practices to large healthcare systems, those reasonable and flexible approaches can vary based on the size of the organization and its complexity, its technical infrastructure related to hardware and software, the potential costs of security measures, and the likelihood and potential risk that e-PHI may be breached (Walsh 2011; AHIMA 2011a).

Risk management, therefore, begins with a risk assessment. Identifying **security threats**, risks, and vulnerabilities, determining how likely it is that any given threat may occur, and estimating the impact of an untoward event are all parts of a risk assessment (Johns 2008, 316). Among the threats to security are human error, such as a data-entry mistake, unauthorized physical access to data, sabotage, power failures, and malfunction of software or hardware (Johns 2008, 316). In addition to the threats and vulnerabilities mentioned above, the organization should also identify how e-PHI is created, managed, stored, and transmitted within the organization and whether vendors or consultants use or maintain e-PHI.

It makes no sense to implement security solutions without first identifying the organization's weaknesses. For example, if the organization is unlikely to experience a catastrophic event such as a tornado, it makes no sense to implement an expensive security solution to protect against such an event. On the other hand, if the facility's employees are connected to the Internet, it makes sense to implement security solutions that will keep hackers out of the facility's computer systems. The organization should also include less obvious sources of risk such as activities by vendors and the use of portable mobile devices to access and store data.

When risks have been identified, it is important to estimate their likelihood of occurring and what their impact on information assets might be. Not all information is of equal importance, so it is essential to determine the value of information to the organization and the consequences of its loss when establishing a risk management program. For example, what impact would a security breach have on quality of care, revenue, service, or organizational image? Several different methodologies can be used to carry out a **risk analysis.** Calculations of risks based on unintentional occurrences such as power failures or data-entry error are usually based on the probability of the specific event occurring. Calculations of risk for intentional acts such as fraud or theft are usually based on such factors as the attractiveness of a system to a perpetrator and the degree of system vulnerability (Johns 2008, 316).

A risk assessment is usually performed by a multidisciplinary team that has specific knowledge about data security and the organization. The first step in the risk assessment is to identify the organization's information assets. This usually includes making an inventory of application software, hardware, networks, and other information assets. Once information assets have been identified, their value to the organization is determined. Value is determined based on a number of factors such as criticality of the asset in daily operations, degree of harm resulting if the asset is not available, legal and regulatory requirements, and loss of revenue should the asset be lost or damaged.

A sample threat assessment matrix is presented in figure 17.3 (Johns 2002, 12). This matrix lists possible security threats and the issues that should be considered for assessing each threat. For example, if the number of users is high, the volume of transactions is high, and the information system is complex, the threat of possible human unintentional error would be high. Risk procedures to manage a threat due to human error should be implemented, such as increased employee training and increased auditing of output for errors.

Incident Detection

Once possible threats are known, it is important to be able to detect whether a threat or incident or intrusion has occurred. **Incident detection** methods should be used to identify both accidental and malicious events. Detection programs monitor the information systems for abnormalities or a series of events that might indicate that a security breach

Figure 17.3. Sample threat assessment matrix

This tool should be used with the Valuation Matrix to determine priority for assignment of security safeguards.				
Application/System				
Threat	**Considerations**	**High**	**Med**	**Low**
Unintentional human error	• Number of users • Daily transactions • Complexity of system use • Level of employee system training			
Programming development	In-house development • Level of system analysis and design methodology • Quality control procedures • Implemented testing procedures • Complexity of system • Number of interfaces • Level of security features Proprietary development • Years in the market • Evaluation reviews • Complexity of system • Vendor reputation • Number of interfaces • Level of security features			
Fraud or theft Employee sabotage	• Contains patient-related data • Contains financial data • Contains proprietary business data • Electronic commerce • Level of security features • Employee satisfaction level • Dial-up lines • Open network			
Loss of physical facilities or infrastructure	• Likelihood of natural disaster • Condition of physical plant • Age and condition of equipment • Maintenance schedule • Reliability of utilities • Level of system redundancy			
Malicious hackers	• Level of company visibility • Patient data • Financial data • Electronic commerce • Buffer overflows • Dial-up lines • Use of open network			
Industrial espionage	• Financial/strategic data • Patient data • Risk management/legal data			

is occurring or has occurred. There are a variety of analytic detection tools and intrusion prevention systems that are used for this purpose.

Incident Response Plan and Procedures

Once a security incident has been identified, there must be a coordinated response to mitigate the incident. An incident response plan includes management procedures and responsibilities to ensure that a quick response is effectively implemented for specific types of incidents. For example, in some instances the plan may call for a "watch and warn" response that includes monitoring and notification of an incident but takes no immediate action. In other instances a "repair and report" response may be instituted. This type of response may be used in the case of a virus attack. A third type of response may be "pursue and prosecute," which would include the monitoring of an attack, the minimization of the attack, the collection of evidence, and the involvement of a law enforcement agency. This last example might be used in instances of suspected identity theft. The specific requirements under the HITECH Act for notifying affected individuals when an information security breach has occurred are discussed later in this chapter and are also addressed in chapter 13.

Regardless of the specific response, all response plans must include seven activities. These include determination that an untoward security event has occurred or is occurring, documentation of the event, notification of the appropriate people that an incident has occurred, containment of the incident, assessment of the scope of damage, removal of the cause of the incident, and recovery of the system (Pipkin 2000, 246–247).

Access Safeguards

Establishing **access safeguards** is a fundamental security strategy. Basically, this means being able to identify which employees should have access to what data. The general practice is that employees should have access only to data they need to do their jobs. For example, an admitting clerk and a healthcare provider would not have access to the same kinds of data.

Determining what data to make available to an employee usually involves identifying classes of information based on the employee's role in the organization. Thus, the organization would determine what information an admitting clerk, for example, would need to know to do his or her job. Thereafter, every individual who works as an admitting clerk would have access to the same information.

Every role in the organization should be identified, along with the type of information required to perform it. This is often referred to as role-based access. Although there are other types of access control strategies, role-based access is probably the one used most often in healthcare organizations. Access to information and information resources (such as computers) must be restricted to those authorized to access the information or the associated resources. This requires that mechanisms be in place to restrict access. There are a number of **access control** mechanisms that can be used. They are discussed later in this chapter. However, the sophistication of the method used should correspond with the value of the information being protected—the more sensitive or valuable the information, the stronger the control mechanisms need to be. Identification, authentication, and authorization are the foundation on which access control mechanisms are based.

Identification

The basic building block of access control is identification of an individual. Usually identification is performed through the username or user number.

Authentication

The second element of access control is **authentication.** Authentication is the act of verifying a claim of identity. There are three different types of information that can be used for authentication: something you know, something you have, or something you are.

Passwords

Examples of *something you know* include such things as a PIN, a **password,** or your mother's maiden name. Passwords are frequently used in conjunction with username. Policies and procedures should be in place to ensure that passwords cannot be easily compromised. For example, passwords should be of a specific length, include special characters and numbers, and should not be words that are included in a dictionary or related to the user's ID or personal information. Even today we find that "password" and "12345" are used as passwords. The policy should include mandatory changes of passwords at specified intervals. These types of restrictions help to limit the chance of an intruder guessing a password or using a program called a password cracker to identify passwords. To help increase security, many computer operating systems will lock out a user ID after a specified number of unsuccessful attempts to gain access to a computer system. In addition, password policies should prohibit users from sharing passwords or writing or displaying passwords. While passwords provide the least amount of security compared to other methods described below, if properly managed and used, they can be an effective security strategy.

Smart Cards and Tokens

Smart cards and token cards are examples of *something you have.* A smart card is a small plastic card with an embedded microchip that can store multiple identification factors for a specific user. Usually a smart card is used in combination with a user identification or password. A one-time password (OTP) token is a small electronic device programmed to generate and display new passwords at certain intervals. An OTP token is usually used in combination with user identification or a password. To access a system, a user puts in an identification code and the OTP token generates a one-time password that is displayed on the token.

Biometrics

Something you are refers to biometrics. Examples of **biometrics** include palm prints, fingerprints, voice prints, and retina (eye) scans.

Two-factor Authentication

Strong authentication requires providing information from two of the three different types of authentication information. For example, something you know plus something you have. This is called two-factor authentication. Examples of two-factor authentication include the use of smart cards or tokens with user identification. Two-factor authentication is a stronger method of protecting data access than user identification with passwords. An example of two-factor identification is being used at Walt Disney World in Florida. Guests insert their park tickets and also have their index finger scanned.

Single Sign-on

Single sign-on allows sign-on to multiple related, but independent, software systems. With this property a user logs in once and gains access to all systems without being prompted to log in again for each of them. Single sign-off is the reverse property whereby a single action of signing out terminates access to multiple software systems.

As different applications and resources support different authentication mechanisms, single sign-on has to internally translate to and store different credentials compared to what is used for initial authentication.

Authorization

The third element of access control is authorization. **Authorization** is a right or permission given to an individual to use a computer resource, such as a computer or to use specific applications and access specific data. It is also a set of actions that gives permission to an individual to perform specific functions such as read, write, or execute tasks.

Authorization to use a computer system is usually addressed through identification and authentication, described previously. Authorization to use specific applications (for example, order entry, coding, and registration) and specific data would be different for different individuals in an organization. For example, employees in the admitting and registration department would not be given the same authorization to computers, programs, and data as nursing care employees.

Usually authorization is managed through special authorization software that uses various criteria to determine if an individual has authorization for access, sometimes referred to as an access control matrix. For example, authorization may be based on not only the individual's identify but also the individual's role (called role-based authorization), physical location of the resource (that is, access to only certain computers), and time of day.

Other Access Controls

CAPTCHA

Systems may require verification that a human, not a computer, is accessing a website or storage portal. A "**c**ompletely **a**utomated **p**ublic **T**uring test to tell **c**omputers and **h**umans **a**part" (CAPTCHA) requires the user to respond to a question that is assumed could not be answered by a machine. A typical example of a CAPTCHA is when access to a site requires the user to type in a string of characters that appears skewed or distorted.

Physical and Administrative Safeguards

Physical safeguards refers to the physical protection of information resources from loss, theft, physical damage, and natural or other disasters. This includes protection and monitoring of the workplace, computing facilities, and any type of hardware or supporting information system infrastructure such as wiring closets, cables, and telephone and data lines.

Equipment should be located in secure locations and protected from natural and environmental hazards and intrusion. Environmental hazards include such things as fire, floods, moisture, temperature variations, and loss of electricity. To protect from natural or environmental hazards, equipment should be housed in structurally sound and safe areas. There should be smoke and fire alarms, fire suppression systems, heat sensors, and appropriate monitored heating and cooling systems in place. Appropriate backup power sources such as uninterruptable power supply (UPS) devices or power generators should be available if a power outage occurs.

To protect from intrusion there should be proper physical separation from the public. Doors, locks, audible alarms, and cameras should be installed to protect particularly sensitive areas such as data centers. Identification procedures should be in place; for example, the use of badges to identify employees. Processes should be instituted for logging out and logging into computer equipment or media. For example, if a data disk or device is being transported or removed from one location to another, there should be a sign-out and sign-in procedure to track access and removal. Furthermore, sign-in/sign-out logs should be in place to track access to sensitive areas such as data centers.

Backup and recovery procedures are also a part of physical security. Backup and recovery should include server, data, and network policies and procedures.

Provisions must also be made to protect workstations that are more exposed to the public. For example, locking devices can be used to prevent removal of computer equipment and other devices and automatic logouts can be used to prevent snooping by unauthorized individuals. Laptops and other mobile devices such as personal digital assistants (PDAs) pose significant threats because they can be easily lost or stolen. Documentation of the custody of such devices must be addressed. One such method is maintaining a custody log that documents who has had custody of the device, the time period of custody, and what files and data were on the laptop during the custody period. Policies and procedures should be in place that cover laptop or mobile device use. Other security mechanisms such as two-factor authentication (discussed previously) and full disk encryption should be used. GPS tracking systems can also be installed on laptops as well as systems to remotely retrieve and delete data, should a computer be lost or stolen. With these features, a computer can be located quickly and appropriate law enforcement officials notified.

In any security program, employee education is one of the best defenses for protection of data and computer resources. Training programs on data security should be conducted at least annually for all employees and cover applicable security responsibilities, policies, and procedures.

Administrative safeguards include policies and procedures that address the management of computer resources. For example, one such policy might direct users to log off the computer system when they are not using it or employ automatic logoffs after a period of inactivity. Other policies include password security (inappropriate sharing, minimum password requirements, change frequencies, and failed login monitoring) and timely removal of terminated employee's system access. Another policy might prohibit employees from accessing the Internet for purposes that are not work-related.

And finally, the organization should have a policy on **Information Technology Asset Disposition** (ITAD) that identifies how all data storage devices are destroyed and purged of data prior to repurposing or disposal.

Software Application Safeguards

Another security strategy is to implement **application safeguards.** These are controls contained in the application software or computer programs. One common **application control** is password management as previously mentioned. It involves keeping a record of end users' identifications and passwords and then matching the passwords to each end user's privileges. Password management ensures that end users can access only the information they have permission to access.

Another type of application control is the edit check. Edit checks help to ensure data integrity by allowing only reasonable and predetermined values to be entered into the computer.

Yet another application control is the audit trail. The audit trail is a software program that tracks every single access to data in the computer system. It logs the name of the individual who accessed the data, the date and time, and the action taken (for example, modifying, reading, or deleting data). Audit trails are usually examined by system administrators who use special analysis software to identify suspicious or abnormal system events or behavior. Because the audit trail maintains a complete log of system activity, it can also be used to help reconstruct how and when an adverse event or failure occurred. This information helps to identify ways to avoid similar problems in the future. Depending on the organization's policy, audit trails are reviewed periodically or on predetermined schedules.

Application controls are important because they are automatic checks that help preserve data confidentiality and integrity.

Network Safeguards

Another important strategy used to guard against security breaches is to implement network safeguards. All kinds of networks are used to transmit healthcare data today, and the data must be protected from intruders and corruption during transmission within and external to the organization. With the widespread use of the Internet, **network controls** also are essential to prevent the threat of hackers. Some common safeguards are discussed below:

Firewalls

A **firewall** (also called a secure gateway) is a part of a computer system or network that is designed to block unauthorized access while permitting authorized communications. It is a software program or device that filters information between two networks, usually between a private network like an intranet and a public network like the Internet. Firewalls allow internal users access to an external network while blocking malicious hackers from damaging internal systems. All messages entering or leaving the private network pass through the firewall, which examines each message and blocks those that don't meet predefined security criteria. A firewall is configured to permit, deny, encrypt, or decrypt computer traffic.

Cryptographic Technologies

Cryptography is a branch of mathematics that is based on the transformation of data by developing ciphers, which are codes that are to be kept secret. Cryptography is used as a tool for data security. Strong cryptography improves the security of information systems and their data. There are several types of cryptographic technologies. Cryptographic technology, such as encryption, digital signatures, and digital certificates are used to protect information in a variety of situations. This includes protecting data when they are in storage (data at rest), on portable devices such as laptops and flash drives, and while they are being transmitted across networks. Three of these technologies used in healthcare are discussed below.

Encryption

Encryption is a method of encoding data so that they are not understood by persons who do not have a key to transform the data into their original form. Data are usually encrypted using some type of algorithm. Data can only be decrypted back to their original form by using a special algorithm. Basically encryption takes the message from one computer and encodes it in a form that only the receiving computer can decode.

One type of encryption is called secret key cryptology. In this method, two or more computers share the same secret key and that key is used to both encrypt and decrypt a message. However, the key must be kept secret. If it is compromised in any way, the security of the data is likely to be eliminated. The best known secret key security is called the data encryption standard (DES) published by NIST.

A common encryption method used over the Internet is a system called Pretty Good Privacy (PGP). PGP uses both a public and a private key, which form a key pair. The public key encrypts the data and the private key decrypts the data. With this type of system there is a registry of public keys, called a certificate authority (described below). If one user wants to send an encrypted message to another, the registry is consulted and the receiving user's public key is used to encrypt the data. Only the recipient, who knows the private key, can decrypt the message into its original form.

Digital Signatures

A **digital signature** or digital signature scheme is a public key cryptography method that ensures that an electronic document such as an e-mail message or text file is authentic.

This means that the receiver knows who created the document and is assured that the document has not been altered in any way since it was created.

In this method data are electronically signed by applying the sender's private key to the data. The digital signature can be stored or transmitted to the data. The signature can then be verified by the receiving party using the public key of the signer.

Digital signatures are sometimes confused with e-signatures. *E-signature* usually means a system for signing or authenticating electronic documents by entering a unique code or password that verifies the identity of the person and creates an individual signature on a document. E-signatures do not necessarily use cryptography.

Digital Certificates

Digital certificates are used to implement public key encryption on a large scale. A digital certificate is an electronic document that uses a digital signature to bind together a public key with an identity such as the name of a person or an organization, their address, and so forth. The certificate can be used to verify that a public key belongs to an individual. An independent source called a certificate authority (CA) acts as the middleman that the sending and receiving computer trusts. It confirms that each computer is who it says it is and provides the public keys of each computer to the other.

Web Security Protocols

Transmission protocols also provide data security. Transport Layer Security (TLS) and its predecessor Secure Sockets Layer (SSL) are based on public key cryptography. These protocols are the most common protocols used to secure communications on the Internet between a web browser and a web server. Versions of these protocols can be used for almost any application but are frequently used for electronic mail, Internet faxing, instant messaging, e-commerce transactions, and voice communications over the Internet (VoIP).

These protocols allow authentication of the server. Once authentication of the server is established, secure communication can begin using symmetric encryption keys. The user's message is encrypted in the user's web browser using an encryption key from the host website. The message is then transported to the host website in encrypted format. Once received by the website, the message is decrypted.

Intrusion Detection Systems

Intrusion detection is the process of identifying attempts or actions to penetrate a system and gain unauthorized access. Intrusion detection can either be performed in real time or after the occurrence of an intrusion. The purpose of intrusion detection is to prevent the compromise of the confidentiality, integrity, or availability of a resource.

Intrusion detection can be performed manually or automatically. Manual intrusion detection might take place by examining log files, audit trails, or other evidence for signs of intrusions. A system that performs automated intrusion detection is called an intrusion detection system (IDS). Procedures should be outlined in the organization's data security plan to determine what actions should be taken in response to a probable intrusion. For example, typical actions to be taken might include notification of appropriate individuals, generating an e-mail alert, and so on.

Business Continuity Plan

What happens when an organization's computer systems are damaged or destroyed by an intentional or unintentional event or a natural disaster such as a flood, tornado, or hurricane as mentioned earlier in the chapter? Even though such an event may be unlikely to occur, organizations must be prepared in the event that one does.

Organizations must develop a **business continuity plan** (BCP) to handle an unexpected computer shutdown caused by an intentional or unintentional event or during a natural disaster. A computer shutdown caused by hackers would be considered an intentional event. A shutdown due to a software error would likely be classified as an unintentional event. Examples of natural disasters include floods, hurricanes, and tornadoes.

Sometimes BCP is also called **contingency and disaster planning.** The BCP typically includes policies and procedures to help the business continue operation during the unexpected shutdown or disaster. It also includes procedures the business can implement to restore its computer systems and resume normal operation after the disaster.

The BCP is based on information gathered during the risk assessment and analysis discussed previously. The risk assessment includes the probability that an unexpected shutdown will occur. Using this information, the BCP is developed based on the following steps (Johns 2008, 317):

1. Identifying the minimum allowable time for system disruption
2. Identifying alternatives for system continuation
3. Evaluating the cost and feasibility of each alternative
4. Developing procedures required for activating the plan

An important part of the BCP is planning how the computer system can be returned to normal operation and ensuring the availability and accuracy of data after a disaster. Restoring system integrity and ensuring that all data are recovered requires that all parts of the system be verified after the disaster has occurred. Usually one system or one component of a system is brought up at a time and processes are verified to ensure that they are working correctly.

The typical contents of a BCP include:

- *Assigning responsibility for development and implementation of the plan:* This includes identifying the responsibilities of the security management team, the emergency operation team, and the damage assessment team and how all teams are coordinated.

- *Determining how a disaster is identified:* This includes the definition of disaster and its identification, notification procedures, identification of disaster cause, and communication procedures.

- *Developing a recovery plan:* For example, outlining the recovery organization and staffing, having in place vendor contracts and backup plans, having plans to recover data affected by the disaster, and having alternate-site contracts in place.

- *Testing the plan:* A plan is only as good as its implementation. The BCP must be tested periodically to ensure that all parts of the plan, from disaster identification to backup and recovery work and run smoothly. (Johns 2008, 317)

Data Quality Control Processes

Ensuring data quality is an essential part of any data security program. The various dimensions of data quality are addressed in chapter 2. Among these dimensions are accuracy, accessibility, comprehensiveness, consistency, currency, definition, granularity, precision, relevancy, and timeliness.

Responsibility for ensuring data quality is shared by many organization stakeholders. For example, data item definition may be the responsibility of the data administrator or those in charge of the data dictionary. Depending on the type of data, determining data granularity may be the responsibility of various department heads or clinical managers. Data accuracy begins with any individual who enters or documents data or systems that capture and provide data such as ICU monitoring systems.

Monitoring and tracking systems that ensure data quality are part of a data security program. All the dimensions of data quality should be addressed in a formal data quality management program. Aspects of such a program are discussed in chapter 2.

Data accessibility, consistency, and definition are three data quality dimensions that are often addressed using computer tools. Data accessibility means that the data are easily obtainable. Computer tools are used to monitor unscheduled computer downtime, determine why failures occurred, and provide data to help minimize future problems.

Data consistency means that data do not change no matter how often or in how many ways they are stored, processed, or displayed. Data values are consistent when the value of any given data element is the same across applications and systems. Procedures are usually developed to monitor data periodically to ensure that they are consistent as they move through computer processes or from one system to another.

Data definition means that data are defined. Every data element should have a clear definition and a range of acceptable values. Data definitions and their values are usually stored in a data dictionary.

Coordinated Security Program

How can the different threats to data security be managed in a coordinated security program? First and most important, someone from inside the organization must be given responsibility for data security. This individual should be someone at the middle or senior management level. As mentioned earlier, he or she is frequently called the chief security officer (CSO). Figure 17.4 lists some of the CSO's functions.

When the data security program with policies and procedures is in place, the CSO is responsible for ensuring that everyone follows them. This is done using monitoring and evaluation systems, usually on an annual basis. Many organizations use outside information systems auditing firms to do their security policy evaluations. In addition to the

Figure 17.4.   Common functions of the chief security officer

• Conducting strategic planning for information system security	• Setting up mechanisms to ensure that data security policies and procedures are followed
• Developing a data and information systems security policy	• Coordinating employee security training
• Developing data security and information systems procedures	• Monitoring audit trails to identify security violations
• Managing confidentiality agreements for employees and contractors	• Conducting risk assessment of enterprise information systems
	• Developing a business continuity plan

yearly audit, the CSO might establish procedures to audit and evaluate current processes randomly.

All data security policies and procedures should be reviewed and evaluated at least every year to make sure they are up-to-date and still relevant to the organization.

Check Your Understanding 17.2

1. Which of the following is a threat to data security?

   A. Encryption
   B. People
   C. Red flags
   D. Access controls

2. An HIT using her password can access and change data in the hospital's master patient index. A billing clerk, using his password, cannot perform the same function. Limiting the class of information and functions that can be performed by these two employees is managed by:

   A. Network controls
   B. Audit trails
   C. Administrative controls
   D. Access controls

3. The patient's address is the same in the master patient index, the electronic health record, laboratory information system, and other systems. This means that the data values are:

   A. Consistent
   B. Accessible
   C. Defined
   D. Granular

4. Data security policies and procedures should be reviewed at least:

   A. Semi-annually
   B. Annually
   C. Every two years
   D. Quarterly

Instructions: Match the terms with the most appropriate description.

5. Employee who makes a typographical mistake

6. Chief security officer

7. Employee confidentiality agreement

8. Identification of most likely security threats

9. Identification of the information that employees need to perform their job functions

10. Edit checks

11. Prevents hacking into a computer system

12. Computer terminals do not face public areas

a. People threat
b. Employee awareness program
c. Network control
d. Risk analysis
e. Access control
f. Application control
g. Physical control
h. Oversight for security program

Data Security Challenges

Breaches

The Office of Civil Rights has been charged with oversight for the Privacy and Security Rule and monitors and investigates reports of **breaches** by covered entities and business associates.

Over a 15-month period ending December 31, 2010, the Office of Civil Rights received approximately 30,500 reports of breaches involving fewer than 500 individuals. An estimated 62,000 people were affected. Although the raw numbers suggest an average of two individuals affected per breach, in reality most breaches involved the information of a single person. Incidents of this nature involved misdirected communications (faxing a record of a patient to the wrong party) and misdirecting claims or mailing records to the incorrect individual. And now because business associates are subject to more stringent uses of e-PHI, they are also now subject to the Rule and according to a recent report by Price-Waterhouse Coopers, of the 11 million people affected by data breaches since September 2009, 55 percent involved business associates (PwC 2011). An analysis of the OCR breach statistics reveals an increase in the number of reported breaches caused by thefts and other losses that affect more than 500 people. Further analysis of the statistics for 2010 and 2011 revealed that a total of 392 breaches involved 19,051,267 individuals with the largest categories of theft and loss. Theft accounted for over 55 percent of the breaches that affected nearly 7.5 million individuals. This analysis revealed a number of breaches (see table 17.1).

One of the largest breaches, according to the Office of Civil Right's website, reported as "other" was in Puerto Rico and was not explained, but other unknown losses involved mostly paper records. One breach of 800,000 people's data was reported as a loss of a portable electronic device and another with more than 1 million affected was a loss of backup tapes by Tricare. This breach involved an employee for a contractor for Tricare who had backup tapes stolen from his car which subsequently resulted in a letter from Congress to Tricare requesting an explanation of the circumstances given the contractor had previous breaches of a similar nature. Congress specifically requested information on data security measures and procedures when employees remove e-PHI from a site and whether encryption procedures were in place or followed. The largest breach in the theft category was due to an EMR breach and involved over 1,700,000 people's data.

The February 2011 AHIMA journal article "Swiped, Not Hacked: After a year of reporting theft remains main cause of breach," reported that lost and stolen laptops, desktops, and network server equipment continues to be the leading cause of large-scale breaches reported to DHHS, not attacks by malicious hackers as most people had believed (AHIMA 2011b).

Poor policies and procedures and monitoring practices are to blame for most employee breaches. A former UCLA Health System employee became the first person in the nation to be sentenced to federal prison for violating HIPAA. Huping Zhou, a licensed cardiothoracic in China before immigrating to the United States, was employed as researcher at the UCLA School of Medicine. He accessed and read confidential medical records of his supervisors and high-profile celebrities according to the US Attorney's Office for the Central District of California, and was fined $2,000 and sentenced to four months in prison.

And in November of 2011, it was reported by Modern Healthcare (www.modern healthcare.com) that Sutter Health, a California-based system, had a desktop computer stolen in the previous month with personal medical information of approximately 4.24 million patients. The data, however, did not include medical records but did include names, addresses, birthdates, phone numbers and other contact information. According

Table 17.1.   OCR breach analysis (2010–2011 data)

Type of Breach	Number of Incidents	Number Affected by Breach
Unauthorized access/disclosure	77	1,055,875
Theft	214	7,453,504
Improper Disposal	21	150,463
Loss (laptop, media lost)	50	7,238,384
Hacking/Intrusion	22	546,923
Other	2	347,479
Unknown	6	2,258,639
Total	**392**	**19,051,267**

to a press release by Sutter Health (www.sutterhealth.org), the computer was company-issued and the data were not encrypted.

Managing Organizational Risk

How vulnerable is health information, and what is the status of data security in healthcare organizations? An ongoing four year HIMSS (Health Information Management Systems Society) Security Survey seeks to identify and report key issues surrounding data security and risk analyses. In the past two years the survey results have been nearly the same with three-quarters of the respondents reporting that they conduct risk analyses (HIMSS. org). Of concern are the 25 percent who do not conduct assessments. Risk assessments are a requirement of HIPAA and have always been a part of good IT practice regardless of HIPAA requirements. Other key findings of the survey included:

- Respondents reported spending 3 percent or less of their IT budget on security and half responded that their budgets increased

- Half of the respondents reported having a CSO or other responsible party in place full time

- Nearly all reported monitoring of EHR information access

- Nearly all reported the use of audit logs for compliance monitoring

- Eighty percent reported sharing of data electronically with external organizations

Since risk analyses are required under HIPAA and Stage 1 of Meaningful Use, the survey should reflect higher numbers of those facilities conducting these analyses. In order for the public to feel safe about their data in electronic form, all organizations must be diligent in performing risk audits.

HIPAA Security Provisions

As mentioned in the introduction to this chapter, the Health Insurance Portability and Accountability Act (HIPAA) was passed in 1996. The act, also called **Public Law 104-191,** includes provisions for insurance reform and administrative simplification. Included in the administrative simplification provisions was a requirement for setting standards to protect health information. Later, in February 2003, the Department of Health and Human Services established security and privacy standards that every healthcare provider, healthcare clearinghouse, and health plan that electronically maintains or transmits patient health information must meet. The compliance date for all but small health plans was April 21, 2005. And in February of 2009, additional changes to the Privacy Law were created as a result of the American Recovery and Reinvestment Act (ARRA) (discussed below).

In July of 2009, enforcement for HIPAA security compliance was moved from the Centers for Medicare and Medicaid Services' Office of Electronic Standards and Security to the **Office for Civil Rights** (OCR). The HITECH Act under ARRA mandated improved enforcement of the Privacy Rule and Security Rule. Privacy and security audits can be conducted of covered entities regardless if they are subject of a complaint or experienced a high-profile incident. Enforcement of HIPAA security must be taken seriously by covered entities and others who must follow HIPAA security rules.

American Recovery and Reinvestment Act of 2009

On February 17, 2009, President Obama signed the American Recovery and Reinvestment Act (ARRA) into law. Parts of the law's revisions broadened privacy and security provisions and now include broader individual rights and protections when third parties handle individually identifiable health information. The provisions of the HITECH Act (chapter 13 covers the changes affecting privacy standards) now include:

- Expanding individuals' rights to access their information and restrict certain types of disclosures of e-PHI to health plans
- Requiring business associates of HIPAA-covered entities to comply with most of the same rules as covered entities
- New limitations on the use and disclosure of PHI for marketing and fundraising
- Prohibiting the sale of e-PHI without patient authorization
- Creation of a Chief Privacy Officer position within the ONC

With regard to the security provisions, the one important change was in the requirements affecting business associates.

As noted in chapter 13, a **business associate** (BA) is a person or organization, other than a member of a covered entity's workforce, that performs functions or activities on behalf of or for a covered entity that involve the use or disclosure of protected health information. Common BAs include consultants, billing companies, transcription companies, accounting firms, and law firms.

With the implementation of the ARRA, several HIPAA security provisions apply to business associates of HIPAA-covered entities (AHIMA 2009). Business associates are directly responsible for instituting these provisions and can be held directly responsible for not complying. Specifically, these include HIPAA security:

- Administrative provisions
- Physical safeguards
- Technical safeguards
- Policies and procedures and documentation requirements

Each of these is discussed in more detail in the following sections.

Another important change that the HITECH Act made was the addition of **breach notification,** which requires both HIPAA-covered entities and noncovered entities (including

PHR vendors) that have custody of e-PHI to identify e-PHI breaches and make appropriate notifications. The privacy aspects of this change are discussed in chapter 13. With regard to security, breach notification has implications for the protection of data by using encryption methods and by using appropriate methods for destruction of data. The technical security issues are discussed later in this chapter under technical safeguards (AHIMA 2009).

HIPAA Security Provisions

Security rule standards are grouped into five categories. These include:

- Administrative safeguards
- Physical safeguards
- Technical safeguards
- Organizational requirements
- Policies and procedures and documentation requirements

The content of each section closely parallels the mechanisms for minimizing security threats discussed earlier in this chapter. Essentially, the HIPAA security provisions follow what have already been established in the information systems field as best practices for the development and implementation of good security policy. Because health information technicians (HITs) should be involved with many aspects of HIPAA security implementation, each of these sections is discussed below using the Security Standards Final Rule (HHS 2003) and draft guidelines provided by HHS regarding risk analyses and security vulnerabilities.

General Rules

The **General Rules** provide the objective and scope for the HIPAA Security Rule as a whole. They specify that covered entities must develop a security program that includes a range of security safeguards that protect individually identifiable health information maintained or transmitted in electronic form. The General Rules include the following:

- *Covered entities must demonstrate and document that they have done the following:*
  - Ensure the confidentiality, integrity, and availability of all electronic protected health information (e-PHI) that is created, received, maintained, or transmitted by the covered entity
  - Identify the flow of e-PHI throughout the organization and who has access at various points
  - Protect e-PHI against any reasonably anticipated threats or hazards to the security or integrity of e-PHI

— Protect e-PHI against any reasonable or anticipated uses or disclosure that are not permitted under the HIPAA Privacy Rule

— Ensure compliance with HIPAA security rules by workforce members

- *Flexibility of approach:* HIPAA allows a covered entity to adopt security protection measures that are appropriate and reasonable for its organization. For example, security mechanisms will be different in complex organizations than in small organizations. Security protections in a large medical facility will be more complex than those implemented in a small group practice. In determining which security measures to use, the following must be taken into account:

— Size, complexity, and capabilities of the covered entity

— Technical infrastructure, hardware, and software capabilities

— Security measure costs

— Probability and criticality of the potential risks to e-PHI

HIPAA requires that covered entities conduct and document organizational and risk assessments in making the determination of which security measures are appropriate in their specific situations. Examples of risk assessment measures were discussed at the beginning of this chapter.

- *Standards:* Standards that covered entities must comply with include those in sections 164.308, 164.310, 164.312, 164.314, and 164.316 of the HIPAA Security Rule. These sections address appropriate screening processes, data backups, authentication and whether and how to utilize data encryption. This means that covered entities must comply with the standards in any of these subparts. Business associates, hybrid entities, and other related entities are also required to comply with these standards.

- *Implementation specifications:* **Implementation specifications** define how standards are to be implemented. Implementation specifications are either "required" or "addressable." The Rule notes that "addressable" does not mean optional. Entities must implement all implementation specifications that are "required." For those implementation specifications that are labeled "addressable," the covered entity must conduct a risk assessment and evaluate whether the specification is appropriate to its environment. If after conducting a risk assessment, the covered entity finds that the specification is not a reasonable and appropriate safeguard for its environment, then the covered entity must:

1. Document why it is not reasonable and appropriate to implement the specification

2. Implement an equivalent alternative method if appropriate. "Addressable" does not mean optional. It means that the covered entity must use reasonable and appropriate measures to meet the standard.

- *Maintenance:* HIPAA requires covered entities and business associates to maintain their security measures. Maintenance requires review and modification, as needed, to comply with the provision of reasonable and appropriate protection of e-PHI.

Administrative Safeguards

Administrative safeguards are documented, formal practices to manage data security measures throughout the organization. Basically, they require the facility to establish a security management process similar to the concepts discussed earlier in this chapter.

The administrative safeguards detail how the security program should be managed from the organization's perspective. Policies and procedures should be written and formalized in a policy manual. The organization should issue a statement of its philosophy on data security. Further, it should outline data security authority and responsibilities throughout the organization. Figure 17.5 shows what an organization's general policy on data security might look like.

The administrative safeguards (164.308 p. 8377-78 of the Rule) include the following standards that must be implemented by covered entities:

- *Security Management Process:* An organization must have a defined security management process. This means that there is a process in place for creating, maintaining, and overseeing the development of security policies and procedures, identifying vulnerabilities and conducting risk analyses, risk management, development of a sanction policy, and review of information system activity.

- *Assigned Security Responsibility:* Each covered entity must designate a security official who has been assigned security responsibility for the development and implementation of the policies and procedures required by the HIPAA Security Rule. Frequently, this individual is given the title of chief security officer (CSO).

- *Workforce Security:* The covered entity must ensure appropriate access to individually identifiable information to workforce members who need to use e-PHI to perform their job duties and must maintain appropriate oversight of authorization and access. Likewise, covered entities must prevent access to information to those who do not need it and have clear procedures of access termination for employees who leave the organization. Sanction policies must also be in place.

- *Information Access Management:* This standard requires covered entities to implement a program of information access management. This includes specific policies and procedures to determine who should have access to what information.

- *Security Awareness Training:* This standard requires the entities to provide security training for all staff.

- *Security Incident procedures:* This standard requires the implementation of policies and procedures to address security incidents.

Figure 17.5. Sample organizational policy on data security

Policy Statement

Background

The State University Hospital relies heavily on computers to meet its operational, financial, and information requirements. These computer systems, related data files, and the information derived from them are important assets of the hospital. A system of internal controls exists to safeguard these assets. Information is processed in a secure environment, and all computer account owners share responsibility for the security, integrity, and confidentiality of information. This policy covers both accidental and intentional disclosure of, or damage to, university information.

Scope

This policy statement applies to the security, integrity, and confidentiality of information obtained, created, or maintained by hospital employees. The definition of information includes paper documents and all computer-related activities involving mainframes, micro- and minicomputers, and service bureaus.

Definitions

Owner/Program Manager: The owner of a collection of information is the person responsible for the business results of that system or the business use of the information. Where appropriate, ownership may be shared by managers of different departments. Ownership of corporate systems is assigned and monitored via the "Profile" system.

Custodian: The custodian is responsible for the processing and storage of the information. For mainframe, micro, and mini applications, the owner or user may retain custodial responsibilities.

User: The user is any person authorized to read, enter, or update information by the owner of the information.

Data: Information stored in any form by the university that is used as a basis for official reasoning, discussion, presentation, or calculation.

Information: Source documents, electronic data files, and any data or reports derived from them.

Responsibilities

Owner: Information processed by a computerized system must have an identified owner, and this assignment must be formally documented. The owner may delegate ownership responsibilities to another individual. The owner of information has the authority and responsibility:

- To judge the value of the information and classify it
- To authorize access and assign custody of information
- To specify controls and communicate the control requirements to the custodian and users of the information
- To determine the statutory requirements regarding retention and privacy of the information, and communicate this information to the custodian

Custodian: The custodian is responsible for the administration of controls as specified by the owner. This includes the responsibility:

- To provide physical and technical safeguards
- To provide procedural guidelines for the users
- To administer access to information
- To evaluate the cost-effectiveness of controls

Figure 17.5. **Sample organizational policy on data security** *(continued)*

> *User:* A user of information has the responsibility:
>
> • To use the information only for the purpose intended by the owner
>
> • To comply with all controls established by the owner and the custodian
>
> • To ensure that classified or sensitive information is not disclosed to anyone without permission of the owner
>
> • To ensure that his or her individual passwords are not disclosed to, or used by, others
>
> • To become familiar with and abide by the Computing Facilities User Guidelines
>
> *Enforcement:* A violation of standards, procedures, or guidelines established pursuant to this policy shall be presented to management for appropriate action and could result in disciplinary action, including expulsion, dismissal, and/or legal prosecution.

- *Contingency Plan:* This standard requires the establishment and implementation of policies and procedures for responding to emergencies or any system failures in systems that contain e-PHI.

- *Evaluation:* A periodic evaluation must be performed in response to environmental or operational changes affecting the security of e-PHI and appropriate improvements in policies and procedures should follow.

- *Business Associate Agreements:* This standard requires business associates to appropriately safeguard information in their possession.

Each of these standards contains required elements as well as those that are addressable. As mentioned in the Implementation section, organizations must comply with the required standards while addressable standards may list two to three options for a facility to consider and they can choose the option that best satisfies the requirement for their environment.

Physical Safeguards

Physical safeguards include the protection of computer systems from natural and environmental hazards and intrusion. Physical safeguards consist of the following also specified in 45 CFR Section 164.308 (HHS 2003):

- *Facility Access Controls:* This includes establishing safeguards to prohibit the physical hardware and computer system itself from unauthorized access while ensuring that proper authorized access is allowed. Similar safeguards are also required to protect the computer system from untoward physical events (for example, fire, flooding, and electrical malfunctions).

- *Workstation Security:* Provisions under workstation security require policies and procedures be in place that document the proper functions to be performed at workstations with access to e-PHI.

- *Device and Media Controls:* This standard requires the facility to specify proper use of electronic media and devices (external drives, backup devices, etc). Covered entities also are required to document the physical attributes of the surroundings of a workstation or a class of workstations that can access e-PHI. Included in this requirement are controls and procedures regarding the receipt and removal of electronic media that contain protected health information and the movement of such data within the facility. The entity must also address procedures for the transfer, removal, or disposal including reuse or redeployment of electronic media. ITAD or information technology asset disposition policies are required under this standard. These policies should address end of life cycle hard drives, laptops, servers, and other media that have contained sensitive data. Because such equipment is often redeployed in an organization, all e-PHI and any other sensitive data must be removed. Before hard drives, servers, or laptops are disposed of, appropriate cleansing or data destruction must be carried out.

Figure 17.6 offers an example of a policy on terminal use.

Technical Safeguards

The **technical safeguard provisions** consist of five broad categories. Essentially, the provisions include those things that can be implemented from a technical standpoint using computer software. These provisions include:

- *Access Controls:* The access controls standard requires implementation of technical procedures to control or limit access to health information. The procedures would be executed through some type of software program. Essentially, this requirement ensures that individuals are given authorization to access only the data they need to perform their jobs. The regulations state that access should be determined by one of three techniques: context-based, role-based, and user-based access schemes. Having procedures in place that determine what data an individual can have access to based on their job duties is an example of an access control.

- *Audit Controls:* The **audit controls** standard requires that procedural mechanisms be implemented that record activity in systems that contain e-PHI and that the output is examined to determine appropriateness of access. This means that organizations must keep documented logs of system access and access attempts. The logs, called **audit trails,** should document who accessed the system, when the access occurred, and what type of activity took place (for example, edit, print, view).

- *Integrity Controls:* The data integrity standard requires covered entities to implement policies and procedures to protect e-PHI from being improperly altered or destroyed. In other words, this standard requires organizations to provide corroboration that their data have not been altered in an unauthorized manner. Data authentication can be substantiated through audit trails and system logs that track users who have accessed and/or modified data via unique identifiers.

Figure 17.6. **Sample policy on terminal use**

Policy on Terminal Controls

Purpose: To prevent unauthorized access to State University data by providing terminal controls

Scope: University terminals

Standard: Proper physical and software control mechanisms shall be in place to control access to and use of devices connected to university computer systems.

Guidelines:

- *Hardware terminal locking:* In areas that are not physically secured, terminals should be equipped with locking devices to prevent their use during unattended periods. The locks should be installed in addition to programmed restrictions, such as automatic disconnect after a given period of inactivity.

- *Operating system identification of terminals:* All terminal activity should be controlled by the operating system, which should be able to identify terminals, whether they are hardwired or connected through communications lines. The operating system should inspect log-on requests to determine which application the terminal user desires. The user should identify an existing application and supply a valid user ID and password combination. If the log-on request is valid, the operating system should make a logical connection between the user and the application.

- *Limitation of log-on attempts:* Limit system log-on attempts from remote terminal devices. More than three unsuccessful attempts should result in termination of the session, generation of a real-time security violation message to the operator and/or the ISO (and log of said message in an audit file), and purging of the input queue of messages from the terminal.

- *Time-out feature:* Ensure that the operating system provides the timing services required to support a secure operational environment. Inactive processes or terminals (in an interactive environment) should be terminated after a predetermined period.

- *Dial-up control:* The communications software should ensure a clean end of connection in all cases, especially in the event of abnormal disconnection.

- *Person or Entity Authentication:* This standard requires that those accessing e-PHI must be appropriately identified and authenticated.

- *Transmission Security:* The Internet and communications networks of many types have become integral parts of most business information systems. Because these networks transmit large amounts of data, there is a good potential for security breaches. Essentially, the controls applicable in **transmission security** are similar to those discussed already. HIPAA requires organizations to have integrity and access controls in place as well as entity authentication and audit trails. For example:

  — Access controls provide protection of sensitive communication transmissions over open or private networks so that the data cannot be easily intercepted and read by parties other than the intended recipient.

  — Access controls ensure that a user has access to what information is needed to do his or her job and nothing else.

In addition, the standard requires the use of **encryption or other similar mechanisms,** when deemed appropriate, for data transmitted over public networks or communication systems. The Security Rule itself does not require encryption, but it could be used or if the facility has another way of accomplishing the security of transmission, it could be used instead of encryption. As discussed earlier, encryption is a process that encodes textual material, converting it to scrambled data that must be decoded in order to be understood. This means that the message is a jumble of unreadable characters and symbols as it is transmitted through the telecommunication network. When the message is received, it is changed to a readable form. Data encryption that provides protection for data going across transmission lines is important because eavesdropping is easily accomplished using devices called sniffers. Sniffers can be attached to networks for the purpose of diverting transmitted data. Protecting data during transmission is only one role of encryption. Passwords stored in a database also may be encrypted. Thus, if a hacker breaks into the password database, the data will be unusable.

Organizational Requirements

This section includes just two standards; one addresses business associates and similar entities and the other addresses general covered entity responsibilities.

- *Business associate or other contracts:* Covered entities must obtain a written contract with business associates or other entities (hybrid or other) who handle e-PHI. The written contract must stipulate that the business associate will implement HIPAA administrative, physical, and technical safeguards and procedures and documentation requirements that safeguard the confidentiality, integrity, and availability of the e-PHI that it creates, receives, maintains, or transmits on behalf of the covered entity. The contract must ensure that any agent, including a subcontractor, agrees to implement reasonable and appropriate safeguards. Specifically, HIPAA requires a business associate to report to the covered entity any security incident or breach of e-PHI of which it becomes aware. The covered entity must authorize termination of the contract if it determines that the business associate has violated a material term of the contract.

- *Covered Entity Responsibilities:* The covered entity must monitor the practices of its business associates and other similar arrangements and take reasonable steps to prevent any breaches and must implement reasonable safeguards to protect e-PHI under its control.

Policies, Procedures, and Documentation Requirements

The Security Rule requires that covered entities and business associates have security policies and procedures and that they be documented in written format. Other information about any actions, assessments, or activities associated with the HIPAA Security Rule also must be in a written format.

- *Policies and procedures:* Entities must implement reasonable and appropriate policies and procedures to comply with the HIPAA security standards, implementation specifications, and other requirements. Policies and procedures should be developed and implemented, taking into account the section on flexibility outlined in the rule.

- *Documentation:* Entities must maintain their security policies and procedures in written form. This includes formats that may be electronic. Any actions, assessments, or activities related to the HIPAA Security Rule also must be documented in a written format.

Documentation must be retained for six years from the date of its creation or the date when it last was in effect, whichever is later. It must be made available to those individuals responsible for implementing security procedures. Further, it must be reviewed periodically and updated, as needed, in response to environmental or organizational changes that affect the security of e-PHI.

HITECH Act Breach Notification Requirements

The HITECH Act requires HIPAA-covered entities to notify affected individuals, and requires business associates to notify covered entities, following the discovery of a breach of unsecured e-PHI. The requirements for breach notification and steps to be taken are covered at length in chapter 13.

Protection measures must be appropriately applied to data in their various forms. These forms include:

- Data in motion—for example, data moving through a network or wireless transmission

- Data at rest—for example, data contained in databases, file systems, or flash drives

- Data in use—for example, data in the process of being created, retrieved, updated, or deleted

- Data disposed—for example, discarded paper records or recycled electronic media

An important aspect of breach notification is awareness of what constitutes **unsecured e-PHI.** Breach notification is required only in instances where there has been a breach of unsecured e-PHI. The HITECH Act defines "unsecured protected health information" as e-PHI that has not been made unusable, unreadable, or indecipherable to unauthorized persons (HHS 2009, 2).

Electronic PHI is considered secure and "rendered unusable, unreadable, or indecipherable to authorized individuals if one or more of the following applies" (AHIMA 2009, 15):

- Electronic PHI has been encrypted as specified in the HIPAA Security Rule and following specified National Institute of Standards and Technology (NIST) publications, or

- The media on which the PHI is stored or recorded have been destroyed in a specified manner.

Encryption is only as secure as the encryption keys used to encrypt and decrypt the data. Therefore, to ensure that encryption keys are not breached, covered entities and business associates should maintain these keys on a separate device from the data that they encrypt and decrypt.

The HITECH provisions require that appropriate methods for destruction of data be in place. E-PHI stored or recorded on paper, film, or other hard-copy media must be shredded or destroyed such that the e-PHI cannot be read or in any way reconstructed. E-PHI stored or recorded on electronic media must be cleared, purged, or destroyed consistent with National Institute of Standards and Technology (NIST) media sanitation guides which include degaussing or completely destroying computer media so that e-PHI cannot be retrieved in any way.

E-PHI must be destroyed in such a way that it cannot be re-created. Examples of destruction methods are provided below:

- Paper record methods of destruction include burning, shredding, pulping, and pulverizing.

- Microfilm or microfiche methods of destruction include recycling and pulverizing.

- Laser discs used in write once-read many document-imaging applications are destroyed by pulverizing.

- Computerized data are destroyed by magnetic degaussing.

- DVDs are destroyed by shredding or cutting.

- Magnetic tapes are destroyed by demagnetizing. (AHIMA 2011a)

Check Your Understanding 17.3

1. Which of the following provides the objective and scope for the HIPAA Security Rule as a whole?

    A. Administrative safeguards
    B. Documentation requirements
    C. General Rules
    D. Physical safeguards

2. Which of the following ensures that procedures are in place to handle an emergency response in the event of an untoward event such as a power outage?

   A. An audit control
   B. A contingency plan
   C. Employee training
   D. Password protection

3. Which of the following ensures that a user has only the information needed to perform his or her job?

   A. Audit controls
   B. Access controls
   C. Person identification forms
   D. Workstation safeguards

4. A visitor sign-in sheet to a computer area is an example of what type of control?

   A. Administrative
   B. Audit
   C. Facility access
   D. Workstation

5. The process that encodes textual material, converting it to scrambled data that must be decoded, is:

   A. An audit trail
   B. An encryption
   C. A password
   D. A physical safeguard

6. According to HIPAA standards, the designated individual responsible for data security:

   A. Must be identified by every covered entity
   B. Is only required in large facilities
   C. Is only required in hospitals
   D. Is not required in small physician office practices

7. Written business associate agreements are required with:

   A. Any company where work is outsourced
   B. Any outside company that handles electronic data
   C. Any outside company that handles electronic PHI
   D. Every outside company

8. Covered entities must retain documentation of their security policies for at least:

   A. Six years
   B. Five years from the date of origination
   C. Six years from the date when last in effect
   D. Six years from the date of the last incident

9. Security policies:

   A. Must be maintained in written format

   B. May be oral agreements between supervisors and employees

   C. May be written or oral

   D. May not be in an electronic form

10. Workforce security awareness and training is required:

   A. For all workforce members

   B. Only for workforce members who handle PHI

   C. Only for workforce members who handle electronic data

   D. Only for workforce members who handle electronic PHI

Forensics

With appropriate policies and procedures in place, it is then the responsibility of the organization and its managers, directors, CSO, and employees with audit responsibilities to review access logs, audit trails, failed logins and other reports generated to monitor compliance with the policies and procedures. These types of events are usually called "trigger events" and include employees viewing (Miaoulis 2011):

- Records of patients with the same last name or address of the employee

- VIP records (celebrities, board members, political figures)

- Records of those involved in high-profile events in the community

- Other employee's records

- Files of minors

- Files of those treated for infectious diseases, sensitive diagnoses such as HIV-AIDS or sexually transmitted diseases

- Records of a spouse (without the same surname)

- Records of terminated employees

- Portions of records of a discipline not consistent with employee's expertise

The organization should have specific policies and monitoring procedures in place to track employee's access via sign-ons and password and periodically audit all reports especially when high-profile incidents occur or VIPs are treated. HIPAA does require a regular review of system activity such as monitoring new user access as they are more likely to view these records than those of longer-term employees; and a review of system access by users in general and testing the access of those employees recently terminated to assure they have, in fact, been removed from access roles. During the Columbine incident in

Colorado, it was determined that several employees without a need to know had accessed victim's records during treatment at a local hospital. Those employees were disciplined since it was prior to HIPAA legislation but nonetheless policies were in place to detect such access. More recently, after news media in Southern California began reporting the birth of octuplets to a single mother from in vitro fertilization, her case received unprecedented media attention. Subsequently, several employees at the hospital where she delivered were disciplined and fined for accessing her records after audit trails revealed unauthorized access.

Enforcement and Accountability

The Privacy and Security Rules include civil penalties and monetary fines for non-adherence. It is the responsibility of a covered entity to develop policies and procedures to ensure compliance with the Rule and to enforce them wherever appropriate. The CSO and others designated in the covered entity must ensure that ongoing monitoring of privacy and security takes place and that breaches are properly reported, investigated, and processed. Mitigation for any breaches that occurred should also be addressed to avoid repetition of the circumstances causing the incident. Additionally, if employees were involved in the breach, appropriate action must be taken. In many of the breaches reported to the Office of Civil Rights, employees were terminated due to the severity of the breach. Each organization must follow its own policies when incidents occur. Sanctions may include disciplinary actions, suspension of access to certain systems or termination of the employee depending on the policies of the organization. Detection of these incidents requires careful monitoring by supervisors, privacy and security officers, and others designated to assist in monitoring systems and networks or those reporting patient complaints of privacy violations.

The Security Program plan for the organization should include the frequency with which these system audits should take place. The plan should address the preparation, documentation, and responses to all audits for review by external auditors as well as internal reviewers. The Security Rule does not specify the frequency of audits, but good IT practices have ongoing monitors in place for many transactions and usually include formal reviews of all elements of the plan on a quarterly basis. As in some of the incidents described previously, high-profile events and people may dictate immediate reviews and monitoring, which continue as long as the event is newsworthy or pertinent to the organization.

External Enforcement

The US Department of Health and Human Services Office of Civil Rights has been charged to enforce the Privacy Rule for covered entities and business associates. Under the Law, they act on complaints that:

- Have taken place after the rules (privacy and security) took effect
- Have been filed against an entity that is required to comply with the Law

- Allege a violation of the Rule (Privacy or Security) took place
- Have been filed within 180 days of the occurrence (or awareness that the alleged violation took place)

The complaint is then investigated by OCR and the covered entity is asked to provide information regarding the complaint. Covered entities are required to comply with any investigation conducted by the OCR or the Department of Justice (DOJ). Most complaints are resolved by the CE who voluntarily corrected policies or procedures or took other actions to mitigate the complaint. Covered entities who do not act in a way that is satisfactory to the OCR may have civil monetary penalties (CMPs) imposed. The complainant is subsequently notified of the resolution of their complaint in writing. Complaints that may be a violation of criminal provisions of the Law may be referred to the Department of Justice for further investigation.

Additionally, the ARRA Act of 2009 (Section 13411) requires HHS to conduct periodic audits to ensure covered entities and business associates are complying with breach notification standards and to identify best privacy and security practices. The identified best practices will be shared with the covered entities and business associates. A pilot of 150 audits of covered entities took place in late 2011 and concluded in December of 2012.

While many of these breaches are privacy violations, as previously discussed, most of these involve a computer, storage devices, or mobile media so security policies and procedures must be consistent with privacy policies and procedures.

Internal Audits

Organizations must conduct their own audits of threats and vulnerabilities and other risks to the compromise or misuse of health data.

An organization's certified EHR that meets the Stage 1 Meaningful Use criteria will also meet HHS audit criteria and may provide enough detailed audit logs to determine if there was an unauthorized access to a patient's record. These built-in audit logs contain literally millions of transaction entries so reviewing these audit logs takes time and skill in reading and interpreting the data.

There are a number of third-party audit tools available which can systematically and automatically analyze the data and generate reports which can then be used to review the data. These tools can be programmed to detect patterns of behaviors of users, detect unauthorized access to a patient's record using pre-written queries (same name as patient, certain dates of service or names of frequent VIP visitors), and present the reports in easy-to-read formats.

Because these audits are resource intensive, organizations frequently only audit access logs and other reports when a problem is reported or suspected. This is not considered best practice and is not consistent with the Privacy and Security Rule requirements. As the Security Rule does not address the frequency for audits, the audit process should be determined by the Chief Security Officer in consultation with the Security Committee, information technology management, and other individuals routinely involved in data scrutiny and report writing. HIPAA requires that covered entities maintain documentation of audits for six years. The documentation should include the review of policies, procedures, and results of past audits including any corrective actions or sanctions that resulted from the audits.

The organization's privacy and security officer should review the results and provide education to other managers and employees about the findings so they will be equipped to understand the findings and any actions that should be taken as a result of such audits.

Organizations should be consistent in their audits and policy revisions. All sanction policies should also be consistent, making sure the sanction fits the incident and that incidents or breaches of a similar nature are handled in the same way with equal sanctions applied. The organization should also develop policies and procedures to address the processing and reporting of any breaches of federal and state laws and educate the workforce including physicians, providers, and all levels of management. The Health Information Technician, as a steward of data and information systems should assist in internal and external audits to the extent possible in order to provide additional assistance to the organization in preventing violations of the privacy and security rules and may also be involved in coordinating and delivering workforce privacy and security training.

Roles and Responsibilities of the Health Information Technician

Why should health information professionals be concerned with data security? As custodians of patient information, they are responsible for ensuring that it is adequately protected from unauthorized use. In addition, they are responsible for ensuring that the data are accurate, complete, and available when needed. After all, if data are incorrect or unavailable when needed, they essentially are useless for patient care.

The HIT's data security role includes being knowledgeable about security threats and measures that protect healthcare data. This role also may include implementing or monitoring compliance with the healthcare organization's security policy and procedures. As a user of health information, the HIT must:

- Respect the privacy and confidentiality of information and ensure that confidential or sensitive information is protected from improper disclosure

- Respect the integrity of information under his or her control and not intentionally develop or use any unauthorized mechanisms to alter or destroy information

- Comply with the legal protection provided by copyright and software licenses to programs and data

- Respect the intended usage for which access to computing resources was granted

- Abide by restrictions to security access and not attempt to subvert or bypass any installed security mechanisms

- Follow incident response procedures and report any security breaches or potential breaches to the appropriate authority
- Ensure that critical data are appropriately backed up
- Understand threats to data and information security

Check Your Understanding 17.4

Instructions: Indicate whether the following statements are true or false (T or F).

1. _____ Trigger events such as the admission of a VIP to a facility should initiate an access control audit.

2. _____ HIPAA does not require a regular review of system activity such as monitoring new user access.

3. _____ The Security Rule does not specify the frequency of system audits.

4. _____ The Health Information Technician can assist in the audit process.

5. _____ An HIT's data security role includes being aware of security threats and other measures to protect data.

Real-World Case

Unauthorized Access/Disclosure from an EHR

The following case appeared on the Office for Civil Rights website (http://www.hhs.gov/ocr) describing a well-known Midwestern medical clinic that was subsequently investigated by the OCR.

An employee inappropriately accessed PHI affecting potentially 1,740 individuals. The category of the breach as reported to the OCR was Unauthorized Access/Disclosure. Following the breach the clinic conducted an investigation, terminated the employee, and re-educated its employees regarding its policies on patient privacy and access to PHI. They also enhanced their supervision and monitoring of employee's access activity and notified the patients they reasonably believed had been affected and offered them identity theft protection services at no cost. They also, as required by the rule, placed the breach notice on their website and in the local newspaper as the breach affected over 500 individuals.

Summary

Every healthcare organization must make the protection of healthcare information a top priority. The cost of security breaches reaches into the billions of dollars every year for American industry in general. For the healthcare industry, these costs include not only potential monetary losses, but can jeopardize patient privacy and affect the quality of care provided.

Health information can be protected through a total security program that combines administrative, technical, and physical safeguards. Each of these controls is equally important in providing a safety net for information. When any one control is lacking, the security program is vulnerable to many potential threats from both within and outside of the healthcare organization.

Health information management professionals are the custodians of patient information. As such, they have a responsibility to protect the integrity and confidentiality of patient information and to assist in monitoring the healthcare facility's compliance with its own data security policies and procedures.

References

American Health Information Management Association. 2009. Analysis of the interim final rule. Breach notification for unsecured protected health information. http://www.ahima.org/dc/documents/AnalysisoftheInterimFinalRulefin_9_11_000.pdf

American Health Information Management Association. 2011a. Retention and Destruction of Health Information. http://library.ahima.org/xpedio/idcplg?IdcService=GET_HIGHLIGHT_INFO &QueryText=xPublishSite+%3cMatches%3e+%60BoK%60+%3cAND%3e+%28%28xSource+%3csubstring%3e+%60AHIMA+Practice+Brief%60+%3cNOT%3e+xSource+%3csubstring%3e+%60Practice+Brief+attachment%60%29+%3cAND%3e+dSecurityGroup+%3csubstring%3e+%60Public%60%29&SortField=xPubDate&SortOrder=Desc&dDocName=bok1_049252&HighlightType=HtmlHighlight&dWebExtension=hcsp

AHIMA. 2011b. "Swiped, Not Hacked: After a Year of Reporting, Theft Remains Main Cause of Breach." *Journal of AHIMA* 82(2).

Department of Health and Human Services. 2003. *Federal Register*. 45 CFR Parts 160, 162, and 164 Health Insurance Reform: Security Standards; Final Rule. http://ecfr.gpoaccess.gov/cgi/t/text/text-idx?c=ecfr&sid=4e7065d0a05080b2b89dabdb6feea751&rgn=div8&view=text&node=45:1.0.1.3.79.3.27.4&idno=45

Department of Health and Human Services. 2009. Guidance and request for comments under section 13402 of the Health Information Technology for Economic and Clinical Health (HITECH) Act, Title XIII of Division A and Title IV of Division B of the American Recovery and Reinvestment Act of 2009 (ARRA) (Pub. L. 111-5).

Goedert, J. 2010. Insurer AvMed sued after data breach. *Health Data Management*. November 17. http://www.healthdatamanagement.com/news/breach-lawsuit-avmed-notification-encryption-hipaa-hitech-41363-1.html

Institute of Medicine. 1991. *The Computer-Based Patient Record: An Essential Technology for Health Care*. Edited by R.S. Dick, E.B. Steen, and D.E. Detmer. Washington, DC: National Academy Press. http://www.nap.edu/openbook.php?isbn=0309055326

Institute of Medicine. 2011. Health IT and Patient Safety: Building safer systems for better care. Consensus Report. http://www.iom.edu/Reports/2011/Health-IT-and-Patient-Safety-Building-Safer-Systems-for-Better-Care.aspx

Johns, M.L. 2002. *HIPAA Security Tool Kit*. Chicago: Holistic Training Solutions.

Johns, M.L. 2008. Privacy and security in health information. In *Electronic Health Records: A Guide for Clinicians and Administrators,* 2nd ed. Edited by J. Carter. Philadelphia: American College of Physicians.

Johnson, E.M. 2009. Data hemorrhages in the health-care sector. Center for Digital Strategies, Tuck School of Business. Hanover, NH: Dartmouth College. http://mba.tuck.dartmouth.edu/digital/Research/ResearchProjects/JohnsonHemorrhagesFC09Proceedingd.pdf

Krigsman, M. 2008. Failed IT causes major Georgia Blue Cross health privacy breach. http://blogs.zdnet.com/projectfailures/?p=945

Miaoulis, W.M. 2011. *Preparing for a HIPAA Security Compliance Assessment*. Chicago: AHIMA.

National Institute of Standards and Technology. 2008. An introduction resource guide for implementing the Health Insurance Portability and Accountability Act (HIPAA) Security Rule. NIST Special Publication 800-66 Revision 1.

Patel, M. 2009. The threat from within. *Risk Management* 56(5):8–9. http://www.rmmag.com/MGTemplate.cfm?Section=RMMagazine&template=Magazine/DisplayMagazines.cfm&AID=3929&ShowArticle=1

Pipkin, D.L. 2000. *Information Security: Protecting the Global Enterprise*. Upper Saddle River, NJ: Prentice Hall.

PwC. 2011. Health industry under-prepared to protect patient privacy; risk of data breaches rise with new access to digital health information, says PwC. http://www.pwc.com/us/en/press-releases/2011/health-industry-under-prepared.jhtml

Ten years after 9/11: A status report on information sharing: Hearing before the Senate Committee on Homeland Security & Governmental Affairs. 2011 (October 11). Testimony of Zoe Budinger and Jeffrey Smith.

US Congress, Office of Technology Assessment. 1993. Protecting privacy in computerized medical information, OTA-TCT-576. Washington, DC: US Government Printing Office.

Walsh, T. 2011 (January). Practice Brief: Security risk analysis and management: An overview (Updated). http://library.ahima.org/xpedio/groups/public/documents/ahima/bok1_048622.hcsp?dDocName=bok1_048622

Additional Resources

American Medical Association. nd. http:/www.ama-assn.org

Department of Health and Human Services. nd. Summary of the HIPAA Security Rule. http://www.hhs.gov/ocr/privacy/hipaa/understanding/srsummary.html

Federal Emergency Management Association. nd. http://www.fema.gov

Health Information Management Systems Society. nd. http://www.himss.org

Modern Health Care. nd. http://www.modernhealthcare.com

Office of Civil Rights/Health & Human Services. nd. http://www.hhs.gov/ocr/

Price Waterhouse Coopers. nd. http://www.pwc.com

Privacy Act of 1974 5 U.S.C. Part 552a. http://www.justice.gov/opcl/privstat.htm

Public Law 104-91: Health Insurance Portability and Accountability Act of 1996. https://www.cms.gov/HIPAAGenInfo/

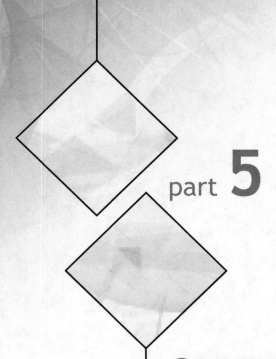

part **5**

Organizational Resources

chapter 18

Principles of Organization and Work Planning

Donald W. Kellogg, PhD, RHIA, CPEHR

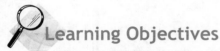

Learning Objectives

- Distinguish between hierarchal and bureaucratic organizational structures
- Identify the roles of the three basic levels of management
- Explain the function of common organization management tools including mission, vision, and values statements; policies; procedures; and organizational charts
- Describe the functions of authority, responsibility, and accountability
- Discuss the fundamentals of leadership
- Discuss the benefits of teamwork in an organization and identify the steps in creating an effective team
- Describe the usual practices for recruitment, orientation, and training for new employees
- Identify effective steps in conducting an interview
- Describe the usual practices for staff retention
- Explain how position descriptions, performance standards, and staff schedules are used as tools in human resource management
- Describe how job descriptions are used in recruitment and hiring
- Discuss the elements of performance management

- Explain the relationship among performance standards, performance review, and performance counseling
- Identify the key steps the supervisor should take in performance counseling or in taking disciplinary action
- Discuss ways that conflict can be minimized in the workplace
- Explain techniques used for staff development
- Distinguish between strategic and operational planning
- Describe the quality improvement cycle and the steps for change
- Explain the budget process and how it relates to organizational and department goals and assumptions
- Describe tools used for planning and managing staff resources
- Explain the processes used in work analysis and design
- Identify the methods for supply management

Key Terms

Accommodating
Accountability
Action steps
Ad hoc committee
Assets
Authority
Avoiding
Board of governors
Board of trustees
Budget assumptions
Bureaucracy
Career planning
Chain of command
Change management
Conflict management
Delegation of authority
Developing stage
Direct costs
Disciplinary action
Employee orientation
Environmental assessment
Ergonomics
Executive management

Executive manager
Executive sponsor
Expenses
Fixed costs
Forming
Grievance management
Hierarchy
Human resources
Indirect costs
Inventory control
Job redesign
Middle management
Middle managers
Mission statement
Mixed costs
Monitoring stage
Norming
Operational plan
Organization
Organizational chart
Performance counseling
Performance evaluations
Performance management

Performance standards	Staff retention
Performing	Staffing analysis
Planning stage	Standing committees
Policy	Storming
Position descriptions	Strategic planning
Procedures	Supervisory management
Process redesign	Supervisory managers
Progressive discipline	Supply management
Quality improvement process	Systems thinking
Rating stage	Team norms
Recruitment	Values statement
Responsibility	Variable costs
Retention	Vision statement
Revenues	Work schedules
Rewarding stage	Workflow analysis

Introduction

Work planning and organization are critical elements in implementing the mission of an organization and achieving its long-term strategic goals and short-term operational goals. These goals are achieved through application of the organization's resources, including its human, financial, and physical **assets.** Supervisors and team leaders contribute directly to managing the organization's resources effectively and efficiently. In other words, they are responsible for ensuring that the organization performs the right activities in the best ways possible to achieve its mission.

In addition to modern management theories, there is the fundamental principle that people accomplish more working collectively than they do working individually. Along with planning tools and methods to monitor resources, team leaders and supervisors can add value on a daily basis to the organizations where they work and the people with whom they work.

Over the past 20 years, a number of industrial management theories have been adapted for use in healthcare organizations, including continuous performance improvement and total quality management (discussed in detail in chapter 11). Generally, the overarching philosophy of modern management emphasizes the needs of customers as the focus of every organization's value system. And *customer* is being defined in the broadest sense to include everyone who receives some sort of service from someone else.

In healthcare organizations, team leaders work on many levels, from supervisors of small functional teams to leaders of cross-functional quality improvement teams. For many supervisors, their leadership role is only one aspect of their job. In contrast, the work of executive-level administrators is entirely managerial. Just as every experienced specialty physician starts out as a medical student, supervisors and directors in healthcare organizations begin their careers by practicing the basics.

This chapter discusses the nature of organizations and the basic elements of team leadership. In addition, it describes management of the organization's **human resources** and the supervisor's role in the organization's recruitment and retention efforts. The fundamentals of work planning and elements of expense management and budgeting also are addressed. Finally, quality improvement within a health information management function is examined.

Theory into Practice

Throughout this chapter Mercy Medical Center (MMC) will be used as a case study to clarify the concepts introduced. As with many medical centers, MMC is being challenged to move from a paper-based medical record to an electronic health record (EHR). Without the financial resources to undertake a full-scale EHR implementation, the leadership of MMC's health information management (HIM) department had to come up with a plan to migrate from the existing paper system in a way that would add value, but temper the investment. Based on input from other departments, it was decided to begin with the implementation of an EHR in the emergency department. A cross-functional team was established to ensure that the information collected in the EHR would provide all the required information for patient care and administrative requirements such as reporting sexually transmitted disease cases to the state Department of Health and completed procedures to MMC's department of billing. Data collected on paper forms were identified and categorized as required, important, or unnecessary. The cross-functional team then mapped those data elements from the forms to the data dictionary in the new EHR system. Additional fields were identified to ensure that all necessary data would be collected. Workflows were determined for all the functions, with the HIM supervisor leading the team in mapping the workflows for administrative reporting and billing. The purpose was to ensure that all data would be collected and available on system-generated reports and to coders for code validation.

When the workflows and data systems had been finalized across all teams and all changes had been made to the EHR, the HIM supervisor was one of the key individuals working with another team to design and implement training for physicians, nurses, and clerical staff in use of the system. Post-implementation, the HIM supervisor performed routine audits of record completion, reinforced training, and suggested system changes.

Principles of Organization

Organization is the planned coordination of the activities of more than one person for the achievement of a common purpose or goal. It is accomplished through the division of labor and function and is based on a **hierarchy** (an arrangement of positions where one is either above, below, or at the same level as another position, see figure 18.2) of authority and responsibility (Schein 1980). Like other types of businesses, healthcare facilities are a type of formal organization. That is, they have established goals and a specific purpose for existing.

Jobs and the people who perform them should be structured in a way that accomplishes the goals of an organization. Some organizational tools are used to communicate the structure, the purpose, and the methods used to accomplish the shared work of the organization's members. Organizations are like sports teams in that they have specific positions, a predefined set of rules, and a goal of winning. Organizations also use communications tools that are similar to a players roster (position descriptions), a rule or playbook (policies and procedures), and a record of wins and losses (a budget and financial records). Although the purpose, structure, and methods vary widely, all healthcare organizations use common systems and tools to achieve their goals.

Nature of Organization

By nature, humans are social creatures. They are biologically designed to live within groups of their own kind. Moreover, they continuously form and reform informal and formal groups of various sizes (two members to billions) and longevity (a few seconds to a few centuries). No two groups have identical purposes, membership, or rules. Therefore, every human group is unique.

There is an endless variety of groups. Groups range from relatively informal friendships, families, and social clubs to extremely formal businesses, educational institutions, and national governments. They can be loose, unstructured, and temporary. An example of an extremely loose, short-term group might be that of a dozen people who planned last year's holiday party. But even the most informal groups have a purpose and a set of more or less well-communicated rules. In this example, the group's purpose was to get from point A to point B. The rules required that the party's activities stay within a framework appropriate for the organization.

Although every group of humans is unique, interactions among humans follow predictable patterns. Human behavior has been studied for untold centuries. Theories on organizational behavior have been offered ever since humans learned how to communicate with each other. Although few principles of organizational behavior go unchallenged, centuries of observation have produced some basic rules. For example, one unchanging principle of organizational behavior seems to be that the group's structure affects the way its members interact with each other. And the structural effects can have both positive and negative consequences for the group as a whole as well as for its individual members.

Organizational Structure

At least until recent decades, formal organizations such as healthcare and manufacturing institutions have tended to be structured as relatively inflexible hierarchies. In a hierarchy, every member of the organization is assigned a specific rank. Each rank, in turn, carries a specific level of decision-making authority as well as specific responsibilities within the institution. Hierarchies are authoritarian in nature. In other words, they are strictly controlled by a powerful elite working at the top of the organization. These few individuals make almost every significant decision on behalf of the entire organization.

Historically, large government institutions have tended to be organized as rigid bureaucratic structures. In a **bureaucracy,** as in a hierarchy, positions within the formal organization are assigned specific ranks. Hierarchical ranks are based on levels of decision-making authority. In contrast, bureaucratic ranks are based on levels of technical expertise.

The purpose of bureaucratic organizations is to conduct highly complex and regulated processes. The structure of the bureaucratic organization reflects the processes it is designed to carry out. Therefore, bureaucracies operate according to well-established and often inflexible rules. Each individual within the bureaucracy is responsible for carrying out only a small, well-defined element of the larger process. The Social Security Administration is a good example of a government bureaucracy. It was created in 1935 with the sole purpose of implementing the Social Security Act.

Both hierarchies and bureaucracies depend on authoritarian **chains of command.** In a traditional chain-of-command structure, one manager oversees the work of many employees, but each employee is accountable to only one boss. The structures of military organizations, for example, are organized around extremely rigid chains of command.

Obviously, management systems and organizational structures have been used by humans working in groups since the beginning of civilization. There is little historical documentation of the management systems in use during ancient times, but the achievements of ancient civilizations reflect their effectiveness. The desert pyramids of Egypt, the Roman aqueducts of western Europe, and the mountain cities of Peru and Chile could not have been realized without systematic planning and organization.

Organizational structure has been studied systematically since the early 20th century. In the following decades, a number of new management theories were suggested and each seems to have required innovations in organizational structure. The period of economic rebuilding after the second World War ushered in the current era of business thinking. Business and management theorists W. Edwards Deming and Joseph M. Juran began developing *modern* management systems in the early 1950s.

Today's management systems are modern in that they are moving away from the traditional authoritarian models that have prevailed since the Industrial Revolution. Most of all, they are modern in that they recognize the potential value of change and treat it as an opportunity rather than as a threat.

Modern management systems are based on the objective statistical analysis of data and information. They emphasize the benefits of sharing authority among employees and managers. They also favor interdisciplinary and cross-functional cooperation and teamwork over bureaucratic regulation and authoritarian control. Modern management systems value continual learning and demand systems thinking (Senge 1990, 6–8). **Systems thinking** is an objective way of looking at work-related ideas and processes. Its goal is to allow people to uncover ineffective patterns of behavior and thinking and then find ways to make lasting improvements.

In large part, modern management systems represent a rejection of the traditional authoritarian, hierarchical, and bureaucratic approaches to organization and management. However, because the traditional systems have been the accepted norm since the Industrial Revolution, they have proved difficult to displace.

Today, management theorists such as Peter Senge continue to lead the movement to establish information-based management systems and team-based organizational structures in all types of business endeavors. Modern quality management philosophies such as continuous quality improvement are based on modern management thinking. Avedis Donabedian, Steven Shortell, and Donald Berwick, among others, are leading the movement to apply modern quality management concepts to healthcare organizations. (Quality management is discussed in detail in chapter 10.)

Management Levels

Managers at all levels of the organization are held directly responsible for handling its resources effectively and efficiently. However, the scope of managerial accountability among supervisors and managers varies considerably. It depends on the size and organization of the facility they work in, the nature of their responsibilities, and their position within their facility.

The fundamental management functions for both large and small healthcare organizations are similar. However, since small healthcare organizations such as physician group practices employ fewer people than large organizations such as hospitals, they have much simpler organizational, operational, and reporting structures. Moreover, unlike large organizations, they are often owned by a single physician or a group of physicians.

Organizations with more than a few employees (for example, 20 or more) usually have three basic levels of management: **supervisory management, middle management,** and **executive management.** In general, supervisory-level managers perform the organization's daily work, middle-level managers monitor and coordinate its ongoing activities, and executive-level managers focus on its future.

Supervisory Management

Supervisory management oversees the organization's efforts at the staff level and monitors the effectiveness of everyday operations and individual performance against preestablished standards. It also ensures that the organization's human assets are used effectively and that its policies and procedures are carried out consistently.

Supervisory managers work in small (2- to 10-person) functional workgroups or teams. They often perform hands-on functions in addition to supervisory functions. They also play an important role in staff training and recruitment or retention efforts. Supervisory managers direct daily work, create work schedules, and monitor the quality of the work and the productivity of the staff. They are important resources in revising procedures and conducting performance reviews because they are familiar with the work of the unit and the performance of individual staff members. Supervisory managers usually have advanced technical skills that allow them to perform the most complex functions of the work team. However, most supervisors have limited financial authority and must seek approval from higher-level managers before spending money or hiring staff. Depending on the size and structure of the organization, HIM supervisors report to another supervisory-level manager or to a department-level manager or assistant manager. Typical titles for HIM professionals in supervisory-level positions in a hospital include file room manager, coding manager, transcription manager, and release of information manager. With the implementation of the EHR, as some positions are eliminated or outsourced these titles may change. However, given that some facilities are still paper-based or using a hybrid system, many of these titles are still relevant.

Effective supervisory managers are extremely important in healthcare, where the greatest part of the organization's resources is expended at the operational level. Labor costs represent the greatest investment the organization makes. Staff and supervisory healthcare workers include nurses, clinical therapists, diagnostic technicians, dietary workers, laboratory workers, environmental support staff, and administrative support staff. Health information technicians (HITs) provide vital administrative services and support patient care by protecting the accuracy and confidentiality of clinical databases and health records. Among other responsibilities, they also ensure the financial health and future of their organizations by providing high-quality clinical coding services.

To lead effectively, every supervisor should have an understanding of the principles and tools used to manage human resources. Many of these tools, such as **position descriptions, performance standards,** and job procedures are discussed later in the chapter.

Middle Management

Middle management is concerned primarily with facilitating the work performed by supervisory- and staff-level personnel as well as by executive leaders. The responsibilities of middle management include:

- Developing, implementing, and revising the organization's policies and procedures under the direction of executive managers
- Executing the organizational plans developed at the board and executive levels
- Providing the operational information that executives need to develop meaningful plans for the organization's future

Typical titles for HIM professionals in middle management include HIM director, compliance manager, director of quality improvement, privacy officer, and director of clinical documentation improvement (CDI).

Middle managers oversee operations of a broader scope in their work as managers or assistant managers of departments or disciplinary functions. For example, they direct health information management, nursing, risk management, and facilities management functions.

Typically, middle managers are responsible for performing a limited number of hands-on analytical and/or decision-making functions related directly to the departments they manage. In an HIM department, for example, an assistant director's responsibilities might include tracking the quality of clinical databases and overseeing coding compliance programs. HIM managers participate on a number of permanent and temporary interdisciplinary committees dealing with subjects that relate to the organization's information resources. They also initiate interdepartmental efforts to address issues that go beyond department-level operations. In small healthcare organizations, the HIM director may play additional managerial roles in risk management, quality management, and/or utilization management. HIM professionals may also have positions of middle management authority outside of the HIM department, such as CDI specialists, quality improvement specialists, and compliance specialists.

Depending on the size and structure of the organization, middle managers in HIM report to a department-level director or an executive manager (vice president) on the organization's senior management team. In an integrated healthcare delivery network, the director of HIM services might report to the vice president of operations (sometimes referred to as the chief operating officer, or COO) or the vice president of information services (sometimes called the chief information officer, or CIO). In a small community hospital, the HIM director might report to the CEO (chief executive officer), the CFO (chief financial officer), or the COO.

Executive Management and Governance

The highest managerial level of the healthcare organization may be divided into two entities: executive management and the governing board. **Executive managers** are employees of the organization. They are hired either by the board or by the organization's CEO with board approval. In publicly owned organizations, board members are elected to their positions by the owners or stockholders. In privately owned organizations, board members are appointed.

Role of Executive Managers

Executive management is primarily responsible for setting the organization's future direction and establishing its strategic plan. To that end, executive management works to ensure that the organization uses its assets wisely, fulfills its current mission, and works toward achieving a meaningful vision for the future. Executive managers oversee broad functions, departments, or groups of departments. Additionally, they are responsible for establishing the policies of healthcare organizations and leading their quality improvement and compliance initiatives. Executive managers also work with other community leaders to make sure that healthcare organizations contribute to the well-being of the communities they serve.

Depending on the complexity of the organization, the titles of executive managers vary. The different titles include CEO, president, executive vice president, senior vice president, vice president, and director. Executive managers may report to other executive managers, to higher-level vice presidents, or to the CEO.

In most organizations, the CEO is the highest-ranking manager. (CEOs sometimes hold more than one title. For example, the head of an organization might have the title president and CEO.) The CEO and/or the president reports directly to the board of directors.

Role of the Governing Board

Healthcare organizations such as hospitals, for-profit healthcare businesses, and integrated healthcare delivery networks are organized as legal entities or corporations. Every state has laws that dictate how corporations are to be structured and run within its jurisdiction. However, all state incorporation laws are consistent in one area: responsibility for the operation of every healthcare organization ultimately lies with its **board of governors, board of trustees,** or board of directors. (The name and structure of the board depend on the profit-making status of the organization, among other factors.) Thus, the board is the final authority in setting the organization's strategic direction, mission and vision, and general philosophy and ethical base.

Typically, the board consists of a chairperson and 10 to 20 board members. It represents the interests of the organization's owners. Any number of different entities may own large healthcare organizations, including federal, state, and local governments; investor groups; educational institutions; and religious organizations. Moreover, healthcare organizations may be owned privately or publicly. In publicly owned entities, investors purchase stock on national and international stock exchanges and receive a share of the profits in the form of dividends.

Roles of Teams and Committees

Like other complex organizations, healthcare facilities often confront problems that cross traditional department lines. At those times, committees or teams may be created to identify issues, set policy, or solve problems. In larger facilities, **standing committees** may exist, such as the medical staff committee, a quality improvement committee, or an infection control committee. Standing committees are put in place to oversee ongoing and cross-functional issues. They are given a broader charge, and committee members are normally appointed for a term that may last one to three years to ensure continuity. Some facilities may have a health information committee or a medical record committee; in other organizations oversight of the information resources may be assigned to one of the other standing committees.

Teams are created to address a more specific issue and generally disband when their work is completed and are referred to as **ad hoc committees.** Teams may be cross-departmental or may be formed within a single department. They should be composed of people who are in the best position to contribute to the charge and communicate the outcome. In the formation of teams, the charge should be carefully considered to ensure clarity of purpose and appropriate results. The charge should consider the amount of authority the team is being given. For instance, a cross-departmental team might be given the charge of investigating alternative sick leave policies but would rarely be given ultimate authority to establish the policy when the decision could have a significant financial impact on the organization. Committees and teams involve more people in decision making, enrich jobs, and develop leadership skills. Fundamentals of team development and organization are discussed later in this chapter and in chapter 11.

Organizational Tools

In today's healthcare organizations, effective management demands that virtually every member of the organization understand its overall purpose. In addition, each member must be prepared to support and foster achievement of that purpose. Mission, vision , and values statements are all effective tools in communicating this information throughout the organization.

Policies and procedures also can be considered organizational tools. *Policies* are written descriptions of the organization's formal positions. *Procedures* are the approved methods for implementing those positions. Together, they spell out what the organization expects employees to do and how they are expected to do it. (Policies and procedures are explained in more detail in the section on human resources management later in this chapter.)

Organizational Charts

An **organizational chart** is a graphic representation of the organization's formal structure. It shows the organization's various activities and the specific members or categories of members assigned to carry them out. The chart for a very small organization might list the actual names of employees or individual position titles. The chart for a very large organization would list the various functional groups or departments responsible for each area of operations.

Traditionally, the reporting relationships between individuals and groups also are indicated according to accepted labeling conventions. For example, a solid line between two elements on a chart indicates a direct reporting relationship and a broken line indicates an indirect reporting relationship. (See figures 18.1, 18.2, and 18.3 for examples of organizational charts developed for different types of healthcare organizations.)

Today's healthcare organizations are somewhat less concerned with official lines of authority. Rather, they are concerned with the interrelationships of workgroups and functions. Individual departments and interdepartmental workgroups sometimes develop detailed organizational charts as a first step in redesigning work processes. The charts then can be used as the basis for creating workflow diagrams and flowcharts. The purpose of these graphic tools is to help work teams visualize current and proposed processes and then suggest and implement improvements.

Some organizations also include organizational charts in their official position (job) descriptions. In this context, the charts put the work of a specific position or employee into the larger context of how the whole organization works as a system of interdependent processes.

Figure 18.1. Sample organizational chart for an acute care hospital with outpatient services

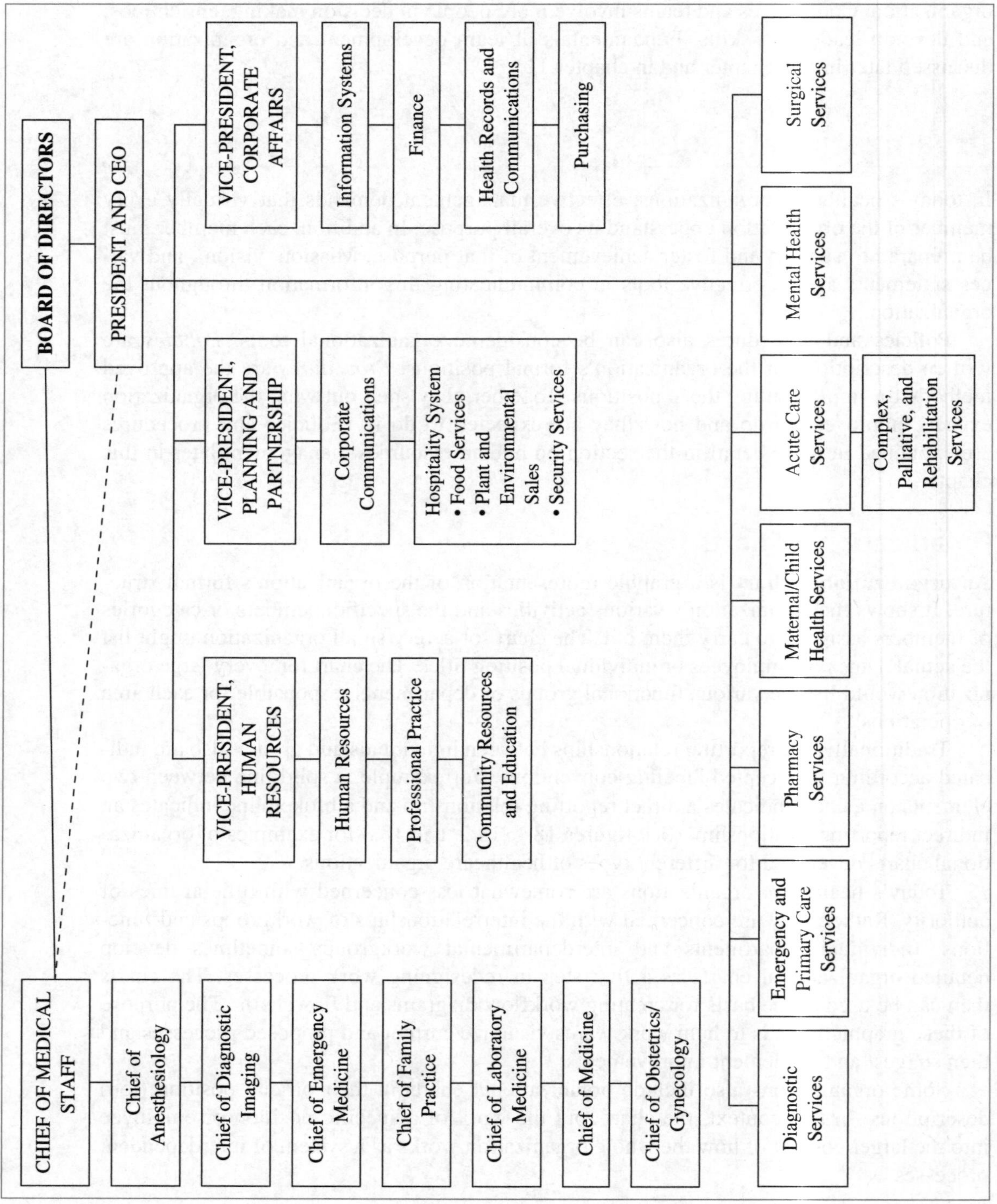

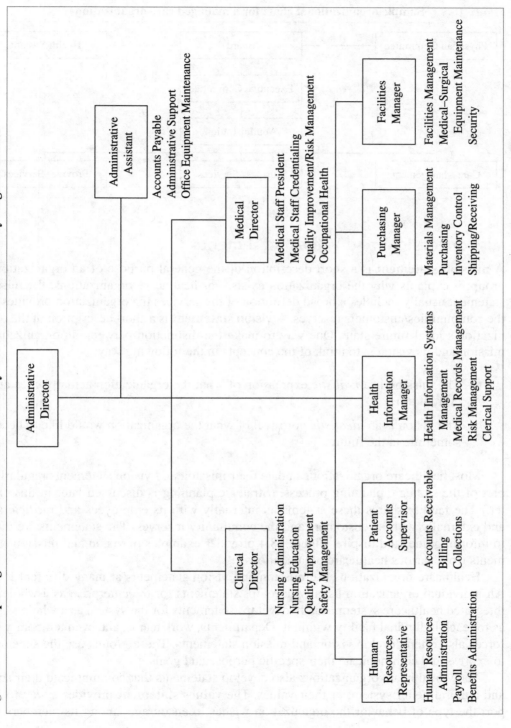

Figure 18.2. Sample organizational chart for an ambulatory care clinic with ambulatory surgical services

Figure 18.3.   **Sample organizational chart for a managed care organization**

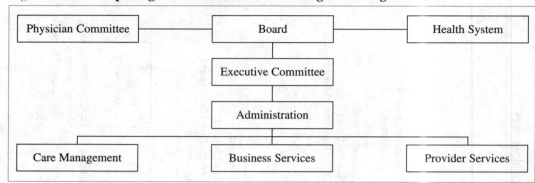

Mission, Vision, and Values Statements

A **mission statement** is a short description of the general purpose of an organization or group; it explains why the organization exists. For healthcare organizations, the mission statement usually includes a broad definition of the services the organization provides and the communities/customers it serves. A **vision statement** is a short description of the organization's ideal future state. One way to make the distinction between an organization's mission and its vision is to think of the concepts in the following way:

- The mission is a *realistic* expression of what the organization actually does at the current time.

- The vision is an *idealistic* portrayal of what the organization would like to become sometime in the future.

Most healthcare organizations update their mission and vision statements regularly as part of the strategic planning process. (Strategic planning is discussed later in this chapter.) The facility shares these statements internally with its employees and medical staff and externally with its customers and the community it serves. The statements are meant to inform, guide, and inspire. Figure 18.4 provides examples of vision and mission statements from various healthcare organizations.

Healthcare organizations use mission and vision statements at many different levels. An individual organization usually develops statements for the enterprise as a whole. An integrated healthcare system usually develops statements for the system as a whole as well as for each individual facility within it. Departments, work teams, and even temporary task forces also often develop vision and mission statements. These groups use the statements to express and communicate their specific purpose and goals.

Many healthcare organizations also develop statements that communicate their social and cultural belief system, or their values. The **values statement** provides a way to support the type of behavior the organization wishes to encourage among its members. For

Figure 18.4.   Sample mission and vision statements

General Hospital Affiliated with a Larger Healthcare System
Lutheran Hospital's **mission** is to improve the health of the communities we serve by providing high-quality services in a responsible and caring way.
Our **vision** is to become the leader in promoting healthy lifestyles in an atmosphere of spiritual support, dignity, compassion, and mutual respect for all.
Community General Hospital
Anytown General Hospital's **mission** is to provide quality health services and technology to meet the changing healthcare needs of the people of southwestern Minnesota.
Anytown General Hospital's **vision** is to become the hospital of choice for residents of Polk, Sunny Isle, and Spring counties, a position we strive to strengthen by our long-term commitment to: • Teamwork   • Service excellence   • Compassionate care   • Cost consciousness   • Continuous improvement
Academic Medical Center
Prairie University Hospital's **mission** is to provide the most up-to-date medical and surgical services available in the three-state area and to train medical students and graduate physicians to meet current and future challenges in healthcare.
Our **vision** is the achievement of healthy communities and progress toward the future of healthcare for Montana, western North Dakota, and northwestern South Dakota.
Specialty Hospital
The **mission** of Women's Hospital of Somewhereville is to meet the healthcare needs of our patients and to exceed their service expectations.
Our **vision** is of a hospital: • Providing services with compassion and kindness   • Striving for performance improvement   • Fostering pride and integrity   • Aiming for increased cost-effectiveness and productivity
Specialty Clinic within an Academic Medical Center
The **mission** of the Midwest Asthma Center is to: • Provide optimal medical care for persons with asthma and related illnesses   • Develop new knowledge about asthma and its management through medical research   • Promote improved understanding about asthma and related illnesses through providing educational programs and materials for our patients, for other healthcare providers, and for the community
The **vision** of the Midwest Asthma Center is to provide the highest quality of integrated comprehensive care for persons with asthma and related illnesses and to be one of the centers of excellence in the world for asthma treatment, research, and education.
Primary Care Physicians' Practice
The **mission** of Coastal Shores Primary Care Associates is to serve the unique needs of individuals and families by providing high-quality, coordinated, primary care medical services through an efficient, accessible, and responsive network of caring providers.
Our **vision** is to be the primary care medical group of choice in the Atlantic County area by delivering high-quality, individualized, and efficient patient care.

example, the American Health Information Management Association (AHIMA) has established the following list of values:

- The public's right to accurate and confidential personal health information
- Innovation and leadership in advancing health information management practices and standards worldwide
- Adherence to the AHIMA Code of Ethics
- Advocacy and interdisciplinary collaboration with other professional organizations

Policies

A **policy** is a clearly stated and comprehensive statement that establishes the parameters for decision making and action. Policies are developed at both the institutional and departmental levels. In both cases, policies should be consistent within the organization. They must be developed in accordance with applicable laws and reflect actual practice. Because they may be used as documentation of intended practice in a lawsuit, policies should be developed very carefully. For example, a policy might state that patients may request to review their health records with a care provider in attendance or in the HIM department. (Examples of HIM policies are found in chapter 8.)

Procedures

A **procedure** is a guide to action and describes how work is done and how policies are carried out. Procedures are instructions that ensure high-quality, consistent outcomes for tasks done, especially when more than one person is involved. (Chapter 8 provides examples of some HIM procedures.)

One of the benefits of developing a procedure is that time is taken to analyze the best possible method of completing a process. This analysis may begin by developing a flowchart to document workflow, decision points, and the flow required to complete a procedure. (Flowcharts are discussed in detail in chapter 11.)

After a flowchart is completed, the steps in the process are written down in order. When more than one person is involved in completing a procedure, each person who performs a task is documented. Anyone generally competent to perform a task should be able to complete it after reading a well-written procedure. This usually takes several drafts that have been reviewed by people who actually perform the work. Moreover, it might be useful to ask someone unfamiliar with the job to try to complete it using the written procedure.

Every procedure should be reviewed at least annually or when the job itself has changed. Today, many procedures within HIM departments are being reviewed and changed as the medical record is moving away from paper-based to an electronic format. The policy may not change, but the procedures of the step-by-step process of how a job is completed will.

Writing a procedure also offers a great opportunity to identify ways to streamline the process. Are supplies available and organized in a way that makes work efficient? Would it be faster to complete one type of task for all the work, or should each job be completed before the next task is begun? Following is an example of the process of logging in requests for information:

1. The receptionist opens all incoming mail daily before 10 a.m. He or she then confirms that the date on the stamp is accurate and stamps all mail in the upper right-hand corner.

2. The receptionist sorts requests for medical information into three categories: legal, medical, or insurance. He or she then counts the requests in each category, clips or binds the requests for each category together, writes the count on a Post-it note, and places the note on the top request of each bundle. The bundles are then delivered to the Release of Information (ROI) inbox. (The inbox is located on the ROI supervisor's desk.)

3. The ROI coordinator picks up medical requests for information from the ROI inbox each morning after 10 a.m. He or she enters the number of requests on a daily work log (an Excel spreadsheet or G:roi/requests/medical).

It would be inefficient for the receptionist to open, date stamp, and deliver each piece of mail individually. However, this example shows how a detailed procedure would be useful in training a new receptionist or ROI coordinator or in providing instructions to anyone needed to perform this task in the regular employee's absence. It also highlights that the receptionist would need to be trained to identify different types of information requestors.

Check Your Understanding 18.1

1. Before I can submit a proposal to a vendor to purchase a new piece of equipment for my department, I need to get it approved. After completion, I give it to my director who reviews and routes it to the vice president. The vice president approves and routes it to the CEO. This movement up the organization's hierarchy is called the:

   A. Bureaucracy
   B. Chain of command
   C. Organizational structure
   D. Organization

2. My job requires me to code as well as perform supervisory functions. Which of the following best describes the management level of my position?

   A. Executive management
   B. Governing board
   C. Supervisory management
   D. Middle management

3. The staff workgroup that I am on has a multidisciplinary make-up. The purpose of the workgroup is ongoing. Which of the following best describes this workgroup?

A. Team
B. Governing board
C. Ad hoc committee
D. Standing committee

4. What organizational tool is used to state the parameters that employees should use when making decisions?

A. Policy
B. Procedure
C. Organizational chart
D. Mission statements

5. What tool might be used to analyze the best method to complete a process?

A. Organizational chart
B. Procedure
C. Mission
D. Vision

Instructions: Indicate whether the following statements are true or false (T or F).

6. _____ Continuous performance and total quality management are examples of industrial management theories.

7. _____ Systems thinking is a subjective way to look at work-related ideas and processes.

8. _____ Ultimate responsibility for the organization's operation lies with its chief executive officer.

9. _____ Today's healthcare organizations are increasingly concerned with official lines of authority.

10. _____ Supervisory management sets the organization's future direction and establishes its goals.

Human Resources

The most important asset of any healthcare organization is its employees. Staff salaries and benefits usually make up most of the organization's operating budget. More critically, however, staff represents the organization to the patients and to other individuals the organization serves. Effective team leadership and supervision of employees leads to improved performance, increased productivity, and reduced expenses. Becoming an effective team leader requires more than developing and using supervisory tools; it requires nurturing a productive working relationship with staff and colleagues.

Effective management of human resources includes team leadership, selecting the right team members, ensuring ongoing performance, and developing people for the future. People work in a variety of configurations within any organization. From a traditional department configuration, where a supervisor or team leader works with a group of employees, to cross-functional teams, committees, and workgroups, performance can be heightened by effective leadership.

Leadership Principles

The term *leadership* has been defined as the "art of mobilizing others to want to struggle for shared aspirations" (Kouzes and Posner 1995, 30). The words *want to* are key to this definition. Leaders inspire and motivate others to choose to follow them instead of using their positions to force compliance. Because of this, leaders can work at any level of an organization. Although some people are more natural leaders than others, leadership can be practiced and learned. According to Kouzes and Posner (1995), leaders:

- Search for opportunities, [challenging] the status quo to improve their organization and realize the vision

- Experiment and take risks, ensuring that they learn from previous mistakes

- Envision the future, imagining new scenarios and developing vision

- Enlist others, attracting others to join them in their pursuit of the future

- Foster collaboration, promoting trust and a shared vision for the future

- Strengthen others by sharing information and power

- Set an example by role-modeling behaviors that make everyone successful

- Achieve small wins, demonstrating success and building commitment to action

- Recognize contributions, linking rewards with performance

- Celebrate accomplishments, taking the time to acknowledge success

There are three key functions that a person accepts when becoming a leader: 1) authority, 2) responsibility, and 3) accountability. **Authority** gives the leader the right to make decisions. Within every group or team, there has to be one person who makes the final decision after weighing all of the options. **Responsibility** is the duty that the leader accepts in making sure that the goal of the team is accomplished. **Accountability** refers to the concept that the leader must acknowledge failure as well as the success of the team efforts.

Effective leaders do not work in isolation; rather, leaders work in teams. Some leadership experts assert that the basic team (group) is the family, a term that is used to mean a basic unit, whether at home or at work. As such, leadership is the property of the group, influenced by the task that the team needs to accomplish and by the group dynamics, which is the environment in which the group works.

Team Leadership

Team leadership is a critical factor in the success of any team. Whether the team is a standing team within a department or a team charged with a specific short-term task, an effective leader can make a big difference in the outcome. Additionally, team leadership is a great opportunity to improve skills, provide professional development, and make a contribution to the organization. Good team leaders not only have a vision, but are also able to communicate that vision to the other members of the team. They create an atmosphere of challenge, commitment, and determination that excites individuals and inspires performance.

A successful team facilitator provides leadership by (Bennett-Woods 1997):

- Creating a purpose and general framework for the project prior to the first meeting

- Encouraging the team to fully discuss the opportunities and potential pitfalls of the task

- Ensuring that all members of the team participate and reach consensus on the purpose

- Establishing specific goals and measurable objectives around which planning can occur and progress can be measured

- Making sure all decisions and plans are consistent with the purpose and goals

- Building trust among team members by emphasizing the unique role and importance of each team member

- Functioning as a cheerleader, reminding team members of the purpose and goals, celebrating achievements, and recognizing the efforts of individual team members

Four steps that occur to make a team functional include forming, storming, norming, and performing (Heinen and Jackson 1976). Team members are selected because of the perceived value they bring to the group **(forming).** When the team members first come together, they may not know their position within the group, nor to what extent they can trust the other members. **Storming** is when team members try to assert and assess their roles within the group. A strong team leader can also reduce the time the group goes through the storming phase by encouraging open dialog while retaining the leadership role. Once everyone knows their team role **(norming),** the team can then be productive and work successfully on the team goals **(performing).** Not every team will need to go through all of these steps, especially if team members already have a working relationship together. Elements of each of these are described below.

Executive Support

Teams do not work in a vacuum. In addition to creating an effective team, the team leader must work to ensure that the organization supports the team by providing appropriate resources and commitment. The key to accomplishing this is to identify and communicate with all the stakeholders. The team leader may do this directly or may enlist the aid of an **executive sponsor.** An executive sponsor is usually a member of senior management who ensures that the team stays on track and communicates its progress to other key leaders. An executive sponsor also may ensure that the team obtains the organizational support, normally time and information, required to accomplish its goal. A key role for the team leader is regular communication with the executive sponsor, manager, or director.

At MMC the decision to provide the EHR in the Emergency Department (ED) had executive support from the chief information officer (CIO) and the chief financial officer (CFO). These two individuals saw that implementing the EHR in one department in the beginning versus all departments at one time had several advantages: it allowed the IT department to test for bugs in both the hardware and software; it allowed management to determine whether the new processes worked efficiently and effectively. In particular, the CFO was interested in looking at the return on investment (ROI) that implementing the EHR would have for the ED facility. These executive champions made sure that the implementation team had the resources (in money, materials, and personnel) to provide optimal results. Without the executive support, the implementation could have run into barriers created by departments whose intent was to protect their own turf, which handicaps the organization in meeting the objectives stated in the strategic plan (see below).

Team Purpose

Not all teams are necessarily effective. For example, a team without a clear purpose could create a product that does not accomplish the work for which it was designed. A leader who dominates the team could reduce its effectiveness and frustrate its members. Members who do not participate, have insufficient expertise, or are unconcerned with success could cause the team to fail. Members who work outside the team or do not support its decisions can create dissension and reduce support for the outcome.

The purpose of the team should be very focused for the task at hand. The purpose should be enlarged to include tasks or goals beyond the reason the team was originally assembled. One of the dangers of teamwork is that the purpose increases as time goes on so that the focus of the team is diluted resulting in a lack of depth over time. The purpose must be clearly understood not only by every team member but also by management so that there is no misunderstanding of the expected outcomes of the team's efforts. A lack of clear purpose can delay essential teamwork as the team members are expecting different outcomes than what management originally intended.

Leading teams is an important part of managing human resources. Careful consideration should be given to creating the team's purpose and composition. Team members need to feel that their work is important and that their contribution makes a difference. A well-run team can be an effective and productive force. A poorly run team can waste time and frustrate and demoralize staff.

Team Selection

Whether selecting a permanent staff team or members of a team for a short-term project, making the right choice is fundamental to the team's success. Putting together a team involves understanding the challenges to be faced and considering all of the perspectives, experience, and knowledge that will be needed. Since the stakes are higher for a hiring decision, additional care should be taken. The members of the team should be selected for what they can contribute to the team. Member selection should not be based purely on job title; rather, team members should be selected for the tasks that they actually can perform and the responsibilities they can carry out. If possible, every stakeholder should have a place on the team. However, in most cases this is not feasible because the team might become too large. The right size of a team depends on the nature of the team's charge. For large-scale projects, a large team is appropriate and then subgroups can be formed to perform the actual work. For smaller projects, no more than 8 to 10 people should be appointed to the team. Any more than 10 individuals on a team and the work becomes bogged down with topics and issues not related to the cross-functional team. Ideally all stakeholders should have representation on the team; however, sometimes the number of stakeholders is too large for efficiently running smaller teams. In that case, the stakeholders that will be most affected by the outcomes of the team's work should be represented on the team.

The team that was selected at MMC for the implementation of the EHR in the Emergency Department contained people identified as being stakeholders in the implementation process. For example, members on the team included the director of the emergency services, an emergency physician whose main interest was medical informatics, an emergency department nurse, the director of the health information management department, representatives from the information technology department, and a project manager who led the team and reported directly back to the facility's chief executive officer (CEO). In some cases the appointments were political (that is, members were appointed solely because of their position) but in most of the other appointments, members were selected based on their knowledge of and experience with the processes to be implemented.

Team/Member Participation

Teams are created to complete specified charges (goals and objectives established by upper-level management). Each team has its own charges and timelines for accomplishing the work assigned.

The biggest advantage of a team over an individual is the team's ability to bring a variety of perspectives and expertise to the issue. The team leader's responsibility is to ensure that each member has the opportunity to contribute. One way to accomplish this is to provide the team with structured tools to assist in their discussion. Developing flowcharts for each technical area being considered can clarify the process and document several perspectives. This activity often identifies unnecessary complexity and miscommunication in any process. Revised flowcharts can be used to describe changes and communicate new workflows. Facilitated brainstorming is another method to engage all members of a team in problem solving by allowing them to be creative in a safe and nonjudgmental exercise.

Teams should meet on a regular scheduled basis, with the time between meetings dependent on the type and amount of independent work required outside of the team meetings. Every member of the team should be willing to dedicate the time required to accomplishing the team's goals. While it is normal that some people may not be able to make every meeting, chronic absenteeism of members will not produce the desired outcomes. Members might also be required to do additional work outside of team meetings. Team members must be willing to perform these tasks, and to attend the meetings prepared to accomplish specific goals.

Team Norms

Team norms are the rules that govern behavior and define what is acceptable and not acceptable for the group. Team norms can promote a higher level of performance that may directly relate to a higher quality of the team outcomes. No employee comes to work to be detrimental to the organization; however, a team without rules or guidelines almost ensures anarchy. Developing the team norms can be a rigorous process as every team member brings different experiences and backgrounds. Examples of team norms include: getting to meetings on time, being prepared with readings or assignments when due, and not criticizing other employee's ideas or comments.

Recruitment, Orientation, and Training

Recruitment is the process of finding, soliciting, and attracting employees. **Retention** is the ability to keep valuable employees from seeking employment elsewhere. This section describes common practices used for staff recruitment, orientation, and training.

Staff Recruitment

Understanding the organization's recruitment and hiring policies or seeking the assistance of human resources is necessary before announcing the vacancy.

There are several ways to advertise a staff opening, both internally and externally. The first thing to consider is whether to promote someone from inside or to look for candidates outside the organization. The advantage to promoting from within is that the act often motivates employees to do well, learn new skills, and work toward advancement. To advertise a vacancy internally, the organization might post it on facility bulletin boards or list it in the organization's newsletter or website. The supervisor or department manager may announce an opening at a routine staff meeting or use any other communication channels available. Management must communicate a promotional opportunity to all staff rather than to the employee who is the most likely candidate. Broad posting is seen as fair and strengthens communication of the underlying message that, whenever possible, internal candidates are considered first.

If the position cannot be filled from within, there are several ways to advertise it externally. For example, the organization might run an ad in a newspaper, post the job on recruitment websites, announce the opportunity at professional meetings, contact people who have previously applied or expressed interest in working at the organization, or work through a recruiter.

In most cases, the approach used depends on the position. For example, the facility might run an ad for a file room position in a local newspaper, but not in a professional journal. On the other hand, the facility might turn to a professional recruiter when trying to fill a department director or experienced coding position.

As in every industry, job seekers looking for professional-level positions in healthcare submit resumes. A resume describes the candidate's educational background and work experience and usually includes information on personal and professional achievements. Candidates also often submit a cover letter describing the type of position in which they are interested. Finally, today, it is common for candidates and organizations to conduct the preliminary screening process through electronic mail.

Most organizations ask every candidate to complete a formal job application. People seeking entry-level positions may be asked to complete an application, but not necessarily to submit a resume.

Employment Interviews

Interviewing is the most important skill that supervisors use in hiring new staff. Failure to adequately prepare for conducting the interview can have serious consequences. Prior to the interview supervisors and managers should read the applicant's resume and think about the questions they need to ask during the interview that are appropriate to the position description.

The interview itself has four basic purposes:

- To obtain information from the applicant about his or her past work history and future goals

- To give information to the applicant about the organization's mission and goals, and the nature of the employment opportunity

- To evaluate the applicant's work experience, attitudes, and personality as a potential fit for the organization

- To give the applicant an opportunity to evaluate the organization as a potential fit for his or her current and future employment goals

A key part of the interview will deal with whether the candidate's education, skills, and experience provide a good fit for the job. Competency-based questions may be asked and a test of their technical skills may be administered.

If the candidate has had previous supervisory experience, it is appropriate to ask scenario-based questions. For example, to ask how the candidate would handle a situation where two employees have a disagreement about a work assignment would be suitable. The answer the candidate gives may provide insight into how the candidate listens, empowers employees, or approaches conflict. For a candidate without supervisory experience, the question can be changed by asking how the situation should be handled or how the candidate has seen such a situation handled effectively by others. The following are some examples of interview questions that can be added to specific questions about a candidate's resume or qualifications for a particular job:

- Why are you looking for a job?

  Beware of candidates who talk negatively about a previous employer. This may signal a lack of responsibility for their own actions and may also indicate how they will talk about your organization in the future.

- Because not everyone in a company is well liked by everyone, what would someone who did not like you have to say?

  The answer may provide insight into how this person gets along with others.

- What has been your biggest mistake at work, and what did you learn from it?

  If the candidate cannot describe a mistake, he or she may lack self-reflection and may not consider mistakes as learning opportunities.

- What criticisms would your previous manager have about you?

  This answer may provide insight into work habits or performance.

All questions during the interview must be focused on the job and the applicant's ability to perform the work. There are some questions that may not be asked during the interview. Listed below are topics that cannot be discussed directly. When in doubt, the Human Resource department should be consulted to determine what is appropriate.

- Nationality
- Religion
- Age
- Marital and family status
- Sexual orientation/gender
- Date of birth
- Anything about children or childcare
- Health and physical abilities
- Is applicant a member of the National Guard or Reserves

Prior to making a hiring decision the candidate's references should be checked. Even though most past employers may not provide a lot of information, the accuracy of the information the candidate has provided, including work history and education, can be confirmed. Candidates can lie on their resumes and applications, so checking references is a relatively easy way to verify that the information provided is true. Generally there are several stages to the interviewing process including a screening interview where candidates are either moved on or eliminated at the beginning of the process based on a set of criteria established prior to the interviewing process, then an interview by a team or committee, and then culminating with an interview with senior management.

Orientation and Training

Once employed, the new employee should complete orientation and job training. One of the key factors in employee satisfaction is feeling knowledgeable and competent. This begins with an effective orientation and training program for new employees. Just as the supervisor prepared for the interview and selection of a new employee, plans must be made to help the new employee learn about the organization, the department, and the job.

Orientation

Most large organizations have a formal new **employee orientation** process. This process may involve a one-on-one session with human resources, group training with new employees from all over the organization, or some form of computer-based training.

Generally, the orientation session addresses the organization's mission and vision, goals, and structure; general employment policies; employee conduct; communication; safety training. Of particular interest to HIM professionals is training on privacy, confidentiality, and how to report privacy violations. It also may include a tour of the facility and cover computer access and responsibilities. If the organization provides this type of orientation, the supervisor must know the material covered and feel comfortable answering any questions or directing the new employee to the appropriate resource for follow-up.

After the general orientation, the employee should attend a departmental orientation in the area in which he or she will work. The departmental orientation should clarify the rules to follow and provide a context for job performance. A departmental orientation checklist might include the following topics:

- Mission and vision
- Goals
- Structure
- Communication policies
- Procedure for requesting time off
- Person to notify in case of absence
- Tour
- Introductions
- Confidentiality policies

- Evaluation process
- Schedules

Job Training

After the new employee has been oriented to the organization and the department, specific job training should be provided. The position description is a good place to begin. This document is usually shared in the interview process, but it takes on new meaning when the employee actually begins work.

The supervisor should first explain why each task in the position description is performed and then review the policies and procedures for the task. This gives the employee information about workflow and available resources. Next, the supervisor should demonstrate how to do the task using the procedure for it. Having observed the supervisor perform the task, the employee should feel comfortable enough to try it. The supervisor now should observe the employee's work, correcting any errors and answering questions. Finally, the employee should be allowed time to work on his or her own. The supervisor should check the new employee's work periodically to ensure the employee understands the training and the work is error free.

The supervisor must be very patient during the first days and schedule adequate time to spend with the new hire. Everyone learns differently and at a different pace. The first days not only establish how the employee will do the job, but also contribute to ongoing relationships. Continued training is essential to ensure that the new employee fully understands the job as this will eliminate rework thereby increasing productivity and ensuring that the position does not have to be refilled due to poor performance.

Staff Retention

It is normal to have a certain level of staff turnover. Employees move, retire, or seek other careers. A supervisor can do little to prevent turnover caused by personal change such as a spouse moving out-of-state or a divorce. However, the supervisor and organizational policies can have an impact on **staff retention.** The following questions should be considered:

- Do organizational policies support continued education either financially or through flexible work schedules?
- Do employees have the opportunity to advance their careers within the organization?
- Are salaries and benefits competitive?
- Do working conditions provide a comfortable and safe environment?

Although a supervisor may have limited influence on these elements of employment, he or she may be able to address other concerns that often cause employees to seek other jobs. For example, employees can become dissatisfied if they feel their work is not appreciated or that they are being treated unfairly. In some cases, they become dissatisfied because they feel overworked, underutilized, or they do not understand how their job contributes to the organization's goals. In other cases, employees may resent being too carefully supervised or working in a constant state of chaos. The challenge to the supervisor is to realize that every employee has different needs. What makes one employee satisfied may not be what another employee requires; in other words, one solution may not fit every situation. The supervisor must find a balance that appeals to each employee and is perceived as being fair. This is no small task. Ways to increase employee morale include recognizing an employee when they have performed a job well, providing a safe and calm work environment, and providing the resources the employee needs to be successful.

Staff turnover is expensive in terms of both lost productivity and recruitment and training costs. To ensure effective management, turnover should be monitored across time and benchmarked with the rest of the organization and/or other organizations in the community or area. Routine satisfaction surveys can help provide information on how employees are feeling about their jobs and insights into how the facility might improve working conditions. The exit interview is another way to obtain information on how employees feel about their jobs and what issues cause them to leave.

Delegation of Authority and Empowerment

Another important part of the manager's function is empowering employees and team members through the **delegation of authority.** The level of authority an employee is given and the types of decisions he or she is empowered to make should be considered when setting the salary for the position and determining its educational and experiential requirements. The responsibilities of the position should be clearly described in the job description. The supervisor can then use the job description in setting performance expectations with individual employees.

Delegating responsibilities and projects to other staff members can greatly benefit managers and supervisors. Delegating authority:

- Frees the team leader to perform more important or complex tasks
- Increases the leader's capacity and productivity
- Reduces delays in decision making
- Develops the staff's capacity and abilities

As a rule, employees should be given as much control as possible over their jobs and the work they perform within their teams. One reason for this is that they usually have the most information about how to improve the processes and productivity in their own areas or address the challenge they have been given. The manager's role is to establish expectations and provide a reason for employees to want to do a better job. This may be accomplished through motivational methods such as recognition or promotion.

When delegating authority, managers should prepare staff members to succeed by:

- Explaining exactly what needs to be done
- Describing clear expectations
- Setting clear deadlines
- Granting authority to make relevant decisions
- Ensuring appropriate communication and reporting
- Providing the resources needed to complete the task

Performance Management

Performance management is the process that businesses use to ensure that goals, as derived from the strategic plan, are being met in the most efficient and effective ways possible. The process includes five stages: planning, monitoring, developing, rating, and rewarding.

In the **planning stage** the organization's goals are defined and it is determined how the performance standards are to be applied at the departmental level. The performance standards need to be measurable, understandable, verifiable, and achievable. It is important to receive input from the employees whose jobs are affected to determine what is feasible and to establish buy-in. This helps ensure that the employees will work hard to achieve the goals.

In the **monitoring stage** the performance standards are monitored continuously. This includes monitoring employee performance and providing feedback so that any changes that need to be made can be implemented during the process rather than waiting until the end.

Training issues regarding introducing a higher skill set or improving work processes to the employee are identified in the **developing stage.** Training also encourages good performance, reinforces job-related skills, and helps the employee stay current on new procedures or technologies.

In the **rating stage** performance evaluations are made so that the organization can ensure that the new procedures are being performed to the optimal limits (see below). This helps the organization determine who the best performers are.

In the **rewarding stage** the organization recognizes employees, either individually or in groups, for excellent performance. This stage is important as the rewards will reinforce good behaviors and encourage other employees to do the same. The rewards can be as simple as a thank you or as elaborate as a gift. What is important to understand about performance management is that it is not a straight-line process. Much like quality improvement, performance management is a circular or spiral process; in other words, performance management is never completed.

As mentioned above a **performance evaluation** is a tool often used to structure discussions regarding individual performance. Usually done on an annual basis, performance reviews include:

- Assessing of the employee's performance compared to performance standards or previously set goals

- Developing job-related goals for the following year

- Developing a plan for professional development

Reviews also may include an employee's self-assessment. In some organizations, other employees may contribute information to the review. In the case of a supervisor, his or her staff may participate in the evaluation. This form of evaluation in which supervisor, peers, and staff contribute is called a 360-degree evaluation.

Many organizations base pay increases on the results of an annual performance review. Whether or not the evaluation affects salary, the annual review is an opportunity to formally discuss accomplishments, development, and new expectations.

Periodic Performance Reviews

Performance management is an ongoing process. Information about performance should be collected regularly and shared with the employee, whether the job is coding records or directing a department. Good performance results should be shared to encourage and reward ongoing success.

Performance issues are rarely resolved by ignoring them. Understanding the cause of problems and working with employees to resolve them is an important supervisory task. Actions that can be taken to improve performance include retraining, streamlining responsibilities, reestablishing expectations, and monitoring progress.

Performance Counseling and Disciplinary Action

When actions taken to improve performance are unsuccessful, more formal counseling and even **disciplinary action** may be required. Most organizations have formal processes in place to ensure that all staff are treated fairly and that employment laws are considered. Supervisors should consult with the human resources department to ensure that any disciplinary actions comply with approved procedures.

The steps described in establishing performance standards, hiring and training employees, and conducting routine performance reviews are all necessary before doing performance counseling or taking disciplinary action. Moreover, steps to improve performance should be taken in all cases.

Performance counseling usually begins with informal counseling or a verbal warning. No record is kept in the employee's file.

Progressive discipline begins with formal documentation of the problem and the steps taken to correct it. Employees may be required to submit an action plan of steps they are committed to take to resolve issues and improve their performance. Execution of the action plan may be binding on the employee, and failure to comply could result in termination.

In other environments, disciplinary actions include suspension from employment without pay, demotion to a job with lower expectations and less pay, or termination. In some cases, more than one of these actions may be taken. Generally, however, suspension and demotion are less popular than the use of binding performance improvement plans because suspension and demotion create a punitive atmosphere. Such punitive actions also affect the morale of other employees and staff. Empowering employees to create a plan of action places the responsibility for performance improvement in their own hands.

Regardless of the counseling or disciplinary actions mandated by the organization, supervisors should take some key steps of their own. They should:

- Be clear and direct with the employee about problems and consequences
- Support the employee's efforts to improve or resolve issues
- Document the steps taken to improve performance
- Follow all organizational policies
- Consult with human resources
- Keep performance issues confidential
- Be consistent with all employees

Conflict Management

Conflicts are inevitable and arise when we feel our values, perspectives, or opinions are being threatened. Not all conflicts are considered a negative in a work environment as they can often be of value as new ideas are raised helping people recognize and benefit from their differences, and can also increase productivity. However, conflict can waste time, reduce productivity, decrease morale, and lead to harmful behavior.

Causes of Conflict

There are many causes of conflict in the workplace including:

- Poor communication. One of the leading causes of employee dissatisfaction and conflict with management is poor communication. Employees want to be informed about changes affecting their jobs and work environment. They want to feel like they are part of the organization. When decisions are made without employee input or the rumor mill provides more information than what is coming from management, employees may feel dissatisfied. As a result morale can drop, and conflicts between management and staff may develop.

- Lack of openness by management or other members of the team. Employees will feel left out if not provided enough information to perform their jobs. This is especially true if the employee feels that management and even other employees on the team are withholding information. It makes them feel that they are not trusted and are considered an outsider to the group.

- Weak leadership. How leadership interacts with employees and management has a significant impact on the workgroup. Leaders should not avoid conflict but work with employees to ensure that everyone follows the team or workplace norms. Avoiding conflict will only accentuate the problem, not solve it.

- Interpersonal interactions with others. How well employees interact with each other has a significant impact on the successful outcomes of a team, a department, or an organization. Personality traits, needs, and wants often conflict with other employees and management.

- Lack of resources. Lack of resources can cause employees to question if management values their work and if sufficient attention is being given to support their job functions.

- Desire for more power. There are times when members of the team want to have more control.

Actions for Minimizing Conflict

Before conflicts actually arise there are steps that can be taken to limit or resolve the potential for conflicts. The first step is to make sure that the job responsibilities are clearly defined and job descriptions and departmental procedures are reviewed regularly with input from the employee. As organizations and departments grow, new jobs are created and new responsibilities are added. What the employee was previously responsible for may not coincide with expanded job responsibilities, leading to the necessity of preparing the employee accordingly.

A leader must also build relationships with the team members so that a level of trust is developed. Employees or team members need to feel they can approach the team leader with issues that concern them, that their concerns will be acknowledged, and that the team leader is willing to find a resolution to the problem. Management should receive regular reports on what their subordinates are working on so that potential issues can be handled prospectively rather than retroactively.

Everyone should have regular training on interpersonal communication and conflict management. The training can take the form of regular meetings so that information from management can be passed down to staff.

Conflict Management Strategies

Conflict management focuses on working with individuals to find a mutually acceptable solution. Listed below are methods for dealing with conflicts in the workplace. Depending on the situation, one or more of these methods can be used. Three positive ways to address conflict are:

- *Compromise:* In this method, both parties must be willing to lose or give up a piece of their position.

- *Control:* In this method, interaction may be prohibited until the employees' emotions are under control. The supervisor also may structure their interactions. For example, he or she can set ground rules for communicating or dealing with specific issues. Another form of controlling is personal counseling. Personal counseling focuses on how people deal with conflict rather than on the cause of disagreements.

- *Constructive confrontation:* In this method, both parties meet with an objective third party to explore their perceptions and feelings. The desired outcome is to produce a mutual understanding of the issues and to create a win-win situation.

Certain behaviors or practices by the manager can make conflict worse. The following management behavior should be avoided:

- *Avoiding:* In this method, one or more of the individuals in conflict chooses to ignore that there is even a problem. The problem is not resolved and stays hidden yet active below the surface.

- *Accommodating:* In this method one party to the conflict gives in and allows the other participant to have their way. While this might resolve the immediate problem, needs are not being met.

If a confrontational situation occurs, the following practices are useful in mitigating the situation:

- Speaking calmly

- Moving the discussion to a more private place away from others

- Listening to the other person's argument or point of view

- Paying attention by nodding your head or repeating/rephrasing what the other person is saying

- Acknowledging points of agreement and disagreement

- Trying to build a consensus

Grievance Management

Grievance management includes the policies and procedures used to handle employee complaints. Employees have the right to disagree with management and can express their opinions in a variety of ways. They should be encouraged to bring problems and concerns directly to their supervisors. If they do not achieve receive satisfaction at that level, the supervisor should explain further options. For example, dissatisfied employees should understand that they can either take their issues to the next management level or discuss them with human resources.

Employees who belong to a union should follow the grievance procedures set by their union. Union contracts usually specify the types of actions employees can take and the time frames for filing grievances. The contracts usually specify time frames for responses and define the formal process for elevating the consideration or resolution of a grievance. Grievances taken to the highest levels will likely have to be resolved through mediation or arbitration.

Each of these steps takes time and can cost money. Therefore, supervisors should try to avoid grievances by maintaining open and effective communication with their staffs.

Employee Development

Employee development refers to the ongoing joint efforts of both the employer and the employee to upgrade the employee's skills, knowledge, and abilities. Healthcare employee development is extremely important and is driven by three conditions:

- The rate of change in healthcare
- The introduction of new technology into the workplace
- The increased demand on maximizing productivity

Donald Super (Super 1955, 1980, 1990) extensively studied employee development and identified the following four stages:

1. *Exploration and trial:* In this stage the employee works with regular guidance and learns to ask for help and take initiative.
2. *Establishment and advancement:* In this stage the staff member has his or her own area of responsibility, works independently, more than likely has a specialization, and can produce significant results.
3. *Mid-career growth, maintenance, decline:* In this stage the employee is responsible for guiding others (it may or may not be in a management position) and uses a large set of technical skills and usually serves as a mentor to others.
4. *Disengagement:* In this stage, the employee will use his or her experiences to provide direction to the organization. The employee may also be preparing to accept a different role; learning to let go of his or her current job in search of something more challenging.

It can be helpful for the employer to evaluate employees based on the stage of development that they are currently at. The employer can then determine how to approach the development process, whether through assigning a mentor, exposing the employee to committee or team work, assigning the employee to temporary assignments that expand the employee's knowledge base, job shadowing, networking, or assigning a career coach. What is important is that the supervisor provides positive and corrective feedback and ensures that there are educational opportunities available for the employee to participate in.

Returning to the example of MMC at the beginning of this chapter, the HIM director needed to identify one of the department coders who could make the transition from coding paper charts to coding from medical information contained within an electronic format. While the medical information is the same, the coder would have to become familiar with both the screen content and where to find specific information. Since this is a pilot project, the director wanted to get the best possible coder available to ensure success on the HIM end of the process. Utilizing the performance management stages, one of the coders stood out as being in stage 3, which meant that this person was comfortable in what he or she was doing, but would also take on the challenge of learning new material and processes. After the coder was selected, it was observed that several of the coders that were not selected expressed their unhappiness at not being selected by spreading rumors that the project was going to fail, slowing down their productivity, and openly defying the coding supervisor. The HIM department director met with the troubled employees and found that it was poor communication on the part of the director in not letting all of the coders know that they would be trained in the new coding system at some point in the future. Using the art of compromise, the director agreed to include the other coders in the training of the new system along with the coder that was originally selected. This made the coders feel that they were appreciated, that management listened to their grievances, and that they were part of the process. The net result was that rather than only training one coder on the new system, several were trained to the benefit of not only the department but to the organization as a whole.

Strategies for Developing Staff Skills

Supervisors are responsible for creating an environment that develops the skills of their staff. No one can make another person learn something, but providing the opportunity for development is critical to creating a successful learner. Following are the three main approaches to training:

- *On-the-job training* provides direct, realistic training in the specific tasks required by the position. The employee's supervisor and peers are available for immediate feedback because they are involved in the training process. On-the-job training can be used with individuals who do not do well in traditional classroom training but can easily handle the work.

- *Information presentation* resembles the traditional classroom approach to education. This approach may include lectures, small group discussions, case studies, audiovisual techniques, and computer-assisted instruction. The training may be offered by the employer, a college or university, professional associations, or for-profit training centers. Information presentation methods range in scope from one-day courses to for-credit college programs. They vary in effectiveness based on the skill being taught, the match of teaching style to learner, and how well the information learned can be applied directly to the job.

- *Action-based methods* of training involve simulations, role-playing, and case studies. Role-playing and simulations give learners the ability to practice new behaviors in a safe environment. Conducted in small group settings, a situation is described and individuals are given roles to act out. In a simulation, learners normally use a defined set of resources to solve a problem in addition to playing a role. Case studies are a more passive form of training. Instead of actually participating in a situation, the learners study how an individual or organization responded to a real-life situation and what the outcomes were.

Regardless of the form of training used, a commitment to ongoing training is critical to maintain and enhance skills, to prepare people for new and higher-level jobs, and to create an interesting and rewarding work environment.

Job Redesign

One way a supervisor can create a positive and rewarding work environment is through **job redesign.** Creatively aligning the needs of the organization with the skills and interests of the employee and then designing the job to meet those needs is job redesign at its best. The reasons to redesign a job may be to introduce new tools or technology, improve a process, use employee skills more effectively, or provide better customer service. Generally, all these outcomes can be addressed through job redesign.

The best way to begin the process of job redesign is to discuss the job with the employee. The supervisor should identify barriers to the employee's current work and areas of frustration. Perhaps the employee feels that he or she is wasting time performing a task at a lower skill level than the rest of the work. Perhaps he or she would like to take on more complex work.

The supervisor should examine the workflow process that includes the employee's job. Does the process involve other tasks the employee could assume? Are there functions in related processes that could be combined into the employee's job? If several people perform similar work, a test or pilot of a new job design might be done with one or two individuals to work out unanticipated problems.

It is important to ensure that training is provided for any new work. Job redesign is one way to initiate or manage change in the workplace, but managing change is an ongoing challenge.

Career Planning and Lifelong Learning

Finding a job is different from planning a career. Although **career planning** may include getting a job, a career extends beyond current job requirements and positions the employee for more challenging and diverse work. When assisting an employee in career planning, supervisors should take the following actions:

- *Lead by example:* They should show how they have enhanced their careers by accepting risk, new challenges, and added responsibilities. Their commitment to lifelong learning should be evident in their actions as job growth requires the addition of new skills and knowledge.

- *Create a supportive environment:* Supervisors should allow time for training and allocate money, whenever possible, to advance the skills of employees. Scheduling must be flexible to allow employees to pursue advanced degrees or continuing education.

- *Provide career counseling:* When possible, supervisors should provide staff with career counseling resources within the organization or connect with community college or university training counselors.

- *Create a partnership:* Supervisors should expect employees to fulfill their commitments when it comes to training and education.

Career planning and lifelong learning are personal. No supervisor can accept responsibility for planning someone else's career. However, through effective leadership, employees can be encouraged and rewarded to see beyond their current job.

Check Your Understanding 18.2

1. The term that defines the right of a leader to make decisions is
    A. Authority
    B. Responsibility
    C. Accountability
    D. Leadership

2. Which of the following is used in the recruitment process?
    A. Monitoring turnover
    B. Conducting reference checks
    C. Holding orientation sessions
    D. Ensuring job training is available

3. Which of the following occurs when a supervisor delegates authority?

   A. Decreases need for performance standards
   B. Reduces the delay in decision making
   C. Eliminates monitoring turnover
   D. Limits staff capabilities

4. In which stage of performance management are performance evaluations conducted?

   A. Planning
   B. Monitoring
   C. Rating
   D. Rewarding

5. In what employee development stage does an employee guide and mentor others?

   A. Exploration and trial
   B. Establishment and advancement
   C. Mid-career growth, maintenance, decline
   D. Disengagement

Instructions: Indicate whether the following statements are true or false (T or F).

6. _____ Performance evaluation is a tool often used to structure discussions regarding team performance.

7. _____ Staff turnover is expensive in terms of lost productivity and recruitment and training costs.

8. _____ Supervisory-level management responsibilities include new employee orientation and training.

9. _____ One thing that teams have in common is that their members are usually from the same department.

10. _____ When redesigning a job, the supervisor should not discuss potential changes with the employee.

Fundamentals of Work Planning

In healthcare organizations, the planning function includes strategic and operational planning. **Strategic planning** generally deals with the organization's long-term approach to the future. Most healthcare organizations' strategic plans apply to activities over at least a five-year period. Operational planning generally deals with the organization's short-term activities. Most healthcare organizations' **operational plans** apply chiefly to the next calendar year.

Strategic Planning

Strategic planning is concerned primarily with how the organization will respond to changes in its external environment in the foreseeable future. Traditionally, the time frame for looking into the future has been 5 to 10 years; however, recently organizations have reduced the planning outlook to 3 to 5 years. These plans take into account environmental factors, which include changes in the organization's external business climate, its competitive status, and/or the broader social and political climate in which it operates.

Strategic planning is an ongoing activity. The output of the strategic planning process is a yearly update and revision of the organization's written strategic plan. The updates focus on action planning for the upcoming year and project plans over several subsequent years.

As noted earlier, primary responsibility for strategic planning lies with the organization's board of directors. However, the board works closely with the executive management team throughout the strategic planning process. In large part, the board depends on the executive staff to provide the information on which the process is based. In turn, the executive team gathers and formulates strategic planning information that was originally collected and analyzed by middle-level managers. As part of their regular management duties, middle-level managers collect a great deal of detailed operational information from the records and databases created by supervisors and staff-level employees.

The strategic planning process is not the same for every organization. Its details vary significantly depending on the type of services the organization provides and its size and structure, corporate structure (for example, for-profit versus not-for-profit), and competitive status. In most healthcare organizations, however, strategic planning involves the following general steps:

1. *Conducting an environmental assessment:* An **environmental assessment** is a collection of information about changes that have occurred in the organization's internal and external environment since the previous year. They may have potentially positive or negative effects on the organization that can be considered threats and/or opportunities for the future. An example of an internal change might include an increased movement toward employee unionization. An external change might be a merger between two of the organization's biggest competitors.

2. *Developing and/or revising the mission and vision statements in response to the environmental assessment:* The organization's mission and vision statements represent broad expressions of its current and future purpose. When the results of the environmental assessment point to a need for fundamental change within the organization, these public statements represent the organization's first acknowledgment and response to that need.

3. *Developing and/or revising the values statements:* The beliefs and values of healthcare organizations usually are rooted in a fundamental respect for the rights and uniqueness of individuals. As such, they do not change significantly from year to year. Changes in the wording or direction of the organization's mission and vision, however, sometimes require a minor rewording of its values statements.

4. *Developing and/or revising the strategic plan for the upcoming year:* In most healthcare organizations, the board's strategic planning committee revises and updates the strategic plan. It works directly with key members of the organization's executive management team to analyze information and trends. Specific strategies for the future are developed on the basis of these trends. The strategic planning committee and executive leaders also work together to make plans for succeeding years. Together, they develop of list of specific recommendations for action.

5. *Revising the strategic plan for the succeeding years in light of the changes made to the plan for the upcoming year:* In addition to devising strategies for the upcoming year, the future strategic plan may need revision. Revisions may be needed to address changes in strategic direction, new regulations that require a long-term response, or economic or technical changes that affect the organization. Frequently, changes in the coming year's plan have a ripple effect on future years.

6. *Developing specific action steps for the upcoming year:* Strategic plans often include a list of specific **action steps** (or plans) the organization should take in the near future. The plans describe projects to be undertaken by board-designated committees or managerial action teams to address threats or opportunities. For example, the strategic planning committee of a private urban hospital might recommend that the hospital initiate a plan to close its emergency department within the next five years. Such a recommendation might be made if the hospital's environmental assessment revealed significant financial losses as a result of providing uncompensated care to uninsured emergency patients.

7. *Discussing the proposed strategic plan with the board of directors and making changes as a result:* In the next step of the strategic planning process, the strategic planning committee communicates its draft plan to the board for comments and reactions. Such discussions are conducted during private meetings of the full board officiated by the board chairman.

8. *Officially documenting the board's approval of the plan:* For the strategic plan to become official, the board must approve it through a legal voting process. The board's actions are then documented in the meeting minutes and become a part of the organization's official records.

9. *Communicating the strategic plan to the administrators and managers:* After the new plan has been accepted by a majority of the board, the executive leadership team communicates it to other executive managers of the organization. In turn, the executive managers provide relevant details of the plan to the departmental or functional managers responsible for carrying out its provisions. Under the leadership of executive and middle managers, project teams are created to develop specific design and implementation plans. These plans bring the board's strategic ideas to reality.

10. *Developing operation plans for the upcoming year on the basis of the action steps and future direction documented in the final strategic plan:* Most organizations develop their timelines for operational planning and budgeting to coincide with the board's strategic planning decisions. Successful implementation of the strategic plan requires investments reflected in the budget and incremental achievement of operational objectives.

In the Theory into Practice example at the beginning of the chapter, MMC used a type of strategic planning scenario assessing strengths, weaknesses, opportunities, and threats referred to as SWOT:

- *Strengths:* Internal attributes of the company that make it successful and provide a competitive advantage. At MCC, one strength is its outreach to the community and advancing health screenings.

- *Weaknesses:* Internal attributes that prevent an organization from being successful. At MCC, an example of a weakness would be the lack of a universal EHR throughout all of the hospital and its outlying clinics.

- *Opportunities:* The external environmental analysis may reveal new opportunities for profit and growth. One opportunity for MCC is the creation of a new cardiac center focusing on early detection and screenings.

- *Threats:* External conditions which may prove harmful to the organization. A major threat for MCC is the progression of healthcare moving away from inpatient care toward more ambulatory experiences.

One of the downfalls of using SWOT is that it can be very time-consuming, which may result in the organization missing opportunities because the strategic plan is not completed in time. Creating a strategic plan requires that the participants allocate enough time and energies to making sure that the strategic plan is well thought out, thorough, and capable of being implemented.

Operational Planning

After the strategic plan is in place and has been communicated to managers and staff, an annual operational plan is established to meet the objectives of the strategic plan. The operational plan has a much more defined time frame, usually one or two years. The organization as a whole may have an operational plan and each department within the organization creates an annual plan that states its goals and objectives. Operational plans are normally tied to budget planning because resources are usually required to meet them.

Departmental planning can be approached in several ways. Information is usually gathered to assess the department's strengths and weaknesses and to identify and prioritize initiatives for the coming year. Customer satisfaction surveys can be developed and the results used in planning. Department supervisors may identify recurrent service or production problems that should be addressed in the operational plan. Reviewing the organization's plans to ensure that the department has the resources to contribute to overall success is an essential step. In addition, opportunities may exist for improving productivity through the replacement of equipment or the streamlining of processes.

Department managers play the key role in assembling the operational plan for a department. Other members of the staff, however, may have a role in compiling information or suggesting process changes within a department and within the framework of the operational plan and priorities.

Supervisors organize the work of their teams by setting short-term (usually daily or weekly) goals. These goals must take into account the overall productivity requirements of both the immediate workgroup and the larger functional workgroup (or department) within which the team operates.

The goal-setting process is relatively straightforward. The supervisor's own manager usually provides information on how much work must be accomplished over the upcoming period of time or which operational improvements need to be implemented. The supervisor then determines how much work each team member must accomplish for the team to keep up with its workload.

Obviously, the team's performance depends on the aggregate performance of its members. The challenge for the supervisor is to ensure that each team member has the training and knowledge to carry out the duties assigned. Therefore, a vital component of organization at the supervisory level is organizing the individual tasks in such a way that the employee assigned to perform each task is qualified to do so.

Expense Budgets

An important part of operational planning is planning for and then managing the expenses of the department or section. Financial control is an ongoing process that begins with a budget or financial plan and continues with ongoing monitoring. Effective financial control creates opportunities for improvements in the use of the organization's resources.

The budget is the primary tool for financial control. It represents the organization's financial plan for the coming time period, in most cases a year. The budget year or fiscal year covers 12 months but may not run from January through December (for example, many academic medical centers run on a July 1 to June 30 fiscal year). Different companies use different fiscal years for a variety of reasons. Budgeting is also a process. It is laying out a plan and then routinely checking actual results against the plan and making adjustments as necessary. Budgeting is part of the overall planning process. A budget should support the goals of the organization, not establish them. However, the reality of available resources may alter the approach or time taken in reaching those goals.

Revenues and Expenses

Budgets can be broken down into revenues and expenses. *Revenues* are monies that will be paid to the organization or income that will be earned by the organization. *Expenses* are monies that will be spent by the organization.

Expenses can be further broken down into fixed costs, variable costs, and **mixed** (semifixed and semivariable) **costs. Fixed costs** are costs that remain the same regardless of how much work is done. Depreciation, space costs or rent, managers' salaries, and general office expenses are all examples of fixed costs. **Variable costs** include employee salaries, materials, and other expenses related to how much work is done. For example, the amount of work to be done in a transcription department determines how many staff members are needed, how much paper will be used, and how many computer supplies will be consumed. There probably will be only one manager regardless of the number of transcriptionists employed. However, the number of supervisors may be semivariable based on whether other shifts are required or whether the supervisor-to-employee ratio becomes too high.

Semifixed costs also change depending upon output, unlike variable costs, but those changes are not proportional. An example of semifixed costs would be when a department relies on part-time employees rather than FTEs to perform tasks within the department. For example, as the amount of transcription increases, the department prefers to hire part-time workers rather than hire full-time FTEs. Once the level of transcription decreases the part-time workers are let go. Fixed, variable, and semivariable costs make up the organization's cost structure. The cost structure can have significant impact on organizational decision making.

Two other types of costs are **direct costs** and **indirect costs.** Direct costs are those that are directly accrued by the department, such as salaries and supplies. Indirect costs are those that are not directly traceable back to the department, such as heating and cooling, electricity, and housekeeping. Some organizations will bill back services to the departments to support non-revenue-generating units. For example, housekeeping may charge a department by how many square feet there are in the area to be maintained.

All the above items involve the operating budget. In addition to operating expense is capital expense. Capital budgets include those items the organization will purchase whose value extends beyond one year. Examples include buildings, equipment, and computers. Unlike operating costs, capital costs are one-time expenses, although payment may be spread out over many years in financial reports and tax returns. Capital costs are fixed and are therefore independent of the level of output.

Budgeting Process

At the departmental level, budgeting usually begins with developing a clear statement of the goals the department wants to achieve in the coming year. Information about the overall organization's budget planning is frequently contained in **budget assumptions.** These assumptions may include an estimation of how revenues will increase or decrease and what limits will be placed on expenses.

HIM functions are largely expense based, with limited revenue in areas such as photocopying records for release to outside parties. In some cases, revenue is generated through charging other departments for services (for example, transcription services). The department manager must understand the budget assumptions before starting the department's budget. Anticipating increased volume within the department is related to the organization's assumptions of volume, although there may not be a direct relationship. Also, any plans to increase or decrease work or any changes in regulations that will affect the operation should be considered at budget time.

Several approaches can be taken to develop a budget. Historical projections are based on looking at prior budgets and actual expense reports and then projecting a percentage increase. This might be useful in cases where there is no anticipated increase in staff, but there is an expected salary increase of 4 percent overall. Another method is called zero-based budgeting. In this approach, each cost is built from scratch without reference to historical information. Each cost is developed based on the number of units required and the price per unit. This works well in areas where costs are highly variable and can be directly related to how much work will be produced in the coming year.

Typically, departments use a combination of approaches. Although salaries and benefits may be increased based on a percentage, the projected cost of certain supplies such as chart folders would be based on actual anticipated usage and price per folder. It is important to verify prices with suppliers prior to budgeting to anticipate any increases. Regardless of the approach taken, managers must thoroughly understand the prior year's budget and year-to-date variations in actual performance before beginning the budget.

Usually, a budget review process is part of developing the overall budget. This may include a formal presentation of the budget to senior management. The department manager should understand the entire budget process and be aware of deadlines for submission of the budget.

Financial Control

Financial control does not end with successful budget presentation. Monitoring ongoing expenses and revenues is an important management responsibility. The budget is a plan. When the actual budget does not match the plan, a variety of actions can be taken. In most organizations, monthly reports detailing revenues and expenses are provided. In addition, reports are generated that compare monthly and year-to-date actual results with the budget. These reports should be reviewed each month to ensure that there are no errors in assigning revenues or expenses to the correct budgets and to monitor actual results from the plan. The manager should:

1. Understand what caused the variation or variance from the budget
2. Determine whether the variance will continue or whether it was a one-time occurrence
3. Determine what actions are necessary to modify future results in order to achieve the overall targets

Staying within the budget is only half the equation. Equally important is completing the objectives set out for the year. Meeting the operational goals is as important as meeting the financial ones. Successful managers keep both in mind as they work to implement the plan.

Supply Management

There is little more frustrating for a supervisor than work coming to a stop because of a shortage of supplies. Imagine a release of information function, still heavily reliant on paper copies, when there is no copy paper. Backlogs build, staff members have to be redeployed, and supplies purchased on short notice are frequently more expensive. **Supply management** can therefore be an extremely important element of controlling overall costs.

Effective Purchasing

The first step in supply management is an effective purchasing process. This may be as straightforward as sitting down with an office supply catalog or as complex as issuing a formal request for proposal (RFP). Matching the right purchasing process to the supply is key in getting the right product at the best price. Standardized general office supplies usually assist in both purchasing and inventory control. Items such as pens, note pads, paper, and all general office supplies should be a compromise between meeting the needs of different staff members and cost. This usually requires a purchasing policy that centralizes ordering authority. The organization as a whole may have contracts or other requirements regarding where supplies are purchased and what supplies are authorized.

In larger types of purchases or customized purchases, an RFP is frequently done to ensure that the required products are purchased at the best price. RFPs are almost always required for other types of purchases such as services or software and contain elements such as requirements, cost, service, and information about the supplying company. Additionally, an RFP may contain a request for references. In the area of supplies, file folders may be purchased through an RFP or some other formal purchase process. The requirements would include specifications for paper weight and color, dividers, fasteners, and so on. As health information moves to new technologies, the types of supplies will require change (for example, electronic storage media may replace file folders).

Inventory Control

One of the key elements of supply management is **inventory control.** Inventory control is the balance between purchasing and storing only the supplies needed. This avoids wasting money or space should the requirements for that supply change or the space available for storage be limited. This type of inventory control is referred to as "just in time" (JIT). With JIT, supplies are only ordered as they are needed, without having a large inventory on site. The biggest issue with JIT inventory control is transportation and availability of the supplies when needed.

Centralized purchasing allows better recordkeeping of how much of an individual supply is used within a given time frame. This information allows the purchaser to better estimate the required on-hand inventory and the amount of time from order placement to order fulfillment. A spreadsheet with all the inventory items, suppliers, current stock, distribution schedule, and cost can be extremely valuable in inventory control. One final purpose for tracking inventory is to identify possible theft of supplies when normal usage rates change for unexplained reasons.

Supplier Relationships

Finally, maintaining a productive relationship with suppliers can help control costs and improve efficiency. Spend time with sales representatives discussing current purchases and suggested alternatives. Encourage representatives to discuss new products or services the company offers. Discuss issues that concern purchasing behavior. For example, taking advantage of volume discounts may not be possible due to storage limitations, but some suppliers can assist by providing storage or offering other solutions. Compare products across suppliers, for both quality and price. Although it may be more convenient to use a single supplier, cost and quality advantages may outweigh the convenience. In addition to communicating with suppliers, discuss product choice and satisfaction with other professional colleagues.

To execute an operational plan, a sound budget and strong supply management are critical, but the biggest factor in success is staffing. Tools are available to help with understanding staffing requirements and planning work that can be adopted by anyone responsible for executing an operational plan.

Staffing

In most healthcare organizations, payroll and benefits consume the most resources. Therefore, adequate time and attention must be paid to the management of human resources. Beyond the financial reason, employees' attitudes and morale affect their ability to perform any task effectively. This becomes even more important when their work involves caring for patients directly or supporting the caregivers.

Large entities such as hospitals, large physician groups, and managed care organizations commonly have a human resources department that acts as a reference and support for supervisors. However, any supervisor must have some understanding of the principles of human resources management to lead effectively.

Staffing Tools

Several tools are used to plan and manage staff resources. For example, position descriptions outline the work and qualifications required by the job. Performance standards establish expectations for how well the job will be done and how much work will be accomplished.

In addition to these basics, supervisors must use work schedules to ensure that there is adequate coverage and staff to complete the required work. Schedules are developed first to provide adequate coverage during the hours the organization or department is open for business.

In hospitals, it is not uncommon to find some part of the HIM department open 24 hours a day, 7 days a week. This enables HIM staff to provide information for admissions to the hospital or emergency department, support discharges and transfers, or handle other tasks requiring full-time coverage. In some organizations, the demand for those services is small enough that business office staff, nursing staff, or emergency department personnel can be cross-trained to perform basic HIM tasks.

Another scheduling consideration is space. Space limitations for workstations or workers in the file room may require scheduling staff to other shifts or days. In addition, staff preferences need to be considered in creating the schedule. Balancing the demands of the organization with individual requests for alternate or flexible start times makes scheduling an important part of the supervisor's responsibility.

When there is an understanding of what the coverage needs are, and any space limitations are considered, the next factor to be considered is workflow. **Workflow analysis** ensures that tasks are done in the most efficient order by considering all the steps in a process and then understanding and documenting how they relate to each other. A workflow diagram is often used as a method of documentation because it clearly depicts each step in the process and can point out dependencies and redundancies.

When an optimal workflow is determined, the amount of work and the staff required to complete it must be considered. In a later section on performance and practice standards, the approach described to determine the performance standard is applied to determine the time required to complete a task. That time is then translated into numbers of full-time equivalents (FTEs) from which staffing assignments can be made.

Written policies and procedures (discussed earlier) explaining staffing requirements and scheduling assist the supervisor in being fair and objective and help the staff understand the rules. The amount of personal time off, as sick leave or vacation, also factors into development of a staff schedule and the overall assessment of staff required. The general rule of thumb is that each staff member will produce 2,080 hours of work in the course of a year (8 hours/day times 5 days/week times 52 weeks/year), not including holidays and vacation time.

An example taken from a physician office practice may be useful. One job that must be done each day is pulling charts on existing patients for upcoming appointments. Space limitations allow only one day to pull the charts and store them outside the main file area. A workflow analysis shows that this task is best done when all the charts are returned to the file at the close of each business day because it is more efficient to pull charts from the main file than to waste time looking for them throughout the clinic. Moreover, until an electronic health record is in place, staff must check for the latest lab reports and update the record prior to the appointment. When this step is done after all the charts are pulled, any missing reports can be printed and attached to the record. Chart filing, pulling, and checking for laboratory work can be done by staff with the same skill level, but the workflow suggests that this function is best performed as operations slow from midafternoon into the evening. Based on volume and time, one person should be able to perform this function routinely each day. However, what happens when that person is on vacation or out for an unanticipated leave? Are other people in the office during the evening? Working alone may create a security concern. Perhaps current staff are unwilling to work evening hours. A variety of possible solutions might be considered. Two part-time employees willing to cover for each other when either was out of the office could share the job. If no other workers currently work evening hours, a group of off-hours tasks could be created (coding, transcription, and so on). The work could be combined into other people's existing tasks and spread at both ends of the day so that some tasks are completed in the afternoon and extended to early evening and others are completed by an early morning shift. There is probably no one right solution, but considering all the elements of staffing is required to create the best solution for a given situation.

Frequently, organizations have some type of position classification system that combines jobs with similar levels of responsibility and qualifications into fair wage ranges and benefit packages. For instance, all supervisors may be classified into one wage and benefit category but have unique job descriptions. These classifications also may determine whether an employee belongs to a union.

Work Schedules

Work schedules are an important tool for the supervisor. Knowing when and what employees will be at work and covering shifts and jobs within the department helps the supervisor manage one of the organization's most costly assets—the employee.

There are several models of work schedules that can be utilized within an HIM department:

- *Standard work week:* In the United States the standard work week is 5 days a week at 8 hours a day. This totals 40 hours a week.

- *Compressed work week:* This model provides the employee with the option of either working 4–10 (4 days of 10 hours per day) or 3–12 (3 days at 12 hours per day). In the case of 4–10 the employee will work 40 hours per week, however, with 3–12 the employee will only work 36 hours per week. The advantage of the compressed work week to the employee is the ability to have 3–4 days off per week. This is ideal for working parents. The disadvantages are the concerns about fatigue and errors on the job.

- *Flextime:* This work schedule model allows the employee to vary their hours within a set time range. For example, if the standard work day is 9 a.m. to 5 p.m., a person on flextime might come to work from 10 a.m. to 6 p.m. The employee is still working five days a week but is able to arrange their hours to better fit their schedule. This is ideal for working parents who need to take a child to school or day care before coming to work or employees who are dependent on public transportation.

When planning the employee work schedule, consider the following:

1. Is the job the employee is performing dictated by the equipment they use? For example, if an employee is copying charts for ROI, will the copier be available when the employee is at work, or will other departments be using the copier?

2. Is the job the employee is performing dictated by external entities? For example, do you have an employee taking minutes at a medical staff or quality improvement meeting and the meeting starts at 7:00 a.m.?

3. Should overlapping shifts be considered to provide continuity as one shift leaves and the other shift begins?

4. Should job sharing be considered where two part-time employees make up one FTE?

5. Are any of the employees on vacation?

6. Will there be any work scheduled that is a significant increase of the average work load? For example, when new coding software is to be implemented, coding staff will need to have training on the new software, yet their job loads will still need to be completed. Do you have coverage?

Position Descriptions

A position, or job, description outlines the work an individual does. It generally consists of four parts: a summary of the position including its purpose, a list of duties, and the qualifications for the job. Position descriptions also contain the title of the job.

Position descriptions are used in the recruitment and interviewing phase to explain the work to prospective candidates. They also enable supervisors or human resources personnel to set appropriate wages for positions and resolve performance problems. The supervisor can use the position description to clarify the tasks the employee is expected to perform.

Generally, job descriptions are needed when:

- An entirely new kind of work is required

- Jobs change and the old description no longer fits the duties

- A change in technology or processes dramatically affects the work to be done

Sometimes top performers outgrow their current descriptions. They may find more efficient ways of doing part of their assigned tasks and/or seek new, more interesting, or more meaningful work. Sometimes employees seek a new or updated job description to support an increase in salary, benefits, or a change in title.

When writing new position descriptions, supervisors may use existing descriptions of similar jobs or interview staff members who are currently performing some of the tasks intended for the new job. They also might ask staff members to keep a diary of how they spend their time for a period that reflects a comprehensive cycle of their work. Staff members with more repetitive daily activities may only need to record their activities for a week. In contrast, staff members with more diverse tasks may need a month to document the scope of their duties.

Performance and Practice Standards

In addition to a position description, performance standards are developed for the key functions of the job. These standards indicate each function's level of acceptable execution. Normally, performance standards are set for both quantity and quality and should be as objective and measurable as possible.

Each organization may have a unique approach to the structure of performance standards, such as in the number of levels of measurement. For example, one function of the coder's job would be to code a certain number of charts per day. Some organizations might have only one level of expected performance (for example, no fewer than 20 charts per day). Others might have several levels of expected performance. For example:

30–35 charts per day	Outstanding
25–29 charts per day	Exceeds expectations
20–24 charts per day	Meets expectations
15–19 charts per day	Needs improvement
Fewer than 14 charts per day	Unsatisfactory

The following example shows how a quality standard might be used as a performance indicator of coding accuracy. For example:

91–95 percent accuracy	Outstanding
86–90 percent accuracy	Exceeds expectations
81–85 percent accuracy	Meets expectations
76–80 percent accuracy	Needs improvement
79 percent or less	Unsatisfactory

In this example, a definition for coding accuracy might be helpful. For example, accurate coding includes capturing accurate codes and sequencing them appropriately for all diagnoses and procedures that affect reimbursement.

Standards that are measurable and relevant to an employee's overall performance are helpful in setting clear expectations. They also are helpful in providing useful feedback. Setting standards may be accomplished in a variety of ways. For example, the supervisor might do one of the following:

1. *Benchmark against industry standards:* Benchmarking is the process of determining what the standards are for a specific type facility; that is, 200-bed hospitals are compared against other 200-bed hospitals and not against 1,000-bed hospitals. The process begins by selecting the function to benchmark. Then look at what similar facilities are doing to increase their performance. Since every facility is unique and not every best practice will work in every facility, judge and select that which is appropriate for your department. Finally, implement and evaluate the best practice to ensure that it did indeed improve performance. AHIMA has produced numerous Best Practice guides that can be accessed through the Body of Knowledge.

2. *Collect data on current performance:* When more than one person is performing a task, the data could be collected over time and averaged. The experience and overall performance of each person must be considered in setting the standard. If there are not enough employees to capture data internally, the supervisor might contact other facilities to establish a standard as long as work conditions are comparable.

3. *Share the standards with any employee who performs that task:* Employees must understand the standards and how information about their performance will be collected.

4. *Determine a collection process:* Quantitative measures can be relatively easy to evaluate. In the preceding coding example, the abstracting system may record how many health charts each staff person codes daily. The average then could be generated over all the charts coded every day. If no automated method of data capture is available, actual work could be tracked manually either daily or for selected periods of time throughout the year. Data on the quality level may be harder to aggregate. Supervisors can check a random sample of work over time or discuss the work with a colleague. Findings from external reviews of work such as audits can be used.

5. *Feedback:* Employees should be given feedback so that they understand how they are performing. The feedback should be given close to the time that the data is collected so that the evaluation is current and relevant as job responsibilities may change between the period of data collection and feedback being provided. Whatever the method, the findings should be reported to staff members on a regular basis so that they clearly understand what is expected of them throughout the year.

Work Analysis and Design

Workflow is the process, progress, or flow of the work within a system. The system generally begins with the input, the process to complete the task (such as staff and tools), and ends with the desired output. Also included in the process is the rate at which it happens. Understanding the workflow within a department is crucial for the supervisor in managing the departmental resources. To understand and control the workflow, the supervisor can perform a workflow analysis and then design the process to be more effective and efficient.

Workflow Analysis

Work analysis is performed to streamline and maximize resources by breaking down the process into its component parts. The key to workflow analysis is to identify any bottlenecks that constrict the flow of the process. The bottleneck can be related to personnel, equipment, or even the process itself. Workflow analysis should be performed anytime new staff is assigned to a process, new tasks are assigned, or when the department matures and takes on new responsibilities. The benefits of performing a workflow analysis are identifying what the organization does, how it does it, and the costs associated with those processes.

Workplace Design

One way to improve workflow within a department is to look at the design of the workplace. Workplaces can create stimulating environments making people more alert, creative, and productive. Workplaces can also be an excellent way to create a community of workers, especially people performing the same function.

When designing an office space, you need to be aware of the placement of staff, flow of traffic, noise, and privacy. The placement of staff should support the job and not have people placed randomly throughout the department wherever a desk was open for the new hire. The grouping of desks also allows coworkers to communicate more easily than if they were spread throughout the department. The aisles between desks and partitions act like the highways of the office and should be wide enough so that two people can pass without touching. It is important in workplace design that traffic flow is highest where people need to be moving around the department and lowest around staffs that need more privacy. Departments should also be designed to manage noise. Try to match people to the appropriate noise level as some people tolerate noise better than others. Try to keep functions that deal with staff using the telephone away from the normal noise in the department (that is, copiers, fax machines, and coffee machines). Try to design the office so that the greater noise areas are in the center of the department while the quieter areas are on the margins. It might be prudent to design social areas (that is, break rooms) away from the main work areas. One method of controlling noise as well as privacy is the use of partitions, which buffer sound in a work area.

Space and Equipment

Employees should have enough space to do their jobs, even if they are job sharing or coming in for a split shift. Work space not only includes access to the equipment they need to perform their tasks but also areas for storage. Work spaces also need to create a sense of personal identity. One way to do this is through the use of partitions, which are a great way to provide privacy and reduce sound, and also provide a wall for staff to post personal items to make the work area more individualized. Another factor that provides support to staff is to have utilities on the work surface rather than buried behind a desk or cubicle. This allows the staff member to place more attention to the task at hand rather than being on hands and knees looking for an outlet or USB port.

Aesthetics

Aesthetics (what appeals to the senses) is an important part of office design that can sometimes be overlooked. To create a productive work environment, staff need to feel a sense of comfort and support from their surroundings. This can be accomplished with the use of light, color, plants, and art work.

When designing work spaces the use of light is fundamental as to how people see and even feel at work. The best type of lighting is natural light, but this is not always possible for all work locations. Overhead fluorescent lights can be too bright or even cause headaches; therefore plan on indirect lighting. Color can either stimulate or sooth, depending on management's desired effect. Some simple rules for the use of color:

- Light colors reflect light and give an open airy look
- Natural colors and textures are relaxing
- Only use bright colors for accents
- Coordinate the colors—bring them to harmony
- Contrast will bring attention

Some staff may feel that plants bring a more relaxing environment to their workstation. Use artwork sparingly around the office. Generally relaxing photographs or artwork is desired. Remember that each staff member is different and may interpret lighting, color, artwork, and even plants differently than others. As a result, a neutral design in the main workplace allows each staff member to individualize their own work area within the organizational and departmental policies and guidelines. Office areas should look clean, professional, and organized.

Ergonomics

Ergonomics is the scientific study of work and space, especially as it pertains to worker productivity. The term human factors is commonly used interchangeably with ergonomics in the United States, but the terms are not the same. While *human factors* is a generalized term used to describe the relationship between humans and machines, ergonomics is focused more on the design and use of equipment in relation to human safety.

Some of the consequences of poorly designed work space, especially with the use of computers, are headaches, eye strain, fatigue, neck and back pain, as well as repetitive stress injuries (carpal tunnel syndrome). Measures that can be taken to reduce computer-related discomfort are:

- Adjust the desk, chair, monitor, and keyboard to the height of each user
- Provide chairs with good lumbar support
- Position computer monitors just below eye level
- Use wrist supports to avoid repetitive stress injuries
- Break up repetitive motion with other activities

- Periodically look away from the monitor to distant objects to avoid eye focusing problems
- Minimize screen glare

Good use of ergonomics can save the organization money by reducing workers' compensation, healthcare expenses, and time off from work.

The following scenario illustrates considerations in workplace design:

Janice is a new member of the MMC HIM management staff. She was specifically hired to increase the department's efficiency and effectiveness as the hospital is converting from paper records to an electronic format. Looking around the department she is horrified to see that while there are defined functional areas (that is, assembly and analysis, coding, release of information), not all of the staff assigned to those areas are physically located within the functional area. For example, one of the newer coders is actually located in the release of information (ROI) section. When asked why, a supervisor noted that the new coder was placed where there was an open desk. Janice also noted that transcription was located in the center of the office space and that coding was located away from the chart completion room. Before jumping in and completely rearranging staff work areas, she is aware that some of the staff have become very attached to their current work spaces and that social groupings have formed that may be difficult to break up. It is obvious to Janice that the current work space assignments are inefficient and are producing bottlenecks in the workflow. What would you do if you were in Janice's shoes?

Work Patterns

The *American Heritage Dictionary* defines a *pattern* as a consistent, characteristic form, style, or method with the most basic patterns being based on repetition and periodicity. When applied to the work setting, a work pattern then becomes the pattern of how work is done within the organization and department. In the office, the work patterns are exhibited by how much time is spent on the telephone, computer, doing paperwork, or talking with neighbors and visitors. When the employee is away from his or her desk the work patterns shift to the length of time the employee is in meetings, at the desks of other staff, in training rooms, or in other parts of the facility. Also, during a normal workday, staff will take breaks and socialize, go to lunch, stretch their legs, and enter and leave the building. All of the motions that a worker does during the day contribute to the work patterns of the department.

For individual tasks, work patterns can be identified and analyzed to make sure that the task is being done in the most efficient method. Often when management sees an employee away from his or her desk it is assumed that the employee is not working; however, the employee may be out collecting data or work materials required for a specialized task. For example, in a paper medical record department, the coder will have to leave his or her desk to return the charts that have been coded and bring back new charts. In tumor registry, staff often have to read the obituaries to see if any of their patients have passed away. To the uninformed it may look like the staff are being unproductive when in reality they are working.

Work Distribution

Work should be distributed according to each of the staff's capabilities and job responsibilities. When analyzing the staff's work distribution it is important to identify what each staff member's responsibilities are and how much time it takes to accomplish each task. In many cases tasks are shared between individuals (that is, job sharing). In this case the percentage of time devoted to a task is identified. There are some jobs where some tasks are easier to perform than other tasks. For example, when coding charts, healthy newborn charts are coded very quickly versus those for patients with congestive heart failure (CHF); therefore, it would not be prudent to rate a coder's job based solely on the number of charts coded unless the different types of charts are divided equally among all of the coders.

Staffing Analysis

Staffing analysis determines the most efficient and effective mix of staff. Historically, time and motion studies were used to calculate the number of staff required in a department. These studies provided information on the amount of time required to complete a task but did not provide information on: 1) are the current practices effective and efficient for the organizational structure; 2) are the individuals working at the appropriate levels; and 3) could alternative processes actually be more beneficial? Essentially, time and motion studies are a snapshot of the situation without truly analyzing the staffing needs.

Before determining the appropriate level of departmental staffing, several questions need to be addressed:

- Is the organization managing its regular staff and overtime costs?
- Is the organization taking advantage of economies of scale?
- Is there an appropriate number of staff to meet policy objectives?
- When should there be an increase or decrease of staff as policy goals and workload changes occur?

When determining staffing levels, management needs to recognize that staffing needs are generally driven by: 1) hours of coverage, and 2) an understanding of the workload. In addition, departmental staffing needs should be determined for the average work load, not for emergencies. So where does the manager start? An evaluation of historical workloads is essential, but also the manager needs to be aware of any expected trends such as moving from a paper to paperless medical record. It is important that the supervisor have clear criteria as to what level is sufficient for staffing.

Check Your Understanding 18.3

1. Strategic planning is concerned primarily with how the organization will respond in the foreseeable future to changes in its:

   A. Long-range goals
   B. Mission statement
   C. Short-term activities
   D. Vision statement

2. In developing the organization's strategic plan, the organization's board of directors works directly with the:

   A. Supervisory-level managers
   B. Executive management team
   C. Staff level employees
   D. First-line employees

3. Which of the following is used to guide and carry out the objectives of an organization's strategic plan?

   A. Performance standards
   B. Inventory management
   C. Operational plan
   D. Organizational charts

4. Supervisors organize the work of their teams by setting what type of goals?

   A. Long-term
   B. Short-term
   C. Strategic
   D. Futuristic

5. Together with inventory control and supplier relationships, which of the following are elements of supply management?

   A. Effective purchasing
   B. Position descriptions
   C. Request for proposals
   D. Job enrichment

6. A new hospital is opening near our hospital. This event would likely be represented in a SWOT analysis as a:

   A. Strength
   B. Weakness
   C. Opportunity
   D. Threat

7. The focus of conflict management is:

    A. Getting personal counseling for the parties involved
    B. Separating the parties involved so that they do not have to work together
    C. Working with the parties involved to find a mutually acceptable solution
    D. Bringing disciplinary action against one party or the other

8. The ultimate goal of constructive confrontation is to:

    A. Encourage employees to file grievances
    B. Prevent interaction between the two parties
    C. Provide one-on-one personal counseling
    D. Create a win-win situation

9. Which of the following is an example of a fixed cost?

    A. Office supplies
    B. Rent
    C. Health record folders
    D. Line level employee salaries

10. Which of the following is a standard work week?

    A. 8 hours a day, 4 days a week
    B. 10 hours days, 4 days a week
    C. 8 hours a day, 5 days a week
    D. 12 hours a day, 3 days a week

Performance and Quality Improvement for HIM Functions

The purpose of efficient health information management is to provide high-quality information for decision making at all levels. Whether it is access to patient-specific information at the point of care or trended data to make planning decisions, information is a key resource to improving care and healthcare delivery. An ongoing performance improvement system for HIM should be in place to ensure that the information service meets the needs of all users. The following discussion is an overview of performance and quality improvement. Chapter 11 provides additional detail on performance and quality improvement methods and techniques.

A Model for Quality Improvement

Most healthcare organizations have an established approach to quality improvement. The HIM function may report in some key indicators to that effort. For instance, the number of incomplete records may be reported as it is an outcome reported to the Joint Commission (TJC). Training and other resources for departmental quality improvement efforts may be available from this organizational program.

A departmental or functional **quality improvement process** includes these steps:

Problem identification

1. Identify key performance measures and possibly future measures where warranted by foreseeable changes to regulatory requirements or introduction of new technologies.
2. Measure current performance.
3. Create a flowchart of the current process.
4. Brainstorm problem areas within the current process.
5. Research all regulatory requirements related to the current process.
6. Compare the current process to the organization's performance standards and/or nationally recognized standards.
7. Conduct a survey to gather customer input on their needs and expectations.
8. Prioritize problem areas for focused improvement.

Process redesign

1. Incorporate findings or changes identified in the research phase of the improvement process.
2. Collect focused data from the prioritized problem areas.
3. Create a flowchart of the redesigned process.
4. Develop policies and procedures that support the redesigned process.
5. Educate involved staff on the new process.
6. Measure for success to identify when new processes are successfully implemented.

Problem Identification

To understand the steps of problem identification or improvement opportunity, consider each one separately.

The first step is to identify key performance measures. These are the ongoing outcomes of the principal activities that affect the overall delivery of HIM services to customers (physicians, the operating room, revenue cycle management team, nursing units, regulatory agencies, or others). Key performance measures may include transcription turnaround, availability of paper or electronic information for admissions or clinic visits, days in accounts receivables, and so on.

Ongoing measuring and monitoring of the key performance measures can signal an interruption or degradation of service that may need to be addressed and is step two in the problem identification process. In most cases, there is an acceptable range of variation that would not signal further investigation or a result may be affected by a known and temporary event (for example, turnaround times could rise because a power outage delayed transcription). Where monitoring demonstrates a significant variation from internal or external benchmarks, further investigation may be warranted.

Creating a flowchart of the current process is a good way to document the process. This should be done with involvement of the staff most directly involved in the process. It is also important to document the process as it really occurs, not as it should happen.

Discussion of the flowchart may uncover redundancies or points of failure in the process. Brainstorming the possible problems with each step in the process (particularly where handoffs are made from one step to another) is useful in collecting a variety of opinions on where the flaws exist. Documenting the current process and then brainstorming potential problems reduce the likelihood of making assumptions of what should be fixed without adequate study.

Consideration should be given to all regulatory requirements of a process. Sometimes deleting a step that seems to be a perfect way to improve efficiency is actually required by regulation. Omission of this step could create a new set of problems in the future. By contrast, sometimes review of a regulation finds that a process previously thought to be required is actually just an artifact of history and can be easily eliminated.

Next, compare the current process with the organization's performance standards or other national benchmarks or best practices. This is where a literature review is very helpful in supplying current information. If no national benchmarks are available, using networking tools to collect information from other organizations about their process and outcomes can add to the analysis.

Conducting a survey of customer expectations and needs can assist quality improvement activities in at least two important ways. First, it provides direct input into the problem or issue under study. Second, it signals the user community that their concerns are important and will help drive the solution.

Finally, prioritize the problem areas for focused improvement. This is necessary in cases where study has determined that there is more than one opportunity for improvement—a common occurrence. Determine which area of focus would have the most impact on customer outcomes or improved efficiency that may indirectly best meet the customer needs.

When the factors that contribute to a process and the opportunities to improve sustained performance are identified and understood, the next focus is process redesign.

Process Redesign

The work of **process redesign** begins with a specific target for improvement activities. The research done during problem identification becomes the basis for considering new approaches to the process. Where best practice information exists in the literature or was identified from other forms of data gathering, it should be applied to the new process.

Additional data may need to be collected about the specific process identified for improvement. Time studies, observations, or other data collection activities may be required to completely understand the reasons for delay, error, or variation.

The next step is to create a new flowchart of the revised process. Again, a flowchart documents each step in the process and clearly communicates the new process to everyone involved. This step helps facilitate the last step in the process, which is to educate staff on the new process.

With the new process in place, the cycle returns to the beginning and data again are routinely collected and monitored. Additional actions still may be necessary to meet the requirements or expectations of the user community. The original process identified additional actions that may be considered for adjustment, and those changes could be put into place when the new process is stabilized. The process of managing the change in any process should not be underestimated as it is critical to the ongoing success of any new system.

It is important to communicate and provide feedback to the employees involved in the process redesign. Failure to provide appropriate information back to the employee will result in inefficient and lost time as work will have to be redone. The communication should be both ways as the employee can also provide feedback to the process redesign team on what is and is not working with the new system.

Change Management

The real work begins at the point of completing the redesign. A flowchart is only a piece of paper until the process that it describes is adopted and fully utilized. In quality improvement activities, **change management** is the key to making improvements happen.

- *Becoming a change agent:* Team leaders should demonstrate a willingness to investigate new ideas, learn new skills, and solve new problems. Only by engaging change will they have the credibility to lead others to accept change.

- *Being available to listen to staff:* Leaders should ask questions to understand staff's anxieties and concerns. This can be done through team meetings and informal discussions. Clearing the air and raising and answering questions can reduce fear of, and resistance to, change.

- *Holding on to the vision:* In times of change and stress, it may seem easier, or maybe even more prudent, to step back from the organization's vision or goal. However, it is during change that leaders must be even more dedicated to achieving their vision. They must demonstrate commitment through actions and then campaign for support of the vision. They should encourage and clarify the vision to others and let their commitment show.

- *Continuing to delegate:* Part of demonstrating commitment and risk taking is to let others share the risk. Only with true ownership of the problem will team members feel they own the solution.

- *Measuring and celebrating success:* When the vision of the future state is clear, it is easy to measure progress toward reaching it. Being able to measure progress is key to maintaining enthusiasm for the journey.

Change can be challenging, energizing, and overwhelming. Preparing to manage change includes making a commitment to quality improvement that is recognized by the entire team.

Check Your Understanding 18.4

1. Which of the following would be part of problem identification in the quality improvement process?

    A. Research all regulatory requirements related to the current process
    B. Educate involved staff on the new process
    C. Develop policies and procedures that support the redesigned process
    D. Collect focused data from the prioritized problem areas

2. Change management includes:

    A. Identifying problems
    B. Being available to listen to staff
    C. Redesigning processes
    D. Educating staff on new processes

3. What could an analysis of a flowchart identify?

    A. Productivity levels
    B. Customer needs
    C. Key performance measures
    D. Redundancies in a process

Instructions: Indicate whether the following statements are true or false (T or F).

4. _____ Quality improvement activities only apply to direct patient care.

5. _____ When leading change, a supervisor should not ask staff questions.

6. _____ Opportunities for improving processes should be prioritized before they are implemented.

7. _____ A customer survey helps communicate the value of the customer's input.

8. _____ Intermittent, focused monitoring is the only way to identify potential improvement opportunities.

Real-World Case

MMC has created a new coding position to handle the increase in workload resulting from the addition of the EHR to the emergency department as well as the implementation of the outpatient prospective payment system for Medicare patients. You are the new supervisor of the outpatient services team with almost 10 years of coding experience. Since being promoted to supervisor, you have never been responsible for interviewing employment candidates. Figure 18.5 shows the resume of one of the numerous candidates applying for a coding specialist position.

Your own manager (the assistant director of the HIM department) has already developed a detailed job description for the new position (figure 18.6). She has promised to help you to get ready for the interviews. Still, you are more than a little nervous about taking on this part of your new job.

Look at the resume and think about the steps you will need to take before interviewing the candidate. What skills are you going to be looking for and how are you going to measure them? Does the resume describe someone you want to interview for your position? How are you going to assess whether the candidate will fit into the current dynamics of your group?

Summary

Organizations are complex and ever changing, whether they are multihospital systems or small group practices. Whether the structure is hierarchical or team based, planning and organizing are important functions in maximizing the organization's assets. Included among those assets are the people who carry out the mission as staff, the teams that come together to solve problems, and the resources they use to perform their work.

As the most critical and costly resource in any healthcare organization, staff members should be organized and led to maximize their contribution. Before the hiring process takes place, effective people management begins with appropriate job design and position description development. Job descriptions, along with effective hiring practices, assist in selecting the best candidates. When hired, ensuring that employees are well oriented and trained begins a working relationship that is fostered through the use of teams, employee empowerment, and staff development planning.

Improving the performance of any organization begins with regular measuring and monitoring. Most improvement activities are incremental and do not create sweeping change on their own, but in combination with other steps and over time, these small steps can have a large impact on the work of the organization. These positive changes create an environment that engages people in their work and allows them to make meaningful contributions.

Figure 18.5.   **Resume for the Real-World Case**

RESUME

Stephen Jeremy Johnsen, RHIT

222 Brickpath Way   Born 1/23/1971
Chicago, ILL 60622   Height 5 ft 9 in
773/222-2222   Weight 180 lb

Goal: Looking for a job that lets me use my education and my
      knowledge of hospital coding and billing
Salary: $30,000+, opportunity for advancement

2000-2001	Coder Lincoln Valley Community Hospital
	I left to move to Chicago to be with my girlfriend
1999	Billing specialist University Medical Center, Champaign, Illinois
	Was here for almost a year; disliked manager; needed more money
1996-1999	Coder Medical Record Temporary Specialists, Urbana, IL
	Worked on and off for temporary agency while I finished my computer programming degree
1994-1999	School Oakwood Community College
	Worked as a orderly to earn money for classes, majored in health information technology (graduated 1996) and computer programming
1989-1992	Army Stationed in South Carolina, Germany, trained as medical corpsman
1989	School, majored in business but dropped out to join Army and earn money for school
1989	Graduated Glenview high school, Computer club, Music Camp, Varsity football, worked in father's landscape business during summers

*References available

Figure 18.6.   Job description for the Real-World Case

Position Description

Position Title: APC Coordinator

**Immediate
Supervisor:**   Director of Health Information Management

General Purpose: The purpose of this position is to create consistency and efficiency in outpatient claims processing and data collection to optimize APC reimbursement and facilitate data quality in outpatient services.

Responsibilities:

- Performs data quality reviews on outpatient encounters to validate the ICD-9-CM, CPT, and HCPCS Level II code and modifier assignments, APC group appropriateness, missed secondary diagnoses and/or procedures, and compliance with all APC mandates and outpatient reporting requirements.

- Monitors medical visit code selection by departments against facility-specific criteria for appropriateness. Assists in the development of such criteria as needed.

- Monitors outpatient service mix reports and the leading medical visit, surgical service, significant procedure, and ancillary APCs assigned in the facility to identify patterns, trends, and variations in the facility's frequently assigned APC groups. Once identified, evaluates the causes of the change, and takes appropriate steps in collaboration with the right department to effect resolution or explanation of the variance.

- Continuously evaluates the quality of clinical documentation to spot incomplete or inconsistent documentation for outpatient encounters that impact the code selection and resulting APC groups and payment. Brings identified concerns to medical staff committee or department managers for resolution.

- Provides and/or arranges for training to facility healthcare professionals on the use of coding guidelines and practices, proper documentation techniques, medical terminology, and disease processes appropriate to the job description and function as it relates to the APC and other outpatient data quality management factors.

- Maintains knowledge of current professional coding certification requirements and promotes recruitment and retention of certified staff in coding positions when possible.

- Reports to the facility Compliance Committee each quarter.

- Abides by the Standards of Ethical Coding as set forth by the American Health Information Management Association and monitors coding staff for violations and reports to the HIM Director when areas of concern are identified. Concerns involving compliance issues are forwarded to the Compliance Committee for action.

Figure 18.6. Job description for the Real-World Case *(continued)*

Position Description—APC Coordinator—Page 2

Responsibilities:
(continued)

- Develops reports and collects and prepares data for studies involving outpatient encounter data for clinical evaluation purposes and/or financial impact and profitability.

- Serves as the facility representative for APCs by attending outpatient coding and reimbursement workshops and bringing back information to the appropriate departments. Communicates any APC updates published in third-party payer newsletters/bulletins and provider manuals to all facility staff that need this information.

- Keeps abreast of new technology in coding and abstracting software and other forms of automation and stays informed about transaction code sets, HIPAA requirements, and other future issues impacting the coding function.

- Demonstrates competency in the use of computer applications and APC Grouper Software, OCE edits, and all coding software and hardware currently in use in the HIM department.

- Performs periodic claim form reviews to check code transfer accuracy from the abstracting system and the chargemaster.

- Evaluates, records, and responds to the Peer Review Organization APC change and/or denial notices. Provides appropriate documentation from required source to the PRO when appealing a PRO decision.

- Monitors outpatient unbilled accounts report for outstanding and/or uncoded outpatient encounters to reduce Accounts Receivable days for outpatients.

- Serves on the Chargemaster maintenance committee.

Qualifications:

- Minimum of associate's degree in a health services discipline. Formal HIM education with national certification, RHIA or RHIT preferred.

- Coding certification required from the American Health Information Management Association or the American Academy of Professional Coders.

- Minimum of five years progressive coding or coding review experience in ICD-9-CM, CPT, and HCPCS with claims processing and/or data management responsibilities a plus.

- Good oral and written communication skills and comprehensive knowledge of the APC structure and regulatory requirements.

- Prefer someone with past auditing experience or strong training background in coding and reimbursement.

References

Bennett-Woods, D. 1997. Team facilitation skills: A step beyond running a good meeting. *Journal of AHIMA* 68(1):20–23.

Heinen, S., and E. Jackson. 1976. A model of task group development in complex organization and a strategy of implementation. *Academy of Management Review* 1(4):98–111.

Kouzes, J.M., and B.Z. Posner. 1995. *The Leadership Challenge.* San Francisco: Jossey-Bass.

Schein, E.H. 1980. *Organizational Psychology,* 3rd ed. Englewood Cliffs, NJ: Prentice-Hall.

Senge, P.M. 1990. *The Fifth Discipline.* New York: Doubleday Currency.

Super, D.E. 1955. Dimensions and measurement of vocational maturity. *Teachers College Record* 57:151–165.

Super, D.E. 1980. A life-span, life-space approach to career development. *Journal of Vocational Behavior* 13:282–298.

Super, D.E. 1990. A life-span, life-space approach to career development. In *Career Choice and Development: Applying Contemporary Theories to Practice,* 2nd ed. Edited by D. Brown and L. Brooks. San Francisco: Jossey-Bass.

Additional Resources

Armstrong, M. 2008. *How to Be an Even Better Manager,* 7th ed. London: Kogan Page.

Cleverley, W.O., and A.E. Cameron. 2007. *Essentials of Health Care Finance,* 6th ed. Boston: Jones and Bartlett.

Cooke, R.A. 2004. *The McGraw-Hill 36-Hour Course in Finance for Nonfinancial Managers,* 2nd ed. San Francisco: McGraw-Hill.

Daley, D.M. 2002. *Strategic Human Resource Management.* Upper Saddle River, NJ: Prentice-Hall.

Dunn, R. 2007. Benchmarking imaging: Making every image count in scanning program. *Journal of AHIMA* 78(6):42–46.

Dunn, R. 2007. *Haiman's Healthcare Management,* 8th ed. Chicago: Health Administration Press.

Gift, R.G., and C.F. Kinney, eds. 1996. *Today's Management Methods: A Guide for the Health Care Executive.* Chicago: American Hospital Publishing.

Hughes, G. 2003. Practice brief: Using benchmarking for performance improvement. *Journal of AHIMA* 74(2):64A–64D.

Martin, D. 1993. *Teamthink: Using the Sports Connection of Develop, Motivate, and Manage a Winning Business Team.* New York: Penguin Group.

Peters, T. 1987. *Thriving on Chaos.* New York: Alfred A. Knopf.

Rosner, B., A. Halcrow, and A. Levins. 2001. *The Boss's Survival Guide.* New York: McGraw-Hill.

chapter 19

Envisioning the Future of the Health Information Management Profession

Bonnie S. Cassidy, MPA, RHIA, FAHIMA, FHIMSS,
2011 President of AHIMA

Introduction

The first decade of the 21st century has been a turbulent time in the HIM profession as the healthcare industry has embarked on some of the greatest transformations in the history of the US healthcare system. The steady stream of change in healthcare and the rapid shift of paradigms challenge and expand the traditional HIM role as the medical record custodian and keeper of clinical information. This necessitates a transformation in the HIM professional. The medical record will cease to be a tangible product or tool as it becomes electronic. Information accuracy and content will continue to be critical; however, clinical information will become intellectual property, organizational capital, and competitive intelligence. Payers, providers, researchers, lawyers, and regulators will require credible information to create knowledge that provides sustainable competitive advantages for their organizations.

These changes have directly impacted health information practice and cannot be done successfully without HIM best practices and leadership. To build best practices and influence policy, the HIM profession is called upon to articulate lessons learned from the implementation of electronic medical records, ICD-10-CM/PCS planning and training, actions taken to achieve meaningful use (MU), computer-assisted coding initiatives, advances in health information exchange, and the introduction of patient-centered care models such as the medical (healthcare) home and accountable care organizations (ACOs).

The health information management (HIM) profession continues to grow and change, becoming highly visible in the national arena as federal laws have evolved to protect patient privacy, to advance technologies which collect and maintain patient data accurately and securely, to adopt classification systems to increase the quality of data in clinical documentation, and to encourage the use of electronic health records as the primary source for monitoring quality of care. This chapter addresses the role of the American Health Information Management Association (AHIMA) as a thought leadership organization that sets strategy on health information governance and influences current and future initiatives which impact the quality of healthcare data and information. As the healthcare industry transitions to new models of care delivery and meaningful use of health information technologies, the opportunities for the HIM profession are wide-ranging and span healthcare, business, government, and many other environments beyond the clinical realm.

The e-HIM Transition

With the widespread adoption of electronic health records and other technology-based information sources and the use of the electronically available data for healthcare management measurement purposes, research functions, and governmental initiatives, health informatics and health information technology are being increasingly utilized in HIM practices in the healthcare industry (Cassidy 2011a).

AHIMA has grown to be a thriving association with over 64,000 members and all HIM professionals now collaborate and learn from each other to strengthen the HIM leadership position in the healthcare industry. AHIMA sought to develop a world-class set of bylaws that strategically align all entities to deliver member value, incorporate association best practices and comply with the evolution of corporate, federal, and state law. AHIMA has set the course for the 21st century with a renewed focus on governance. The AHIMA Board of Directors sets strategy. In 2011, the AHIMA bylaws were rewritten to reflect the strategic thinking for future generations of HIM professionals. By design, AHIMA has clearly articulated in the bylaws that the Board of Directors governs the association and the House of Delegates governs the HIM profession (Cassidy 2011b). See figure 19.1 for the key roles of the AHIMA Board of Directors and the AHIMA House of Delegates.

As the American healthcare industry moves forward with health information technology (HIT) adoption, providers need the skills and expertise of health information management professionals to support the implementation and achievement of MU of electronic health records. The migration to electronic health records (EHRs) changes the design and operations of traditional HIM departments. These changes add complexity to the

Figure 19.1.   **Key roles of the AHIMA Board of Directors and the AHIMA House of Delegates**

Board of Directors	House of Delegates
Fiduciary Responsibility	Set Code of Ethics
Strategy Development and Oversight	Conduct Environmental Scanning
Authority over Governing Documents	Vet Professional and Practice Issues, Proposed Resolutions
Fiscal and Financial Management	Recommend Action to the Board

management of health information. HIM professionals are now assuming new responsibilities that, in addition to a solid foundation in health data and information systems concepts and principles, require advanced education and experience in leadership and management skills, as well as a solid understanding of the capabilities of information technologies. Roles will continue to evolve, and opportunities await HIM professionals who evaluate and enhance their expertise to keep pace with changing practice.

AHIMA continues to influence policy and position the HIM professionals as the qualified experts in electronic health record (EHR) clinical content in the industry today. In this transition to e-HIM, HIM professionals serve a broad range of roles: planning, organizing, and managing clinical content, integrity, accessibility, use, and protection. HIM professionals are now project managers who identify work process improvements, employ implementation techniques, and lead efforts to redefine information management practices in healthcare organizations. HIM professionals work at the convergence of people, processes, regulations, organizational structure, standards, and system design.

Given the magnitude of change occurring in the ways health information systems and technology is deployed within organizations, expectations of executives make it clear that the HIM department is responsible for the successful creation of the emerging digital and virtual HIM department (Cassidy 2011a). HIM professionals are transforming all HIM functions to e-HIM functions. The role of the HIM professional is growing toward being an effective change agent and champion for EHR deployment. With the emergence of electronic systems, the HIM department has a greater capability to be virtual, employing and contracting with offsite staff to create the strongest team possible. They are analyzing and visualizing both documented and undocumented intradepartmental and interdepartmental information management functions to understand the current and envision (or establish) the future state of the HIM services within the organization, while ensuring that HIM best practices and standards such as privacy, the legal health record, data quality, and information integrity are consistently maintained.

AHIMA's top 10 tenets, shown in figure 19.2, for managing the transition from paper to EHRs are critical to the successful evolution of managing health information. Transitioning health information services to this virtual environment offers many operational and financial advantages. New HIM roles will be prominent and positioned throughout a healthcare organization: for example, project managers, EHR system managers, and workflow and data analysts. Privacy coordinators, different from privacy officers, will act as directors, creating policy, implementing programs, and directing the goals. At the same time, the health information department will continue to serve as the primary location for assuring the quality of documentation in the patient record, maintaining the organization's legal patient record, for responding to authorized requests for release of patient information, and envision new and as yet unseen roles that will be necessary to the effective management of health information in the future. Some examples of developing and anticipated new roles are: information technology, information workflow designer, data exchange manager, EHR content manager, EMPI data integrity analyst, corporate record manager, clinical data analyst, and health information exchange (HIE) privacy gatekeeper. However, every HIM function performed to support the paper health record today will be re-engineered. This will challenge HIM directors and managers to not only manage new workflow processes, but for geographically diverse integrated healthcare systems and to enable interoperability, to do so remotely. For it to be successful, this transformation to the virtual management of health information requires active engagement of healthcare executives in support of their HIM teams (Cassidy 2011a).

Changing Times: HIM and ICD-10-CM/PCS

How well the healthcare industry implements and executes the strategic and tactical tasks for the ICD-10-CM/PCS, ICD-11, and SNOMED CT transformation will go a long way in determining the future state and success of the HIM profession. HIM involvement with disease classifications and nomenclatures can be traced back to the early 20th century. The HIM profession has been the recognized expert and leader in data collection,

Figure 19.2.   **AHIMA's top ten tenets for transitioning from paper to electronic health records**

1. The EHR must be part of an organization's vision and strategic plan. As part of this plan, the organization should have a standard definition for the legal health record.

2. The organization must ensure that adequate leadership, consultation, staff training, equipment, policies and procedures, and funding or other resources are in place to support EHR development.

3. Organizations must establish a legal health record steering committee to guide the organization from a paper to an electronic environment. This group must be empowered to make proactive and constructive changes. Its members should include department managers from health information management; risk, quality, or compliance management; medical staff; nursing; ancillary departments; IT; and the privacy officer.

4. The legal health record steering committee must develop and publish policies and procedures for operating in the paper state, hybrid state, and electronic state and include long-term archive, purge, retention, and destruction guidelines.

5. HIM professionals must participate actively in the development and implementation of the EHR, given the significant operational management effects on workflow within HIM and their role as custodians of the legal health record.

6. There must be a formal process for approving EHR software and hardware to ensure that it can support the organization's operational needs adequately for the paper, hybrid, and electronic medical record.

7. There must be a formal process for managing forms, paper, electronic, hybrid, and system-generated records, including input, output, and versioning of document content and access.

8. There must be a formal process and written guidelines addressing access, confidentiality, security, print control, spoliation mitigation, disclosure, and e-discovery.

9. A complete record inventory of all existing storage and management of paper, hybrid, shadow (duplicate), and electronic records must be maintained by all healthcare organizations.

10. The facility must develop a policy for retention and destruction of medical records, regardless of whether paper, hybrid, or electronic medical records are used.

Source: AHIMA 2010b.

classification, and reporting since Grace Whiting Myers, founder of the association known today as AHIMA, served on the Committee on Uniform Nomenclature that developed a disease classification system based on etiological groupings. HIM's history is rich with HIM professionals that helped develop the Standard Nomenclature of Disease (SNDO), a forerunner of the widely used clinical terminology SNOMED CT. The medical record professionals working in US hospitals in the mid-20th century were responsible for collecting and reporting disease and procedure information from medical records using SNDO. HIM professionals have an outstanding track record as leaders in employing classification standards consistently, and will maintain that track record through the processes of change that reflect and support medicine's cutting edge. America needs the highest confidence that health information management is ready for this challenge (Cassidy 2011c).

Changing Times: HIM and Patient-Centered Care

Organizations practicing patient-centered care recognize that a patient is an individual to be cared for, not a medical condition to be treated. Patient-centered care is offered in a setting where each patient is viewed as a unique person, with diverse needs. Patients and families are partners and have knowledge and expertise that is essential to their care. Care that is truly patient centered considers patients' cultural traditions, their personal preferences and values, their family situations, and their lifestyles. It makes patients and their loved ones an integral part of the care team who collaborate with healthcare professionals in making clinical decisions. Patient-centered care puts responsibility for important aspects of self-care and monitoring in patients' hands—along with the tools and support they need to carry out that responsibility. Patient-centered care ensures that transitions between providers, departments, and healthcare settings are respectful, coordinated, and efficient. When care is patient centered, unneeded and unwanted services can be reduced.

The new and exciting unique role for HIM is to create HIM governance guidelines and policies for healthcare organizations that address the access to understandable health information and take on the challenge and responsibility for providing access to that information. Patient-centered care is the core of a high-quality healthcare system and a necessary foundation for safe, effective, efficient, timely, and equitable care.

The Institute of Medicine's 2001 report, *Crossing the Quality Chasm: A New Health System for the 21st Century*, called for healthcare systems that respect patients' values, preferences and expressed needs; coordinate and integrate care across boundaries of the system; provide the information, communication, and education that people need and want; and guarantee physical comfort, emotional support, and the involvement of family and friends.

Health Information Exchange (HIE), which is the mobilization of healthcare information electronically across organizations within a region, community, or hospital system, is a requirement for achieving the highest standards of quality and continuity of patient care. HIE initiatives today focus on technology, interoperability, standards utilization and harmonization. With a patient-centered care focus, the HIEs will provide access to the right clinical information to the right person at the right time.

A healthcare organization cannot achieve success in providing patient-centered care without an HIM infrastructure of governance including policies, procedures, guidelines, and protocols that address access to medical information (electronic, paper, or hybrid medical records), personal health records, electronic communications to and from physicians and other providers, and patient education information (Cassidy 2011d).

Employment Outlook for HIM Professionals

The industry today is faced with a major challenge—not enough HIM professionals to help implement and manage health IT. There is a growing need for many HIM professionals in many new roles and functions. Radical change is required to transform a primarily paper-based system to a totally electronic, interoperable healthcare industry. Health IT must enable providers to achieve quality and efficiency in and of the services they provide (Cassidy 2011e).

There exists a dispersion of HIM roles throughout healthcare facilities. HIM professionals still play important roles but are no longer living in a silo or are associated with one particular department. HIM professionals are playing key roles in information technology, decision support, identity management, revenue cycle management, risk management, privacy and security, clinical documentation improvement, case management, and many other areas throughout an enterprise. This is a new way of practicing that has positive potential implications for new HIM education models and competition in the job market. One major area of importance is integrity of the HIM certification process and the value that the industry has placed on the AHIMA certifications. All are well recognized in the industry and with that comes an understanding that those credentialed individuals will deliver results. AHIMA's certifications are:

- Registered Health Information Administrator (RHIA)
- Registered Health Information Technician (RHIT)
- Certified Coding Associate (CCA)
- Certified Coding Specialist (CCS)
- Certified Coding Specialist—Physician-based (CCS-P)
- Certified Health Data Analyst (CHDA)
- Certified in Healthcare Privacy and Security (CHPS)
- Certified Documentation Improvement Practitioner (CDIP)

AHIMA leaders have played an active role in initiatives aimed at increasing the much needed healthcare informatics and information management workforce, including the HIT workforce community college and university-based education programs funded by the Office of the National Coordinator of HIT. The Office of the National Coordinator for

Health Information Technology (ONC) has identified numerous roles that widen the scope of HIM, requiring expertise throughout an organization. Some of the roles are listed in figure 19.3.

HIM Expertise

HIM professionals are experts in data content standardization and have the necessary skills and competencies to advance improved validation, capture, analysis, and output of information for quality and patient safety initiatives. HIM professionals must lead all efforts on data governance, data standardization, data capture validation and maintenance, and data capture, analysis, and output. MU takes HIM work to the next level. It is what people in the HIM profession have been working toward for all these decades—patient access to data so consumers can be more informed and involved in their own healthcare, improving the timeliness, comprehensiveness of health information, accuracy, and reliability of documentation and data, leveraging the use of technology to really improve the quality of care and the efficiency of the care delivery process.

HIM professionals are the ideal candidates to lead organizational HIM initiatives while at the same time playing a pivotal role in the information capturing process and system improvement measures. HIM professionals are able to provide data related to serious adverse events, present on admission indicators, and hospital-acquired conditions, and they are equipped to analyze and interpret these data and participate in the patient safety teams that conduct root-cause analyses and develop action plans for improvement (Cassidy 2011f).

As with all professions that must adapt to changes, HIM professionals must continue to learn, and HIM professionals are challenged to continuously upgrade their skills and expertise to keep pace and be successful in the new e-HIM practice. Healthcare executives, ever mindful of the need to empower and advance their workforce, should place a high priority on empowering HIM professionals as key leaders in EHR implementation and management (AHIMA 2010a).

Future Roles of HIM Professionals

According to the Bureau of Labor Statistics 2010–2011 Occupational Outlook Handbook "employment of medical and health services managers is expected to grow 16 percent

Figure 19.3.   Roles that widen the scope of HIM

• Workflow and information management redesign specialist	• Trainer
• Clinician or practitioner consultant	• Public health leader
• Implementation support specialist	• Health information exchange specialist
• Implementation manager	• Privacy and security officer
• Technical and software support	• Research and development scientist

Source: ONC 2011.

from 2008 to 2018, faster than the average for all occupations." In addition, only 38 percent of medical and health service managers work in hospitals. Nineteen percent of these positions indicate opportunities in physician offices or nursing or residential care facilities. Additional opportunities are available in home health, government facilities, outpatient facilities, insurance payer groups, or community healthcare facilities.

Strategic thinking and research brought about the development and refinement of the HIM core model that focuses on the current state and future state of the HIM profession in all areas of education, research, influencing policy, and establishing best practices and standards in HIM. (Refer to chapter 1 for more information on the HIM core model.) To keep pace, HIM professionals must understand the principles of change management and transition management, and the impact of the EHR on core HIM practices. Some related items include the following items published in the *Journal of AHIMA*.

- e-HIM Practice Transformation (AHIMA 2011)
- Forces of Change: The Growth of Data Drives Demand for Data Management (Rollins 2010)
- Managing the Transition from Paper to EHR (AHIMA 2010b)

Health information management (HIM) roles are evolving with the transformation from paper to electronic health information and medical record management. Some of the HIM functions tied to paper-based systems will disappear. Many HIM functions will be transformed to accommodate electronic systems and new roles will emerge. This transformation of HIM best practices requires streamlining and standardizing workflow and work processes, implementing new techniques, and redesigning (redefining) information management practices. As HIM professionals are managing health information in the digital world, new challenges and issues arise. For each of these new issues, there are often new process workflows designed that require specialized talent and expertise.

Some of the new roles that have emerged as a result of achieving the MU of EHRs include, but are not limited to, those listed in figure 19.4. HIM professionals are the workforce members most suited to address these needs. They have deep understanding of information management, coding, data integrity, and information workflow.

Figure 19.4.   New roles that have emerged as a result of achieving the MU of EHRs

• Identity coordinator or master patient index (MPI) coordinator	• Applications systems analyst
	• Regulatory analyst
• Content management coordinator (working with IT on documentation)	• Regulatory manager
• Electronic medical record (EMR) integrity specialist	• Associate director for record design and management
• Compliance analyst (privacy and documentation audits)	• Physician educator

The HIM core model illustrates new roles including business change manager, EHR system manager, IT training specialist, business process engineer, clinical vocabulary manager, workflow and data analyst, consumer advocate, clinical alerts and reminders manager, clinical research coordinator, privacy coordinator, enterprise application specialist, and many more. The primary roles of the HIM professional in the future state are focused on five main functional areas of health information (AHIMA 2011):

1. Data capture, validation, and maintenance
2. Data and information analysis, transformation, and decision support
3. Information dissemination and liaison
4. Health information resource management and innovation
5. Information governance and stewardship

These five main functional areas of HIM professionals have a common theme of protecting and managing health information. The primary ethical obligation of the HIM professional is to protect the privacy of confidential patient information that includes oversight of health information systems and health records, the quality of information, and disclosure of information.

Information governance and stewardship are gaining significant attention within the healthcare industry. Data governance is the high level organizational framework or enterprise-wide infrastructure of accountability and responsibility that define the purpose for collecting data, ownership of data, and intended use of data. One of the critical success factors within the domain of data governance is data stewardship. Data stewardship focuses on the details of data quality management: the processes, workflows, and policies and procedures that support the capture and maintenance of accurate and complete data. A central concept of data stewardship is accountability. The role of data steward should be a formal responsibility within the organization for assuring appropriate use of data, and with liability for inappropriate use.

Health data stewardship has taken on great practical urgency because of the increase in availability of electronic health data; growing recognition of the value of electronic data in improving healthcare and population health; the acceleration in the use of information and communication technology; and awareness of the potential risks associated with incorrect or inappropriate uses of health data. Health data stewardship supports the benefits to society of using individuals' personal health information to improve understanding of health and healthcare while at the same time respecting individuals' privacy and confidentiality. As such, health data stewardship is a key responsibility of HIM professionals who strive to ensure the knowledgeable and appropriate use of data derived from individuals' personal health information.

When thinking about the role of an HIM professional serving as the designated data steward of an organization, one must revisit the AHIMA Code of Ethics. The very core values associated with data stewardship are contained in the profession's Code of Ethics.

The specific principles within the Code of Ethics most closely aligned with the responsibilities of a data steward are:

- Advocate, uphold, and defend the individual's right to privacy and the doctrine of confidentiality in the use and disclosure of information.

- Preserve, protect, and secure personal health information in any form or medium and hold in the highest regards health information and other information of a confidential nature obtained in an official capacity, taking into account the applicable statutes and regulations.

- Facilitate interdisciplinary collaboration in situations supporting health information practice.

- Refuse to participate in or conceal unethical practices or procedures and report such practices.

One of the key HIM guiding principles is to facilitate interdisciplinary collaboration in situations supporting health information practice. HIM professionals are the primary drivers of raising awareness to the entire enterprise when it comes to the safeguarding of personal health data and information. HIM professionals fully recognize that data stewardship is not simply a technology solution; it is the term used to define the people, policies, procedures, and technologies necessary to complement the data governance model (Cassidy 2011g).

Vision of the HIM Professional in the C-suite

As a profession, HIM professionals use of technology and data analytic tools to facilitate better patient care delivery, inform policy leaders, and move into the 21st century and beyond. To meet the needs of various healthcare organizations in their use of emerging technologies HIM professionals need to be involved at an executive level where decisions are made regarding the design, implementation, and use of technology from a systems approach. From an operational perspective this would suggest involvement in the adoption and implementation of systemwide technology; the use of data to improve patient care and reduce cost; and a role as leaders who define future policies and procedures as they relate to the privacy and security of the organization (Cassidy 2011h).

Growing the HIM profession requires a focus on both those who are beginning their education as well as those already in the workforce. It is important to offer current professionals educational opportunities for growth and development that can lead to decision-making positions within healthcare organizations. As the HIM profession evolves and expertise in information governance is recognized, new career paths that move the current workforce into executive level decision-making positions will be taking place (Cassidy 2011h). There are many possibilities and opportunities for HIM professionals to move into the C-suite, a term used to indicate the "chief" or C-leadership level of an organization that includes the chief executive officer (CEO), chief information officer (CIO), chief financial officer (CFO), and many other organizational leaders.

The chief executive officer (CEO) is the guiding force of an organization. CEOs are expected to be more business-centric than to practice in any particular functional area—extensive expertise in HIM, IT, data quality, clinical needs, and workflow processes, as well as leadership ability, are key qualities in CEOs in healthcare-related fields. HIM professionals are particularly well-suited to become chief information officers (CIOs), a role that encompasses a perspective of the total organization, an orientation to information processes across the organization, and an understanding of the ways that the organization can effectively use its growing stores of data (Groysberg et al. 2011). HIM professionals who have enterprise-wide responsibility are sometimes referred to as chief health information officers.

There are many possibilities and opportunities for HIM professionals to advance. The creation of a chief knowledge officer position within the C-Suite is one example of a development that would further senior-level positions and advancement opportunities. Another direction for HIM professionals who have expertise in reimbursement is to become a chief revenue cycle officer. Healthcare is in the middle of an information evolution with the convergence of the ICD-10-CM/PCS, ARRA/HITECH, and Meaningful Use EHR initiatives. The explosion of information fuels a vision for care developed by payers and regulators that is predicated on the mitigation of preventable complications, readmissions, and untoward events across the continuum of care. The aggressive transition to the EHR powered by the MU program will further promote the use of healthcare information. The proliferation and use of health information will intensify even further throughout the industry as information and technology evolve.

The goal of organizations will be to access and use the right information at the right time so the right decisions are made at the right level.

Summary

The American Recovery and Reinvestment Act and HITECH Act of 2009, along with the nation's transition to ICD-10-CM/PCS have put the spotlight on the HIM profession, and it is up to the HIM professionals to deliver. Federal, state, and industry initiatives have given HIM professionals a unique opportunity to leverage strengths and demonstrate the ability to deliver value-added services to an organization (Cassidy 2011b). Achieving excellence and MU of electronic health information only comes with a commitment to applying professional HIM principles that guide the development of organizational HIM policy and EHR governance.

Throughout healthcare, industry models for cost reductions, clinical outcomes, pay-for-performance, competitive advantage, and best practice are the result of improved technology and expanded data assets. As information and technology become richer and more sophisticated, they will create the need within healthcare organizations for a systematic approach to converting data and information into knowledge for strategic value.

The goal of organizations will be to access and use the right information at the right time so the right decisions are made at the right level. HIM professionals are the workforce members most suited to address this need. They have deep understanding of information management, coding, data integrity, and information workflow (Cassidy 2011h).

Healthcare executives and employers in the second decade of the 21st century are counting on HIM professionals to lead the transition to managing health information in an electronic environment; actively involved in information technology (HIT) adoption; creating strategy, managing implementations with new workflows and seeing that the organization demonstrates MU while properly planning for the monumental transition to ICD-10-CM/PCS; and developing policy and practices to govern the capture, maintenance, and use of electronic patient data to meet the needs of a host of authorized healthcare data users.

These are revitalizing times in the history of the health information management profession. It is a time for HIM professionals to come together to promote and advance the values which serve as the foundation of professional practice—a time for HIM professional's voices to be heard (Cassidy 2011b). It is a time for HIM leadership to continue evolving best practices that assure the privacy, security, accuracy and value of health information in the electronic healthcare industry. HIM is uniquely qualified to lead the initiative for successful ICD-10-CM/PCS implementation and establishing strategies for implementing computer-assisted coding.

The new HIM core model focuses on the current and future state of the HIM profession in all areas of education, research, influencing public policy, and establishing best practices and standards in HIM (Cassidy 2011i). It is important that HIM professionals continuously improve, make changes, and make significant contributions to support the healthcare system's growing need for high-quality healthcare data and information resources. The HIM professionals must continue to passionately promote HIM education, best practices, standards, policy, and research, and continue to provide services for today while being visionary in setting the bar for the future.

This is the greatest transformation in the history of the healthcare system and cannot be done successfully without leadership (Cassidy 2011j). With electronic health information's widening availability, great advances in medicine are not only possible, they are mandatory for the exchange of healthcare information and affordable quality healthcare worldwide.

References

American Health Information Management Association. 2010a. e-HIM® practice transformation (updated). *Journal of AHIMA* 81(8):52–55.

American Health Information Management Association. 2010b. Managing the transition from paper to EHRs. *Journal of AHIMA* 81(11).

American Health Information Management Association. 2011. A core model for the HIM future. Chicago: AHIMA. http://library.ahima.org/xpedio/groups/public/documents/ahima/bok1_049283. pdf

Cassidy, B.S. 2011a. President's message: Stepping into new e-HIM® roles: The e-HIM® transition changes HIM roles and responsibilities. *Journal of AHIMA* 82(9):10.

Cassidy, B.S. 2011b. President's message: Leading the e-HIM® transformation. *Journal of AHIMA* 82(1):10.

Cassidy, B.S. 2011c. President's message: Taking coding to the next level: HIM's long coding history can help transform the industry with ICD-10. *Journal of AHIMA* 82(7):10.

Cassidy, B.S. 2011d. President's message: Embracing patient-centered care and its roles. *Journal of AHIMA* 82(2):10.

Cassidy, B.S. 2011e. President's message: Embracing the ICD-10 transition. *Journal of AHIMA* 82(6):10.

Cassidy, B.S. 2011f. President's message: Taking the lead on meaningful use: Program goals align with HIM expertise and objectives. *Journal of AHIMA* 82(10):10.

Cassidy, B.S. 2011g. President's message: Data governance—HIM's sweet spot. *Journal of AHIMA* 82(4):10.

Cassidy, B.S. 2011h. Teaching the future: An educational response to the AHIMA core model. *Journal of AHIMA* 82(10):34–38.

Cassidy, B.S. 2011i. President's message: A year of progress: Outstanding advancements on 2011 strategic initiatives. *Journal of AHIMA* 82(11): expanded online version.

Cassidy, B.S. 2011j. President's message: Investing in your future: Professional development enables HIM to transition with changing healthcare landscape. *Journal of AHIMA* 82(8):10.

Groysberg, B., L.K. Kelly, and B. MacDonald. 2011. The new path to the C-suite. *Harvard Business Review* 89(3). http://hbr.org/2011/03/the-new-path-to-the-c-suite/ar/1

Institute of Medicine. 2001. Committee on Quality of Health Care in America. *Crossing the Quality Chasm: A New Health System for the 21st Century.* Washington, DC: National Academy Press.

Office of the National Coordinator for Health Information Technology. 2011. Get the facts about health IT workforce development program. Hyattsville, MD: HHS.

Rollins, Genna. 2010. Forces of Change: The Growth of Data Drives Demand for Data Management. *Journal of AHIMA* 81(10):28–32.

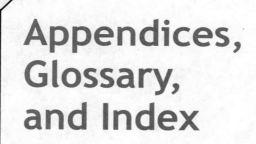

Appendices, Glossary, and Index

Sample HIM Position Descriptions

The following position descriptions and related articles may be found in the AHIMA website at http://ahima.org. In some cases, access is restricted to AHIMA members. (Some descriptions are included in more than one category.) The website is regularly updated to reflect current and emerging practice areas.

Role	Job Title
Management	Health Information Director, Health Information Management Supervisor, Project Manager
Data management	Specialist, Clinical Data Specialist, Data Quality Manager, Data Resource Administrator, Data Analyst, EHR Data Integrity Analyst
EHR	Clinical Analyst, Clinical Applications Coordinator, Clinical Project Manager, Senior Project Manager, Clinical Research Associate, Clinical Vocabulary Manager, Compliance and Privacy Officer—eHealth, Enterprise Applications Specialist, Health Systems Specialist, Health Information Services, Department Technician Information Privacy Coordinator, Integration Architect (Implementation), Optical Imaging Coordinator, Process Improvement Engineer, Records and Information Coordinator, Risk Management Specialist, Senior Document Coordinator, Solution Analyst, Solution Consultant, Systems Analyst *See: EHR career opportunities: Sample HIM job descriptions*
Emerging roles	Clinical Data Specialist, Data Quality Manager, Data Resource Administrator, Health Information Manager for Integrated Systems, Information Security Manager, Patient Information Coordinator, Research and Decision Support Specialist *See: Evolving HIM careers: Seven roles for the future*

General	Educator, Health Information Management Director, HIM Domain Manager, Medical Staff Coordinator, Patient Information Coordinator, Risk Manager, Utilization Management Director
Privacy and security	Compliance and Privacy Officer—eHealth, Compliance and Regulatory Management Officer, Compliance Manager/Director/Officer, Copy Service Manager, Corporate Compliance Director, Disclosure Coordinator, Information Officer/Chief Information Officer, Information Security Manager, Information Services Manager, Medical Records Manager, Patient Accounts Manager, Privacy Officer/Chief Privacy Officer, Release of Information Coordinator, Security Manager/Director/Officer *See: Success at every level: A career ladder for privacy officers*
Quality	Quality Improvement Director

Sample Notice of Health Information Practices

This notice describes how information about you may be used and disclosed and how you can get access to this information. Please review it carefully.

Understanding Your Health Record/Information

Each time you visit a hospital, physician, or other healthcare provider, a record of your visit is made. Typically, this record contains your symptoms, examination and test results, diagnoses, treatment, and a plan for future care or treatment. This information, often referred to as your health or medical record, serves as a:

- basis for planning your care and treatment;
- means of communication among the many health professionals who contribute to your care;
- legal document describing the care you received;
- means by which you or a third-party payer can verify that services billed were actually provided;
- tool in educating health professionals;
- source of data for medical research;
- source of information for public health officials charged with improving the health of the nation;
- source of data for facility planning and marketing; and
- tool with which we can assess and continually work to improve the care we render and the outcomes we achieve.

Understanding what is in your record and how your health information is used helps you to:

- ensure its accuracy;
- better understand who, what, when, where, and why others may access your health information; and
- make more informed decisions when authorizing disclosure to others.

Your Health Information Rights

Although your health record is the physical property of the healthcare practitioner or facility that compiled it, the information belongs to you. You have the right to:

- request a restriction on certain uses and disclosures of your information as provided by 45 CFR 164.522;
- obtain a paper copy of the notice of information practices upon request;
- inspect and copy your health record as provided for in 45 CFR 164.524;
- amend your health record as provided in 45 CFR 164.528;
- obtain an accounting of disclosures of your health information as provided in 45 CFR 164.528;
- request communication of your health information by alternative means or at alternative locations; and
- revoke your authorization to use or disclose health information except to the extent that action has already been taken.

Our Responsibilities

This organization is required to:

- maintain the privacy of your health information;
- provide you with a notice as to our legal duties and privacy practices with respect to information we collect and maintain about you;
- abide by the terms of this notice;
- notify you if we are unable to agree to a requested restriction; and
- accommodate reasonable requests you may have to communicate health information by alternative means or at alternative locations.

We reserve the right to change our practices and to make the new provisions effective for all protected health information we maintain. Should our information practices change, we will mail a revised notice to the address you've supplied us.

We will not use or disclose your health information without your authorization, except as described in this notice.

For More Information or to Report a Problem

If you have questions and would like additional information, you may contact the Director of Health Information Management at (444) 111-1111.

If you believe your privacy rights have been violated, you can file a complaint with the Director of Health Information Management or with the Secretary of Health and Human Services. There will be no retaliation for filing a complaint.

Examples of Disclosures for Treatment, Payment, and Health Operations

We will use your health information for treatment. For example: Information obtained by a nurse, physician, or other member of your healthcare team will be recorded in your record and used to determine the course of treatment that should work best for you. Your physician will document in your record his/her expectations of the members of your healthcare team. Members of your healthcare team will then record the actions they take and their observations. In this way your physician will know how you are responding to treatment.

We will also provide your physician or a subsequent healthcare provider with copies of various reports that should assist him/her in treating you once you're discharged from this hospital.

We will use your health information for payment. For example: A bill may be sent to you or a third-party payer. The information on or accompanying the bill may include information that identifies you, as well as your diagnosis, procedures, and supplies used.

We will use your health information for regular health operations. For example: Members of the medical staff, the risk or quality improvement manager, or members of the quality improvement team may use information in your health record to assess the care and outcomes in your case and others like it. This information will then be used in an effort to continually improve the quality and effectiveness of the healthcare and service we provide.

Other Uses or Disclosures

Business Associates: There are some services provided in our organization through contacts with business associates. Examples include physician services in the Emergency Department and Radiology, certain laboratory tests, and a copy service we use when making copies of your health record. When these services are contracted, we may disclose your health information to our business associates so that they can perform the job we've asked them to do and bill you or your third-party payer for services rendered. So that your health information is protected, however, we require the business associate to appropriately safeguard your information.

Directory: Unless you notify us that you object, we will use your name, location in the facility, general condition, and religious affiliation for directory purposes. This information may be provided to members of the clergy and, except for religious affiliation, to other people who ask for you by name.

Notification: We may use or disclose information to notify or assist in notifying a family member, a personal representative, or another person responsible for your care of your location and general condition.

Communication with Family: Health professionals, using their best judgment, may disclose to a family member, another relative, a close personal friend, or any other person you identify health information relevant to that person's involvement in your care or payment related to your care.

Research: We may disclose information to researchers when their research has been approved by an institutional review board that has reviewed the research proposal and established protocols to ensure the privacy of your health information.

Funeral Directors: We may disclose health information to funeral directors consistent with applicable law to carry out their duties.

Organ Procurement Organizations: Consistent with applicable law, we may disclose health information to organ procurement organizations or other entities engaged in the procurement, banking, or transplantation of organs for the purpose of tissue donation and transplant.

Marketing: We may contact you to provide appointment reminders or information about treatment alternatives or other health-related benefits and services that may be of interest to you.

Fund-Raising: We may contact you as part of a fund-raising effort.

Food and Drug Administration (FDA): We may disclose to the FDA health information relative to adverse events with respect to food, supplements, products and product defects, or post-marketing surveillance information to enable product recalls, repairs, or replacement.

Workers' Compensation: We may disclose health information to the extent authorized by, and to the extent necessary to comply with, laws relating to workers' compensation or other similar programs established by law.

Public Health: As required by law, we may disclose your health information to public health or legal authorities charged with preventing or controlling disease, injury, or disability.

Correctional Institution: Should you be an inmate of a correctional institution, we may disclose to the institution, or agents thereof, health information necessary for your health and the health and safety of other individuals.

Law Enforcement: We may disclose health information for law enforcement purposes as required by law, or in response to a valid subpoena.

Federal law makes provision for your health information to be released to an appropriate health oversight agency, public health authority, or attorney, provided that a workforce member or business associate believes in good faith that we have engaged in unlawful conduct or have otherwise violated professional or clinical standards and are potentially endangering one or more patients or workers or the public.

My signature below indicates that I have been provided with a copy of the notice of privacy practices.

_____
Signature of Patient or Legal Representative

Date:

If signed by legal representative, relationship to patient _____

Effective Date:

Distribution: Original to provider; copy to patient

Source: AHIMA. 2002 (November). Practice brief (updated): Notice of information practices. *Journal of American Health Information Management Association.* Available online at http://ahima.org.

The above form is not meant to encompass all the various ways in which any particular facility may use health information. For example, those who use protected health information for fund-raising or marketing will want to add those types of disclosures. It is intended to get readers started insofar as developing their own notices. As with any form of this nature, the document should be reviewed and approved by legal counsel prior to implementation.

Check Your Understanding Key

 Chapter 1

1.1
1. C
2. B
3. C
4. A
5. A
6. D
7. B
8. B

1.2
1. C
2. B
3. B
4. D
5. D

 Chapter 2

2.1
1. B
2. C
3. D
4. B
5. C

6. T
7. F
8. F
9. F
10. F

2.2

1. A
2. D
3. C
4. B
5. A
6. F
7. F
8. F
9. T
10. F

2.3

1. A
2. D
3. D
4. B
5. D
6. A
7. B
8. D
9. E
10. C

 # Chapter 3

3.1

1. B
2. D
3. C
4. B
5. B
6. A
7. B

3.2

1. B
2. A
3. C
4. A
5. C
6. B
7. D
8. A

3.3

1. B
2. A

3. C
4. B
5. C
6. B
7. C
8. D
9. B
10. C

3.4

1. A
2. C
3. C
4. A
5. B
6. A
7. A
8. B

Chapter 4

4.1
1. D
2. D
3. B
4. A
5. C
6. B
7. B
8. D
9. B
10. C

4.2
1. B
2. B
3. B
4. D
5. D
6. C
7. A
8. A
9. D

Chapter 5

5.1
1. bacillary, bacilluria, bacillus, back
2. abortus infection, anthracis infection, coli, infection
3. a. P
   b. D
   c. D
   d. P
   e. D
   f. P

5.2
1. benign
2. malignant, metastatic
3. malignant, primary
4. carcinoma in situ

5.3
1. evaluation and management
2. medicine
3. surgical
4. anesthesia
5. pathology & laboratory
6. radiology
7. category III codes

5.4
1. e
2. a
3. b

5.5
1. T
2. T
3. F
4. F
5. T

5.6
1. F
2. T
3. T
4. T
5. T

5.7
1. F
2. F
3. F

4. F
5. T

Chapter 6

6.1
1. B
2. B
3. B
4. C
5. D
6. A

7. C
8. C

6.2
1. B
2. D
3. D
4. C
5. A

6.6
1. C
2. A
3. B
4. B
5. B

6.3
1. B
2. A
3. D
4. C
5. D

6.7
1. B
2. A
3. B
4. D
5. A
6. C
7. C
8. A
9. A
10. A
11. B
12. D
13. B
14. B
15. A

6.4
1. D
2. B
3. C
4. D
5. A

6.5
1. B
2. D
3. C
4. A
5. D
6. D

6.8
1. C
2. B
3. C
4. T
5. T

6. F	
7. T	
8. T	

6.9	1. A
	2. B
	3. A
	4. D

5. A	
6. C	
7. D	
8. T	p. 303
9. T	p. 302
10. T	p. 304
11. F	p. 305–306

✓ Chapter 7

7.1	1. B
	2. A
	3. D
	4. A
	5. A
	6. A
	7. A
	8. C
	9. B
	10. D

7.2	1. B
	2. D
	3. D
	4. B
	5. B

7.3	1. C
	2. C
	3. B
	4. C
	5. A

7.4	1. C
	2. D
	3. C

4. D	
5. B	

7.5	1. A
	2. A
	3. D
	4. B
	5. C
	6. B
	7. B
	8. F
	9. T
	10. T

7.6	1. C
	2. A
	3. D
	4. B
	5. A

7.7	1. B
	2. C
	3. B
	4. B
	5. D
	6. T

7.	F	5.	B
8.	T	6.	D
9.	T	7.	A
10.	F	8.	C

7.8
1.	A	9.	A
2.	A	10.	B
3.	B	11.	A
4.	C	12.	A

 # Chapter 8

8.1
1.	A	6.	B
2.	D	7.	A
3.	A	8.	A
4.	T	9.	C
5.	F		
6.	T		
7.	F		

8.3
1.	D
2.	C

8.2
1.	B	3.	A
2.	D	4.	F
3.	A	5.	T
4.	A	6.	F
5.	C	7.	T

 # Chapter 9

9.1
1.	Discrete	7.	Continuous
2.	Continuous	8.	Discrete
3.	Discrete	9.	Continuous
4.	Continuous	10.	Discrete
5.	Discrete	11.	Discrete
6.	Discrete	12.	Continuous

13. Discrete

14. Discrete

15. Continuous

9.2   1. ratio

2. proportion

3. rate

9.3   1. a. $(150 + 20) - 15 = 155$

b. $[(150 + 20) - 15] + 2 = 157$

c. $[(150 + 20) - 15] + 2 = 157$

2. a. $(14 + 5) - 3 = 16$

b. $[(14 + 5) - 3] + 1 = 17$

3. a. (10 remaining + 1 from the ESD + 1 from Surgery + 1 from Medicine) – 1 patient to Medicine unit = 12

b. [((10 remaining + 1 from ESD + 1 from Surgery + 1 from Medicine) – 1 patient to Medicine unit)] + 1 A&D = 13

9.4   1. Medicine $36 \times 30 = 1,080$
$(580/1,080) \times 100 = 53.7$

Surgery $42 \times 30 = 1,260$
$(689/1,260) \times 100 = 54.7$

Pediatric $18 \times 30 = 540$
$(232/540) \times 100 = 43.0$

Psychiatric $35 \times 30 = 1,050$
$(889/1,050) \times 100 = 84.7$

Obstetrics $10 \times 30 = 300$
$(222/300) \times 100 = 74.0$

Newborn $15 \times 30 = 450$
$(222/450) \times 100 = 49.3$

2. $580 + 689 + 232 + 889 + 222 + 222 = 2,834$

$36 + 42 + 18 + 35 + 10 + 15 = 156$

$156 \times 30 = 4,680$

$(2,834/4,680) \times 100 = 60.6$

3. January–June $31 + 28 + 31 + 30 + 31 + 30 = 181$

$181 \times 156 = 28,236$

$(15,672/28,236) \times 100 = 55.5$

July–December $31 + 31 + 30 + 31 + 30 + 31 = 184$

$184 \times 200 = 36,800$

$(25,876/36,800) \times 100 = 70.3$

Total $15,672 + 25,876 = 41,548$

$28,236 + 36,800 = 65,036$

$(41,548/65,036) \times 100 = 63.9$

9.5   1. a. $72 + 70 + 72 + 136 + 32 + 81 + 68 + 80 + 63 + 84 = 758$

b. $72 + 70 + 72 + 136 + 32 + 81 + 68 + 80 + 63 + 84 = 758$

$12 + 10 + 12 + 17 + 8 + 9 + 11 + 10 + 14 + 12 = 115$

c. $72 + 70 + 72 + 136 + 32 + 81 + 68 + 80 + 63 + 84 = 758$

$12 + 10 + 12 + 17 + 8 + 9 + 11 + 10 + 14 + 12 = 115$

$758/115 = 6.6$

9.6
1. $(20 \times 100)/1{,}250 = 1.60\%$
2. $[(20 - 3) \times 100]/(1{,}250 - 3) = 1{,}700/1{,}247 = 1.36\%$
3. $(4 \times 100)/(155 + 4) = 400/159 = 2.52\%$
4. $(2 \times 100)/155 = 1.29\%$
5. $[(20 + 2) \times 100]/(1{,}250+2) = 2{,}200/1{,}252 = 1.76\%$
6. $(1 \times 100)/155 = 0.65\%$

9.7
1. $(12/25) \times 100 = 48\%$
2. $(12/(25-2)) \times 100 = 52\%$
3. $(13/(25 + 1)) \times 100 = 50\%$

9.8
1. $(6 \times 100)/57 = 10.5\%$
2. $(57 \times 100)/149 = 38.3\%$
3. MS-DRG 179
$1.0088 \times 5 = 5.0440$
MS-DRG 187
$1.0620 \times 2 = 2.1240$
MS-DRG 189
$1.3455 \times 3 = 4.0365$
MS-DRG 194
$0.9976 \times 1 = 0.9976$
MS-DRG 208
$2.2358 \times 1 = 2.2358$
MS-DRG 280
$1.8313 \times 3 = 5.4939$
MS-DRG 299
$1.4045 \times 2 = 2.8090$
MS-DRG 313
$0.5404 \times 4 = 2.1616$
MS-DRG 377
$1.6149 \times 1 = 1.6149$
MS-DRG 391
$1.0958 \times 1 = 1.0958$
MS-DRG 547
$0.7475 \times 1 = 0.7475$
MS-DRG 552
$0.7937 \times 1 = 0.7937$

MS-DRG 684
$0.6746 \times 1 = 0.6746$
MS-DRG 812
$0.7751 \times 2 = 1.5502$
MS-DRG 872
$1.1155 \times 1 = 1.1155$
MS-DRG 918
$0.5839 \times 1 = 0.5839$

$5 + 2 + 3 + 1 + 1 + 3 + 2 + 4 + 1 + 1 + 1 + 1 + 1 + 2 + 1 + 1 = 30$

$5.0440 + 2.1240 + 4.0365 + 0.9976 + 2.2358 + 5.4939 + 2.8090 + 2.1616 + 1.6149 + 1.0958 + 0.7475 + 0.7937 + 0.6746 + 1.5502 + 1.1155 + 0.5839 = 33.0785$

$33.0785/30 = 1.1026$

4. Nosocomial infection

9.9
1. A
2. E
3. J
4. K
5. F
6. D
7. G
8. I
9. H
10. B
11. C

9.10
1. $(1{,}203{,}812/148{,}660{,}898) \times 10{,}000 = 81$ deaths per 10,000 population
2. $(1{,}219{,}699/152{,}962{,}259) \times 10{,}000 = 79.7$ deaths per 10,000 population

3. $(1,203,812 + 1,219,699)/$
   $(148,660,898 +$
   $152,962,259) \times 10,000 =$
   $(2,423,511/301,623,157)$
   $\times 10,000 = 80.3$ deaths
   per 10,000 population

4. $50,105/21,618,734 =$
   $.00232 \times 10,000 = 23.18$

5. $(29,501 + 70,230)/$
   $(21,542,555 +$
   $22,279,847) \times 10,000 =$
   $(99,731/43,822,402) \times$
   $10,000 = 22.8$ deaths per
   10,000 population

9.11

1. Incidence: used to
   compare the frequency of
   disease in populations
   Prevalence: the
   proportion of persons in
   a population who have
   a particular disease at a
   specific point in time or
   over a specified period of
   time.

2. Notifiable disease:
   one for which regular,
   frequent, and timely
   information on individual
   cases is considered
   necessary to prevent and
   control disease

3. $(189,000/301,623,157)$
   $\times 100,000 = 62.7$ new
   cases per 100,000
   population

9.12

1. table
2. pie
3. line
4. bar
5. histogram
6. boxplot
7. scatter chart

9.13

1. $2,450 + 2,540 + 2,300 +$
   $2,715 + 2,400 + 2,750 +$
   $2,815 + 1,735 + 1,800 +$
   $2,485 + 2,600 + 2,540 +$
   $1,720 + 2,780 + 2,640 =$
   $36,270/15 = 2,418$

2. 1,720, 1,735, 1,800,
   2,300, 2,400, 2,450,
   2,485, **2,540**, 2,540,
   2,600, 2,640, 2,715,
   2,750, 2,780, 2,815

3. 1,720, 1,735, 1,800,
   2,300, 2,400, 2,450,
   2,485, **2,540, 2,540**,
   2,600, 2,640, 2,715,
   2,750, 2,780, 2,815

4. $2,815 - 1,720 = 1,095$
5. 1,396,147.1
6. 373.7

9.14

1. Bell shaped and
   symmetrical about mean.

2. Skewness is the
   horizontal stretching of
   a frequency distribution
   to one side or the other
   so that one tail is longer
   than the other.

3. Kurtosis is the
   vertical stretching of a
   distribution

9.15

1. 25 minutes $\times$ 400 records
   $= 10,000$ minutes
   10,000 minutes/60
   minutes in one hour $=$
   $166.66 = 166.67$ hours
   166.7/37.5 productive
   hours $= 4.4$ FTEs

2. $\$10.23 \times 40 = 4,092 \times 52$
   $= \$21,278.40$

Chapter 10

10.1	1. A
	2. C
	3. A
	4. F
	5. F
	6. T
10.2	1. B
	2. D
	3. D
	4. T
	5. F
	6. T
10.3	1. B
	2. A
	3. C

	4. F
	5. T
	6. T
10.4	1. A
	2. A
	3. D
	4. F
	5. F
	6. T
10.5	1. A
	2. C
	3. D
	4. C
	5. A

 Chapter 11

11.1	1. D
	2. D
	3. B
	4. A
	5. B
	6. A
	7. D
	8. F
	9. F
	10. T
11.2	1. D
	2. D

	3. C
	4. B
	5. B
	6. C
	7. D
	8. B
	9. E
	10. A
11.3	1. B
	2. B
	3. C
	4. D

	5. C		8. C
	6. D		9. B
	7. C	11.6	1. C
	8. B		2. D
	9. E		3. A
	10. A		4. B
11.4	1. D		5. D
	2. A		6. C
	3. D		7. E
	4. A		8. A
	5. A		9. B
	6. T		10. D
	7. T	11.7	1. D
	8. T		2. C
	9. F		3. B
	10. F		4. B
11.5	1. B		5. D
	2. D		6. F
	3. C		7. T
	4. B		8. T
	5. D		9. F
	6. D		10. T
	7. A		

Chapter 12

12.1	1. C	12.2	1. E, B, D, A, F, G, C
	2. A	12.3	1. B
	3. A		2. A
	4. C		3. F
	5. B		4. T
	6. B		5. C
	7. C		6. D
	8. A		7. A
	9. D		8. B

✓ Chapter 13

13.1
1. D
2. B
3. C
4. D
5. C

13.2
1. A
2. B
3. D
4. D
5. C
6. B
7. D
8. D
9. D
10. A

13.3
1. D
2. C
3. A
4. C
5. B

13.4
1. A
2. A
3. C
4. A
5. B
6. D
7. D
8. A
9. B
10. B
11. B

12. A
13. D
14. D
15. D
16. D
17. A
18. C
19. A
20. D
21. D
22. B
23. D
24. D
25. A
26. B
27. C
28. D
29. D
30. D
31. C
32. C
33. C

13.5
1. B
2. A
3. D
4. D
5. B
6. B
7. C
8. A
9. B
10. B

Chapter 14

14.1	1. D	3. F	
	2. B	4. T	
	3. B	5. F	
	4. D	6. T	
	5. A	7. T	
14.2	1. D	8. T	
	2. B	9. T	
	3. E	**14.5**	1. C
	4. A		2. E
14.3	1. A		3. G
	2. B		4. D
	3. B		5. J
	4. D		6. B
	5. C		7. I
	6. 3, 4, 1, 9, 7, 11, 13, 15, 6, 16, 14, 8, 5, 10, 12, 2		8. H
			9. A
14.4	1. F		10. F
	2. T		

Chapter 15

15.1	1. C	**15.2**	1. B
	2. D		2. C
	3. C		3. A
	4. C		4. D
	5. C		5. C
	6. F		6. B
	7. T		7. D
	8. F		8. A
	9. T		9. C
	10. T		10. E

15.3   1. D
2. D
3. C
4. B
5. D

15.4   1. C
2. C
3. A
4. A
5. D

 Chapter 16

16.1   1. A
2. B
3. A
4. A
5. C
6. T
7. T
8. T
9. F
10. T

16.2   1. B
2. A
3. C
4. B
5. B
6. T
7. F
8. T
9. F
10. T

16.3   1. D
2. C
3. C
4. D
5. B

16.4   1. B
2. B
3. C
4. D
5. A
6. A
7. D
8. B
9. E
10. C

16.5   1. C
2. B
3. C
4. B
5. D

Chapter 17

17.1
1. A
2. D
3. B
4. T
5. T
6. T
7. F
8. T

17.2
1. B
2. D
3. A
4. B
5. A
6. H
7. B
8. D
9. E
10. F

11. C
12. G

17.3
1. C
2. B
3. B
4. C
5. B
6. A
7. C
8. C
9. A
10. A

17.4
1. T
2. F
3. T
4. T
5. T

Chapter 18

18.1
1. B
2. C
3. D
4. A
5. B
6. T
7. F
8. F
9. F
10. F

18.2
1. A
2. B
3. B
4. C
5. C
6. F
7. T
8. T
9. T
10. F

18.3

1. A
2. B
3. C
4. B
5. A
6. D
7. C
8. B
9. B
10. C

18.4

1. A
2. B
3. D
4. F
5. F
6. T
7. T
8. F

Glossary

Abbreviated Injury Scale (AIS): A set of numbers used in a trauma registry to indicate the nature and severity of injuries by body system

Abstracting: 1. The process of extracting information from a document to create a brief summary of a patient's illness, treatment, and outcome 2. The process of extracting elements of data from a source document or database and entering them into an automated system

Accept assignment: A term used to refer to a provider's or a supplier's acceptance of the allowed charges (from a fee schedule) as payment in full for services or materials provided

Acceptance testing: Final review during EHR implementation to ensure that all tests have been performed and all issues have been resolved; usually triggers the final payment for the system and when a maintenance contract becomes effective

Access control: 1. A computer software program designed to prevent unauthorized use of an information resource 2. The process of designing, implementing, and monitoring a system for guaranteeing that only individuals with a legitimate need are allowed to view or amend specific data sets

Access report: Report that provides a list of individuals who accessed the patient information during a given period

Accession number: A number assigned to each case as it is entered in a cancer registry

Accession registry: A list of cases in a cancer registry in the order in which they were entered

Accommodating: In business, the practice whereby one party in a conflict or disagreement gives in to the other party as a temporary solution

Accountability: Responsibility for a specific activity

Accountable Care Organization (ACO): An organization of healthcare providers accountable for the quality, cost, and overall care of Medicare beneficiaries who are assigned and enrolled in the traditional fee-for-service program

Accounts receivable (A/R): Records of the payments owed to the organization by outside entities such as third-party payers and patients

Accreditation: 1. A voluntary process of institutional or organizational review in which a quasi-independent body created for this purpose periodically evaluates the quality of the entity's work against preestablished written criteria 2. A determination by an accrediting body that an eligible organization, network, program, group, or individual complies with applicable standards

Accreditation Association for Ambulatory Health Care (AAAHC): A professional organization that offers accreditation programs for ambulatory and outpatient organizations such as single- and multispecialty group practices, ambulatory surgery centers, college/university health services, and community health centers

Accreditation Commission for Health Care (ACHC): A private nonprofit accreditation organization offering accreditation services for home health, hospice, and alternate site healthcare such as infusion nursing, and home/durable medical equipment supplies

Accreditation organization: A professional organization that establishes the standards against which healthcare organizations are measured and conducts periodic assessments of the performance of individual healthcare organizations

Accreditation standards: Preestablished statements of the criteria against which the performance of participating healthcare organizations will be assessed during a voluntary accreditation process

Accredited Standards Committee X12N (ASC X12N): A committee of the National Standards Institute that develops and maintains standards for the electronic exchange of business transactions, such as 837—Health Care Claim, 835—Health Care Claim Payment/Advice, and others

Action steps: Specific plans an organization intends to accomplish in the near future as an effort toward achieving its long-term strategic plan

Active membership: Individuals interested in the AHIMA purpose and willing to abide by the Code of Ethics are eligible for active membership; active members in good standing shall be entitled to all membership privileges including the right to vote

Activities of daily living (ADL): The basic activities of self-care, including grooming, bathing, ambulating, toileting, and eating

Actor: The role a user plays in a system

Acute care: Medical care of a limited duration that is provided in an inpatient hospital setting to diagnose and/or treat an injury or a short-term illness

Acute care prospective payment system (PPS): The reimbursement system for inpatient hospital services provided to Medicare and Medicaid beneficiaries that is based on the use of diagnosis-related groups as a classification tool

Ad hoc committee: A group of individuals who join together to solve a particular task or problem

Administrative controls: Policies and procedures that address the management of computer resources

Administrative information systems: A category of healthcare information systems that supports human resources management, financial management, executive decision support, and other business-related functions

Administrative law: A body of rules and regulations developed by various administrative entities empowered by Congress; falls under the umbrella of public law

Administrative provisions: Documented, formal practices to manage data security measures throughout the healthcare organization

Administrative services only (ASO) contract: An agreement between an employer and an insurance organization to administer the employer's self-insured health plan

Administrative simplification: A term referring to HIPAA's attempt to streamline and standardize the healthcare industry's nonuniform and seemingly chaotic business practices, such as billing

Admissibility: The condition of being admitted into evidence in a court of law

Admission-discharge-transfer (ADT): The name given to the computer systems in healthcare facilities that register and track patients

Admission utilization review: A review of planned services (intensity of service) and/or a patient's condition (severity of illness) to determine whether care must be delivered in an acute care setting

Advance Beneficiary Notice of Noncoverage (ABN): A statement signed by the patient when he or she is notified by the provider, prior to a service or procedure being done, that Medicare may not reimburse the provider for the service, wherein the patient indicates that he will be responsible for any charges

Advance directive: A legal, written document that describes the patient's preferences regarding future healthcare or stipulates the person who is authorized to make medical decisions in the event the patient is incapable of communicating his or her preferences

Affinity grouping: A technique for organizing similar ideas together in natural groupings

Affordable Care Act: Also known as Patient Protection and Affordable Care Act (PPACA). A federal statute that was signed into law on March 23, 2010. Along with the Health Care and Education Reconciliation Act of 2010 (signed into law on March 30, 2010), the Act is the product of the healthcare reform agenda of the Democratic 111th Congress and the Obama administration

Age Discrimination in Employment Act: Federal legislation that prohibits employment discrimination against persons between the ages of 40 and 70 and restricts mandatory retirement requirements except where age is a bona fide occupational qualification

Agency for Healthcare Research and Quality (AHRQ): The branch of the United States Public Health Service that supports general health research and distributes research findings and treatment guidelines with the goal of improving the quality, appropriateness, and effectiveness of healthcare services

Aggregate data: Data extracted from individual health records and combined to form de-identified information about groups of patients that can be compared and analyzed

Aggregate information system: The combining of various data sets in order to compile overview or summary statistics

Alert fatigue: When an excessive number of alerts are used in an information system, users may get tired of looking at the alerts and ignore them.

All patient DRGs (AP-DRGs): A case-mix system developed by 3M and used in a number of state reimbursement systems to classify non-Medicare discharges for reimbursement purposes

Allied health professional: A credentialed healthcare worker who is not a physician, nurse, psychologist, or pharmacist (for example, a physical therapist, dietitian, social worker, or occupational therapist)

Alphabetic filing system: A system of health record identification and storage that uses the patient's last name as the first component of identification and his or her first name and middle name or initial for further definition

Alphanumeric filing system: A system of health record identification and storage that uses a combination of alphabetic letters (usually the first two letters of the patient's last name) and numbers to identify individual records

Ambulatory care information system: A type of information system used to support ambulatory care

Ambulatory payment classification (APC) system: Hospital outpatient prospective payment system (HOPPS); the classification is a resource-based reimbursement system; the payment unit is the ambulatory payment classification group (APC group)

Ambulatory payment classification group (APC group): Basic unit of the ambulatory payment classification (APC) system. Within a group, the diagnoses and procedures are similar in terms of resources used, complexity of illness, and conditions represented. A single payment is made for the outpatient services provided. APC groups are based on HCPCS/CPT codes. A single visit can result in multiple APC groups. APC groups consist of five types of service: significant procedures, surgical services, medical visits, ancillary services, and partial hospitalization. The APC group was formerly known as the ambulatory visit group (AVG) and ambulatory patient group (APG).

Ambulatory surgery center (ASC): Under Medicare, an outpatient surgical facility that has its own national identifier; is a separate entity with respect to its licensure, accreditation, governance, professional supervision, administrative functions, clinical services, recordkeeping, and financial and accounting systems; has as its sole purpose the provision of services in connection with surgical procedures that do not require inpatient hospital-ization; and meets the conditions and requirements set forth in the Medicare Conditions of Participation

American Academy of Professional Coders: The American Academy of Professional Coders provides certified credentials to medical coders in physician offices, hospital out-patient facilities, ambulatory surgical centers, and in payer organizations

American Association for Accreditation of Ambulatory Surgery Facilities (AAAASF): An organization that sets standards for accrediting ambulatory surgical facilities

American Association of Health Plans (AAHP): The trade organization for health main-tenance organizations, preferred provider organizations, and other network-based health plans created by the merger of the Group Health Association of America and the American Managed Care and Review Association

American Association of Medical Colleges (AAMC): The organization established in 1876 to standardize the curriculum for medical schools in the United States and to pro-mote the licensure of physicians

American Association of Medical Record Librarians (AAMRL): The name adopted by the Association of Record Librarians of North America in 1944; precursor of the **American Health Information Management Association**

American College of Healthcare Executives (ACHE): The national professional organi-zation of healthcare administrators that provides certification services for its members and promotes excellence in the field

American College of Radiology-National Electrical Manufacturers Association (ACR-NEMA): The professional organization (ACR) and trade association (NEMA) that work collaboratively to develop digital imaging standards

American College of Surgeons (ACS): The scientific and educational association of sur-geons formed to improve the quality of surgical care by setting high standards for surgical education and practice

American Correctional Association: An organization that developed basic accreditation standards for healthcare in correctional facilities

American Health Information Management Association (AHIMA): The professional membership organization for managers of health record services and healthcare informa-tion systems as well as coding services; provides accreditation, certification, and educa-tional services

American Hospital Association (AHA): The national trade organization that provides education, conducts research, and represents the hospital industry's interests in national legislative matters; membership includes individual healthcare organizations as well as individual healthcare professionals working in specialized areas of hospitals, such as risk management

American Medical Association (AMA): The national professional membership organization for physicians that distributes scientific information to its members and the public, informs members of legislation related to health and medicine, and represents the medical profession's interests in national legislative matters

American Medical Record Association (AMRA): The name adopted by the American Association of Medical Record Librarians in 1970; precursor of the **American Health Information Management Association**

American National Standards Institute (ANSI): The organization that accredits all U.S. standards development organizations to ensure that they are following due process in promulgating standards

American Nurses Association (ANA): The national professional membership association of nurses that works for the improvement of health standards and the availability of healthcare services, fosters high professional standards for the nursing profession, and advances the economic and general welfare of nurses

American Osteopathic Association (AOA): The professional association of osteopathic physicians, surgeons, and graduates of approved colleges of osteopathic medicine that inspects and accredits osteopathic colleges and hospitals

American Recovery and Reinvestment Act of 2009 (ARRA): Previously known as the stimulus bill or HR 1. The actions related to health information technology are spread throughout the law; however, the bulk of the items are in Title XIII—Health Information Technology; also called Health Information Technology for Economic and Clinical Health Act or HITECH

American Society for Healthcare Risk Management (ASHRM): The professional society for healthcare risk management professionals that is affiliated with the American Hospital Association and provides educational tools and networking opportunities for its members

American Society for Testing and Materials (ASTM): A national organization whose purpose is to establish standards on materials, products, systems, and services

Americans with Disabilities Act of 1990: Federal legislation that makes it illegal to discriminate against individuals with disabilities in employment, public accommodations, public services, transportation, and telecommunications

Ancillary systems: Electronic systems that generate clinical information (such as laboratory information systems, radiology information systems, pharmacy information systems, and so on)

Anesthesia report: The report that notes any preoperative medication and response to it, the anesthesia administered with dose and method of administration, the duration of administration, the patient's vital signs while under anesthesia, and any additional products given the patient during a procedure

APC grouper: Software programs that help coders determine the appropriate ambulatory payment classification for an outpatient encounter

Appeal: A request for reconsideration of a negative claim decision

Appellate court: In a state court system, the court that hears appeals of final judgments from state trial courts

Application controls: Security strategies, such as password management, included in application software and computer programs

Application service provider (ASP): A third-party service company that delivers, manages, and remotely hosts standardized applications software via a network through an outsourcing contract based on fixed monthly usage or transaction-based pricing

Application software: Software designed to assist a user in performing either a single task or multiple, related tasks

Arbitration: A proceeding in which disputes are submitted to a third party or a panel of experts outside the judicial trial system

Architecture: The configuration, structure, and relationships of hardware (the machinery of the computer including input/output devices, storage devices, and so on) in an information system

Artificial intelligence: High-level information technologies used in developing machines that imitate human qualities such as learning and reasoning

Assembler: A computer program that translates assembly-language instructions into machine language

Assembly language: A second-generation computer programming language that uses simple phrases rather than the complex series of switches used in machine language

Assets: The human, financial, and physical resources of an organization

Association of Record Librarians of North America (ARLNA): Organization formed 10 years after the beginning of the hospital standardization movement whose original objective was to elevate the standards of clinical recordkeeping in hospitals, dispensaries, and other healthcare facilities; precursor of the **American Health Information Management Association**

Association for Healthcare Documentation Integrity (AHDI): Formerly the American Association for Medical Transcription (AAMT), the AHDI has a model curriculum for formal educational programs that includes the study of medical terminology, anatomy and physiology, medical science, operative procedures, instruments, supplies, laboratory values, reference use and research techniques, and English grammar

ASTM International: Formerly known as the American Society for Testing and Materials, a system of standards developed primarily for various EHR management processes

ASTM Standard E1384-02a: Standard that identifies the content and structure for EHRs, covering all types of healthcare services, including acute care hospitals, ambulatory care, skilled nursing facilities, home healthcare, and specialty environments

Attending Physician Statement (APS): The standardized insurance claim form created in 1958 by the Health Insurance Association of America and the American Medical Association

Audit controls: A method for monitoring attempts to gain access to a computer information system

Audit log (audit trail): "A chronological set of computerized records that provides evidence of information system activity (log-ins and log-outs, file accesses) that is used to determine security violations" (Harris, S. 2005. *CISSP Exam Guide.* New York: McGraw-Hill/Osborne)

Auditing: The performance of internal and/or external reviews (audits) to identify variations from established baselines (for example, review of outpatient coding as compared with CMS outpatient coding guidelines)

Authenticate: Confirm by signing

Authentication: 1. The process of identifying the source of health record entries by attaching a handwritten signature, the author's initials, or an electronic signature 2. Proof of authorship that ensures, as much as possible, that log-ins and messages from a user originate from an authorized source

Authority: The right to make decisions and take actions necessary to carry out assigned tasks

Authorization: The granting of permission to disclose confidential information; as defined in terms of the HIPAA Privacy Rule, an individual's formal, written permission to use or disclose his or her personally identifiable health information for purposes other than treatment, payment, or healthcare operations

Authorization to disclose information: An authorization that allows the healthcare facility to verbally disclose or send health information to other organizations; *See* **authorization**

Autodialing system: A method used to automatically call and remind patients of upcoming appointments

Automated drug dispensing machines: System that makes drugs available for patient care

Autonomy: A core ethical principle centered on the individual's right to self-determination that includes respect for the individual; in clinical applications, the patient's right to determine what does or does not happen to him or her in terms of healthcare

Autopsy report: Written documentation of the findings from a postmortem pathological examination

Average daily census: The mean number of hospital inpatients present in the hospital each day for a given period of time

Average length of stay (ALOS): The mean length of stay for hospital inpatients discharged during a given period of time

Avoiding: In business, a situation where two parties in conflict ignore that conflict

Back-end speech recognition: Specific use of SRT in an environment where the recognition process occurs after the completion of dictation by sending voice files through a server

Balance billing: A reimbursement method that allows providers to bill patients for charges in excess of the amount paid by the patients' health plan or other third-party payer (not allowed under Medicare or Medicaid)

Balanced Budget Refinement Act (BBRA) of 1999: The amended version of the Balanced Budget Act of 1997 that authorizes implementation of a per-discharge prospective payment system for care provided to Medicare beneficiaries by inpatient rehabilitation facilities

Bar chart: A graphic technique used to display frequency distributions of nominal or ordinal data that fall into categories

Barcode: Machine-readable code, appearing as a series of lines, that represents specific information

Barcode-enabled devices: Devices used throughout healthcare facilities that are designed to use barcodes for increased accuracy; *See* **barcoding technology**

Barcode medication administration record (BC-MAR): Systems that identify the right patient and right drug to be given at the right time, in the right dose, and via the right route

Barcoding technology: A method of encoding data that consists of parallel arrangements of dark elements, referred to as bars, and light elements, referred to as spaces, and interpreting the data for automatic identification and data collection purposes

Bar graph: *See* **bar chart**

Bed count (complement): The number of inpatient beds set up and staffed for use on a given day

Bed count day: A unit of measure that denotes the presence of one inpatient bed (either occupied or vacant) set up and staffed for use in one 24-hour period

Bed turnover rate: The average number of times a bed changes occupants during a given period of time

Benchmarking: An analysis process that is based on comparison

Bench trial: A trial in which a judge reviews the evidence and makes a determination, without a sitting jury

Beneficence: A legal term that means promoting good for others or providing services that benefit others, such as releasing health information that will help a patient receive care or will ensure payment for services received

Best of breed: A vendor strategy used when purchasing an EHR that refers to system applications that are considered the best in their class

Best of fit: A vendor strategy used when purchasing an EHR in which all the systems required by the healthcare facility are available from one vendor

Billing system: Information system that generates bill for healthcare services performed

Bioethics: A field of study that applies ethical principles to decisions that affect the lives of humans, such as whether to approve or deny access to health information

Biometrics: The physical characteristics of users (such as fingerprints, voiceprints, retinal scans, iris traits) that systems store and use to authenticate identity before allowing the user access to a system

Blanket authorization: An authorization for the release of confidential information from a certain point in time and any time thereafter

Blue Cross and Blue Shield (BC/BS): The first prepaid healthcare plans in the United States; Blue Shield plans traditionally cover hospital care and Blue Cross plans cover physicians' services

Blue Cross and Blue Shield Federal Employee Program (FEP): A federal program that offers a fee-for-service plan with preferred provider organizations and a point-of-service product

Board of directors: The elected or appointed group of officials who bear ultimate responsibility for the successful operation of a healthcare organization; *See* **board of governors**

Board of governors (board of trustees): The elected or appointed group of officials who bear ultimate responsibility for the successful operation of a healthcare organization

Board of trustees: *See* **board of directors**

Boxplot: Tool in the form of a graph that displays a five-number data summary

Brainstorming: A group problem-solving technique that involves the spontaneous contribution of ideas from all members of the group

Breach: A violation of the law

Breach notification: HITECH Act Rule that requires both HIPAA-covered entities and business associates to identify unsecured PHI breaches and notify the involved parties of the breach

Bubble chart: A type of scatter plot with circular symbols used to compare three variables; the area of the circle indicates the value of a third variable

Budget: A plan that converts the organization's goals and objectives into targets for revenue and spending

Bugs: Problems in software that prevent the smooth application of a function

Bundled payments: A category of payments made as lump sums to providers for all healthcare services delivered to a patient for a specific illness and/or over a specified time period; they include multiple services and may include multiple providers of care

Bureaucracy: A formal organizational structure based on a rigid hierarchy of decision making and inflexible rules and procedures

Bus: A type of hardware that controls the flow of commands between the central processor and other components

Bus topology: Type of network design

Business associate: According to the HIPAA Privacy Rule, an individual (or group) who is not a member of a covered entity's workforce but who helps the covered entity in the performance of various functions involving the use or disclosure of patient-identifiable health information

Business associate agreement: A written and signed contract that allows covered entities to lawfully disclose protected health information to business associates such as consultants, billing companies, accounting firms, or others that may perform services for the provider, provided that the business associate agrees to abide by the provider's requirements to protect the information's security and confidentiality

Business continuity plan: A program that incorporates policies and procedures for continuing business operations during a computer system shutdown; sometimes called **contingency and disaster planning**

Business intelligence: The end product or goal of knowledge management

Business process: A set of related policies and procedures that are performed step by step to accomplish a business-related function

Business-to-business (B2B): Transaction(s) between businesses—for example, between a wholesaler and a retailer

Business-to-customer (B2C): Transactions between businesses and public consumers

Capital budget: The allocation of resources for long-term investments and projects

Capitation: A method of healthcare reimbursement in which an insurance carrier prepays a physician, hospital, or other healthcare provider a fixed amount for a given population without regard to the actual number or nature of healthcare services provided to the population

Care pathways: A care-planning tool similar to a clinical practice guideline that has a multidisciplinary focus emphasizing the coordination of clinical services; *Also called* **clinical algorithm**; *See* **clinical pathway**; **critical path or critical pathway**

Care plan: The specific goals in the treatment of an individual patient, amended as the patient's condition requires, and the assessment of the outcomes of care; serves as the primary source for ongoing documentation of the resident's care, condition, and needs

Career planning: Looking beyond simply getting a job to position oneself for more challenging and diverse work in the long term

Case definition: A method of determining criteria for cases that should be included in a registry

Case fatality rate: The total number of deaths due to a specific illness during a given time period divided by the total number of cases during the same period

Case finding: A method of identifying patients who have been seen and/or treated in a healthcare facility for the particular disease or condition of interest to the registry

Case management: 1. The ongoing, concurrent review performed by clinical professionals to ensure the necessity and effectiveness of the clinical services being provided to a patient 2. A process that integrates and coordinates patient care over time and across multiple sites and providers, especially in complex and high-cost cases 3. The process of developing a specific care plan for a patient that serves as a communication tool to improve quality of care and reduce cost

Case mix: 1. A description of a patient population based on any number of specific characteristics, including age, gender, type of insurance, diagnosis, risk factors, treatment received, and resources used 2. Set of categories of patients (type and volume) treated by a healthcare organization and representing the complexity of the organization's caseload

Case-mix groups (CMGs): The 97 function-related groups into which inpatient rehabilitation facility discharges are classified on the basis of the patient's level of impairment, age, comorbidities, functional ability, and other factors

Case-mix group (CMG) relative weights: Factors that account for the variance in cost per discharge and resource utilization among case-mix groups

Case-mix index (CMI): The average relative weight of all cases treated at a given facility or by a given physician, which reflects the resource intensity or clinical severity of a specific group in relation to the other groups in the classification system; calculated by dividing the sum of the weights of diagnosis-related groups for patients discharged during a given period divided by the total number of patients discharged

Categorically needy eligibility groups: Categories of individuals to whom states must provide coverage under the federal Medicaid program

Causation: In law, a relationship between the defendant's conduct and the harm that was suffered

Cause-and-effect diagram: An investigational technique that facilitates the identification of the various factors that contribute to a problem; *See also* **fishbone diagram**

Cause-specific death rate: The total number of deaths due to a specific illness during a given time period divided by the estimated population for the same time period

Census: The number of inpatients present in a healthcare facility at any given time

Centers for Disease Control and Prevention (CDC): A group of federal agencies that oversee health promotion and disease control and prevention activities in the United States

Centers for Medicare and Medicaid Services (CMS): The division of the Department of Health and Human Services that is responsible for developing healthcare policy in the United States and for administering the Medicare program and the federal portion of the Medicaid program; called the Health Care Financing Administration (HCFA) prior to 2001

Certificate of destruction: A document that constitutes proof that a health record was destroyed and that includes the method of destruction, the signature of the person responsible for destruction, and inclusive dates for destruction

Certification: 1. The process by which a duly authorized body evaluates and recognizes an individual, institution, or educational program as meeting predetermined requirements 2. An evaluation performed to establish the extent to which a particular computer system, network design, or application implementation meets a prespecified set of requirements

Certification Commission on Health Information Technology (CCHIT): An effort initiated by the private sector to evaluate and potentially test EHR products against specific criteria, drawn from the HL7 standard EHR system functionality

Certified Document Improvement Professional: An individual who has achieved specialized skills in documentation improvement

Certified Tumor Registrar (CTR): An individual who has achieved specialized skills in the cancer registry

Chain of command: A hierarchical reporting structure within an organization

Change agent: An individual within an organization whose primary responsibility is to facilitate change

Change control: The process of performing an impact analysis and obtaining approval before modifications to the project scope are made

Change management: The formal process of introducing change, getting it adopted, and diffusing it throughout the organization

Charge capture: The process of collecting all services, procedures, and supplies provided during patient care

Chargemaster: A financial management form that contains information about the organization's charges for the healthcare services it provides to patients

Chart conversion: An EHR implementation activity in which data from the paper chart are converted into electronic form

Chart deficiency system: A software system designed to allow the HIM department to electronically track and manage documentation omissions from the health record

Checksheet: A tool that permits the systematic recording of observations of a particular phenomenon so that trends or patterns can be identified

Chief executive officer (CEO): The senior manager appointed by a governing board to direct an organization's overall management

Chief financial officer (CFO): The senior manager responsible for the fiscal management of an organization

Chief information officer (CIO): The senior manager responsible for the overall management of information resources in an organization

Chief information security officer (CISO): A recently created position that is responsible for overseeing the development, implementation, and enforcement of a healthcare organization's security policies, managing the security of all patient-identifiable information, whether stored in paper-based or computer-based systems

Chief medical informatics officer (CMIO): A relatively new position within the information services organizational structure, typically held by a member of the medical staff and responsible for, among other things, leading EMR system implementation, engaging healthcare professionals in the system's development and use, and leading the group designated to serve as the central governance forum for establishing the healthcare organization's clinical IS priorities

Chief nursing officer (CNO): The senior manager (usually a registered nurse with advanced education and extensive experience) responsible for administering patient care services

Chief operating officer (COO): Individual who oversees the healthcare organization's internal operations, usually including direct patient care services, but not financial or information-related services

Chief privacy officer: A position that (1) oversees activities related to the development, implementation, and maintenance of, and adherence to, organizational policies and procedures regarding the privacy of and access to patient-specific information and (2) ensures compliance with federal, state, and accrediting body rules and regulations concerning the confidentiality and privacy of health-related information

Civilian Health and Medical Program of the Uniformed Services (CHAMPUS): A federal program providing supplementary civilian-sector hospital and medical services beyond that which is available in military treatment facilities to military dependents, retirees and their dependents, and certain others

Civilian Health and Medical Program-Veterans Affairs (CHAMPVA): The federal healthcare benefits program for dependents of veterans rated by the Veterans Administration as having a total and permanent disability, for survivors of veterans who died from

VA-rated service-connected conditions or who were rated permanently and totally disabled at the time of death from a VA-rated service-connected condition, and for survivors of persons who died in the line of duty

Claim: Itemized statement of healthcare services and their costs provided by a hospital, physician's office, or other healthcare provider; submitted for reimbursement to the healthcare insurance plan by either the insured party or by the provider

Claims attachment: Additional information that is submitted with a claim for healthcare services provided

Claims data: Information required to be reported on a healthcare claim for service reimbursement

Claims management: A function related to risk management that enables an organization to track descriptive claims information (incidents, claimants, insurance, demands, dates, and so on), along with data on investigation, litigation, settlement, defendants, and subrogation

Class: The higher-level abstraction of an object that defines its properties and operations

Classification system: 1. A system for grouping similar diseases and procedures and organizing related information for easy retrieval 2. A system for assigning numeric or alphanumeric code numbers to represent specific diseases and/or procedures

Client: A patient who receives behavioral or mental health services

Client/server architecture: A computer architecture in which multiple computers (clients) are connected to other computers (servers) that store and distribute large amounts of shared data

Clinic outpatient: A patient who is admitted to a clinical service of a clinic or hospital for diagnosis or treatment on an ambulatory basis

Clinical coding: The process of assigning numeric or alphanumeric classifications to diagnostic and procedural statements

Clinical Document Architecture (CDA): An HL7 XML-based document markup standard for the electronic exchange model for clinical documents (such as discharge summaries and progress notes)

Clinical data repository (CDR): A central database that focuses on clinical information

Clinical data warehouse (CDW): A database that makes it possible to access data from multiple databases and combine the results into a single query and reporting interface; also called a **data warehouse**

Clinical decision support (CDS): The process in which individual data elements are represented in the computer by a special code to be used in making comparisons, trending results, and supplying clinical reminders and alerts

Clinical decision support system (CDSS): A special subcategory of clinical information systems that is designed to help healthcare providers make knowledge-based clinical decisions

Clinical Document Architecture (CDA): HL7 electronic exchange model for clinical documents (such as discharge summaries and progress notes)

Clinical documentation system: The process in which individual data elements are represented in the computer by a special code to be used in making comparisons, trending results, and supplying clinical reminders and alerts

Clinical information system (CIS): A category of a healthcare information system that includes systems that directly support patient care

Clinical messaging: The function of electronically delivering data and automating the workflow around the management of clinical data

Clinical pathway: A tool designed to coordinate multidisciplinary care planning for specific diagnoses and treatments

Clinical practice guideline: A detailed, step-by-step guide used by healthcare practitioners to make knowledge-based decisions related to patient care and issued by an authoritative organization such as a medical society or government agency; *See* **clinical protocol**

Clinical privileges: The authorization granted by a healthcare organization's governing board to a member of the medical staff that enables the physician to provide patient services in the organization within specific practice limits

Clinical protocol: Specific instructions for performing clinical procedures established by authoritative bodies, such as medical staff committees, and intended to be applied literally and universally; *See* **clinical practice guideline**

Clinical quality assessment: The process for determining whether the services provided to patients meet predetermined standards of care

Clinical trial: A controlled research study involving human subjects that is designed to evaluate prospectively the safety and effectiveness of new drugs, tests, devices, or interventions

Clinical vocabulary: A formally recognized list of preferred medical terms

Clinician: A healthcare provider, including physicians and others who treat patients

Closed-loop medication management: Information systems used to provide patient safety when ordering and administering medications

Cloud computing: Information systems that use the Internet to access data

CMS-1500: The universal insurance claim form developed and approved by the American Medical Association and the Centers for Medicare and Medicaid Services; physicians use it to bill Medicare, Medicaid, and private insurers for services provided.

Code of ethics: A statement of ethical principles regarding business practices and professional behavior

Coding and abstracting systems: Information system used to assign code numbers and enter key information from the health record.

Coding specialist: The healthcare worker responsible for assigning numeric or alphanumeric codes to diagnostic or procedural statements

Coinsurance: Cost-sharing in which the policy or certificate holder pays a preestablished percentage of eligible expenses after the deductible has been met

Collaborative Stage Data Set: A new standardized neoplasm staging system developed by the American Joint Commission on Cancer

Collective bargaining: The negotiating process between an employer and a labor union, usually regarding working conditions, wages, and so on

Column/field: A basic fact within a table, such as LAST_NAME, FIRST_NAME, and date of birth

Commission for the Accreditation of Birth Centers: A group that surveys and accredits freestanding birth centers

Commission on Accreditation for Health Informatics and Information Management Education (CAHIIM): The accrediting organization for educational programs in health informatics and information management

Commission on Accreditation of Rehabilitation Facilities (CARF): A private, not-for-profit organization that develops customer-focused standards for behavioral healthcare and medical rehabilitation programs and accredits such programs on the basis of its standards

Commission on Certification of Health Informatics and Information Management (CHIIM): An independent body within AHIMA that serves the public and the profession by establishing and enforcing standards for the initial certification and certification maintenance of health informatics and information management professionals

Common Formats Version 1.1: Tracking system used to report patient safety events

Common-cause variation: The source of variation in a process that is inherent within the process

Communications technology: Computer networks in an information system

Communities of Practice (CoP): A web-based electronic network for communication among members of the American Health Information Management Association

Community-acquired infection: An infectious disease contracted as the result of exposure before or after a patient's period of hospitalization

Community Health Accreditation Program: A group that surveys and accredits both home healthcare and hospice organizations

Comorbidity: A medical condition that coexists with the primary cause for hospitalization and affects the patient's treatment and length of stay

Comparative information: Information having identical attributes from different organizations or facilities that can be used for comparison purposes

Compiler: 1. A type of software that looks at an entire high-level program before translating it into machine language 2. A third-generation programming language

Complaint: A written legal statement from a plaintiff that initiates a civil lawsuit

Complete EHR: Under meaningful use, EHR technology that has been developed to meet, at a minimum, all applicable certification criteria adopted by the Secretary of HHS

Compliance: 1. The process of establishing an organizational culture that promotes the prevention, detection, and resolution of instances of conduct that do not conform to federal, state, or private payer healthcare program requirements or the healthcare organization's ethical and business policies 2. The act of adhering to official requirements

Compliance program guidance: The information provided by the Office of the Inspector General of the Department of Health and Human Services to help healthcare organizations develop internal controls that promote adherence to applicable federal and state guidelines

Complication: A medical condition that arises during an inpatient hospitalization (for example, a postoperative wound infection)

Component state associations (CSAs): Component state associations are part of the volunteer structure of AHIMA and are organized in every state, the District of Columbia, and the Commonwealth of Puerto Rico. The purpose of each component state association shall be to promote the mission and purpose of AHIMA in its state.

Computer-assisted coding (CAC): Utilizes natural language processing (NLP) and algorithmic software to electronically analyze entire medical charts to pre-code with both CPT procedure and ICD-9 diagnostic nomenclatures

Computer-based patient record (CPR): An electronic patient record housed in a system designed to provide users with access to complete and accurate data, practitioner alerts and reminders, clinical decision support systems, and links to medical knowledge; *See* **electronic health record**

Computer output to laser disk/enterprise report management (COLD/ERM): Technology that electronically stores documents and distributes them with fax, e-mail, web, and traditional hard-copy print processes

Computer virus: A software program that attacks computer systems and sometimes damages or destroys files

Computerized provider order entry (CPOE): Systems that allow physicians to enter medication or other orders and receive clinical advice about drug dosages, contraindications, or other clinical decision support; sometimes called computerized physician order entry

Computers on wheels (COWs): Laptops or computers mounted on rolling stands used for input throughout a facility

Concurrent review: A review of the health record while the patient is still hospitalized or under treatment

Concurrent utilization review: An evaluation of the medical necessity, quality, and cost-effectiveness of a hospital admission and ongoing patient care at or during the time that services are rendered

Conditions for Coverage: Standards applied to facilities that choose to participate in federal government reimbursement programs such as Medicare and Medicaid; *See* **Conditions of Participation**

Conditions of Participation: The administrative and operational guidelines and regulations under which facilities are allowed to take part in the Medicare and Medicaid programs; published by the Centers for Medicare and Medicaid Services, a federal agency under the Department of Health and Human Services; also called **Conditions for Coverage**

Confidentiality: A legal and ethical concept that establishes the healthcare provider's responsibility for protecting health records and other personal and private information from unauthorized use or disclosure

Configuration management: The process of keeping a record of changes made in an EHR system as it is being customized to the organization's specifications

Conflict management: A problem-solving technique that focuses on working with individuals to find a mutually acceptable solution

Consent: A means for residents to convey to healthcare providers their implied or expressed permission to administer care or treatment or to perform surgery or other medical procedures

Consent directive: A process by which patients may opt in or opt out of having their data exchanged in the HIE

Consent to treatment: Legal permission given by a patient or a patient's legal representative to a healthcare provider that allows the provider to administer care and/or treatment or to perform surgery and/or other medical procedures

Consistent federated model (of HIE): Health information exchange model where there is no centerilized storage of patient data

Consolidated Health Informatics (CHI) initiative: The effort to achieve CHI through federal agencies spearheaded by the Office of National Coordinator for Health Information Technology

Constitutional law: The body of law that deals with the amount and types of power and authority that governments are given

Consultation rate: The total number of hospital inpatients receiving consultations for a given period divided by the total number of discharges and deaths for the same period

Consultation report: Health record documentation that describes the findings and recommendations of consulting physicians

Consumer informatics: The field of information science concerned with the management of data and information used to support consumers by consumers (the general public) through the application of computers and computer technologies

Contextual: The condition of depending on the parts of a written or spoken statement that precede or follow a specified word or phrase and can influence its meaning or effect

Contingency and disaster planning: *See* **business continuity plan**

Continued-stay utilization review: A periodic review conducted during a hospital stay to determine whether the patient continues to need acute care services

Continuity of care document (CCD): In the exchange of information with other providers and the patient, the CCD combines the content that physicians have agreed should be included in patient referrals with a means to format that data for electronic transmission.

Continuity of care record (CCR): Documentation of care delivery from one healthcare experience to another

Continuity plan: A business plan to resume services after an interruption

Continuous improvement: *See* **continuous quality improvement**

Continuous quality improvement (CQI): 1. A management philosophy that emphasizes the importance of knowing and meeting customer expectations, reducing variation within processes, and relying on data to build knowledge for process improvement 2. A continuous cycle of planning, measuring, and monitoring performance and making knowledge-based improvements

Continuous variable: Discrete variables measured with sufficient precision

Continuum of care: The range of healthcare services provided to patients, from routine ambulatory care to intensive acute care

Contraindication: Medication should not be prescribed due to another medication or condition

Controlled vocabulary: A predefined set of terms and their meanings that may be used in structured data entry or natural language processing to represent expressions

Coordination of benefits (COB) transaction: The electronic transmission of claims and/or payment information from a healthcare provider to a health plan for the purpose of determining relative payment responsibilities

Core data elements/core content: A small set of data elements with standardized definitions often considered to be the core of data collection efforts

Core measure: Standardized performance measure developed to improve the safety and quality of healthcare (for example, core measures are used in the Joint Commission on Accreditation's ORYX initiative)

Corporate negligence: The failure of an organization to exercise the degree of care considered reasonable under the circumstances that resulted in an unintended injury to another party

Cost-benefit analysis: A process that uses quantitative techniques to evaluate and measure the benefit of providing products or services compared to the cost of providing them

Cost outlier: Exceptionally high costs associated with inpatient care when compared with other cases in the same diagnosis-related group

Cost outlier adjustment: Additional reimbursement for certain high-cost home care cases based on the loss-sharing ratio of costs in excess of a threshold amount for each home health resource group

Council on Certification: An arm of AHIMA that today fulfills the role of the Board of Registration, a certification board instituted in 1933 to provide a baseline by which to measure qualified medical record librarians

Counterclaim: In a court of law, a countersuit

Court order: An official direction issued by a court judge and requiring or forbidding specific parties to perform specific actions

Courts of appeal: A branch of the federal court system that has the power to hear appeals on the final judgments of district courts

Covered entity: According to the HIPAA Privacy Rule, any health plan, healthcare clearinghouse, or healthcare provider that transmits specific healthcare transactions in electronic form

Credentialing: The process of reviewing and validating the qualifications (degrees, licenses, and other credentials) of physicians and other licensed independent practitioners, for granting medical staff membership to provide patient care services

Critical pathway: The sequence of tasks that determines the project finish date

Cross-claim: In law, a complaint filed against a codefendant

Crude birth rate: The number of live births divided by the population at risk

Crude death rate: The total number of deaths in a given population for a given period of time divided by the estimated population for the same period of time

Cryptography: The art of keeping data secret through the use of mathematical or logical functions that transform intelligible data into seemingly unintelligible data and back again

Current Procedural Terminology (CPT): A comprehensive, descriptive list of terms and numeric codes used for reporting diagnostic and therapeutic procedures and other medical services performed by physicians; published and updated annually by the American Medical Association

Curriculum: A prescribed course of study in an educational program

Customer: An internal or external recipient of services, products, or information

Daily inpatient census: The number of inpatients present at census-taking time each day, plus any inpatients who were both admitted and discharged after the census-taking time the previous day

Dashboards: Reports of process measures to help leaders know what is currently going on so that they can plan strategically where they want to go next; sometimes called **scorecards**

Data: The dates, numbers, images, symbols, letters, and words that represent basic facts and observations about people, processes, measurements, and conditions

Data abstracts: A defined and standardized set of data points or elements common to a patient population that can be regularly identified in the health records of the population and coded for use and analysis in database management systems

Data accessibility: The extent to which healthcare data are obtainable

Data accuracy: The extent to which data are free of identifiable errors

Data availability: The extent to which healthcare data are accessible whenever and wherever they are needed

Data center: Where the hardware and software for the electronic information systems are held

Data comparability: The standardization of vocabulary such that the meaning of a single term is the same each time the term is used in order to produce consistency in information derived from the data

Data comprehensiveness: The extent to which healthcare data are complete

Data confidentiality: The extent to which personal health information is kept private

Data consistency: The extent to which healthcare data are reliable

Data conversion: The task of moving data from one data structure to another, usually at the time of a new system installation

Data currency: The extent to which data are up-to-date; *See* **data timeliness**

Data definition: The specific meaning of a healthcare-related data element

Data dictionary: A descriptive list of the data elements to be collected in an information system or database whose purpose is to ensure consistency of terminology

Data element: An individual fact or measurement that is the smallest unique subset of a database

Data Elements for Emergency Department Systems (DEEDS): A data set designed to support the uniform collection of information in hospital-based emergency departments

Data exchange standards: Protocols that help ensure that data transmitted from one system to another remain comparable

Data granularity: The level of detail at which the attributes and values of healthcare data are described

Data integrity: 1. The extent to which healthcare data are complete, accurate, consistent, and timely 2. A security principle that keeps information from being modified or otherwise corrupted either maliciously or accidentally

Data mart: A well-organized, user-centered, searchable database system that usually draws information from a data warehouse to meet the specific needs of users

Data mining: The process of extracting information from a database and then quantifying and filtering discrete, structured data

Data precision: The extent to which data have the values they are expected to have

Data quality management: A managerial process that ensures the integrity (accuracy and completeness) of an organization's data during data collection, application, warehousing, and analysis

Data relevancy: The extent to which healthcare-related data are useful for the purpose for which they were collected

Data security: The process of keeping data safe from unauthorized alteration or destruction

Data set: A list of recommended data elements with uniform definitions that are relevant for a particular use

Data standard: Data standards are the agreed upon specifications for the values acceptable for specific data fields

Data stewardship: The responsibilities and accountabilities associated with managing, collecting, viewing, storing, sharing, disclosing, or otherwise making use of personal health information

Data timeliness: Concept of data quality that involves whether the data is up-to-date and available within a useful time frame; *See* **data currency**

Data type: A technical category of data (text, numbers, currency, date, memo, and link data) that a field in a database can contain

Data warehouse: A database that makes it possible to access data from multiple databases and combine the results into a single query and reporting interface

Data warehousing: A type of system used to analyze data for decision-making purposes

Database: An organized collection of data, text, references, or pictures in a standardized format, typically stored in a computer system for multiple applications

Database management system (DBMS): Computer software that enables the user to create, modify, delete, and view the data in a database

Decision support system (DSS): A computer-based system that gathers data from a variety of sources and assists in providing structure to the data by using various analytical models and visual tools in order to facilitate and improve the ultimate outcome in decision-making tasks associated with nonroutine and nonrepetitive problems

Deemed status: An official designation indicating that a healthcare facility is in compliance with the Medicare Conditions of Participation; to qualify for deemed status, facilities must be accredited by the Joint Commission on Accreditation of Healthcare Organizations or the American Osteopathic Association.

Defendant: In civil cases, an individual or entity against whom a civil complaint has been filed; in criminal cases, an individual who has been accused of a crime

Deficiency slip: A device for tracking information (for example, reports) missing from a paper-based health record

Deidentified information: Health information from which all names and other identifying descriptors have been removed to protect the privacy of the patients, family members, and healthcare providers who were involved in the case

Delegation of authority: The assignment of authority or responsibility

Delinquent record: An incomplete record not finished or made complete within the time frame determined by the medical staff of the facility

Demographic information: Information used to identify an individual, such as name, address, gender, age, and other information linked to a specific person

Department of Health and Human Services (HHS): The cabinet-level federal agency that oversees all of the health- and human-services–related activities of the federal government and administers federal regulations

Department of Health and Human Services Office for Civil Rights (OCR): Agency within the Department of Health and Human Services responsible for civil rights and health privacy rights law enforcement

Deposition: A method of gathering information to be used in a litigation process

Descriptive statistics: A set of statistical techniques used to describe data such as means, frequency distributions, and standard deviations; statistical information that describes the characteristics of a specific group or a population

Designated record set: A group of records maintained by or for a covered entity that may include patient medical and billing records; the enrollment, payment, claims adjudication, and cases or medical management record systems maintained by or for a health plan; or information used, in whole or in part, to make patient care–related decisions

Destruction: 1. The act of breaking down the components of a health record into pieces that can no longer be recognized as parts of the original record; for example, paper records can be destroyed by shredding, and electronic records can be destroyed by magnetic degaussing. 2. The ablation of benign, premalignant, or malignant tissues, by any method, with or without curettement, including local anesthesia, and not usually requiring closure

Developing stage: In performance management, the stage during which opportunities for improving work processes or employee skills are identified

Diagnosis-related groups (DRGs): A unit of case-mix classification adopted by the federal government and some other payers as a prospective payment mechanism for hospital inpatients in which diseases are placed into groups because related diseases and treatments tend to consume similar amounts of healthcare resources and incur similar amounts of cost; in the Medicare and Medicaid programs, one of more than 500 diagnostic classifications in which cases demonstrate similar resource consumption and length-of-stay patterns

Diagnostic codes: Numeric or alphanumeric characters used to classify and report diseases, conditions, and injuries

***Diagnostic and Statistical Manual of Mental Disorders, Fourth Revision, Text Revision* (DSM-IV-TR):** The 2004 text revision of the *Diagnostic and Statistical Manual of Mental Disorders, Fourth Revision,* with updated clinical terms, but very few coding changes

Diagnostic studies: Laboratory and other tests performed to help diagnose a patient

Digital certificate: An electronic document that establishes a person's online identity

Digital dictation: A process in which vocal sounds are converted to bits and stored on computer for random access

Digital images: Data provided in a computer-readable format

Digital Imaging and Communication in Medicine (DICOM): A standard that promotes a digital image communications format and picture archive and communications systems for use with digital images

Digital signature: An electronic signature that binds a message to a particular individual and can be used by the receiver to authenticate the identity of the sender

Direct costs: Resources expended that can be identified as pertaining to specific goods and/or services (for example, medications pertain to specific patients)

Direct cutover conversion: The abrupt, immediate implementation of a new system to replace an existing system

Discharge abstract system: A data repository (usually electronic) used for collecting information on demographics, clinical conditions, and services in which data are condensed from hospital health records into coded data for the purpose of producing summary statistics about discharged patients

Discharge planning: The process of coordinating the activities related to the release of a patient when inpatient hospital care is no longer needed

Discharge summary: A summary of the resident's stay at the long-term care facility that is used along with the postdischarge plan of care to provide continuity of care for the resident upon discharge from the facility

Discharge utilization review: A process for assessing a patient's readiness to leave the hospital

Disciplinary action: Action taken to improve unsatisfactory work performance or behavior on the job

Discounting: The application of lower rates of payment to multiple surgical procedures performed during the same operative session under the outpatient prospective payment system; the application of adjusted rates of payment by preferred provider organizations

Discovery: *See* **discovery process**

Discovery process: The pretrial stage in the litigation process during which both parties to a suit use various strategies to identify information about the case, the primary focus of which is to determine the strength of the opposing party's case

Discrete data: Data that represent separate and distinct values or observations; that is, data that contain only finite numbers and have only specified values

Discrete variable: A dichotomous or nominal variable whose values are placed into categories

Disease index: A list of diseases and conditions of patients sequenced according to the code numbers of the classification system in use

Disease management (DM): 1. A more expansive view of case management in which patients with the highest risk of incurring high-cost interventions are targeted for standardizing and managing care throughout integrated delivery systems 2. A program focused on preventing exacerbation of chronic diseases and on promoting healthier life styles for patients and clients with chronic diseases

Disease registry: A centralized collection of data used to improve the quality of care and measure the effectiveness of a particular aspect of healthcare delivery

District court: The lowest tier in the federal court system, which hears cases involving felonies and misdemeanors that fall under federal statute and suits in which a citizen of one state sues a citizen of another state

Diversity jurisdiction: Refers to district court cases that involve suits where a citizen of one state sues a citizen of another state and the amount in dispute exceeds $75,000

DNV (Det Norske Veritas): An independent international organization that began offering hospital accreditation services in the United States in 2008

Document imaging: The practice of electronically scanning written or printed paper documents into an optical or electronic system for later retrieval of the document or parts of the document if parts have been indexed

Document imaging management system: Information system that allowed a paper document to be scanned and displayed.

DRG grouper: A computer program that assigns inpatient cases to diagnosis-related groups and determines the Medicare reimbursement rate

Drug knowledge database: A database of information about drugs

Dual core (vendor strategy): A vendor strategy in which one vendor primarily supplies the financial and administrative applications and another vendor primarily supplies the clinical applications

Duplicate medical record number: The situation in which a patient that already has a medical record number is assigned a new number

Duty: Obligation

E codes (external cause of injury code): A supplementary ICD-9-CM classification used to identify the external causes of injuries, poisonings, and adverse effects of pharmaceuticals

Edit: A condition that must be satisfied before a computer system can accept data

e-health: The application of e-commerce to the healthcare industry, including electronic data interchange and links among healthcare entities

Electronic data interchange (EDI): A standard transmission format using strings of data for business information communicated among the computer systems of independent organizations

Electronic document/content management (ED/CM): A type of electronic document management system that uses methods such as bar coding on the forms to identify specific content

Electronic document management system (EDMS): A storage solution based on digital scanning technology in which source documents are scanned to create digital images of the documents that can be stored electronically on optical disks

Electronic funds transfer (EFT): Process of moving money electronically

Electronic health record (EHR): An electronic record of health-related information on an individual that conforms to nationally recognized interoperability standards and that can be created, managed, and consulted by authorized clinicians and staff across more than one healthcare organization

Electronic medical record (EMR): An electronic record of health-related information on an individual that can be created, gathered, managed, and consulted by authorized clinicians and staff within a single healthcare organization

Electronic medication administration record (E-MAR): A system designed to prevent medication errors by checking a patient's medication information against his or her barcoded wristband

Electronic prescribing (e-Rx): When a prescription is written from the personal digital assistant and an electronic fax or when an actual electronic data interchange transaction is generated that transmits the prescription directly to the retail pharmacy's information system

Electronic protected health information (ePHI): Electronically transmitted protected health information that is required to comply with the Privacy Rule

Electronic remittance advice (ERA): A classification of payment information from third-party payers that is communicated electronically

Electronic (enterprise) report management (ERM): Systems that capture data from print files and other report-formatted digital documents, such as e-mail, e-fax, instant messages, web pages, digital dictation, and speech recognition and store them for subsequent viewing

Electronic signature authentication (ESA): A system that requires the author of a document to sign onto a patient record using a user ID and password, reviews the document to be signed, and indicates approval

Eligibility verification: Confirmation of insurance status

Emergency Maternal and Infant Care Program (EMIC): The federal medical program that provides obstetrical and infant care to dependents of active-duty military personnel in the four lowest pay grades

Emergency patient: A patient who is admitted to the emergency services department of a hospital for the diagnosis and treatment of a condition that requires immediate medical, dental, or allied health services in order to sustain life or to prevent critical consequences

Employee orientation: The process in which employees are introduced to an organization and a new job

Employer-based self-insurance: An umbrella term used to describe health plans that are funded directly by employers to provide coverage for their employees exclusively in which employers establish accounts to cover their employees' medical expenses and retain control over the funds but bear the risk of paying claims greater than their estimates

Encoded: Converted into code

Encoder: Specialty software used to facilitate the assignment of diagnostic and procedural codes according to the rules of the coding system

Encounter: The professional, direct personal contact between a patient and a physician or other person who is authorized by state licensure law and, if applicable, by medical staff bylaws to order or furnish healthcare services for the diagnosis or treatment of the patient; face-to-face contact between a patient and a provider who has primary responsibility for assessing and treating the condition of the patient at a given contact and exercises independent judgment in the care of the patient

Encryption: The process of transforming text into an unintelligible string of characters that can be transmitted via communications media with a high degree of security and then decrypted when it reaches a secure destination

Enterprise content and record management (ECRM): The combination of methodologies and processes for maintaining and utilizing data from all departments of a healthcare facility

Enterprise master person/patient index (EMPI): An index that provides access to multiple repositories of information from overlapping patient populations that are maintained in separate systems and databases

Enterprise-wide system: A computer-based system that manages the data for all departments of a business

Environmental assessment: External—a collection of information about changes that have occurred in the healthcare industry as well as the broader U.S. economy during a specified time period; internal—a collection of information about changes that have occurred within an organization during a specified time period

Episode-of-care (EOC) reimbursement: A category of payments made as lump sums to providers for all healthcare services delivered to a patient for a specific illness and/or over a specified time period; also called **bundled payments** because they include multiple services and may include multiple providers of care

e-Prescribing (e-Rx): Enables prescriptions to be checked for drug contraindications and sent directly to a retail pharmacy of the patient's choosing

Equal Employment Opportunity Act: The 1972 amendment to the Civil Rights Act of 1964 prohibiting discrimination in employment on the basis of age, race, color, religion, sex, or national origin

Equal Pay Act of 1963: The federal legislation that requires equal pay for men and women who perform substantially the same work

Ergonomics: A discipline of functional design associated with the employee in relationship to his or her work environment, including equipment, workstation, and office furniture adaptation to accommodate the employee's unique physical requirements so as to facilitate efficacy of work functions

Essential Medical Data Set (EMDS): A recommended data set designed to create a health history for an individual patient treated in an emergency service

Ethernet: A popular protocol (format) for transmitting data in local area networks

Ethical agent: An individual who promotes and supports ethical behavior

Ethical decision making: The process of requiring everyone to consider the perspectives of others, even when they do not agree with them

Ethicist: An individual trained in the application of ethical theories and principles to problems that cannot be easily solved because of conflicting values, perspectives, and options for action

Ethics: A field of study that deals with moral principles, theories, and values; in healthcare, a formal decision-making process for dealing with the competing perspectives and obligations of the people who have an interest in a common problem

Evidence-based medicine: Healthcare services based on clinical methods that have been thoroughly tested through controlled, peer-reviewed biomedical studies

E-visits: Non-face-to-face interaction between patient and provider

Exclusive provider organization (EPO): Hybrid managed care organization that provides benefits to subscribers only when healthcare services are performed by network providers; sponsored by self-insured (self-funded) employers or associations and exhibits characteristics of both health maintenance organizations and preferred provider organizations

Executive information system (EIS): An information system designed to combine financial and clinical information for use in the management of business affairs of a healthcare organization

Executive management: The managerial level of an organization that is primarily responsible for setting the organization's future direction and establishing its strategic plan

Executive manager: A senior manager who oversees a broad functional area or group of departments or services, sets the organization's future direction, and monitors the organization's operations

Executive sponsor: An individual who helps a team leader keep the team on track and sometimes ensures that the team obtains the organizational support required to accomplish its goal

Expenses: Amounts that are charged as costs by an organization to the current year's activities of operation

Expert knowledge-based information system: Information system that assists physicians and other healthcare providers in the diagnosis and treatment of a patient

Expert system: A type of information system that supports the work of professionals engaged in the development or evaluation of complex activities that require high-level knowledge in a well-defined and usually limited area

Explanation of Benefits (EOB): A statement issued to the insured and the healthcare provider by an insurer to explain the services provided, amounts billed, and payments made by a health plan

Express contract: Agreement between physician and patient that is specifically articulated

Expressed consent: The spoken or written permission granted by a patient to a healthcare provider that allows the provider to perform medical or surgical services

Extended care facility: A healthcare facility licensed by applicable state or local law to offer room and board, skilled nursing by a full-time registered nurse, intermediate care, or a combination of levels on a 24-hour basis over a long period of time

Extensible markup language (XML): A standardized computer language that allows the interchange of data as structured text

External customers: Individuals from outside the organization who receive products or services from within the organization

External review (audit): A performance or quality review conducted by a third-party payer or consultant hired for the purpose

Extranet: A system of connections of private Internet networks outside an organization's firewall that uses Internet technology to enable collaborative applications among enterprises

Facilities management: The functional oversight of a healthcare organization's physical plant to ensure operational efficiency in an environment that is safe for patients, staff, and visitors

Facility-based registry: A registry that includes only cases from a particular type of healthcare facility, such as a hospital or clinic

Facility-specific system: A computer information system developed exclusively to meet the needs of one healthcare organization

FAHIMA: *See* **Fellowship Program**

Fair and Accurate Credit Transactions Act (FACTA): Law passed in 2003 that contains provisions and requirements to reduce identity theft

Fair Labor Standards Act of 1938 (FLSA): The federal legislation that sets the minimum wage and overtime payment regulations

False Claims Act: Federal legislation stipulating that an individual may file claim (for example, against a hospital) for up to 10 years after an incident has occurred

Federal Employees' Compensation Act (FECA): The legislation enacted in 1916 to mandate workers' compensation for civilian federal employees, whose coverage includes lost wages, medical expenses, and survivors' benefits

Federal Trade Commission (FTC): An independent federal agency tasked with dealing with two areas of economics in the United States: consumer protection and issues having to do with competition in business

Federated model (of HIE): Model of health information exchange where there is not a centralized database of patient information

Fee schedule: A list of healthcare services and procedures (usually CPT/HCPCS codes) and the charges associated with them developed by a third-party payer to represent the approved payment levels for a given insurance plan; also called table of allowances

Fee-for-service basis: A method of reimbursement through which providers retrospectively receive payment based on either billed charges for services provided or on annually updated fee schedules; also called fee-for-service reimbursement

Fellowship Program: Program of earned recognition for AHIMA members who have made significant and sustained contributions to the HIM profession through meritorious service, excellence in professional practice, education, and advancement of the profession through innovation and knowledge sharing

Fetal autopsy rate: The number of autopsies performed on intermediate and late fetal deaths for a given time period divided by the total number of intermediate and late fetal deaths for the same time period

Fetal death (stillborn): The death of a product of human conception before its complete expulsion or extraction from the mother regardless of the duration of the pregnancy

Fetal death rate: A proportion that compares the number of intermediate and/or late fetal deaths to the total number of live births and intermediate or late fetal deaths during the same period of time

Financial indicators: A set of measures designed to routinely monitor the current financial status of a healthcare organization or of one of its constituent parts

Financial information system: The accounting/financial programs and data necessary for running a healthcare facility

Firewall: A computer system or a combination of systems that provides a security barrier or supports an access control policy between two networks or between a network and the Internet

Fiscal year: Any consecutive 12-month period an organization uses as its accounting period

Fishbone diagram: A performance improvement tool used to identify or classify the root causes of a problem or condition and to display the root causes graphically; also called **cause-and-effect diagram**

Fixed costs: Resources expended that do not vary with the activity of the organization; for example, mortgage expenses do not vary with patient volume

Flat file: Early form of database where data is stored in plain text file

Flexibility of approach: Condition under HIPAA in which a covered entity can adopt security protection measures that are appropriate for its organization

Flowchart: A graphic tool that uses standard symbols to visually display detailed information, including time and distance, of the sequential flow of work of an individual or a product as it progresses through a process

Food and Drug Administration (FDA) Health Services Research: The federal agency responsible for controlling the sale and use of pharmaceuticals, biological products, medical devices, food, cosmetics, and products that emit radiation, including the licensing of medications for human use

Force-field analysis: A performance improvement tool used to identify specific drivers of, and barriers to, an organizational change so that positive factors can be reinforced and negative factors reduced

Foreign key: A key attribute used to link one entity/table to another

Forming: The first of four steps in assembling a functional team

Fraud and abuse: The intentional and mistaken misrepresentation of reimbursement claims submitted to government-sponsored health programs

Free-text data: Data that are narrative in nature

Frequency distribution: A table or graph that displays the number of times (frequency) a particular observation occurs

Frequency polygon: A type of line graph that represents a frequency distribution

Front-end speech recognition: The specific use of speech recognition technology in an environment where the recognition process occurs in real time (or near-real time) as dictation takes place

Full-time equivalent employee: A statistic representing the number of full-time employees as calculated by the reported number of hours worked by all employees, including part-time

General Rules: HIPAA data security provisions that provide the objective and scope for the HIPAA security rule as a whole

Geographic practice cost index (GPCI): An index developed by the Centers for Medicare and Medicaid Services to measure the differences in resource costs among fee schedule areas compared to the national average in the three components of the relative value unit: physician work, practice expenses, and malpractice coverage

Global payment: A form of reimbursement used for radiological and other procedures that combines the professional and technical components of the procedures and disperses payments as lump sums to be distributed between the physician and the healthcare facility

Global surgery payment: A payment made for surgical procedures that includes the provision of all healthcare services, from the treatment decision through postoperative patient care

Graphical user interface (GUI): A style of computer interface in which typed commands are replaced by images that represent tasks; for example, small pictures (icons) that represent the tasks, functions, and programs performed by a software program

Grievance management: The policies and procedures used to handle employee complaints

Gross autopsy rate: The number of inpatient autopsies conducted during a given time period divided by the total number of inpatient deaths for the same time period

Gross death rate: The number of inpatient deaths that occurred during a given time period divided by the total number of inpatient discharges, including deaths, for the same time period

Ground rules: An agreement concerning attendance, time management, participation, communication, decision making, documentation, room arrangements and cleanup, and so forth, that has been developed by PI team members at the initiation of the team's work

Group health insurance: A prepaid medical plan that covers the healthcare expenses of an organization's full-time employees

Group model HMO: A type of health plan in which an HMO contracts with an independent multispecialty physician group to provide medical services to members of the plan

Group practice without walls (GPWW): A type of managed care contract that allows physicians to maintain their own offices and share administrative services

Groupware: An Internet technology that consolidates documents from different information systems within an organization into a tightly integrated workflow

Hard-coding: The process of attaching a CPT/HCPCS code to a procedure located on the facility's chargemaster so that the code will automatically be included on the patient's bill

Hardware: The machines and media used in an information system

Health Care Quality Improvement Program (HCQIP): A quality initiative begun in 1992 by the Health Care Financing Administration and implemented by peer review organizations that uses patterns of care analysis and collaboration with practitioners, beneficiaries, providers, plans, and other purchasers of healthcare services to develop scientifically based quality indicators and to identify and implement opportunities for healthcare improvement

Health Information and Management Systems Society: A national membership association that provides leadership in healthcare for the management of technology, information, and change

Health information exchange (HIE): A plan in which health information is shared among providers

Health information exchange organization (HIEO): An organization that supports, oversees, or governs the exchange of health-related information among organizations according to nationally recognized standards

Health information management (HIM): An allied health profession that is responsible for ensuring the availability, accuracy, and protection of the clinical information that is needed to deliver healthcare services and to make appropriate healthcare-related decisions

Health information services department: The department in a healthcare organization that is responsible for maintaining patient care records in accordance with external and internal rules and regulations

Health information technology (HIT): The technical aspects of processing health data and records, including classification and coding, abstracting, registry development, storage, and so on

Health Information Technology Expert Panel (HITEP): Panel charged to create a better link between current quality measurement and EHR reporting capabilities

Health Information Technology for Economic and Clinical Health (HITECH) Act: Part of the American Recovery and Reinvestment Act of 2009, the HITECH Act includes requirements for standards development and for investment in health information technology infrastructure and strengthens federal privacy and security law; meant to increase the momentum of developing and implementing the EHR by 2014

Health Insurance Portability and Accountability Act of 1996 (HIPAA): The federal legislation enacted to provide continuity of health coverage, control fraud and abuse in healthcare, reduce healthcare costs, and guarantee the security and privacy of health information. The act limits exclusion for preexisting medical conditions, prohibits discrimination against employees and dependents based on health status, guarantees availability of health insurance to small employers, and guarantees renewability of insurance to all employees regardless of size of employer. Public Law 104-191, also known as the Kassebaum-Kennedy Law

Health IT Policy Committee: An HHS advisory committee that recommends the policy framework for the development and adoption of a nationwide health information infrastructure

Health IT Standards Committee: An HHS advisory committee that recommends standards, implementation specifications, and certification criteria for the electronic exchange and use of health information

Health Level Seven (HL7): A standards development organization accredited by the American National Standards Institute that addresses issues at the seventh, or application, level of healthcare systems interconnections

Health maintenance organization (HMO): Entity that combines the provision of healthcare insurance and the delivery of healthcare services, characterized by: (1) an organized healthcare delivery system to a geographic area, (2) a set of basic and supplemental health maintenance and treatment services, (3) voluntarily enrolled members, and (4) predetermined fixed, periodic prepayments for members' coverage

Health record: A paper- or computer-based tool for collecting and storing information about the healthcare services provided to a patient in a single healthcare facility; also called a patient record, medical record, resident record, or client record, depending on the healthcare setting

Health record number: A unique numeric or alphanumeric identifier assigned to each patient's record upon admission to a healthcare facility

Health savings accounts (HSAs): Savings accounts designed to help people save for future medical and retiree health costs on a tax-free basis; part of the 2003 Medicare bill; also called medical savings accounts

Health services research: Research conducted on the subject of healthcare delivery that examines organizational structures and systems as well as the effectiveness and efficiency of healthcare services

Health systems agency (HSA): A type of organization called for by the Health Planning and Resources Development Act of 1974 to have broad representation of healthcare providers and consumers on governing boards and committees

Healthcare claims and payment/advice transaction: An electronic transmission sent by a health plan to a provider's financial representative for the purpose of providing information about payments and/or payment processing and information about the transfer of funds

Healthcare Common Procedure Coding System (HCPCS): An alphanumeric classification system that identifies healthcare procedures, equipment, and supplies for claim submission purposes; the three levels are as follows: I, *Current Procedural Terminology* codes, developed by the AMA; II, codes for equipment, supplies, and services not covered by *Current Procedural Terminology* codes as well as modifiers that can be used with all levels of codes, developed by CMS; and III (eliminated December 31, 2003, to comply with HIPAA), local codes developed by regional Medicare Part B carriers and used to report physicians' services and supplies to Medicare for reimbursement

Healthcare Cost and Utilization Project (HCUP): A group of healthcare databases and related software tools developed through collaboration by the federal government, state governments, and industry to create a national information resource for patient-level healthcare data

Healthcare Effectiveness Data and Information Set (HEDIS): A set of performance measures developed by the National Commission for Quality Assurance that are designed to provide purchasers and consumers of healthcare with the information they need to compare the performance of managed care plans

Healthcare informatics standards: Guidelines developed to standardize data throughout the healthcare industry (for example, developing uniform terminologies and vocabularies)

Healthcare Information Technology Standards Panel (HITSP): An organization developed under the auspices of the American National Standards Institute (ANSI) to address interoperability in healthcare by harmonizing health information technology standards

Healthcare Integrity and Protection Data Bank (HIPDB): A database maintained by the federal government to provide information on fraud-and-abuse findings against U.S. healthcare providers

Healthcare provider: A provider of diagnostic, medical, and surgical care as well as the services or supplies related to the health of an individual and any other person or organization that issues reimbursement claims or is paid for healthcare in the normal course of business

Hierarchy: An authoritarian organizational structure in which each member is assigned a specific rank that reflects his or her level of decision-making authority within the organization

Hierarchical database: Type of database that allows duplicate data

Hill-Burton Act: The federal legislation enacted in 1946 as the Hospital Survey and Construction Act to authorize grants for states to construct new hospitals and, later, to modernize old ones

Histocompatibility: The immunologic similarity between an organ donor and a transplant recipient

Histogram: A graphic technique used to display the frequency distribution of continuous data (interval or ratio data) as either numbers or percentages in a series of bars

Home Assessment Validation and Entry (HAVEN): A type of data-entry software used to collect Outcome and Assessment Information Set (OASIS) data and then transmit them to state databases; imports and exports data in standard OASIS record format, maintains agency/patient/employee information, enforces data integrity through rigorous edit checks, and provides comprehensive online help

Home health agency (HHA): A program or organization that provides a blend of home-based medical and social services to homebound patients and their families for the purpose of promoting, maintaining, or restoring health or of minimizing the effects of illness, injury, or disability

Home health information system: An information system designed to support the care provided at a home health organization

Home health prospective payment system (HH PPS): The reimbursement system developed by the Centers for Medicare and Medicaid Services to cover home health services provided to Medicare beneficiaries

Home health resource group (HHRG): A classification system with 80 home health episode rates established to support the prospective reimbursement of covered home care and rehabilitation services provided to Medicare beneficiaries during 60-day episodes of care

Home healthcare: The medical and/or personal care provided to individuals and families in their place of residence with the goal of promoting, maintaining, or restoring health or minimizing the effects of disabilities and illnesses, including terminal illnesses

Hospice: An interdisciplinary program of palliative care and supportive services that addresses the physical, spiritual, social, and economic needs of terminally ill patients and their families

Hospice care: The medical care provided to persons with life expectancies of six months or less who elect to forgo standard treatment of their illness and to receive only palliative care

Hospital-acquired conditions: Select, reasonably preventable conditions for which hospitals do not receive additional payment when one of the conditions was not present on admission

Hospital-acquired infection: An infection acquired by a patient while receiving care or services in a healthcare organization

Hospital-acquired (nosocomial) infection rate: The number of infections that occur in a hospital's various patient care units on a continuous basis

Hospital ambulatory care: All hospital-directed preventive, therapeutic, and rehabilitative services provided by physicians and their surrogates to patients who are not hospital inpatients

Hospital autopsy: A postmortem (after death) examination performed on the body of a person who has at some time been a hospital patient by a hospital pathologist or a physician of the medical staff who has been delegated the responsibility

Hospital autopsy rate: The total number of autopsies performed by a hospital pathologist for a given time period divided by the number of deaths of hospital patients (inpatients and outpatients) whose bodies were available for autopsy for the same time period

Hospital death rate: The number of inpatient deaths for a given period of time divided by the total number of live discharges and deaths for the same time period

Hospital discharge abstract system: A group of databases compiled from aggregate data on all patients discharged from a hospital

Hospital (nosocomial) infection rate: The number of infections that occur in a hospital's various patient care units on a continuous basis

Hospital information system (HIS): The comprehensive database containing all the clinical, administrative, financial, and demographic information about each patient served by a hospital

Hospital inpatient: A patient who is provided with room, board, and continuous general nursing services in an area of an acute care facility where patients generally stay at least overnight

Hospital inpatient autopsy: A postmortem (after death) examination performed on the body of a patient who died during an inpatient hospitalization by a hospital pathologist or a physician of the medical staff who has been delegated the responsibility

Hospital newborn inpatient: A patient born in the hospital at the beginning of the current inpatient hospitalization

Hospital outpatient: A hospital patient who receives services in one or more of a hospital's facilities when he or she is not currently an inpatient or a home care patient

Hospital Standardization Program: An early twentieth-century survey mechanism instituted by the American College of Surgeons and aimed at identifying quality-of-care problems and improving patient care; precursor to the survey program offered by the Joint Commission on Accreditation of Healthcare Organizations

Hospitalist: Physician employed by teaching hospitals to play the role that admitting physicians fulfill in hospitals that are not affiliated with medical training programs

Hospitalization insurance (Medicare Part A): A federal program that covers the costs associated with inpatient hospitalization as well as other healthcare services provided to Medicare beneficiaries

House of Delegates: An important component of the volunteer structure of the American Health Information Management Association that conducts the official business of the organization and functions as its legislative body

Human–computer interface: The device used by humans to access and enter data into a computer system, such as a keyboard on a PC, personal digital assistant, voice recognition system, and so on

Human resources: The employees of an organization

Hybrid health record: A combination of paper and electronic records; a health record that includes both paper and electronic elements

Hybrid record: A health record that includes both paper and electronic elements

Identifier standards: Recommended methods for assigning unique identifiers to individuals (patients and clinical providers), corporate providers, and healthcare vendors and suppliers

Identity matching algorithm: Process used to identify any patient for whom data are to be exchanged

Imaging technology: Computer software designed to combine health record text files with diagnostic imaging files

Implementation specifications: Descriptions that define how HIPAA standards are to be implemented

Implied consent: The type of permission that is inferred when a patient voluntarily submits to treatment

Implied contract: Type of agreement between physician and patient that is created by actions

Incidence: The number of new cases of a specific disease

Incidence rate: A computation that compares the number of new cases of a specific disease for a given time period to the population at risk for the disease during the same time period

Incident/occurrence report: A quality/performance management tool used to collect data and information about potentially compensable events (events that may result in death or serious injury)

Indemnity plans: Health insurance coverage provided in the form of cash payments to patients or providers

Identity management: In the master patient index, policies and procedures that manage patient identity, such as prohibiting the same record number for duplicate patients or duplicate records for one patient

Identity matching algorithm: Rules established in an information system that predicts the probability that two or more patients in the database are the same patient

Independent practice association (IPA): An open-panel health maintenance organization that provides contract healthcare services to subscribers through independent physicians who treat patients in their own offices; the HMO reimburses the IPA on a capitated basis; the IPA may reimburse the physicians on a fee-for-service or a capitated basis

Index: An organized (usually alphabetical) list of specific data that serves to guide, indicate, or otherwise facilitate reference to the data

Indian Health Service (IHS): The federal agency within the Department of Health and Human Services that is responsible for providing federal healthcare services to American Indians and Alaska natives

Indirect costs: Resources expended that cannot be identified as pertaining to specific goods and/or services (for example, electricity is not allocable to a specific patient)

Individual: According to the HIPAA Privacy Rule, a person who is the subject of protected health information

Individually identifiable health information: According to HIPAA privacy provisions, that information that specifically identifies the patient to whom the information relates

Infant mortality rate: The number of deaths of individuals under one year of age during a given time period divided by the number of live births reported for the same time period

Infection control: A system for the prevention of communicable diseases that concentrates on protecting healthcare workers and patients against exposure to disease-causing organisms and promotes compliance with applicable legal requirements through early identification of potential sources of contamination and implementation of policies and procedures that limit the spread of disease

Inferential statistics: 1. Statistics that are used to make inferences from a smaller group of data to a large one 2. A set of statistical techniques that allows researchers to make generalizations about a population's characteristics (parameters) on the basis of a sample's characteristics

Information: Factual data that have been collected, combined, analyzed, interpreted, and/or converted into a form that can be used for a specific purpose

Information kiosk: A computer station located within a healthcare facility that patients and families can use to access information

Information resource management: A concept that assumes that information is a valuable resource that must be managed, regardless of the form it takes or the medium in which it is stored

Information services department: *See* **health information services department**

Information system (IS): An automated system that uses computer hardware and software to record, manipulate, store, recover, and disseminate data (that is, a system that receives and processes input and provides output); often used interchangeably with **information technology (IT)**

Information technology (IT): Computer technology (hardware and software) combined with telecommunications technology (data, image, and voice networks); often used interchangeably with **information system (IS)**

Injury (harm): In a negligence lawsuit, one of four elements, which may be economic (hospital expenses and loss of wages) and noneconomic (pain and suffering), that must be proved to be successful

Injury Severity Score (ISS): An overall severity measurement maintained in the trauma registry and calculated from the abbreviated injury scores for the three most severe injuries of each patient

Inpatient: A patient who is provided with room, board, and continuous general nursing services in an area of an acute care facility where patients generally stay at least overnight

Inpatient admission: An acute care facility's formal acceptance of a patient who is to be provided with room, board, and continuous nursing service in an area of the facility where patients generally stay at least overnight

Inpatient bed occupancy rate (percentage of occupancy): The total number of inpatient service days for a given time period divided by the total number of inpatient bed count days for the same time period

Inpatient discharge: The termination of hospitalization through the formal release of an inpatient from a hospital

Inpatient hospitalization: The period during an individual's life when he or she is a patient in a single hospital without interruption except by possible intervening leaves of absence

Inpatient psychiatric facility (IPF): A healthcare facility that offers psychiatric medical care on an inpatient basis; CMS established a prospective payment system for reimbursing these types of facilities using the current DRGs for inpatient hospitals

Inpatient rehabilitation facility (IRF): A healthcare facility that specializes in providing services to patients who have suffered a disabling illness or injury in an effort to help them achieve or maintain their optimal level of functioning, self-care, and independence

Inpatient Rehabilitation Validation and Entry (IRVEN): A computerized data-entry system used by inpatient rehabilitation facilities

Inpatient service day (IPSD): A unit of measure equivalent to the services received by one inpatient during one 24-hour period

Inputs: Data entered into a hospital system (for example, the patient's knowledge of his or her condition, the admitting clerk's knowledge of the admission process, and the computer with its admitting template are all inputs for the hospital's admitting system)

Institute of Electrical and Electronics Engineers (IEEE): A national organization that develops standards for hospital system interface transactions, including links between critical care bedside instruments and clinical information systems

Institute of Medicine (IOM): A branch of the National Academy of Sciences whose goal is to advance and distribute scientific knowledge with the mission of improving human health

Institutional Review Board: An administrative body that provides oversight for the research studies conducted within a healthcare institution

Insured: A holder of a health insurance policy

Insurer: An organization that pays healthcare expenses on behalf of its enrollees

Integrated delivery network (IDN): *See* **integrated delivery system**

Integrated delivery system (IDS): A system that combines the financial and clinical aspects of healthcare and uses a group of healthcare providers, selected on the basis of quality and cost management criteria, to furnish comprehensive health services across the continuum of care; *See* **integrated provider organization**

Integrated health record format: A system of health record organization in which all the paper forms are arranged in strict chronological order and mixed with forms created by different departments

Integrated health records: *See* **integrated health record format**

Integrated provider organization (IPO): An organization that manages the delivery of healthcare services provided by hospitals, physicians (employees of the IPO), and other healthcare organizations (for example, nursing facilities); *See* **integrated delivery system**

Integrity: The state of being whole or unimpaired

Integrity constraints: Limits placed on the data that may be entered into a database

Intensity-of-service screening criteria: Preestablished standards used to determine the most efficient healthcare setting in which to safely provide needed services

Intentional tort: A circumstance where a healthcare provider purposely commits a wrongful act that results in injury

Interface: The zone between different computer systems across which users want to pass information (for example, a computer program written to exchange information between systems or the graphic display of an application program designed to make the program easier to use)

Internal customers: Individuals within the organization who receive products or services from an organizational unit or department

International Classification of Diseases, Ninth Revision, Clinical Modification (ICD-9-CM): A classification system used in the United States to report morbidity and mortality information

International Classification of Diseases, Tenth Revision, Clinical Modification (ICD-10-CM): The planned replacement for ICD-9-CM, volumes 1 and 2, developed to contain more codes and allow greater specificity

International Classification of Diseases, Tenth Revision, Procedure Coding System (ICD-10-PCS): A separate procedure coding system that would replace ICD-9-CM, volume 3, intended to improve coding accuracy and efficiency, reduce training effort, and improve communication with physicians

International Classification of Diseases for Oncology, Third Edition (ICD-O-3): A system used for classifying incidences of malignant disease

International Health Terminology Standards Development Organization: A company based in Denmark that is responsible for maintaining SNOMED International (formerly known as the Systematized Nomenclature of Human and Veterinary Medicine), a method for encoding data variables when physicians enter data into a history and physical exam template

Internet: An international network of computer servers that provides individual users with communications channels and access to software and information repositories worldwide

Interoperability: The ability, generally by adoption of standards, of systems to work together

Interpreter: A type of communications technology that converts high-level language statements into machine language one at a time

Interrater reliability: A measure of a research instrument's consistency in data collection when used by different abstractors

Interval-level data: Data with a defined unit of measure, no true zero point, and equal intervals between successive values; *See* **ratio-level data**

Intranet: A private information network that is similar to the Internet and whose servers are located inside a firewall or security barrier so that the general public cannot gain access to information housed within the network

Intrusion detection: The process of identifying and repelling attempts by unauthorized parties to gain access to a company's proprietary data

Inventory control: The balance between purchasing and storing needed supplies and not wasting money or space should the requirements for those supplies change or the space available for storage be limited

Investor-owned hospital chain: Group of for-profit healthcare facilities owned by stockholders

ISO 9000 Certification: An internationally agreed-upon set of generic standards for quality management systems established by the International Standards Organization

Issues management: The process of resolving unexpected occurrences (for example, the late delivery of needed supplies or an uncorrected system problem)

Job redesign: The process of realigning the needs of the organization with the skills and interests of the employee and then designing the job to meet those needs (for example, in order to introduce new tools or technology or provide better customer service)

Joinder: In a countersuit, a third party against whom the defendant files a complaint

Joint Commission (TJC): A private, not-for-profit organization that evaluates and accredits hospitals and other healthcare organizations on the basis of predefined performance standards; formerly known as the Joint Commission on Accreditation of Healthcare Organizations (JCAHO)

Judicial law: The body of law created as a result of court (judicial) decisions

Jurisdiction: The power and authority of a court to hear and decide specific types of cases

Justice: The impartial administration of policies or laws that takes into consideration the competing interests and limited resources of the individual or groups involved

Key field: An explanatory notation that uniquely identifies each row in a database table; *See* **primary key**

Knowledge database: A database that not only manages raw data but also integrates them with information from various reference works; *See* **data repository**

Knowledge management system (KMS): A type of system that supports the creation, organization, and dissemination of business or clinical knowledge and expertise to providers, employees, and managers throughout a healthcare enterprise

Laboratory information system (LIS): An information system that collects, stores, and manages laboratory tests and their respective results. The LIS can speed up access to test results through improved efficiency from various locations, including anywhere in the hospital, the physician's office, or even the clinician's home.

Language translator: A software system that translates a program written in a particular computer language into a language that other types of computers can understand

Legal health record: Documents and data elements that a healthcare provider may include in a response to a legally permissible request for patient information

Length of stay (LOS): The total number of patient days for an inpatient episode, calculated by subtracting the date of admission from the date of discharge

Liability: 1. A legal obligation or responsibility that may have financial repercussions if not fulfilled. 2. An amount owed by an individual or organization to another individual or organization.

Licensure: The legal authority or formal permission from authorities to carry on certain activities that by law or regulation require such permission (applicable to institutions as well as individuals)

Line graph: A graphic technique used to illustrate the relationship between continuous measurements; consists of a line drawn to connect a series of points on an arithmetic scale; often used to display time trends

Litigation: A civil lawsuit or contest in court

Local area network (LAN): A network that connects multiple computer devices via continuous cable within a relatively small geographic area

Logical Observations, Identifiers, Names and Codes (LOINC): A database protocol developed by the Regenstrief Institute for Health Care aimed at standardizing laboratory and clinical codes for use in clinical care, outcomes management, and research

Long-term care hospital (LTCH): A hospital with an average length of stay of 25 days or more

Long-term care information system: Information system designed to support the care provided in a long-term care facility

Low-utilization payment adjustment (LUPA): An alternative (reduced) payment made to home health agencies instead of the home health resource group reimbursement rate when a patient receives fewer than four home care visits during a 60-day episode

Machine language: Binary codes made up of zeroes and ones that computers use directly to represent precise storage locations and operations

Mainframe: A computer architecture built with a single central processing unit to which dumb terminals and/or personal computers are connected

Mainframe architecture: The term used to refer to the configuration of a mainframe computer

Major diagnostic category (MDC): Under diagnosis-related groups (DRGs), one of 25 categories based on single or multiple organ systems into which all diseases and disorders relating to that system are classified

Major medical insurance: Prepaid healthcare benefits that include a high limit for most types of medical expenses and usually require a large deductible and sometimes place limits on coverage and charges (for example, room and board)

Malfeasance: A wrong or improper act

Malware: Short for malicious software, this is software designed to invade another person's or business's computer system with malicious intent.

Managed care: 1. Payment method in which the third-party payer has implemented some provisions to control the costs of healthcare while maintaining quality care 2. Systematic merger of clinical, financial, and administrative processes to manage access, cost, and quality of healthcare

Managed care organization (MCO): A type of healthcare organization that delivers medical care and manages all aspects of the care or the payment for care by limiting providers of care, discounting payment to providers of care, and/or limiting access to care

Management information system (MIS): A computer-based system that provides information to a healthcare organization's managers for use in making decisions that affect a variety of day-to-day activities

Management service organization (MSO): An organization, usually owned by a group of physicians or a hospital, that provides administrative and support services to one or more physician group practices or small hospitals

Management support information systems: Systems that provide information primarily to support manager decision making

Master patient index (MPI): A list or database created and maintained by a healthcare facility to record the name and identification number of every patient who has ever been admitted or treated in the facility

Materials management system: Information system that manages the supplies and equipment within a facility

Maternal death rate: For a hospital, the total number of maternal deaths directly related to pregnancy for a given time period divided by the total number of obstetrical discharges for the same time period; for a community, the total number of deaths attributed to maternal conditions during a given time period in a specific geographic area divided by the total number of live births for the same time period in the same area

Maternal mortality rate: The rate that measures deaths associated with pregnancy for a community for a specific period of time

Mean: A measure of central tendency that is determined by calculating the arithmetic average of the observations in a frequency distribution

Meaningful use: Term used in the ARRA/HITECH legislation for providers to qualify for incentives for using EHR. There are three types of requirements for meaningful use: (1) use of certified EHR technology in a meaningful manner (for example, electronic prescribing); (2) that the certified EHR technology is connected in a manner that provides for the electronic exchange of health information to improve the quality of care; and (3) that, in using certified EHR technology, the provider submits information on clinical quality measures (42 CFR Parts 412)

Median: A measure of central tendency that shows the midpoint of a frequency distribution when the observations have been arranged in order from lowest to highest

Mediation: In law, when a dispute is submitted to a third party to facilitate agreement between the disputing parties

Medicaid: An entitlement program that oversees medical assistance for individuals and families with low incomes and limited resources; jointly funded between state and federal governments

Medical device: Instruments that collect or supply health information

Medical foundation: Multipurpose, nonprofit service organization for physicians and other healthcare providers at the local and county level; as managed care organizations, medical foundations have established preferred provider organizations, exclusive provider organizations, and management service organizations, with emphases on freedom of choice and preservation of the physician-patient relationship

Medical Group Management Association (MGMA): A national organization composed of individuals actively engaged in the business management of medical groups consisting of three or more physicians in medical practice

Medical history: A record of the information provided by a patient to his or her physician to explain the patient's chief complaint, present and past illnesses, and personal and family medical problems; includes a description of the physician's review of systems

Medical identity theft: Occurs when an individual's health information is misrepresented and used by an unauthorized individual to obtain healthcare goods, services, or money to which they are neither eligible nor entitled

Medical Literature Analysis and Retrieval System Online (MEDLINE): A computerized, online database in the bibliographic Medical Literature Analysis and Retrieval System (MEDLARS) of the National Library of Medicine

Medical malpractice: The professional liability of healthcare providers in the delivery of patient care

Medical staff bylaws: A collection of guidelines adopted by a hospital's medical staff to govern its business conduct and the rights and responsibilities of its members

Medical staff classifications: The organization of physicians in a healthcare facility; typical medical staff classifications include active, provisional, honorary, consulting, courtesy, and medical resident assignments

Medical staff privileges: Permission granted to provide clinical services in a healthcare facility based on the credentials of the individual and limited to a specific scope of practice

Medical transcription: The conversion of verbal medical reports dictated by healthcare providers into written form for inclusion in patients' health records

Medically needy option (Medicaid): An option in the Medicaid program that allows states to extend eligibility to persons who would be eligible for Medicaid under one of the mandatory or optional groups but whose income and/or resources fall above the eligibility level set by their state

Medicare: A federally funded health program established in 1965 to assist with the medical care costs of Americans 65 years of age and older as well as other individuals entitled to Social Security benefits owing to their disabilities

Medicare Administrative Contractor (MAC): Newly established contracting entities that will administer Medicare Part A and Part B as of 2011; MACs will replace the carriers and fiscal intermediaries

Medicare Advantage (Medicare Part C): Optional managed care plan for Medicare beneficiaries who are entitled to Part A, enrolled in Part B, and live in an area with a plan; types include health maintenance organization, point-of-service plan, preferred provider organization, and provider-sponsored organization; formerly Medicare+Choice

Medicare carrier: A health plan that processes Part B claims for services by physicians and medical suppliers (for example, the Blue Shield plan in a state)

Medicare Conditions of Participation or Conditions for Coverage: A publication that describes the requirements that institutional providers (such as hospitals, skilled nursing facilities, and home health agencies) must meet to receive reimbursement for services provided to Medicare beneficiaries

Medicare fee schedule (MFS): A feature of the resource-based relative value system that includes a complete list of the payments Medicare makes to physicians and other providers

Medicare prospective payment system: *See* **acute care prospective payment system**, **home health prospective payment system**, and **skilled nursing facility prospective payment system**

Medicare Provider Analysis and Review (MEDPAR) File: A collection of data from reimbursement claims submitted to the Medicare program by acute care hospitals and skilled nursing facilities that is used to evaluate the quality and effectiveness of the care being provided

Medicare severity diagnosis-related groups (MS-DRGs): The U.S. government's 2007 revision of the DRG system, the MS-DRG system better accounts for severity of illness and resource consumption

Medicare Summary Notice (MSN): A summary sent to the patient from Medicare that summarizes all services provided over a period of time with an explanation of benefits provided

Medication administration system: Information system designed to support the administration of medications safely

Medication Five Rights: The right drug, in the right dose, through the right route, at the right time, and to the right patient

Medication reconciliation: Process that monitors and confirms that the patient receives consistent dosing across all facility transfers, such as on admission, from nursing unit to surgery, and from surgery to intensive care unit (ICU)

Medigap: A private insurance policy that supplements Medicare coverage

Mesh topology: A network in which every device on the network is physically connected to every other device on the same network

Message format standards: Protocols that help ensure that data transmitted from one system to another remain comparable

Metadata: Descriptive data that characterize other data to create a clearer understanding of their meaning and to achieve greater reliability and quality of information

Microcomputer: A personal computer characterized by its relatively small size and fast processing speed

Middle digit filing system: A numeric filing system in which the middle digits are used as the finding aid to organize the filing system

Middle management: The management level in an organization that is concerned primarily with facilitating the work performed by supervisory- and staff-level personnel

Middle managers: The individuals in an organization who oversee the operation of a broad scope of functions at the departmental level or who oversee defined product or service lines

Migration path: A series of steps required to move from one situation to another

Minicomputer: A small, mainframe computer

Minimum Data Set (MDS) for Long-Term Care: The instrument specified by the Centers for Medicare and Medicaid Services that requires nursing facilities (both Medicare certified and/or Medicaid certified) to conduct a comprehensive, accurate, standardized, reproducible assessment of each resident's functional capacity

Minimum Data Set Version 3.0 (MDS 3.0): A federally mandated standard assessment form that Medicare- and/or Medicaid-certified nursing facilities must use to collect demographic and clinical data on nursing home residents

Minimum necessary standard: A stipulation of the HIPAA Privacy Rule that requires healthcare facilities and other covered entities to make reasonable efforts to limit the patient-identifiable information they disclose to the least amount required to accomplish the intended purpose for which the information was requested

Misfeasance: Relating to negligence, improper performance during an otherwise correct act

Mission: The defined purpose for which a group of people or an organization joins forces to accomplish specific goals

Mission statement: A short description of an organization's or group's general purpose for existing

Mixed costs: Costs that are part variable and part fixed

Mode: A measure of central tendency that consists of the most frequent observation in a frequency distribution

Modular EHR: EHR product meets only one or more but not all of the requirements of a certified EHR

Monitoring stage: In performance management, the stage during which established performance standards are continuously checked for any additional need corrections

Morality: A composite of the personal values concerning what is considered right or wrong in a specific cultural group

Moral values: A system of principles by which one guides one's life, usually with regard to right or wrong

Morbidity: A term referring to the state of being diseased (including illness, injury, or deviation from normal health); the number of sick persons or cases of disease in relationship to a specific population

Mortality: 1. A term referring to the incidence of death in a specific population 2. The loss of subjects during the course of a clinical research study

MS-DRG Grouper: A computer program that assigns inpatient cases to Medicare severity diagnosis-related groups and determines the Medicare reimbursement rate

Multi-dimensional database: A database specifically designed to handle data organized into a data structure with numerous dimensions

Multivoting technique: A decision-making method for determining group consensus on the prioritization of issues or solutions

National Alliance for Health Information Technology (NAHIT): A partnership of government and private sector leaders from various healthcare organizations working to use technology to achieve improvements in patient safety, quality of care, and operating performance; founded in 2002

National Cancer Registrars Association (NCRA): An organization of cancer registry professionals that promotes research and education in cancer registry administration and practice

National Center for Health Statistics (NCHS): The federal agency responsible for collecting and disseminating information on health services utilization and the health status of the population in the United States

National Commission on Correctional Health Care: An accreditation organization that maintains comprehensive standards for healthcare in correctional facilities throughout the United States

National Committee for Quality Assurance (NCQA): A private, not-for-profit accreditation organization whose mission is to evaluate and report on the quality of managed care organizations in the United States

National Committee on Vital and Health Statistics (NCVHS): A public policy advisory board that recommends policy to the National Center for Health Statistics and other health-related federal programs

National conversion factor (CF): A mathematical factor used to convert relative value units into monetary payments for services provided to Medicare beneficiaries

National Correct Coding Initiative (NCCI): A series of code edits on Medicare Part B claims

National Council for Prescription Drug Programs (NCPDP): An organization that develops standards for exchanging prescription and payment information

National Drug Codes (NDC): Codes that serve as product identifiers for human drugs, currently limited to prescription drugs and a few selected over-the-counter products

National health information infrastructure (NHII): An infrastructure proposed by the National Committee on Vital and Health Statistics in 2002 that would be a set of technologies, standards, applications, systems, values, and laws that support all facets of provider healthcare, individual health, and public health; also called a national health information network

National Health Information Network (NHIN): Provides the technology to support the national health information infrastructure

National Institute for Standards and Technology (NIST): An agency of the US Department of Commerce, NIST was founded in 1901 as the nation's first federal physical science research laboratory

National Institutes of Health (NIH): Federal agency of the Department of Health and Human Services comprising a number of institutes that carry out research and programs related to certain types of diseases, such as cancer

National Labor Relations Act: Federal legislation that provides, among other things, procedures for union representation and prohibits unfair labor practices by unions, such as coercing nonstriking employees, and by employers, such as interference with the union selection process and discrimination against employees who support a union

National Library of Medicine (NLM): The world's largest medical library and a branch of the National Institutes of Health

National patient safety goals (NPSGs): Goals issued by the Joint Commission on Accreditation of Healthcare Organizations to improve patient safety in healthcare organizations nationwide

National Practitioner Data Bank (NPDB): A data bank established by the federal government through the 1986 Health Care Quality Improvement Act that contains information on professional review actions taken against physicians and other licensed healthcare practitioners, which healthcare organizations are required to check as part of the credentialing process

National provider identifier (NPI): An eight-character alphanumeric identifier used to identify individual healthcare providers for Medicare billing purposes

National Uniform Billing Committee (NUBC): The national group responsible for identifying data elements and designing the CMS-1500

National Uniform Claim Committee (NUCC): The national group that replaced the Uniform Claim Form Task Force in 1995 and developed a standard data set to be used in the transmission of noninstitutional provider claims to and from third-party payers

National Vaccine Advisory Committee (NVAC): A national advisory group that supports the director of the National Vaccine Program

Nationwide Health Information Network (NHIN): System that links various healthcare information systems together, allowing patients, physicians, healthcare institutions, and other entities nationwide to share clinical information privately and securely

Natural language: A fifth-generation computer programming language that uses human language to give people a more natural connection with computers

Natural language processing (NLP): A field of computer science and linguistics concerned with the interactions between computers and human (natural) languages that converts information from computer databases into readable human language

Need-to-know principle: The release-of-information principle based on the minimum necessary standard that means that only the information needed by a specific individual to perform a specific task should be released

Negligence: A legal term that refers to the result of an action by an individual who does not act the way a reasonably prudent person would act under the same circumstances

Net autopsy rate: The ratio of inpatient autopsies compared to inpatient deaths calculated by dividing the total number of inpatient autopsies performed by the hospital pathologist for a given time period by the total number of inpatient deaths minus unautopsied coroners' or medical examiners' cases for the same time period

Net death rate: The total number of inpatient deaths minus the number of deaths that occurred less than 48 hours after admission for a given time period divided by the total number of inpatient discharges minus the number of deaths that occurred less than 48 hours after admission for the same time period

Network: 1. A type of information technology that connects different computers and computer systems so that they can share information 2. Physicians, hospitals, and other providers who provide healthcare services to members of a managed care organization; providers may be associated through formal or informal contracts and agreements.

Network controls: A method of protecting data from unauthorized change and corruption during transmission among information systems

Network model HMO: Program in which participating HMOs contract for services with one or more multispecialty group practices

Network protocol: A set of conventions that governs the exchange of data between hardware and/or software components in a communications network

Network provider: A physician or another healthcare professional who is a member of a managed care network

Newborn: An inpatient who was born in a hospital at the beginning of the current inpatient hospitalization

Newborn autopsy rate: The number of autopsies performed on newborns who died during a given time period divided by the total number of newborns who died during the same time period

Nomenclature: A recognized system of terms used in science or art that follows preestablished naming conventions; a disease nomenclature is a listing of the proper name for each disease entity with its specific code number

Nominal group technique: A group process technique that involves the steps of silent listing, recording each participant's list, discussing, and rank ordering the priority or importance of items

Nominal-level data: Data that fall into groups or categories that are mutually exclusive and with no specific order (for example, patient demographics such as third-party payer, race, and sex); also called categorical data

Nonfeasance: A type of negligence meaning failure to act

Nonmaleficence: A legal principle that means do no harm

Nonparticipating providers: A healthcare provider who did not sign a participation agreement with Medicare and so is not obligated to accept assignment on Medicare claims

Nonrepudiation: Limits an EHR's user's ability to deny (repudiate) the origination, receipt, or authorization of a data exchange by that user

Normal distribution: A theoretical family of continuous frequency distributions characterized by a symmetric bell-shaped curve, with an equal mean, median, and mode, any standard deviation, and with half of the observations above the mean and half below it

Norming: The third of the four steps in forming a functional team, during which each team member comes to understand his or her role

North American Association of Central Cancer Registries (NAACCR): A national organization that certifies state, population-based cancer registries

Nosocomial (hospital-acquired) infection: An infection acquired by a patient while receiving care or services in a healthcare organization; *See* **hospital-acquired infection**

Nosology: The branch of medical science that deals with classification systems

Notice of privacy practices: A statement (mandated by the HIPAA Privacy Rule) issued by a healthcare organization that informs individuals of the uses and disclosures of patient-identifiable health information that may be made by the organization, as well as the individual's rights and the organization's legal duties with respect to that information

Notifiable disease: A disease that must be reported to a government agency so that regular, frequent, and timely information on individual cases can be used to prevent and control future cases of the disease

Numeric filing system: A system of health record identification and storage in which records are arranged consecutively in ascending numerical order according to the health record number

Nursing information system (NIS): Information system that assists in the planning and monitoring of overall patient care and documents the nursing care provided to a patient

Nursing vocabularies: A classification system used to capture documentation on nursing care

Object: The basic component in an object-oriented database that includes both data and their relationships within a single structure

Object-oriented database (OODB): A type of database that uses commands that act as small, self-contained instructional units (objects) that may be combined in various ways

Object-relational database: A type of database (both object-oriented and relational) that stores both objects and traditional tables

Occasion of service: A specified identifiable service involved in the care of a patient that is not an encounter (for example, a lab test ordered during an encounter)

Occupational Safety and Health Act (OSHA) of 1970: The federal legislation that established comprehensive safety and health guidelines for employers

Occurrence screening: A risk management technique in which the risk manager reviews the health records of current and discharged hospital inpatients with the goal of identifying potentially compensable events

Office of the National Coordinator (ONC) for Health Information Technology: Office that provides leadership for the development and implementation of an interoperable health information technology infrastructure nationwide to improve healthcare quality and delivery

Omnibus Budget Reconciliation Act (OBRA): Federal legislation passed in 1987 that required the Health Care Financing Administration (now renamed the Centers for Medicare and Medicaid Services) to develop an assessment instrument (called the resident assessment instrument) to standardize the collection of patient data from skilled nursing facilities

Online analytical processing (OLAP): A data access architecture that allows the user to retrieve specific information from a large volume of data

Operating rules: Rules that further explain the standards so their use is consistent across health plans

Operating system: Processes that are affected by what is going on around them and must adjust as the environment changes

Operation index: A list of the operations and surgical procedures performed in a healthcare facility that is sequenced according to the code numbers of the classification system in use

Operation support systems (OSS): An information system that facilitates the operational management of a healthcare organization

Operational budget: A type of budget that allocates and controls resources to meet an organization's goals and objectives for the fiscal year

Operational plan: The short-term objectives set by an organization to improve its methods of doing business and achieve its planned outcomes

Operative report: A formal document that describes the events surrounding a surgical procedure or operation and identifies the principal participants in the surgery

Opportunity for improvement: A healthcare structure, product, service, process, or outcome that does not meet its customers' expectations and, therefore, could be improved

Opt-in/opt-out: Patients' choices for having their data exchanged in the HIE

Ordinal-level data: Data with inherent order and with higher numbers usually associated with higher values; also called ordinal data or ranked data

Organization: The planned coordination of the activities of more than one person for the achievement of a common purpose or goal

Organizational chart: A graphic representation of an organization's formal structure

ORYX initiative: A Joint Commission on Accreditation of Healthcare Organizations initiative that supports the integration of outcomes data and other performance measurement data into the accreditation process

Out-of-pocket expenses: Healthcare costs paid by the insured (for example, deductibles, copayments, and coinsurance) after which the insurer pays a percentage (often 80 or 100 percent) of covered expenses

Outcomes and Assessment Information Set (OASIS-C): A standard core assessment data tool developed to measure the outcomes of adult patients receiving home health services under the Medicare and Medicaid programs

Outguide: A device used in paper-based health record systems to track the location of records removed from the file storage area

Outpatient: A patient who receives ambulatory care services in a hospital-based clinic or department

Outpatient code editor (OCE): A software program linked to the Correct Coding Initiative that applies a set of logical rules to determine whether various combinations of codes are correct and appropriately represent the services provided

Outpatient prospective payment system (OPPS): The Medicare prospective payment system used for hospital-based outpatient services and procedures that is predicated on the assignment of ambulatory payment classifications

Outpatient visit: A patient's visit to one or more units located in the ambulatory services area (clinic or physician's office) of an acute care hospital in which an overnight stay does not occur

Outputs: The outcomes of inputs into a system (for example, the output of the admitting process is the patient's admission to the hospital)

Overlap: Situation in which a patient is issued more than one medical record number from an organization with multiple facilities

Overlay: Situation in which a patient is issued a medical record number that has been previously issued to a different patient

Packaging: A payment under the Medicare outpatient prospective payment system that includes items such as anesthesia, supplies, certain drugs, and the use of recovery and observation rooms

Palliative care: A type of medical care designed to relieve the patient's pain and suffering without attempting to cure the underlying disease

Parallel approach conversion: A process whereby both an old information technology system and a new IT system run in parallel for a period of time before completely converting to the new technology

Pareto chart: A bar graph that includes bars arranged in order of descending size to show decisions on the prioritization of issues, problems, or solutions

Partial hospitalization: A term that refers to limited patients stays in the hospital setting, typically as part of a transitional program to a less intense level of service; for example, psychiatric and drug and alcohol treatment facilities that offer services to help patients reenter the community, return to work, and assume family responsibilities

Password: A series of characters that must be entered to authenticate user identity and gain access to a computer or specified portions of a database

Pathology report: A type of health record or documentation that describes the results of a microscopic and macroscopic evaluation of a specimen removed or expelled during a surgical procedure

Patient account number: A number assigned by a healthcare facility for billing purposes that is unique to a particular episode of care; a new account number is assigned each time the patient receives care or services at the facility

Patient acuity staffing: The number of nurses and other care provides is based on how sick the patient is.

Patient advocacy: The function performed by patient representatives (sometimes called ombudsmen) who respond personally to complaints from patients and/or their families

Patient assessment instrument (PAI): A standardized tool used to evaluate the patient's condition after admission to, and at discharge from, the healthcare facility

Patient care charting system: A system in which caregivers enter data into health records

Patient-Centered Medical Home (PCMH): A program to provide comprehensive primary care that partners physicians with the patient and their family to allow better access to healthcare and improved outcomes

Patient financial system (PFS): Information system that manages patient accounts

Patient history questionnaire: A series of structured questions to be answered by patients to provide information to clinicians about their current health status

Patient-identifiable data: Personal information that can be linked to a specific patient, such as age, gender, date of birth, and address

Patient portal: Information system that allows patient to login to obtain information, register and perform other functions.

Patient Protection and Affordable Care Act: A federal statute that was signed into law on March 23, 2010. Along with the Health Care and Education Reconciliation Act of 2010 (signed into law on March 30, 2010), the Act is the product of the healthcare reform agenda of the Democratic 111th Congress and the Obama administration

Patient safety: The condition of a patient being safe from harm or injury

Patient Self-Determination Act (PSDA): The federal legislation that requires healthcare facilities to provide written information on the patient's right to issue advance directives and to accept or refuse medical treatment

Patient-specific/identifiable data: Personal information that can be linked to a specific patient, such as age, gender, date of birth, and address

Patient-specific information: *See* **patient-specific/identifiable data**

Patient's bill of rights: The protections afforded to individuals who are undergoing medical procedures in hospitals or other healthcare facilities; also referred to as patient rights

Payback period: A financial method used to evaluate the value of a capital expenditure by calculating the time frame that must pass before inflow of cash from a project equals or exceeds outflow of cash

Payer of last resort: A Medicaid term that means that Medicare pays for the services provided to individuals enrolled in both Medicare and Medicaid until Medicare benefits are exhausted and Medicaid benefits begin

Payment status indicator (PSI): An alphabetic code assigned to CPT/HCPCS codes to indicate whether a service or procedure is to be reimbursed under the Medicare outpatient prospective payment system

Peer review organization (PRO): Until 2002, a medical organization that performs a professional review of medical necessity, quality, and appropriateness of healthcare services provided to Medicare beneficiaries; now called quality improvement organization (QIO)

Percentage of occupancy: *See* **inpatient bed occupancy rate**

Performance counseling: Guidance provided to an individual in an attempt to improve his or her work performance

Performance evaluations: Reviews of employee job performance

Performance improvement (PI): The continuous study and adaptation of a healthcare organization's functions and processes to increase the likelihood of achieving desired outcomes

Performance indicators: Measures used by healthcare facilities to assess the quality, effectiveness, and efficiency of their services

Performance management: Encompasses all activities necessary to ensure that a company's stated goals are met in the most efficient manner

Performance standards: The stated expectations for acceptable quality and productivity associated with a job function

Performing: The fourth of the four steps in forming a functional team, at which point each team member is in a position to work toward achieving the team's stated goals

Peripheral: Any hardware device connected to a computer (for example, a keyboard, mouse, or printer)

Per member per month (PMPM): *See* **per patient per month**

Per patient per month (PPPM): A type of managed care arrangement by which providers are paid a fixed fee in exchange for supplying all of the healthcare services an enrollee needs for a specified period of time (usually one month but sometimes one year)

Personal digital assistant (PDA): A hand-held microcomputer, without a hard drive, that is capable of running applications such as e-mail and providing access to data and information, such as notes, phone lists, schedules, and laboratory results, primarily through a pen device

Personal health record (PHR): An electronic record of health-related information on an individual that conforms to nationally recognized interoperability standards and that can be drawn from multiple sources while being managed and controlled by the individual

Personal representative: Person with legal authority to act on a patient's behalf

Petition for writ of certiorari: A document filed with the U.S. Supreme Court, asking for a review of a lower court's findings

Pharmacy benefits manager (PBM): The vendor selected by the Bureau of Workers' Compensation to process outpatient medication bills submitted electronically

Pharmacy information system: System that assists care providers in ordering, allocating, and administering medication; focuses on patient safety issues, especially medication errors and providing optimal patient care

Phased approach conversion: A process whereby separate elements of a new information technology system are implemented over a period of time

Physical access controls: 1. Security mechanisms designed to protect an organization's equipment, media, and facilities from physical damage or intrusion 2. Security mechanisms designed to prevent unauthorized physical access to health records and health record storage areas

Physical examination report: Documentation of a physician's assessment of a patient's body systems

Physical safeguards: Measures such as locking doors to safeguard data and computer programs from undesired occurrences and exposures

Physical security: The safeguarding of data from loss, theft, or other disasters

Physical topology: The method by which data flows through a company's network

Physician champion: An individual who assists in communicating and educating medical staff in areas such as documentation procedures for accurate billing and appropriate EHR processes

Physician-hospital organization (PHO): An integrated delivery system formed by hospitals and physicians (usually through managed care contracts) that allows for cooperative activity but permits participants to retain some level of independence

Physician index: A list of patients and their physicians that is usually arranged according to the physician code numbers assigned by the healthcare facility

Physician's orders: A physician's written or verbal instructions to the other caregivers involved in a patient's care

Physician Quality Reporting System (PQRS): An incentive payment system for eligible professionals who satisfactorily report data on quality measures for covered professional services furnished to Medicare beneficiaries; formerly known as the Physician Quality Reporting Initiative (PQRI)

Picture archiving and communications system (PACS): An integrated computer system that obtains, stores, retrieves, and displays digital images (in healthcare, radiological images)

Pie chart: A graphic technique in which the proportions of a category are displayed as portions of a circle (like pieces of a pie)

Plaintiff: The group or person who initiates a civil lawsuit

Plan-do-study-act (PDSA) cycle: A performance improvement model designed specifically for healthcare organizations

Planning stage: In performance management, the stage during which specific goals and performance standards are defined

Point of care (POC): The place or location where the physician administers services to the patient

Point-of-care charting: A system whereby information is entered into the health record at the time and location of service

Point-of-care documentation: A system whereby information is entered into the health record at the time and location of service

Point-of-service (POS) plan: A type of managed care plan in which enrollees are encouraged to select healthcare providers from a network of providers under contract with the plan but are also allowed to select providers outside the network and pay a larger share of the cost

Policies: 1. Governing principles that describe how a department or an organization is supposed to handle a specific situation 2. Binding contracts issued by a healthcare insurance company to an individual or group in which the company promises to pay for healthcare to treat illness or injury

Policyholder: An individual or entity that purchases healthcare insurance coverage

Population-based registry: A type of registry that includes information from more than one facility in a specific geopolitical area, such as a state or region

Population-based statistics: Statistics based on a defined population rather than on a sample drawn from the same population

Portals: Special web pages that offer secure access and entry of data upon authorization of the owner of the page

Position description: A document that outlines the work responsibilities associated with a job

Postneonatal mortality rate: The number of deaths of persons aged 28 days up to, but not including, one year during a given time period divided by the number of live births for the same time period

Postoperative infection rate: The number of infections that occur in clean surgical cases for a given time period divided by the total number of operations within the same time period

Potentially compensable event: An event that may result in financial liability for a healthcare organization, for example, an injury, accident, or medical error

Practice guidelines: Protocols of care that guide the clinical care process

Practice management system (PMS): Software designed to help medical practices run more smoothly and efficiently

Preadmission utilization review: A type of review conducted before a patient's admission to an acute care facility to determine whether the planned service (intensity of service) or the patient's condition (severity of illness) warrants care in an inpatient setting

Precertification: Process of obtaining approval from a healthcare insurance company before receiving healthcare services

Preemption: In law, the principle that a statute at one level supersedes or is applied over the same or similar statute at a lower level, for example, the federal HIPAA privacy provisions trump the same or similar state law with certain exceptions

Preferred provider organization (PPO): A managed care arrangement based on a contractual agreement between healthcare providers (professional and/or institutional) and employers, insurance carriers, or third-party administrators to provide healthcare services to a defined population of enrollees at established fees that may or may not be a discount from usual and customary or reasonable charges

Premium: Amount of money that a policyholder or certificate holder must periodically pay an insurer in return for healthcare coverage

Present on admission (POA): A condition present at the time of inpatient admission

Prevalence rate: The proportion of people in a population who have a particular disease at a specific point in time or over a specified period of time

Primary care manager (PCM): The healthcare provider assigned to a TRICARE enrollee

Primary care physician (PCP): 1. The physician who provides, supervises, and coordinates the healthcare of a member and who manages referrals to other healthcare providers and utilization of healthcare services both inside and outside a managed care plan 2. The physician who makes the initial diagnosis of a patient's medical condition

Primary data source: A record developed by healthcare professionals in the process of providing patient care

Primary key: *See* **key field**

Principal diagnosis: The disease or condition that was present on admission, was the principal reason for admission, and received treatment or evaluation during the hospital stay or visit

Principal procedure: The procedure performed for the definitive treatment of a condition (as opposed to a procedure performed for diagnostic or exploratory purposes) or for care of a complication

Print file: Output from a computer system that generates a file containing an image of information that can be printed

Prior authorization: Process of obtaining approval from a healthcare insurance company before receiving healthcare services

Privacy: The quality or state of being hidden from, or undisturbed by, the observation or activities of other persons or freedom from unauthorized intrusion; in healthcare-related contexts, the right of a patient to control disclosure of personal information

Privacy officer: The individual responsible for the development and implementation of an organization's privacy policies and procedures

Privacy standards: Rules, conditions, or requirements developed to ensure the privacy of patient information

Private law: The collective rules and principles that define the rights and duties of people and private businesses

Problem list: A list of illnesses, injuries, and other factors that affect the health of an individual patient, usually identifying the time of occurrence or identification and resolution

Problem-oriented health record: Patient record in which clinical problems are defined and documented individually

Procedural codes: The numeric or alphanumeric characters used to classify and report the medical procedures and services performed for patients

Procedures: The steps taken to implement a policy

Process improvement: A series of actions taken to identify, analyze, and improve existing processes

Process indicators: Specific measures that enable the assessment of the steps taken in rendering a service

Process redesign: The second step in a quality improvement process in which the findings in the research phase are identified, focused data from the prioritized problem areas are collected, a flowchart of the redesigned process is created, policies and procedures are developed, and staff are educated on the new process

Processes: The day-to-day tasks and methods utilized in a standardized procedure to accomplish the provision by an individual or organization of products and services to its customers

Productivity indicators: A set of measures designed to routinely monitor the output and quality of products and/or services provided by an individual, an organization or one of its constituent parts

Productivity: A unit of performance defined by management in quantitative standards

Productivity software: A type of computer software used for word-processing, spreadsheet, and database management applications

Professional component (PC): 1. The portion of a healthcare procedure performed by a physician 2. A term generally used in reference to the elements of radiological procedures performed by a physician

Professional standards review organization (PSRO): An organization responsible for determining whether the care and services provided to hospital inpatients were medically necessary and met professional standards in the context of eligibility for reimbursement under the Medicare and Medicaid programs

Programming language: A set of words and symbols that allows programmers to tell the computer what operations to follow

Progress notes: The documentation of a patient's care, treatment, and therapeutic response that is entered into the health record by each of the clinical professionals involved in a patient's care, including nurses, physicians, therapists, and social workers

Progressive discipline: A four-step process for shaping employee behavior to conform to the requirements of the employee's job position that begins with a verbal caution and progresses to written reprimand, suspension, and dismissal upon subsequent offenses

Proportion: A type of ratio in which the elements included in the numerator also must be included in the denominator

Proportionate mortality ratio (PMR): The total number of deaths due to a specific cause during a given time period divided by the total number of deaths due to all causes

Proprietary vocabulary: A controlled vocabulary that is formally approved by an organizatino such as a vendor that developed the vocabulary

Prospective payment system (PPS): A type of reimbursement system that is based on preset payment levels rather than actual charges billed after the service has been provided; specifically, one of several Medicare reimbursement systems based on predetermined payment rates or periods and linked to the anticipated intensity of services delivered as well as the beneficiary's condition; *See* **acute care prospective payment system**, **home health prospective payment system**, **outpatient prospective payment system**, and **skilled nursing facility prospective payment system**

Prospective utilization review: A review of a patient's health records before admission to determine the necessity of admission to an acute care facility and to determine or satisfy benefit coverage requirements

Protected health information (PHI): Under HIPAA, all individually identifiable information, whether oral or recorded in any form or medium, that is created or received by a healthcare provider or any other entity subject to HIPAA requirements

Protocol: In healthcare, a detailed plan of care for a specific medical condition based on investigative studies; in medical research, a rule or procedure to be followed in a clinical trial; in a computer network, a protocol is used to address and ensure delivery of data

Provider: Physician, clinic, hospital, nursing home, or other healthcare entity (second party) that delivers healthcare services

Public assistance: A monetary subsidy provided to financially needy individuals

Public health: An area of healthcare that deals with the health of populations in geopolitical areas, such as states and counties

Public health services: Services concerned primarily with the health of entire communities and population groups

Public law: A type of legislation that involves the government and its relations with individuals and business organizations

Public Law 104-191: The alternate name for the Health Insurance Portability and Accountability Act (HIPAA) passed in 1996; *See* **Health Insurance Portability and Accountability Act of 1996**

Purged records: Patient health records that have been removed from the active file area

Quality: The degree or grade of excellence of goods or services, including, in healthcare, meeting expectations for outcomes of care

Quality Data Model (QDM): Model that describes clinical concepts in a standardized format

Quality improvement organization (QIO): An organization that performs medical peer review of Medicare and Medicaid claims, including review of validity of hospital diagnosis and procedure coding information; completeness, adequacy, and quality of care; and appropriateness of prospective payments for outlier cases and nonemergent use of the emergency room; until 2002, called peer review organization

Quality improvement process: An approach undertaken to improve healthcare delivery that involves two principal steps: problem identification and process redesign

Quality indicator: A standard against which actual care may be measured to identify a level of performance for that standard

Quantitative analysis: A review of the health record to determine its completeness and accuracy

Radio-frequency identification: An automatic recognition technology that uses a device attached to an object to transmit data to a receiver and does not require direct contact

Radiology information system (RIS): A system that collects, stores, and provides information on radiological tests such as ultrasound, magnetic resonance imaging, and positron emission tomography

Range: A measure of variability between the smallest and largest observations in a frequency distribution

Rate: A measure used to compare an event over time; a comparison of the number of times an event did happen (numerator) with the number of times an event could have happened (denominator)

Rating stage: In performance management, the fourth of five steps during which specific performance criteria are evaluated

Ratio: 1. A calculation found by dividing one quantity by another 2. A general term that can include a number of specific measures such as proportion, percentage, and rate

Ratio-level data: Data with a defined unit of measure, a real zero point, and with equal intervals between successive values; also called ratio data; *See* **interval-level data**

Read Codes: The former name of the United Kingdom's CTV3 codes; named for James Read, the physician who originally devised the system to organize computer-based patient data in his primary care practice

Record completion: The process whereby healthcare professionals are able to access, complete, and/or authenticate a specific patient's medical information

Record locator service (RLS): A service that indicates where a given patient may have health information using probability equations

Record processing: The processes that encompass the creation, maintenance, and updating of each patient's medical record

Record reconciliation: The process of assuring that all the records of discharged patients have been received by the HIM department for processing

Recovery room report: A type of health record documentation used by nurses to document the patient's reaction to anesthesia and condition after surgery; also called recovery room record

Recruitment: The process of finding, soliciting, and attracting employees

Red Flag Rules: A set of FTC regulations that require certain entities to develop and implement identity theft prevention programs

Red flags: Suspicious documents, information, or behaviors that indicate the possibility of identity theft

Redundant arrays of independent (or inexpensive) disks (RAID): A method of ensuring data security

Reengineering: Fundamental rethinking and radical redesign of business processes to achieve significant performance improvements

Referred outpatient: An outpatient who is provided special diagnostic or therapeutic services by a hospital on an ambulatory basis but whose medical care remains the responsibility of the referring physician

Regional health information organization (RHIO): A health information organization that brings together healthcare stakeholders within a defined geographic area and governs health information exchange among them for the purpose of improving health and care in the community

Registered Health Information Administrator (RHIA): A type of certification granted after completion of an AHIMA-accredited four-year program in health information management and a credentialing examination

Registered Health Information Technician (RHIT): A type of certification granted after completion of an AHIMA-accredited two-year program in health information management and a credentialing examination

Registration: The act of enrolling

Registration-Admission, Discharge, Transfer (R-ADT): A type of administrative information system that stores demographic information and performs functionality related to registration, admission, discharge, and transfer of patients within the organization

Registry: A collection of care information related to a specific disease, condition, or procedure that makes health record information available for analysis and comparison

Rehabilitation Act: Federal legislation passed in 1973 to protect handicapped employees against discrimination

Rehabilitation services: Health services provided to assist patients in achieving and maintaining their optimal level of function, self-care, and independence after some type of disability

Reimbursement: Compensation or repayment for healthcare services

Relational database: A type of database that stores data in predefined tables made up of rows and columns

Relative value unit (RVU): A number assigned to a procedure that describes its difficulty and expense in relationship to other procedures

Release of information (ROI): The process of disclosing patient-identifiable information from the health record to another party

Release of information system: Information system used when disclosing patient-identifiable information from the health record to another party

Remittance advice (RA): An explanation of payments (for example, claim denials) made by third-party payers

Remote patient monitoring device: A device that enables a healthcare provider to monitor and treat a patient from a remote location

Report card: A method used by managed care organizations (and other healthcare sectors) to report cost and quality of care provided

Request for information (RFI): A written communication often sent to a comprehensive list of vendors during the design phase of the systems development life cycle to ask for general product information

Request for proposal (RFP): A type of business correspondence asking for very specific product and contract information that is often sent to a narrow list of vendors that have been preselected after a review of requests for information during the design phase of the systems development life cycle

Requisition: A request from an authorized health record user to gain access to a medical record

Resident assessment instrument (RAI): A uniform assessment instrument developed by the Centers for Medicare and Medicaid Services to standardize the collection of skilled nursing facility patient data; includes the Minimum Data Set 3.0, triggers, and resident assessment protocols

Resident assessment protocol (RAP): A summary of a long-term care resident's medical condition and care requirements

Resident Assessment Validation and Entry (RAVEN): A type of data-entry software developed by the Centers for Medicare and Medicaid Services for long-term care facilities and used to collect Minimum Data Set assessments and to transmit data to state databases

Resource Utilization Groups, Version IV (RUG-IV): A case-mix–adjusted classification system based on Minimum Data Set assessments and used by skilled nursing facilities

Resource-based relative value scale (RBRVS): A Medicare reimbursement system implemented in 1992 to compensate physicians according to a fee schedule predicated on weights assigned on the basis of the resources required to provide the services

Respite care: A type of short-term care provided during the day or overnight to individuals in the home or institution to temporarily relieve the family home caregiver

Responsibility: The accountability required as part of a job, such as supervising work performed by others or managing assets or funds

Results management: Results retrieval technology that permits viewing of data by type and manipulation of several different types of data; also referred to as results management systems

Results retrieval: A lookup system that enables a user to access several different types of data from different source systems through a single application screen

Retention: 1. The process whereby inactive health records are stored and made available for future use in compliance with state and federal requirements 2. The ability to keep valuable employees from seeking employment elsewhere

Retention schedule: A time line for various records retention based on factors such as federal and state laws, statutes of limitations, age of patient, competency of patient, accreditation standards, AHIMA recommendations, and operational needs

Retraction: Removal of a document from standard view within an electronic document management system (EDMS)

Retrospective payment system: Type of fee-for-service reimbursement in which providers receive recompense after health services have been rendered

Retrospective review: The part of the utilization review process that concentrates on a review of clinical information following patient discharge

Retrospective utilization review: A review of records some time after the patient's discharge to determine any of several issues, including the quality or appropriateness of the care provided

Return on investment: The financial analysis of the extent of value a major purchase will provide

Revenue Audit Contractor (RAC): Organization contracted to detect and correct improper payments in the Medicare Fee for Service (FFS) program

Revenue codes: A three- or four-digit number in the chargemaster that totals all items and their charges for printing on the form used for Medicare billing

Revenue cycle management (RCM): The supervision of all administrative and clinical functions that contribute to the capture, management, and collection of patient service revenue, with the goals of accelerated cash flow and lowered accounts receivable

Revenues: The charges generated from providing healthcare services; earned and measurable income

Rewarding stage: In performance management, the fifth of five stages during which individual employees are rewarded for exceptional achievement

Right-to-work laws: Federal legislation dealing with labor rights (examples include workers' compensation, child labor, and minimum wage laws)

Ring topology: A computer circuit/networking arrangement where each computer is connected to two others, forming a signal path in the shape of a ring

Risk: 1. The probability of incurring injury or loss 2. The probable amount of loss foreseen by an insurer in issuing a contract 3. A formal insurance term denoting liability to compensate individuals for injuries sustained in a healthcare facility

Risk analysis: An assessment of possible security threats to the organization's data

Risk assessment: *See* **risk analysis**

Risk management (RM): A comprehensive program of activities intended to minimize the potential for injuries to occur in a facility and to anticipate and respond to ensuing liabilities for those injuries that do occur

Risk management program: *See* **risk management**

Root-cause analysis: A technique used in performance improvement initiatives to discover the underlying causes of a problem

Row/record: A set of columns or a collection of related data items in a table

Rules and regulations: Operating documents that describe the rules and regulations under which a healthcare organization operates

Run chart: A type of graph that shows data points collected over time and identifies emerging trends or patterns

RxNorm: A clinical drug nomenclature developed by the Food and Drug Administration, the Department of Veterans Affairs, and HL7 to provide standard names for clinical drugs and administered dose forms

Safety management: A system for providing a risk-free environment for patients, visitors, and employees

Scales of measurement: A reference standard for data collection and classification; *See* nominal-level data, ordinal-level data, interval-level data, and ratio-level data

Scatter diagram: A graph that visually displays the linear relationships among factors

Scatter plot: A visual representation of data points on an interval or ratio level used to depict relationships between two variables

Scorecards: Reports of outcomes measures to help leaders know what they have accomplished; sometimes called dashboards

Screen prototype: A sketch of the user interface of each screen that is anticipated in a project

Secondary data source: Data derived from the primary patient record, such as an index or a database

Secondary release of information: A type of information release in which the initial requester forwards confidential information to others without obtaining required patient authorization

Secondary storage: The permanent storage of data and programs on disks or tapes

Security: 1. The means to control access and protect information from accidental or intentional disclosure to unauthorized persons and from unauthorized alteration, destruction, or loss 2. The physical protection of facilities and equipment from theft, damage, or unauthorized access; collectively, the policies, procedures, and safeguards designed to protect the confidentiality of information, maintain the integrity and availability of information systems, and control access to the content of these systems

Security breach: A violation of the policies or standards developed to ensure security

Security management: The oversight of facilities, equipment, and other resources, including human resources and technology, to reduce the possibility of harm to or theft of these assets of an organization

Security program: A plan outlining the policies and procedures created to protect healthcare information

Security standards: Statements that describe the processes and procedures meant to ensure that patient-identifiable health information remains confidential and protected from unauthorized disclosure, alteration, and destruction

Security threat: A situation that has the potential to damage a healthcare organization's information system

Sequence diagram: A systems analysis tool for documenting the interaction between an actor and the information system

Serial numbering system: A type of health record identification and filing system in which patients are assigned a different but unique numerical identifier for every admission

Serial-unit numbering system: A health record identification system in which patient numbers are assigned in a serial manner but records are brought forward and filed under the last number assigned

Server: A type of computer that makes it possible to share information resources across a network of client computers

Server failover: At least two if not more servers are performing the same processing on data simultaneously

Server redundancy: Situation where two servers are duplicating effort

Severity-of-illness screening criteria: Standards used to determine the most appropriate setting of care based on the level of clinical signs and symptoms that a patient shows upon presentation to a healthcare facility

Shared systems: Systems developed by data-processing companies in the 1960s and 1970s to address the computing needs of healthcare organizations that could not afford, or chose not to purchase, their own mainframe computing systems

Single sign-on: A type of technology that allows a user access to all disparate applications through one authentication procedure, thus reducing the number and variety of passwords a user must remember and enforcing and centralizing access control

Six Sigma: Disciplined and data-driven methodology for getting rid of defects in any process

Skilled nursing facility (SNF): A long-term care facility with an organized professional staff and permanent facilities (including inpatient beds) that provides continuous nursing and other health-related, psychosocial, and personal services to patients who are not in an acute phase of illness but who primarily require continued care on an inpatient basis

Skilled nursing facility prospective payment system (SNF PPS): A per-diem reimbursement system implemented in July 1998 for costs (routine, ancillary, and capital) associated with covered skilled nursing facility services furnished to Medicare Part A beneficiaries

SOAP: An acronym for a component of the problem-oriented medical record that refers to how each progress note contains documentation relative to subjective observations, objective observations, assessments, and plans

Social Security Act of 1935: The federal legislation that originally established the Social Security program as well as unemployment compensation, and support for mothers and children; amended in 1965 to create the Medicare and Medicaid programs

Software: A program that directs the hardware components of a computer system to perform the tasks required

Source-oriented health record: *See* source-oriented health record format

Source-oriented health record format: A system of health record organization in which information is arranged according to the patient care department that provided the care

Special-cause variation: An unusual source of variation that occurs outside a process but affects it

Specialty software: A type of applications software that performs specialized, niche functions such as encoding or drawing and painting

Speech dictation: Method of collecting information in an information system through the spoken word

Speech recognition: Situation where speech is converted to text on a screen

Staff model HMO: A type of health maintenance that employs physicians to provide healthcare services to subscribers

Staff retention: The process of keeping valued employees on the job and reducing turnover

Staffing analysis: Study performed to determine the most efficient and cost-effective staff mix

Staffing level: The number of employees

Stage of the neoplasm: A classification of malignancies (cancers) according to the anatomic extent of the tumor, such as primary neoplasm, regional lymph nodes, and metastases

Stakeholder: An individual within the company who has an interest in, or is affected by, the results of a project

Standard: 1. A scientifically based statement of expected behavior against which structures, processes, and outcomes can be measured 2. A model or example established by authority, custom, or general consent or a rule established by an authority as a measure of quantity, weight, extent, value, or quality

Standard deviation: A measure of variability that describes the deviation from the mean of a frequency distribution in the original units of measurement; the square root of the variance

Standard of care: An established set of clinical decisions and actions taken by clinicians and other representatives of healthcare organizations in accordance with state and federal laws, regulations, and guidelines; codes of ethics published by professional associations or societies; regulations for accreditation published by accreditation agencies; usual and common practice of equivalent clinicians or organizations in a geographical region

Standard vocabulary: A vocabulary that is accepted throughout the healthcare industry

Standards and Interoperability (S&I) Framework: A standard used to support interoperability of data

Standards development organizations (SDOs): Private or government agencies involved in the development of healthcare informatics standards at a national or international level

Standing committees: Committees that are put in place to oversee ongoing and cross-functional issues (examples include the medical staff committee, a quality improvement committee, or an infection control committee)

Star topology: An information technology structure in which each computer is connected to a central, or hub, computer, through which all information passes

State Children's Health Insurance Program (SCHIP): The children's healthcare program implemented as part of the Balanced Budget Act of 1997; sometimes referred to as the Children's Health Insurance Program, or CHIP

State workers' compensation insurance funds: Funds that provide a stable source of insurance coverage for work-related illnesses and injuries and serve to protect employers from underwriting uncertainties by making it possible to have continuing availability of workers' compensation coverage

Statistical process control chart: A type of run chart that includes both upper and lower control limits and indicates whether a process is stable or unstable

Statutory law: Written law established by federal and state legislatures

Stem and leaf plots: A visual display that organizes data to show its shape and distribution, using two columns with the stem in the left-hand column and all leaves associated with that stem in the right-hand column; the "leaf" is the ones digit of the number, and the other digits form the "stem"

Storage and retrieval: A healthcare facility's method for safely and securely maintaining and archiving individual patient health records for future reference

Storage area network (SAN): Storage devices organized into a network so that they can be accessible from any server in the network

Storage management: System used to manage the SAN, keep track of where data are stored, and move older data to less expensive, but still accessible, storage locations

Storage management software: Software used to manage the SAN, keep track of where data are stored, and move older data to less expensive, but still accessible, storage locations

Storming: The second of four steps that occur when creating a functional team, storming occurs when individual team members examine their role within the group

Straight numeric filing system: A health record filing system in which health records are arranged in ascending numerical order

Strategic decision making: A type of decision making that is usually limited to individuals, such as boards of directors, chief executive officers, and top-level executives, who make decisions about the healthcare organization's strategic direction

Strategic decision support system: *See* **decision support system (DSS)**

Strategic information systems planning: A process for setting IS priorities within an organization; the process of identifying and prioritizing IS needs based on the organization's strategic goals with the intent of ensuring that all IS technology initiatives are integrated and aligned with the organization's overall strategic plan

Strategic planning: A disciplined effort to produce fundamental decisions that shape and guide what an organization is, what it does, and why it does it

Structure and content standards: Common data elements and definitions of the data elements to be included in an electronic patient record

Structure indicators: Quality indicators that measure the attributes of an organizational setting, such as number and qualifications of staff, adequacy of equipment and facilities, and adequacy of organizational policies and procedures

Structured brainstorming: A group problem-solving technique wherein the team leader asks each participant to generate a list of ideas for the topic under discussion and then report them to the group in a nonjudgmental manner

Structured data: Binary, computer-readable data

Structured input (SI): Information that has been organized to allow identification and separation of the context of the information from its content

Structured query language (SQL): A fourth-generation computer language that includes both DDL and DML components and is used to create and manipulate relational databases

Student membership: AHIMA membership category for students enrolled in an AHIMA accredited or approved program

Subacute care: A type of step-down care provided after a patient is released from an acute care hospital (including nursing homes and other facilities that provide medical care, but not surgical or emergency care)

Subject matter jurisdiction: Pertaining to district courts, jurisdiction to hear cases involving felonies and misdemeanors that fall under federal statutes

Subjective, objective, assessment, plan (SOAP): Documentation method that refers to how each progress note contains documentation relative to subjective observations, objective observations, assessments, and plans

Subpoena ad testificandum: A command to appear at a certain time and place to give testimony on a certain matter

Subpoena duces tecum: A written document directing individuals or organizations to furnish relevant documents and records

Summons: An instrument used to begin a civil action or special proceeding and is a means of acquiring jurisdiction over a party

Supercomputer: The largest, fastest, and most expensive type of computer that exists today

Supervisory management: Management level that oversees the organization's efforts at the staff level and monitors the effectiveness of everyday operations and individual performance against preestablished standards

Supervisory managers: Managers who oversee small (2- to 10-person) functional workgroups or teams and often perform hands-on functions in addition to supervisory functions

Supplemental medical insurance (SMI) (Medicare Part B): A voluntary medical insurance program that helps pay for physicians' services, medical services, and supplies not covered by Medicare Part A

Supply management: Management and control of the supplies used within an organization

Supreme Court: The highest court in the U.S. legal system; hears cases from the U.S. Courts of Appeals and the highest state courts when federal statutes, treaties, or the U.S. Constitution is involved

Surgical operation: One or more surgical procedures performed at one time for one patient via a common approach or for a common purpose

Surgical procedure: Any single, separate, systematic process upon or within the body that can be complete in itself; is normally performed by a physician, dentist, or other licensed practitioner; can be performed either with or without instruments; and is performed to restore disunited or deficient parts, remove diseased or injured tissues, extract foreign matter, assist in obstetrical delivery, or aid in diagnosis

System: A set of related and highly interdependent components that are operating for a particular purpose

System build: The creation of data dictionaries, tables, decision support rules, templates for data entry, screen layouts, and reports used in a system

System design: The second phase of the systems development life cycle

System implementation: The third phase of the systems development life cycle

System maintenance and evaluation: The final phase of the systems development life cycle

System planning and analysis: The first phase of the systems development life cycle

System software: The platform on which all applications reside and function

System testing: A type of testing performed by an independent organization to identify problems in information systems

Systematized Nomenclature of Human and Veterinary Medicine (SNOMED): A comprehensive clinical vocabulary developed by the College of American Pathologists that is the most promising set of clinical terms available for a controlled vocabulary for healthcare; now known as SNOMED International

Systemized Nomenclature of Medicine Clinical Terminology (SNOMED CT): A concept-based terminology consisting of more than 110,000 concepts with linkages to more than 180,000 terms with unique computer-readable codes

Systems development life cycle (SDLC): A model used to represent the ongoing process of developing (or purchasing) information systems

Systems thinking: An objective way of looking at work-related ideas and processes with the goal of allowing people to uncover ineffective patterns of behavior and thinking and then finding ways to make lasting improvements

Table: An organized arrangement of data, usually in columns and rows

Tax Equity and Fiscal Responsibility Act of 1982 (TEFRA): The federal legislation that modified Medicare's retrospective reimbursement system for inpatient hospital stays by requiring implementation of diagnosis-related groups and the acute care prospective payment system

Team norms: The rules, both explicit and implied, that determine both acceptable and unacceptable behavior for a group

Technical component (TC): The portion of radiological and other procedures that is facility based or nonphysician based (for example, radiology films, equipment, overhead, endoscopic suites, and so on)

Telecommunications: Voice and data communications

Telehealth: A telecommunications system that links healthcare organizations and patients from diverse geographic locations and transmits text and images for (medical) consultation and treatment

Telematics: The use of telecommunications and networks to share information among patients and a healthcare providers located in at different locations/sites

Telesurgery: The use of telecommunication technologies and computers to exchange healthcare information and to provide services to clients at another location

Template: A pattern used in computer-based patient records to capture data in a structured manner

Temporary Assistance for Needy Families (TANF): A federal program that provides states with grants to be spent on time-limited cash assistance for low-income families, generally limiting a family's lifetime cash welfare benefits to a maximum of five years and permitting states to impose other requirements

Terminal-digit filing system: A system of health record identification and filing in which the last digit or group of digits (terminal digits) in the health record number determines file placement

Textual: A term referring to the narrative nature of much of clinical documentation to date

Thick client: Information system will full processing capabilities

Thin client: A computer with processing capability but no persistent storage (disk memory) that relies on data and applications on the host it accesses to be able to process data

Third-party payer: An insurance company (for example, Blue Cross/Blue Shield) or healthcare program (for example, Medicare) that reimburses healthcare providers (second party) and/or patients (first party) for the delivery of medical services

Tort: An action brought when one party believes that another party caused harm through wrongful conduct and seeks compensation for that harm

Total length of stay (discharge days): The sum of the days of stay of any group of inpatients discharged during a specific period of time

Traditional fee-for-service reimbursement: A reimbursement method involving third-party payers who compensate providers after the healthcare services have been delivered; payment is based on specific services provided to subscribers

Transaction: 1. Units of work performed against a database management system that are treated in a coherent and reliable way independent of other transactions. A database transaction is atomic, consistent, isolated and durable. Examples of healthcare transactions are the entry of a medication order for a patient, the retrieval of a lab result for a patient, and the posting of temperature for a patient 2. The individual events or activities that provide the basic input to the accounting process

Transaction standards: Standards that support the uniform format and sequence of data during transmission from one healthcare entity to another

Transaction-processing system (TPS): A computer-based information system that keeps track of an organization's business transactions through inputs (for example, transaction data such as admissions, discharges, and transfers in a hospital) and outputs (for example, census reports and bills)

Transactional database: See clinical data repository

Transcription: The process of deciphering and typing medical dictation

Transcriptionist: A specially trained typist who understands medical terminology and translates physicians' verbal dictation into written reports

Transfer record: A review of the patient's acute stay along with current status, discharge and transfer orders, and any additional instructions that accompanies the patient when he or she is transferred to another facility; also called a **referral form**

Transparency: The degree to which individual patients are made aware of how their personal health information is or has been dispersed to secondary medical databases

Traumatic injury: A wound or injury included in a trauma registry

Treatment, payment, and operations (TPO): Term used in the HIPAA Privacy Rule pertaining to broad activities under normal treatment, payment, and operations activities, important because of the rule's many exceptions to the release and disclosure of personal health information

Trial court: The lowest tier of state court, usually divided into two courts: the court of limited jurisdiction, which hears cases pertaining to a particular subject matter or involving crimes of lesser severity or civil matters of lower dollar amounts; and the court of general jurisdiction, which hears more serious criminal cases or civil cases that involve large amounts of money

TRICARE: The federal healthcare program that provides coverage for the dependents of armed forces personnel and for retirees receiving care outside military treatment facilities in which the federal government pays a percentage of the cost; formerly known as the Civilian Health and Medical Program of the Uniformed Services

TRICARE Extra: A cost-effective preferred provider network TRICARE option in which costs for healthcare are lower than for the standard TRICARE program because a physician or medical specialist is selected from a network of civilian healthcare professionals who participate in TRICARE Extra

TRICARE Prime: A TRICARE program that provides the most comprehensive healthcare benefits at the lowest cost of the three TRICARE options, in which military treatment facilities serve as the principal source of healthcare and a primary care manager is assigned to each enrollee

TRICARE Standard: A TRICARE program that allows eligible beneficiaries to choose any physician or healthcare provider, which permits the most flexibility but may be the most expensive

Turnkey system: A computer application that may be purchased from a vendor and installed without modification or further development by the user organization

UB-04: *See* **Uniform Bill-04**

UB-92 (CMS-1450): A Medicare form used for standardized uniform billing

Unbundling: The practice of using multiple codes to bill for the various individual steps in a single procedure rather than using a single code that includes all of the steps of the comprehensive procedure

Unified Medical Language System (UMLS): A program initiated by the National Library of Medicine to build an intelligent, automated system that can understand biomedical concepts, words, and expressions and their interrelationships

Unified modeling language (UML): A common data-modeling notation used in conjunction with object-oriented database design

Uniform Ambulatory Care Data Set (UACDS): A data set developed by the National Committee on Vital and Health Statistics consisting of a minimum set of patient/client-specific data elements to be collected in ambulatory care settings

Uniform Bill-04 (UB-04): The single standardized Medicare form for standardized uniform billing, scheduled for implementation in 2007 for hospital inpatients and outpatients; this form will also be used by the major third-party payers and most hospitals

Uniform Hospital Discharge Data Set (UHDDS): A core set of data elements adopted by the U.S. Department of Health, Education, and Welfare in 1974 that are collected by hospitals on all discharges and all discharge abstract systems

Unit numbering system: A health record identification system in which the patient receives a unique medical record number at the time of the first encounter that is used for all subsequent encounters

Unintended consequence: An event that occurs that was not expected

Uninterruptable power supply (UPS): Source of power that allows equipment or information systems to work when the power source is unavailable

Unstructured brainstorming method: A group problem-solving technique wherein the team leader solicits spontaneous ideas for the topic under discussion from members of the team in a free-flowing and nonjudgmental manner

Unstructured data: Nonbinary, human-readable data

Upcoding: The practice of assigning diagnostic or procedural codes that represent higher payment rates than the codes that actually reflect the services provided to patients

Use case diagram: A systems analysis technique used to document a software project from a user's perspective

Use, disclosures, and requests: Three types of situations in which personal health information is handled: use, which is internal to a covered entity or its business associate; disclosure, which is the dissemination of PHI from a covered entity or its business associate; and requests for PHI made by a covered entity or its business associate

Uses and disclosures: Referring to the use and disclosure of a patient's personal health information

Usual, customary, and reasonable (UCR) charges: Method of evaluating providers' fees in which the third-party payer pays for fees that are usual in that provider's practice; customary in the community; and reasonable for the situation

Utility program: A software program that supports, enhances, or expands existing programs in a computer system, such as virus checking, data recovery, backup, and data compression

Utilization management (UM): 1. The planned, systematic review of the patients in a healthcare facility against care criteria for admission, continued stay, and discharge 2. A collection of systems and processes to ensure that facilities and resources, both human and nonhuman, are used maximally and are consistent with patient care needs

Utilization management organization: An organization that reviews the appropriateness of the care setting and resources used to treat a patient

Utilization review (UR): The process of determining whether the medical care provided to a specific patient is necessary according to preestablished objective screening criteria at time frames specified in the organization's utilization management plan

Utilization Review Act: The federal legislation that requires hospitals to conduct continued-stay reviews for Medicare and Medicaid patients

V codes: A set of ICD-9-CM codes used to classify occasions when circumstances other than disease or injury are recorded as the reason for the patient's encounter with healthcare providers

Values statement: A short description that communicates an organization's social and cultural belief system

Variable costs: Resources expended that vary with the activity of the organization, for example, medication expenses vary with patient volume

Variablility: The dispersion of a set of measures around the population mean

Variance: A measure of variability that gives the average of the squared deviations from the mean; in financial management, the difference between the budgeted amount and the actual amount of a line item; in project management, the difference between the original project plan and current estimates

Vendor system: A computer system developed by a commercial company not affiliated with the healthcare organization

Version control: The process whereby a healthcare facility ensures that only the most current version of a patient's health record is available for viewing, updating, and so forth

Veterans Health Administration: The component of the U.S. Department of Veterans Affairs that implements the medical assistance program of the VA

Virtual HIM: Health information management function that takes place outside of a traditional office setting

Virtuoso teams: Group of experts brought together to address an issue or situation.

Vision statement: A short description of an organization's ideal future state

Vital statistics: Data related to births, deaths, marriages, and fetal deaths

Vocabulary standards: A common definition for medical terms to encourage consistent descriptions of an individual's condition in the health record

Voice recognition technology: A method of encoding speech signals that do not require speaker pauses (but uses pauses when they are present) and of interpreting at least some of the signals' content as words or the intent of the speaker

Voir dire: The process of jury selection

Voluntary Disclosure Program: A program unveiled in 1998 by the Office of the Inspector General (OIG) that encourages healthcare providers to voluntarily report fraudulent conduct affecting Medicare, Medicaid, and other federal healthcare programs

Web services architecture (WSA): An emerging architecture that utilizes web-based tools to permit communication among different software applications

Wide area network (WAN): A computer network that connects devices across a large geographical area

Wireless network: Any type of computer network that is not connected by cables of any kind

Wireless on wheels (WOWs): Notebook computers mounted on carts that can be moved through the facility by users

Work schedules: The process by which facility managers ensure that each department is has adequate personnel to properly complete all assigned tasks

Workers' compensation: The medical and income insurance coverage for certain employees in unusually hazardous jobs

Workflow: Any work process that must be handled by more than one person

Workflow analysis: A technique used to study the flow of operations for automation

Workflow and process management: Ensures that the components work together to achieve their intended purpose.

Workforce members: Employees, volunteers, trainees, and other persons who work under the direct control of a HIPAA-covered entity, regardless of whether they are paid by the covered entity

Workstation: A computer designed to accept data from multiple sources in order to assist in managing information for daily activities and to provide a convenient means of entering data as desired by the user at the point of care

World Health Organization (WHO): The United Nations specialized agency for health, established on April 7, 1948, with the objective, as set out in its constitution, of the attainment by all peoples of the highest possible levels of health; responsible for the International Statistical Classification of Diseases & Related Health Problems (ICD-10)

Index

AHIMA PRESS EXAM PREP
TRUST AHIMA FOR YOUR EXAM PREP SOLUTIONS.

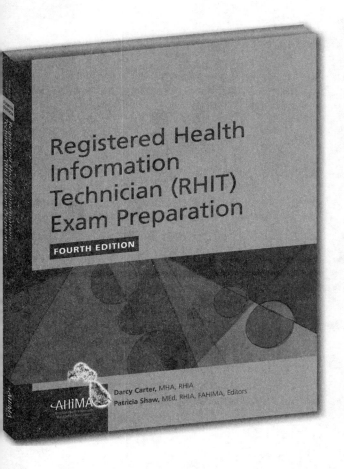

Whether you're still learning or ready to test your skills, *Registered Health Information Technician (RHIT) Exam Preparation* challenges, motivates, and guides you all the way to exam day. Also, the Fourth Edition includes online assessments that include practice exams that can be customized to test strengths and weaknesses working within your time constraints.

Confidently prepare for the Registered Health Information Technician (RHIT) exam with AHIMA.

Registered Health Information Technician (RHIT) Exam Preparation

Order Information
Prod. No. AB105012 • ISBN: 9781584263852
Aprox. 312 pages • Softcover © 2012

learn more, ▷ visit ahima.org/certification/exam.aspx and select the exam preparation publication that fits your need.

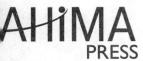

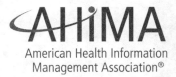

American Health Information
Management Association®

EXPLORE YOUR FUTURE IN HIM
on AHIMA's HIM Career Map!

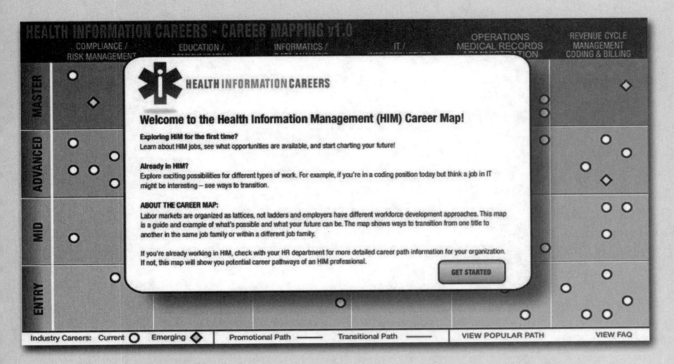

This interactive and visual representation of the job roles that making up the health information management (HIM) profession and the career pathways associated with them can help you chart your future success!

- Find out what education, skills, and credentials you need to start or advance your career
- Build your career path—where do you want to be in five years and how can you make it happen?
- Check out HIM job roles, job descriptions, salary data, and more
- See emerging roles in HIM to better understand where the field is headed

Visit the HIM Career Map today to learn more!
hicareers.com/careermap

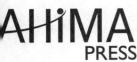

AHIMA
PRESS

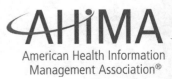

AHIMA
American Health Information
Management Association®